CURRENT THERAPY IN EQUINE MEDICINE 3

N. EDWARD ROBINSON, Ph.D., M.R.C.V.S.

Matilda R. Wilson Professor of Large Animal Clinical Sciences
Michigan State University College of Veterinary Medicine
East Lansing, Michigan

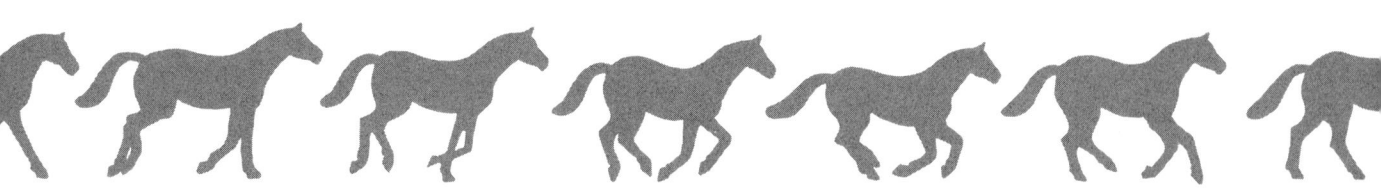

PHILADELPHIA, LONDON, TORONTO, MONTREAL, SYDNEY, TOKYO

CURRENT THERAPY IN EQUINE MEDICINE

3

W.B. SAUNDERS COMPANY Harcourt Brace Jovanovich, Inc.

W. B. SAUNDERS COMPANY
Harcourt Brace Jovanovich, Inc.

The Curtis Center
Independence Square West
Philadelphia, Pennsylvania 19103

Editor: Linda Mills

Current Therapy in Equine Medicine ISBN 0-7216-3475-3

Copyright © 1992 by W. B. Saunders Company.

All rights reserved. No part of this publication may be reproduced or transmitted in any form or by any means, electronic or mechanical, including photocopy, recording, or any information storage and retrieval system, without permission in writing from the publisher. ISSN 1058-8884.

Printed in Mexico.

Last digit is the print number: 9   8   7   6   5   4   3   2

Dedicated to

Pat

lifelong friend, trusted confidante, and fellow veterinarian,
who understands that the successful veterinarian
must integrate humane care of the animal
with the needs of the owner

and to

Emily and Sarah

for making everything worthwhile

Current Therapy in Equine Medicine

CONSULTING EDITORS

N. EDWARD ROBINSON
Therapeutics

GLENN F. ANDERSON
Duties of a Veterinarian

DALLAS O. GOBLE
Special Problems of Draft Horses and Mules

ALICIA BERTONE
Musculoskeletal Diseases

MICHAEL J. MURRAY
Alimentary Tract Diseases

RICHARD P. HACKETT
NORMAN G. DUCHARME
Upper Airway Diseases

ANDREW F. CLARKE
Lower Respiratory Tract Diseases

FRANCIS D. GALEY
Toxicology

VIRGINIA B. REEF
Cardiovascular Diseases

BENJAMIN J. DARIEN
Foal Diseases

DEBRA DEEM MORRIS
Hematopoietic Diseases

RICHARD M. DEBOWES
JUDY H. COX
Neurological Diseases

MARY B. GLAZE
Ocular Diseases

THOMAS J. DIVERS
Urinary Tract Diseases

GORDON L. WOODS
Reproduction

DIANE BEVIER
Skin Diseases

SARAH L. RALSTON
Nutrition

WILLIAM W. LAEGREID
Exotic Diseases

ELISABETH MORRIS
Assessment of Performance Problems

CONTRIBUTORS

HENRY S. ADAIR, M.S., D.V.M.
Assistant Professor of Surgery, Department of Rural Practice, University of Tennessee College of Veterinary Medicine, Knoxville, Tennessee.
Common Lameness Problems of the Draft Horse

GREGG P. ADAMS, D.V.M., Ph.D.
Research Associate, Department of Veterinary Science, University of Wisconsin, Madison, Wisconsin.
Ultrasonographic Evaluation of the Mare's Reproductive Tract

DOUGLAS ALLEN, Jr., D.V.M., M.S., Diplomate A.C.V.S.
Chief of Staff, Large Animal Clinic. Associate Professor, Department of Large Animal Medicine, College of Veterinary Medicine, University of Georgia, Athens, Georgia.
Duodenitis—Proximal Jejunitis

LANCE L. ALLEN, D.V.M., B.S.
President, Agri-Risk Services, Inc. President, International Livestock Adjusting Company, Inc., Kansas City, Missouri.
The Veterinarian's Role in Insurance

THOMAS H. ALLISON, D.V.M., J.D.
Cleveland, Ohio.
Selected Medical-Legal Considerations in the Practice of Equine Medicine; The Veterinarian as a Witness

GLENN F. ANDERSON, F.D.V.M.
Owner, Equine Veterinary Associates, Broken Arrow, Oklahoma.
Purchase Examination of the Performance Horse

FRANK M. ANDREWS, D.V.M., M.S., Diplomate A.C.V.I.M.
Assistant Professor, Department of Rural Practice, University of Tennessee College of Veterinary Medicine. Section Head, Veterinary Teaching Hospital, University of Tennessee College of Veterinary Medicine, Knoxville, Tennessee.
Seizures and Narcolepsy

E. MURL BAILEY, Jr., D.V.M., M.S., Ph.D., Diplomate A.B.V.T
Professor, Department of Veterinary Physiology and Pharmacology, College of Veterinary Medicine, Texas A&M University, College Station, Texas.
Management of Toxicoses; Industrial Toxicants

M. BAILEY, B.V.Sc., Ph.D., M.R.C.V.S.
Research Assistant, Department of Veterinary Medicine, University of Bristol, Bristol, England.
Lung Parasites

AUBREY N. BAIRD, D.V.M., M.S.
Assistant Professor of Large Animal Surgery and Medicine, Auburn University College of Veterinary Medicine, Auburn, Alabama.
Rectal Tears

BARRY A. BALL, D.V.M., Ph.D., Diplomate A.C.T.
Assistant Professor of Theriogenology, Cornell University Veterinary Medical Teaching Hospital, Ithaca, New York.
Embryonic Loss

JOY BARBET, B.S., D.V.M., Diplomate, A.C.V.D.
Adjunct Assistant Professor, University of Florida, Gainesville, Florida. Referral Practice in Dermatology, Seminole Veterinary Hospital, Sanford, Florida. Referral Practice in Dermatology, Sunshine Animal Hospital, Tampa, Florida.
Culicoides Hypersensitivity

GARY M. BAXTER, V.M.D., M.S., Diplomate, A.C.V.S.
Assistant Professor of Surgery, Colorado State University. Large Animal Surgeon, Colorado

x / CONTRIBUTORS—continued

State University Veterinary Teaching Hospital, Fort Collins, Colorado.
Laminitis

WARREN L. BEARD, D.V.M., M.S., Diplomate A.C.V.S.
Assistant Professor, Department of Veterinary Clinical Sciences, College of Veterinary Medicine, The Ohio State University, Columbus, Ohio.
Developmental Orthopedic Disease

VAL RICHARD BEASLEY, D.V.M., Ph.D.
Associate Professor of Toxicology, University of Illinois College of Veterinary Medicine, Urbana-Champaign, Illinois.
Equine Leukoencephalomalacia/Hepatosis and Stachybotryotoxicosis

RICHARD M. BEDNARSKI, D.V.M., M.S., Diplomate A.C.V.A.
Associate Professor, Department of Clinical Sciences, The Ohio State University College of Veterinary Medicine. Section Head Anesthesiology, The Ohio State University Medical Teaching School, Columbus, Ohio.
Chemical Restraint of the Standing Horse

BILL BERNARD, D.V.M., Diplomate A.C.V.I.M.
Internist, Rood and Riddle Equine Hospital, Lexington, Kentucky.
Pericardial Disease

ALICIA L. BERTONE, D.V.M., Ph.D.
Assistant Professor, The Ohio State University. Equine Orthopedic Surgeon, Ohio State Veterinary Hospital, Columbus, Ohio.
Infectious Synovitis; Noninfectious Synovitis

JOSEPH J. BERTONE, D.V.M., M.S.
Assistant Professor, Department of Clinical Sciences, The Ohio State University College of Veterinary Medicine, Columbus, Ohio.
Nutritional Secondary Hyperparathyroidism; Differential Diagnoses of Lameness: Nutritional, Toxic, Metabolic, and Other Conditions; Togaviral Encephalatides: Alphavirus (Eastern and Western) Equine Encephalitis

LINDA L. BLYTHE, D.V.M., Ph.D.
Clinical Neurologist, Oregon State University College of Veterinary Medicine, Corvallis, Oregon.
Degenerative Myeloencephalopathy

MARY GARDINER BOY, M.S., V.M.D.
Lecturer, Large Animal Medicine, University of Pennsylvania School of Veterinary Medicine, New Bolton Center, Kennett Square, Pennsylvania.
Cystitis and Pyelonephritis

LAWRENCE R. BRAMLAGE, D.V.M., M.S.
Adjunct Associate Professor, The Ohio State University. Equine Surgeon, Rood and Riddle Equine Hospital, Lexington, Kentucky.
Medical Treatment of Tendinitis

GARY W. BRANDT, D.V.M., M.S., Diplomate A.C.T.
Assistant Professor of Equine Theriogenology and Medicine, Kansas State University College of Veterinary Medicine, Manhattan, Kansas.
Hypocalcemic Tetany

BARBARA D. BREWER, M.A., D.V.M., Diplomate A.C.V.I.M., Diplomate A.C.V.E.C.C.
Associate Professor of Large Animal Medicine, College of Veterinary Medicine, University of Florida, Gainesville, Florida.
Identification and Early Management of the High-Risk Neonatal Foal

DENNIS E. BROOKS, D.V.M., Ph.D., Diplomate A.C.V.O.
Associate Professor of Ophthalmology, University of Florida. Service Chief, Ophthalmology, Departments of Large and Small Animal Clinical Sciences, College of Veterinary Medicine, University of Florida, Gainesville, Florida.
Glaucoma

TED A. BROOME, D.V.M.
Resident, Department of Large Animal Clinical Sciences, College of Veterinary Medicine, University of Florida, Gainesville, Florida.
Hemophilia; Warfarin Toxicosis

CHRISTOPHER M. BROWN, B.S., B.V.Sc., Ph.D., M.R.C.V.S., Diplomate A.C.V.I.M.
Professor, Large Animal Clinical Sciences, Michigan State University College of Veterinary Medicine, East Lansing, Michigan.
Dysphagia; Neonatal Maladjustment Syndrome

GORDON W. BRUMBAUGH, D.V.M., Ph.D.
Associate Professor, Texas A&M University College of Veterinary Medicine, College Station, Texas.
Toxicity of Pharmacological Agents

WILLIAM J. BURKHOLDER, D.V.M.
Graduate Research Assistant, Virginia-Maryland Regional College of Veterinary Medicine. Clinical Nutrition Service, Veterinary Medical Teaching Hospital, Virginia-Maryland Regional College of Veterinary Medicine, Blacksburg, Virginia.
Enteral Nutritional Support of Sick Horses

E. SUSAN CLARK, D.V.M., Ph.D., Diplomate A.C.V.I.M.
Assistant Professor of Large Animal Medicine, University of Georgia Large Animal Teaching Hospital, Athens, Georgia.
Pharmacologic Management of Colic; Duodenitis—Proximal Jejunitis; Urinary Incontinence

ANDREW F. CLARKE, B.V.Sc., Ph.D., M.R.C.V.S.
Director, Equine Research Centre, University of Guelph, Guelph, Ontario, Canada
Environmental Monitoring in Relation to Equine Respiratory Disease; Chronic Obstructive Pulmonary Disease; Exercise-Induced Pulmonary Hemorrhage

CHRYSANN COLLATOS, V.M.D.
Resident, Large Animal Medicine, College of Veterinary Medicine, University of Georgia, Athens, Georgia.
Bacterial Endocarditis; Lymphoproliferative and Myeloproliferative Disorders

STEVEN B. COLTER, D.V.M., Diplomate A.C.V.I.M. (Neurology)
Rocky Mountain Veterinary Neurology Clinic, Fort Collins, Colorado.
Tail Alterations in Show Horses

JUDY H. COX, D.V.M., M.S., Diplomate A.C.V.I.M.
Associate Professor, Department of Clinical Sciences, College of Veterinary Medicine, Kansas State University, Manhattan, Kansas.
Neurological Examination; Rabies; Neuromuscular Disorders

C. P. COYNE, D.V.M., Ph.D.
Assistant Professor of Equine Internal Medicine, College of Veterinary Medicine, Kansas State University, Manhattan, Kansas.
Neurological Examination; Cerebrospinal Fluid Collection and Analysis

A. MORRIE CRAIG, Ph.D.
Toxicologist, Oregon State University College of Veterinary Medicine, Corvallis, Oregon.
Degenerative Myeloencephalopathy

SANDRA S. CURRAN, D.V.M., M.S.
Private Practitioner, Gillett, Wisconsin.
Diagnosis of Fetal Gender by Ultrasonography

BENJAMIN J. DARIEN, D.V.M., M.S., Diplomate A.C.V.I.M.
Assistant Professor, Large Animal Medicine, Oregon State University College of Veterinary Medicine, Corvallis, Oregon.
Hemostasis in the Newborn Foal; Septic Arthritis and Osteomyelitis

MICHAEL DAVIDSON, D.V.M., Diplomate A.C.V.O.
Assistant Professor of Ophthalmology, Department of Companion Animal and Special Species Medicine, North Carolina State University College of Veterinary Medicine, Raleigh, North Carolina.
Anterior Uveitis

RICHARD M. DeBOWES, D.V.M., M.S.
Associate Professor of Equine Surgery, Kansas State University College of Veterinary Medicine. Associate Head, Department of Clinical Sciences, Kansas State University College of Veterinary Medicine, Manhattan, Kansas.
Common Malformations and Congenital Abnormalities of the Central Nervous System; Trauma of the Brain and Spinal Cord

FREDERIK J. DERKSEN, D.V.M., Ph.D., Diplomate A.C.V.I.M.
Professor, Department of Large Animal Clinical Sciences, College of Veterinary Medicine, Michigan State University, East Lansing, Michigan.
Pulmonary Function Tests

JOSEPH A. DiPIETRO, D.V.M., M.S.
Professor, Parasitology Division, Departments of Veterinary Pathology and Equine Medicine and Surgery Section, Department of Veterinary Clinical Medicine, University of Illinois College of Veterinary Medicine, Urbana, Illinois.
Internal Parasite Control Programs

THOMAS J. DIVERS, D.V.M., Diplomate A.C.V.I.M.
Associate Professor of Medicine, New York State College of Veterinary Medicine, Cornell University, Ithaca, New York.
Hepatic Disease; Urinary Tract Neoplasia; Acute Renal Failure

PATRICK M. DIXON, M.V.B., Ph.D., M.R.C.V.S.
Lecturer, Department of Veterinary Clinical Studies, University of Edinburgh Royal Dick

xii / CONTRIBUTORS—*continued*

School of Veterinary Studies, Easter Bush, Roslin, Midlothian, Scotland.
Therapeutics of the Respiratory Tract

WILLIAM J. DONAWICK, D.V.M., Diplomate A.C.V.S.
Mark Whittier and Lila Griswold Allam Professor of Surgery, The George D. Widener Hospital for Large Animals, University of Pennsylvania School of Veterinary Medicine, New Bolton Center, Kennett Square, Pennsylvania.
Jugular Vein Thrombophlebitis

NORMAND G. DUCHARME, D.V.M., M.Sc.
Associate Professor of Surgery, Department of Clinical Sciences, New York State College of Veterinary Medicine. Head, Large Animal Clinic, Veterinary Medical Teaching Hospital, Cornell University College of Veterinary Medicine, Ithaca, New York.
Dynamic Pharyngeal Collapse

WENDY M. DUCKETT, D.V.M., M.S., Diplomate A.C.V.I.M.
Assistant Professor, Department of Food Animal and Equine Medicine, College of Veterinary Medicine, North Carolina State University, Raleigh, North Carolina.
Verminous Myelitis

ROBERT W. DUNSTAN, D.V.M., M.S.
Associate Professor of Pathology, College of Veterinary Medicine, Michigan State University, East Lansing, Michigan.
Skin Biopsies in the Diagnosis of Inflammatory Skin Diseases

JOAN DZIEZYC, D.V.M.
Assistant Professor, Department of Small Animal Medicine and Surgery, Texas A&M University College of Veterinary Medicine, College Station, Texas.
Cataracts

WILLIAM C. EDWARDS, D.V.M., M.S.
Professor of Medicine and Surgery, Oklahoma State University College of Veterinary Medicine, Stillwater, Oklahoma.
Toxicologic Implications of Sudden, Unexplained Death

VALERIE A. FADOK, D.V.M., Ph.D., Diplomate A.C.V.D.
Research Associate, Department of Medicine, National Jewish Center, Denver, Colorado.
Appendicular Inflammatory Disorders

BERNARD F. FELDMAN, D.V.M., Ph.D.
Director of Immunology Laboratory. Director of Comparative Hemostasis Laboratory. Professor of Veterinary Clinical Hematology and Biochemistry, Department of Pathobiology, Virginia-Maryland Regional College of Veterinary Medicine, Virginia Polytechnic Institute and State University, Blacksburg, Virginia.
Hemostasis in the Newborn Foal

CLARA K. FENGER, D.V.M.
Resident, Equine Medicine, College of Veterinary Medicine, The Ohio State University, Columbus, Ohio.
Diseases of the Nasal Passages

PAMELA L. FERRANTE, D.V.M., M.S.
John Lee Pratt Fellow in Animal Nutrition, Department of Animal Science, College of Agriculture and Life Sciences, Virginia Polytechnic Institute and State University, Blacksburg, Virginia.
Ergogenic Diets and Nutrients

CAROL S. FOIL, M.S., D.V.M., Diplomate A.C.V.D.
Associate Professor, Department of Veterinary Clinical Sciences, Louisiana State University School of Veterinary Medicine. Veterinary Dermatologist, Chief of Service, Veterinary Teaching Hospital and Clinics, Louisiana State University School of Veterinary Medicine, Baton Rouge, Louisiana.
Control of Ectoparasites

LANE FOIL, Ph.D.
Professor, Veterinary Entomology, Louisiana State University School of Medicine, Baton Rouge, Louisiana.
Control of Ectoparasites

TROY S. FORD, D.V.M., Diplomate A.C.V.S.
Assistant Professor, Department of Large Animal Medicine and Surgery, Texas Veterinary Medical Center, Texas A&M University College of Veterinary Medicine, College Station, Texas.
Obstruction and Rupture of the Urinary Tract

JONATHAN H. FOREMAN, D.V.M., M.S.
Associate Professor, University of Illinois College of Veterinary Medicine, Urbana, Illinois.
Bacterial Meningitis and Cerebral Abscesses; Hematological and Endocrine Changes During Exercise

CONTRIBUTORS—continued

LINDA A. FRANK, M.S., D.V.M.
Senior Resident, University of Florida College of Veterinary Medicine, Gainesville, Florida.
Dermatophytosis

JOHN FREESTONE, B.V.Sc., F.R.C.V.S., M.A.C.V.Sc., Diplomate A.C.V.I.M.
Associate Professor of Equine Medicine, Louisiana State University School of Veterinary Medicine, Baton Rouge, Louisiana.
Anhidrosis

FRANCIS D. GALEY, D.V.M., Ph.D., Diplomate A.B.V.T.
Assistant Professor of Clinical Diagnostic Veterinary Toxicology, California Veterinary Diagnostic Laboratory System, University of California School of Veterinary Medicine, Davis, California.
Diagnostic Toxicology

RICHARD H. GALLEY, D.V.M.
Willow Park, Texas.
The Veterinarian's Role in Racing

SARAH Y. GARDNER, D.V.M.
Graduate Assistant, Department of Anatomy, Physiological Sciences and Radiology, North Carolina State University College of Veterinary Medicine, Raleigh, North Carolina.
Jugular Vein Thrombophlebitis

TAM GARLAND, D.V.M.
Veterinary Clinical Associate, Department of Physiology and Pharmacology, College of Veterinary Medicine, Texas A&M University, College Station, Texas.
Management of Toxicoses; Industrial Toxicants

DONNA M. GATEWOOD, D.V.M.
Instructor, Department of Laboratory Medicine, Kansas State University College of Veterinary Medicine, Manhattan, Kansas.
Dermatologic Conditions of the Penis and Prepuce

DENNIS R. GEISER, B.S., D.V.M., Diplomate A.B.V.P. (Equine)
Associate Professor, College of Veterinary Medicine, University of Tennessee. Large Animal Anesthesiologist, Neonatal Intensive Care, University of Tennessee Veterinary Teaching Hospital, Knoxville, Tennessee.
Chemical Restraint and Anesthesia of the Draft Horse; Respiratory Support of the Newborn Foal

LISA GIFT, D.V.M.
Chief Resident in Equine Surgery, Kansas State University College of Veterinary Medicine, Manhattan, Kansas.
Common Malformations and Congenital Abnormalities of the Central Nervous System; Trauma of the Brain and Spinal Cord

MARY B. GLAZE, D.V.M., M.S., Diplomate A.C.V.O.
Associate Professor of Veterinary Ophthalmology, Department of Veterinary Clinical Sciences, Louisiana State University School of Veterinary Medicine. Veterinary Ophthalmologist, Louisiana State University Veterinary Teaching Hospital and Clinics, Baton Rouge, Louisiana.
Corneal Stromal Abscesses

DALLAS O. GOBLE, D.V.M., Diplomate A.C.V.S.
Associate Professor of Surgery, College of Veterinary Medicine, University of Tennessee. Head of Clinic, Department of Rural Practice, University of Tennessee College of Veterinary Medicine, Knoxville, Tennessee.
Upper Respiratory Problems of the Draft Horse

ELEANOR M. GREEN, D.V.M., Diplomate A.C.V.I.M., Diplomate A.B.V.P.
Associate Professor of Equine Medicine, Equine Internal Medicine, University of Missouri College of Veterinary Medicine, Columbia, Missouri.
Esophageal Obstruction

RICHARD P. HACKETT, D.V.M., M.S.
Associate Professor of Surgery, Department of Clinical Sciences, Cornell University College of Veterinary Medicine. Chief, Section of Surgery, Veterinary Medical Teaching Hospital, Cornell University College of Veterinary Medicine, Ithaca, New York.
The Significance of Arytenoid Cartilage Movement

JOHN C. HALIBURTON, D.V.M., Ph.D.
Head, Diagnostic Toxicology, Texas Veterinary Medical Diagnostic Laboratory, Amarillo, Texas.
Toxicologic Implications of Sudden, Unexplained Death

A. L. HALLOWELL, D.V.M.
Private Practitioner, Auburn, Washington.
Management of Twin Pregnancy

CONTRIBUTORS—continued

JOANNE HARDY, D.V.M., M.S., Diplomate A.C.V.S.
Clinical Instructor, Department of Veterinary Clinical Sciences, The Ohio State University, Columbus, Ohio.
Sesamoiditis and Suspensory Desmitis

DAN L. HAWKINS, D.V.M., M.S.
Assistant Professor, Large Animal Surgery, University of Florida College of Veterinary Medicine, Gainesville, Florida.
Diseases of the Guttural Pouches

PETER F. HAYNES, D.V.M., M.S.
Professor of Veterinary Surgery, Louisiana State University School of Veterinary Medicine. Equine Service Chief, Louisiana State University Veterinary Teaching Hospital and Clinics. Director, Equine Clinical Research, Louisiana State University School of Veterinary Medicine, Baton Rouge, Louisiana.
Epiglottic Entrapment and Cysts; Pharyngeal Lymphoid Hyperplasia and Pharyngeal Stricture

ANN C. HENDERSON, B.S.
Editor/Large Animal Veterinarian, Watt Publishing Company, Mount Morris, Illinois.
The Veterinarian's Role in Insurance

MICHELLE M. HENRY, D.V.M., Ph.D., Diplomate A.C.V.I.M.
Clinical Instructor, Department of Large Animal Medicine, University of Georgia College of Veterinary Medicine, Athens, Georgia.
Diagnostic Approach to Anemia; Blood Loss Anemia; Anemia Due to Inadequate Erythropoiesis; Hemolytic Anemia

KATRIN HINRICHS, D.V.M., Ph.D.
Assistant Professor, Tufts University School of Veterinary Medicine, North Grafton, Massachusetts.
Embryo Transfer

HAROLD F. HINTZ, Ph.D.
Professor of Animal Nutrition, Cornell University, Ithaca, New York.
Enteroliths; Nutrition and Skin Diseases; Nutrient Requirements

LYNN ROLLAND HOVDA, D.V.M., M.S.
Equine Medicine, Equine Hospitals, Inc., Hastings, Minnesota.
Neonatal Septicemia

DAVID J. JASKO, D.V.M., Ph.D.
Assistant Professor of Clinical Sciences, Colorado State University College of Veterinary Medicine and Biomedical Sciences, Fort Collins, Colorado.
Stallion Seminal Characteristics and Fertility

BILL J. JOHNSON, D.V.M., Diplomate A.C.V.P.
Assistant Professor of Clinical Diagnostic Pathology, University of California. Pathologist and Section Head of Pathology, California Veterinary Diagnostic Laboratory System, Davis, California.
Forensic Necropsy

KERRY L. KETRING, D.V.M., Diplomate A.C.V.O.
Owner, All Animal Eye Clinic, Cincinnati, Ohio.
Visual Impairment

THOMAS R. KLEI, Ph.D.
Professor of Parasitology, Department of Veterinary Microbiology and Parasitology, Louisiana State University School of Veterinary Medicine, Baton Rouge, Louisiana.
Ivermectin in Dermatologic Disorders

DEBRA A. KNIGHT, M.S., Ph.D.
Clinical Research Associate, Ross Laboratories, Columbus, Ohio.
Developmental Orthopedic Disease

DONALD P. KNOWLES, D.V.M., Ph.D.
Veterinary Medical Officer, United States Department of Agriculture, Agricultural Research Service, Washington State University. Assistant Professor, Washington State University, Pullman, Washington.
Babesiosis

RALPH C. KNOWLES, D.V.M.
Salisbury, Maryland.
International Transport of Horses

CATHERINE W. KOHN, V.M.D.
Associate Professor, Department of Veterinary Clinical Sciences, College of Veterinary Medicine, The Ohio State University, Columbus, Ohio.
Junctional Mechanobullous Disease in Belgian Foals

CONTRIBUTORS—continued

NORBERT KOPF, Dr. Med. Vet. Univ.-Doz.
Universitätsdozent für Chirurgie and Augenheilkunde an der Universitätsklinik für Chirurgie und Augenheilkunde der Veterinärmedizinischen Universität Wien. Universitätslektor für "Abdominalchirurgie des Pferdes" an der Universitätsklinik für Chirurgie and Augenheilkunde der Veterinärmedizinischen Universität Wien: Praktischer Tierarzt. Privatpraxis in Wien, Breitensee, Austria.
Rectal Examination of the Colic Patient

GREGG KORTZ, D.V.M.
Resident, Neurology/Neurosurgery, University of California Veterinary Medical Teaching Hospital, Davis, California.
Equine Herpes Myeloencephalopathy

DAVID S. KRONFELD, M.V.Sc., Ph.D., D.Sc., Diplomate A.C.V.N., Diplomate A.C.V.I.M.
The Paul Mellon Distinguished Professor of Agriculture and Professor of Veterinary Medicine, Virginia Polytechnic Institute and State University, Blacksburg, Virginia.
Ergogenic Diets and Nutrients

WILLIAM W. LAEGREID, D.V.M., Ph.D.
Research Leader, Molecular Pathology, Plum Island Animal Disease Center, United States Department of Agriculture, Agricultural Research Service, Greenport, New York.
African Horse Sickness; Other Exotic Diseases

JEAN LAMB, D.V.M.
Private Practitioner, Lexington, Kentucky.
Pericardial Disease

J. DANIEL LAVACH, D.V.M., M.S., Diplomate A.C.V.O.
Eye Clinic for Animals, Garden Grove, California.
Ocular Neoplasia

DESMOND P. LEADON, M.A., M.V.B., M.Sc., F.R.C.V.S.
Irish Equine Centre, Johnston, Naas, County Kildare, Ireland.
Clinical Pathology Data

PATRICK H. LEBLANC, D.V.M., M.S., Diplomate A.C.V.A.
Assistant Professor, The Michigan State University, East Lansing, Michigan.
Regional Anesthesia

WILLIAM B. LEY, D.V.M., M.S., Diplomate A.C.T.
Associate Professor of Equine Production Management Medicine, Virginia-Maryland Regional College of Veterinary Medicine, Virginia Polytechnic Institute and State University, Blacksburg, Virginia.
Prefoaling Management of the Mare and Induction of Parturition

WILLIAM A. LINDSAY, D.V.M.
Associate Professor, Large Animal Surgery, University of Wisconsin Veterinary Medical Teaching Hospital, Madison, Wisconsin.
Ethmoidal Hematoma

ROBERT J. MACKAY, B.V.Sc. Ph.D.
Assistant Professor, Department of Large Animal Clinical Sciences, University of Florida College of Veterinary Medicine, Gainesville, Florida.
Endotoxemia

TIM MAIR, B.V.Sc., Ph.D., M.R.C.V.S.
Private Veterinary Practitioner, Kent, England.
Diagnostic Techniques for Lower Respiratory Tract Diseases

MARK D. MARKEL, D.V.M., Ph.D.
Assistant Professor of Surgery, University of Wisconsin School of Veterinary Medicine, Madison, Wisconsin.
Diseases of the Spine

CELIA M. MARR, B.V.M.S., M.V.M., Ph.D., M.R.C.V.S.
Clinical Associate, New Bolton Center, University of Pennsylvania School of Veterinary Medicine. Emergency Service Clinician, The George D. Widener Hospital, New Bolton Center, Kennett Square, Pennsylvania.
Acquired Valvular Heart Disease

MICHAEL T. MARTIN, D.V.M., M.S.
Associate Professor, Equine Field Service, Texas A & M University, College Station, Texas.
Veterinary Services for Horse Shows

MARIA D. MASRI, M.V.Z., M.S.
Visiting Assistant Professor, Department of Large Animal Medicine, College of Veterinary Medicine, University of Florida, Gainesville, Florida.
Mycotoxic Encephalomalacia

HILARY K. MATTHEWS, D.V.M.

Medical Resident, University of Tennessee College of Veterinary Medicine, Knoxville, Tennessee.

Seizures and Narcolepsy

NORA S. MATTHEWS, D.V.M.

Assistant Professor, Department of Small Animal Medicine and Surgery, Texas A&M University, College Station, Texas.

General Anesthesia; Sedation and Anesthesia of Mules and Donkeys

SARAH MAXWELL, B.S., D.V.M., M.S.

Resident, Veterinary Ophthalmology, Kansas State University College of Veterinary Medicine, Manhattan, Kansas.

Neurological Causes of Blindness

STEPHEN A. MAY, M.A., Vet.M.B., Ph.D., D.V.R., Cert.C.O., M.R.C.V.S.

Lecturer in Equine Orthopaedics, Department of Veterinary Clinical Science, University of Liverpool, Leahurst, England.

Anti-Inflammatory Agents

REBECCA McCONNICO, D.V.M.

Resident, Large Animal Internal Medicine, North Carolina State University College of Veterinary Medicine. Resident, Large Animal Internal Medicine, North Carolina State University Veterinary Teaching Hospital, Raleigh, North Carolina.

Tetanus

SUE M. McDONNELL, Ph.D., A.B.S.Cert.

Lecturer, Section of Reproductive Studies, University of Pennsylvania School of Veterinary Medicine. Head, Reproductive Behavior Laboratory, University of Pennsylvania School of Veterinary Medicine, New Bolton Center, Kennett Square, Pennsylvania.

Sexual Behavior Dysfunction in Mares; Sexual Behavior Dysfunction in Stallions

THOMAS R. MILLER, D.V.M., M.S., Diplomate A.C.V.O.

Assistant Professor, University of Florida College of Veterinary Medicine. Staff Ophthalmologist, University of Florida Medical Teaching Hospital, Gainesville, Florida.

Punctate Keratitis

NICHOLAS J. MILLICHAMP, B.Vet.Med., Ph.D., Diplomate A.C.V.O., D.V.Ophthal.

Department of Small Animal Medicine and Surgery, College of Veterinary Medicine, Texas A&M University, College Station, Texas.

Cataracts

CECIL P. MOORE, D.V.M., M.S., Diplomate A.C.V.I.M.

Associate Professor, Department of Veterinary Medicine and Surgery, University of Missouri. Head, Ophthalmology Service, University of Missouri Veterinary Medical Teaching Hospital, Columbia, Missouri.

Ocular Discharge; Corneal Ulceration

DEBRA DEEM MORRIS, D.V.M., M.S.

Associate Professor of Large Animal Medicine, College of Veterinary Medicine, University of Georgia Veterinary Medical Teaching Hospital, Athens, Georgia.

Disseminated Intravascular Coagulation; Idiopathic Thrombocytopenia; Vasculitis

ELISABETH MORRIS, D.V.M.

Assistant Professor, Large Animal Medicine, Tufts University School of Veterinary Medicine, North Grafton, Massachusetts.

Introduction to Performance Evaluation; Dynamic Endoscopy of the Upper Airway; Fitness Testing

JENNIFER A. MUMFORD, B.Sc., Ph.D.

Head, Department of Infectious Diseases, Equine Research Station, Animal Health Trust, Newmarket, England.

Respiratory Viral Disease

MIKE MURPHY, D.V.M., Ph.D.

Assistant Professor, Department of Veterinary Diagnostic Medicine, University of Minnesota College of Veterinary Medicine, St. Paul, Minnesota.

Toxic Plants

MICHAEL J. MURRAY, D.V.M., M.S., Diplomate A.C.V.I.M.

Assistant Professor, Marion DuPont Scott Equine Medical Center, Virginia-Maryland Regional College of Veterinarian Medicine, Virginia Polytechnic Institute and State University. Chief, Internal Medicine Service, Leesburg, Virginia.

Diagnostic Procedures for Evaluation of the Alimentary System; Gastroduodenal Ulceration; Acute Colitis

CONTRIBUTORS—continued

JONATHAN M. NAYLOR, B.Sc., B.V.Sc., Ph.D., Diplomate A.C.V.I.M., Diplomate A.C.V.N.
Professor, Department of Veterinary Internal Medicine, University of Saskatchewan. Clinician, Western College of Veterinary Medicine, University of Saskatchewan, Saskatoon, Saskatchewan, Canada.
Nutritional Management in Disease

FRANK A. NICKELS, D.V.M., M.S.
Associate Professor, Department of Large Animal Clinical Sciences, College of Veterinary Medicine, Michigan State University, East Lansing, Michigan.
Arytenoid Chondritis

ALAN J. NIXON, B.V.Sc, M.S.
Associate Professor, Large Animal Orthopedic Surgery, Cornell University College of Veterinary Medicine, Ithaca, New York.
Intra-Articular Medication

KAREN A. NYROP, D.V.M., M.S.
Equine Practitioner, Phoenix, Arizona.
Cutaneous Mastocytosis

MICHAEL W. O'CALLAGHAN, B.V.Sc., M.Sc.V., Ph.D., M.R.C.V.S.
Associate Professor of Radiology, Tufts University School of Veterinary Medicine, North Grafton, Massachusetts.
Imaging of the Lower Airways

EDGAR A. OTT, B.S., M.S., Ph.D.
Professor of Animal Nutrition, Animal Sciences Department, University of Florida, Gainesville, Florida.
Nutritional Factors in Developmental Orthopedic Disease

JOHNATHAN E. PALMER, V.M.D., Diplomate A.C.V.I.M.
Assistant Professor of Medicine, University of Pennsylvania, New Bolton Center, Kennett Square, Pennsylvania.
Potomac Horse Fever

JOHN R. PASCOE, B.V.Sc., Ph.D., Diplomate A.C.V.S.
Associate Professor, Department of Veterinary Medical Surgery, University of California. Chief, Equine Surgery Service, University of California Veterinary Medical Teaching Hospital, Davis, California.
Upper Airway Flow Dynamics

JOHN W. PAUL, D.V.M., M.S.
Manager, Professional Services, Hoechst-Roussel Agri-Vet Company, Somerville, New Jersey.
Clinical Field Trials

ERWIN G. PEARSON, D.V.M., M.S., Diplomate A.C.V.I.M.
Professor, Large Animal Internal Medicine, Oregon State University Veterinary Teaching Hospital, Corvallis, Oregon.
Hepatic Diseases in Foals

PAMELA A. PINTCHUK, D.V.M.
Resident, Large Animal Medicine, Equine Emphasis, University of California School of Veterinary Medicine, Davis, California.
Botulism

FRANK S. PIPERS, D.V.M., Ph.D.
Tufts University School of Veterinary Medicine, North Grafton, Massachusetts.
Congenital Cardiovascular Disorders; Electrophysiologic Responses to Exercise

JOHN PRINGLE, D.V.M., D.V.Sc.
Associate Professor, Department of Health Management, University of Prince Edward Island Atlantic Veterinary College, Charlottetown, Canada.
Emergency Treatment of the Traumatized Horse

JERRY R. RAINS, M.S., D.V.M., Diplomate A.C.T.
Assistant Professor, Veterinary Medicine and Surgery, Oklahoma State University. Professional Services Specialist, Hoechst-Roussel Agri-Vet Company, Kansas City, Missouri.
The Veterinarian's Role in Insurance

MERL F. RAISBECK, D.V.M., M.S., Ph.D.
Associate Professor of Veterinary Toxicology, University of Wyoming, Laramie, Wyoming.
Feed-Associated Poisoning

SARAH L. RALSTON, V.M.D., Ph.D., Diplomate A.C.V.N.
Assistant Professor, Department of Animal Sciences, Cook College, Rutgers University, New Brunswick, New Jersey.
Diagnosis of Common Mineral Imbalances

JOHN REAGOR, Ph.D.
Head, Department of Toxicology, Texas Veterinary Medical Diagnostic Laboratory, Texas A&M University, College Station, Texas.
Toxic Plants

CONTRIBUTORS—continued

VIRGINIA B. REEF, D.V.M.

Associate Professor of Medicine in the Widener Hospital, University of Pennsylvania. Director, Large Animal Cardiology and Diagnostic Ultrasonography, University of Pennsylvania, New Bolton Center, Kennett Square, Pennsylvania.

Cardiovascular Problems Associated with Poor Performance; Myocardial Disease; Ultrasonographic Evaluation and Diagnosis of Foal Diseases; Evaluation of Tendons and Ligaments

MATTHEW REEVES, B.V.Sc., M.S., M.R.C.V.S., Diplomate A.C.V.S.

Lecturer, Section of Epidemiology and Public Health, University of Pennsylvania School of Veterinary Medicine, New Bolton Center, Kennett Square, Pennsylvania.

Risk and Prognostic Factors in Colic

JOHANA M. REINER, V.M.D., Diplomate A.C.V.I.M.

Lecturer, New Bolton Center, University of Pennsylvania, School of Veterinary Medicine, New Bolton Center, Kennett Square, Pennsylvania.

Cardiac Arrhythmias

DEAN W. RICHARDSON, D.V.M.

Assistant Professor of Surgery, University of Pennsylvania, School of Veterinary Medicine, New Bolton Center, Kennett Square, Pennsylvania.

Degenerative Joint Disease

MALCOLM C. ROBERTS, B.V.Sc., Ph.D., F.R.C.V.S., F.A.C.V.Sc.

Professor of Equine Medicine and Head, Department of Food Animal and Equine Medicine. Equine Clinician, Veterinary Teaching Hospital, North Carolina State University College of Veterinary Medicine, Raleigh, North Carolina.

Chronic Eosinophilic Dermatitides

JAMES T. ROBERTSON, D.V.M., Diplomate A.C.V.S.

Associate Professor, Equine Surgery, College of Veterinary Medicine, The Ohio State University, Columbus, Ohio.

Diseases of the Nasal Passages

SHEILAH A. ROBERTSON, B.V.M.S., Ph.D., Diplomate A.C.V.A.

Assistant Professor, Department of Large Animal Clinical Sciences, College of Veterinary Medicine, Michigan State University.

Sedation and General Anesthesia of the Foal

N. EDWARD ROBINSON, B.Vet.Med., M.R.C.V.S., Ph.D.

Matilda R. Wilson Professor, Department of Large Animal Clinical Sciences, College of Veterinary Medicine, Michigan State University, East Lansing, Michigan.

Table of Drugs: Approximate Doses; Interstate Shipping of Horses

YVES ROSSIER

Assistant Professor, University of Montreal Veterinary School, Quebec, Canada.

Renal Tubular Acidosis

LINDA K. SCHLATER, D.V.M., M.S., Diplomate A.C.V.M. (Bacteriology), Diplomate A.C.V.P.M.

Head, Aerobic Bacteriology Section, Biologics Bacteriology Laboratory, United States Department of Agriculture, Animal and Plant Health Inspection Service, National Veterinary Services Laboratories, Ames, Iowa.

Glanders; Meliodosis

L. MICHAEL SCHMALL, D.V.M., M.S.

Assistant Professor, Department of Veterinary Clinical Sciences, The Ohio State University, Columbus, Ohio.

Fluid and Electrolyte Therapy

DANNY W. SCOTT, D.V.M., Diplomate A.C.V.D.

Professor of Medicine, New York State College of Veterinary Medicine, Cornell University, Ithaca, New York.

Staphyloccal Skin Disease

LEON SCRUTCHFIELD, D.V.M., M.S.

Associate Professor, Large Animal Medicine and Surgery. Chief, Field Services, Veterinary Teaching Hospital, Texas A&M University College of Veterinary Medicine, College Station, Texas.

Veterinary Services for Horse Shows

HOWARD J. SEEHERMAN, Ph.D., V.M.D.

Assistant Professor of Large Animal Surgery and Head of Large Animal Surgery Section and Director of Equine Sports Medicine, Tufts University School of Veterinary Medicine, North Grafton, Massachusetts.

Gait Analysis; Evaluation of Bone

SUSAN D. SEMRAD, V.M.D., Ph.D.
Assistant Professor, Large Animal Internal Medicine, University of Wisconsin, Madison, Wisconsin.
Peritonitis; Neurological Examination of the Neonatal Foal; Gastrointestinal Diseases of the Neonatal Foal

PATRICIA L. SERTICH, M.S., V.M.D., Diplomate A.C.T.
Lecturer, Section of Reproductive Studies and Head, Hoffman Center for Reproductive Studies, New Bolton Center, University of Pennsylvania School of Veterinary Medicine, Kennett Square, Pennsylvania.
Persistent Estrus: Fact or Fiction?

SUSAN SHAFTOE, V.M.D., Diplomate A.C.V.I.M.
Clinical Assistant Professor, University of Wisconsin School of Veterinary Medicine, Madison, Wisconsin.
Neurological Examination of the Neonatal Foal; Gastrointestinal Diseases of the Neonatal Foal

R. STEWART SHOEMAKER, D.V.M.
Assistant Professor, Equine Surgery Section and Coordinator Equine Treadmill, Louisiana State University School of Veterinary Medicine, Baton Rouge, Louisiana.
Epiglottic Entrapment and Cysts; Pharyngeal Lymphoid Hyperplasia and Pharyngeal Stricture

ROBERT E. SHOPE, M.D.
Professor of Epidemiology, Yale University School of Medicine, New Haven, Connecticut.
Japanese Encephalitis

JANA M. SMITH, D.V.M., M.S.
Clovis Equine Clinic, Clovis, California.
Vestibular Disease

JACK R. SNYDER, D.V.M., Ph.D., Diplomate A.C.V.S.
Assistant Professor, Department of Surgery, University of California School of Veterinary Medicine, Davis, California.
Physical and Laboratory Evaluation of the Horse with Colic; Nonstrangulating and Strangulating Obstruction of the Ascending Colon Enteroliths

MITCHELL D. SONG, D.V.M.
Chief Dermatology Resident, University of California School of Veterinary Medicine, Davis, California.
Skin Biopsies in the Diagnosis of Inflammatory Skin Diseases

VICTOR C. SPEIRS, B.V.Sc., M.V.Sc.
Professor and Head, Equine Surgery, University of Berne Klinik fur Nutztiere und Pferde Tierspital, Berne, Switzerland.
Diseases of the Paranasal Sinuses

MICHAEL S. SPENSLEY, D.V.M.
Project Manager, Department of Pharmaceutical Development, Solvay Animal Health Inc., Mendota Heights, Minnesota.
Preventive Medicine Programs

SHARON J. SPIER, D.V.M., Ph.D.
Assistant Professor, Department of Medicine, University of California School of Veterinary Medicine, Davis, California.
Hyperkalemic Periodic Paralysis; Physical and Laboratory Evaluation of the Horse with Colic; Nonstrangulating Obstruction of the Ascending Colon

SHAUNA L. SPURLOCK, D.V.M., M.S.
Private Practitioner, Spurlock Equine Associates, Lovettsville, Virginia.
Parenteral Nutrition

SUSAN M. STOVER, D.V.M., Ph.D.
Assistant Professor, Department of Anatomy, University of California School of Veterinary Medicine, Davis, California.
Dorsal Metacarpal Disease

KENNETH E. SULLINS, D.V.M., M.S., Diplomate A.C.V.S.
Associate Professor of Surgery, Marion DuPont Scott Equine Medical Center, Leesburg, Virginia.
Strangulating and Nonstrangulating Obstruction of the Small Intestine

TERRY D. SWANSON, D.V.M.
Vice President, Littleton Large Animal Clinic, Littleton, Colorado.
The Veterinarian's Responsibilities at Trail Rides

CORRINE RAPHEL SWEENEY, D.V.M.
Assistant Professor of Medicine, University of Pennsylvania School of Veterinary Medicine,

New Bolton Center, Kennett Square, Pennsylvania.
Pleuropneumonia

LLOYD P. TATE, Jr., V.M.D.
Associate Professor of Equine Surgery and Service Chief, North Carolina State University College of Veterinary Medicine, Raleigh, North Carolina.
Lasers in Dermatology

FRANK G. R. TAYLOR, B.V.Sc., Ph.D., M.R.C.V.S.
Lecturer in Equine Medicine, Langford House, University of Bristol, Bristol, England.
Strangles

TEX TAYLOR, D.V.M.
Professor, Chief of Surgery, Department of Large Animal Medicine and Surgery, Texas A&M University, College Station, Texas.
Sedation and Anesthesia of Mules and Donkeys

CRAIG D. THATCHER, D.V.M., Ph.D.
Assistant Professor and Production Management Medicine and Clinical Nutrition Service, Veterinary Medical Teaching Hospital, Virginia-Maryland Regional College of Veterinary Medicine, Blacksburg, Virginia.
Enteral Nutritional Support of Sick Horses

LARRY J. THOMPSON, D.V.M., Diplomate A.B.V.T.
Clinical Toxicologist, Diagnostic Laboratory, Cornell University College of Veterinary Medicine, Ithaca, New York.
Heavy Metal Toxicosis

PETER J. TIMONEY, M.V.B., Ph.D., F.R.C.V.S.
Professor, Department of Veterinary Science, Maxwell H. Gluck Equine Research Center, University of Kentucky, Lexington, Kentucky.
Contageous Equine Metritis

JOSIE L. TRAUB-DARGATZ, D.V.M., M.S.
Associate Professor, Colorado State University College of Veterinary Medicine, Fort Collins, Colorado.
Biliary Disorders

ERIC TULLENERS, D.V.M., Diplomate A.C.V.S.
Chief of Large Animal Surgery and Assistant Professor of Surgery, University of Pennsylvania School of Veterinary Medicine, New Bolton Center, Kennett Square, Pennsylvania.
Laser Surgery for Upper Respiratory Disorders

TRACY A. TURNER, D.V.M., M.S.
Surgeon and Director of Sports Medicine, Rochester Equine Clinic, Rochester, New Hampshire.
Muscular Disorders; Navicular Syndrome

WENDY E. VAALA, V.M.D.
Lecturer, University of Pennsylvania School of Veterinary Medicine, New Bolton Center, Kennett Square, Pennsylvania.
Nutritional Management of the Critically Ill Neonate

STEPHANIE J. VALBERG, D.V.M., Ph.D.
Resident, Large Animal Medicine, Veterinary Medical Teaching Hospital, University of California School of Veterinary Medicine, Davis, California.
Evaluation of Muscle

DIRK K. VANDERWALL, D.V.M.
Graduate Assistant, Department of Animal and Veterinary Science, University of Idaho, Moscow, Idaho.
Age-Related Ovulatory Dysfunction

DICKSON D. VARNER, D.V.M., M.S.
Associate Professor, Department of Large Animal Medicine and Surgery, Texas A&M University College of Veterinary Medicine, College Station, Texas.
Handling of Stallion Semen

PAMELA C. WAGNER, D.V.M., M.S.
Professor, Oregon State University College of Veterinary Medicine. Surgeon, Veterinary Teaching Hospital, Oregon State University College of Veterinary Medicine, Corvallis, Oregon.
Septic Arthritis and Osteomyelitis

ROBERT D. WALKER, M.S., Ph.D.
Professor of Microbiology and Public Health, Michigan State University College of Veterinary Medicine. Section Chief, Bacteriology/Mycology, Animal Health Diagnostic Laboratory, Michigan State University, East Lansing, Michigan.
Antimicrobial Chemotherapy

THOMAS E. WALTON, D.V.M., Ph.D.

Adjunct Professor of Veterinary Science, University of Wyoming, Laramie, Wyoming. Affiliate Faculty in Microbiology, Colorado State University, Fort Collins, Colorado.

Venezuelan Equine Encephalitis

MICHAEL V. WARD, D.V.M.

Director of Clinical Programs, North America, Japan, Europe, Baxter Health Care Corporation. Vice President of Product Development, Hemovet Veterinary Transfusion and Blood Processing, Irvine, California.

Parenteral Nutrition

BARBARA J. WATROUS, D.V.M., Diplomate A.C.V.R.

Associate Professor of Radiology, Veterinary Teaching Hospital, College of Veterinary Medicine, Oregon State University, Corvallis, Oregon.

Septic Arthritis and Osteomyelitis

JAMES A. WEBER, M.S.

Graduate Student, Department of Animal and Veterinary Sciences, University of Idaho, Moscow, Idaho.

Ultrasonographic Evaluation of Accessory Sex Gland Structure and Function in the Stallion

SIMON J. WHEELER, B.V.Sc., Ph.D., M.R.C.V.S.

Assistant Professor of Neurology, Department of Companion Animal and Special Species Medicine. Neurologist, Veterinary Teaching Hospital, North Carolina State University College of Veterinary Medicine, Raleigh, North Carolina.

Peripheral Neuropathies

SUSAN L. WHITE, D.V.M., M.S., Diplomate A.C.V.I.M.

Associate Professor, Large Animal Internal Medicine, University of Georgia College of Veterinary Medicine, Athens, Georgia.

Passive Transfer of Immunity to Foals

ROBERT H. WHITLOCK, D.V.M., Ph.D.

Marilyn A. Simpson Professor of Equine Medicine, Department of Clinical Studies, University of Pennsylvania School of Veterinary Medicine, New Bolton Center, Kennett Square, Pennsylvania.

Polyuria; Chronic Renal Failure

DAVID A. WILKIE, D.V.M., M.S., Diplomate A.C.V.O.

Assistant Professor, Department of Veterinary Clinical Sciences, The Ohio State University, Columbus, Ohio.

Ocular Injuries

M. AMY WILLIAMS, D.V.M., M.S., Diplomate A.B.V.P.

Assistant Professor of Equine Medicine, Department of Large Animal Medicine and Surgery, Auburn University College of Veterinary Medicine, Auburn, Alabama.

Risk Factors Associated with Developmental Orthopedic Disease

LISA WILLIAMSON, D.V.M., M.S., Diplomate A.C.V.I.M.

Assistant Professor, Department of Large Animal Medicine, College of Veterinary Medicine, University of Georgia, Athens, Georgia.

Blood and Plasma Therapy

W. DAVID WILSON, B.V.M.S., M.S., M.R.C.V.S.

Associate Professor, Department of Medicine. Senior Clinician, Equine Field Service Section, Large Animal Medicine Service, Veterinary Medical Teaching Hospital, University of California School of Veterinary Medicine, Davis, California.

Preventive Medicine Programs; Foal Pneumonia

GORDON L. WOODS, D.V.M., Ph.D., Diplomate A.C.T.

Professor, Department of Animal and Veterinary Sciences, University of Idaho, Moscow, Idaho.

Age-Related Ovulatory Dysfunction; Management of Twin Pregnancy; Ultrasonographic Evaluation of Accessory Sex Gland Structure and Function in the Stallion

KATHLEEN YVORCHUK, D.M.V.

Assistant Professor, Equine Field Service, Department of Veterinary Clinical Sciences, Kansas State University College of Veterinary Medicine, Manhattan, Kansas.

PREFACE

Editing each new edition of *Current Therapy in Equine Medicine* provides me with an opportunity to review the progress that has been made in equine medicine over the past four or five years. The challenge is to continue to include the common and important medical problems while at the same time including material on newer diagnostic techniques and therapies—all within 900 or so pages.

In this edition, as before, there are sections on diseases of each of the organ systems, including a new section on medical problems of the musculoskeletal system. Other new sections emphasize the changes in equine practice, the influence of technology, and the "shrinking" world. The burgeoning number of pharmaceuticals necessitated a section on therapeutics. The section on the duties of a veterinarian reflects the increasing legal responsibilities of practice and advises what is expected when a practitioner agrees to undertake certain duties. Exotic diseases are included because the movement of horses and people around the globe increases the likelihood that these diseases may be seen by the practitioner. The use of the high-speed treadmill and imaging techniques for diagnosis is described in "Assessment of Athletic Performance."

As with previous editions, this book is written for the practitioner and veterinary student. In general, each article contains a description of clinical signs, confirmatory tests, and therapy of a disease. Authors have provided their best opinions of routes of drug administration and dosage schedules. Each article was also reviewed by a consulting editor, who initially suggested the content of the section.

I am extremely indebted to the consulting editors and authors for the dedication they showed to the production of this book. As a result of their efforts, we were able to produce this edition in less time than previous ones so that the information is indeed current.

Current Therapy in Equine Medicine 3 is not meant to be a complete reference on all diseases of the horse and should not be judged as such. Topics and authors change with each edition of the book. In recognition of this changing emphasis and of the excellent material in earlier editions, we have cross-referenced the index of the new volume 3 with *Current Therapy in Equine Medicine 2*.

My work in East Lansing would have been much more difficult without the editorial assistance of Victoria Kingsbury, who put manuscripts in final format for the publisher; Doug Clarke; Cheryl Gahrs; Carol Kuzma; and Emily Robinson, who checked the references. The staff of W. B. Saunders and Editorial Services of New England maintained their high standards and were totally cooperative and supportive. Linda Mills, Lorraine B. Kilmer, Frank Polizzano, and John Fitzpatrick deserve special thanks for keeping the book on schedule.

N. EDWARD ROBINSON

Current Therapy in Equine Medicine

NOTICE

Equine medicine is an ever-changing field. But as new research and clinical experience grow, changes in treatment and drug therapy become necessary or appropriate. The authors and editors of this work have carefully checked and verified drug dosages to assure that dosage information is precise and in accord with standards accepted at the time of publication. Readers are advised, however, to check the product information currently provided by the manufacturer of each drug to be administered to be certain that changes have not been made in the recommended dose or in the contraindications for administration. This is of particular importance in regard to new or infrequently used drugs. Recommended dosages for animals are sometimes based on adjustments in the dosage that would be suitable for humans. Some of the drugs mentioned have been given experimentally by the authors. Others have been used in dosages greater than those recommended by the manufacturer. In these kinds of cases, the authors have reported on their own considerable experience. It is the responsibility of those administering a drug, relying on their professional skill and experience, to determine dosages, the best treatment for the patient, and whether the benefits of giving a drug justify the attendant risk. The editors cannot be responsible for misuse or misapplication of the material in this work.

THE PUBLISHER

CONTENTS

Section 1 THERAPEUTICS
N. Edward Robinson, *Consulting Editor*

ANTIMICROBIAL CHEMOTHERAPY *Robert D. Walker*	1
ANTI-INFLAMMATORY AGENTS *Stephen A. May*	14
FLUID AND ELECTROLYTE THERAPY *L. Michael Schmall*	18
CHEMICAL RESTRAINT OF THE STANDING HORSE *Richard M. Bednarski*	22
REGIONAL ANESTHESIA *Patrick H. LeBlanc*	25
GENERAL ANESTHESIA *Nora S. Matthews*	28
EMERGENCY TREATMENT OF THE TRAUMATIZED HORSE *John Pringle*	32
PREVENTIVE MEDICINE PROGRAMS *W. David Wilson and Michael S. Spensley*	35
INTERNAL PARASITE CONTROL PROGRAMS *Joseph A. DiPietro*	51

Section 2 DUTIES OF A VETERINARIAN
Glenn F. Anderson, *Consulting Editor*

SELECTED MEDICAL-LEGAL CONSIDERATIONS IN THE PRACTICE OF EQUINE MEDICINE *Thomas H. Allison*	57
THE VETERINARIAN AS A WITNESS *Thomas H. Allison*	61
THE VETERINARIAN'S ROLE IN INSURANCE *Lance L. Allen, Jerry R. Rains, and Ann C. Henderson*	65
PURCHASE EXAMINATION OF THE PERFORMANCE HORSE *Glenn F. Anderson*	68
INTERNATIONAL TRANSPORT OF HORSES *Ralph C. Knowles*	72
CLINICAL FIELD TRIALS *John W. Paul*	74
VETERINARY SERVICES FOR HORSE SHOWS, *Michael T. Martin and Leon Scrutchfield*	76
THE VETERINARIAN'S ROLE IN RACING *Richard H. Galley*	78
THE VETERINARIAN'S RESPONSIBILITIES AT TRAIL RIDES *Terry D. Swanson*	80

Section 3 SPECIAL PROBLEMS OF DRAFT HORSES AND MULES
Dallas O. Goble, *Consulting Editor*

COMMON LAMENESS PROBLEMS OF THE DRAFT HORSE *Henry S. Adair*	85
UPPER RESPIRATORY PROBLEMS OF THE DRAFT HORSE *Dallas O. Goble*	92
CHEMICAL RESTRAINT AND ANESTHESIA OF THE DRAFT HORSE *Dennis R. Geiser*	95

SEDATION AND ANESTHESIA OF MULES AND DONKEYS   *Nora S. Matthews and Tex Taylor* 101

Section 4   MUSCULOSKELETAL DISEASES
Alicia Bertone, *Consulting Editor*

DEVELOPMENTAL ORTHOPEDIC DISEASE   *Warren L. Beard and Debra A. Knight* 105
DISEASES OF THE SPINE   *Mark D. Markel* 109
MUSCULAR DISORDERS   *Tracy A. Turner* 113
HYERKALEMIC PERIODIC PARALYSIS   *Sharon J. Spier* 117
NUTRITIONAL SECONDARY HYPERPARATHYROIDISM   *Joseph J. Bertone* 119
DIFFERENTIAL DIAGNOSES OF MEDICAL LAMENESS: NUTRITIONAL, TOXIC, METABOLIC, AND OTHER CONDITIONS   *Joseph J. Bertone* 123
INTRA-ARTICULAR MEDICATION   *Alan J. Nixon* 127
INFECTIOUS SYNOVITIS   *Alicia L. Bertone* 131
NONINFECTIOUS SYNOVITIS   *Alicia L. Bertone* 134
DEGENERATIVE JOINT DISEASE   *Dean W. Richardson* 137
SESAMOIDITIS AND SUSPENSORY DESMITIS   *Joanne Hardy* 140
DORSAL METACARPAL DISEASE   *Susan M. Stover* 143
MEDICAL TREATMENT OF TENDINITIS   *Lawrence R. Bramlage* 146
NAVICULAR SYNDROME   *Tracy A. Turner* 149
LAMINITIS   *Gary M. Baxter* 154
APPENDICULAR INFLAMMATORY DISORDERS   *Valerie A. Fadok* 161

Section 5   ALIMENTARY TRACT DISEASE
Michael J. Murray, *Consulting Editor*

DIAGNOSTIC PROCEDURES FOR EVALUATION OF THE ALIMENTARY SYSTEM   *Michael J. Murray* 167
DYSPHAGIA   *Christopher M. Brown* 171
ESOPHAGEAL OBSTRUCTION   *Eleanor M. Green* 175
GASTROINTESTINAL ULCERATION   *Michael J. Murray* 184
PHYSICAL AND LABORATORY EVALUATION OF THE HORSE WITH COLIC   *Sharon J. Spier and Jack R. Snyder* 190
RECTAL EXAMINATION OF THE COLIC PATIENT   *Norbert Kopf* 196
PHARMACOLOGIC MANAGEMENT OF COLIC   *E. Susan Clark* 201
RISK AND PROGNOSTIC FACTORS IN COLIC   *Matthew Reeves* 206
DUODENITIS—PROXIMAL JEJUNITIS   *Douglas Allen, Jr. and E. Susan Clark* 211
STRANGULATING AND NONSTRANGULATING OBSTRUCTION OF THE SMALL INTESTINE   *Kenneth E. Sullins* 214
NONSTRANGULATING AND STRANGULATING OBSTRUCTION OF THE ASCENDING COLON   *Jack R. Snyder and Sharon J. Spier* 218
ENTEROLITHS   *Harold F. Hintz and Jack R. Snyder* 223
ENDOTOXEMIA   *Robert J. MacKay* 225
RECTAL TEARS   *Aubrey N. Baird* 232
PERITONITIS   *Susan D. Semrad* 236
ACUTE COLITIS   *Michael J. Murray* 244
POTOMAC HORSE FEVER   *Jonathan E. Palmer* 250
HEPATIC DISEASE   *Thomas J. Divers* 253
BILIARY DISORDERS   *Josie L. Traub-Dargatz* 259

Section 6 UPPER AIRWAY DISEASES
Richard P. Hackett and Normand G. Ducharme, *Consulting Editors*

DISEASES OF THE NASAL PASSAGES *James T. Robertson and Clara K. Fenger* 265
DISEASES OF PARANASAL SINUSES *Victor C. Speirs* 271
ETHMOIDAL HEMATOMA *William A. Lindsay* 274
DISEASES OF THE GUTTURAL POUCHES *Dan L. Hawkins* 275
EPIGLOTTIC ENTRAPMENT AND CYSTS *R. Stuart Shoemaker and Peter F. Haynes* 281
PHARYNGEAL LYMPHOID HYPERPLASIA AND PHARYNGEAL STRICTURE *R. Stuart Shoemaker and Peter F. Haynes* 282
DYNAMIC PHARYNGEAL COLLAPSE *Normand G. Ducharme* 283
THE SIGNIFICANCE OF ARYTENOID CARTILAGE MOVEMENT *Richard P. Hackett* 285
ARYTENOID CHONDRITIS *Frank A. Nickels* 289
UPPER AIRWAY FLOW DYNAMICS *John R. Pascoe* 291
LASER SURGERY FOR UPPER RESPIRATORY DISORDERS *Eric Tulleners* 294

Section 7 LOWER RESPIRATORY TRACT DISEASES
Andrew F. Clarke, *Consulting Editor*

DIAGNOSTIC TECHNIQUES FOR LOWER RESPIRATORY TRACT DISEASES *Tim Mair* 299
THERAPEUTICS OF THE RESPIRATORY TRACT *Patrick M. Dixon* 303
ENVIRONMENTAL MONITORING IN RELATION TO EQUINE RESPIRATORY DISEASE *Andrew F. Clarke* 310
RESPIRATORY VIRAL DISEASE *Jenny A. Mumford* 316
STRANGLES *Frank G. R. Taylor* 324
PLEUROPNEUMONIA *Corrine Raphel Sweeney* 327
CHRONIC OBSTRUCTIVE PULMONARY DISEASE *Andrew F. Clarke* 329
LUNG PARASITES *M. Bailey* 332
EXERCISE-INDUCED PULMONARY HEMORRHAGE *Andrew F. Clarke* 335

Section 8 TOXICOLOGY
Francis D. Galey, *Consulting Editor*

DIAGNOSTIC TOXICOLOGY *Francis D. Galey* 337
TOXICOLOGIC IMPLICATIONS OF SUDDEN, UNEXPLAINED DEATH *John C. Haliburton and William C. Edwards* 340
FORENSIC NECROPSY *Bill J. Johnson* 344
MANAGEMENT OF TOXICOSES *E. Murl Bailey, Jr. and Tam Garland* 346
TOXICITY OF PHARMACOLOGICAL AGENTS *Gordon W. Brumbaugh* 353
INDUSTRIAL TOXICANTS *E. Murl Bailey, Jr. and Tam Garland* 358
HEAVY METAL TOXICOSIS *Larry J. Thompson* 363
FEED-ASSOCIATED POISONING *Merl F. Raisbeck* 366
TOXIC PLANTS *Mike Murphy and John Reagor* 372
EQUINE LEUKOENCEPHALOMALACIA/HEPATOSIS AND STACHYBOTRYOTOXICOSIS *Val Richard Beasley* 377

Section 9 CARDIOVASCULAR DISEASE
Virginia B. Reef, *Consulting Editor*

CARDIOVASCULAR PROBLEMS ASSOCIATED WITH POOR PERFORMANCE *Virginia B. Reef* .. 381
CARDIAC ARRHYTHMIAS *Johanna M. Reimer* 383

MYOCARDIAL DISEASE   *Virginia B. Reef* 393
ACQUIRED VALVULAR HEART DISEASE   *Celia M. Marr* 396
BACTERIAL ENDOCARDITIS   *Chrysann Collatos* 399
PERICARDIAL DISEASE   *Bill Bernard and Jean Lamb* 402
JUGULAR VEIN THROMBOPHLEBITIS   *Sarah Y. Gardner and William J. Donawick* 406
CONGENITAL CARDIOVASCULAR DISORDERS   *Frank S. Pipers* 408

Section 10 FOAL DISEASES
Benjamin J. Darien, *Consulting Editor*

IDENTIFICATION AND EARLY MANAGEMENT OF THE HIGH-RISK NEONATAL FOAL   *Barbara D. Brewer* 411
NEUROLOGICAL EXAMINATION OF THE NEONATAL FOAL   *Susan Shaftoe and Susan D. Semrad* 414
ULTRASONOGRAPHIC EVALUATION AND DIAGNOSIS OF FOAL DISEASES   *Virginia B. Reef* .. 417
PASSIVE TRANSFER OF IMMUNITY TO FOALS   *Susan L. White* 422
HEMOSTASIS IN THE NEWBORN FOAL   *Benjamin J. Darien and Bernard F. Feldman* .. 427
NEONATAL MALADJUSTMENT SYNDROME   *Christopher M. Brown* 432
NEONATAL SEPTICEMIA   *Lynn Rolland Hovda* 435
HEPATIC DISEASE IN FOALS   *Erwin G. Pearson* 442
GASTROINTESTINAL DISEASES OF THE NEONATAL FOAL   *Susan D. Semrad and Susan Shaftoe* 445
SEPTIC ARTHRITIS AND OSTEOMYELITIS   *Pamela C. Wagner, Barbara J. Watrous and Benjamin J. Darien* 455
RISK FACTORS ASSOCIATED WITH DEVELOPMENTAL ORTHOPEDIC DISEASE   *M. Amy Williams* 462
FOAL PNEUMONIA   *W. David Wilson* 466
SEDATION AND GENERAL ANESTHESIA OF THE FOAL   *Sheilah A. Robertson* 474
RESPIRATORY SUPPORT OF THE NEWBORN FOAL   *Dennis R. Geiser* 478

Section 11 HEMATOPOIETIC DISEASES
Debra Deem Morris, *Consulting Editor*

DIAGNOSTIC APPROACH TO ANEMIA   *Michelle M. Henry* 487
BLOOD LOSS ANEMIA   *Michelle M. Henry* 492
ANEMIA DUE TO INADEQUATE ERYTHROPOIESIS   *Michelle M. Henry* 494
HEMOLYTIC ANEMIA   *Michelle M. Henry* 495
HEMOPHILIA   *Ted A. Broome* 501
WARFARIN TOXICOSIS   *Ted A. Broome* 502
DISSEMINATED INTRAVASCULAR COAGULATION   *Debra Deem Morris* 504
IDIOPATHIC THROMBOCYTOPENIA   *Debra Deem Morris* 507
VASCULITIS   *Debra Deem Morris* 510
LYMPHOPROLIFERATIVE AND MYELOPROLIFERATIVE DISORDERS   *Chrysann Collatos* 513
BLOOD AND PLASMA THERAPY   *Lisa Williamson* 517

Section 12 NEUROLOGICAL DISEASES
Richard M. DeBowes and Judy H. Cox, *Consulting Editors*

NEUROLOGICAL EXAMINATION   *C. P. Coyne and Judy Cox* 521
CEREBROSPINAL FLUID COLLECTION AND ANALYSIS   *C. P. Coyne* 527

COMMON MALFORMATIONS AND CONGENITAL ABNORMALITIES OF THE CENTRAL NERVOUS
   SYSTEM   *Richard M. DeBowes and Lisa Gift* 530
TRAUMA OF THE BRAIN AND SPINAL CORD   *Richard M. DeBowes and Lisa Gift* 535
TETANUS   *Rebecca McConnico* 540
BOTULISM   *Pamela A. Pintchuk* 542
RABIES   *Judy H. Cox* 545
TOGAVIRAL ENCEPHALITIDES: ALPAHVIRUS (EASTERN AND WESTERN) EQUINE
   ENCEPHALITIS   *Joseph J. Bertone* 547
EQUINE HERPES MYELOENCEPHALOPATHY   *Gregg Kortz* 550
BACTERIAL MENINGITIS AND CEREBRAL ABSCESSES   *Jonathan H. Foreman* 552
PROTOZOAL MYELOENCEPHALITIS   *Kathleen Yvorchuk* 554
VERMINA MYELITIS   *Wendy M. Duckett* 556
MYCOTOXIC ENCEPHALOMALACIA   *Maria D. Masri* 558
DEGENERATIVE MYELOENCEPHALOPATHY   *Linda L. Blythe and A. Morrie Craig* 559
SEIZURES AND NARCOLEPSY   *Frank M. Andrews and Hilary K. Matthews* 561
HYPOCALCEMIC TETANY   *Gary W. Brandt* 566
POLYNEURITIS EQUI   *Kathleen Yvorchuk* 569
NEUROMUSCULAR DISORDERS   *Judy Cox* 571
NEUROLOGICAL CAUSES OF BLINDNESS   *Sarah Maxwell* 573
VESTIBULAR DISEASE   *Jana M. Smith* 575
PERIPHERAL NEUROPATHIES   *Simon J. Wheeler* 577
TAIL ALTERATIONS IN SHOW HORSES   *Steven B. Colter* 579

Section 13   OCULAR DISEASES
Mary B. Glaze, *Consulting Editor*

OCULAR DISCHARGE   *Cecil P. Moore* 583
OCULAR INJURIES   *David A. Wilkie* 587
ANTERIOR UVEITIS   *Michael Davidson* 592
CORNEAL STROMAL ABSCESSES   *Mary B. Glaze* 594
CORNEAL ULCERATION   *Cecil P. Moore* 596
PUNCTATE KERATITIS   *Thomas R. Miller* 599
CATARACTS   *Joan Dziezyc and Nicholas J. Millichamp* 601
GLAUCOMA   *Dennis E. Brooks* 602
OCULAR NEOPLASIA   *J. Daniel Lavach* 604
VISUAL IMPAIRMENT   *Kerry L. Ketring* 608

Section 14   URINARY TRACT DISEASE
Thomas J. Divers, *Consulting Editor*

OBSTRUCTION AND RUPTURE OF THE URINARY TRACT   *Troy S. Ford* 613
CYSTITIS AND PYELONEPHRITIS   *Mary Gardiner Boy* 616
URINARY INCONTINENCE   *E. Susan Clark* 618
POLYURIA   *Robert H. Whitlock* 620
URINARY TRACT NEOPLASIA   *Thomas J. Divers* 623
ACUTE RENAL FAILURE   *Thomas J. Divers* 623
RENAL TUBULAR ACIDOSIS   *Yves Rossier* 627
CHRONIC RENAL FAILURE   *Robert H. Whitlock* 628

Section 15 REPRODUCTION
Gordon L. Woods, *Consulting Editor*

SEXUAL BEHAVIOR DYSFUNCTION IN MARES *Sue M. McDonnell*	633
EMBRYO TRANSFER *Katrin Hinrichs*	637
PERSISTENT ESTRUS: FACT OR FICTION? *Patricia L. Sertich*	641
AGE-RELATED OVULATORY DYSFUNCTION *Dirk K. Vanderwall and Gordon L. Woods*	643
EMBRYONIC LOSS *Barry A. Ball*	644
ULTRASONOGRAPHIC EXAMINATION OF THE MARE'S REPRODUCTIVE TRACT *Gregg P. Adams*	648
MANAGEMENT OF TWIN PREGNANCY *A. L. Hallowell and Gordon L. Woods*	657
DIAGNOSIS OF FETAL GENDER BY ULTRASONOGRAPHY *Sandra S. Curran*	660
PREFOALING MANAGEMENT OF THE MARE AND INDUCTION OF PARTURITION *William B. Ley*	664
SEXUAL BEHAVIOR DYSFUNCTION IN STALLIONS *Sue McDonnell*	668
STALLION SEMINAL CHARACTERISTICS AND FERTILITY *David J. Jasko*	671
HANDLING OF STALLION SEMEN *Dickson D. Varner*	674
ULTRASONOGRAPHIC EVALUATION OF ACCESSORY SEX GLAND STRUCTURE AND FUNCTION IN THE STALLION *James A. Weber and Gordon L. Woods*	678

Section 16 SKIN DISEASES
Diane Bevier, *Consulting Editor*

SKIN BIOPSIES IN THE DIAGNOSIS OF INFLAMMATORY SKIN DISEASES *Robert W. Dunstan and Mitchell D. Song*	683
NUTRITION AND SKIN DISEASES *Harold F. Hintz*	686
CONTROL OF ECTOPARASITES *Lane Foil and Carol Foil*	688
CULICOIDES HYPERSENSITIVITY *Joy Barbet*	693
IVERMECTIN IN DERMATOLOGIC DISORDERS *Thomas R. Klei*	696
DERMATOPHYTOSIS *Linda A. Frank*	698
STAPHYLOCOCCAL SKIN DISEASE *Danny W. Scott*	700
CUTANEOUS MASTOCYTOSIS *Karen A. Nyrop*	702
ANHIDROSIS *John Freestone*	703
JUNCTIONAL MECHANOBULLOUS DISEASE IN BELGIAN FOALS *Catherine W. Kohn*	705
CHRONIC EOSINOPHILIC DERMATITIDES *Malcolm C. Roberts*	706
DERMATOLOGIC CONDITIONS OF THE PENIS AND PREPUCE *Donna M. Gatewood*	708
LASERS IN DERMATOLOGY *Lloyd P. Tate, Jr.*	711

Section 17 NUTRITION
Sarah L. Ralston, *Consulting Editor*

NUTRIENT REQUIREMENTS *Harold F. Hintz*	715
DIAGNOSIS OF COMMON MINERAL IMBALANCES *Sarah L. Ralston*	717
NUTRITIONAL FACTORS IN DEVELOPMENTAL ORTHOPEDIC DISEASE *Edgar A. Ott*	720
ENTERAL NUTRITIONAL SUPPORT OF SICK HORSES *William J. Burkholder and Craig D. Thatcher*	724
PARENTERAL NUTRITION *Shauna L. Spurlock and Michael V. Ward*	732
NUTRITIONAL MANAGEMENT IN DISEASE *Jonathan M. Naylor*	736
NUTRITIONAL MANAGEMENT OF THE CRITICALLY ILL NEONATE *Wendy E. Vaala*	741

Section 18 EXOTIC DISEASES
Willaim W. Laegreid, *Consulting Editor*

AFRICAN HORSE SICKNESS *William W. Laegreid*	753
BABESIOSIS *Donald P. Knowles, Jr.*	756
CONTAGIOUS EQUINE METRITIS *Peter J. Timoney*	757
GLANDERS *Linda K. Schlater*	761
MELIOIDOSIS *Linda K. Schlater*	762
JAPANESE ENCEPHALITIS *Robert E. Shope*	764
VENEZUELAN EQUINE ENCEPHALOMYELITIS *Thomas E. Walton*	765
OTHER EXOTIC DISEASES *William W. Laegreid*	768

Section 19 ASSESSMENT OF PERFORMANCE PROBLEMS
Elisabeth Morris, *Consulting Editor*

INTRODUCTION TO PERFORMANCE EVALUATION *Elisabeth Morris*	771
DYNAMIC ENDOSCOPY OF THE UPPER AIRWAY *Elisabeth Morris*	774
PULMONARY FUNCTION TESTS *Frederick J. Derksen*	777
IMAGING OF THE LOWER AIRWAYS *Michael W. O'Callaghan*	779
ELECTROPHYSIOLOGIC RESPONSES TO EXERCISE *Frank S. Pipers*	783
GAIT ANALYSIS *Howard J. Seeherman*	786
EVALUATION OF BONE *Howard J. Seeherman*	791
EVALUATION OF TENDONS AND LIGAMENTS *Virginia B. Reef*	796
EVALUATION OF MUSCLE *Stephanie J. Valberg*	799
FITNESS TESTING *Elisabeth Morris*	802
HEMATOLOGICAL AND ENDOCRINE CHANGES DURING EXERCISE *Jonathan H. Foreman*	807
ERGOGENIC DIETS AND NUTRIENTS *Pamela L. Ferrante and David S. Kronfeld*	809

Section 20 APPENDICES

TABLE OF DRUGS: APPROXIMATE DOSES *N. Edward Robinson*	815
CLINICAL PATHOLOGY DATA *Desmond P. Leadon*	822
INTERSTATE SHIPMENT OF HORSES *N. Edward Robinson*	829

INDEX	833

Section 1

THERAPEUTICS

Edited by N. Edward Robinson

Antimicrobial Chemotherapy
Robert D. Walker, EAST LANSING, MICHIGAN

Successful antimicrobial chemotherapy in the horse involves unique challenges not encountered in other animal species. The reasons for this include the size of the horse; poor absorption of orally administered antimicrobial agents; the temperament of horses, especially when subjected to long-term parenteral therapy; the short list of antimicrobial agents approved for use in horses; the lack of pharmacokinetic data for the various antimicrobials that are used; the increasing number of bacterial agents that are known to cause disease in the horse; and the ability of many of these organisms to develop resistance to the currently available drugs. Because of the ever-changing world of the bacterial pathogen in relation to these problems, the attending clinician needs to understand the host-bacterium-antimicrobial agent interaction. Such an understanding provides a better chance of successfully treating infectious disease processes of bacterial etiology.

BACTERIAL COLONIZATION

Beginning at birth an incredible number and diverse type of bacteria rapidly colonize all cutaneous and most mucosal surfaces exposed to the external environment. These indigenous flora, composed of both aerobic and anaerobic bacteria, develop a "win-win" relationship with the host. The host provides a favorable environment and nutrients for microbial growth, while the bacteria provide the host with nutrients through their metabolic activities and protect the host from exogenous organisms. The indigenous flora attaches to cutaneous and mucosal surfaces by means of fimbriae, a glycocalyx, or both. The glycocalyx also serves as a reservoir of nutrients and trace minerals and protects the bacteria from toxic substances such as antibiotics and antibodies. The bacterial glycocalyx is believed to be a fundamental factor in the development of disease; bacteria protected by the glycocalyx are more resistant to phagocytosis and antimicrobial chemotherapy.

FACTORS INVOLVED IN THE DEVELOPMENT OF DISEASE

Disease is a breakdown in the symbiotic relationship between the microbe and the host. Factors contributing to this disruption include the administration of antimicrobial chemotherapeutic agents, the administration of corticosteroids causing an immune dysfunction, primary or secondary immune dysfunction due to other causes, penetrating wounds, abrasive actions, malnutrition, physical or emotional stress, and surgical procedures.

Factors that stress the host defense system alter receptor sites on mucosal surfaces, which in turn alters the population of bacteria colonizing these surfaces and results in decreased ability of the phagocytic cells to find and destroy bacteria that may gain access to protected areas. Surgical procedures and penetrating injuries also disrupt the vascular bed, resulting in tissue damage, accumulation of extravascular fluids, and a reduced oxidation-reduction potential. The more prolonged the surgical procedures or the more severe the tissue injury, the greater is the suppressive effect on the host immune system, the greater is the tissue damage, and the more susceptible is the host to infection. Bacterial factors required for the development of disease include introduction into susceptible body tissue in sufficient numbers, the ability to resist or evade host defense mechanisms, the ability to metabolize and proliferate in host tissue, and the ability to produce substances that disrupt the normal function of host cells and tissue.

Basically, bacteria produce disease by invading tissues or producing toxins (including metabolic byproducts that are injurious to host cells), or both. By knowing that the development of an infectious disease process occurs as a result of host immune dysfunction or as a result of exposure to a sufficient concentration of bacteria that have the potential to cause disease, or both, the role of the clinician in treating these infectious disease processes becomes obvious. That is, the clinician must supply supportive therapy to the host to bolster its immune system, reduce the population of bacteria and their toxic metabolic byproducts at the site of infection, and reduce the ability of the bacteria to multiply long enough to allow the host's defenses to mount a successful counter-offensive. The nature and extent of supportive therapy depend on the nature and location of the infectious disease process. Generally, nutritional support, fluid therapy, and reduced stress are all supportive of the host immune system. Reduction of the population of bacteria and their toxins usually requires surgical debridement and/or drainage. Flushing of the infected site with copious amounts of sterile fluids can also reduce the population of bacteria. The primary purpose of these fluids is to reduce bacterial concentrations. Addition of substances toxic to the bacteria, such as Betadine, may also damage host cells and provide more nutrients for the surviving bacteria. Preventing bacterial replication requires the use of antimicrobial agents to which the invading microorganism is susceptible. For maximum effect, these agents must reach and be maintained at therapeutic concentration at the site of infection for the appropriate length of time.

ANTIMICROBIAL CHEMOTHERAPY

A few basic concepts should be considered regarding the use of antimicrobial agents. When used intelligently and judiciously, antimicrobial agents are invaluable; when used inappropriately, they can endanger the life of the animal being treated. This is done by neglecting appropriate therapy, making the patient more susceptible to colonization by fungi or multiresistant bacteria, or by selecting for resistant pathogenic bacteria. For example, colitis can result from the use of tetracyclines or lincosamides, and the growth of anaerobic bacteria in polymicrobial infections may be enhanced following the use of aminoglycosides as a single agent.

Under most circumstances antibiotics do not eliminate an infection. The purpose of antimicrobial chemotherapy is to slow the rate of proliferation of the invading bacteria long enough to allow the host to mount a successful counter-offensive. Thus, the weaker the host, or the more compromised its immune response, the more accurate and aggressive the antimicrobial therapy must be. In other words, when an infectious disease process such as endocarditis or meningitis develops, because these disease processes are life-threatening and the white cell population has limited access to these infected sites, bactericidal agents that kill the bacteria would be more appropriate than bacteriostatic agents that merely inhibit their growth.

In vitro bacterial growth curves show four phases of growth. The shape and length of the curve are dictated by the size of the inoculum, the incubation temperature, the supply of nutrients available, and the build-up of toxic metabolites. In vivo growth involves a different set of circumstances. Generally speaking, the length of time before clinical disease manifests itself depends on the size of the inoculum, the virulence of the organism, and the immune status of the host. The larger the inoculum, the more virulent the organism, or the more immunosuppressed the host, the quicker clinical disease is manifested. Once the organisms gain access to the site of infection, there is a steady influx of nutrients from body fluid or lysis of host cells and a steady outflow of toxic metabolites away from the site of bacterial proliferation. Under these conditions, there are no defined growth phases. In fact, at any given time there may be 1,000, 10,000, 100,000 or more bacteria dividing. Generally, the more acute the infectious process, the more bacteria will be undergoing cell division and the more susceptible the infectious process will be to those antimicrobial agents that require bacterial proliferation for inhibitory action. Even in chronic infections there is still bacterial proliferation.

Approximately 70 per cent of infectious disease processes are adequately dealt with by the host's defenses. The other 30 per cent require accurate antimicrobial chemotherapy with a few requiring aggressive chemotherapy. Unfortunately, one cannot empirically know whether or not an infectious process falls into the 70 per cent or the 30 per cent category. Consequently, each case must be approached as potentially being in the 30 per cent category. In other words, each infectious disease process must be treated individually. Appropriate antimicrobial chemotherapy provides an optimal concentration of the appropriate antibiotic at the site of infection, in active form, for the appropriate length of time.

CHOOSING AN ANTIBIOTIC

In choosing the appropriate antibiotic, one must consider (1) the identity of the infecting organism, (2) its antimicrobial susceptibility profile, (3) the nature and site of the infectious disease process, and (4) the pharmacokinetic parameters (host factors) associated with the chosen antimicrobial agent, such as route of administration, tissue distribution, and rate of elimination.

The etiological agent may be identified by several methods. Previous clinical experience can provide insight as to the most likely organism causing the infection, such as *Streptococcus equi* causing strangles (Table 1). A Gram stain of properly collected material is a simple, inexpensive, and useful means to identify not only the presence of but also the morphological features of microorganisms in body fluids that are normally sterile, such as transtracheal washes, pleural and peritoneal fluids, and urine, especially in acute infections. However, in some infectious disease processes a Gram stain may fail to reveal any bacteria. Because there are usually so few bacteria in cerebrospinal fluid, joint fluid, or fluid from chronic infections, it is difficult to identify them by staining techniques. Gram stains of stool specimens may provide useful information in cases of clostridial diarrhea, where large gram-positive rods appear as the predominant organisms, replacing the normal gram-negative rod flora. The presence of polymorphonuclear leukocytes (PMNs) in gram-stained stool smears is suggestive of bacterial gastroenteritis, such as that induced by *Salmonella*, invasive *E. coli*, or *Campylobacter*, as PMNs are not found in stools of patients with viral gastroenteritis, toxicities, or noninvasive *E. coli* infection.

If neither clinical experience, the site of infection, nor a Gram stain provides insight into the etiological agent, definitive identification may be made by collecting the appropriate specimen and submitting it for culture evaluation. When this procedure is used, it is imperative that proper specimen collection techniques or instruments be employed. One only has to consider the ubiquitousness of the microorganisms in the equine environment to gain an appreciation of this. For example, transtracheal washes performed in a horse that has just finished eating hay will yield bacteria and the fungi associated with the hay in addition to the respiratory pathogen. Under most circumstances, determining which isolate is the contaminant and which is the pathogen is difficult.

Once the etiological agent has been determined, the next task is to identify an appropriate antibiotic. Generally, susceptibility testing is unnecessary for all clinical isolates from all infectious processes. For example, β-haemolytic *Streptococcus* is routinely susceptible to penicillin G, as are all anaerobes except *Bacteroides* spp. Thus, when these organisms are isolated in pure culture, there is no need to test their susceptibility to other drugs. Susceptibility testing is generally required on all other clinically important isolates from properly collected specimens, especially those from animals with serious or life-threatening infections, polymicrobial infections, or infections involving bacteria that are traditionally multiply drug-resistant. The commonly used disk-diffusion method is simple to perform and is relatively inexpensive (less than $4 per isolate). However, at best it provides only semiqualitative information (susceptible, moderately susceptible, resistant) concerning the susceptibility of the isolate, and those values are based on the pharmacokinetics of the antimicrobial agents in humans. The disk-diffusion method is also of no value for slow-growing fastidious or anaerobic bacteria. Quantitative data, actual minimal inhibitory concentrations (MIC), may be obtained by using various commercially available microdilution susceptibility test panels. These test systems incorporate serial dilutions of antimicrobial agents in broth cultures and measure the concentration of drug required to inhibit the growth of the bacteria under standardized, controlled laboratory conditions. The lowest concentration of the antimicrobial agent that prevents visible growth after four to 24 hours of incubation is known as the MIC. While these techniques result in quantitative data, the results indicate the concentration of drug required to inhibit the bacteria, not kill it. Rarely, if ever, do the same conditions under which the tests were run also exist in vivo. To the contrary, in an infectious disease process where there is purulent material, reduced oxygen, decreased

TABLE 1. EMPIRICAL THERAPY FOR INFECTIOUS DISEASE PROCESSES OF BACTERIAL ETIOLOGY

Site of Infection	Possible Pathogen	First-Choice Antimicrobial(s)	Alternate Antimicrobial(s)
Upper respiratory tract	*Streptococcus equi*	Penicillin G	Ampicillin, amoxicillin
	Staphylococcus aureus	Oxacillin	Cephalothin°
	Pseudomonas aeruginosa	Gentamicin	Amikacin
	Actinobacillus suis-like	Trimethoprim-sulfa	Cephalothin°
Lower respiratory tract	*Streptococcus zooepidemicus*	Penicillin G	Ampicillin, amoxicillin
	Rhodococcus equi	Erythromycin + rifampin	Penicillin + gentamicin
	Staphylococcus aureus	Oxacillin + rifampin	Cephalothin°
	Actinobacillus equuli	Trimethoprim-sulfa	Cephalothin°, gentamicin
	Bordetella bronchiseptica	Trimethoprim-sulfa	Gentamicin
	Pseudomonas aeruginosa	Gentamicin	Amikacin
	Salmonella spp.	Trimethoprim-sulfa	Amoxicillin
	Gram-negative anaerobes	Metronidazole	Chloramphenicol
Gastrointestinal tract	*Salmonella* spp.†	Trimethoprim-sulfa	Amoxicillin
	Actinobacillus equuli	Trimethoprim-sulfa	Chloramphenicol
	Rhodococcus equi	Erythromycin + rifampin	Penicillin + gentamicin
	Clostridium perfringens	Penicillin G	Chloramphenicol
	Ehrlichia risticii	Oxytetracycline	Minocycline
Integumentary system	Group C *Streptococcus*	Penicillin G	Ampicillin
	Coagulase-positive *Staphylococcus*‡	Oxacillin	Cephalothin°
	Pseudomonas aeruginosa	Gentamicin	Amikacin
	Dermatophilus congolensis§	Iodine	
Skeletal system	Group C *Streptococcus*	Penicillin G	Ampicillin
	Staphylococcus aureus	Oxacillin	Cephalothin°
	Brucella spp.	Tetracycline + streptomycin	Trimethoprim-sulfa
	Actinobacillus equuli	Gentamicin	Cephalothin, trimethoprim-sulfa
	Actinomyces bovis	Penicillin G	Ampicillin, amoxicillin
	Pseudomonas aeruginosa	Gentamicin	Amikacin
	Nocardia asteroides	Trimethoprim-sulfa	Triple sulfa
	Ehrlichia risticii	Oxytetracycline	Minocycline
Vascular system	Group C *Streptococcus*	Penicillin G	Ampicillin
	Escherichia coli	Gentamicin	Cephalothin°
	Salmonella spp.	Gentamicin	Ampicillin, amoxicillin
	Actinobacillus equuli	Gentamicin	Trimethoprim-sulfa, cephalothin
Lymphatic system	*Streptococcus equi*	Penicillin G	Ampicillin
	Corynebacterium pseudotuberculosis	Penicillin G	Ampicillin, amoxicillin
	Rhodococcus equi	Erythromycin + rifampin	Penicillin + gentamicin
Reproductive tract‖	*Streptococcus zooepidemicus*	Penicillin G	Ampicillin
	Streptococcus equisimilis	Penicillin G	Ampicillin
	Klebsiella pneumoniae	Ceftiofur	Trimethoprim-sulfa
	Pseudomonas aeruginosa	Gentamicin	Amikacin
	Actinobacillus equuli	Gentamicin	Trimethoprim-sulfa, cephalothin
Abscesses¶	*Streptococcus zooepidemicus*	Penicillin G	Ampicillin
	Streptococcus equisimilis	Penicillin G	Ampicillin
	Coagulase-positive *Staphylococcus*	Oxacillin	Cephalothin°
	Escherichia coli	Gentamicin	Cephalothin°
	Klebsiella pneumoniae	Ceftiofur	Trimethoprim-sulfa
	Pseudomonas aeruginosa	Gentamicin	Amikacin
	Fusobacterium spp.	Penicillin G	Metronidazole
	Bacteroides spp.	Metronidazole	Chloramphenicol

°Represents all first generation cephalosporins.
†Antimicrobial chemotherapy for intestinal salmonellosis is generally not warranted.
‡Approximately 50 per cent of the coagulase-positive *Staphylococcus* isolates in veterinary medicine are β-lactamase positive. Primary species in the horse are *S. aureus* and *S. intermedius*.
§Infections caused by *Dermatophilus congolensis* are best treated with topical iodine and moving the horse to a dry environment.
‖In previously untreated mares, β-haemolytic streptococci are the most common isolates, whereas in previously treated mares, gram-negative bacteria, which require in vitro susceptibility testing, are more common.
¶Abscesses may be polymicrobial infections involving aerobic and anaerobic bacteria. When therapy is initiated early such infections, including pleuritis and peritonitis, should respond to drainage and high doses of ceftiofur and metronidazole.

pH, or necrotic tissue, the concentration of drug required to inhibit the growth of the bacteria may be severalfold higher than the MIC determined in vitro. To compensate for the differences between in vitro and in vivo conditions the rule of thumb is that the peak serum level of the chosen antibiotic should be greater than four times the MIC. In light of this, the use of such data loses its value unless one knows the pharmacokinetic behavior of the chosen drug. For example, if the MIC data indicate that it takes 2 μg per ml of ampicillin to inhibit *Staphylococcus aureus*, should ampicillin be used? If it is known that ampicillin dosed at 4.4 mg per kg produces a peak serum concentration of 6 μg per ml, the drug should not be used. On the other hand, if the MIC was 0.1, a positive clinical response could be expected. Thus, without knowledge of the peak serum or tissue concentrations of the various drugs in the horse, MIC data are of limited value. Because most of the commercially available systems have been developed for use in human medicine, most of the drugs available for testing are very expensive for use in the horse. On the other hand, two companies, Sensititer* and Vitek,† have begun addressing the antimicrobial needs of veterinary medicine. While evaluations are in the preliminary stage, the products offer promise for quality products in the future.

Susceptibility test results must be interpreted in light of the organism isolated, the testing procedure used, the antibiotic's tissue distribution, toxicity potential, mode of action, and cost. It is often difficult to determine if the organism isolated from a clinical specimen is a pathogen requiring antimicrobial chemotherapy or a contaminant that is best ignored. This decision becomes even more difficult when the organism isolated is considered part of the normal flora as well as a pathogen. Results that may help to incriminate the isolate as a pathogen include the isolation of one or two organisms in large numbers or the presence of numerous neutrophils. The absence of neutrophils, the presence of only a few bacteria, or the presence of multiple bacterial species in equal numbers could (but does not always) indicate contamination, possibly due to a poorly collected specimen. In addition, the testing procedure used to determine the susceptibility profile of the isolate can provide erroneous results if the laboratory performing the tests does not adhere to quality control standards outlined for the tests or if the company producing the susceptibility panels has not developed the product with proper quality control.

While the etiological agent may be susceptible to several antimicrobial agents, not all such agents may reach or be maintained at therapeutic concentrations at the site of infection for a sufficient length of time. The tissue distribution of the antibiotic is dictated by its formulation, lipid solubility, state of ionization, and protein-binding capacity. The route of administration also contributes to the peak concentration of drug that reaches the site of infection. Most antimicrobial agents that are administered orally, especially to the horse, have lower serum and tissue concentration curves than do drugs administered parenterally. The vascularity at the site of administration can also affect the rate of absorption. Injections into neck muscle produce peak serum concentrations faster than injections into gluteal muscles, which in turn provide faster absorption than do subcutaneous injections. The intravenous (IV) administration of drugs ensures that the total dose enters the systemic circulation, with the shape of the serum and tissue concentration curves being dictated by the rate of infusion and elimination.

The nature and site of the infectious process can also have an effect on the success of the antimicrobial agent. Many antibiotics, such as the aminoglycosides, diffuse into abscesses very poorly. Some are also inactivated by purulent exudate, low pH, low oxidation-reduction potential, and necrotic debris associated with abscesses. Thus, the goal of antimicrobial therapy is to select an antibiotic that exhibits good antibacterial activity against the infecting organism and has the ability to diffuse rapidly into the infected area in a high concentration and in an active form. When the antibiotic is given early in the infectious process and maintained at the site of the infection at a concentration above the MIC of the infecting organism, the chance for therapeutic success is enhanced. On the other hand, antibiotics that are absorbed slowly, diffuse poorly, are inactivated by factors associated with the infectious process, are given at too low a dose or improper dosing frequency, or are only moderately effective against the infectious agent usually result in therapeutic failure.

To enhance the possibility of therapeutic success, the clinician needs to understand the advantages and limitations of the antibiotics that are currently available. The remainder of this chapter describes many antimicrobial agents currently marketed in the United States. Dosages and routes of administration are given in Table 2. While very few of these drugs have been approved for use in the horse and many of

---

*Microbiological Systems, Westlake, OH
†Vitek Systems, Hazelwood, MO

TABLE 2. SELECTED ANTIBIOTICS AND SUGGESTED DOSAGE REGIMENS

Antibiotic Generic (Trade) Names	Suggested Dosage	Route	Frequency
Aminoglycosides*			
Streptomycin and dihydrostreptomycin	11 mg/kg	IM, SC	q 12 hrs
Neomycin†	Horse: 1 gm	PO	q 6 hrs
	2 gm	PO	q 12 hrs
	Foal: 0.5 gm	PO	q 6 hrs
	1.5 gm	PO	q 12 hrs
Gentamicin‡	2–4 mg/kg	IV, IM, SC	q 6–8 hrs
Kanamycin	7.5 mg/kg	IV, IM	q 8 hrs
Amikacin	3.7 mg/kg	IM, SC	q 6 hrs
	7.0 mg/kg	IM, SC	q 12 hrs
	2 gm/200 ml	IU	
Tobramycin	1.0–1.7 mg/kg (human dose)	IV, IM	q 8 hrs
Netilmicin§	Adult: 4–6 mg/kg/day	IV, IM	q 8–12 hrs
	Young: 5–8 mg/kg	IV, IM	q 8–12 hrs
	Neonate: 2–3 mg/kg	IV, IM	q 12 hrs

*When given IV, aminoglycosides should be administered slowly. If renal function is impaired, dosage interval should be increased or dosage decreased.
†Because of its toxicity, neomycin should never be given IV, IM, or SC.
‡Recent studies have indicated that a single, total daily dose of gentamicin (i.e., 4–6 mg/kg administered q 24 hrs), and possibly other aminoglycosides, may be equal to or better than multiple doses.
§In very serious infections, netilmicin may be administered at 7.5 mg/kg/day for up to 48 hours.

Antibiotic Generic (Trade) Names	Suggested Dosage	Route	Frequency
Cephalosporins*			
First Generation:			
Cephalothin (Keflin)	20–40 mg/kg	IV, IM	q 6–8 hrs
Cephapirin (Cefadyl)	30 mg/kg	IV, IM	q 4–6 hrs
Cefazolin (Ancef)	15 mg/kg	IV, IM	q 8–12 hrs
Cephalexin (Keflex)	10–30 mg/kg	PO	q 6–8 hrs
Cefadroxil (Duricef)	22 mg/kg	PO	q 12 hrs
Second Generation:			
Cefamandole (Mandol)	10–30 mg/kg	IV, IM	q 4–8 hrs
Cefonicid (Monicid)	10–15 mg/kg	IV, IM	q 24 hrs
Ceforanide (Precef)	5–10 mg/kg	IV, IM	q 12 hrs
Cefotetan (Cefotan)	15–30 mg/kg	IV, IM	q 12 hrs
Cefoxitin (Mefoxin)	30–40 mg/kg	IM	q 6–8 hrs
Cefuroxime (Zinacef)	25–50 mg/kg	IV, IM	q 8 hrs
Cefuroxime axetil (Ceftin)	250–500 mg/kg	PO	q 12 hrs
Cefaclor (Ceclor)	20–40 mg/kg	PO	q 8 hrs
Third Generation:			
Cefotaxime (Claforan)	25–50 mg/kg	IV, IM	q 8–12 hrs
Cefoperazone (Cefobid)	30–50 mg/kg	IV, IM	q 8–12 hrs
Ceftizoxime (Cefizox)	25–50 mg/kg	IV, IM	q 8–12 hrs
Ceftriaxone (Rocephin)	25–50 mg/kg	IV, IM	q 12 hrs
Ceftazidime (Fortum)	25–50 mg/kg	IV, IM	q 12 hrs
Ceftiofur (Naxcel)	1–2 mg/kg	IM	q 12–24 hrs
Moxalactam (Moxam)	50 mg/kg	IV, IM	q 8 hrs
Cefixime (Suprax)	400 mg/kg	PO	q 8 hrs

*Dosages listed are general guidelines only and may vary considerably, depending on the product or disease condition. Oral cephalosporins are not absorbed in adult horses. Except for ceftiofur, the dosages listed for the second- and third-generation cephalosporins are human doses. A cefamycin (cefoxitin) is included with the cephalosporins for convenience.

Antibiotic Generic (Trade) Names	Suggested Dosage	Route	Frequency
Macrolides*			
Erythromycin	25 mg/kg	PO	q 8 hrs
	2.5–5.0 mg/kg	IV	q 6–8 hrs
Tylosin	10 mg/kg	IM	q 12 hrs

*Produce swelling and pain at injection site. When erythromycin and tylosin are administered PO, IV, or IM, there is rapid absorption and diffusion into tissues and fluids (including liver, pleural, and peritoneal fluids), bile (unobstructed), and borderline absorption and diffusion in the middle ear cavity and cerebrospinal fluid (only with inflamed meninges).

TABLE 2. SELECTED ANTIBIOTICS AND SUGGESTED DOSAGE REGIMENS *Continued*

Antibiotic Generic (Trade) Names	Suggested Dosage	Route	Frequency
Benzyl Penicillins			
Penicillin V	110,000 mg/kg	PO	q 6–12 hrs
Sodium penicillin G°	10,000–50,000 IU/kg (1 unit = 0.6 µg)	IV, IM	q 6 hrs
Potassium penicillin G†	10,000–50,000 IU/kg	IV, IM	q 6 hrs
	20,000 IU/kg	PO	q 6 hrs
Procaine penicillin G‡	20,000–50,000 IU/kg	IM, SC	q 12 hrs
Benzathine penicillin G§	10,000–40,000 IU/kg	IM	q 48–72 hrs

°May add to sodium load.
†May produce hyperkalemia. IM administration may result in delayed absorption. PO absorption is unreliable in the horse.
‡Never administer IV. Contraindicated in horses that are scheduled to race.
§Never administer IV. The use of this drug may result in tissue concentrations below the MIC of the infecting organism, thus prolonging the infection or contributing to a relapse.

Antibiotic Generic (Trade) Names	Suggested Dosage	Route	Frequency
Aminobenzyl Penicillins			
Ampicillin sodium	25–100 mg/kg	IV	q 6 hrs
Ampicillin trihydrate	11–22 mg/kg	IM	q 12 hrs
Amoxicillin sodium	10–22 mg/kg	IM	q 8 hrs
Penicillinase-Resistant Penicillins			
Methicillin°	25 mg/kg	IM	q 4–6 hrs
Nafcillin	10 mg/kg	IM	q 6 hrs
Cloxacillin	10 mg/kg	IM	q 6 hrs
Dicloxacillin	10 mg/kg	IM	q 6 hrs
Floxacillin	10 mg/kg	IM	q 6 hrs
Oxacillin	20–50 mg/kg	IV, IM	q 8–12 hrs

°Not stable in solution.

Antibiotic Generic (Trade) Names	Suggested Dosage	Route	Frequency
Carboxy Penicillins			
Carbenicillin sodium°	50–80 mg/kg	IV, IM	q 8–12 hrs
Carbenicillin indanyl†	20–30 mg/kg	PO	q 8 hrs
Ticarcillin‡	40–80 mg/kg	IV, IM	q 8 hrs

°Often synergistic with aminoglycosides.
†Therapeutic levels reached in the bladder only.
‡For severe infections the higher dose is recommended. Given intrauterine, 6 gm in 250 ml sterile saline.

Antibiotic Generic (Trade) Names	Suggested Dosage	Route	Frequency
Aminoacetylureido Penicillins			
Pipercillin°	35–50 mg/kg†	IV, IM	q 4–6 hrs
	20–30 mg/kg‡	IV, IM	q 6–8 hrs
	15–20 mg/kg§	IV, IM	q 6–12 hrs
Azlocillin or mezlocillin°	50–75 mg/kg†	IV	q 6 hrs
	35–50 mg/kg‡	IV	q 6 hrs
	25–30 mg/kg§	IV	q 6 hrs

°Intravenous dose may be administered in 3- to 5-minute intervals. IM administration may cause irritation. Dosage based on human dose.
†For septicemia, nosocomial pneumonia, intra-abdominal, aerobic and anaerobic gynecological, skin and soft tissue, lower respiratory tract, and skeletal infections.
‡For complicated urinary tract infections.
§For uncomplicated urinary tract infections.

Antibiotic Generic (Trade) Names	Suggested Dosage	Route	Frequency
Potentiated Sulfonamide			
Trimethoprim-Sulfadiazine	15 mg/kg (injectable)	IV	q 12 hrs
	15 mg/kg (oral)	PO	q 12 hrs
	36 mg/kg (paste)	PO	q 12 hrs
	2.4–4.9 gm	Intrauterine	q 24 hrs
Tetracyclines			
Oxytetracyclines°	Foals: 10–20 mg/kg	PO	q 8–12 hrs
	Horse: 10 mg/kg	IV°	q 12–24 hrs
Doxycycline	3 mg/kg	PO	q 12 hrs
Minocycline	3 mg/kg	PO	q 12 hrs

°Shock may occur when given IV in the horse. Diarrhea is common in the horse.

TABLE 2. SELECTED ANTIBIOTICS AND SUGGESTED DOSAGE REGIMENS *Continued*

Antibiotic Generic (Trade) Names	Suggested Dosage	Route	Frequency
	Other Antibiotics		
Chloramphenicol	Foal: 4–10 mg/kg	IM	q 6–8 hrs
	Horse: 25–50 mg/kg	IM	q 4–6 hrs
	Horse: 50 mg/kg	PO	q 6 hrs
Metronidazole°	15 mg/kg then	IV, PO	q 6–8 hrs
	7.5 mg/kg		
Nitrofurantoin	3 mg/kg	IM	q 12 hrs
Polymyxin B	10,000 units/kg	PO	q 6 hrs
Colistin	2,500 units/kg	IV, IM†	q 6 hrs
Rifampin	10–20 mg/kg	PO‡	q 24 hrs
Vancomycin	Adult: 15 mg/kg	IV§	q 12 hrs
	7.5 mg/kg	PO‖	q 6–8 hrs
	Young: 20 mg/kg	IV§	q 12 hrs
	10 mg/kg	PO‖	q 6–8 hrs
Imipenem	15 mg/kg	IV	q 4–6 hrs

°Administer for a maximum of 7 to 10 days.
†IM injections are painful. IV dosages should be given over a 5-minute period or by continuous drip. This drug is rarely, if ever, used systemically in veterinary medicine.
‡When given PO, is well absorbed in fasting state (food produces delayed and lower peak level). Parenteral formulation is not available in the United States.
§After reconstitution in water, the required dose should be diluted in 160–200 mls of 5% dextrose or 0.9% saline.
‖Is not absorbed from the gastrointestinal tract. Primary use is for clostridial enteritis.

them are very expensive, several may represent the only choice available for treating an infectious disease process caused by a multiresistant bacterium. In addition, as new drugs are tried and found to be successful, empirical therapy begins to become rational therapy, allowing for the development of new therapeutic strategies.

A final consideration is that the most expensive antimicrobial agent is the one that results in therapeutic failure. Using $200 worth of antibiotic and having the horse die is more expensive than using $400 worth of antibiotic to obtain a healthy horse.

ANTIMICROBIAL AGENTS

AMINOGLYCOSIDES

Aminoglycoside antibiotics represent a class of antibiotics with a wide spectrum of bactericidal activity against both gram-positive and gram-negative aerobic bacteria. However, their use should be restricted to treating infections caused by susceptible gram-negative bacteria. Because of their low lipid solubility, the aminoglycosides and spectinomycin (an aminocytocyl) are poorly absorbed from the gastrointestinal (GI) tract and have restricted distribution to tissues outside the vascular bed, including mammary tissue. Aminoglycosides are also inactivated in purulent material and require an oxidative transport system to carry them across the bacterial cytoplasmic membrane. Thus, infections involving anaerobic or microaerophilic conditions would decrease the effectiveness of the aminoglycosides against all bacteria present, regardless of their in vitro susceptibility results. All aminoglycosides have the potential to cause oto- and nephrotoxicity. Predisposing factors associated with these toxicities include prior aminoglycoside therapy, dehydration, current or previous kidney disease, and concurrent therapy with a drug that may enhance their toxicity, such as furosemide.

When given IV, aminoglycosides should be administered slowly. If renal function is impaired, the dosage interval should be increased or the dosage decreased.

Streptomycin and Dihydrostreptomycin

The only clinical indication for using streptomycin or dihydrostreptomycin in the treatment of infections caused by gram-positive bacteria is for enterococcal infections, and then in combination with β-lactam antibiotics such as benzyl penicillin or aminobenzyl penicillin (gentamicin is an alternative). For infections caused by gram-negative bacteria, streptomycin and dihydrostreptomycin are only effective against certain species; thus, in vitro testing is necessary before initiating therapy. When expense is not a consideration, gentamicin is generally preferred because of less toxicity and less likelihood of the bacteria developing resistance. An exception might be brucellosis, rare in the horse, for which streptomycin (or gentamicin) in combination with tetracycline is the therapy of choice.

Neomycin

Neomycin is a medium-spectrum antibiotic with activity against both gram-positive (*Streptococcus* spp. are usually resistant) and gram-negative bacteria (*Pseudomonas aeruginosa* is usually resistant). Neomycin has activity against *Mycobacterium tuberculosis* and *Treponema* spp. Because neomycin is so nephrotoxic, clinical indications for this drug are restricted to those infections that can be treated topically, such as eye or ear infections. Neomycin may also be used to treat enteritis caused by susceptible organisms, but it has been associated with villous atrophy in calves.

Gentamicin

Gentamicin is highly active against a wide range of gram-negative bacteria. Its activity against gram-positive bacteria is somewhat restricted in that in vitro tests may indicate that *Streptococcus* spp. are susceptible, whereas in vivo they may not respond to the treatment. The only accepted use for gentamicin in treating gram-positive infections is in enterococcal infections when used in combination with a β-lactam antibiotic such as ampicillin or amoxicillin. Like all aminoglycosides, gentamicin is inactivated by purulent exudates. This occurs primarily in the presence of lysed PMNs; the PMN's nucleic acids are the major component to which the gentamicin binds.

Kanamycin

Kanamycin diffuses into body tissues better than all other aminoglycosides except amikacin. There are no clinical indications for the use of kanamycin in treating infections caused by gram-positive bacteria. There are members of all species of clinically important gram-negative bacteria that have acquired resistance to kanamycin; thus, its use should be restricted to treating only those infections where in vitro testing indicates susceptibility. All *Pseudomonas aeruginosa* strains are resistant to kanamycin.

Amikacin

Amikacin is active against aerobic gram-negative bacilli, including many strains that are resistant to gentamicin and tobramycin. In structure and pharmacology it is very similar to kanamycin. Currently there are no clinical indications for using amikacin to treat infections caused by gram-positive bacteria. For treating infections caused by gram-negative bacteria, the use of amikacin should be reserved for gentamicin- and tobramycin-resistant isolates. Resistance to amikacin by gram-negative bacteria is uncommon, and resistance rarely develops among susceptible organisms.

Tobramycin

Tobramycin is a newer aminoglycoside. Its spectrum of activity, potency, and pharmacology is similar to that of gentamicin, except there is increased activity against *Pseudomonas aeruginosa* and somewhat decreased activity against certain other gram-negative bacteria. Thus, except for *Pseudomonas aeruginosa*, all gentamicin-resistant organisms are also resistant to tobramycin. For these reasons, the use of tobramycin should be restricted to isolates of *Pseudomonas aeruginosa* proven to be sensitive to tobramycin and resistant to gentamicin. There are no clinical indications for the use of tobramycin for treating infections caused by gram-positive bacteria.

Netilmicin

Netilmicin is very similar to gentamicin in its structure and spectrum of activity. Animal studies have indicated that it may be less toxic than the other aminoglycosides. Because its spectrum of activity is so similar to that of gentamicin, amikacin, and tobramycin, the use of netilmicin should be restricted to those organisms whose antibiograms indicate that netilmicin is the drug of choice.

CEPHALOSPORINS

Cephalosporins are broad spectrum in that they are effective against both gram-positive and gram-negative bacteria. All cephalosporins are bactericidal. Cephalosporins have two principal advantages over penicillins: (1) they have a greater ability to penetrate the outer envelope of gram-negative bacteria, which allows them to gain access to the cell wall target sites (penicillin-binding proteins); and (2) the cephalosporins are generally much less susceptible to hydrolysis by the β-lactamase that is produced by some staphylococci. Their susceptibility to the β-lactamase produced by gram-negative bacteria varies among the cephalosporins. There are currently three classes of cephalosporins. These classifications are based primarily on increased activity against gram-negative bacteria. This increase in gram-negative activity is often at the expense of activity against gram-positive bacteria.

First-Generation Cephalosporins

Cephalosporins should rarely be considered the primary drug of choice and their use should be restricted to treating infections caused by susceptible organisms in the respiratory tract, skin, urinary tract, soft tissue infections, osteomyelitis, and joint infections. While most gram-positive bacteria encountered in veterinary medicine are susceptible, *Enterococcus* spp. are resistant. The susceptibility of gram-negative bacteria to the first-generation cephalosporins varies among the different species and thus requires in vitro testing.

Second-Generation Cephalosporins

Second-generation cephalosporins offer a slightly extended spectrum against gram-negative bacteria compared to first-generation cephalosporins. However, because of their greater expense with little or no clinical advantage over other cephalosporins or other agents to which the bacteria may be susceptible, they are of limited value in equine medicine. Cefoxitin, a cefamycin, has good activity against anaerobic bacteria such as *Bacteroides fragilis* and has been shown to produce excellent results when used to treat polymicrobial infections caused by susceptible aerobic and anaerobic bacteria. Its expense limits its value in equine medicine.

Third-Generation Cephalosporins

Third-generation cephalosporins generally exhibit a limited spectrum of activity against aerobic and anaerobic gram-positive bacteria and an extended spectrum of activity against gram-negative bacteria, including *Ps. aeruginosa*. Of all the third-generation cephalosporins on the market today, only one has been approved for use in veterinary medicine, ceftiofur sodium.* Ceftiofur has been approved for the treatment of bovine respiratory diseases caused by *Pasteurella haemolytica*, *Pasteurella multocida*, and *Haemophilus somnus*. Ceftiofur is also active against many other species of bovine and equine pathogens, including many anaerobic bacteria. Ceftiofur is not active against *Ps. aeruginosa*.

CHLORAMPHENICOL

Chloramphenicol inhibits the growth of a wide range of gram-positive and gram-negative bacteria, including anaerobic gram-positive and gram-negative bacteria. It is also effective against *Rickettsia*, *Coxiella* and *Chlamydia*. *Pseudomonas aeruginosa* is usually resistant to chloramphenicol; therefore, susceptibility testing should always be performed before treating *Pseudomonas* infections with this drug. Resistance to chloramphenicol may also occur among the Enterobacteraciae (*Escherichia coli*, *Klebsiella pneumoniae*, *Enterobacter* spp., and so forth)

---

*Ceftiofur sodium (Naxcel), The Upjohn Company, Kalamazoo, MI

during the course of therapy. Chloramphenicol is one of the most active antimicrobial agents against anaerobic bacteria. Anaerobes are rarely resistant to chloramphenicol; resistance usually occurs among bacteria belonging to the genus *Bacteroides*. Triamphenicol, an analogue of chloramphenicol, is not currently available for use in the United States. Its antibacterial activity is similar to that of chloramphenicol, but unlike chloramphenicol, this drug has not been associated with aplastic anemia. In regard to aplastic anemia, practitioners should be aware that skin exposure to chloramphenicol may result in aplastic anemia in susceptible people.

4-QUINOLONES

Nalidixic Acid

The only use of nalidixic acid is as a urinary antiseptic, since therapeutic serum and tissue levels are never achieved. The rapid development of resistance, even during therapy, greatly limits its usefulness.

Enrofloxacin, Ciprofloxacin, and Norfloxacin

Enrofloxacin, ciprofloxacin, and norfloxacin are stable derivatives of nalidixic acid and are referred to as the fluoroquinolones. These compounds represent a new group of antimicrobial agents with bactericidal activity against a broad array of bacteria including multiresistant gram-negative rods such as *Ps. aeruginosa*. They have limited activity against gram-positive bacteria, especially the streptococci, and have no activity against anaerobic bacteria. Enrofloxacin is the only drug currently approved for use in veterinary medicine. Because of poor absorption and arthritic toxic effects, the fluoroquinolones cannot be used in horses.

IMIPENEM

Imipenem (N-formimidoyl thienamycin) represents a new class of β-lactam antibiotics, the carbapenems. It is highly bactericidal against a broad spectrum of bacteria, including almost all aerobic and anaerobic gram-positive and gram-negative equine bacterial pathogens. Imipenem is marketed for IV use in humans under the name of Primaxin. Primaxin is a combination of imipenem and cilistatin. Cilistatin reduces hydrolysis of imipenem by the kidneys, thus producing higher concentrations of the active drug in the urine, and reduces the nephrotoxicity of imipenem, especially when administered at higher doses. In human medicine, imipenem has a half-life of 1 hour. In our limited experience with this drug in the horse, we found it to be well tolerated when administered IV, over a 20-minute period, at 15 mg per kg. However, by 3 to 4 hours after dosing, serum concentrations of the drug could no longer be detected.

Lincosamides (Clindamycin and Lincomycin)

Clindamycin is a derivative of lincomycin with better pharmacokinetic parameters and antibacterial activity in vitro than lincomycin. Both are bacteriostatic, lipid soluble, and widely distributed throughout the body, including bone. Pseudomembranous colitis following oral and parenteral administration of these drugs has been demonstrated in humans and cats and is suspected in horses and rabbits. Thus, both lincomycin and clindamycin are contraindicated in horses because of the potential of severe colitis.

Macrolides

The macrolides are bacteriostatic, lipid-soluble antimicrobial agents that diffuse readily throughout the body tissues, including bone. These drugs are useful for treatment of infections caused by *Staphylococcus* spp. resistant to benzyl and aminobenzyl penicillins.

Erythromycin

Erythromycin has antibacterial activity similar to that of the older penicillins with additional activity against *Mycoplasma* spp., *Chlamydia* spp., and *Rickettsia*.

Spiramycin

Spiramycin exhibits antibacterial activity similar to that of erythromycin. This antibiotic is concentrated in body fluids, where it produces much higher concentrations than in serum. Because of this, it is considered a good drug to treat pneumonia caused by susceptible organisms, reaching therapeutic tissue levels even though serum levels are low.

Tylosin

Tylosin is marketed for use in veterinary medicine only. Because there are no disks available for susceptibility testing, erythromycin disks are used. Though very little data are available, it is generally assumed that the pharmacokinetic parameters of erythromycin and tylosin are similar.

Tilmicosin

Tilmicosin is a new macrolide antibiotic that is currently under investigation for treating bovine respiratory diseases caused by *Pasteurella* spp.

Metronidazole

Metronidazole is the first and best known of the imidazole derivatives. Tinidazole and ornidazole are currently under investigation and should become available in the near future. Aerobic bacteria are not affected by metronidazole; however, they may be affected by the metabolic products produced by anaerobic bacterial metabolism of metronidazole.

Over 90 per cent of clinically important anaerobic bacteria are susceptible to metronidazole, including *Bacteroides fragilis*, but excluding *Propionibacterium* and *Actinomyces*. Clinical indications include (1) polymicrobial infections involving aerobic and anaerobic bacteria, for which metronidazole is given in conjunction with aminoglycosides, potentiated sulfas, or ceftiofur; (2) infections caused by β-lactamase–producing anaerobic bacteria; and (3) serious, life-threatening infections, such as endocarditis or meningitis, involving anaerobic and aerobic bacteria for which a bacteriologic cure is necessary; under such circumstances metronidazole should be used in combination with an appropriate β-lactam antibiotic.

Nitrofurantoin

Because nitrofurantoin only achieves therapeutic concentrations in the urine (not serum or tissues), its only use is as a urinary antisepsis agent.

Penicillins

Benzyl Penicillins

The benzyl penicillins include sodium penicillin G, potassium penicillin G, procaine penicillin G, benzathine penicillin G, and penicillin V. When organisms are susceptible, penicillin has traditionally been the drug of choice because of its potency, narrow spectrum, and remarkably few adverse effects. Penicillins inhibit cell wall synthesis in multiplying bacteria, which ultimately results in cell death. At sub-MIC levels there is abnormal cell formation, resulting in enhanced phagocytosis by host phagocytic cells. All gram-positive cocci, except penicillinase-producing *Staphylococcus* spp. and some *Enterococcus* spp., are susceptible to penicillins. Most anaerobes are considered susceptible, except β-lactamase–producing *Bacteroides* spp. such as *B. fragilis*. Most gram-negative bacteria associated with infectious disease processes in the horse are resistant to benzyl penicillins. The penicillins are bug-drug concentration dependent; thus, the more active the infection, the higher the initial dose should be.

Aminobenzyl Penicillins

The aminobenzyl penicillins (ampicillin and amoxicillin) are broad-spectrum penicillins with increased activity against gram-negative bacteria but are slightly less active than penicillin G against gram-positive bacteria and anaerobic bacteria. Unfortunately, acquired resistance to these drugs is making them less effective.

Ampicillin has increased activity against many gram-negative bacteria and *Enterococcus* spp. For susceptible gram-positive bacteria, a benzyl penicillin should be the drug of choice.

Ampicillin/sulbactam is a β-lactamase–resistant ampicillin product marketed for IV use in humans. The sulbactam molecule binds to plasmid-mediated bacterial β-lactamases, thus preventing the destruction of the ampicillin molecule. This increases the effectiveness of the aminobenzyl penicillins against resistant bacteria such as *E. coli* and *Klebsiella pneumoniae* but has no effect against bacteria such as *Ps. aeruginosa*.

Amoxicillin has antibacterial activity similar to that of ampicillin. Some studies have suggested that it is more rapidly lethal to susceptible bacteria than ampicillin. In animals other than the horse, amoxicillin administered orally is more completely absorbed than ampicillin, thus producing higher serum levels for an equivalent dose and therefore allowing t.i.d. rather than q.i.d. dosing. This more complete absorption may also account for the reported lower incidence of diarrhea with amoxicillin as compared to ampicillin.

Clavamox is a β-lactamase–resistant amoxicillin-clavulanic acid product. The clavulanic acid binds to and inactivates plasmid-mediated β-lactamases, thus increasing the effectiveness of amoxicillin against some β-lactamase–producing bacteria. Clavamox is not effective against *Ps. aeruginosa*. This drug is available as an oral preparation only.

Penicillinase-Resistant Penicillins

The *only* indication for penicillinase-resistant penicillins (methicillin, nafcillin; isoxazolyl penicillins [oxacillin, floxacillin, cloxacillin, dicloxacillin]) is in the treatment of, and in certain situations, prophylaxis against, staphylococcal infections. As with the other penicillins, the penicillinase-resistant penicillins are not well absorbed from the GI tract of the adult horse. Following parenteral administration, the tissue levels of penicillinase-resistant penicillins are similar to those of penicillin G.

Carboxy Penicillins

The carboxy penicillins were the first penicillins with anti-*Pseudomonas* activity; they include carbenicillin (sodium and indanyl sodium), ticarcillin, and timentin.

Carbenicillin is a semisynthetic penicillin that, like ampicillin, is inactivated by penicillinase. Its use is confined to the treatment of known *Morganella morganii, Proteus vulgaris, Providencia rettgeri, Enterobacter,* and *Ps. aeruginosa* infections, and in certain circumstances, severe gram-negative sepsis. In very high doses it is active against anaerobes, including *Bacteroides fragilis*, but offers no clear-cut advantage over other currently recommended therapy for anaerobic infections. Because of its low potency, large doses must be administered to be effective. However, carbenicillin has an extremely low toxicity and can therefore be used effectively and safely at large doses. Sodium carbenicillin is not adequately absorbed with oral administration. Indanyl sodium carbenicillin is marketed for oral use but only reaches therapeutic concentrations in the urine.

Ticarcillin is very similar to carbenicillin. On a weight-for-weight basis, it is somewhat more active than carbenicillin, especially against *Ps. aeruginosa*. However, for most other organisms (e.g., *E. coli, Enterobacter* spp., *Proteus* spp., and *Bacteroides fragilis*) the activity of ticarcillin is very similar to that of carbenicillin and equivalent doses should be used. Relative cost should be an important consideration in choosing ticarcillin or carbenicillin.

Timentin is a combination of ticarcillin plus clavulanic acid. This product has similar pharmacokinetics as ticarcillin. This combination has increased activity against plasmid-mediated β-lactamase–producing bacteria such as *Staphylococcus aureus, Klebsiella pneumoniae,* and *Bacteroides fragilis*.

Aminoacetyl (Ureido) Penicillins

The aminoacetyl penicillins are the second generation of anti-pseudomonas penicillins; they include pipercillin, azlocillin, and mezlocillin.

Pipercillin is a semisynthetic derivative of aminobenzyl penicillin and has been shown to be two to eight times more potent than carbenicillin and ticarcillin against *Escherichia coli, Enterobacter* spp., *Proteus mirabilis, Klebsiella pneumoniae, Citrobacter, Acinetobacter, Salmonella* spp., and *Pseudomonas* strains. For example, 70 per cent of *Pseudomonas* strains are susceptible to 100 µg of carbenicillin, whereas 100 per cent are susceptible to 20 µg of pipercillin.

Azlocillin is a semisynthetic broad-spectrum acylureido penicillin for IV administration. Its indication is primarily for treatment of serious infections caused by *Ps. aeruginosa*. In vitro studies have shown that azlocillin is four to 16 times more active against *Pseudomonas* than carbenicillin and two to four times more active than ticarcillin.

Mezlocillin is very similar to azlocillin in spectrum of activity and pharmacokinetics but is currently less expensive.

Polymyxin B and Colistin

This class of drugs has been displaced by the aminoglycosides and extended spectrum penicillins for the recalcitrant gram-negative bacteria. Polymyxin B and colistin are very nephrotoxic. They have a narrow spectrum with activity restricted to the gram-negative bacteria. Absorption from the GI tract is slow and they are nephrotoxic. Parenteral use should be restricted to severe urinary tract or systemic infections caused by susceptible coliforms or *Ps. aeruginosa*.

Rifampin

Rifampin has a wide spectrum of antibacterial activity. While its major clinical use in the past was as part of combination therapy for the treatment of mycobacterial disease, it has also been found to work synergistically with antibacterial drugs for enhanced treatment of bacterial infections caused by such bacteria as *Rhodococcus equi* and *Staphylococcus aureus*. Because resistance to rifampin can develop during therapy, it should *never* be used as a single agent.

Sulfonamides

As a single therapeutic agent, sulfonamides should not be used in the horse.

Potentiated Sulfonamides

Potentiated sulfonamides consist of trimethoprim (a diaminopyrimidine) in combination with a variety of sulfonamides in a fixed ratio of 1 part trimethoprim to 5 parts sulfa. Examples include sulfamethoxazole, Septra®,* Bactrim®,† sulfadiazine, Tribrissen®,‡ and Di-Trim®.§

Trimethoprim-sulfadiazine has been used to treat a variety of infectious disease processes in the horse, including meningitis caused by gram-negative bacteria, salmonellosis, acute urinary tract infections, and bacterial infections of the upper and lower respiratory tract. Because the mechanism of action of the trimethoprim-sulfonamide combination is a two-step inhibition of bacterial folic acid synthesis, the presence of purulent material neutralizes the effect of this drug combination. Thus, in infections involving necrotic tissue or purulent material, such as anaerobic infections, these products will be less effective.

Tetracyclines

There are two classes of tetracyclines, the natural and the semisynthetic or synthetic tetracyclines. The natural tetracyclines include oxytetracycline, chlortetracycline, and demeclocycline. The synthetic tetracyclines include tetracycline, doxycycline, minocycline, rolitetracycline, and methacycline. The use of tetracycline in the immature animal can cause browning of the teeth, while in the adult horse it may lead to antibiotic-induced enteritis. Because of this, the tetracyclines should not be used for the treatment of bacterial infections in the horse, with few exceptions. Oxytetracycline is the drug of choice for the treatment of Potomac Valley Fever caused by *Ehrlichia risticii*, equine ehrlichiosis, and mycoplasma infections such as *Mycoplasma felis* pleuritis. The use of doxycycline and minocycline by equine practitioners may be on the increase as both drugs have the potential to be very rapidly absorbed and have a longer serum half-life than other tetracyclines. Doxycycline is excreted primarily through bile, whereas minocycline is excreted primarily through the kidneys.

Vancomycin

Vancomycin is a parenteral agent with excellent activity against gram-positive organisms. However, because of its toxicity and expense, it should not be considered unless penicillin, cephalosporins, and other classes of drugs cannot be used.

Supplemental Readings

Brumbaugh, G. W.: Rational selection of antimicrobial drugs for treatment of infections of horses. Vet. Clin. North Am. (Equine Pract. Clin. Pharmacol.), 3:191–220, 1987.

Hirsh, D. C., and Jang, S. S.: Antimicrobic susceptibility of bacterial pathogens from horses. Vet. Clin. North Am. (Equine Pract. Clin. Pharmacol.), 3:181–190, 1987.

Nordström, L., Ringberg, H., Cronberg, S., Tjernström, O., and Walder, M.: Does administration of an aminoglycoside in a single daily dose affect its efficacy and toxicity? J. Antimicrob. Chemother. 25:159–173, 1990.

Paterson, P. Y.: Introduction to infectious diseases. *In* Youmans, G. P. (ed.): The Biologic and Clinical Basis of Infectious Diseases, 3rd ed. Philadelphia, W. B. Saunders Co., 1985, pp. 2–7.

Prescott, J. F., and Baggot, J. D.: Antimicrobial Therapy in Veterinary Medicine. Boston, Blackwell Scientific Publications, 1988.

Youmans, G. P.: Host-bacteria interactions: External defense mechanisms. *In* Youmans, G. P. (ed.): The Biologic and Clinical Basis of Infectious Diseases, 3rd ed. Philadelphia, W. B. Saunders Co., 1985, pp. 8–17.

Youmans, G. P.: Host-bacteria interactions: Nonimmunologic internal defense mechanisms. *In* Youmans, G. P. (ed.): The Biologic and Clinical Basis of Infectious Diseases, 3rd ed. Philadelphia, W. B. Saunders Co., 1985, pp. 18–24.

Youmans, G. P.: Host-bacteria interactions: Immunological defense mechanisms. *In* Youmans G. P. (ed.): The Biologic and Clinical Basis of Infectious Diseases, 3rd ed. Philadelphia, W. B. Saunders Co., 1985, pp. 25–34.

---

*Septra, Burroughs-Wellcome Co., Research Triangle Park, NC
†Bactrim, Roche Labs, Nutley, N.J.
‡Tribrissen, Coopers Animal Health Inc., Kansas City, KS
§Di-Trim, Syntex Animal Health, West Des Moines, IA

Anti-Inflammatory Agents

Stephen A. May, LEAHURST, ENGLAND

Inflammation is a healing process. It is common to all body tissues that have suffered injury, and ideally it should lead to resolution or repair. This means that, unlike the situation with antibiotics or anthelmintics, which are clearly targeted toward organisms that are harmful to the host, the case for intervention in the inflammatory process with pharmacological agents is not straightforward. Inflammation may be beneficial or it may be aberrant and harmful, and the decision on whether or not to use anti-inflammatory drugs will depend on the subjective judgment of the clinician as to which situation predominates in the disease process in an individual animal.

In general, anti-inflammatory agents have a role to play in two broad categories of abnormal response. The first category includes those situations in which inflammation is inappropriate and not associated with defense or healing. In the horse, allergic diseases are the main conditions that fall into this category, but autoimmune conditions are recognized with increasing frequency. The second broad category of abnormal response includes those situations in which inflammation is appropriate but excessive: either too large an overall response, as in endotoxic shock, where inflammatory mediators such as tumor necrosis factor may kill the animal producing them; or too long-lasting, as in various forms of joint disease, where persistent inflammation results in continued degradation of articular cartilage. When deciding to intervene in an undesirable inflammatory response, the clinician should remember also that the effectiveness of the therapy will be compromised if the inciting stimulus remains. Infection needs to be controlled and allergens, irritants, and foreign bodies removed if the response to therapy is to be permanent. Otherwise, animals are likely to relapse when treatment is terminated, necessitating, in some cases, continuous administration of these agents.

In assessing the effect of anti-inflammatory drugs on disease processes, it is important to remember that pain is one of the cardinal signs of inflammation. Apparent improvement in the condition of an animal may relate more to the analgesic properties of these agents than to a general anti-inflammatory effect. This is particularly true with the nonsteroidal anti-inflammatory drugs. These are potent inhibitors of the production of eicosanoids, in particular prostaglandin E_2, which probably accounts for their ability to relieve pain. However, nonsteroidal anti-inflammatory drugs are much less effective at reducing leukocyte infiltration into inflammatory foci and controlling edema formation. It is easy for the clinician to assume, wrongly, that improvement following nonsteroidal anti-inflammatory drug therapy relates to disease modification and consequential pain relief rather than to a direct analgesic effect.

For the purposes of discussion, the anti-inflammatory agents are best divided into three groups: the corticosteroids, the classic nonsteroidal anti-inflammatory drugs, and other, miscellaneous agents. The classic nonsteroidal anti-inflammatory drugs are the drugs that inhibit cyclooxygenase (prostaglandin synthetase) and thus prevent the production of the prostaglandins and thromboxanes. The miscellaneous group includes agents that have different anti-inflammatory properties from drugs in the other two groups. At present, these are mainly antiarthritic agents.

CORTICOSTEROIDS

Glucocorticoids are the most effective of the anti-inflammatory agents in clinical use because they affect all aspects of the inflammatory response. It has been suggested that, in part, this relates to their ability to stimulate the production of proteins with antiphospholipase A activity, and that these lipocortins prevent the release of the precursors involved in the synthesis of the prostaglandins, thromboxanes, leukotrienes, and platelet-activating factor. In addition to reducing pain, edema formation, and leukocyte infiltration, glucocorticoids have a marked effect on anabolism. Tissue repair is retarded, and the synthesis of tissue matrix, such as proteoglycan molecules, is inhibited. Therefore, even where steroids are not directly catabolic, they may result in tissue degradation by affecting the balance between synthesis and breakdown.

Within the categories of abnormal inflammatory response outlined above, glucocorticoids are most useful in the treatment of inappropriate inflammatory responses. These include allergic conditions such as *Culicoides* hypersensitivity (sweet itch) and urticarial reactions, and autoimmune conditions such as purpura haemorrhagica and immune-mediated joint disease. Wher-

TABLE 1. RECOMMENDED DOSES OF GLUCOCORTICOID

Glucocorticoid	Dosage	Example and Route
Betamethasone	0.02–0.1 mg/kg	Betamethasone sodium phosphate IV, IM; betamethasone IM
Dexamethasone	0.02–0.1 mg/kg	Dexamethasone sodium phosphate IV, IM; dexamethasone acetate IM
Flumethasone	0.002–0.008 mg/kg	Flumethasone, IM
Methylprednisolone	0.2–0.7 mg/kg	Methylprednisolone acetate, IM
Prednisolone	0.2–1.0 mg/kg	Prednisolone, IM
Triamcinolone	0.02–0.1 mg/kg	Triamcinolone acetonide, IM

ever possible, the cause of the problem should be removed at the time that therapy is initiated. The ideal way to manage a *Culicoides*-sensitive individual is to remove that individual from the environment in which it is being bitten! However, this is often not practical.

A list of glucocorticoids used in the systemic treatment of these conditions is given in Table 1. The particular drug chosen will depend on the personal preference of the clinician. Factors that affect this decision include the severity of the condition being treated, the anticipated duration of therapy, and the convenience of administration. In general, treatment should be for the least possible time at as low a dose as possible. If prolonged administration is anticipated, alternate-day dosing (in the early mornings) with a short-acting steroid such as prednisolone is recommended in an attempt to minimize adrenal suppression (Table 2). Even so, if treatment is continued for several weeks, it is advisable to withdraw the drug gradually over an additional 1 to 3 weeks.

Sometimes it is difficult to ensure regular treatment, and an owner may prefer the single use of a long-acting steroid. A typical situation is a mild case of sweet itch, for which the animal may need only one intramuscular injection of methylprednisolone acetate at the first signs of the problem to remain relatively free of signs for the whole of the *Culicoides* biting season. Slightly more severe cases may be controlled by a second injection given 4 weeks after the first.

The use of glucocorticoids in the horse in conditions involving an excessive inflammatory response is more controversial. In laboratory animals, these agents are effective at controlling experimentally induced forms of shock, provided they are given before the onset of the shock state. The use of steroids once shock is established is much more disappointing, and, in endotoxic shock in the horse, they appear to have no advantage over the nonsteroidal anti-inflammatory drug flunixin meglumine. If the decision is made to use steroids as an adjunct to other therapy in any form of shock, it must be remembered that only doses 10 to 50 times the recommended dose for other conditions are likely to affect the clinical outcome. This is up to 2 gm of dexamethasone, which would be 20 50-ml vials of dexamethasone sodium phosphate, 2 mg per ml.

A number of glucocorticoid formulations exist for the intra-articular therapy of equine degenerative joint disease. Such treatment will produce dramatic symptomatic relief of this condition, but will equally dramatically suppress anabolic processes within the articular tissues. Particularly if horses are worked before cartilage collagen and proteoglycan synthesis has returned to normal, this can lead to accelerated degenerative changes, so-called steroid arthropathy. Therefore, the main candidates for steroid therapy of degenerative joint disease are animals in which short-term relief of lameness is more important than a long working career.

One other factor that needs to be considered when the use of glucocorticoids is contemplated in the horse is the ability of these agents to cause laminitis. This may relate in part to the ability of steroids to amplify the vasoconstrictive effects of epinephrine and serotonin, and in part to their effects on the synthesis of structural molecules at

TABLE 2. DURATION OF ACTION OF GLUCOCORTICOID FORMULATIONS

Rapid onset (duration of action that of free steroid)
Soluble esters, given IV
  Betamethasone sodium phosphate
  Dexamethasone sodium phosphate
  Prednisolone sodium succinate
  Methylprednisolone sodium succinate

Free steroid (kinetic data incomplete for the horse)
Prednisolone t½(horse) 2 h.; adrenal suppression over by 24 hr after 0.6 mg/kg prednisolone succinate IV
Dexamethasone t½(horse) 53 min.; adrenal suppression for 4–5 days following 0.05 mg/kg dexamethasone IV or IM

Long duration of action (dependent on solubility)
Insoluble esters, given IM
  Dexamethasone acetate
  Methylprednisolone acetate
  Triamcinolone acetonide
  Prednisolone acetate (at 0.6 mg/kg IM, induces adrenal suppression for about 3 weeks)

the laminar junction. For this reason alone, the equine clinician should avoid the trivial use of glucocorticoids. In addition, although a number of formulations still include laminitis as one indication for their use, it is now generally accepted that steroids are contraindicated in the treatment of all forms of laminitis.

NONSTEROIDAL ANTI-INFLAMMATORY DRUGS

The common feature of the drugs in this group is their ability to inhibit cyclooxygenase (prostaglandin synthetase) and thus inhibit the production of the prostaglandins and the thromboxanes. This explains the antipyretic and analgesic effects of the nonsteroidal anti-inflammatory drugs, and also their more limited anti-inflammatory effects.

Endogenous pyrogens, such as interleukin-1, tumor necrosis factor, and interferon-gamma, stimulate hypothalamic production of prostaglandin E_2, and this results in elevation of the hypothalamic thermal set-point. Nonsteroidal anti-inflammatory drugs reverse this process. Therefore, nonsteroidal anti-inflammatory drugs will only be effective in pyrexia related to a raised set-point. They will have no effect where pyrexia is related to defective heat loss, as in heat stroke.

At an inflammatory focus, prostaglandin E_2 is probably important in amplifying the pain-inducing effects of mediators such as histamine and bradykinin, and it may also affect the body's ability to discriminate between benign and noxious stimuli. For instance, touch, normally a nonpainful sensation, may be perceived as painful in the presence of prostaglandin E_2. Nonsteroidal anti-inflammatory drugs exert their analgesic effect by preventing the production of prostaglandin E_2.

Although the prostaglandins and the thromboxanes are important in the early vascular events in acute inflammation, other inflammatory mediators such as the leukotrienes are probably more important in the recruitment of leukocytes to inflammatory foci, and interleukin-1 may be important in the control of subsequent connective tissue remodeling. Thus, the cyclooxygenase-inhibiting ability of the nonsteroidal anti-inflammatory drugs will have little effect on these aspects of the inflammatory process. However, not all of the anti-inflammatory properties of the individual nonsteroidal anti-inflammatory drugs can be attributed to cyclooxygenase inhibition. They may, to a variable extent, have additional anti-inflammatory activity. For instance, relative to their ability to inhibit prostaglandin synthesis, naproxen is much more effective in the inhibition of leukocyte migration than phenylbutazone in laboratory animals. Unfortunately, similar information is not available on meclofenamic acid and flunixin meglumine.

The restricted anti-inflammatory activity of the nonsteroidal anti-inflammatory drugs explains their relative lack of efficacy in allergic and autoimmune conditions. However, they are extremely useful in two other areas. The first is in providing analgesia, where pain is a significant part of the inflammatory process. This includes conditions such as acute laminitis, severe joint sprains, and severe muscle and tendon injuries. It also includes the chronic pain associated with degenerative joint disease. However, the clinician should be cautious about the use of nonsteroidal anti-inflammatory drugs in animals if subsequent medical therapy with sodium hyaluronate or polysulfated glycosaminoglycan is contemplated. Under such circumstances the joint disease may be aggravated, making the second therapy less effective. Recommended doses and routes of administration for the nonsteroidal anti-inflammatory drugs are given in Table 3.

The second area in which nonsteroidal anti-inflammatory drugs are important is in the treatment of endotoxin-related systemic inflammation (endotoxic shock). In other inflammatory conditions, it is the extravascular processes such as edema, leukocyte migration, and tissue remodeling that are of clinical concern. Endotoxic shock differs from other forms of inflammation in that the intravascular components of inflammation are more important than its extravascular consequences. This means that the ability of the nonsteroidal anti-inflammatory drugs to inhibit the production of the vasoactive prostaglandins and thromboxanes can be utilized, and their relatively restricted activity gives them advantages over the corticosteroids. The nonsteroidal anti-inflammatory drugs do not interfere with wound

TABLE 3. DOSES OF NONSTEROIDAL ANTI-INFLAMMATORY DRUGS

Drug	Dosage	Route
Acetylsalicylic acid	25–35 mg/kg q 12 hr	PO
Dipyrone	5–22 mg/kg	IM, IV
Flunixin meglumine	1.1 mg/kg q 24 hr (Anti-endotoxic dose, 0.25 mg/kg)	PO, IM, IV
Meclofenamic acid	2.2 mg/kg q 24 hr	PO
Naproxen	10 mg/kg q 12 hr	PO
Phenylbutazone	2–4 mg/kg q 12 hr	PO, IV

Typical recommended doses for a course of treatment with phenylbutazone: day 1, 4.4 mg/kg q 12 hr; days 2–5, 2.2 mg/kg q 12 hr; followed by 2.2 mg/kg q 24 hr.

healing, which is important following colic surgery, and they do not compromise the body's ability to defend itself against infection, important when endotoxemia may be associated with bacteremia. Both flunixin meglumine and phenylbutazone moderate the biochemical and clinical abnormalities identified in experimental endotoxemia in the horse. In the case of flunixin, a beneficial clinical effect is obtained with a dose of 0.25 mg per kg, as opposed to the recommended dose of 1.0 mg per kg (see Table 3).

The nonsteroidal anti-inflammatory drug used most widely in the horse is phenylbutazone. Although much has been learned about its toxicity in humans and the horse in recent years (see *Current Therapy in Equine Medicine 2*, p. 118) (phenylbutazone has been withdrawn from use in humans in the United Kingdom), this has not altered the general impression that phenylbutazone is a relatively safe drug when used in the horse at recommended doses. However, care must always be taken with the use of all these agents in young, old, and sick animals, where drug catabolism may be retarded. The clinician should think about using lower doses and, if possible, increasing the time interval between doses. It is no coincidence that most of the adverse reactions caused by the use of these agents in humans have occurred following their use in old people. In addition, it should be remembered that just as the modes of action of the nonsteroidal anti-inflammatory drugs are similar, so are their toxic effects, and that these are additive when different agents are used together. Particular caution should be taken against the unwitting use of a nonsteroidal anti-inflammatory drug with a combination product, such as hyoscine/dipyrone* or methindizate/dipyrone,† and if insufficient analgesia is obtained with the recommended dose of a nonsteroidal anti-inflammatory drug the use of a different type of analgesic, such as an opiate, should be considered.

MISCELLANEOUS AGENTS

There are currently three agents in use in various parts of the world that are aimed at modifying the disease process in degenerative joint disease. These are sodium hyaluronate, polysulfated glycosaminoglycan,‡ and pentosan sulfate.§

---

*Buscopan Compositum, Boehringer Ingelheim, Bracknell, England.
†Isaverin, Bayer, Bury St. Edmunds, England.
‡Adequan, Luitpold Pharmaceuticals, Shirley, NY.
§Anarthron-H, RWR Veterinary Products, Agnes Bank, NSW, Australia.

The mode of action of these drugs varies, but they are all aimed at returning the synovial environment to normal. It is hoped that this will reverse the disease process in early joint disease and arrest or retard the disease process in more advanced disease. Individual response is variable, but, provided degenerative joint disease is identified as the cause of the lameness sufficiently early, these agents are an advance on steroids and nonsteroidal anti-inflammatory drugs in providing disease-oriented rather than sign-oriented (symptomatic) therapy. The recommended dose of sodium hyaluronate, which is given by the intra-articular route, varies according to the manufacturer (Table 4) and is probably affected by the presence of contaminants and preservatives in the product. The dose may be repeated at weekly intervals until a satisfactory response is obtained or until it is decided that the treatment has failed. If at any stage the next injection fails to improve on the result of the previous injection, the chances of further improvement are slim. The recommended treatment regimen for polysulfated glycosaminoglycan is 250 mg given intra-articularly at weekly intervals for 5 weeks. Alternatively, 500 mg may be given intramuscularly every 4 days for a total of seven injections. Polysulfated glycosaminoglycan has the theoretical advantage over sodium hyaluronate in that it inhibits enzymes likely to be important in the degradation of articular cartilage. However, it may aggravate the inflammatory process in the presence of significant synovitis. Therefore, polysulfated glycosaminoglycan is to be preferred in the less inflammatory forms of degenerative joint disease, and sodium hyaluronate in the more inflammatory forms. In addition, sodium hyaluronate may be useful as an adjunct to other therapy in the treatment of infective arthritis and tenosynovitis, whereas polysulfated glycosaminoglycan would be contraindicated (see p. 128).

TABLE 4. DOSES OF SODIUM HYALURONATE PREPARATIONS

Drug, Manufacturer	Dosage
Equron, Solvay	10 mg/joint for small joints 20 mg/joint for large joints
Hyalovet, Fort Dodge Hylartil, Fisons Hylartin V, Pharmacia Hyvisc, MedChem Products	20 mg/joint for small joints (radiocarpal, intercarpal, metacarpophalangeal, interphalangeal) 40 mg/joint for large joints (tibiotarsal, femorotibial, femoropatellar)
Remobilase, Arnolds	50 mg/joint
Synacid, Schering	50 mg/joint

The author has no experience of the use of pentosan sulfate. The recommended dose is 250 mg given by intra-articular injection, and its mode of action is probably similar to that of polysulfated glycosaminoglycan. Repeat injections can be administered at 7- to 10-day intervals, but two treatments are usually sufficient.

Supplemental Readings

Higgins, A. J., and Lees, P.: The acute inflammatory process, arachidonic acid metabolism and the mode of action of anti-inflammatory drugs. Equine Vet. J., 16:163, 1984.

Lees, P., and Higgins, A. J.: Clinical pharmacology and therapeutic uses of non-steroidal anti-inflammatory drugs in the horse. Equine Vet. J., 17:83, 1985.

May, S. A., Lees, P., Higgins, A. J., and Sedgwick, A. D.: Inflammation: A clinical perspective. Vet. Record, 120:514, 1987.

Moore, J. N.: Nonsteroidal antiinflammatory drug therapy for endotoxemia: We're doing the right thing, aren't we? Comp. Cont. Ed. Pract. Vet., 11:741, 1989.

Toutain, P. L., and Brandon, R. A.: Steroidal anti-inflammatory agents in the horse: Pharmacokinetics and action on the adrenal gland. In Ruckebusch, Y., Toutain, P.-L., and Koritz, G. D. (eds.): Veterinary Pharmacology and Toxicology. Westport, CT, AVI Publishing Co. Inc., 1983, pp. 353–366.

Fluid and Electrolyte Therapy

L. Michael Schmall, COLUMBUS, OHIO

In equine medicine clinical conditions that require fluid and electrolyte therapy are frequently encountered and of critical importance to the success or failure of treatment. The goal of fluid and electrolyte therapy is to increase vascular volume in an attempt to restore and maintain cardiovascular function, and correct tissue hydration and electrolyte and acid-base imbalances. Intravenous (IV) fluids may be necessary on a short-term basis, as replacement, or may be required for prolonged periods. In the latter situations not only replacement but maintenance requirements need to be considered. Additionally, fluids are often a vehicle for IV administration of medications.

This chapter focuses on the compartmental distribution of water and electrolytes, the clinical and clinicopathologic assessment of fluid and electrolyte requirements, the development of a plan for fluid and electrolyte therapy, including specific types of fluids and indications for their use, and routes of administration. The discussion does not consider specific disease entities, which are addressed in detail elsewhere.

WATER AND ELECTROLYTE DISTRIBUTION

Approximately 60 per cent of adult and up to 80 per cent of neonatal total body weight consists of water that is freely distributed by osmotic forces between the intracellular (ICF) and extracellular (ECF) fluid compartments. ICF accounts for approximately two-thirds and ECF for one-third of total body water. ECF may be further subdivided into plasma volume and interstitial fluid, lymph, and transcellular fluid, respectively accounting for approximately 8 to 12 per cent and 15 per cent of total body weight. ECF osmolality is maintained primarily by sodium and chloride ions, while intracellular osmotic forces are a function of potassium and phosphates. Disturbances in water balance result from either increased loss, decreased intake, or a combination of these two factors. Decreased volume of either the ICF or ECF is associated with changes in osmotic forces and a redistribution of water between the two compartments. For instance, acute loss of fluid from the extracellular compartment increases the effective osmolality and water moves from the intracellular space until osmotic equilibrium is reestablished.

As already mentioned, significant differences exist in the ionic composition of each compartment. Sodium is the major cation in the ECF and is responsible for maintenance of the extracellular osmotic forces and fluid volume. Serum sodium concentrations are routinely used to estimate alterations in body sodium stores but may not be reliable. Serum sodium is dependent on the exchangeable sodium content of the ECF, the exchangeable potassium content of the ICF, and total body water (TBW), and can be defined by the following relationship:

$$\text{Serum Na}^+ = \frac{\text{Exchangeable Na}^+ + \text{Exchangeable K}^+}{\text{TBW}}.$$

Therefore, hypernatremia, in which a relative water deficit exists, may be due to losses in TBW, sodium or potassium excess, or a combination of these factors. Hyponatremia, in which a relative water excess is present, can be due to sodium or potassium loss or TBW excess. Clinically, hypernatremia has been defined as a sodium concentration greater than 146 mEq per L, while hyponatremia is present when the sodium concentration is less than 132 mEq per L. Typically, hyponatremic states occur in diarrheal conditions, where massive losses of fluid and electrolyte are followed by partial replacement of fluid requirements through oral intake of water. Hypernatremic states are infrequently encountered but may occur with overzealous fluid therapy.

Potassium is the major intracellular cation, with only 2% of total body stores present in the ECF. As such, plasma potassium concentrations are of limited value in estimating total body potassium. Potassium ions produce the osmotic force necessary for maintaining ICF volume in a manner analogous to sodium in the ECF. Hyperkalemia is unusual in the horse unless it occurs in association with impaired renal function or severe acidosis. Hypokalemia is more frequently encountered, particularly in anorectic horses and foals with secretory diarrheal diseases. Large decreases in potassium concentration are often indicative of severe acid-base imbalances and may be manifested by alterations in neuromuscular conduction and myocardial function. Potassium deficits are readily replaced once horses resume eating sufficient quantities of hay.

Chloride and bicarbonate are the major anions in the ECF and exhibit a reciprocal relationship. Hypochloremia is usually the result of increased loss via the gastrointestinal tract, either with diarrhea or duodenitis-proximal jejunitis, or from massive losses due to sweating. Bicarbonate functions as a major buffering system and to that extent reflects acid-base imbalances; marked decreases in bicarbonate concentration accompany moderate to severe acidotic states. However, IV sodium bicarbonate solutions should be used with caution since excessive administration may cause the development of persistent metabolic alkalosis, hypernatremia, hyperosmolality, and hypokalemia.

ASSESSMENT OF FLUID REQUIREMENTS

The initial steps in the treatment of horses with fluid and electrolyte deficits include collection of a history and complete physical examination. Dehydration is assessed clinically using several variables such as decreased skin turgor, muscular weakness, dry oral mucous membranes, and decreased urine production. Unfortunately, recognizable changes in these clinical parameters are not evident until fluid deficits approach approximately 5 per cent of body weight. In an adult horse weighing 450 kg, fluid deficits may reach 20 liters before becoming clinically apparent. Clinically, dehydration is usually evaluated subjectively and is graded as mild, moderate, or severe. Generally, mild losses are 5 to 7 per cent, moderate losses are 8 to 10 per cent, and severe losses are 10 per cent or greater of total body weight. Fluid losses are also frequently accompanied by signs of hypovolemic shock: decreased jugular distensibility, increased capillary refill time, cold extremities, increased heart rate, and reduced pulse pressure. Packed cell volume (PCV) and total plasma protein concentration (TPP) are two commonly used laboratory indicators of dehydration. However, these two parameters can be affected by other factors that must be taken into account. Significant changes in PCV can be produced by splenic contraction and release of marginated erythrocytes. Conditions where there is significant protein loss will affect the validity of using TPP to evaluate hydration status. Creatinine and blood urea nitrogen (BUN) concentrations are also frequently increased in horses with significant acute fluid losses and are used diagnostically. These data are of limited value individually and must be viewed in the overall context of the animal's condition and other laboratory findings.

Acid-base imbalances often occur with conditions for which fluid therapy is indicated and are reflected in bicarbonate concentration. Clinically, metabolic acidosis occurs most frequently in association with obstructive gastrointestinal disease, diarrhea, and renal failure. Increased base loss, increased acid, primarily lactate, production, and reduced peripheral perfusion contribute to the acidosis in these situations. Respiratory compensation and decreased P_{CO_2} may be noted in acidotic horses. Polyionic solutions or solutions containing high concentrations of bicarbonate (5 per cent $NaHCO_3$) are most commonly used for correction of this condition. It is advisable to assess the degree of acidosis prior to the administration of large quantities of bicarbonate-containing solutions. Hypochloremic metabolic alkalosis is usually observed in horses after endurance exercise and with early intestinal obstruction. Treatment should be directed at replacement of chloride deficits with potassium and sodium salts.

Samples for blood gas evaluation should be collected anaerobically in heparinized syringes and may be stored on ice for up to 4 hours prior to analysis. Although desirable, laboratory facilities equipped with blood gas analytic capabilities are not always available. In these instances the Harleco procedure for total CO_2 determinations offers an alternative for assessment of bicarbonate. Approximately 95 per cent of the total CO_2 content of blood is considered to be bicarbonate. Total CO_2 is decreased in acidosis and increased in alkalosis.

FORMULATION OF A FLUID THERAPY PLAN

It is essential that a therapeutic fluid plan be developed as soon as possible to avoid complications associated with large or continued fluid losses. The quantity of fluid and rate of administration are dependent on clinical presentation. For instance, horses with diarrhea frequently require rapid IV administration of large volumes of fluids. Less critical conditions would require a less aggressive approach. Often a portion of the existing deficit is rapidly replaced, with the remainder given more slowly over several hours. The volume of fluid for replacement can be calculated using the following formula:

$$\text{Fluid deficit (L)} = \text{Clinical dehydration (\%)} \times \text{Body weight (kg)}.$$

This quantity is in addition to maintenance requirements of 50 to 100 ml per kg per day.

Clinicopathologic data consisting of hematocrit and total plasma protein, sodium, chloride, and potassium concentrations aid in the selection of the proper fluid. Additional data such as calcium, BUN, creatinine, and glucose concentrations and blood gas analysis are also of benefit. With the exception of conditions in which potassium administration is contraindicated, polyionic solutions are the fluid of choice.

Potassium supplementation via the IV route should be approached with some caution and should be considered only after deficits have been confirmed by laboratory analysis. If potassium concentrations are less than 3 mEq per L or if the horse is unable to eat, potassium can be supplemented in fluids at 20 to 40 mEq per L. Administration rate should not exceed 0.5 mEq per kg per hour. If oral administration is chosen, potassium can be supplemented at 40 gm per 450 kg twice daily.

Bicarbonate supplementation is frequently used for correction of a metabolic acidosis, generally when bicarbonate concentration is less than 10 to 12 mEq per L. Deficits can be calculated using the following equation:

$$HCO_3^- \text{ (mEq/L)} = 0.4 \times \text{Body weight (kg)} \times \text{Base deficit}.$$

Sodium bicarbonate precursors are included in polyionic solutions that are given IV. If bicarbonate deficits require greater amounts, 5 per cent sodium bicarbonate may be used. It should be kept in mind that each liter of 5 per cent sodium bicarbonate supplies 600 mEq of sodium, which will have a bearing on total fluid and electrolyte requirements.

TYPES OF FLUIDS

In general, the types of fluids available can be divided into two categories, crystalloids and colloids. Because of economic considerations and the potential for adverse reactions, colloids such as dextran and hydroxyethyl starch are not extensively utilized in the horse. Both commercially prepared and fresh horse plasma have been used with some success by some clinicians but have not gained widespread acceptance. Equine plasma is indicated in situations where continued protein losses are occurring or where continued fluid therapy has resulted in dilution of plasma protein concentration below 4 gm per dl and subcutaneous edema has developed. More recently equine plasma containing high concentrations of antibodies specific to gram-negative endotoxin has also become available. As with the other colloids, expense may become an issue when these products are used.

Crystalloids are the most commonly used therapeutic fluid in the horse. The ionic composition of fluids used routinely is listed in Table 1. Polyionic solutions, represented by lactated Ringer's solution, and isotonic (0.9 per cent) sodium chloride are used most often. The composition of the polyionic fluids closely resembles that of the ECF. This type of crystalloid remains largely confined to the extracellular space and provides significant expansion of the plasma volume, which may in turn improve tissue perfusion and correct an existing metabolic acidosis. Disadvantages include hemodilution and decreases in total plasma protein concentration. Isotonic sodium chloride is frequently referred to as "normal" or "physiologic" saline, although it is not similar to the ECF. A relative excess of sodium compared to chloride is present in this solution. This fluid is best suited when deficits of electrolytes relative to water are present. In selected instances where sodium and chloride concentrations remain below normal after rehydration, double- and triple-strength saline solutions can be used. As with the polyionic fluids, significant decreases in packed cell volume and total protein concentrations may occur when saline is administered.

Other solutions include both 5 per cent dextrose and 5 per cent sodium bicarbonate. Dex-

TABLE 1. IONIC COMPOSITION OF CRYSTALLOID SOLUTIONS

	Na (mEq/L)	Cl (mEq/L)	K (mEq/L)	Bicarbonate/ Precursor (mEq/L)	Ca (mEq/L)	Mg (mEq/L)	Dextrose (gm/dl)
Polyionic solutions							
Lactated Ringer's	130	109	4	28 (L)	3		
Normosol R°	140	98	5	50 (A, G)			
Plasma-Lyte A†	140	98	5	50 (A, G)	3		
Isolyte E‡	140	103	10	57 (A, C)	5	3	
Physiologic saline	154	154					
5% Dextrose							50
5% Sodium Bicarbonate	600			600			
7% Sodium Chloride	1200	1200					

Abbreviations: L, lactate; A, acetate; G, gluconate; C, citrate.
°Abbott Laboratories, North Chicago, IL.
†Baxter Laboratories, Deerfield, IL.
‡McGraw Laboratories, Santa Ana, CA.

trose-containing solutions are best used in conditions in which the animal's metabolic needs are not being met through voluntary intake. Although by no means all of the metabolic requirements can be met, administration of glucose may provide significant benefit to horses in shock. This condition is characterized by increased glucose utilization. Dextrose therapy is also frequently used for nutritional support of the neonatal foal, which has limited energy reserves. Dextrose should be given at a rate that does not result in prolonged hyperglycemia. Overdosing of glucose may result in diuresis, increased dehydration, and decreased plasma sodium concentrations.

Sodium bicarbonate solutions should be used only in circumstances characterized by a severe metabolic acidosis. Because of the instability of bicarbonate, polyionic solutions contain bicarbonate precursors such as lactate or pyruvate. Treatment with polyionic solutions will affect bicarbonate concentrations and will also frequently improve peripheral perfusion and produce a marked reduction in acid-base abnormalities. The existence of an acidosis should be established prior to the administration of amounts greater than 2 liters of 5 per cent sodium bicarbonate. Overdosing with sodium bicarbonate can lead to a persistent metabolic alkalosis and respiratory depression.

Recent studies have indicated that small volumes, 4 to 6 ml per kg of hypertonic, 3 to 7 per cent sodium salts, alone or in combination with dextran, have significant resuscitative benefits in both animal models of shock and in human clinical trials. Specifically, 4 ml per kg of 7 per cent NaCl has been shown to restore systemic blood pressure, cardiac output, and stroke volume to preshock levels. These improvements are transient but can be prolonged through the combination of 7 per cent NaCl in 6% Dextran 70. One advantage to this form of therapy lies in the small volume and relative ease of administration. The average 450-kg horse requires only 1800 ml of a 7 per cent solution of sodium chloride, well within the range that can be given in field situations. Other advantages are the rapid response, which may be superior to that of isotonic fluids, and the ease of preparation of this fluid. These solutions should be used only for immediate resuscitative effects; continued monitoring and replacement of existing deficits with isotonic fluids is necessary. These solutions have been used experimentally in the horse and function as in other species. However, the paucity of clinical data limits recommendation for routine use at this time.

ROUTE AND RATE OF ADMINISTRATION

Fluid administration in the horse is limited to oral and IV routes. Oral fluid administration is advisable only when intestinal absorptive processes are intact. This approach is most successfully used in animals in which dehydration is associated with exercise, such as horses competing in endurance events; in mild to moderate cases of exertional rhabdomyolysis; or in cases of anorexia or colic, in which large volumes are not required. In these situations relatively large quantities of electrolyte-containing solutions can be rapidly administered. Repeated dosing at 30- to 60-minute intervals with 5 to 10 liters is recommended. Commercially packaged combinations of electrolytes and glucose designed for oral use are readily available.

Unfortunately, in many instances where fluids are critically needed, such as in colic or diarrhea, fluid therapy via the gastrointestinal system is not an option. The IV route is therefore the route most commonly used and provides the most immediate benefit to the horse. Systems for the administration of large volumes of fluid are available and are relatively easy to use. Requirements include an IV catheter and fluid administration line. Several types of catheters are available; the choice depends on factors such as duration of fluid administration and the potential for development of complications. Most commonly used are the 14- and 16-gauge Teflon, silicone elastomer, and polyurethane catheters. The latter two are of greater benefit in animals in which thrombosis formation is a major concern and where fluids may be administered for long periods of time. The jugular vein is readily accessible and is routinely used for most fluid administration. However, thrombosis of the jugular veins and obstruction of venous return can lead to severe swelling of the head. For this reason the lateral thoracic vein is often selected in horses at high risk for the development of thrombosis. The cephalic and saphenous vein are also potential routes for IV fluid administration. Strict adherence to aseptic technique cannot be overemphasized and is essential if catheter patency is to be maintained. Catheters should be checked frequently and flushed with an appropriate anticoagulant solution such as heparinized saline. The catheter should be removed if any evidence of thrombosis, infection, or reaction at the catheter site is observed.

The volume of fluids necessary to effectively resuscitate horses in severe states of hypovolemic or endotoxic shock is often on the order of 20 to 40 liters and can be as great as 80 to 100 liters during the first 2 to 3 days of hospitalization. Fluid amounts of 60 to 90 ml per kg are frequently administered during the first hour to small animals and humans in shock. Such volumes are difficult to achieve in the horse. Using two IV catheters and fluid pumps, 10 to 20 liters of fluid may be given over a one hour period, followed by maintenance administration at a slower rate.

Supplemental Readings

Carlson, G. P.: Fluid therapy. In Robinson, N. E. (ed.): Current Therapy in Equine Medicine. Philadelphia, W. B. Saunders Co., 1983, pp. 311–318.
Carlson, G. P.: Fluid therapy in horses with acute diarrhea. Vet. Clin. North Am., 1(2):313–330, 1979.
Rose, R. J.: A physiological approach to fluid and electrolyte therapy in the horse. Equine Vet. J., 13:7, 1981.
Rose, R. J.: Electrolytes: Clinical applications. Vet. Clin. North Am., 6(2):281–294, 1990.
Spier, S. J., Snyder, J. R., and Murray, M. J.: Fluid and electrolyte therapy for gastrointestinal disorders. In Smith, B. P. (ed.): Large Animal Internal Medicine. St. Louis, C. V. Mosby Co., 1990, pp. 708–714.

Chemical Restraint of the Standing Horse

Richard M. Bednarski, COLUMBUS, OHIO

The practitioner of equine medicine frequently performs a variety of procedures that require a calm, tractable horse. A partial list of procedures facilitated by chemical restraint includes ocular, oral, and rectal examinations and diagnostic procedures such as respiratory tract endoscopy, transtracheal wash, radiography, and ultrasonography. Standing surgical procedures such as laceration repair, wound debridement, cast removal, castration, tenectomy, and tenotomy and procedures involving joints are also possible in the properly sedated horse. Drugs or drug combinations that produce analgesia and sedation are useful in these situations. Many standing surgical procedures require concurrent epidural or regional infiltration of local anesthetics in addition to chemical restraint. Despite continued research and development, there is no drug available that produces perfect sedation and analgesia without also producing some undesirable side effects, such as cardiopulmonary depression or ataxia. For this reason, various sedatives, tranquilizers, and opioids have been tried in combination. Drugs and drug combinations commonly used for chemical restraint of the standing horse are listed in Table 1.

α_2-AGONISTS

Xylazine and more recently detomidine are most frequently used for chemical restraint of

TABLE 1. DRUGS USEFUL FOR CHEMICAL RESTRAINT OF THE STANDING HORSE

Drug	Intravenous Dosage* (mg/kg)
Phenothiazines	
Acepromazine	0.04–0.06
Promazine	0.5–1.0
	1.0–2.0 (oral granules)
Alpha$_2$ agonists	
Xylazine	0.5–1.0
Detomidine	0.01–0.04
Combinations	
Acepromazine / xylazine	0.02 / 0.6
Acepromazine / butorphanol	0.04 / 0.02
Acepromazine / meperidine	0.04 / 0.6
Xylazine / butorphanol	0.8 / 0.02
Xylazine / morphine	0.6 / 0.6
Opioid antagonist	
Naloxone	1–2 µg/kg

*Intramuscular dosages are 1.5 to 2 times intravenous dosages.

the horse. Both have sedative, analgesic, and muscle relaxant properties. Xylazine and detomidine differ primarily in potency and duration of action. They produce sedation by stimulating central nervous system (CNS) α_2-adrenergic receptors. The onset of action after intravenous administration is almost immediate (1 to 3 minutes), whereas the onset is within 3 to 5 minutes after intramuscular administration. Peak sedative effects occur approximately 15 minutes following administration. The sedative effects and duration of action are dose dependent. Generally xylazine's duration of action is 30 to 60 minutes, whereas that of detomidine is 60 to 150 minutes. The analgesic effects generally last one-half to two-thirds the duration of sedation. Sedation is characterized by lack of or reduced responses to painful stimuli or sound. However, horses can be aroused from sedation, particularly by sudden movement or loud noises. The horse's head is extended and lowered, and there is dose-related ataxia. The penis characteristically drops from the sheath. Sweating, either generalized or local around the site of intramuscular administration, frequently occurs. Although direct controlled comparisons are lacking, detomidine appears to provide relatively greater analgesia and sedation than xylazine. For example, restraint for procedures involving the rear limbs is frequently possible with detomidine alone, whereas xylazine is often supplemented with other sedatives, tranquilizers, or opioids to achieve a comparable effect.

α_2-Agonists characteristically produce a dose-dependent decrease in cardiac output. Cardiac output typically decreases by 50 per cent after recommended doses of α_2-adrenoceptor agonists as a result of bradycardia and vasoconstriction. The vasoconstriction results from peripheral α_2-receptor activation. Bradycardia results from centrally mediated decreased sympathetic nervous system activity and a centrally induced increase in parasympathetic tone. The bradycardia is reversed by glycopyrrolate or atropine. First- or second-degree heart block is commonly induced; however, preexisting heart block is usually not aggravated after xylazine administration. The cardiovascular effects are well tolerated in healthy horses; however, the increased vascular resistance and decreased cardiac output can be significant problems in horses with limited cardiac reserves, such as those with circulatory shock or primary myocardial disease. Doses should be reduced in these animals. Both detomidine and xylazine produce a dose-dependent depression of arterial oxygenation, characterized by a decreased partial pressure of arterial oxygen (Pa_{O_2}). This is a result of ventilation-perfusion mismatching and not hypoventilation, since Pa_{CO_2} typically remains unchanged or is only slightly increased. Ventilation is characterized by a reduced frequency and increased tidal volume. Breathing frequently becomes noisy due to relaxation of the laryngeal and pharyngeal musculature and to passive congestion of the upper airway resulting from the prolonged head-down posture. The α_2-agonists can contribute to profound respiratory depression if they are used prior to induction of general anesthesia. The α_2-agonists decrease propulsive activity of the distal but not proximal bowel, increase segmental intestinal motility, and decrease intestinal blood flow. These effects are of no consequence in the normal animal. The effects in animals with a compromised intestine are unknown. Other notable α_2-agonist effects include insulin suppression and an associated hyperglycemia. Frequency of urination and urine volume are increased. These effects are associated with a lowered urine specific gravity. Increased urine production apparently is not related to glucosuria. A suppression of ADH release or another unidentified factor may be responsible. The α_2-agonists should be used cautiously in dehydrated patients in which diuresis is undesirable. Xylazine causes increased uterine motility due to an oxytocin-like effect. Until these effects are better defined, the α_2-agonists should be used cautiously in horses in advanced pregnancy.

PHENOTHIAZINE TRANQUILIZERS

Acepromazine and promazine are the phenothiazine tranquilizers commonly used in the horse. The phenothiazine tranquilizers are useful alone to facilitate transport of reluctant horses or to calm a horse prior to introduction into a new environment. These drugs are not good analgesics or muscle relaxants so they are usually combined with opioids or sedatives for chemical restraint of the standing horse. Another reason for their infrequent use as the sole agent for standing restraint is the 15- to 30-minute lapse to onset to action, even following intravenous administration. Their duration of action is variable but typically lasts 1 to 3 hours. Despite a calm appearance, horses can, without warning, overcome the apparent tranquilization.

The phenothiazine tranquilizers inhibit sensory transmission through the reticular activating system and basal ganglia of the CNS. They decrease dopamine and 5-hydroxytryptamine concentrations within the CNS. Phenothiazine tranquilizers characteristically produce mental calming. The horse appears slightly relaxed and unconcerned with its surroundings. There is some muscle relaxation and ataxia, and the head is slightly lowered. A flaccid, prolapsed penis is present in the male. Priapism occasionally occurs following phenothiazine use and may necessitate medical and occasionally surgical intervention. Because of this phenothiazine tranquilizers should be used cautiously in male animals. Most reported instances of priapism have followed relatively high phenothiazine doses.

The phenothiazine tranquilizers induce vasodilation due to peripheral α-adrenergic receptor blockade and central suppression of sympathetic nervous system activity. This results in a decrease in systemic blood pressure and an unchanged or increased cardiac output in the normal healthy horse. Phenothiazines should be used cautiously in hypovolemic or extremely excited horses because of the potential for development of clinically significant hypotension. Hypotension is manifested by weakness, ataxia, tachycardia, tachypnea, sweating, and sometimes excitement. Treatment is with an intravenous crystalloid solution such as lactated Ringer's solution administered to effect. The respiratory effects of the phenothiazines are not dramatic. Usually the respiratory rate is decreased and the tidal volume is increased.

OPIOIDS

The opioid agonists and agonist-antagonists have been used in the horse for analgesia and in combination with sedatives and tranquilizers for pain relief and for standing restraint. Opioids are relatively potent analgesics. Analgesia is produced by stimulation of opioid receptors located within the CNS and peripheral nervous system. Compared to the α_2-agonists, opioids are not as effective against peripheral and visceral pain. This has been demonstrated in pain models involving cecal balloon inflation, tooth pulp electrical stimulation, and peripheral limb heat. Opioid receptor activation is associated with various degrees of sedation in many species; however, opioid receptor stimulation in the horse is associated with CNS excitement, particularly in higher doses. For this reason opioids are rarely used alone for chemical restraint of the standing horse. This dose-dependent excitement is manifested by pacing, pawing, and sweating, which often continue for 1 to 2 hours after administration. Horses with abdominal pain that receive opioids often appear sedated as a result of the pain relief.

The cardiopulmonary effects of opioids are variable and depend on the opioid dose and the animal's condition. Higher dosages associated with excitement induce increases in heart rate and respiratory rate. Heart rate and respiratory rate usually decrease in horses in pain after opioid administration, probably because of the accompanying analgesia. The combination of an opioid with a sedative or tranquilizer usually does not induce significant cardiopulmonary depression in young healthy horses.

Opioids induce segmental contraction and a decrease of propulsive motility of the gastrointestinal tract. This results in initial defecation followed by a variable period, often hours, of fecal dehydration and retention.

CLINICAL USE OF CHEMICAL RESTRAINT

The drug or drugs selected for chemical restraint depend on the procedure to be performed; the animal's temperament, age, and physical status; and the available facilities and assistance. For example, a young horse that is difficult to handle may require the same dosage and combination of drugs for a nonpainful oral examination that an older, calm animal would require for an extensive and painful wound debridement. Lack of assistance for concurrent physical restraint will require the use of a relatively more potent drug, dose, or drug combination.

The phenothiazine tranquilizers, because of their relatively slow onset, long duration of action, and low cost, are usually selected to provide long-term calming for such procedures as transporting horses. An oral promazine preparation is available for this purpose. Phenothiazine tranquilizers are useful when combined with xylazine or with certain opioids for profound CNS depression and analgesia. The combination of acepromazine and xylazine produces profound sedation and is suitable for calming extremely aggressive or nervous horses. Phenothiazine-opioid combinations are suitable for procedures such as joint medication because ataxia following phenothiazine use is relatively mild. Acepromazine-meperidine was one of the first tranquilizer-opioid combinations described. It is still widely used because of its efficacy and safety. Butorphanol, because of its excellent cardiopulmonary stability and because its purchase and use are not subject to federal narcotics regulations, is often combined with acepromazine or the α_2-agonists. Procedures such as castration, wound debridement, and tenectomies and tenotomies are facilitated by the xylazine-butorphanol combination.

The α_2-agonists are useful for mild short-term as well as potent long-term restraint. Detomidine is well suited for use in lengthy procedures requiring maximum analgesia and restraint. Xylazine in recommended dosages provides relatively less analgesia and sedation than detomidine. This can be an advantage, however, in all but very long or painful procedures since return to the presedation level of consciousness is more rapid following xylazine administration. Xylazine has been combined with opioids to increase its utility for very painful procedures. The combination of xylazine and butorphanol or xylazine and morphine produces excellent short to medium duration sedation and analgesia. These combinations are associated with excellent cardiopulmonary stability.

Occasionally horses will recover from tranquilizer-opioid combinations with some degree of excitement or agitation. This is attributed to lingering opioid effects. This behavior can be suppressed by administering additional tranquilizer or by administering the opioid antagonist naloxone.

Supplemental Readings

Muir, W. W.: Drugs used to produce standing chemical restraint in horses. Vet. Clin. North Am. (Large Anim. Pract.), 3:17–44, 1981.

Muir, W. W.: Tranquilizers, sedatives and muscle relaxants. *In* Mansmann, R. A., and McAllister, E. S. (eds.): Equine Medicine and Surgery, 3rd ed. Santa Barbara, Calif., American Veterinary Publishing, 1982, pp. 250–257.

Jochle, W., and Hamm, D.: Sedation and analgesia with Domosedan (detomidine hydrochloride) in horses: Dose response studies on efficacy and its duration. Acta. Vet. Scand., 82:69, 1986.

Clarke, K. W., and Taylor, P. M.: Detomidine: A new sedative for horses. Equine Vet. J., 18:366, 1986.

Regional Anesthesia
Patrick H. LeBlanc, EAST LANSING, MICHIGAN

For over a century local anesthetics have been used to reduce the pain associated with surgery. The first local anesthetic used for this purpose was cocaine; however, its addictive property limited its therapeutic utility. In 1905, procaine, another ester-type local anesthetic, was originally synthesized. Procaine is nonaddictive and remains the prototype for many local anesthetic compounds used today. Lidocaine, the first amide-type local anesthetic, was introduced four decades later. The principal advantages of lidocaine—its rapid onset, greater efficacy, longer duration of action, and lack of addictive potential—made this compound the standard to which all local anesthetics are compared. Most local anesthetics synthesized since lidocaine have been of the amide class.

Local anesthesia is attractive because it is inexpensive and relatively safe. Organ toxic effects from local anesthetic agents are rare. Complications associated with local anesthetics are related to overdosage. Systemic signs of local anesthetic overdosage (12 mg per kg) include changes in central nervous system (CNS) activity such as excitement or depression, muscle tremors, and hypotension at extremely high doses. Since a large quantity of drug (approximately 300 ml) is required to produce these effects in the average-sized adult horse, these complications are very rare. Local anesthetic–induced changes in CNS activity are more common in smaller horses or foals, in which a relative overdosage can occur more easily. Overdosage with local anesthetic agents administered in the caudal epidural space may cause motor paralysis, hind limb weakness, ataxia, and recumbency. The horse that becomes recumbent following a caudal epidural injection of a local anesthetic should be kept sedated to avoid self-injury until the animal is capable of standing.

An intrinsic vasodilator activity of local anesthetic compounds increases their absorption by the vascular system and therefore limits their duration of action. Prolongation of anesthetic effect is possible by reducing this vasodilation. The duration of local anesthesia can be doubled by including a vasoconstrictive substance (1:200,000 epinephrine) in the solution. This concentration of epinephrine may be achieved by adding 0.1 ml of 1:1,000 epinephrine to 20 ml of the local anesthetic. Because mepivacaine has little intrinsic vasodilator effect, its action is not augmented or prolonged by the addition of epinephrine.

TOPICAL AND LOCAL ANESTHESIA

The topical application of some local anesthetics such as tetracaine and lidocaine to a mucosal surface can produce effective analgesia. Lidocaine gel has been applied topically to facilitate equine urethral catheterization. Application of lidocaine to the equine larynx has been described as a useful adjuvant to intubation of foals. Topical anesthesia has an important indication in ophthalmology. The topical agents work well, but they cause transient stinging and conjunctival hyperemia. The most commonly used agents are 0.5 per cent proparacaine and 0.5 per cent tetracaine hydrochloride. These agents possess similar potency and cause the least amount of corneal injury. A combination of 0.5 per cent proparacaine and 0.25 per cent fluorescein dye is available and useful when topical anesthesia and fluorescein staining are indicated. The topical agents can be applied directly from the bottle or through a tuberculin syringe. Three or four applications of these agents are necessary at 1-minute intervals to completely desensitize the cornea.

Local anesthetics applied to normal skin cause little or no anesthetic effect. A combination product currently under investigation (EMLA, Astra Pharmaceuticals) has been used effectively on intact infant, porcine, and canine skin. This combination of lidocaine and prilocaine in a eutectic mixture may have potential future applications for minor surgical procedures in the horse.

The subcutaneous injection of a local anesthetic solution is a technique used chiefly for desensitizing the spermatic cord during standing castration, removal of small skin tumors, and suturing wounds. Infected wounds may have reduced tissue pH, thus compromising the onset and effectiveness of analgesia. The principal advantage of this technique is its relative ease of use. Large volumes of the local anesthetic may be required, so overdosage and toxicity are potential disadvantages of the infiltration technique, especially in small horses and foals. As a rule of thumb, 1 ml of solution is required per 1 cm of incision.

REGIONAL ANESTHESIA

FACE

The auriculopalpebral and supraorbital nerves provide motor and sensory innervation, respectively, to the equine upper eyelid (Fig. 1). A combination of the auriculopalpebral block and the supraorbital nerve block is sufficient for most minor surgical procedures involving the equine upper eyelid. The auriculopalpebral nerve is blocked by injection with a 22-gauge, 2.5-cm hypodermic needle inserted at the posterior edge of the zygomatic arch. This nerve is located at the slight depression on the temporal portion of the zygomatic arch. Five ml of 2 per cent lidocaine is injected into this area in a fan-shaped pattern. The supraorbital nerve emerges through the supraorbital foramen, which is located on the supraorbital process approximately 6 cm dorsal to the medial canthus of the eye (see Fig. 1). With a 22-gauge, 2.5-cm hypodermic needle, 3 ml of 2 per cent lidocaine is injected into the foramen and 2 ml is injected at the opening of this foramen and the overlying subcutaneous tissues. A sterile ophthalmic gel should be applied to the desensitized cornea, because the protective blink response is lost following these techniques.

The infraorbital nerve emerges from the infraorbital foramen just under the nasolabialis muscle (see Fig. 1). Blocking this nerve can facilitate minor surgical procedures involving the upper lip, nostrils, and upper teeth to the level of the first molar. Injection of 3 to 5 ml of 2 per cent lidocaine into the bony lip of the foramen is made through a 20- to 22-gauge, 5-cm needle. To desensitize the face, lower eyelid, and upper teeth to the level of the first molar, the 5-cm needle is inserted its entire length into the infraorbital foramen and 5 ml of 2 per cent lidocaine is deposited.

The mental nerve emerges from the mental foramen on the lateral aspect of the ramus of the mandible in the middle of the interdental space (see Fig. 1). Blocking this nerve produces analgesia of the lower lip and incisors. A 22-gauge, 2.5-cm needle is advanced into the mental foramen and 5 ml of 2 per cent lidocaine is injected. To block the lower teeth to the level of the first

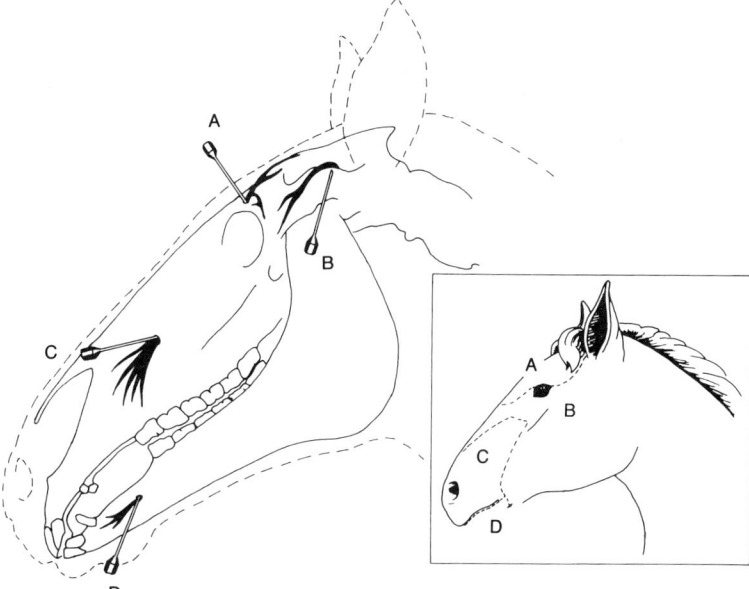

Figure 1. Proper needle placement for blocking the following nerves: *A*, supraorbital; *B*, auriculopalpebral; *C*, infraorbital; and *D*, mental. Inset shows sensory fields supplied by *A*, the supraorbital, *C*, the infraorbital, and *D*, the mental nerve.

molar, a 5-cm needle is inserted its entire length into the mental foramen and 5 ml of 2 per cent lidocaine is injected.

FLANK

Occasionally flank analgesia is required in standing horses to facilitate certain surgical procedures such as ovariectomy, exploratory laparotomy, and intestinal biopsy. This type of analgesia is performed with either an infiltrative technique or the paravertebral nerve block. Infiltrative anesthesia is accomplished by injecting the local anesthetic through an 18- to 22-gauge, 3.5-cm needle at multiple sites along the proposed incision line to desensitize the superficial layer. If lidocaine is used, the peritoneum is anesthetized with approximately 60 ml of lidocaine injected through a 7.5- to 10-cm 18-gauge needle. Alternatively, the paravertebral nerve block can be used to desensitize a larger area of the flank using less local anesthetic. Two 15-ml injections of 2 per cent lidocaine are made approximately 10 cm from midline at the three sites. The superficial branches of the nerves are blocked beginning with T18, which is located between the caudal border of the last rib and the distal end of the first lumbar transverse process. The deep branches of this nerve are blocked by injection with an 18-gauge, 5- to 7.5-cm needle after the superficial block is successful. The needle is advanced ventrally until the peritoneum is perforated. Positive signs of correct needle placement are loss of resistance to further needle advancement and, occasionally, a hissing sound as negative pressure is relieved. The needle is then withdrawn slightly to a position within the musculature where the deep branches of the vertebral nerves are located. At this point, the second 15-ml dose of local anesthetic is deposited. The superficial and deep branches of L1 and L2 are blocked in a similar manner between the first and second lumbar transverse processes and the second and third lumbar transverse processes, respectively. Flank analgesia may persist for up to 2 hours when this technique is used.

PERINEUM

Caudal epidural analgesia is useful for procedures that require analgesia of the tail, perineal skin, anus, rectum, vulva, and vagina. Proper use of this technique will also reduce the abdominal straining that may be associated with dystocia. The injection site for this technique is in the midline between the first and second coccygeal vertebrae. This space is located by palpation of the first movable joint caudad to the sacrum during dorsoventral manipulation of the tail. The space also corresponds to 5 to 7 cm craniad to the beginning of the long tail hairs (Fig. 2). Following aseptic preparation of the skin over the injection site, a sterile 18- to 21-gauge, 3.5-cm hypodermic needle is inserted perpendicular to the skin. The hub of the needle is then filled with the local anesthetic solution and the needle slowly advanced toward the epidural space. Once this space is penetrated, the solution will be aspirated from the hub, owing to negative pressure within the epidural space. Occasionally a hissing sound is heard. Lack of resistance to 10 ml of air and no evidence of blood on aspiration are two additional indicators of proper needle location.

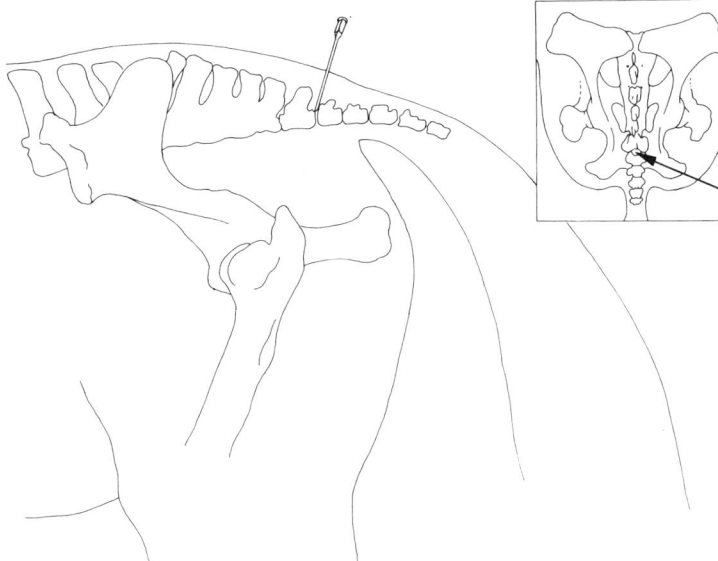

Figure 2. Proper needle placement for injecting the caudal epidural space of a horse. The needle is located in the first coccygeal interspace.

The amount of local anesthetic injected is dependent upon the specific agent used, the size of the horse, and the area to be desensitized. In a 450-kg horse, approximately 7 ml of 2 per cent lidocaine should be sufficient to achieve analgesia of the rectum, vagina, and urethra in a standing animal for approximately 60 minutes. For a similar area of analgesia with a slightly longer duration of action, 5 ml of 2 per cent mepivacaine is adequate. Injection of 10 ml of 2 per cent lidocaine will desensitize a larger perineal area for a slightly longer duration, but the potential for hind limb weakness is greater.

Xylazine (0.17 mg per kg, diluted to a 10-ml volume with saline) injected into this space produces analgesia similar to that achieved with lidocaine but without the same degree of motor weakness. This technique has a wide margin of safety, since only mild and transient ataxia of little clinical significance was reported when xylazine at double this dose (0.35 mg per kg) was administered to ponies. In clinical situations this technique appears to produce a much longer duration of action (up to 4 hours) than could be expected for lidocaine. The onset of analgesia is longer for xylazine than for lidocaine (30 vs. 10 minutes). A common side effect of epidurally administered xylazine is a dermatome of sweat that corresponds to the area of analgesia.

Supplemental Readings

Lumb, W. V., and Jones, E. W.: Local anesthetic agents. *In* Lumb, W. V., Jones, E. W. (eds.): Veterinary Anesthesia, 2nd ed. Philadelphia, Lea & Febiger, 1984, pp. 357–370.

Skarda, R. T.: Local and regional analgesia. *In* Short, C. E. (ed.): Principles and Practice of Veterinary Anesthesia, 1st ed. Baltimore, Williams & Wilkins Co., 1987, pp. 91–133.

General Anesthesia

Nora S. Matthews, COLLEGE STATION, TEXAS

PREOPERATIVE ASSESSMENT AND PLAN

This chapter provides an overview of techniques used for general anesthesia. However, before considering what drugs to use, one should always ask the question: Is general anesthesia necessary and indicated? If an elective procedure is to be performed, is the horse healthy enough to withstand it? If an emergency procedure is necessary, could it be performed with chemical restraint or analgesia while the horse is standing? The practitioner cannot answer these questions unless the patient's physical condition and history have been evaluated. This evaluation may consist only of a physical examination or may include laboratory tests, electrocardiography, and so forth, but, simple or extensive, some form of assessment should be performed. It is also wise and helpful to know as much as possible about the horse's temperament, medical history, recent medications, and herd health history, since all of these factors may affect the choice or dose of anesthetic drugs.

For routine elective anesthesia, it is recommended to fast the horse for 12 hours (water is allowed), accurately estimate body weight (by weight tape or weighing) to allow drug calculation, and place an intravenous (IV) catheter. If an endotracheal tube will be placed, the horse's mouth should be washed out so that feed is not transferred into the trachea.

An anesthetic plan should be formulated based on the type and duration of the surgical procedure, physical status of the horse, equipment, facilities, and help available. It is important to be prepared for anticipated problems (for instance, to have drugs drawn up for redosing if needed). In addition, it is wise to have emergency drugs available and to be familiar with their dosages (Table 1).

INDUCTION AND MAINTENANCE WITH INJECTABLE AGENTS

There is no "perfect" anesthetic: the results will depend as much on the skill and judgment of the administrator as on the drug combination itself. Individual variations in response are normal rather than the exception, so the veterinarian must remain flexible about the drugs used, rather than becoming regimented toward drug combinations. However, there are two basic drug combinations, with variations, that will provide effective anesthesia in most situations.

The first type of combination uses xylazine* with ketamine†: xylazine is administered at 1.1 mg per kg IV to produce "adequate" sedation. The horse's head will droop to its knees if sedation is adequate. Ketamine is then administered at 2.2 mg per kg IV. Recumbency usually occurs within 1 minute and is smooth if the head is controlled to prevent the horse from rolling backward or falling on its nose. The horse will usually remain recumbent for about 20 minutes, and then will stand smoothly after briefly sitting in

---

*Rompun, Haver-Lockhart, Shawnee, KS
†Ketaset, Aveco Co. Inc., Fort Dodge, IA

TABLE 1. EMERGENCY DRUGS FOR HORSES

Problem	Treatment Drug	Concentration	Dose for 450-kg Horse
Hypotension	a) Administer or increase rate of fluid administration and lighten plane of anesthesia *If no results, try:*	1 or 5 L bags	4.5–9.0 L lactated Ringer's solution given rapidly IV
	b) Calcium chloride or Cal-Dextro #2 *If no effect, go to:*	100 mg/ml	1–2 gm given slowly to effect; 100 ml diluted into 5 L of lactated Ringer's solution, monitor heart rate and rhythm
	c) Dobutamine or	12.5 mg/ml	50 mg into 500 ml 5% dextrose in water, 1 drop/sec (10 drops/ml)
	Dopamine	40 mg/ml	40 mg into 500 ml 5% dextrose in water, 1–3 drops/sec
Bradycardia (HR < 25 bpm)	Atropine or	15 mg/ml	0.5–3 ml IV
	Glycopyrrolate	0.2 mg/ml	10–12 ml IV
Tachyarrhythmias or premature ventricular contractions	a) Stop inotropic drugs (if being administered)		
	b) Lidocaine (without epinephrine)	20 mg/ml	10–20 ml IV; may need to redose
Shock	a) Increase rate of fluid administration, decrease depth of anesthesia		Lactated Ringer's solution, up to 40 L, or hypertonic saline (7.5% NaCl; 2.5 L)
	b) Prednisolone sodium succinate	500 mg/vial	1–2 gm IV
	Flunixin meglumine (endotoxic shock)	50 mg/ml	10 ml IV
Asystole	Epinephrine	1:1000	5–10 ml IV or intracardiac (intratracheal administration is effective route in dogs, humans; volume of dilution and efficacy in horses unknown)

sternal posture. If sedation is not adequate after xylazine, or if an extra 5 to 10 minutes of recumbency is desired, butorphanol‡ (0.044 mg per kg IV) may be administered with the xylazine before ketamine, or diazepam§ (0.03 to 0.04 mg per kg IV) may be administered with the ketamine. Either drug will improve the quality of induction and recovery, especially in nervous horses, and significantly increase the recumbency time produced by one dose. Recumbency time can be extended to about 60 minutes by redosing with one fourth to one half of the original dose of xylazine and/or ketamine. The cardiovascular depression produced by xylazine is additive so that additional doses of xylazine should be given cautiously. Ketamine alone is often enough to prolong anesthesia.

A combination of xylazine-ketamine-guaifenesin° may also be used to extend anesthesia following induction with xylazine-ketamine. The mixture is made by adding 500 mg of xylazine and 1000 mg of ketamine to 1 liter of 5 per cent guaifenesin, which is dripped at a rate of 2.75 ml per kg body weight per hour, or slowly to effect. Anesthesia is easily maintained for up to 1 hour, and recoveries are good. Use of an IV catheter is recommended since guaifenesin is irritating if administered perivascularly.

Detomidine† (0.02 to 0.04 mg per kg IV) has been used prior to ketamine (2.2 mg per kg IV) to produce anesthesia. Since the onset of sedation is slower with detomidine than with xylazine, the practitioner should allow 8 to 10 minutes for sedation before administering ketamine. Recumbency time will be similar to that seen with xylazine and ketamine, so there is no particular advantage to this combination over the xylazine-ketamine combination.

The combination of tiletamine-zolazepam‡ (1.1 mg per kg of the combination IV) has also been used, following xylazine (1.1 mg per kg IV) premedication, for short-term anesthesia. Recumbency time is usually about 10 minutes longer than with the other combinations; however, there may be more stumbling during recovery because of the long-lasting muscle incoordination produced by the zolazepam. This product may be useful in darts to capture wild equids because it is a powder and may be reconstituted with xylazine into a small volume. For intramuscular administration the dose of both the xylazine and the tiletamine-zolazepam combination should be doubled.

The second type of combination uses thiamylal° (4.4 mg per kg) with guaifenesin, following premedication with xylazine (0.2 mg per kg IV) or acepromazine (0.05 mg per kg IV). Guaifenesin (10 per cent) is administered rapidly through a catheter until the horse is wobbly, then about three quarters of the calculated dose of thiamylal is administered as a bolus. Alternatively, the thiamylal may be combined with 1 liter of 5 per cent guaifenesin and administered rapidly through a 10- to 12-gauge catheter or from a pressurized bottle. Induction of a 450-kg horse requires approximately 400 to 600 ml. Anesthesia can be maintained by slowly dripping the remaining mixture to effect. The major advantage of this combination is that the drugs are given "to effect," which allows for more variation to account for differences in the individual or its condition. The disadvantage is that during induction the horse will be wobbly for the longer period of time required for large volume administration.

Anesthesia should not be maintained for more than 45 to 60 minutes with injectable techniques because of hypoventilation and hypoxemia associated with recumbency and anesthesia in horses. If possible, oxygen should be supplemented by nasal insufflation of 10 to 15 L per minute. Precautions should also be taken to avoid myopathy or neuropathy associated with recumbency in horses. These precautions include removing the halter while the horse is recumbent, pulling both lower limbs forward, padding the hip and shoulder with foam or inner tubes, supporting the upper limbs, avoiding tying or taping limbs in extreme flexion or extension, and minimizing the animal's contact with hard surfaces whenever possible.

INHALANT ANESTHESIA

For procedures taking longer than 45 to 60 minutes, inhalant anesthesia with halothane or isoflurane is recommended. Inhalational anesthesia requires familiarity with more equipment (a vaporizer, inhalant anesthesia machine, oxygen source, endotracheal tube) and their appropriate use, as well as a working knowledge of the inhalant agents and their uptake and distribution. The reader should consult the references for necessary information (which is beyond the scope of this chapter). Many problems with inhalant anesthesia may be avoided if the practitio-

---

‡Torbugesic, Fort Dodge Labs., Fort Dodge, IA
§Valium, Roche, Nutley, NJ
°Guaifenesin U.S.P., Chemical Products Manufacturing Corp., St. Joseph, MO
†Dormosedan, Norden Labs., Lincoln, NE
‡Telazol, A. H. Robins, Richmond, VA

°Biotal, Bioceutic, St. Joseph, MO

ner uses good quality equipment that is regularly serviced and calibrated by a qualified service representative.

MONITORING

Effective monitoring is critical to providing safe anesthesia (which means safe for the horse as well as for the surgeon). It is often very difficult, if not impossible, to maintain the patient in a plane of anesthesia that provides adequate analgesia and immobilization for surgery while facilitating the rapid recovery that is desirable in the horse. Heart rate and rhythm are not quick to change with depth of anesthesia, as in other species, so any change must be considered an indicator of a major disturbance preceding a crisis such as a cardiac arrest. Muscle relaxation is very dependent on what drugs have been used and is generally poor with ketamine, even when the degree of unconsciousness and immobilization are adequate. It is desirable to see normal mucous membrane color and capillary refill time, but these indices may not change rapidly enough to be good warning signals of significant problems.

Eye signs, respiratory rate and pattern, and blood pressure are the most useful indicators of anesthetic depth in the horse. The anesthetist should maintain a corneal reflex with inhalant anesthesia, and palpebral and corneal reflexes with injectable anesthetics. Nystagmus may be maintained throughout the procedure if ketamine has been used. Spontaneous tearing usually indicates a very light, nonsurgical plane of anesthesia.

Respiratory rate and rhythm will be influenced by the drugs administered. Both respiratory rate and tidal volume will be depressed immediately after induction, and both rate and depth will increase as anesthesia lightens. Respiratory rate may be irregular when ketamine is used: several breaths will be followed by periods of breath-holding. Spontaneous "sighing" is an indication that the plane of anesthesia is very light, but should not be confused with agonal breaths, which imply death or impending death.

Blood pressure, measured directly or indirectly, is the best early warning system, since it increases as anesthesia lightens and decreases as the anesthesia becomes deeper. Although one should palpate the pulse, pulse pressure may not accurately reflect the presence or absence of hypotension. Since hypotension is associated with postoperative myositis as well as more severe consequences, it is important to monitor and support blood pressure. Even for short procedures, this can be accomplished inexpensively either indirectly, using a Doppler Ultrasonic Flow Detector, or directly, using an anaeroid manometer. The anaeroid manometer available from medical supply houses is connected to an 18- or 20-gauge Teflon catheter percutaneously placed into a peripheral artery using an extension set, three-way stopcock, and another extension set. The extension set closest to the catheter is filled with heparinized saline that, when the stopcock is opened, will partially fill the extension set connected to the manometer. Compliance of the tubing will allow only the mean arterial pressure to be measured. With the manometer zeroed at the level of the horse's heart, this pressure should be maintained above 60 to 70 mm Hg. Treatment of hypotension includes lightening the plane of anesthesia, administering fluid, and use of inotropic drugs (see Table 1).

Supplemental Readings

Grandy, J. L., and Hodgson, D. S.: Anesthetic considerations for emergency equine abdominal surgery. Vet. Clin. North Am. (Equine Pract.), 4:67–78, 1988.
Greene, S. A., Thurmon, J. C., Tranquilli, W. J., and Benson, G. J.: Cardiopulmonary effects of continuous intravenous infusion of guaifenesin, ketamine and xylazine in ponies. Am. J. Vet. Res., 47:2364, 1986.
Hall, L. W.: General anesthesia: Fundamental considerations. Vet. Clin. North Am. (Large Anim. Pract.), 3:3–15, 1981.
Riebold, T. W., and Wolz, G. C.: Large animal anesthesia: Monitoring equine patients. Anim. Health Technician, 3:101, 1982.

Emergency Treatment of the Traumatized Horse

John Pringle, CHARLOTTETOWN, PRINCE EDWARD ISLAND, CANADA

Traumatic injuries to horses are everyday occurrences in equine practice and successful management of the traumatized horse is often the main criterion by which clients judge the skills of their veterinarian. Horses sustain injuries in many ways, including impalement on sharp objects such as fencing material, wire cuts, kicks, trailer accidents, stable fires, collisions with solid objects, or falls. The diagnosis of trauma is usually readily apparent. The veterinarian attending a traumatized horse must perform initial life-saving measures, as well as make a rapid assessment of the prognosis for future function as expected by the client. Skin lacerations and puncture wounds may be alarming to the owner, but they seldom threaten the life or function of the horse. However, other types of trauma, such as head injuries, may produce minimal external damage, yet may have caused severe or irreparable damage.

ABCD OF TRAUMA

Management of all cases of trauma should begin with an initial ABCD examination (*A*irways, *B*reathing, *C*irculation, *D*isability), which will ensure that underlying life-threatening problems are not overlooked. For example, a horse burned in a stable fire may be more in need of respiratory support or fluid therapy than attention to the obvious skin burns.

AIRWAYS

Airway patency is of paramount importance. Mandibular and pharyngeal trauma, or burns to the upper airways incurred during stable fires, may result in inspiratory distress. Nasotracheal intubation with an endotracheal tube (18- or 20-mm diameter) or a nasogastric tube will create an air passage and provide temporary relief of upper airway obstruction. However, if inspiratory distress is severe, the clinician should not hesitate to perform a tracheostomy. This will allow time for more thorough assessment of the nature of and appropriate treatment of the upper airway problem.

BREATHING

In the presence of respiratory distress despite adequate upper airway function, the clinician should evaluate the lower respiratory tract for pneumothorax or hemothorax, particularly if there is evidence of chest trauma with concurrent rib fracture, or subcutaneous thoracic emphysema. Clinical examination may determine an absence of lung sounds on the affected side, or a hollow or abnormally dull sound on chest percussion, but the differences may be subtle and impossible to distinguish in a clinical setting. In such cases, thoracocentesis will confirm the presence of blood or air in the pleural space. If either is present, the pleural cavity should be evacuated, using a one-way flutter valve in the case of pneumothorax, or a teat cannula and syringe in the case of hemothorax. This allows lung expansion and, with hemothorax, may prevent the subsequent development of fibrous adhesions in the pleural space. Intranasal oxygen administration is only minimally useful, as pulmonary problems in the acutely traumatized patient are usually mechanical in nature. If respiratory distress continues despite the above corrective measures, ventilatory support may be required. Although difficult to perform in the conscious adult horse, a crude form of positive end-expiratory pressure (PEEP) can be achieved by supplying oxygen through a tracheostomy tube, via a demand valve, and restricting expiratory air flow to prevent alveolar collapse.

CIRCULATION

Once breathing is considered to be stable, circulatory support is the next priority. Blood loss from skin lacerations is difficult to measure accurately, and while it can appear profuse, it is seldom clinically significant. Life-threatening internal hemorrhage due to blunt trauma, although common in small animals, is rare in the horse. The onset of systemic signs of shock through blood loss may not become evident until up to 30 per cent of the blood volume (10 to 12 liters in a 500-kg horse) is lost. Some injuries, such as burns incurred in stable fires, can induce massive fluid losses into the burned tissue, and result in hypovolemic shock. Clinical signs of hemorrhagic or hypovolemic shock include increased heart rate, decreased pulse strength, pale mucous membranes with prolonged capillary refill time, cool extremities, patchy sweating, slowly filling jugular veins, muscular weakness, and depression.

External bleeding should be controlled with application of direct pressure over a sterile dressing. Time taken to ligate vessels is unnecessary; one should preferentially concentrate on replacement of lost fluids, as the primary problem will be hypovolemia. Both hemorrhagic and hypovolemic shock can be treated similarly with isotonic electrolyte solutions administered IV at the rate of one blood volume, 35 to 40 liters in a 500-kg horse, per hour initially (see also p. 18). In the case of massive blood loss, whole blood administered at 15 to 25 ml per kg is the treatment of choice. Up to 8 liters of whole blood can safely be removed from a healthy mature horse. Cross-matching is both unnecessary for the first transfusion and often impractical in a practice situation. A potential alternative to blood transfusion in hemorrhagic shock is hypertonic saline (7.5 per cent NaCl, 2400 mOsm per L) at 4 ml per kg IV, given over 5 to 10 minutes, followed by administration of appropriate volumes of crystalloids. Experimentally, hypertonic saline rapidly expands the plasma volume by distributing throughout the extracellular fluid space and draws water from the intracellular fluid space by osmotic forces. Some of its advantages are the small volume needed to restore plasma volume, minimal net water administration, stimulation of cardiac contractility, and peripheral vasodilation. However, its use is contraindicated in the setting of impaired renal function. Clinical improvement from hypovolemia will be accompanied by a decrease in heart rate, improved jugular filling, increased pulse pressure, improved capillary refill time, and warming of extremities.

Disability

Once the respiratory and cardiovascular functions have been stabilized, the horse should be examined for other injuries, such as neurologic damage or fractures, which may limit full recovery.

CENTRAL NERVOUS SYSTEM TRAUMA

Injuries to the head or spinal cord in horses may be mild or may carry grave consequences despite early and intensive therapy. Trauma to the head can result from a variety of circumstances, most commonly from falling over backward, running into solid objects, or a kick from another horse. Damage to neural tissue is often a combination of direct disruption of the neural tissue and subsequent hemorrhage and tissue swelling, leading to poor perfusion and hypoxia. The consequences are particularly severe when the swelling is confined within the rigid cranium.

Cranial trauma is manifested by three main clinical syndromes: cerebral, midbrain, and medullary-inner ear syndromes. The cerebral syndrome is characterized by temporary loss of consciousness and lateralization of subsequent signs, such as circling to the affected side and blindness with intact pupillary light reflexes. In the midbrain syndrome there is coma followed by severe depression, with pupils asymmetric and poorly reactive to light. The medullary-inner ear syndrome, which is often a consequence of trauma to the back of the head due to falling over backward, results in facial and vestibular nerve deficits, with depression and weakness if there is a central component.

Trauma to the spinal cord is usually precipitated by a fall or a collision with a solid object. The C1 to T2 region is most commonly affected, but damage can occur at any site in the spinal cord. Signs are usually nonprogressive and, depending on the site of the lesion, may include hind end paresis and ataxia, tetraplegia/tetraparesis, and/or urinary and fecal incontinence.

Diagnosis

There is usually ample evidence, either from direct observation or circumstantially, that trauma has occurred. Skull or cervical radiographs may be warranted, but cerebrospinal fluid (CSF) collection is contraindicated in situations with increased CSF pressure, and laboratory test results seldom influence the choice of treatment.

Therapy

Pathophysiologic events, and therefore treatment goals, of brain and spinal cord injury are similar and are aimed at reducing central nervous system (CNS) swelling and maintaining blood flow to the damaged area. The thrashing or delirious horse should be sedated with low IV doses of pentobarbital° at 5 mg/kg or acepromazine† at 0.05 mg/kg, although the latter may lower the seizure threshold. α_2-Agonists such as xylazine‡ or detomidine§ should be used with caution as they can cause transient hypertension if given IV, which could exacerbate nervous system hemorrhage and consequently cause further respiratory depression. Seizures can be treated with diazepam∥ IV (0.1 mg per kg for foals; 0.05

°Somnopentyl Injection, Pitman Moore Inc., Washington Crossing, NJ
†Atravet, Fort Dodge Laboratories, Fort Dodge, IA
‡Rompun, Mobay Animal Health, Haver Division, Mission, KS
§Dormosedan, Norden Laboratories, Lincoln, NE
∥Valium, Hoffman-LaRoche Inc., Nutley, NJ

to 0.2 mg per kg for adult horses) and repeated as required. Horses with significant neurologic signs should be treated for CNS edema with glucocorticoids, such as dexamethasone° at 0.1 to 0.2 mg per kg IV, repeated every 4 to 6 hours for 1 to 4 days, to decrease CNS edema and intracranial pressure. There is, however, a risk of inducing laminitis in adult horses, and the benefits of glucocorticoids for CNS trauma, even at massive doses, have been questioned. If the horse is recumbent and comatose, additional treatment, as follows, may be necessary. Hyperosmolar fluids, such as 20% mannitol,† given IV at 0.25 to 1.0 g per kg over 20 minutes, will decrease CNS tissue swelling for 1 to 2 hours. This can be repeated every 6 to 12 hours if there is clinical improvement. Naloxone,‡ an opioid antagonist, may also reduce subsequent CNS damage by antagonizing endogenous opioid-associated compromise of microcirculatory blood flow. Additionally, dimethylsulfoxide§ (DMSO), although its use is controversial and of unproven efficacy, may reduce CNS swelling and inflammation. It should be given slowly IV as a 10 per cent solution in 0.9 per cent saline or 5 per cent dextrose, at 1 gm per kg, and repeated up to 6 times in 72 hours. Cases of cranial trauma in which clinical signs deteriorate or compressed skull fractures are present may require surgical decompressive craniotomy. Time alone, however, will be necessary to predict the extent of the horse's recovery. For further information on CNS trauma, see the suggested readings and other sections in this text.

FRACTURES

The emergency treatment of fractures in horses is restricted to initial assessment and support prior to transport to a veterinary hospital, the objective being to immobilize the affected limb, thereby preventing further trauma to associated nerves, vessels, soft tissues, and bone at the fracture site. The fracture site should be examined for vascular integrity, distal nerve function, and the presence of comminution. Fractures of the scapula, humerus, and femur, or those severely comminuted fractures are usually not amenable to repair; however, where clinical findings are equivocal, the horse should not be destroyed until radiographic findings are available.

THERAPY

The ability to adequately immobilize the fractured limb at an early stage is a major factor in successful management of these cases. Pain can be relieved with xylazine (0.5 to 1 mg per kg IV or intramuscularly) or butorphanol° (0.02 to 0.1 mg per kg IV), and facilitates patient examination as well as application of support materials prior to transport. Compound fractures should be cleansed with sterile saline and covered with a topical dressing before the support is applied. Antibiotics should be given for all but closed fractures with only minor soft tissue trauma. Because the distractive forces acting on the equine limb are extreme, immobilization should be done with the most rigid device possible. A resin cast is the most desirable as it will allow close approximation of the limb contours and sets quickly to a strong, reasonably light support. Alternatives are a modified Robert Jones bandage splinting with PCV piping, or heavy metal mass of metasplint type of supports. The support *must* incorporate the joint above and below the fracture site, or the device will simply exacerbate the damage through exaggerated lever arm forces at the fracture site. Before the horse is transported, support bandages should be applied to the other limbs. The use of low trailers with the horse facing the rear may reduce the stresses of loading and unloading as well as additional stresses of ensuring secure footing during transport.

OTHER INJURIES

Other traumatic injuries, such as cuts, punctures, and abrasions, tend to be self-limiting and can be treated topically. The exception is corneal trauma, in which the cornea should be stained with fluorescein† to assess the integrity of the epithelium. If corneal ulceration is present, treatment should begin immediately with topical atropine‡ given every 12 hours or until the pupil is dilated, and antibiotics, such as gentamicin§ drops, should be given every 6 hours. Severe corneal lacerations may require surgical repair. Once the immediate problems are controlled,

---

°Dexamethasone Sterile Solution, Beecham Laboratories, Bristol, TN
†Mannitol, Abbott Labs., North Chicago, IL
‡Narcan, Dupont Pharmaceuticals, Wilmington, DE
§DOMOSO Solution, Syntex Animal Health, West Des Moines, IA

°Torbugesic, Fort Dodge Laboratories, Fort Dodge, IA
†Fluor-I-Strip, Ayerst Laboratories, New York, NY
‡Isopto Atropine Ophthalmic Drops, Alcon Laboratories, Fort Worth, TX
§Gentocin Ophthalmic Solution, Schering Animal Health, Union, NJ

convalescent care and a more complete medical evaluation can be initiated.

EUTHANASIA

If trauma has resulted in an indisputably hopeless prognosis, such as a compound fracture of a long bone or evisceration and gross contamination of the abdominal contents, the horse should be euthanized as soon as possible. Shooting the horse in the head, which is the method of choice in the United Kingdom, is both humane and instantly effective. A close-range shot to the head with a small-gauge shotgun (.410, 28-gauge or 20-gauge) is preferred; larger gauge shotguns or high-powered rifles are more likely to cause visible tissue destruction, and the latter is subject to potentially dangerous ricochet. Ideally, the projectile should reach the brain stem and destroy the control centers of respiration and circulation. This is best accomplished with the gun aimed perpendicular to the frontal bone at the intersection of lines drawn between each eye and its contralateral ear. For aesthetic reasons, many clients prefer euthanasia of their horse by injection of a lethal substance, such as pentobarbital given IV at 110 mg per kg. If a minimum of agonal movement is desired, or if transport of the injured horse out of sight of curious onlookers is deemed appropriate, the horse can first be anesthetized with xylazine (1.1 mg per kg IV) followed in 5 minutes with ketamine (2.2 mg per kg IV), or guaifenesin as a 5 to 15 per cent solution until the horse is relaxed, followed by 2 gm* of thiamylal. Once the horse is anesthetized or away from the crush of curious onlookers, pentobarbital (110 mg per kg IV) can be administered. While some advocate the use of succinyl choline or magnesium sulfate IV for destruction of a horse, these products should not be used as the sole agent for euthanasia, as they merely rely on paralysis of the animal's respiratory muscles and death through suffocation. However, should there be *any* question of the potential for survival of the horse, a decision on euthanasia should be delayed until initial life-saving measures are instituted and a thorough evaluation of the nature of the injuries and the animal's prognosis can be completed.

Supplemental Readings

Becht, J. L., and Gordon, B. J.: Blood and plasma therapy. *In* Robinson, N. E. (ed.): Current Therapy in Equine Medicine, 2nd ed. Philadelphia, W. B. Saunders Co., 1987, pp. 317–322.
Bitterman, H., Triolo, J., and Lefer, A. M.: Use of hypertonic saline in the treatment of hemorrhagic shock. Circ. Shock, 21:271–283, 1987.
Demling, R. H.: Pathophysiology of burn injury. *In* Richardson, J. D., Polk, H. C., Flint, L. M. (eds.): Trauma: Clinical Care and Pathophysiology. Chicago, Year Book Medical Publishers, 1987, pp. 132–144.
Ferguson, J. G.: Trauma and critical care of the large animal patient. *In* Zaslow, I. M. (ed.): Veterinary Trauma and Critical Care. Philadelphia, Lea & Febiger, 1984, pp. 419–446.
Lavach, J. D.: Large Animal Ophthalmology. St. Louis, C. V. Mosby Co., 1990.
Lewis, F. R., and Trunkey, D. D.: Emergency department care. *In* Trunkey, D. D., and Lewis, F. R. (eds.): Current Therapy of Trauma 1984–1985. St. Louis, C. V. Mosby Co., 1984, pp. 7–9.
Martin, L., Kaswan, R., and Chapman, W.: Four cases of traumatic optic nerve blindness in the horse. Equine Vet. J., 18:133–137, 1986.
Mayhew, I. G.: Large Animal Neurology. Philadelphia, Lea & Febiger, 1989, pp. 139–144, 129–130, 266–271.
Stewart, R. H.: Central nervous system trauma. Vet. Clin. North Am. (Equine Pract.), 3:371–377, 1987.
Wingfield, W. E., and Henik, R. A.: Treatment priorities in cases of multiple trauma. Semin. Vet. Med. Surg. (Small Anim.), 3:193–201, 1988.

---

*In a 500-kg horse.

Preventive Medicine Programs
W. David Wilson, DAVIS, CALIFORNIA
Michael S. Spensley, MENDOTA HEIGHTS, MINNESOTA

The role of the veterinarian in preventive medicine programs for horses should extend beyond the traditional function of vaccination and periodic deworming to embrace all aspects of the care and use of horses that affect their health and welfare. Effective preventive medicine requires not only knowledge of epidemiology, medicine, and preventive strategies but also a thorough understanding of sound management, husbandry, and horsemanship and an appreciation of the economics of the industry and individual enterprise being served. The marked variation in the type and sophistication of horse enterprises, and the fact that many people become horse owners without formal training or experience in horse management and husbandry, make for a very broad range of client needs. Because client expectations vary tremendously, the goals of any program should be mutually defined by the client and veterinarian from the outset. Breeding farms and training stables are run as businesses for profit, so preventive measures should be economically beneficial. This goal is not incompatible with the obligation of the veterinarian to promote the welfare of his or her patients. Although considerable financial constraints also exist with regard to backyard pleasure horses, the main goal in preventive medicine programs is often different and cost-effectiveness is more difficult to judge. Realistic goals of a preventive medicine program might include increasing the quantity or quality of horses produced (thus increasing profitability); improving the overall health status and useful life expectancy, thereby increasing client enjoyment of show or pleasure horses; minimizing treatment costs and time out of work associated with preventable diseases or injuries; and minimizing pain and suffering experienced by horses. Complete prevention of disease, however, is an unrealistic expectation.

The rapid increase in the population of horses has not been matched by an increase in the number of experienced horsemen. Successful preventive medicine programs thus incorporate client education and promote good communication between horsemen, veterinarians, and others, such as farriers, who offer services to horse owners. The veterinarian plays a central role in educating horse owners in good management and preventive medicine strategies. The veterinarian frequently needs to take the lead in offering advice, rather than simply responding to problems as they arise. Depending on the level of experience of the client and the training required, it may be possible to maintain the educational aspects of a program during regularly scheduled visits. However, it is usually not possible to provide new horse owners with sufficient information in this manner, and most owners of pleasure horses currently are unwilling to pay for individual client consultation and education. Most clients will attend evening or weekend continuing education lectures or demonstrations, especially if they are well illustrated with appropriate case examples. Newsletters, which double as timely reminders for routine procedures, also provide a useful avenue for client education. Directing clients to appropriate books and lay publications often results in effective and efficient time utilization. Regular "sit-down" consultations with large breeding farm or performance barn clients are helpful for continued fine-tuning of a program and often result in considerable overall time saving for the veterinarian. The goal of these educational endeavors should be to develop an informed clientele that understands and appreciates good veterinary care and the value of preventive medicine. Educated and understanding clients make veterinary practice more enjoyable and rewarding.

Despite wide variation in the specifics of individual preventive medicine programs, they all include the following elements: client education, infectious disease prevention, parasite control, nutrition and feeding management, dental care, prevention and early detection of lameness or musculoskeletal injury (including foot care and shoeing), breeding and reproductive management, foal care, conditioning and training, recognition and initial treatment of emergencies, prepurchase examination, facilities and pasture planning and management, appropriate diagnosis and treatment of illness or injury, and maintenance of medical records.

CLIENT EDUCATION

The prepurchase examination (see p. 68) is often the first contact between the veterinarian and a potential client and can be important in establishing the framework for a mutually rewarding future relationship. Prepurchase examinations provide a useful and cost-effective service by helping clients to avoid buying horses that are unlikely to fulfill their expectations or that have problems that will need constant attention. The scope of the examination may vary with the age, sex, fitness, value, and intended use of the horse, but in each case the expectations of the owner should be addressed realistically to reduce the potential for misunderstanding and future disputes. For novice owners, establishing whether the horse is physically and mentally suited to the client and to its intended use is important. During the prepurchase examination the knowledge and experience of the buyer should be assessed and appropriate advice should be offered regarding preventive health care and sources of continuing education.

Many pleasure horse owners express an interest in breeding their mare to produce a foal. This may be a sound economic decision based on the previous performance or genetic superiority of the mare, but frequently the rationale hinges on a sentimental desire to rear a foal. The veterinarian should take an active role in counseling horse owners regarding the desirability of breeding the mare, bearing in mind the age, reproductive history, and genetic quality of the mare, anticipated stallion and boarding fees, veterinary fees, available facilities and personnel, experience of the client, anticipated value and use of the foal, and the reality that breeding the mare during a given season carries a less than 50 per cent chance that in 3 years' time the breeding will result in a horse that is suitable to break and train for riding. Clients who choose to breed their mare should be directed to sources of information on the care and feeding of the pregnant mare, foaling management, recognition of normal and abnormal parturition, normal foal behavior, and care of the lactating mare and foal. The veterinarian should be actively involved in this educational process and in monitoring the mare and foal. The mare should be examined after foaling to detect and treat complications that may adversely affect her health or future reproductive potential. A thorough physical examination of the foal should be aimed at detecting congenital or acquired abnormalities or infection and to ensure that adequate passive transfer of colostral antibodies is achieved (see p. 422).

Veterinarians are frequently asked for advice on the design and construction of facilities for horses. Appropriate advice can have a significant impact on horse health and safety as well as improving the efficiency of the enterprise and working conditions for the veterinarian. While the specific needs of individual enterprises vary tremendously, there are many important considerations common to many circumstances. Barns and paddocks should be situated to take advantage of terrain to optimize drainage, shelter, and natural ventilation as well as providing vantage points from which a large portion of the farm can be easily viewed. Paddocks and access roads should be laid out in such a way that horses can be easily and safely moved between paddocks and to the barns. Paddocks should be constructed with safe and durable fencing materials and should have round or angled corners to reduce the risk of horses sustaining injuries while running alongside fences. Depending on the layout of access roads, it may be helpful to include catch pens in one corner of the paddock to facilitate restraint of groups of horses for routine procedures. Double fencing of paddocks reduces transmission of contagious diseases. When horses are fed as a group in paddocks, sufficient space should be provided for each horse to reduce fighting and ensure that dominant individuals do not unduly affect the feed intake of more submissive horses. Feeders should be elevated above ground level to reduce ingestion of sand and infective parasite eggs. It is helpful to have feed racks that can be moved to reduce poaching of the land, mud accumulation in wet weather, and dusty conditions in dry weather. Alternatively, permanent feeders can be placed on a solid base, such as concrete or packed crushed rock, and under a roof to reduce problems with mud and dust. Other dust control measures such as pasture irrigation, frequent pasture rotation, and avoidance of overcrowding are extremely important for the prevention of pneumonia and other respiratory tract infections of foals in arid climates.

Barns should be constructed with due consideration for ventilation, temperature regulation, dust control, drainage, lighting, the space requirements of different types of horses, ease of cleaning and access, facilities for restraint and performance of procedures, ease of observation, prevention of disease transmission, and safety for horses and personnel. Floors should be constructed of nonslip material and stall divisions should prevent direct contact between horses in adjacent stalls. Feed and bedding should be stored in an air space separate from that occupied by horses to reduce dust accumulation. Similarly, riding arenas, a frequent source of dust and fungal spores, should be physically separate from stabling facilities. On breeding farms in particular, it is advisable to have a separate receiving barn for outside horses as well as an isolation barn for sick horses. The ability to provide timed artificial lighting for groups of mares as well as individual horses is also important on breeding farms.

INFECTIOUS DISEASE PREVENTION

Infectious disease prevention should be directed toward reducing challenge as well as enhancing resistance through vaccination and other measures. Programs that rely solely on vaccination often fail or are less than optimally effective because tenuous resistance can be overridden by massive challenge. Educating clients in the early recognition of signs of disease and the costs associated with treatment, sequelae, and time lost from training will help them understand the need for a comprehensive approach to infectious disease control. Clients should be taught how to take the temperature, pulse, and respiratory rates of their horses and to recognize normal attitude and behavior. The prevalence of infectious disease in horse populations tends to increase with the number and concentration of horses on a farm, movement of horses on and off the farm, and with external environmental and management influences. The conditions on breeding farms, in performance horse and show horse barns, and at racetracks are ideal for the transmission of infectious diseases, particularly respiratory tract infections.

On breeding farms, the movement of horses from different sources on and off the farm for breeding and sales, the mix of horses of different ages, and the high proportion of young susceptible animals and pregnant mares pose special problems. The risk of acquiring infection can be reduced by maintaining distinct groups by age and function. Resident mares and foals should be kept separate from weanlings, yearlings, horses in training, and visiting mares. Visiting mares should Coggins-test negative for equine infectious anemia and should be appropriately vaccinated and dewormed prior to arrival. They should be received and maintained in barns and paddocks separate from the farm population. New arrivals should be received in an isolation barn physically separated from the remainder of the farm. Separate equipment and preferably separate personnel should be used in this facility. During the 30-day quarantine period, horses should be monitored for signs of contagious disease, including daily recording of rectal temperature, and any prophylactic procedures not performed prior to arrival should be completed during this period. Foaling mares being sent for breeding to a distant breeding farm should be shipped 6 to 8 weeks before foaling. This will allow exposure to resident pathogens at the farm of destination in time for the mare to mount an immune response and concentrate antibodies in the colostrum to improve passive protection of the foal. Mares being shipped short distances for breeding can be transported during estrus, without the foal, and returned to the farm on the same day to reduce the risk of the foal acquiring infection.

Regardless of the type of equine enterprise being considered, any horse that becomes ill with a potentially contagious disease should be promptly isolated, preferably in an air space separate from the remainder of the herd, for at least 10 days following complete abatement of clinical signs of disease. Separate utensils should be used and, if separate personnel are not available to treat and care for sick horses, these horses should be tended to after other horses on the farm. Stalls that have housed sick horses should be thoroughly cleaned, disinfected, allowed to dry, and left empty for as long as possible before being used by other horses. This approach is particularly important when dealing with organisms such as *Streptococcus equi*, which can survive in a protected moist environment for several months.

Vaccination forms an imporant part of the overall control program for infectious diseases in most horse enterprises. The decision to use a particular vaccine in a herd depends on the risk of acquiring infection and on the medical and economic consequences of infection versus the efficacy, cost, and potential side effects of the vaccination program. The risk of acquiring infection will depend on geographic location, season, type of enterprise, and, particularly, on management measures taken to reduce challenge by infectious agents. In performance horses, the goal is generally to minimize time spent out of training to maximize earning potential. Under these circumstances an enforced period of rest due to infectious disease would have much more significant economic consequences than a similar recommendation for a barren brood mare or a backyard horse. On the other hand, many owners of backyard horses will diligently vaccinate against even low-risk diseases, despite the expense involved, in order to keep their horses healthy.

The efficacy of vaccines directed against different diseases is highly variable, and there may be some variation in the efficacy of vaccines from different manufacturers. Vaccination is unlikely to confer more durable protection than that resulting from recovery from natural disease, especially when the vaccination route (usually intramuscular [IM]) is different from the route of natural infection. The efficacy and durability of protection induced by parenteral vaccines directed against respiratory tract pathogens are frequently questioned. This may reflect the fact that immunity following natural infection with these pathogens is short-lived and that local immune responses at the level of the respiratory mucous membrane may be very important for effective protection. In general, parenterally administered inactivated vaccines do not induce good mucosal immune responses. The immune response of individuals in a population is variable; thus, not all individuals in the population are protected to an equal extent or for an equal duration. Animals with a low level of immunity may resist a modest challenge but succumb to a heavier or more virulent challenge.

Passive transfer of antibodies via colostrum should be exploited in immunization programs for foals by the administration of booster doses of vaccine to mares during the last 6 weeks of gestation. Foals are more competent immunologically at birth than the young of many other species, but their response to antigens is generally poorer than that of adult horses. In addition, the presence of maternal antibody may attenuate or completely block a primary response, especially when modified live vaccines are used, since vaccines of this type generally rely on distribution and replication of vaccinal virus to increase antigenic mass in order to induce an adequate immune response.

Disease control programs should be tailored to the individual farm with consideration of the age, type, number, use, stocking density, and value of the horses, and the facilities, management, geographic location, and potential exposure to individual diseases. The expectations of the owners should be addressed realistically, bearing in mind the efficacy of available vaccines and the level of management owners are willing to devote to reducing disease challenge. Completion of a primary vaccination series and administration of booster doses should be timed to precede likely exposure. All animals in the herd should be vaccinated on the same schedule, whenever possible, to simplify record keeping, gain economic benefit from bulk purchases, and maximize the benefit from an individual visit by the veterinarian. More important, this approach maximizes the level of herd immunity so that transmission blocks are established that minimize replication of infectious agents, thereby protecting the animals in the herd that respond poorly to vaccination. Strict attention should be paid to the recommendations of the manufacturer for vaccine storage, handling, and administration to maximize its efficacy. Above all, good, readily accessible records should be kept, detailing which vaccines were administered and on what date. Hand-written individual horse records are appropriate for smaller enterprises, whereas calendar-based computerized records can improve efficiency in large herds. Owners should be encouraged to send copies of the vaccination and health maintenance records with horses leaving the farm for sales, training, or breeding and should request copies of the records of all horses entering the farm.

The availability of approved biologicals limits the diseases that can be included in a vaccination program. Vaccines are currently available in North America to aid in the prevention of tetanus; Eastern, Western, and Venezuelan encephalomyelitis; influenza A-equi-1 and A-equi-2 infection; equine herpesvirus 1 and equine herpesvirus 4 infection; strangles; rabies; Potomac horse fever; botulism; equine viral arteritis; and anthrax. Information concerning available biologicals and the recommendations of the manufacturers for their use are presented in Tables 1 and 2. For some diseases, particularly respiratory tract infections, the recommendations of the manufacturer may not be completely effective in disease prevention, necessitating modification of the recommended protocols. General guidelines for the use of the most frequently indicated equine vaccines under various management and geographic conditions are presented in Table 3.

All horses, regardless of their state or country of residence, should be vaccinated against tetanus since the causal organism is ubiquitous, the disease is expensive to treat and has a high mortality rate, and available vaccines (toxoids) are safe and effective. Active immunization with tetanus toxoid reduces the need to use tetanus antitoxin. Administration of tetanus antitoxin is associated with an increased risk of inducing fatal serum hepatitis. Tetanus antitoxin should be reserved for use in foals from mares that did not receive booster immunizations late in pregnancy and for horses with an unknown vaccination history that sustain a wound or undergo surgery. Every attempt should be made to ascertain the vaccination history of an injured horse before administration of tetanus antitoxin is elected. Active immunization with tetanus toxoid can be combined with passive immunization with tetanus antitoxin in injured unvaccinated horses by administration of the two biologicals at separate sites. A second dose of tetanus toxoid administered 4 weeks later will complete the primary immunization series.

In the United States, severe outbreaks of Western equine encephalomyelitis (WEE) have been recorded in the western and midwestern states, with sporadic cases in the Northeast and Southeast, whereas the distribution of Eastern equine encephalomyelitis (EEE) is restricted to the eastern and southeastern states. Consequently, most horses in the United States are at risk during the insect vector season and should be vaccinated with a bivalent encephalomyelitis vaccine. Annual revaccination of horses with bivalent WEE and EEE products in the spring, prior to the peak insect vector season, is recommended for all horses in endemic areas. Although no longer specifically recommended by vaccine manufacturers, many veterinarians in southern states in which insect vectors, particularly mosquitos, are active year-round prefer to vaccinate horses biannually. Annual encephalomyelitis immunization can conveniently be combined with tetanus and, where appropriate, influenza and rhinopneumonitis revaccination using polyvalent combination vaccines (see Table 2).

Routine vaccination of horses against Venezuelan equine encephalomyelitis (VEE) is not recommended since the disease has not occurred in this country for almost 20 years and is not cur-

Text continued on page 47

TABLE 1. MANUFACTURERS' RECOMMENDATIONS FOR USE OF EQUINE IMMUNIZING AGENTS/BIOLOGICALS

Disease	Etiologic Agent	Type of Product	Sample Product	Manufacturer	Dose	Route	Age for Primary Series	Regimen for Primary Series	Regimen for Revaccination	Comments
Anthrax	*Bacillus anthracis*	Nonencapsulated, live bacterial spores	Anthrax vaccine	Colorado Serum Co.	1 ml	SC		2 doses, 2–3 wk apart	Annual	Vaccinate 4 wk prior to potential exposure. Placing a horse in a dark stall for 10 days of rest may be beneficial. Local reactions may occur. Do not administer antibiotics within 1 wk of vaccination.
		Nonencapsulated, live bacterial spores	Thraxol-2	Cutter	2 ml	SC				
Botulism	*Clostridium botulinum* type B toxin	Toxoid	Bot Tox-B	Neogen Biologics	2 ml	IM		3 doses at least 4 wk apart	Annual	In pregnant mares, administer booster 2–4 wk before parturition. Protects only against botulism caused by *Clostridium botulinum* type B.
Equine encephalomyelitis	Bivalent vaccines: WEE°, EEE†	Inactivated chicken tissue culture origin	Encevac	Haver	1 ml	IM		2 doses, 3–4 wks apart	Annual	Time primary series and boosters to precede mosquito season.
		Inactivated chicken tissue culture origin	Encephaloid IM	Fort Dodge	1 ml	IM		2 doses, 3 wk apart	Annual	Time primary series and boosters to precede mosquito season.
	Trivalent vaccines: WEE, EEE, VEE	Inactivated chicken tissue culture origin (WEE, EEE); porcine tissue culture origin (VEE)	Cephalovac (VEW)	Coopers/Pitman-Moore	2 ml	IM		2 doses, 3–4 wk apart	Annual	Time primary series and boosters to precede mosquito season.
		Inactivated tissue culture origin	Triple-E	Solvay/Connaught	1 ml	IM		2 doses, 2–4 wks apart	Annual or if exposure threatened	Time primary series and boosters to precede mosquito season.

Disease	Antigen	Type	Trade name	Manufacturer	Dose	Route	Min. age	Primary	Booster	Comments
Equine viral arteritis	Equine arteritis virus	Modified live equine cell line origin	Arvac	Fort Dodge	1 ml	IM	>6 wk	1 dose	Annual	Vaccinate stallions at least 3 wk prior to breeding season. Vaccinate mares as maidens or while open at least 3 wk prior to breeding. Pregnant mares should not be vaccinated. Prior authorization by state veterinarian required. Permit may be necessary. Regulations vary with state. Vaccinated horses may be ineligible for export due to seroconversion.
Equine influenza	Equine influenza: A-equi-1 and A-equi-2	Inactivated canine cell line origin	Equicine II with Havolgen	Haver	1 ml	IM		2 doses, 3–4 wk apart	Annual	Contains Prague-56 (A_1) and Miami-63 (A_2) strains.
		Inactivated allantoic fluid of embryonated chicken eggs	Fluvac	Fort Dodge	1 ml	IM		2 doses, 2–4 wk apart	Annual	Contains Prague-56 (A_1), Lexington-63 (A_2) and Kentucky-81 (A_2) strains.
			Inflogen	Solvay/Connaught	1 ml	IM		2 doses, 2–4 wk apart	Annual	Contains Detroit-64 (A_1) and Milford-64 (A_2) strains.
		Inactivated viral cell line origin	Equi-Flu	Coopers/Pitman-Moore	1 ml	IM		2 doses, 3–4 wk apart	Annual	Contains Newmarket-79 (A_1) and Brentwood-79 (A_2) strains.
		Inactivated	Flumune	SmithKline Beecham	1 ml	IM		2 doses, 3 wk apart	Annual	Contains Prague 56 (A_1) and Miami-63 (A_2) strains.

Vaccination immediately prior to an athletic event or show is to be avoided since transient, usually self-limiting, febrile responses may occur following influenza vaccination. Protection following vaccination is serviceable but may be short-lived in the face of heavy challenge with virulent virus. More frequent booster immunization at intevals of 2–6 months may be required to prevent influenza under these circumstances.

Rabies	Rabies virus	Inactivated cell line origin	Imrab	Pitman-Moore	2 ml	IM	>3 mo	1 dose	Annual	
		Inactivated porcine cell line origin	Rabguard-TC	SmithKline Beecham	1 ml	IM	>3 mo	1 dose	Annual	
		Inactivated cell line origin	Rabvac 3	Solvay	2 ml	IM	>3 mo	1 dose	Annual	

TABLE 1. MANUFACTURERS RECOMMENDATIONS FOR USE OF EQUINE IMMUNIZING AGENTS/BIOLOGICALS *Continued*

Disease	Etiologic Agent	Type of Product	Sample Product	Manufacturer	Dose	Route	Age for Primary Series	Regimen for Primary Series	Regimen for Revaccination	Comments
Rhinopneumonitis	Equine herpesvirus I	Inactivated	Pneumabort K	Fort Dodge	2 ml	IM	Postweaning	2 doses, 3–4 wk apart	Young horses: 6 months after primary series, annually thereafter. Pregnant mares: repeat doses during 5th, 7th and 9th months of gestation	Vaccinate open and maiden mares at the same time as pregnant mares. For mares beyond the 5th month of gestation when vaccination is initiated, vaccinate on presentation and every 2 months thereafter until foaling.
		Modified live equine cell line origin	Rhinomune	SmithKline Beecham	1 ml	IM	3 months	2 doses, 4–8 wk apart	Biannual or prior to expected exposure annually	Vaccinate pregnant mares after the second month of gestation. Approved for use in pregnant mares, but no label claim for prevention of EHV-1 abortion.
	Equine herpesvirus-1 and equine herpesvirus-4	Inactivated bivalent tissue culture origin	Prestige with Havlogen	Haver	2 ml	IM		2 doses, 4–6 wks apart	Annually or any time exposure is imminent. Foals should receive a booster dose 6 months after primary series.	Approved for pregnant mares but no label claim for prevention of EHV-1 abortion.
Strangles	*Streptococcus equi*	Inactivated whole bacteria	Equibac II	Fort Dodge	2 ml	IM	3 months	3 doses at 2–4 wk intervals	Annual	Administration more frequently than 1 dose per year may increase the risk of anaphylaxis. Contraindicated in infected animals and in those incubating the disease.
		Inactivated bacterial M-protein extract	Strepguard Stranglevac	Haver Cutter	1 ml	IM	3 months	2 doses, 3–4 wk apart	Annual or when epidemic conditions exist or exposure is imminent	If foals less than 3 months old are vaccinated, an extra dose at 6 months of age or at weaning is recommended.
		Inactivated, bacterial M-protein extract	Strepvac II	Coopers/Pitman-Moore	1 ml	IM	3 months	3 doses at 3-wk intervals	Annual or prior to anticipated exposure	Foals vaccinated when less than 3 months old should receive an additional dose at 6 months or at weaning.

Potomac horse fever	Ehrlichia risticii	Inactivated	PHF-VAX	Schering	1 ml	IM	2 doses, 3–4 wks apart	Biannual	Efficacy may be improved by administration of 2 doses annually prior to period of peak challenge.
		Inactivated	Potomavac	Pitman-Moore/Rhone Merieux	1 ml	IM	2 doses, 3–4 wks apart	Annual	
Tetanus	Clostridium tetani	Toxoid (inactivated)	Tetanus toxoid	Fort Dodge, Franklin	1 ml	IM	2 doses, 4–8 wk apart	Annual	
			Super-Tet	Haver, Cutter	1 ml	IM	2 doses, 3–4 wk apart	Annual	
			Tetanus toxoid	Schering	1 ml	IM	2 doses, 3–4 wk apart	Annual	
			Tetanus toxoid	Colorado Serum Co.	1 ml	IM or SC	2 doses, 4 wk apart	Annual	
			Unitox	Coopers/Pitman-Moore	1 ml	IM or SC	2 doses, 4 wk apart	Annual	
		Antitoxin	Tetanus antitoxin	Ceva	1500 units	IM or SC			Administer on exposure of unimmunized animals or those with an unknown vaccination status. Fatal serum hepatitis has been observed following administration of tetanus antitoxin to horses.
				Fort Dodge	1500 units	IM or SC			
				Haver	1500 units	IM or SC			
				Colorado Serum Co.	1500 units	IM or SC			
				Coopers/Pitman-Moore	1500–4500 units	IM or SC			

° = Western equine encephalomyelitis.
† = Eastern equine encephalomyelitis.

TABLE 2. MANUFACTURERS RECOMMENDATIONS FOR USE OF COMBINATION VACCINES

Antigens Included	Sample Product	Manufacturer	Dose	Route	Age at Primary Series	Regimen for Primary Series	Regimen for Booster doses	Comments
Influenza A_1 and A_2 (inactivated) + Equine herpesvirus-4 (inactivated)	Fluvac (EHV-4)	Fort Dodge	1 ml	IM	>3 mo	2 doses, 4–6 wk apart	Annually or at any time epidemic conditions exist or exposure is likely.	Foals vaccinated before 3 months of age should be given a 3rd dose 4–6 wk after the 2nd dose to complete the primary series.
Influenza A_1 and A_2 (inactivated) + Equine herpesvirus-1 (modified live)	Rhino-Flu	SmithKline Beecham	1 ml	IM	>3 mo	2 doses, 3 wk apart	Annually or whenever epidemic conditions exist or exposure is likely.	As above.
Influenza A_1 and A_2 (inactivated) + Equine herpesvirus-1 (inactivated) + Equine herpesvirus-4 (inactivated)	Prestige II with Havlogen	Haver	1 ml	IM		2 doses 4–6 wks apart	Annually or any time exposure is imminent.	No label claim for prevention of EHV-1 abortion. Foals should receive booster 6 mos after primary series.
Encephalomyelitis (inactivated EEE, WEE) and tetanus toxoid	Equiloid	Fort Dodge	1 ml	IM		2 doses, 4–8 wk apart	Annual	
	Encevac-T	Haver	1 ml	IM		2 doses, 3–4 wk apart	Annual	
	Double-ET	Solvay/Connaught	1 ml	IM		2 doses, 2–4 wk apart	Annual	
	Cephalovac EWT	Coopers/Pitman-Moore	2 ml	IM		2 doses, 4–6 wk apart	Annual	
Encephalomyelitis (inactivated EEE, WEE, VEE) and tetanus toxoid	Triple-ET	Solvay/Connaught	1 ml	IM		2 doses, 2–4 wk apart	Annual or in face of potential exposure	
	Cephalovac VEWT	Coopers/Pitman-Moore	2 ml	IM		2 doses, 4–6 wk apart	Annual	

PREVENTIVE MEDICINE PROGRAMS—*continued*

Encephalomyelitis (inactivated EEE, WEE), influenza A₁ and A₂ (inactivated) and tetanus toxoid	Encevac TC-4	Haver	1 ml	IM		2 doses, 3–4 wk apart	Annual
	Fluvac EWT	Fort Dodge	1 ml	IM		2 doses, 4–8 wk apart	Annual
	Equi-Flu EWT	Coopers/Pitman-Moore	2 ml	IM		2 doses, 4–6 wk apart	Annual
	Double-EFT	Solvay/Connaught	1 ml	IM		2 doses, 2–4 wk apart	Annual
	Flumune EWT	SmithKline Beecham	2 ml	IM	>3 mo	2 doses, 3 wk apart	Annual
Encephalomyelitis (inactivated EEE, WEE, VEE), influenza A₁ and A₂ (inactivated) and tetanus toxoid	Triple-EFT	Solvay/Connaught	1 ml	IM		2 doses, 2–4 wk apart	Annual
Influenza A₁ and A₂ (inactivated) and tetanus toxoid	Fluvac T	Fort Dodge	1 ml	IM		2 doses, 4–8 wk apart	Annual
	Inflogen-T	Solvay/Connaught	1 ml	IM		2 doses, 2–4 wk apart	Annual
Influenza A₁ and A₂ (inactivated), equine herpesvirus 1 (modified live), tetanus toxoid	Rhino-Flu T	SmithKline Beecham	2 ml	IM	>3 mo	2 doses, 3 wk apart	Annual
Influenza A₁ and A₂ (inactivated), EHV-1 (modified live), EEE and WEE (inactivated), tetanus toxoid	Rhino-Flu EWT	SmithKline Beecham	2 ml	IM	>3 mo	2 doses, 3 wk apart	Annual

TABLE 3. RECOMMENDED IMMUNIZING SCHEDULE FOR USE OF THE MOST COMMONLY INDICATED VACCINES IN HORSES

Disease/Vaccine	Foals/Weanlings	Yearlings*	Performance Horses*	Pleasure Horses*	Brood Mares*	Comments
Tetanus toxoid	1st dose: 3 mo 2nd dose: 4 mo	Annual	Annual	Annual	Annual, 3–5 wk before foaling	Conveniently administered in combination with EEE, WEE, influenza ($\pm$EHV-1)
EEE, WEE	1st dose: 3 mo 2nd dose: 4 mo	Annual, spring	Annual, spring	Annual, spring	Annual, 3–6 wk before foaling	Conveniently administered in combination with tetanus and influenza ($\pm$EHV-1)
Influenza	1st dose: 1–3 mo 2nd dose: 2–4 mo 3rd dose: 3 mo (See Comments) Repeat at 3-mo intervals	Every 3 mo	Every 3 mo	Biannually with added boosters prior to likely exposure	At least biannually with one booster timed 3–6 wk prefoaling	If primary series is started before 3 months of age, a 3-dose primary series is necessary. Use combination vaccine for pre-foaling and spring boosters.
Rhinopneumonitis† (EHV-1 and EHV-4)	1st dose: 2–3 mo 2nd dose: 3–4 mo 3rd dose: 4 mo (See Comments) Repeat at 3 mo intervals	Every 3 mo	Every 3 mo	Optional; biannually if elected	5th, 7th and 9th month of gestation (inactivated EHV-1 vaccine)	If primary series is started before 3 months of age, a 3-dose primary series is necessary.
Rabies	1st dose: 3–4 mo 2nd dose: 4–5 mo	Annual	Annual	Annual	Annual, before breeding	Use in endemic areas.
Strangles	1st dose: 8–12 wk 2nd dose: 11–15 wk 3rd dose: 14–18 wk (depending on product used) 4th dose: Weaning (6–8 mo)	Biannual	Optional; biannual if risk high	Optional; biannual if risk high	Biannual with one dose timed 3–6 wk prefoaling	Vaccines containing M-protein extract are preferred over whole cell vaccines. Use when endemic conditions exist or risk is high.

*Assuming primary series was completed during foalhood. Otherwise follow label directions for primary immunization. Stallions and barren mares should follow the same program as brood mares with biannual rhinopneumonitis booster vaccination substituted for rhinopneumonitis program recommended for pregnant mares.
†Products containing EHV-4 may be indicated in foals, weanlings, yearlings, performance horses, and pleasure horses because a large proportion of EHV respiratory infections are caused by EHV-4.

rently considered to pose a significant threat to horses in the United States (see p. 765). In addition, seropositivity for VEE may preclude export to certain countries. Previous requirements for VEE vaccination of horses entering Texas, in order to maintain a buffer zone of vaccinated horses, have been discontinued.

Vaccination against influenza is recommended for all horses that have significant exposure to horses from outside facilities, such as at breeding farms, racetracks, training centers, boarding stables, shows, and similar athletic events. Influenza epizootics tend to cycle every few years on a worldwide basis through exposed susceptible populations. Morbidity rates during outbreaks may approach 100 per cent. Solid immunity following natural infection does not persist for more than 1 year, and influenza viruses, particularly influenza A-equi-2, tend to show antigenic drift between epizootics. Consequently, available vaccines, all of which are inactivated and administered by IM injection, do not appear to induce durable protection in the field setting when the recommendations of manufacturers for annual revaccination are followed. Veterinarians have increased the frequency of vaccination of high-risk populations to as often as 2-month intervals, even though there is good evidence to suggest that influenza vaccination in the face of a high titer will inhibit development of an optimal anamnestic response. A similar situation appears to occur when foals younger than 4 months of age from immunized dams are vaccinated with influenza vaccines. A suitable compromise appears to be a 6-month interval for revaccination of adult horses at moderate risk and a 3-month interval for horses at high risk. When primary vaccination of foals is initiated before 4 months of age, a three-dose rather than two-dose series should be used.

Recent developments in the manufacture of influenza vaccines have focused on antigen presenting systems or adjuvants that will enhance the immune response, and on the issue of antigenic drift. Mutations within the hemagglutinin antigens have led to significant antigenic drift of A-2 viruses away from the Miami-63 prototype. Although antibodies to prototype virus cross-neutralize recent drifted isolates, this cross-reacting antibody is less efficient and less durable in its effect than is strain-specific antibody directed against the homologous strain; thus, frequent vaccination is necessary. In addition, primary vaccination with one strain of A-2 virus may reduce the antibody response to drifted field or vaccinal viral strains that may be encountered later. These findings have led the World Health Organization to recommend inclusion of representatives of drifted A-2 virus in current vaccines. Several manufacturers have responded by including A-2 strains such as Kentucky-81, Fontainbleau-79 or Brentwood-79 in their vaccines, while others have preferred to preserve the antigenic mass of Miami-63 virus in the vaccine and enhance the immune response by modifying adjuvant systems.

Some horses suffer a transient, self-limiting systemic reaction of unknown etiology, characterized by pyrexia, inappetence, and depression after influenza vaccination. Thus it is inadvisable to vaccinate horses for influenza within 7 to 10 days of an event. However, for horses that have not received a booster within 3 months prior to anticipated exposure, it is recommended that a booster be administered 2 to 3 weeks before the high-risk circumstances are encountered.

Published data regarding the efficacy of vaccines for prevention of rhinopneumonitis (equine herpesvirus 1, EHV-1) infection show variation in results, but there are good data to indicate that the incidence of abortion storms caused by EHV-1 has declined significantly since the introduction and widespread use of EHV-1 vaccines in the United States. Vaccination of pregnant mares is highly recommended even though 100 per cent protection is not achieved. Sporadic abortions and rare abortion storms do occur in vaccinated mares. Of the three vaccines currently approved for use in pregnant mares in the United States, only the inactivated univalent vaccine carries a label claim for the prevention of abortion. Label recommendations call for administration of this vaccine during the 5th, 7th, and 9th months of gestation. Many practitioners also administer a dose during the 3rd month of gestation, although the efficacy and necessity of this approach have not been critically evaluated. Until recently, all EHV-1 vaccines were prepared from subtype 1 virus, which is responsible for almost all recorded abortions but for only a small proportion of outbreaks of respiratory disease due to EHV-1. The majority of isolates from foals and older horses with respiratory disease are heterologous EHV-1, subtype 2 virus (EHV-4). Vaccination of foals and young horses to prevent respiratory infections has relied on the induction of cross-reactive antibody using either modified-live or inactivated vaccines containing EHV-1, subtype 1 virus. The short duration of protection afforded by this strategy has necessitated frequent revaccination at 2- to 3-month intervals to achieve acceptable protection against respiratory infections. Many horse owners prefer to accept and manage this respiratory tract disease rather than subject their young horses to the stress and expense of this program. Others find that the incidence of pneumonia in foals and of upper respiratory tract infections in yearlings and young horses in training is reduced by intensive immunization programs that target EHV-1 and influenza. New vaccines containing inactivated EHV-4 virus in combination with inactivated influenza A-1 and A-2 viruses have recently been approved for use in the prevention of respiratory infections with these viruses. These vaccines seem appropriate in view of the changes in the understanding of the epidemiology and pathogenesis of EHV infections. Since EHV-1 and EHV-4 infections are endemic in many horse populations, the immunizing effect of multiple infections or vaccination tends to reduce the severity of respiratory disease, often to a subclinical level, in mature nonpregnant horses. Thus, frequent vaccination of nonpregnant mature horses with EHV-1 vaccines generally is not indicated. Available vaccines make no claim to prevent the neurological form of EHV-1 infection.

The efficacy of approved, parenterally administered vaccines for prevention of strangles has been questioned by veterinarians. Outbreaks of strangles have occurred in horses vaccinated according to the manufacturer's recommendations. In addition, strangles vaccines are associated with a higher rate of local and systemic side effects than are most biologicals used in horses. Reactions appear to be more common with whole cell bacterins than with subunit M-protein vaccines. While parenteral vaccination does not stimulate a significant nasopharyngeal secretory antibody response, which appears to be important in preventing infection, the systemic antibody response appears to attenuate the severity and duration of clinical signs of disease. In addition, morbidity rates may also be reduced. In view of these findings, routine use of current strangles vaccines is not recommended except on premises, particularly breeding farms, where strangles is a persistent endemic problem or for horses that are being transported to such high-risk facilities. On breeding farms, efforts should be concentrated on preventing infections in foals and weanlings by vaccinating brood mares with approved products during the last 3 to 6 weeks of gestation, then starting foal vaccination at 2 to 3 months of age. Because a significant number of foals do not show a serological response to primary immunization, an additional dose at 6 months of age or at weaning is recommended. Thereafter, annual or, preferably, biannual revaccination is indicated. Strangles vaccination of pleasure or performance horses kept in low-risk situations is not routinely recommended.

Other vaccines are used for horses on a more limited basis reflecting the regional incidence of certain diseases or the sporadic occurrence of disease outbreaks. The three rabies vaccines currently approved for use in horses in the United States are inactivated, cell-line origin products that appear to be safe and effective. Their use is recommended when horses are kept in proximity to habitats of wild animal populations that maintain sylvatic rabies. The animal species that serve as the reservoir for infection vary in different parts of the world but typically include skunks, raccoons, foxes, badgers, and bats. Rural, particularly wooded, areas constitute the highest risk. Rabies vaccination of pregnant mares is not recommended, pending data on safety during gestation. Foals can be vaccinated beginning at 3 months of age. Nonapproved modified live rabies vaccines should not be used in horses.

Potomac horse fever (equine monocytic ehrlichiosis), originally described as a sporadic disease affecting horses residing near the Potomac River in Maryland, has been confirmed clinically or serologically in the majority of states in the United States and in several other countries. The disease does not appear to be directly contagious from horse to horse, and it is likely, although not proven, that an insect vector is involved in disease transmission. The high rate of serious complications and mortality associated with this disease justifies vaccination of horses residing in or traveling to endemic areas, using one of the two inactivated *Ehrlichia risticii* bacterins now available in the United States. A two-dose primary series administered 3 to 4 weeks apart, followed by boosters at 6-month intervals, has been shown to be a safe and effective approach. Vaccination should be timed to precede peak potential challenge during the summer months (midwestern and eastern states) or fall, winter, and spring (California coastal foothill areas).

Of the eight antigenically distinct toxins produced by subtypes of *Clostridium botulinum*, types B and C are associated with the majority of botulism outbreaks in horses. A toxoid directed against *C. botulinum* type B is approved for use in horses in the United States. Its main indication is to prevent toxicoinfectious botulism (Shaker foal syndrome), a significant problem in foals in Kentucky and in the mid-Atlantic seaboard states. After a three-dose primary series, annual boosters should be administered. In pregnant mares, the annual booster should be given 2 to 4 weeks prior to parturition to provide passive protection for the foal during the high-risk neonatal period.

The modified-live equine viral arteritis (EVA) vaccine is approved for use in stallions and open mares for prevention of EVA, under strict supervision of the U.S. Department of Agriculture and

State veterinarians. Use of this vaccine was initiated to control the recent EVA outbreak in Kentucky, particularly transmission from carrier stallions to unaffected mares. Vaccination induces seroconversion and may interfere with testing requirements for export. Blood tests that provide evidence that the horse was seronegative prior to vaccination may be helpful in resolving disputes.

Anthrax vaccine is a suspension of live, nonencapsulated spores of *Bacillus anthracis* used for active immunization of horses in endemic areas. A two-dose primary series followed by annual revaccination appears to provide adequate protection. Anthrax vaccines, which are administered subcutaneously, are frequently associated with local and occasionally systemic reactions.

Despite the frequent and repeated use of vaccines in horses, significant systemic reactions are uncommon. Anaphylaxis occurs infrequently but constitutes a life-threatening emergency requiring prompt treatment with epinephrine (5 ml of a 1:10,000 dilution IV) or, in less acute situations, 1 to 2 ml of a 1:1,000 dilution IM or SC). Local irritant tissue reactions occur more frequently, particularly when polyvalent combination vaccines and strangles vaccines are used. These reactions are usually self-limiting, but resolution can be promoted by the parenteral or oral administration of nonsteroidal anti-inflammatory drugs (NSAIDs), topical application of warm compresses or drawing agents, and gentle exercise. Because significant reactions in the neck muscles may make the horse reluctant to lower or raise the head, feed and water buckets should be positioned accordingly. The incidence of local reactions can be reduced by administration of the vaccine deep in the semimembranosus or semitendinosus muscles of the hind leg rather than in the neck, and by giving the horse the opportunity to exercise. Additionally, horses that repeatedly react to combination vaccines may benefit from administration of an NSAID before administration of the vaccine, administration of the individual antigenic components separately in different sites, or use of a different brand of vaccine.

PARASITE CONTROL AND NUTRITION

Parasite control and nutrition are extremely important components of the overall health maintenance program for horses. Minimizing the parasite load by diligent pasture and stable management as well as by continuous or periodic use of anthelmintics, at intervals determined by regular fecal examinations, is important to maintain the health and feed efficiency of horses and to reduce the incidence of serious gastrointestinal diseases such as colic. Parasite control programs (see p. 51), and nutrition and feeding management (see p. 715) are discussed elsewhere in this and previous editions of *Current Therapy in Equine Medicine*.

DENTAL CARE

Dental care is an important but frequently neglected part of health maintenance programs for horses. Dental prophylaxis should begin with the postfoaling examination of the newborn foal, at which time malocclusions and congenital abnormalities of the lips, tongue, palate, maxilla, mandible, and gums can be detected and appropriate genetic counseling and early treatment can be pursued. Incisor and premolar occlusion should be inspected again at 6 to 8 months of age, at which time the deciduous incisors should be erupted. Prognathism (parrot mouth), the most common malocclusion in horses, can be improved or corrected by initiating treatment with bite plates at this time. Thereafter, routine dental examinations at 6-month intervals throughout the life of the horse should be directed toward identifying and correcting retained deciduous teeth; maleruption of permanent teeth; supernumerary teeth; injuries to the jaws, teeth, cheek, gums, or tongue; lesions caused by oral foreign bodies and grass awns; enamel points; premolar and molar hooks; malocclusion; abnormalities of wear; cracked or missing teeth; excessive tartar build-up; and periodontal disease. Many of the severe, often untreatable malocclusions and wear abnormalities seen in older horses can be effectively prevented by regular dental inspection and prophylaxis. In addition, feed utilization and general body condition are better maintained and the incidence of gastrointestinal disorders is minimized when routine dental care is practiced.

If routine removal of wolf teeth before horses enter training is practiced, the procedure is best completed before the horse is 2 years old, and preferably between 12 and 18 months of age, since the periodontal membrane is relatively easily broken down at this time. Retained deciduous incisor or premolar teeth may interfere with eruption of permanent teeth, resulting in maleruption, delayed or arrested eruption, and, in the case of lower premolar teeth, deformation, infection, and fistula formation in the mandible. In addition, the sharp edges of fully or partially shed dental caps may lacerate the tongue or cheeks, causing quidding or bitting problems. For this reason, caps retained more than a few months after the predicted eruption date of the permanent tooth or caps causing obvious problems should be extracted. Deciduous incisor teeth that have not been shed after eruption of the corresponding permanent incisor should also be extracted, since they frequently impinge on the lip.

Enamel points, which develop in most horses on the buccal edge of the maxillary cheek teeth and on the lingual edge of the lower cheek teeth, should be removed by routine floating. Many parrot-mouthed horses and some with normal incisor occlusion also develop hooks on the rostral surface of the upper first cheek tooth (second premolar) or on the caudal edge of the lower sixth cheek tooth (third molar), or both, due to inadequate wear from the opposing tooth. The resulting tendency for caudal displacement of the mandible will exacerbate bite abnormalities and perhaps create other dental problems if these hooks are not regularly detected and removed. Canine teeth occasionally become excessively long or sharp and may cause bitting problems which necessitate filing to shorten and round off the offending tooth or teeth (see *Current Therapy in Equine Medicine 2*, p. 6).

PREVENTION AND DETECTION OF LAMENESS

Many orthopedic problems and lamenesses result from inadequate foot care or from improper trimming and shoeing. Advice to the client and farrier on current or developing problems, particularly foot imbalances, and establishment of a good working relationship between the veterinarian and farrier are very important. Foals should be trained from birth to accept having their feet picked up and trimmed. The limbs of foals should be carefully examined during the postfoaling examination to detect early signs of infection, foot abnormalities, and congenital flexural or angular limb deformities. Mild angular and flexural deformities frequently benefit from corrective trimming initiated during the first week of life and continued at 1- to 2-week intervals until correction is achieved. More severe abnormalities may require further diagnostic evaluation, including radiography, and the institution of corrective measures such as application of glue-on shoes, splinting, casting, or surgical intervention in addition to corrective trimming in order to achieve correction. The limbs and feet of foals should be inspected and the feet trimmed if necessary at intervals of no more than 6 weeks in order to optimize the development of normal feet and minimize secondary limb deformities. This approach also trains the foal to accept having the feet worked on and allows early detection and correction of developmental angular and flexural limb deformities. In particular the treatment of carpal valgal deformities and club-foot are much more successful when initiated during the first few months of life rather than when the foal is approaching 1 year of age. A 6-week interval is suitable for trimming and, when appropriate, shoeing of weanlings, yearlings, and older horses, although some horses will require a shorter interval between trimming. Overgrowth of the feet increases susceptibility to infective conditions such as thrush and exaggerates imbalances created by poor conformation, asymmetric hoof growth or improper trimming. The resulting abnormal weight-bearing increases the likelihood of secondary damage to the joints and soft tissue structures in the foot and limbs during exercise.

Supplemental Readings

Anon.: Compendium of equine immunizing agents. American Association of Equine Practitioners, 1987.

Anon.: Guidelines for vaccination of horses. J. Am. Vet. Med. Assoc., *185*:32–34, 1984.

Ardans, A.: Immunoprophylaxis in the horse. J. Am. Vet. Med. Assoc., *181*:1150–1153, 1982.

Haines, J. M.: Preventive medicine in equine practice. J. Am. Vet. Med. Assoc., *174*:396–398, 1979.

Onions, D.: Equine herpesvirus: New approaches to an old problem. Equine Vet. J., *23*:6–7, 1991.

Timoney, J. F.: Protecting against "strangles": A contemporary view. Equine Vet. J., *20*:392–396, 1988.

Wood, J. M.: Antigenic variation of equine influenza: A stable virus. Equine Vet. J., *20*:316–318, 1988.

Internal Parasite Control Programs

Joseph A. DiPietro, URBANA, ILLINOIS

Controlling endoparasites is an essential part of an effective equine preventive medicine program for all horses and is especially beneficial in young horses. Young horses are more likely to be adversely affected by parasites than adults, and parasite control allows them to develop and grow to their full potential. Adequately controlling parasites in horses also results in a decreased incidence of colic.

EQUINE ANTHELMINTICS

Currently several different anthelmintics or anthelmintic combinations are approved for use in horses in the United States (Table 1). With the exception of piperazine and trichlorfon they are broad-spectrum antinematodal drugs. Piperazine is often used in combination with benzimidazoles to improve efficacy against benzimidazole-resistant small strongyles. Trichlorfon, dichlorvos, and ivermectin are effective boticides. Ivermectin has the broadest spectrum of activity, including bots, nematodes, migratory stages of *Strongylus vulgaris* and *Parascaris equorum*, and cutaneous stages of nematodes.

A population, approximately 10 species, of small strongyles has been described as benzimidazole and probenzimidazole resistant. Benzimidazole-resistant small strongyles are widespread throughout the United States. Most anthelmintics other than the benzimidazoles and probenzimidazoles are effective against benzimidazole-resistant small strongyles (see Table 1). Numerous recommendations have been made about how anthelmintics should be rotated based on drug class to minimize problems with existing resistant populations of small strongyles and to prevent further development of resistance. Currently, two recommendations are most common: frequent rotation of anthelmintics within a year and rotation of anthelmintics at yearly intervals. Conflicting results have been reported as to which strategy is most likely to increase the development of strongyle resistance. Slow rotation of anthelmintics may select for populations of parasites against which the selected anthelmintic is not highly effective. For example, pyrantel pamoate or levamisole-piperazine mixtures, although highly effective against benzimidazole-resistant small strongyles, may select for *S. edentatus* based on their moderate activity (63 to 70 per cent) against this large strongyle. Frequent rotation of anthelmintics, if selected appropriately, would cancel out such weaknesses. Because of ivermectin's distinct benefit as compared to other anthelmintics in the treatment of larval stages of large strongyles and *P. equorum*, its use should not be precluded based on the possible development of resistant strongyles. Either approach to the rotation of anthelmintics may be used. It is important that the practitioner be comfortable with whichever approach is used; the approach used should be based on experience with parasite control programs on a particular farm or in a geographic location.

How an anthelmintic is administered has little bearing on its effectiveness. In general, as long as the following criteria are met, regardless of the route of administration (stomach tube, intraoral, or mixed with feed), effective deworming should occur.

1. The correct amount of dewormer must be administered based on an accurate estimation of the horse's weight.
2. Dose consumption and/or retention must be complete.
3. The anthelmintic selected must be highly effective against the parasites infesting the horse.
4. The anthelmintic must be approved for use via the route of administration selected.

The route of administration selected is best left to the practitioner's discretion based on the patient, economics, and client preference.

PARASITE CONTROL PROGRAMS

Equine parasite control programs are intended to reduce parasite transmission by minimizing contact between horses and infective stages of parasites in their environment. Consequently, horses on control programs are less likely to suffer damage or clinical disease due to parasitic infestations. Appropriate utilization and selection of effective anthelmintics, sound management practices to reduce parasite transmission, and assessment of parasite control are essential components of a complete equine parasite control

TABLE 1. DOSAGE, SAFETY, METHOD OF ADMINISTRATION, AND EFFICACY OF EQUINE ANTHELMINTICS

Drug Class	Anthelmintic	Relative Onset of Action	Dosage (mg/kg)	Safety Index*	Method	Mean Efficacy (%)†					Effective Against BZM-Resistant Small Strongyles
						Bots	P. equorum	Strongyles		O. equi	
								Large	Small		
Simple heterocyclic	Piperazine	Fast	88–110§	17	S	0	97	5–50	95	50	Yes
Benzimidazole	Thiabendazole	Slow	44–88‖	13	S,F,O	0	42	97	95	95	No
Benzimidazole	Mebendazole	Slow	8.8	45	S,F,O	0	97	80–97	87	97	No
Benzimidazole	Fenbendazole	Slow	5–10‖	200	S,F,O	0	95	95–97	97	97	No
Benzimidazole	Oxfendazole	Slow	10	10	S,F,O	0	95	97	97	97	No
Benzimidazole	Oxibendazole	Slow	10–15	60	S,O	0	95	97	97	97	No
Imidazothiazole-simple heterocyclic	Levamisole-piperazine	Fast‡	8/88¶	<3	S	0	100	63–97	97	90	Yes
Tetrahydropyrimidine	Pyrantel pamoate	Slow	6.6	20	S,F,O	0	95	70–97	95	65	Yes
Organophosphate	Trichlorfon	Fast	40	1	S,O	95	97	0	0	95	—
Organophosphate	Dichlorvos resin pellet	Fast	35	3	F	90	97	75–97	90	95	Yes
Probenzimidazole	Febantel	Slow	6	33	S,F,O	0	97	97	97	97	No
Avermectin	Ivermectin	Slow	0.2	10	S,O	99	100	100	100	100	Yes

Abbreviations: S = stomach tube, F = feed, O = orally as paste or drench, BZM = benzimidazole.
*Safety index = (Dose at which symptoms first appear)/(Minimim therapeutic dose).
†Applies to susceptible parasites only. Resistant populations may be encountered, especially small strongyles.
‡Due to piperazine.
§As piperazine base.
‖Higher doses required for P. equorum.
¶As levamisole/piperazine base.

program. All-encompassing recommendations for control programs across the wide range of climatic conditions in the United States cannot be made. Programs developed for different areas of the United States should be based specifically on parasite epidemiology, past experiences, management practices, and economics in a region.

Deworming programs for adult horses are primarily aimed at controlling bots and large and small strongyles. Programs for horses less than 1 year of age are primarily aimed at controlling *P. equorum*, bots, and large and small strongyles. Tapeworm and *Strongyloides westeri* control is necessary on facilities with a prior history of infestations.

INTERVAL PROGRAMS

Interval parasite control programs have been recommended since the mid-1960s. They consist of routine administration of dewormers at predetermined intervals throughout the year (Tables 2 and 3). The appropriate interval is determined by fecal examinations carried out at 2-week intervals following treatment during the first year of the program or is implemented based on prior experiences in the area under similar conditions. Field studies in the central United States have shown that an interval of 6 to 8 weeks is generally appropriate. This is based on the length of time that parasite egg suppression occurs after treatment—marked reductions occur for 4 weeks, with small increases occurring from 5 to 6 weeks, and marked increases during weeks 7 to 8.

TABLE 2. EXAMPLE OF INTERVAL DEWORMING PROGRAM FOR ADULT HORSES IN NORTH CENTRAL UNITED STATES

Month	Example of Anthelmintic	Efficacy Desired
February	Pyrantel pamoate	Nematodes
April	Oxibendazole	Nematodes
May	Fenbendazole and piperazine	Nematodes
July	Ivermectin	Nematodes and bots
September	Pyrantel pamoate	Nematodes
November	Ivermectin	Nematodes° and bots

°Includes immature/arterial stages of *S. vulgaris*.

TABLE 3. EXAMPLE OF INTERVAL DEWORMING PROGRAM FOR FOALS WITH AVERAGE BIRTH DATE IN FEBRUARY IN NORTH CENTRAL UNITED STATES

Age (Mo)	Example of Anthelmintic	Efficacy Desired
2	Ivermectin	Nematodes°
4	Oxibendazole	Nematodes
6	Pyrantel pamoate	Nematodes
8	Ivermectin	Nematodes and bots°
10	Pyrantel pamoate	Nematodes
12	Ivermectin	Nematodes and bots°

°Includes migrating stages of *P. equorum* and/or immature/arterial stages of *S. vulgaris*.

Adult Horses

In most cases, six dewormings yearly aimed at strongyle control are the framework for a complete interval deworming program (see Table 2). Additionally, to control bot infestations, boticides should be administered at least two times per year: once about 1 month after the first bot egg is noticed on the hair coat of horses, and once after the end of the botfly season. In some areas of the United States, additional bot treatments should be administered where botfly activity is severe or exceeds 6 months in length.

Foals

Interval deworming programs for foals (see Table 3) should include six dewormings at 2-month intervals beginning at 8 weeks of age. Routine anthelmintic therapy is begun at 8 weeks of age, because that is when immature and mature adult stages of *P. equorum* are commonly first present in the small intestine. On large farms, averaging the age of all foals housed together to calculate dates for anthelmintic administration is easier, promotes compliance, and is more economical than deworming based on exact ages. After reaching 1 year of age, horses should be placed on a deworming program suitable for adults.

On facilities where *S. westeri* is a clinical problem it may be controlled by treatment of the foals with ivermectin or oxibendazole (15 mg per kg) at an average of 3 weeks of age. Additional control of *S. westeri* may be achieved by treating mares within 12 hours post partum with ivermectin, which reduces milk-borne and consequent environmental transmission of *S. westeri*. Routine deworming of mares within 12 hours following parturition is beneficial in reducing the incidence of other nematode infections in their foals as well. Mares are the primary souce of infective stages of parasites for foals. Deworming mares shortly after foaling decreases the transmission of parasites to the foals during the periparturient period. Subsequent deworming of mares concurrent with deworming of the foals should further reduce the transmission of parasites to foals.

Additional benefit to foals can be derived from ivermectin treatment because of its high efficacy against mature and immature adult *P. equorum* and migratory stages of *P. equorum* in the lungs and liver. To avoid the likelihood of treatment complications such as impactions or intestinal rupture, treatment of foals with heavy or severe *P. equorum* infestations should not be done with anthelmintics that act quickly. Compounds that act slowly (see Table 1), such as the tetrahydropyrimidines, avermectins, or the benzimidazoles, are less likely to cause complications.

Seasonal Programs

A newer approach to the control of strongyles is the seasonal control program (Table 4). This program aims treatments strategically at times of the year when anthelmintic-susceptible, egg-producing adult strongyles occur in peak numbers. The spring rise in numbers of adult strongyles and *Strongylus* egg counts is well documented in climates similar to those in the northern two-thirds of the United States. Strategic treatments administered in the spring and early summer have successfully blocked the spring rise in egg counts and decreased the transmission of strongyles during the following grazing season. This approach can only be used where climatic conditions are such that a seasonal rise in strongyle egg production is known to occur. At least one treatment per year in the fall (after botfly activity is over) with a boticide is needed to limit damage caused by bots. In fact, an additional bot treatment in July or August, except in the very northerly United States, may be indicated.

Seasonal control programs should be less expensive than interval programs and may decrease the likelihood of anthelmintic-resistant strains of parasites developing. Whether they are as effective in the long term in controlling strongyles as interval programs is not yet fully known. Because the seasonal approach to control is only aimed at controlling strongyles and bots, it should not be used for horses less than 1 year of age.

Daily Anthelmintic Feeding Programs

Administration of 2.64 mg per kg of pyrantel tartrate* on a daily basis is effective in the prevention of *S. vulgaris* infections and control of large strongyles, small strongyles (adults and fourth-stage larvae in the intestine), pinworms, and ascarids (adults and fourth-stage larvae in the intestine). Daily treatment with pyrantel tartrate kills larvae prior to their migration, and adult worms and larvae in the intestine. Where peak periods of transmission of strongyles are known to occur seasonally, pyrantel tartrate may be fed to decrease the establishment of infections during only that period of the year. For example, in the northern United States, where

TABLE 4. EXAMPLE OF SEASONAL DEWORMING PROGRAM FOR ADULT HORSES IN NORTH CENTRAL UNITED STATES

Month	Example of Anthelmintic	Efficacy Desired
May	Ivermectin	Nematodes°
July	Ivermectin	Nematodes° and bots
December	Ivermectin	Nematodes° and bots

°Includes immature/arterial stages of *S. vulgaris*.

---

*Purina Horse and Colt Wormer, Purina Mills, Inc., St. Louis, MO.

strongyle fecal egg counts increase in the spring, pyrantel would be fed from approximately March through October. Larvicidal treatment with ivermectin at the beginning and end of the feeding period would further enhance control of nematodes, as well as provide adequate control of bots. Foals may be started on daily anthelmintic feeding programs once they consistently consume their grain ration.

Tapeworm Control

Some beneficial control of tapeworms can be achieved with the manufacturer's recommended dosages of pyrantel pamoate (6.6 mg per kg is 85 per cent effective). Better control can be achieved with double the label dosage of pyrantel pamoate (13.2 mg per kg is 100 per cent effective). Benefit from chemotherapy can be optimized by treatment 2 weeks prior to and at the conclusion of the grazing season.

ENVIRONMENTAL CONTROL

Additional parasite control beyond that achieved by routine administration of anthelmintics may be obtained by implementing management practices that further decrease the number of infective stages of parasites in the environment. Management practices that enhance parasite control include the following:

1. Routine removal of feces from stalls, pastures and paddocks.
2. Proper disposal of manure. Manure should not be spread on pastures unless it has been composted for over 1 year.
3. Regular rotation of pastures and avoidance of overstocking.
4. Quarantine of all new additions. Fecal examination and appropriate treatment with nonbenzimidazole anthelmintics before intermingling with other horses.
5. Prevention of fecal contamination of feed and water.
6. Harrowing pastures during the driest and hottest season of the year.
7. Deworming all horses housed together at the same time.
8. Performing fecal examinations regularly to evaluate parasite control.

EVALUATION OF CONTROL PROGRAMS

Complete parasite control programs should be carefully and routinely evaluated by performing fecal examinations. Qualitative examination techniques (see Table 4) are preferred because they are easier to perform than quantitative examinations and are less likely to produce false negative results (Table 5).

Fecal examination of at least 10 per cent of the horses should be carried out a minimum of two to three times per year, 14 days after the horses are dewormed, because most horses should not be passing parasite eggs 14 days after treatment with a dewormer. If environmental control is adequate and the dewormers used are highly effective, less than 10 per cent of the samples obtained should contain parasite eggs. The following possible causes should be considered if more than 10 per cent of the samples contain parasite eggs: improper anthelmintic administration, parasite reinfection, anthelmintic-resistant parasites, improper anthelmintic selection, or maturation of non-anthelmintic-sensitive immature stages of parasites between the time of treatment and the day fecal samples are obtained. Once identified, proper recommendations should be made to avoid such treatment failures in the future.

When treatment failures are identified by qualitative fecal examination, quantitative fecal examinations (modified McMaster's technique) should be performed to determine the relative risk of transmission. The same number of horses should be used in both the qualitative and quantitative examinations. Eggs per gram counts should be determined prior to anthelmintic treatment and at 2-week intervals during the period between treatments. Parasite egg per gram counts do not correlate well with parasite burdens, but do give an indication of potential contamination of the horse's environment with in-

TABLE 5. QUALITATIVE FECAL EXAMINATION TECHNIQUE

1. With a tongue depressor, press 2 to 5 gm of feces mixed with approximately 10 ml of water through a tea strainer into a suitable container.
2. Remove strainer and discard its contents. Pour fecal suspension from the container into a test tube.
3. Centrifuge at 1500 rpm for 10 minutes.
4. Decant the supernatant from test tube.
5. Add Sheather's solution until the test tube is two-thirds full. Stir with an applicator stick until well resuspended.
6. Fill remainder of test tube with Sheather's solution until a small meniscus forms.
7. Place a coverslip on top of the test tube.
8. Centrifuge at 1500 rpm for 10 minutes or let stand for more than 30 minutes.
9. Remove the coverslip and place on microscope slide.
10. Scan slide at 100× magnification for parasite eggs.
11. Results are reported as positive or negative.

fective stages of parasites and thus an assessment of parasite transmission potential. Ideally, *Strongylus* egg counts should be less than 100 per gm at all times. Additional information about anthelmintic resistance may be determined from quantitative fecal examinations by comparing pre- and post-anthelmintic treatment *Strongylus* egg counts. If egg counts determined 2 weeks after treatment remain at or near pretreatment levels, anthelmintic-resistant parasites are the most likely cause.

Supplemental Readings

DiPietro, J. A., Klei, T. R., and French, D. D.: Contemporary topics in equine parasitology. Compend. Cont. Ed. *12*:713, 1990.

DiPietro, J. A., and Todd, K. S.: Anthelmintics used in treatment of parasitic infections of horses. Vet. Clin. North Am. (Equine Pract.), 3:1, 1987.

Herd, R. P.: Internal parasites. *In* Robinson, N. E. (ed.): Current Therapy in Equine Medicine 2. Philadelphia, W. B. Saunders Co., 1987, pp. 323–336.

Herd, R. P. (ed.): Parasitology. Vet. Clin. North Am. (Equine Pract.), 2, 1986.

Section 2

DUTIES OF A VETERINARIAN

Edited by Glenn F. Anderson

Selected Medical-Legal Considerations in the Practice of Equine Medicine

Thomas H. Allison, CLEVELAND, OHIO

It goes without saying that veterinarians are legally and ethically required to practice competent veterinary medicine in a professional manner. The legal duty arises from veterinary practice acts and the administrative rules and regulations governing the practice of veterinary medicine, and from the case law of the various jurisdictions. The ethical duty arises from the American Veterinary Medical Association's Princples of Veterinary Medical Ethics and from one's own personal and professional ethical beliefs.

It is not possible to discuss all of the legal ramifications of the practice of equine medicine in this chapter. Therefore, selected medical-legal considerations attendant on the practice of equine medicine will be discussed, including maintenance of complete and accurate medical records, the confidentiality of patient information, and the appropriate response to subpoenas for patient medical information. It is not possible in a format such as this to provide an exhaustive presentation of the law, across all jurisdictions, on these several topics. The following discussion is intended to convey general information on selected topics of interest to practitioners of equine medicine. It should not be used as a substitute for legal counseling in specific situations. Readers should not act on the information presented without professional legal guidance.

MEDICAL RECORDS/DOCUMENTATION

Aside from the patient itself, the medical record is the most important item in the care and treatment of that patient. Not only are complete and accurate medical records vital to proper patient care, they are also of great medical-legal significance. Lawsuits alleging veterinary malpractice are won or lost on the basis of the medical records. If the records are complete and accurate the lawsuit may be avoided entirely, or at least placed in a defensible position. However, if the records are not complete and accurate, the attorney representing the plaintiff horse owner has a better chance of convincing the jury that sloppy record keeping equates with a less than acceptable standard of veterinary care. Finally, the old axiom, "if it is not in the record, it was not done," is as true today as ever.

Complete and accurate medical records should contain all of the pertinent information necessary to provide acceptable care and treatment to the patient. In some states, the requirements for adequate medical records are specifically set forth in the practice act or administrative rules governing veterinary practice. It is suggested that the patient's medical record include the following: (1) results of the veterinarian's history and examination, (2) laboratory test results, (3) original radiographs, (4) reports from consulting veterinarians, (5) consent forms or documentation of the owner's "informed consent," (6) any correspondence received from the owner or any third party regarding the particular patient, and the veterinarian's response to that correspondence, (7) copies of any forms or other materials submitted to any insurance company, whether an application for insurance or a report concerning the animal's health care or death, and (8) records received from prior treating veterinarians.

In general, the medical record is the property of the individual practitioner or the professional veterinary group. However, the information in the medical record is the property of the horse's owner. Because this information belongs to the owner and is accessible to him or her upon request, medical records should be written and maintained in a totally objective manner. The record should show the pertinent medical facts obtained and observed by the practitioner. Personal comments not bearing directly on patient care should not be included in the medical record. The practitioner should avoid nonfactual, judgmental statements of opinion about the care and treatment provided by the owner, trainer, or any prior treating veterinarians. Also to be avoided are vague phrases such as "ate fair."

The practitioner's notes concerning any patient should include a complete and accurate history and a factual description of the results of the physical examination. On the basis of that information, a list of tentative differential diagnoses should be noted. A plan for further diagnostic studies should be described. Finally, the initial treatment information should be recorded. As the treatment progresses or subsequent examinations are conducted, new factual data should be entered in the medical chart and changes in diagnosis or treatment should be documented.

The record should contain either a written consent form signed by the client authorizing the treatment to be undertaken or a notation that the veterinarian has discussed the treatment plan with the client, all of the owner's questions have been answered, and the owner has consented. Further, it is important to document the owner's refusal to consent to treatment or testing that has been discussed and advised.

All medications administered should be noted in the chart, including the name of the medication, dose, route of administration, date and time of administration, and the initials of the person giving the medication.

Medical records should be written legibly and only standard abbreviations used. This is especially important in practices where more than one veterinarian may be involved in the horse's health care or where technicians provide certain care and treatment. To avoid inadvertent errors in treatment, the practitioner must be sure that all persons involved in the horse's care thoroughly understand, upon reviewing a clear, concise, legible record, what treatment is to be administered. A veterinarian's credibility will be attacked on the witness stand if his notes are so illegible that even he cannot read them. Plaintiff's counsel will attempt to convince the jury that sloppy record keeping means substandard care was given.

It is important to adequately document repeat observations of a hospitalized patient or an ambulatory patient seen on a repeated basis. The facts of those examinations should be clearly noted and the date and time of the observations recorded. It is little comfort to a veterinarian on the witness stand to know that he or she saw a patient between the hours of midnight and 6:00 A.M. when there is no documentation in the medical record to substantiate that testimony and plaintiff's counsel is able to convince a jury that the animal was not observed during that period of time and was actually found dead at 6:00 A.M.

Incorrect entries in a medical record will occur and are the result of simple human error. An error in documentation in a patient's chart does not constitute inappropriate veterinary care. However, failure to detect and correct that error may subject a veterinarian to liability. Veterinarians should review patient records and note and correct any errors in the medical chart. Do not obliterate, erase, scratch out, or use correction fluid to correct an error in a medical chart.

For example, if an animal's temperature was 100.4° F and it was inadvertently written as 104° F, this inadvertent error should be corrected. Simply draw a single line through the incorrect entry, write the word "error," and initial the corrected entry. If inadvertent mistakes are corrected in this manner, no allegation can be made that the records were tampered with. Do not change medical records in any other manner, and never attempt to alter medical records after notice of a potential claim has been received or a lawsuit has been filed. To do so could subject the practitioner to damages far beyond what would have been recovered and, in some states, could subject the veterinarian to liability for punitive damages, punishment for intentional wrongdoing.

It is recommended that these guidelines for documenting patient care and treatment be followed whether the animal is hospitalized or seen on an ambulatory basis. Although it is more difficult to maintain complete records on ambulatory patients, some attempt should be made to create a medical record for ambulatory care and treatment that will provide a sound basis not only for acceptable veterinary care, but also for avoiding or defending a claim of malpractice.

Keeping and maintaining complete and accurate medical records is not a task that most practitioners enjoy. Generally, the attitude is that spending a great amount of time in record keeping takes away from the practitioner's opportunity to provide actual patient care. However, in this day and age, when medical records may well become evidence in a claim or lawsuit alleging veterinary negligence, it is vital that legible, complete, and accurate medical records be maintained.

CONFIDENTIALITY

The original medical record is the property of the practicing veterinarian; however, the information in that record is the property of the horse's owner. In that regard, the veterinarian owes a duty to his client not to disclose this confidential patient information to anyone without the consent of the owner.

Many states have specific statutes and case law regarding the requirement of physician-patient confidentiality. Although this area of the law is not well developed in veterinary medicine, it is reasonable to assume that in situations involving alleged breach of confidentiality, the law of the particular jurisdiction will be borrowed directly from the human arena and the veterinarian may be found liable for breach of confidentiality. With the exception of members of the same practice involved in providing care for the horse, it is recommended that a veterinarian never discuss an animal's condition with anyone other than the owner, or the owner's authorized agent, without the express consent of the owner, preferably in writing.

Because the information in the medical record is the property of the animal's owner, in general it must be released to the owner upon request. It is suggested that requests for medical records be made in writing and signed by the owner. This suggestion applies whether the owner personally wants a copy of the record or whether the record is being sent to another veterinarian.

Do not release original medical records, including the results of laboratory tests and original radiographs. Copies of the written medical chart and all other information should be provided to the owner upon request. It is advised that the original radiographs not be given to the owner, but rather copies supplied if the owner wants them personally. If the medical record including the radiographs is to be sent to another veterinarian, it is generally acceptable to provide the other veterinarian with the original radiographs, on condition that they be returned to the original practitioner after review.

The practitioner must beware of potential breaches of client confidentiality when conducting a prepurchase physical examination on a horse for a prospective buyer when that particular animal has been the veterinarian's patient and the seller a client. It is suggested that under these circumstances the practitioner not agree to conduct the purchase examination for the prospective buyer unless the seller-client provides written authorization allowing the examining veterinarian to consider the animal's medical history as the practitioner knows it to be and specifically authorizes the veterinarian to release all of the information in his possession to the prospective buyer.

SUBPOENAS FOR MEDICAL RECORDS

Veterinarians increasingly find themselves in receipt of a subpoena for their medical records on a particular horse. Subpoenas are documents issued at the request of a party to a lawsuit commanding a person to produce certain materials or to appear and give testimony. Technically, a subpoena requiring a person to produce books, papers, records, and other tangible items is known as a *subpoena duces tecum*. A subpoena requiring a person to appear and give testimony is a *subpoena ad testificandum*. Depending on the jurisdiction, the subpoenas may be issued by the clerk of the court in which the lawsuit is pending or by notary publics as designated officers of the court.

Although specifically governed by the law of the particular jurisdiction, in general the appropriate action to take in response to a subpoena for medical records depends on who is requesting those records. Determining who is requesting the records by subpoena before releasing them is necessary because of the confidential nature of the information contained in those records. Remember, no one has a right to that information except the horse's owner.

Most states have statutes dealing with the release of human medical records in various legal situations. Again, this area of law in veterinary medicine is not well developed; however, it is likely that the principles applicable to obtaining human medical records by subpoena in the particular jurisdiction will be applied to veterinary medical records.

When the practitioner receives a subpoena for medical records, it means that a lawsuit has been filed and someone is requesting the court to require the production of those records. Depending on the exact nature of the lawsuit, the records could be requested by the animal's owner, a defendant veterinarian in a malpractice action brought by the owner, or some other party involved in a lawsuit with the owner in which the horse's health is an issue in the case.

On receipt of a subpoena requesting production of a horse's medical records, the first question that must be answered is who is requesting those records. This question can usually be answered by reviewing the subpoena to determine whether it has been issued by the attorney for the horse's owner or by some other party's attorney. The telephone number of the attorney issuing the subpoena is usually provided on the subpoena, and a telephone call to that attorney should shed some light on exactly who has requested the records and whether the owner has consented to the release of information.

Although it is unusual to receive a subpoena for records from a horse's owner, because the owner is entitled to a copy of those records, if you determine that the subpoena was issued by the owner's attorney, then the records should be copied and provided to that attorney on receipt of a signed authorization. Alternatively, the owner or his attorney may want to inspect the original record. If that is the case, the practitioner should arrange a mutually convenient time and place for that inspection. The practitioner should not turn over the original records to anyone. The practitioner or someone designated by the practitioner should be present at all times when the original record is inspected, and the entire original record should be returned to that person on completion of inspection.

It is more likely that the subpoena will be issued by someone other than the owner's attorney. If the lawsuit is one for malpractice against another veterinarian and the practitioner has treated the involved horse either before or after the defendant veterinarian, then the defendant veterinarian's attorney may be attempting to obtain the records regarding that horse. Notwithstanding any desire the practitioner may have to assist the defendant veterinarian's attorney, the horse's medical records should not be released to that attorney and the care and treatment of the horse should not be discussed with that attorney unless the horse's owner has provided written authorization for release of such information. Release of information without written authorization could subject the practitioner to liability for breach of confidentiality.

Medical records may also be subpoenaed by a party other than the owner in a lawsuit that does not involve allegations of professional negligence against another veterinarian. As above, the same guidelines apply. No information should be released or discussed with the attorney for someone other than the owner until a written authorization permitting the practitioner to release medical information is provided by the owner. The practitioner should not take the representations of anyone regarding the owner's permission to release medical information on a particular horse but should insist on a written authorization form signed by the owner permitting release of medical information.

The stated guidelines for responding to a subpoena are subject to the laws of the individual jurisdiction. If the practitioner is uncertain how to respond, he or she should consult a personal attorney before releasing any medical information. Additionally, it may be necessary to involve the personal attorney to arrange a mutually convenient time and place for allowing inspection of the original medical records.

The Veterinarian as a Witness

Thomas H. Allison, CLEVELAND, OHIO

Owing to the number of lawsuits involving issues of equine health and equine veterinary care, it is likely that at some point a practitioner of equine medicine will be asked or ordered to serve as a witness. The practitioner may be asked or ordered to provide testimony as a fact witness or may be asked to provide expert review and serve as an expert witness.

In a lawsuit involving equine health issues the practitioner may be asked or ordered to give testimony as a fact witness. For instance, in lawsuits by horse owners against trainers, farm managers, horse transportation companies, and others responsible for the horse's care that involve allegations of harm or injury to a horse, a practitioner who treated the horse before or after the injury resulting in the lawsuit may be asked or ordered to give testimony regarding the facts of his examination and treatment.

In veterinary malpractice actions, the practitioner may be ordered to testify as a fact witness or requested to testify as an expert witness. In almost all veterinary malpractice actions, the defendant veterinarian will testify in his or her case at trial and could also be required by the rules of court to give deposition testimony or to testify on cross-examination in the plaintiff horse owner's case at trial.

In a veterinary malpractice lawsuit alleging negligence against another veterinarian, a practitioner who treated the horse before or after the treatment rendered by the allegedly negligent veterinarian may also be ordered, by subpoena, to provide deposition testimony and to testify at trial regarding the facts of his examination and treatment.

In lawsuits alleging veterinary malpractice and in other lawsuits involving equine health care issues, the practitioner may be requested by either plaintiff or defendant to review the facts of the case and to render an expert opinion regarding equine health care issues. It is fair to say that one cannot be ordered to become an expert witness. When the practitioner is requested to testify as an expert, the decision to become involved in the case is entirely a voluntary one and the practitioner may decline to review the case and provide expert testimony.

With these general comments in mind, the following discussion focuses on the peculiarities of testifying as a fact witness and providing expert review and testimony, and offers some general guidelines for providing sworn testimony at a deposition or trial.

FACT WITNESS TESTIMONY

The equine practitioner may be asked to provide fact witness testimony regarding the care and treatment of an animal in malpractice actions and other cases. In such a situation, if either party believes that the veterinarian's knowledge of the horse's health condition would be helpful to the case, then it is probable that the veterinarian will be ordered, by way of subpoena, to provide deposition testimony. As will be discussed in greater detail below, a deposition is a relatively informal legal proceeding at which the person providing the testimony, the *deponent,* is placed under oath and asked questions by the attorney ordering the deposition. If the veterinarian is not a party to the lawsuit, in almost all instances the party's right to conduct the deposition will be enforced by a court order, the subpoena.

It is important to remember that if the lawsuit is one for veterinary malpractice against another practitioner, and the veterinarian with knowledge of the horse's condition is subpoenaed for deposition, the deponent veterinarian will not be represented by an attorney unless he or she obtains one. Incidents have occurred in which a veterinarian, not originally a defendant in a malpractice action, was deposed regarding the care and treatment of the involved horse. Then, after the deposition was conducted without the veterinarian's personal attorney present, the veterinarian was named as a new defendant in the lawsuit. Therefore, it is suggested that if a practitioner is subpoenaed for deposition in a case and is not a defendant, a personal attorney be contacted before the practitioner offers testimony.

The facts of the non-party practitioner's care and treatment of the horse should be discussed with that practitioner's attorney, as well as knowledge of the facts that resulted in the lawsuit. In this manner, the deponent's personal attorney can determine whether it is in the deponent's best interests to have personal counsel present when giving the deposition. This same suggestion also applies if the veterinarian has any reason to believe that the deposition testimony in a nonmalpractice case could result in being named as a defendant in that lawsuit.

Whether or not a veterinarian has been deposed as a fact witness, testimony at trial may be requested on behalf of either party. If the veterinarian is called to testify as a "friendly" witness, a witness with facts supporting the requesting party's case, it is not essential that a subpoena be issued requiring the practitioner's appearance at trial. However, in almost all instances, even with friendly witnesses, the party requesting the veterinarian's testimony will issue a subpoena requiring the practitioner's appearance, to protect the client's interests in the event some situation should occur that would prevent the veterinarian from appearing in court to give testimony. Usually, the requesting party's attorney will inform the witness that the subpoena will be issued as a matter of court procedure.

Prior to offering trial testimony on behalf of a party, the veterinarian should meet with the attorney for the party requesting testimony, in order to prepare to give direct testimony at trial and to prepare for potential cross-examination by the opposing party's attorney.

EXPERT WITNESS REVIEW AND TESTIMONY

A plaintiff horse owner in a lawsuit alleging veterinary malpractice, and in some nonmalpractice lawsuits involving equine health care issues, will be required to utilize expert veterinary medical testimony to prove the case. Therefore, it is entirely possible that at some point in a professional career, an equine practitioner may be asked by a plaintiff horse owner or a defendant veterinarian to serve as an expert witness in a veterinary malpractice case, or to serve as an expert witness on equine health care issues in nonmalpractice actions.

In veterinary malpractice actions, the plaintiff horse owner has a burden of proving, by a preponderance of the evidence, (1) the applicable standard of practice that should have been used by the veterinarian in the care and treatment of the horse, (2) that the veterinarian deviated from this standard of care, and (3) that the deviation was the proximate or legal cause of harm or injury to the plaintiff or the plaintiff's personal property, the horse. Further, almost all jurisdictions require that the plaintiff's proof as to these matters be provided by expert veterinary medical testimony offered by another veterinarian.

In a nonmalpractice action, a veterinarian might be called on to offer an expert opinion regarding certain equine health issues. For instance, in an action against a horse transportation company or farm manager for injury to a horse in their custody and control, expert veterinary medical testimony may be required to prove that the care provided by the horse transportation company or the farm manager was the proximate or legal cause of the alleged injury.

It is important to realize that a veterinarian cannot be ordered or compelled to provide expert testimony. There is no legal duty to serve as an expert witness for either party. The decision to serve as a reviewing expert is entirely a matter of personal choice. It must be understood, however, that service as a reviewing expert in any lawsuit is a significant undertaking and must be entered into with a full understanding of the responsibilities of an expert witness and the legal process to which the expert will be subjected. The following discussion briefly describes an expert's responsibilities and the legal process related to expert testimony, to enable the practitioner to decide whether or not to serve as an expert.

First, service as an expert witness may, depending on the complexity of the case, require a substantial amount of the practitioner's time. It may involve additional time away from the practice of veterinary medicine to meet with the attorney requesting the expert review, perform medical research, give deposition testimony, and even testify at trial. The reviewing expert must be committed to allocating a sufficient amount of time to provide a thorough review of the case and perform these various responsibilities.

Second, the expert's review of the case should include all of the medical records involved in the lawsuit. Further, transcripts of all relevant depositions should be reviewed.

Third, the expert may need to spend some time reviewing the appropriate veterinary medical literature, and will need to meet with the attorney engaging the services and discuss the medical issues in the case, opinions, and the basis for those opinions. To properly prepare for trial, the attorney must become familiar with the medical issues involved in the case. The attorney will rely, in part, on the expert witness to provide the necessary education on those medical issues.

A fourth consideration in deciding whether to serve as an expert witness is the practitioner's familiarity with the specific medical issues involved in the particular case. Although most jurisdictions would allow any licensed veterinarian to testify on any aspect of veterinary medicine, an expert's knowledge of the specific subject matter involved in the case, including expertise and experience in that area, will determine how credible the expert's testimony will be and how highly his or her opinions will be regarded by the jury. If an expert is testifying out of his or her area of expertise, the opposing party's attorney will use the expert's lack of knowledge, expertise, and experience in that specific area to attack credibility and attempt to convince the jury that the expert's opinions have no value. For instance, if the case involves allegations of misdiagnosis of a soft tissue injury by the use of diagnostic ultrasound and the expert has no experience with that diagnostic modality, the opposing party's attorney will use that lack of experience to attack the expert's opinions in the case.

A practitioner is not required to serve as an expert witness when asked to do so. If the practitioner has the time and expertise necessary to offer an expert review, then an agreement to offer expert review and testimony may be made with the requesting attorney. One area of that agreement concerns professional fees. The reviewing expert should be compensated for professional time spent as a reviewing expert. It is suggested that the expert charge an hourly fee for professional time. The reviewing expert should keep accurate records of all time spent reviewing the materials relevant to the case, discussing the case with the attorney, and preparing for and giving deposition or trial testimony.

The primary function of a reviewing expert is to act as an objective, unbiased reviewer of the facts of a particular case and to offer an expert opinion based on knowledge, training, and experience in that subject matter area. The practitioner should not undertake the review if he or she has a personal relationship with the plaintiff horse owner, defendant veterinarian, or other defendant. Because the reviewer should be offering totally objective opinions, the opposing party's attorney will attempt to represent any personal relationship as bias toward the party on whose behalf the expert is testifying and will attempt to convince the jury that the opinions should not be given consideration for that reason.

In order to reach an opinion, the expert must review and analyze all pertinent information, including medical records; all deposition transcripts, not only those of the plaintiff and defendant but also those of all fact witnesses and the opposing party's expert; and all pertinent veterinary medical literature. If the reviewing expert requires further information to form an opinion, that information should be requested from the attorney who retained the expert.

After the initial review of all available information, the veterinarian should arrange to discuss the case with the engaging attorney. That discussion must set forth the expert's honest, objective opinions of the case. It is just as important for the attorney to know about unfavorable opinions of the case as it is favorable ones. For this reason, it is suggested that the expert not put opinions in writing until after the case has been thoroughly discussed with the retaining attorney, who will then request a written report. This precaution is necessary because in many jurisdictions the court rules provide that any written information received by the attorney may be obtainable by the opposing party during the process of discovery. Conversations, however, are not discoverable.

Following the discussion, the expert may be asked to set forth opinions in writing. Generally, this written report will be provided to the opposing party.

After the report is provided to the opposing party, it is likely that the opposing party will want to take the expert's deposition. Further, if the case is not settled, it is probable that the expert will be asked to provide live testimony at trial. Some basic guidelines for providing sworn testimony during a deposition or at trial follow.

GUIDELINES FOR OFFERING SWORN TESTIMONY

Whether a practitioner is called to give deposition or trial testimony as a fact or an expert witness, the process of offering sworn testimony is similar. Both fact witnesses and expert witnesses can be ordered to provide deposition testimony during the discovery phase of the lawsuit. In the discovery period, the parties are given the opportunity to learn everything they can about the other party's case, including what their witnesses will say at trial.

A deposition is a legal proceeding, governed by court rules, whereby the opposing party can take the sworn testimony of a fact or expert witness. The people present at a deposition include a court reporter to administer the oath and take down everything that is said during the deposition, the opposing party's attorney, who will ask questions during the deposition, and the attorney for the party being deposed or who retained the expert. Further, the actual parties to the lawsuit have the right to be present at all depositions and may choose to attend.

At the beginning of the deposition, the person giving the testimony, the deponent, is placed under oath and sworn to tell the truth by the court reporter. The attorney requesting the deposition asks questions to learn everything possible about a fact witness's recollection of the events involved in the lawsuit or an expert witness's background, experience, training, knowledge of the subject matter area, knowledge of the specific facts of the case, and opinions and the basis for those opinions.

The practitioner who is a fact witness and is not a party to the lawsuit must retain personal counsel in order to be represented by an attorney during the deposition. Further, an expert is not represented by an attorney at the deposition, although the attorney for the retaining party will be present to ensure that the client's interests are protected and in so doing will aid the expert during the deposition.

The deponent who is a party to the lawsuit or who is offering expert testimony should meet with the representing or engaging attorney to prepare for testimony. If the deponent is a non-party fact witness, he should determine through discussions with personal counsel whether to be represented by an attorney at the deposition and should be prepared to give deposition testimony, whether the attorney is present or not.

Before a party gives any testimony at trial, that party's attorney should prepare him or her to offer direct testimony and for the probable cross-examination by the opposing party's attorney. An expert witness should also be prepared to offer direct testimony and be cross-examined at trial.

Whether offering sworn testimony at deposition or at trial, the cardinal rule is to tell the truth. Only through truthful answers can a case be resolved on the basis of the facts. As well as being entirely truthful, answers should also be as fair and accurate as possible. With those requirements in mind, it is important to realize that how the truth is told may be very significant. This is a primary reason for being adequately prepared by the attorney prior to offering sworn testimony.

In addition to telling the truth fairly and accurately, certain other suggestions will make the process more comfortable. First, answer all questions directly and do not volunteer any information. A witness is obligated to answer all questions to the best of recollection; however, it is almost always harmful to volunteer information. Simply answer the question asked. The witness does not have any obligation to help the attorney asking questions on cross-examination during a deposition or at trial.

A witness should never answer a question that is not fully understood. If the witness is unsure of exactly what is being asked, he or she should simply request the attorney to repeat or rephrase the question.

A witness should never guess at the answer to a question. "I do not know" and "I do not remember" are complete and truthful answers to many questions. However, there is a difference between the two. "I do not know" is generally interpreted to mean that the witness never knew, whereas "I do not remember" means that the witness knew at one time but does not remember at that moment of the deposition or trial. Importantly, in order to preserve the opportunity to have further recall later, if that should happen, it is best to state, "I do not recall at this time." The credibility of a witness who answers in this manner will not be subject to attack later if the witness does recall further information.

Most lawyers operate on the principle that they can obtain more information by being nice than by being obnoxious. However, some attorneys use the hard-line technique to intimidate a witness into giving them information. Court rules prevent an attorney from being overly obnoxious or disrespectful to a witness. However, any witness may be subject to a certain amount of uncomfortable questioning. Never lose your temper. To do so will result in answers that may be incorrect and are probably not the best answers that could be given to certain questions.

If a witness discovers during the course of a deposition that a previous answer was incorrect, then an effort should be made to correct that answer. It is entirely appropriate to inform the questioning attorney that the answer to the question given 5 minutes ago about a certain subject was incorrect and then simply state the correct answer for the record.

The court reporter takes down everything said during the deposition. In that regard, as well as correcting known incorrect answers, the witness should speak clearly and answer all questions orally, rather than with nods of the head, so that there is no question as to what has taken place.

During the deposition, attorneys may make objections to questions that are asked. If any lawyer objects to a question, the witness waits until the objection is completed before answering the question. Many times the objections are to the form of the question; for instance, it may actually be two questions and it will create inaccuracy to try to answer them with a single answer. Other questions may be confusing or misleading. Always listen to what is being said during the objection, because it may provide information about why the question was inappropriate. Beware of "summary questions," those that attempt to summarize previous testimony. Whenever an attorney summarizes previous testimony and then asks for a yes or no answer as to whether that is correct, listen very carefully to make sure that the testimony has not been misquoted.

Finally, at the end of the deposition the witness should be instructed about the right to read the deposition transcript for accuracy. It is suggested that this right to review the transcript never be waived. For the sake of complete accuracy, it is better to review the transcript and make any necessary corrections, because the sworn testimony obtained during a deposition may be utilized during trial to show that the witness has changed answers or altered testimony in some way, and, therefore, should not be believed.

The Veterinarian's Role in Insurance

Lance L. Allen, KANSAS CITY, MISSOURI
Jerry R. Rains, KANSAS CITY, MISSOURI
Ann C. Henderson, MOUNT MORRIS, ILLINOIS

Many veterinarians regard equine mortality insurance examinations and claims as necessary evils. All too often the veterinarian, especially a mixed-practice veterinarian, receives little compensation for this service and feels that dealing with insurance companies and client claims is expensive and inconvenient. The basis for these feelings is usually an unpleasant past experience. A better understanding of the responsibilities of each party and the legal obligations of the owner and the veterinarian is necessary if this service is to be seen in a different light.

OBTAINING COVERAGE

In most cases the horse owner may choose which veterinarian will provide routine care and conduct the pre-insurance examination. During the examination it is the owner's responsibility to disclose all known previous illnesses or injuries of the horse to the attending practitioner. The veterinarian then examines the horse and completes a Veterinary Certificate of Examination for Equine Mortality Insurance (Fig. 1).

The type of questions and information the veterinarian must provide will vary from insurance company to insurance company, but most forms contain similar questions about the horse's health. In addition, the veterinarian may be asked to assist with a positive identification by completing schematic drawings on the application or providing a photograph. The form must be completed to the veterinarian's best knowledge and ability.

The insurance company reviews the pre-insurance examination to determine insurability. Pre-existing or chronic diseases may be excluded from coverage, but that does not necessarily mean that all coverage will be denied. For example, a veterinarian may simply remark "colic surgery performed Jan. 1985 and again in Jan. 1987. Treated again in May, 1987; resolved without surgery. Suggested routine deworming to prevent future colic." A more detailed statement by the practitioner helps clarify the condition. Such an animal may be granted full coverage or coverage with a colic exclusion, depending on the company. The practitioner is not making an insurability decision but rather is providing information that will allow the insurance company to make that decision. Questions such as "In your opinion, is this animal insurable?" should be left to the company. The company may contact the veterinarian with specific questions regarding the previous health of the horse. It is important to have the permission of the owner before giving any animal health information to the company. Overlooking a seemingly minor defect may jeopardize future claims and have legal ramifications.

POLICY RESPONSIBILITY

Under the typical policy, the owner agrees to seek needed veterinary care and notify the insurance company or a company-appointed adjustor in the case of injury, illness, or accident. If the injury or illness is not life-threatening, the

Veterinary Certificate of Examination for Equine Mortality Insurance

The purpose of this examination is to identify and examine the involved horse in accordance with this certificate, and to report the medical facts obtained by the examination to the insurance company. This Veterinary Certificate of Examination for Mortality Insurance is NOT a statement of insurability or serviceability for any intended use.

Horses being examined should be observed in motion. This certificate should be completed by the examining veterinarian to the best of his knowledge and ability as a licensed veterinarian.

I, _____ , do hereby certify that I am a graduate veterinarian and hold a current license to practice veterinary medicine in the State of _____ and that I have this date examined:

Name: _____ Breed: _____

Age: _____ Color: _____ Sex: _____ Tattoo: _____

Sire: _____ Dam: _____

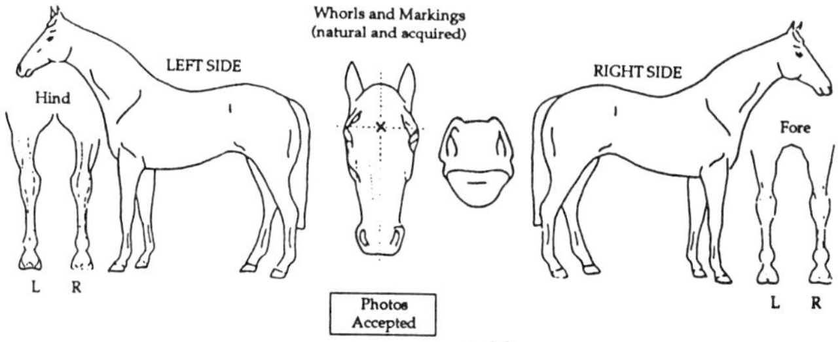

Whorls and Markings (natural and acquired)

LEFT SIDE — Hind L R   RIGHT SIDE — Fore L R

Photos Accepted

Owner: _____ Address: _____

Temperature: _____ °F   Pulse: _____ b/min   Respiration: _____ b/min

Is horse a bleeder?	Yes ☐	No ☐	NTMK ☐
Has horse been nerved?	Yes ☐	No ☐	NTMK ☐
Eyes clinically normal?	Yes ☐	No ☐	
Heart and lungs auscultated?	Yes ☐	No ☐	
If male, are both testicles palpable?	Yes ☐	No ☐	
Has horse been castrated?	Yes ☐	No ☐	

If so, when? _____

If surgery has been performed, has horse clinically recovered? Yes ☐ No ☐ *(Explain below)*

In your opinion, is there any clinical evidence of lameness, or significant conformational defects or other pathological conditions? Yes ☐ No ☐ *(Explain below)*

Does this horse manifest clinical evidence of contagious or infectious disease? Yes ☐ No ☐ *(Explain below)*

Any history or clinical evidence of other surgery? Yes ☐ No ☐ NTMK ☐
Any colic within last six months? Yes ☐ No ☐ NTMK ☐
If, mare, is she reported to be pregnant? Yes ☐ No ☐ NTMK ☐
Date of last pregnancy exam? _____

Any knowledge or clinical evidence of contagious or infectious disease on the premises within the last 60 days? Yes ☐ No ☐ *(Explain below)*

Any clinical evidence of objectionable vices or habits? Yes ☐ No ☐ *(Explain below)*

In your opinion or to your knowledge, are there any additional medical facts that should be brought to the attention of the company? Yes ☐ No ☐ *(Explain below)*

Has official EIA test been run? Yes ☐ No ☐
Date: _____ Results: _____ Lab: _____

If any surgery has been performed, describe type of surgery: _____

Explanation of abnormal findings and/or additional comments? _____

Date: _____ Time: _____ (of examination)

Signed: _____
           Veterinarian   Address: _____

Phone: _____

I certify that I have no knowledge contrary to the above statements.

Signed: _____
           Owner/Agent   Address: _____

Date: _____ Phone: _____

Figure 1. Sample mortality insurance certificate.

insurance company must be notified before treatment begins. If the veterinarian feels the animal's life is in danger, treatment may begin immediately. It is up to the owner to make all policy guidelines known to the practitioner. Without exception, the veterinarian and owner must follow the guidelines for appropriate care as described in the policy or risk claim denial.

Direct discussions between the insurance company or its adjustor and the veterinarian early in the treatment process can prevent costly misunderstandings. Before treatment is begun the insurance company may ask for a history of the animal and for an indication of intended treatment. The insurer may approve the attending veterinarian's treatment, ask for a second opinion, or ask that the animal be referred to another veterinarian or clinic.

The veterinarian should note that if the services are associated with third-party liability, depending on the client's ability to pay, the practitioner may have to finance care until the client can recover from the liable party. In some instances this will depend on the client's ability to win a legal dispute regarding liability.

EUTHANASIA

In the event the attending veterinarian determines the horse cannot be returned to good health, euthanasia may become an option. In almost all instances, the company holding the insurance policy must agree prior to humane destruction for a claim to be valid. Most insurance companies recognize the American Association of Equine Practitioners guidelines for determining when humane destruction is indicated. The veterinarian should consider the following points: Is the condition chronic or incurable? With respect to the immediate condition, is the prognosis for life hopeless? Is the horse a hazard to itself or its handlers? Will the horse require continuous medication for relief of pain for the remainder of its life? Justification for euthanasia of a horse for humane reasons should be based on medical, not economic, considerations; the same criteria should be applied to all horses regardless of age, sex, or potential value.

In some cases local laws will play a part in the destruction of an injured or sick horse. Under some state statutes, failure to end the life of a suffering animal is a misdemeanor. Veterinarians need to familiarize themselves with the local and state laws in their area. This information is available from local animal control facilities, humane societies, or the clerk of the court.

Once the decision has been made to euthanize an insured horse, telephone authorization should be obtained from the insurance company's representative. The patient's records should contain the authorizing person's name, phone number, and the date and time of the conversation.

THE POSTMORTEM EXAMINATION

In order to process an owner's claim a necropsy is usually required by the insurance company. Practitioners should be aware that, even though a company has asked for a necropsy, serious problems of liability can occur if the owner's property rights to the animal's body are not respected. In most cases the carcass should not be examined or disposed of without an owner's authorization. In addition, the intentional, arbitrary, or negligent disposal of an animal that has been undergoing veterinary care is likely to produce questions regarding its death.

When the cause of death is known, the postmortem examination can include only those areas pertinent to the cause of death. Where the cause of death is less certain, most adjustors and companies require that specific procedures be followed and samples taken. If the practitioner lacks the time or expertise necessary for a thorough postmortem examination, that fact should be made clear. The insurance company may offer suggestions or ask for referral to a diagnostic center.

Expenses for specialists, additional postmortem examinations, and tests beyond what would be considered normal are the prerogative and, in most cases, the financial responsibility of the insurance company.

PREPARATION

At the time of the postmortem examination, the insurance company or adjustor may stipulate which samples will be taken and what procedures will be followed (see p. 344). The veterinarian should be prepared to supply the following information:

- Date and name of person or agency contacted before performing necropsy.
- Date and time of necropsy.
- Names of witnesses to necropsy, if any.
- Description of the animal, including any photographs of characteristic features of the animal. This may include tattoos, ear tags, brands, or other markings. Written statements and tape-recorded observations made during the necropsy are helpful. A video-

TABLE 1. MATERIALS FOR POSTMORTEM SAMPLE COLLECTION AND IDENTIFICATION
Magic Markers
Pint and quart size glass jars with lids
Aluminum foil to seal jars
10% formalin
Whirlpack plastic bags
Styrofoam containers
Swabs with transport media for certain bacteriology and virology specimens

If the cause of death is not readily apparent, extra tissue samples should be retained for future toxicology studies (see Table 2).

TABLE 2. TISSUE AND FLUIDS NEEDED FOR TOXICOLOGIC STUDIES
Urine (all available or 500 ml)
Serum with clot removed
Heart blood (250–500 ml)
Other body fluids
Brain (½ in formalin and ½ frozen)
Liver (0.5–1.0 kg)
Spleen (0.5–1.0 kg)
Heart (0.5–1.0 kg)
Stomach contents (1 kg)
Intestinal contents (1 kg)
Intact eyeball
Lung (1 kg)

Additional nonanimal samples of feed, water, bedding, suspect poisonous plants, and miscellaneous specimens, such as suspect chemicals and pesticides, are helpful. After the samples have been retained, an owner release form should be prepared so the diagnostic information can be sent to the insurance company.

tape of the necropsy is an excellent method of recording the exact findings.

The insurer may also ask for a recent health history. The practitioner should be prepared to provide the following information:

- Dates and types of vaccinations administered.
- Medication records for the past 30 days.
- History of clinical signs, behavior, contact with other animals.
- Conditions of surroundings, evidence of struggle, or other predeath signs.

When performing a necropsy it is critical that the veterinarian have the proper materials available for sample collection (Tables 1 and 2).

LEGAL RESPONSIBILITY

Insurance companies rarely sue veterinarians unless the insurance company uncovers intentional misrepresentations or an agreement of misrepresentation between the veterinarian and policyholder. This misrepresentation may occur during the pre-insurance examination or any time thereafter. Veterinarians' understanding of their role in equine insurance will greatly reduce their liability exposure.

Supplemental Readings

Edwards, W. C., and Johnson, B. J.: Equine insurance examinations. Equine Pract. 8(6):19–22, 1986.
The veterinary role in equine insurance. American Association of Equine Practitioners Newsletter, September 1985.
Henderson, A.: Equine insurance. Large Anim. Vet. 44(5):17, 1989.
Rains, J., and Allen, L.: Choosing equine insurance: Ratings and reputation count. Mod. Horse Breed. 6(3):27, 1989.
Rains, J., and Allen, L.: Reading the fine print. Mod. Horse Breed. 6(4):28, 1989.
Rains, J., and Allen, L.: Variations on the theme of insurance. Mod. Horse Breed. 6(2):26, 1989.

Purchase Examination of the Performance Horse

Glenn F. Anderson, BROKEN ARROW, OKLAHOMA

This chapter addresses the philosophy, intent, and performance of purchase examinations. Evaluation of stallions and mares as breeding animals will not be discussed.

A purchase examination is most often requested by the buyer prior to purchase of the horse, but veterinarians may be asked to evaluate a horse recently acquired so that the owner can make an informed decision regarding the horse's future. Problems may have surfaced that prompt the new owner to attempt to return the horse to the seller. For example, the horse may exhibit lameness, respiratory noise, ocular problems, or other problems that were not apparent to the buyer at the time of purchase. The old axiom, "Let the buyer beware!" is being challenged in the courts of many states. These situations can prove very challenging for the veterinarian. Therefore, it is important that the veterinarian understand the buyer's or owner's expectations of the purchase examination. These expectations, and the limitations of the examination, should be discussed with the buyer to avoid future misunderstandings and litigation against the examiner. The examining veterinarian should have direct communication with the buyer, as agents for both the buyer and seller may misinterpret or intentionally misinform the buyer in an attempt to secure their commission.

The purchaser must understand that horses do not pass or fail purchase examinations. The purpose of the examination should be to discover existing or potential medical problems and to interpret them in light of the horse's intended use. This enables the potential buyer to make an informed decision regarding purchase of this individual horse. The examining veterinarian must be familiar with the horse's intended use before he or she can interpret the significance of the examination findings. If the veterinarian has no knowledge or experience with a particular breed or sport, he or she should decline the opportunity to examine the horse. A veterinarian unaware of the breed association's rules can easily be placed in a compromising position, leading to misunderstandings, disappointments, embarrassments, and litigation. It is far better to recognize limitations and decline the examination than to have shortcomings pointed out in a court of law by the plaintiff's attorney. It is not the veterinarian's responsibility to determine the suitability of a horse for a given use. It is, however, this author's opinion that veterinarians have a responsibility to discuss a potentially dangerous situation, as veterinarians are increasingly being held liable for human injury inflicted on owners by their horses. The prospective buyer should be made aware that an aggressive, undisciplined horse could inflict serious injury on an inexperienced child or others. Many first-time owners are not aware of these potential dangers, and the seller often is not the best source of this information.

Two areas of particular concern are whether the horse has been in regular work at the intended use prior to examination, and whether or not the horse is under any medications that could influence the examination findings. There are various ways to address these concerns. The seller may be asked to sign a statement regarding previous exercise history and nonadministration of medications. Drug testing may be undertaken, realizing the limitations regarding intra-articular and undetectable medications. The horse may be placed in the purchaser's or examining veterinarian's care for a mutually agreed-upon period of time prior to the examination. This is the best option, and 72 hours is the minimum time period recommended. Liability questions must be addressed before this option is chosen. Insurance for full mortality and loss of use is available on a short-term basis to cover the buyer or examining veterinarian. It must be recognized that many chronic lameness problems seemingly resolve with rest only to recur when the horse is put back to work. If a horse must be examined after a significant period of inactivity, the purchaser should be made aware of the risks involved.

Veterinarians engaged in purchase examinations should develop a thorough and systematic approach to examination of the performance horse. A routine should be established to avoid overlooking any existing or potential problems that could adversely affect the horse at its intended use. Modern technology does not substitute for a thorough clinical evaluation.

Ideally, the examination should begin after the horse has been allowed to stand in the stall overnight rather than after it has been warmed up, as many lameness problems improve as the horse is exercised and are most noticeable when the horse is first brought out of its stall in the morning. It is not the purpose of this chapter to offer a checklist for purchase examinations; however, several points need to be made. Every square inch of the horse's exterior should be examined visually and manually, with emphasis on symmetry, swelling, swelling of joints or synovial sheaths, pain on digital palpation, and areas of increased heat. The mouth, nares, ears, eyes, anus, sheath or vagina, and other body orifices should be observed for abnormal odor or discharge. The eyes should be examined and any deviations from normal noted. Remember to assess vision, as a blind eye may appear grossly normal. The thorax should be thoroughly auscultated before and after work, as should the larynx and trachea. The horse's response to flexion, extension, torsion, and palpation of accessible joints should be noted.

The feet must be carefully evaluated, as modern acrylics and horseshoeing techniques can disguise many serious injuries or defects such as quarter cracks, club feet, and dished anterior hoof walls. Good quality hoof testers applied conscientiously are mandatory. Horses that are shod with pads cannot be properly evaluated until shoes and pads have been removed. If this is the case, the feet should be evaluated after the horse has been observed on the longe line and at

70 / PURCHASE EXAMINATION OF THE PERFORMANCE HORSE—*continued*

EQUINE VETERINARY ASSOCIATES

9101 S. Garnett · Tulsa, OK 74133 · (918) 252-7407

RECORD OF EXAMINATION OF A HORSE FOR PURCHASE   TICKET #

Issued: _____Name_____ _____Address_____

At the request of _____Name_____ I have examined the horse described

below, the property of _____Name_____ _____Address_____ at ___Place of Exam___

on ___Date & Time___. Intended use: _____

Horse: Name _____ Breed/Type _____ Sex _____

Color _____ Height _____ Weight _____ Age _____ Registration #/Tattoo _____

Brands/Acquired Markings _____

WHORLS/WHITE MARKINGS

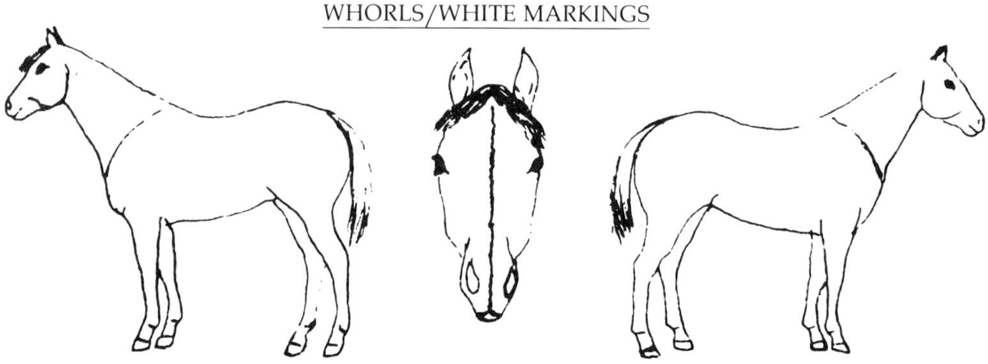

Int. Parasite Control _____ Immunizations _____ E.I.A. _____
At the time of the examination, the following findings were noted: _____

_____
_____
_____
_____
_____
_____
_____
_____
_____
_____
_____
_____
_____
_____
_____
_____

The above statements are based on the clinical exam performed on this date. If the purchaser requires a warranty regarding non administration of drugs prior to examination, exact height and weight, freedom of vices, performance ability, etc., he should obtain such from the seller as these matters are not the responsibility of the veterinarian.

Signed _____

Figure 1. Sample form for use in purchase examination.

work. If the seller will not grant permission for shoes to be removed, this should be noted, and the buyer should be aware that the examination will be compromised. The horse should be observed moving in both directions on the longe line over safe footing. It is ideal to have both deep footing and hard surface available, as some problems are exacerbated by one, while others will worsen on the other. An incline is useful, as certain lamenesses, such as high suspensary desmitis and intermittent upward fixation of the patella, are much more obvious when the horse trots downhill.

After the horse has been observed on the longe line, it should be worked at its intended use in harness. Many problems such as subtle lameness, inspiratory noise, and anhydrosis become apparent only during work. The horse should be worked at least until the heart rate doubles from resting level. After work, it should be cooled and reexamined on the longe line. Flexion tests are usually done after the initial work on the longe line.

Additional diagnostic tests such as radiography, endoscopy, ultrasonography, electrocardiography, electromyography, rectal examination, hematology, and various enzyme or chemistry assays should be done according to the buyer's wishes and the clinical indications for their need. If additional diagnostic tests are recommended by the examiner but declined by the buyer or refused by the seller, this should be noted in the record.

Radiography is the most commonly employed and potentially confusing of the ancillary tests used in purchase evaluations. Questions frequently arise as to which areas should be routinely radiographed, how many views are necessary to properly evaluate the area, and what constitutes an incidental finding rather than a clinically relevant lesion. I do not routinely recommend radiography as part of a purchase examination unless the clinical evaluation indicates a need for it. Interpretation of radiographic changes is very difficult in the absence of clinical signs. This is particularly true with regard to the navicular bone and the distal joints of the tarsus. Many useful athletes are needlessly condemned by clinically silent radiographic "lesions" found at the time of purchase examination. If radiographs are taken, they must include sufficient views of the area being evaluated. Radiographs must be of diagnostic quality and be properly labeled. Poor quality radiographs are worse than none at all, and do nothing to elevate the veterinarian's public image.

Endoscopic findings must be evaluated with caution, as recent work with video endoscopes and high-speed treadmills have questioned the validity of endoscopic evaluation at rest. These limitations should be explained to the potential buyer. The seller's permission is required for any diagnostic procedure. If the buyer requests tests not available to the examining veterinarian, every effort should be made to refer the buyer to a facility where the tests can be performed.

Recording and reporting the findings of the purchase examination are of utmost importance. I use a printed report form for this purpose (Fig. 1). A copy of the form is given to the buyer, and a copy is retained for the hospital files. The horse is identified on the form, the preventive medicine history or lack of same is noted, witnesses to the examination are listed, and examination findings are recorded as the examination proceeds. All deviations from normal (including blemishes and conformation defects) are noted. After the examination and the form are completed, all findings are discussed with the buyer. Veterinarians are usually asked at this point whether or not the horse should be purchased. The veterinarian does not have the responsibility to answer this question. The prospective buyer may be advised to use a balance sheet concept to make this decision. The buyer should list all of the positive things about the horse, for example, size, color, training, temperament, cost, and the like, on one side of the sheet and all of the negative points on the other. The buyer should then be able to make an informed decision regarding purchase of the horse. Remember that the information generated during the course of the purchase examination is confidential and should not be discussed with others unless the buyer has granted permission.

Veterinarians are often asked to examine a horse owned by one of their clients. A conflict of interest can arise if the buyer is not aware of the situation or if the seller, buyer, or veterinarian is not comfortable with the arrangement. If the examining veterinarian has prior medical knowledge of the horse, this should be discussed with both buyer and seller. If the seller does not wish to disclose this information to the buyer, I would decline to examine the horse.

Purchase examinations performed in a conscientious manner provide opportunities to showcase the veterinarian's knowledge and expertise, as well as an opportunity to elevate the public image of equine practice. They can also invite disaster. Good communication and record keeping, a thorough and unhurried examination, and honesty are the fundamentals for successful purchase examinations.

International Transport of Horses

Ralph C. Knowles, SALISBURY, MARYLAND

The development of jet aircraft has allowed people and horses to move extensively internationally. Horses are truly an international commodity. It is not uncommon for horse owners, brokers, and transport companies to seek animal health guidance and services from veterinarians who are equine practitioners. The following paragraphs are written from the perspective of a veterinarian practicing in the United States. The major concerns can be separated into those involving Equidae intended for importation into the United States and those involving equine stock offered for export to foreign countries.

IMPORTATION CONSIDERATIONS

The Veterinary Services section of the Animal and Plant Health Inspection Services, United States Department of Agriculture (USDA), has the responsibility of regulating the health requirements for Equidae being imported or exported. A summary of equine import requirements follows.

In general, all horses to be imported require a properly executed health certificate either signed by or endorsed by a salaried veterinarian of the country of origin. The health certificate should state that the horses have:

1. been in that country for 60 days immediately preceding importation. If the horses have not been in the country for 60 days, they are to be accompanied by a like certificate issued by a full-time salaried veterinary officer of the national government of each country in which the horses have been during the 60 days immediately preceding shipment to the United States;
2. been inspected and found free of contagious diseases and, insofar as can be determined, exposure thereto during the 60 days immediately preceding exportation;
3. not been vaccinated with live or attenuated or inactivated vaccine during the 14 days immediately preceding exportation;
4. not been on premises where African horse sickness, dourine, glanders, surra, epizootic lymphangitis, ulcerative lymphangitis, equine piroplasmosis, equine infectious anemia (EIA), contagious equine metritis (CEM), or Venezuelan equine encephalomyelitis (VEE) has occurred during the 60 days immediately preceding exportation, nor have these diseases occurred on any adjoining premises during this same period of time;
5. not been in a country where CEM is known to exist, nor have had any contact, breeding or otherwise, with horses from such a country, for the 12 months preceding exportation. The countries considered to have CEM are United Kingdom, Ireland, France, West Germany, Italy, Belgium, Austria, Denmark, Sweden, Japan, Netherlands, Norway, Yugoslavia, and Switzerland.

Horses from Mexico originating from known fever tick areas shall be chute inspected and treated once with an approved acaricide if free of fever ticks. Horses found to be infested with fever ticks will be denied entry. Horses from countries other than Canada and Mexico shall require quarantine at a USDA-approved quarantine center and must test negative for dourine, glanders, equine piroplasmosis, and EIA within a minimum time of 3 days, except that:

1. African horses require 60 days in quarantine to prevent the introduction of African horse sickness.
2. Horses from CEM countries over 731 days of age, except geldings, require negative tests and treatment prior to importation. A permit issued by the import staff is required along with additional testing and treatment in approved states after the federal quarantine release.
3. Horses from South America (except Argentina), Central America, and the West Indies shall spend a minimum of 7 days of quarantine with temperatures taken twice daily to detect a febrile response that could be attributed to VEE.
4. A pre-entry screening test for equine piroplasmosis is recommended for all horses except those from Canada.

As may be appreciated, certain changes in the animal health status can occur in foreign countries. It is, therefore, advisable to consult with the federal veterinarian in your state concerning current animal health requirements relating to horse stock offered for importation into the United States.

EXPORTATION CONSIDERATIONS

Horses and other Equidae to be exported from the United States must be examined and certified by an accredited veterinarian and be moved to a USDA-designated export facility. Details concerning these export qualifying steps follow.

An accredited veterinarian is a licensed veterinarian who has completed certain steps to qualify for approval by the USDA to do animal health regulatory work. For animals offered for export from the United States, the USDA complies with the animal health requirements of the receiving foreign country. Therefore, before going to the farm or stable to examine an animal intended for export, it is necessary to contact the federal veterinarian in charge in that state to determine what laboratory tests or vaccinations are required by the country of destination.

All animals intended for exportation to a foreign country other than Mexico or Canada shall be accompanied from the state of origin of the export movement to the port of embarkation by a U.S. origin health certificate. All animals intended for exportation to Mexico or Canada shall be accompanied from the state of origin of the export movement to the border of the United States by a U.S. origin health certificate. The origin health certificate shall certify that the animals were inspected within 30 days prior to the date of the movement of the animals for export and were found to be "sound, healthy, and free from evidence of communicable disease and exposure thereto." The origin health certificate shall be endorsed by an authorized Veterinary Services veterinarian in the state of origin, and shall include any test results added by such authorized Veterinary Services veterinarian (any added test results shall be initialed by such authorized Veterinary Services veterinarian). The origin health certificate shall individually identify the animals in the shipment as to species, breed, sex, and age, and, if applicable, shall also show registration name and number, tattoo markings, or other natural or acquired markings.

All animals in each export shipment, except animals intended for export to Mexico or Canada, shall have been inspected and tested prior to the movement of the export shipment to the export inspection facility. All animals in each export shipment intended for export to Mexico or Canada shall have been inspected and tested prior to the movement of the animals from the state of origin.

All samples for tests required for exportation of animals shall be taken by an inspector or an accredited veterinarian in the state of origin of the export movement. Such samples shall be taken and tests made within the 30 days prior to the date of movement of the animals for export from the premises of origin. The origin health certificate accompanying animals shall include a statement from the issuing accredited veterinarian or inspector that the means of conveyance or container has been cleaned and disinfected with a disinfectant approved by the USDA since last used for animals and prior to loading, or that the carrier or container has not previously been used in transporting animals.

The USDA maintains a list of approved ports of embarkation. To determine the location of the most practical port for a given shipment the practitioner should contact the federal veterinarian in charge for his or her state. Most horse owners engage a broker or transport agent when moving animals internationally. These agents are usually located in port cities such as New York City, Miami, and Los Angeles. Because they are knowledgeable regarding the requirements of moving animals internationally, it is advisable to communicate with them in advance of an intended shipment concerning shipping times and availability of space on international carriers or in animal quarantine stations.

Supplemental Reading

U.S. Government Document: Code of Federal Regulations, Title 9: Animals and Animal Products, Part 91, Jan. 1, 1988.

Clinical Field Trials

John W. Paul, SOMERVILLE, NEW JERSEY

Animal drugs are regulated by the Food and Drug Administration/Center for Veterinary Medicine (FDA/CVM), referred to herein as the Agency. This authority was vested in the Agency by the Food, Drug and Cosmetic Act of 1938 and its various amendments (the Act). The original Act required that adequate data be submitted to the Agency prior to marketing a new animal drug to establish the safety of the new drug under the labeled conditions of use. Subsequently, this mandate was expanded by the Kefauver-Harris Amendments of 1962 to also require the establishment of efficacy of a new drug prior to FDA marketing approval. In the case of new drugs intended for use in food animals, the Agency also requires substantial evidence that harmful drug or metabolic residues are not present in edible tissues for human consumption. At this time, horses are not generally used for human food in the United States. If this custom should change, then extensive drug residue studies in horses would be required for new drugs. Currently, new drugs for horses are labeled with the warning, *"Do not use in horses intended for food."*

The Act requires that the efficacy of a new animal drug be established in at least two adequate and well-controlled trials; one of these trials is to be a clinical trial in at least three different geographic locations where the new drug is evaluated under intended conditions of use. In addition to the efficacy data gathered in clinical trials, clinical investigators are required to carefully monitor and evaluate animals treated with the new drug for expected or unexpected adverse reactions. Clinical trials also serve to evaluate the feasibility of label instructions and use of the product under field and clinic conditions. Shipment of the investigational drug for use in these trials must be under the provisions of an exemption from the Act referred to as an Investigational New Animal Drug Application (INADA). The Act prohibits interstate shipments of new animal drugs for investigational use unless certain conditions are met, such as proper labeling, proper records, and the like.

Once the drug sponsor has collected, analyzed, and assembled the safety and efficacy data as well as information relating to components and composition, manufacturing and quality control procedures, an environmental impact analysis, tissue residues if required, and a draft label, the New Animal Drug Application (NADA) is submitted to the FDA/CVM for exhaustive and critical review. The sponsor is not permitted to market the new drug until the Agency has determined that all available data support the safety and efficacy of the drug under intended conditions of use. At that time the final labeling is agreed upon and the sponsor is notified in writing that the NADA is approved. Subsequently, the Agency's decision is published in the Federal Register and the approval becomes officially listed in the Code of Federal Regulations. This Agency approval process applies not only to new chemical entities but also to any change in formulation, manufacturing process, packaging, or use conditions.

With the foregoing overview of the regulatory process of new animal drugs, the responsibilities of veterinarians as clinical investigators will be outlined. It should be clear that the entire process of new drug development, including clinical investigations by independent investigators, is strictly regulated by the FDA/CVM.

SETTING UP THE CLINICAL TRIAL

The first involvement a practitioner or clinician may have with the drug development process might be to provide expert advice to the sponsor on protocol design for a meaningful and realistic clinical trial. The protocol may be submitted by the sponsor to the FDA/CVM for comments; if it is agreed that the protocol will result in the collection of adequate data to allow the Agency to conclusively review the NADA, the sponsor holds discussions with the prospective clinical investigators to determine if an investigator is fully qualified and has the ability to conduct the trial. It is the sponsor's responsibility to be certain that each investigator fully understands the protocol and the federal regulations that apply to his or her involvement in the trial. At this point a written agreement between the sponsor and the investigator must be drawn up, specifying that the veterinarian is able and willing to conduct the trial strictly in accordance with the protocol. Only after reaching this agreement, which includes the number of animals to be used in the study, and signing of a Statement of Clinical Investigation and notifying the FDA/CVM of claimed investigational exemption for a New Animal Drug, is the sponsor permitted to ship test substances for the trial.

The test substances will depend on the type of control to be used in the clinical trial. The Act provides for three types of controls: (1) historical controls, in which the outcome of a disease is highly predictable (for example, rabies leads to death); (2) active controls, in which the new drug is compared to a currently approved drug; and (3) placebo controls, in which the new drug is compared to the administration of an inactive look-alike substance, or untreated controls are used in lieu of placebo. If historical or untreated controls are used or if the animal is to serve as its own control, for example in anthelmintic trials, where fecal egg counts are expected to be different before and after treatment, adequate supplies of only the new drug are provided to the investigator. With active controls or placebo control trials, the identity of the substances must be disguised (blinded) to the clinical evaluator. If the test drug looks exactly like the active control or placebo, the packages of the two substances are labeled A and B or 1 and 2 and are administered according to a random numbers scheme. If the test substance looks different from the active or placebo control, blinding is accomplished by another qualified person administering the test substances according to a random scheme while the clinical investigator evaluates the animals and test results and collects data, without knowing which treatment was administered.

CONDUCTING THE TRIAL

The clinical trial is initiated by the investigator selecting only the animal patients as provided in the protocol and treating the animals as described above. For ethical and legal reasons, the investigator should fully discuss the trial with the owners of the animals and receive written and informed consent to allow their animals to be entered in the trial; financial considerations, if any, should also be agreed upon. No claims can be made as to efficacy or safety of the New Animal Drug. Only animals owned by persons who agree to submit the animals for follow-up examinations and agree to manage the animals as specified by the protocol should be entered in the trial. If adverse reactions occur, the sponsor monitor should be notified immediately. Follow-up evaluations must be performed on schedule and all data must be collected. If case report forms are used, they must be filled out correctly and completely and confirmed by the signature of the investigator. A designated monitor for the sponsor is required to visit the test site at least once and preferably several times during the trial. The monitor should review each case report form for completeness and accuracy and to make sure the protocol is being followed precisely. Deviation from the protocol could invalidate the trial, causing lost time in the approval process and, in severe cases, possible FDA/CVM action against the investigator. The investigator must maintain a drug inventory with records of when and how much drug was received and used. The monitor will also inventory the test supplies and reconcile the inventory with the amounts shipped to and used by the investigator. Also, the monitor will make sure that all adverse reactions are fully documented, evaluated, and the exact cause determined, if possible. Investigators should also be prepared for visits by FDA/CVM inspectors during or after the trial for verification of protocol adherence, proper data collection, and accountability of test substance records.

CONCLUDING THE TRIAL

The clinical investigator should conclude the trial within the time frame agreed upon in the Sponsor/Investigator Agreement. All case report forms or other reports should be audited by the investigator for accuracy and completeness, and submitted to the sponsor in a timely fashion. The investigator is required by the Act to maintain a file of all case reports, including supportive data for 2 years after termination of the investigation or approval of the NADA, whichever is later. All clinical supplies must be reconciled with the amounts shipped and used in the trial; remaining supplies should be returned to the sponsor or disposed of per instructions of the sponsor. An FDA/CVM inspector may show up to review records long after the trial has been concluded, so careful record keeping is important for the clinical investigator.

CONCLUSION

Clinical trials are a very important part of the development and approval of new animal drugs. Veterinarians who participate in the scientific endeavor of clinical trials as part of new drug development must realize their responsibility and be prepared to adhere to the protocol, keep accurate records, and use the experimental drug only as provided in the protocol. Most clinical investigators find their work to be challenging and professionally rewarding; however, those who do not play by the rules are often frustrated and embarrassed.

Veterinary Services for Horse Shows

Michael T. Martin, COLLEGE STATION, TEXAS
Leon Scrutchfield, COLLEGE STATION, TEXAS

Veterinarians are involved in at least two areas of service and responsibility at horse shows, as official show veterinarians or attending veterinarians, and may be involved in three additional areas of activity: enforcement of the Horse Protection Act of 1970, collection of samples for drug and medication testing, and enforcement of state regulatory requirements.

OFFICIAL SHOW VETERINARIAN

The official show veterinarian is employed by and responsible to show management. The show veterinarian's primary function is to serve as professional consultant and advisor on all veterinary matters affecting the show. The veterinarian must have an in-depth understanding of all show rules and any state or federal regulations pertaining to veterinary services for the show. All horse shows are governed by a set of rules that dictate or affect veterinary services. The rule book of the American Horse Show Association (AHSA) clearly states the duties of the official show veterinarian. Other governing rule books are likely to be less specific. Not all rule books contain the same veterinary requirements, and more than one rule book may be in effect at a show. Therefore, the veterinarian must determine from management what rules pertain to a particular show and must know what the duties and responsibilities of the position are. The American Association of Equine Practitioners' (AAEP) *Guide for Veterinary Service and Judging of Equestrian Events,* 4th edition, suggests the following guidelines for official veterinarians:

1. Learn in advance which rule books govern the show, then understand and strictly adhere to all applicable rules contained therein. Give special attention to all drug and medication rules.

2. Do not assume or accept duties or responsibilities that are not specifically those of a veterinarian and of the veterinary position in which you are serving.

3. When called into a show ring to observe a horse for soundness, observe several horses in the same manner in addition to the one under question by the judge. Do not place a hand on a horse being observed or follow any other procedure that will allow spectators to conclude which horse and what ailment is suspected. Erroneous conclusions based on such action can be financially disastrous for the owner of the horse.

4. Give a horse the benefit of the doubt regarding soundness in the show ring, but be consistent and do not be lenient because it is in first or second place or in a stake class.

5. Maintain liaison with the show steward and judges and be available if your service in the show ring is requested by either.

6. Discuss the soundness and qualities of competing horses only with the judge and then only when requested. You will be sufficiently misquoted even without contributing information for the gossip mill.

7. Provide or allow vigorous appropriate treatment for all horses with minor injuries or problems that may safely continue to show.

8. Be fair, consistent, and firm in issuing *scratch certificates* and do not accept fees for issuing them. Owners for various reasons may request a scratch certificate on a horse which if used entitles them to receive a refund on the horse's entry fee. Show management expects and wants as few horses scratched as possible. Scratch certificates should be issued only when in the professional judgment of the official veterinarian a horse for reasons of injury or health is not in satisfactory physical condition to show. There are no other considerations.

9. Anticipate, be prepared, and have show management adequately equipped and prepared to promptly care for horses with broken legs, freak accidents, acute colic, and other emergency situations in the show ring and on the show grounds.

10. Establish liaison at once with all other veterinarians assigned to or practicing on the show grounds and ensure appropriate coordination for all veterinary services.

11. If responsible for any emergency service, leave word with show management so that you can be reached at any time.

12. In communications with show management, establish in advance your compensation and responsibilities. The AHSA rule book indicates that an official veterinarian should receive consideration and remuneration comparable to

that paid other show officials. If the intent is to provide free service for a benefit or charity show, the preferred procedure is to have management compensate you in full for service and you in turn pass the amount to the charity as a personal contribution. This places the worth of your time and services in proper perspective for all concerned and also gives appropriate credit for your charitable contribution.

13. Do not drink alcoholic beverages, including beer, while on duty or during show hours. As an exhibitor put it, "Even a smell is too much because when I smell liquor on an official, I smell incompetence and irresponsibility."

14. Avoid argumentative discussion about your decisions with exhibitors. If one should press on embarrassingly, the show steward should be immediately advised so that he or she may remind the offender to maintain composure and comply with show rules.

15. Be cooperative and helpful to all other show officials and exhibitors, but remember which veterinary hat or hats you are wearing and do not assume or accept responsibilities other than those assigned to the office you represent. The veterinarian should keep the horse's welfare at the highest priority. This helps keep the sport in a highly competitive arena.

ATTENDING VETERINARIAN

The attending veterinarian has the role of private practitioner on the horse show grounds. This individual's responsibility is much the same as that of a practitioner on a race track who is employed by individual owners or trainers to examine and/or treat specific problems of show horses. Management of the individual show will usually contact a veterinarian who has some experience with show horses and list that person's name as being on call during the show. This is usually done as a courtesy to the exhibitors, who may be unfamiliar with the veterinary support in the area. The attending veterinarian should be prepared to provide the following information or services for a fee:

1. Examine and treat sick or injured horses.
2. Be available on a 24-hour call basis during the show, and be prepared to refer any horses requiring intensive care to a hospital.
3. Communicate treatment options to the owner or trainer so that the drug and medication rules of the specific horse show organizations can be followed.

The AAEP policy discourages dual roles, whereby one individual serves as both official veterinarian and attending veterinarian. However, at many shows the veterinarian is required to assume both roles as it is too expensive for management to contract with two different veterinarians.

TESTING VETERINARIAN

A testing veterinarian may be present at certain horse shows. Various equine breed associations and disciplines provide for periodic blood and/or urine testing to enforce their individual drug and medication rules. Contracts between associations and a specific veterinarian govern these services as to how and which animals are to be tested at a given show or event. A number of breed associations or disciplines have employed veterinarians to provide this service:

1. American Horse Shows Association
2. American Quarter Horse Association
3. American Paint Horse Association
4. Palomino Horse Breeders of America
5. Appaloosa Horse Club
6. Woman's Professional Rodeo Association

The AHSA represents 23 breeds of horses and/or disciplines of equestrian competition, and its Drug and Medication Program affects some 2500 horse shows and events in the United States annually. The AHSA testing program is the most extensive in the United States. More information can be gained by contacting John G. Lengel, DVM, Drugs and Medications Program, American Horse Shows Association, Inc., 3780 Ridge Mill Drive, Columbia, OH 43026; 800/633-2472.

OTHER VETERINARY ROLES

Veterinarians may be involved in horse shows as employees of the USDA or as a Designated Qualified Person under the Horse Protection Act. Public Law 91-540, the Horse Protection Act, was enacted in December 1970 and amended by Public Law 94-360 in July 1976. Congress intended this law to prevent the showing of sored Tennessee Walking Horses, but the Act protects all horses. Breeds with an animated gait (American Saddlebred, fox trotters, racing horses, Tennessee Walking Horses) are inspected by USDA representatives for evidence of violations of the Act.

The Act places several responsibilities on horse show management. The Act is enforced by veterinarians from the Animal and Plant Health Inspection Service of the USDA. The 1976 amendment provided for self-regulation by industry via the Designated Qualified Person (DQP) program. The DQP is licensed by horse industry associations. Veterinarians are eligible for licensing as a DQP if they are accredited in any state by the USDA and are (1) a member of the AAEP, (2) a large animal practitioner with substantial equine experience, and (3) knowledgeable about equine lameness caused by soring. Veterinarians responsible for enforcing the Act at a show should fully understand USDA rules and regulations. Information can be obtained from the USDA (APHIS), Federal Building, 6505 Belcrest Road, Hyattsville, MD 20782, or from the APHIS area office. By appointing a DQP and following his findings, show management is relieved of responsibility under the provisions of the Act.

Veterinarians representing a state or federal agency may be present at a show to enforce animal disease regulations. These veterinarians usually are under contract by show management to enforce entry requirements to the show grounds. The specific state or federal agency whose regulations govern entry to the grounds provides the rules, and the veterinarian or representative checks certificates of inspection, health certificates, or any laboratory test that may come under entry requirements for horse shows.

In summary, veterinary services for horse shows fall into one or a combination of the five areas of responsibility outlined above. It is important for the veterinarian at a given show to know the duties and the rules that must be followed. These responsibilities are very visible, and it is important that no conflict of interest arise when dual roles are accepted. Horse shows are an important aspect of the equine industry and a place where the equine practitioner can play a vital part.

Supplemental Readings

Guide for Veterinary Service and Judging of Equestrian Events, 3rd ed. Lexington, Kentucky, American Association of Equine Practitioners, 1984.

Guide for Veterinary Service and Judging of Equestrian Events, 4th ed. Lexington, Kentucky, American Association of Equine Practitioners, 1991, pp. 32–63.

The Veterinarian's Role in Racing

Richard H. Galley, WILLOW PARK, TEXAS

The veterinarian has occupied many roles in horse racing in the history of the sport. Initially this role was limited to the care of the race horse, but today it has been expanded to include other duties. While exceptions do exist, the role of the veterinarian in racing is usually either as a racetrack practitioner or as a regulatory veterinarian.

THE RACETRACK PRACTITIONER

The racetrack practitioner may expect to encounter the same array of medical problems as a practitioner in other types of equine practice, with racing injuries and conditions of the equine athlete predominating. When deciding on therapy, the racetrack practitioner must consider the rules of racing in a given racing jurisdiction. Often these rules, formulated by racing commissioners, preclude the use of certain modern therapeutic medications. The reasons for the prohibition of certain substances are varied. The medication may have properties that might alter the outcome of a race, allow an unfit or injured horse to race, or interfere with testing of post race samples of blood or urine. Prohibiting these types of medication on the racetrack is easily justified. Certain racing jurisdictions also prohibit other medications that do not possess the properties mentioned above and thereby place the practicing veterinarian in a difficult situation when deciding on a course of therapy.

The practitioner must adhere to the highest standards of professional and ethical practice while conforming to the rules of racing in a given racing jurisdiction. It is mandatory to be informed of the rules of racing, the clearance times of the medications that are permitted, and the capabilities of the racing chemist. This enables proper selection of medications and provision of correct advice to clients regarding medications and any possible rule violations. Communication between the practitioner and the regulatory veterinarians is vital to both the success of a controlled medication program and the optimal treatment of horses. Unfortunately, this communication is better in some jurisdictions than in others. The practitioner should also attempt to establish communications with the racing commissioners in the racing state. This serves not only to help educate the commissioners but also to avoid any undesirable conflicts in the medication rules when they are considered by the commission.

THE REGULATORY VETERINARIAN

The duties of the veterinarian who is involved in the regulatory aspect of the racing industry are usually divided into two categories: those of the racing commission or state veterinarian, and those of the association or track veterinarian.

THE RACING COMMISSION VETERINARIAN

The racing commission veterinarian or the "state veterinarian" administers the rules of racing as they concern veterinary medicine and advises the racing commission regarding rules of racing as they pertain to the medication and care of the racehorse. Many racing commission veterinarians have no previous experience in racing and are placed in the extremely difficult position of advising a group of individuals who rarely have any knowledge of medication as it pertains to the racehorse. Fortunately, organizations such as the American Association of Equine Practitioners provide expertise and assistance in these situations.

This advisory capacity becomes of particular importance as the laboratories of racing chemists become more proficient in detecting a larger number of substances for a much longer period of time after their administration. The commission veterinarian must be able to advise the commission intelligently regarding the detection of even a trace amount of a drug in a given sample. Questions such as "Was the drug present in an amount that was pharmacologically active?" and "Did the drug influence the outcome of the race?" must be addressed. The veterinarian must often obtain additional information in order to adequately address such questions. Communication with the racing chemist and laboratory personnel can ease the exchange of important information. The commission veterinarian must, however, keep in mind that one of the primary functions of all racing commissions is to ensure and preserve the integrity of racing.

The commission veterinarian is also in charge of the test barn, where responsibilities include the collection of the post race blood or urine samples from those horses designated by the racing officials, maintenance of security in the sampling procedure, proper identification of the samples, and assurance that the samples are transported to the testing laboratory in a safe and timely fashion. The commission veterinarian often is also responsible for the administration of the exercise-induced pulmonary hemorrhage (EIPH) or bleeder program. This might include the certification of the horses that are afflicted with EIPH, as well as supervision of the administration of the various EIPH medications permitted for use in almost all of the parimutual racing jurisdictions.

Further duties might include witnessing the required necropsy examination of any horses that die or are euthanized on the racetrack. This is required in an attempt to establish the cause of death for the racing commission. The horse must be properly identified and such portmortem samples taken as may be deemed necessary by the commission veterinarian.

The commission veterinarian must establish lines of communication with practicing veterinarians. While this is a responsibility of both parties, it is helpful if the practicing veterinarians feel that they may approach the commission veterinarian for advice or questions. Communication allows the commission veterinarian to fulfill the responsibility of informing the practicing veterinarian about the rules of racing that pertain to the practice of veterinary medicine.

THE ASSOCIATION VETERINARIAN

The racing association or track veterinarian is employed by the racetrack or the racing association that is sponsoring the race meet. The association or track veterinarian is usually mandated by state statute for a racetrack handling in excess of $100,000 daily. Considerable clinical experience and racing background are desirable attributes for this position. It should be pointed out that the American Association of Equine Practitioners considers it a conflict of interest for a veterinarian who is practicing on a given racetrack to act as the association veterinarian for the same track.

The primary responsibility of the association veterinarian is to ensure the health, soundness, and suitability of the horses entered to race. This necessitates the examination of every horse entered to race. In some jurisdictions this is done at the horse's stable in the morning hours prior to the race. In other jurisdictions the examination is conducted in the paddock area just before the horses are saddled. Emphasis should always be placed on the welfare of the horse by preventing an injury from occurring or worsening.

Decisions in this regard place the association veterinarian in a very difficult position, because the management will exert pressure to retain a full field of horses and thus maintain the greatest possible parimutuel handle. Thus, when the association veterinarian recommends the "scratching" or withdrawal of a horse that is unfit to race, it is often viewed with disfavor by the employer. Prior clinical and racing experience makes the justification of these decisions much easier.

The association veterinarian also is required to accompany the horses to the starting gate prior to the start of the race and to be available for advice and determination of racing suitability in the event of an accident at the starting gate. At the gate, the association veterinarian can also observe the horses following a period of warm-up for any lameness or unsoundness that may have become pronounced since the initial examination.

The association veterinarian directs the activities surrounding the care of an injured horse until it is removed from the racetrack and under the care of the practicing veterinarian. The association veterinarian often is first on the scene and may have to administer emergency therapy. This requires prior organization of emergency equipment and the availability of competent, previously trained personnel. Drugs, emergency equipment such as splinting devices, and a horse ambulance should be available at all times, enabling an immediate response at the site of a breakdown or racing injury. The association veterinarian and the practicing veterinarians should cooperate in handling and managing these injuries. In cases of breakdown injuries where humane considerations necessitate euthanasia, it is often the responsibility of the association veterinarian to perform the euthanasia. The decision as to whether euthanasia is necessary is often a difficult one. Factors such as the value of the horse, the insurance status of the horse (see p. xx), the severity of the injury, and the finality of the euthanasia must all be carefully considered. Communication and cooperation between the practitioner and the association veterinarian become very important in these situations.

Supplemental Reading

Guidelines for handling the acutely injured horse. In Guide to Veterinary Service and Judging of Equestrian Events. Lexington, Kentucky, American Association of Equine Practitioners, 1991.

Guide to Veterinary Service and Judging of Equestrian Events. Lexington, Kentucky, American Association of Equine Practitioners, 1991, pp. 78–89.

The Veterinarian's Responsibilities at Trail Rides

Terry D. Swanson, LITTLETON, COLORADO

Trail rides are organized to achieve a variety of objectives, commonly for pleasure, for competition, and to test endurance. Pleasure rides consist of 1 or more days of relatively nonstrenuous work by horses that may not be as well conditioned or prepared as horses competing in competitive or endurance rides. The veterinarian's responsibility is to protect each horse from being overstressed and to provide necessary veterinary care.

Competitive rides are conducted over a specific trail and must be completed in a specified amount of time. They may be 1 to 3 days in duration. The work load is generally greater than in pleasure riding but less than in endurance riding. The horses are judged on their soundness, conditioning, and other criteria established by the ride management or sanctioning group. In addition to protecting and caring for the horses, a veterinarian is also part of the judging team. Usually it is not reasonable for one veterinarian to perform both roles.

Endurance rides cover a specific trail of 50 to 100 miles. The horse that finishes in the shortest time in an acceptable condition is the winner. Veterinary responsibilities include control and protection of each horse's stress levels and providing necessary veterinary care.

To be certain that the best veterinary care is provided, a veterinarian who is knowledgeable about the type of ride must be involved in the management and planning of such rides. Adequate veterinary care of trail horses requires careful and detailed planning to ensure that essential personnel and materials will be available in remote locations. Four-wheel-drive vehicles

TABLE 1. EQUIPMENT AND MEDICATIONS REQUIRED BY THE VETERINARY TEAM AT A TRAIL RIDE

Equipment
Twitch
Towels
Halter and lead
Stethoscope
Thermometer
Refractometer
Syringes and needles
IV catheters
Stomach tube and pump
Bucket, cup, and brush
IV tubes
Bandage material (including splint)

Medication
Water (drinking and cooling)
Intravenous electrolyte fluid (40 liters)
Oral electrolytes
Ice (in extreme heat)
Mineral oil
Local anesthetics
Surgical pack and suture materials
Ophthalmic medication
Wound medications
Injectable medications:
    Analgesics
    Antibiotics
    Sedatives
    Corticosteroids
    Calcium solution
    Nonsteroidal anti-inflammatories
        Phenylbutazone
        Flunixin meglumine
Dioctyl sodium sulfosuccinate (DSS)
Euthanasia solution

---

or pack animals may be used to transport personnel and equipment. Preride arrangements for hauling sick and injured animals from remote regions are also important. A communication system for members of the veterinary team is helpful to relay information about individuals that are being closely monitored. Table 1 lists suggested equipment and medications.

MONITORING STRESS

The veterinarian may have several roles, especially on a small ride, including management, trail layout, monitoring the stress levels of each horse, treating sick horses, and scoring or judging the performance of the horses on the ride. The most vital of these roles are monitoring and controlling stress levels and providing therapy. The ride management must understand that these are the veterinarian's primary responsibilities. To be sure the ride will not be disrupted, to allow adequate monitoring, and to treat as needed, the veterinary responsibilities must be handled by a veterinary team.

The team consists of one to several veterinarians and a host of technically trained individuals who can monitor heart rate, respiratory rate, and body temperature, make observations, and assist with intensive care. The number of team members depends on the number of horses on the ride, the stressfulness of the ride, the remoteness of checkpoints, and environmental conditions such as heat and humidity.

The goal of the veterinary team is to identify significantly stressed horses and rest or remove them from competition before they become fatigued. Identification of the stressed horse is based on the evaluation of the heart rate recovery at rest stops and close observation of the clinical attitude of each horse on the trail or at rest stops.

Signs of Stress

The heart rate recovery during rest periods is affected by the horse's preride physical condition, the difficulty of the ride just prior to the checkpoint, and the environmental temperature and humidity. Horses that are able to cope with the stresses will have a heart rate of less than 70 beats per minute within 10 to 15 minutes of reaching a checkpoint.

Failure to recover is an indication of serious stress, and the horse must be further evaluated before it is allowed to continue on the trail. The exact parameters will vary according to the difficulty of the remaining trail and the environmental conditions. The clinical signs of excessive stress or fatigue include a change of mental attitude indicated by a lack of interest in surroundings, lack of appetite, lack of thirst, loss of intestinal activity for more than 30 minutes, abdominal pain, loss of anal tone, a respiratory rate higher than the heart rate, body temperature over 103° F (39.4°C), muscle fasciculation and trembling, unwillingness to move, an incoordinated or irregular gait, absence of sweat or the presence of dry, sticky sweat, injected mucus membranes, capillary refill time greater than 2.5 seconds, and synchronous diaphragmatic flutter. A respiratory rate greater than heart rate is especially significant if the heart rate is still elevated; panting respiration may be an effort to cool the body.

When any of the above signs are noted, a review and evaluation of the affected individual is indicated. The seriousness of the condition is indicated by the severity of the observations and ranges from minor stress to complete exhaustion. Once it is established that the horse is significantly stressed, a course of action must be outlined.

TREATMENT OF STRESS

Options for treating stress include allowing the horse to continue under close observation after an extended rest period, removal from competition and allowing the horse to walk to camp, hauling the horse to camp, or administering emergency care on the spot.

It is important for the veterinarian to take charge of the situation. The rider must understand the veterinary concerns and the reasons for these concerns. The rider needs to understand the goals and rationale of the treatment plan and the consequences if the plan is not followed. Most experienced riders monitor their horses closely, know if their horse is seriously stressed, and appreciate the veterinarian's concern and help. However, the intensity of competition can be such a driving force for the rider that prudent judgment concerning the horse is difficult.

Horses that show excessive signs of stress are dehydrated, have electrolyte imbalances, and lack energy. Horses with mild signs respond to rest in the shade if it is available, controlled drinking of electrolyte-enriched water, and moderate amounts of roughage. Electrolyte-enriched water is prepared by adding 1 level tablespoon each of common salt (NaCl) and Lite salt* (NaCl + KCl) to 1 gallon (4 liters) of water. This provides 107 mEq per L sodium, 28 mEq per L potassium, and 135 mEq per L chloride.

Although synchronous diaphragmatic flutter is observed in stressed trail horses, it does not always indicate a severe level of stress. Synchronous diaphragmatic flutter is contraction of the diaphragm synchronous with the heart. It is associated with electrolyte imbalance and is treated with IV calcium (100 to 300 ml of 20 per cent calcium borogluconate) or glucose (50 to 100 gm per hour), or both. Some horses with synchronous diaphragmatic flutter can continue on the trail uneventfully, others cannot. This condition must therefore be considered important and further evaluation of the individual is indicated.

Cases of moderate fatigue need more active intervention, such as oral administration of electrolyte-enriched fluids, which can be isotonic or hypotonic, and mild analgesic medication if abdominal pain is noted. Special attention to hydration is vital if any hypotensive medications such as acepromazine are used. Nonsteroidal anti-inflammatory medications are also helpful, provided tissue perfusion is adequate.

---

*Morton Thiokol, Chicago, IL

WHAT TO USE

Intravenous (IV) fluid therapy with polyionic fluids (12 to 24 liters) is usually indicated in severely stressed horses. Saline contains appropriate proportions of sodium and chloride to replace sweat losses. Alkaline products such as lactated Ringer's solution should be avoided, because most trail-stressed horses are alkalotic. If muscle fasciculations are present, adding 300 ml of 23 per cent calcium gluconate (100 ml per L) to the fluids is indicated. Also, adding KCl, 10 mEq per L, may be helpful, because sweating depletes the body of sodium, potassium, chloride, calcium, and magnesium (see *Current Therapy in Equine Medicine 2*, p. 482).

Severe exhaustion is not hard to recognize and may easily progress to a more complicated metabolic disease with neurological complications and renal shutdown. Massive and rapid fluid therapy (40 to 80 liters) is the most important tool available. Electrolytes and glucose may be added as indicated above. Electrolyte-enriched fluids administered by nasogastric tube are helpful if the stomach is emptying.

If the body temperature is 105° F (40.6°C) or more, cooling the body with cold water is indicated. Water should be concentrated on the head by use of soaked towels, and on the legs with water bandages. In extreme cases, cold water enemas are also helpful. Cooling large muscle mass areas of the body at one time should be avoided, as this may precipitate muscle spasms.

The horse's response to therapy depends on rehydration, establishing proper electrolyte balance, and providing minimum energy levels. The signs of clinical improvement must be the guidelines for response, since laboratory support is not readily available. Patience and a steady attitude by the veterinarian are very important. Response to hydration is best indicated by mucus membranes. They become pink, there is loss of capillary injection, adequate moistness is present, and capillary refill time is less than 2 seconds. Proper electrolyte balance lowers the heart rate, improves intestinal activity, improves muscular strength, and reduces muscular spasms. Return of adequate energy levels may be indicated by improved mental alertness, willingness to travel, and more coordinated muscular activity.

INJURIES

Horses with lameness or physical injuries also need attention. After these conditions are evaluated and treated, a judgment is made as to whether the horse can continue the ride. If the problem is minor and not expected to worsen with continued riding, the horse may continue with careful monitoring. However, painful conditions such as mild lameness may over a period of time add significantly to the stress of the horse, and a metabolic disease may be an unexpected and unwelcome complication of a relatively minor problem.

Supplemental Readings

Guide for Veterinary Service and Judging of Equestrian Events, 4th ed. American Association of Equine Practitioners, Lexington, KY.

Judge's Manual. North American Trail Ride Conference, 1505 E. San Martin Ave., San Martin, CA 95046.

Veterinarian's Handbook. American Endurance Ride Conference, 701 High Street, Suite 201, Auburn, CA 95603.

Section 3

SPECIAL PROBLEMS OF DRAFT HORSES AND MULES

Edited by Dallas O. Goble

Common Lameness Problems of the Draft Horse

Henry S. Adair, KNOXVILLE, TENNESSEE

Even though most lameness problems that occur in light breeds also occur in draft breeds, the size of draft horses often makes diagnosis and therapy difficult and challenging. Additionally, because of their body size, a minor problem in lighter breeds may be a major problem in the draft horse. This section describes the more common lamenesses in the draft breed and practical approaches to diagnosis and therapy.

LAMINITIS

Laminitis can be acute or chronic. Acute laminitis lasts for 72 hours after the onset of Obel grade I lameness, in which the horse repeatedly lifts its feet every few seconds. After 72 hours, laminitis is said to be chronic. The duration of laminitis, as well as the degree of third phalanx rotation, is important when considering the mode of therapy.

The etiology of laminitis is similar in the draft breeds and light breeds. Vascular events such as vasoconstriction and arteriovenous shunting within the vasculature supplying the digit are considered responsible for the laminar ischemia that develops during acute laminitis. Disease processes that may lead to these vascular events include grain overload, retained placenta, endotoxemia, and systemic illness or trauma.

CLINICAL SIGNS

Clinical signs include increased amplitude of digital pulses, increased heat in the hoof, front feet placed forward of their normal position ("camped-out stance"), and shifting weight between limbs. Untreated, the condition may progress to Obel grade IV lameness, in which the horse refuses to move, is recumbent, and appears unwilling to rise unless forced. Radiographs of the foot may show no rotation of the pedal bone, severe rotation, or sinking of the pedal bone within the hoof. Poor hoof quality and large body size may predispose draft horses to the latter problem.

THERAPY

It is critical to identify any underlying disease and treat accordingly. Failure to do so will result in progression of the laminitis. When the horse is first examined, radiographs should be taken of all involved feet for future comparison. A common complication in the draft horse suffering from laminitis is myositis due to abnormal stance or prolonged recumbency. Even in relatively mild laminitis, euthanasia is sometimes necessary because of the onset of severe myositis. Therapy should include prevention of myositis in addition to treatment of laminitis.

The goal of therapy during acute stages of laminitis is to restore or maintain blood flow to the laminar bed. Vasoactive drugs that may be useful include acepromazine maleate° (0.05 mg per kg given intramuscularly [IM] t.i.d.), isoxsuprine hydrochloride† (0.66 mg per kg per os [PO] b.i.d.), and phenoxybenzamine hydrochloride.‡ Phenoxybenzamine (1 mg per kg diluted in 500 ml of saline and given intravenously [IV] twice with a 12-hour interval) provides alpha-adrenergic blockade for 72 hours. Additionally, dimethyl sulfoxide§ (1 gm per kg IV) given once or twice daily for 3 days has proven to be clinically beneficial. Phenylbutazone‖ (4.4 mg per kg PO b.i.d.) should be administered for its anti-inflammatory and analgesic properties. Sodium heparin¶ (100 units per kg IV q.i.d.) may be given to possibly reduce microthrombi formation. Flunixin meglumine# (0.25 mg per kg IM t.i.d.) should be given if endotoxemia is suspected.

Radiographs are taken as clinically indicated to monitor progression of the disease. If accumulation of fluid between the third phalanx and hoof wall is noted, 8-mm holes should be drilled into the fluid pocket to relieve pressure and prevent further dissection of the laminae. The exposed laminae should be protected with a clean bandage. Exercise should be limited to 5 to 10 minutes of hand walking every 2 to 3 hours as long as severe pain is not apparent. The diet is limited to grass or mixed legume hay. Frog supports are beneficial and may be attached to the foot with tape or cast material. Alternatively, the horse should be placed in a stall bedded with sand. It is not recommended that shoes be applied or removed during the acute phase of laminitis. If significant improvement is not noted within 72 hours, the condition is classified as refractory or chronic laminitis.

Therapy for refractory or chronic laminitis is directed toward pain relief and stabilization of the third phalanx. Vasodilator therapy is usually unrewarding because the vascular damage has already occurred. The minimum dose of nonsteroidal anti-inflammatory drugs that provides pain relief should be used. Radiographs are repeated at 10- to 14-day intervals to monitor the progression of the disease. The horse should continue to be bedded on sand to provide support of the pedal bone. If laminar necrosis is severe, resection of the anterior hoof wall will allow debridement and drainage. Support of the hoof wall may be necessary if the resection requires removal of a large section of hoof wall. The application of heart bar shoes is extremely difficult in the draft horse and should only be attempted under radiographic guidance and with the aid of a skilled farrier. A useful alternative is to fashion a heart bar pad out of ½-inch-thick rubber matting and attach it to the hoof with fiberglass casting material.° The cast should not enclose the sole of the hoof. The apex of the frog support should end ⅜ inch from the apex of the frog. Care should be taken to avoid sole contact except on the frog. Trimming of the foot should be directed toward realignment of the third phalanx with the ground surface, while not placing undue stress on the deep digital flexor tendon. DL-Methionine† (10 to 20 gm daily) may be added to the diet to provide disulfide bond substrate. In some chronic cases deep digital flexor tenotomy at the midmetacarpal/metatarsal level may be indicated to counteract the stresses placed on the third phalanx by the tendon. The importance of supportive care during this period cannot be overemphasized. The prognosis for return to previous function is extremely poor, and euthanasia may be necessary in protracted cases.

OSSIFICATION OF LATERAL CARTILAGES

Ossification of the lateral cartilages of the third phalanx of the foot, or sidebone, is common in draft breeds. The exact etiology is unknown; however, continual concussion at the quarters, direct trauma, poor conformation, poor shoeing, and unbalanced trimming are contributing factors.

°PromAce, Fort Dodge Labs., Fort Dodge, IA
†Isoxsuprine, Rugby Lab., Rockville Centre, NY
‡Dibenzyline, Smith Kline & French Labs., Philadelphia, PA
§DOMOSO, Syntex, West Des Moines, IA
‖Phenylbutazone, Burns Vet Supply, Oakland, CA
¶Heparin sodium, Rugby Labs., Rockville Centre, NY
#Banamine, Schering Corp, Kenilworth, NJ

°Zim-Flex, Zimmer, Warsaw, IN
†Methio-Vet, Vet-A-Mix, Inc., Shenandoah, IN

CLINICAL SIGNS

The disease is most commonly observed in the forelimbs. Sidebone is generally nonpainful; however, pain may occur during acute stages when the cartilages are undergoing ossification or have fractured. Lameness may also be observed when the cartilaginous ossification is complete, limiting expansion of the hoof.

Diagnosis, which should eliminate other disease processes, is based on physical examination, diagnostic nerve blocks, and radiographs. Pain, swelling, and increased heat over the affected cartilages are common findings. Many horses will show lameness when working on hard surfaces or when turned. Unilateral or bilateral palmar digital nerve blocks or direct infiltration over the affected cartilage will usually improve the lameness.

THERAPY

Therapy varies according to the stage of disease. Cartilages that are undergoing ossification benefit from rest and nonsteroidal anti-inflammatory drugs. Expansion of the hoof by thinning the quarters or vertically grooving the hoof wall near the coronary band on the affected side may be beneficial. The toe should also be rolled to decrease the motion of the distal interphalangeal joint. If the horse is to be shod, the toe of the shoe should be rolled, the shoe slippered, and the last nail hole left open. Cases that are chronic and not fractured may benefit from counterirritation.

Small proximal fractures of the lateral cartilages are best managed by surgical removal of the fractured fragment. Secondary centers of ossification should not be confused with a fracture. Following removal of the cartilages, the limb should be immobilized until all inflammation has subsided. Large fragments are best managed with conservative therapy involving rest. The limb should be immobilized for a period of 4 to 6 weeks or until all signs of inflammation have subsided, after which the hoof should be shod with a bar shoe with side clips. The horse should be kept in confinement and shod in this manner for 6 to 8 months, after which light work may be resumed. Generally a fibrous rather than an osseous union will form and separation may recur. These cases and those that are refractory to other modes of therapy may benefit from a palmar digital neurectomy.

HOOF CRACKS

Hoof cracks can be divided into two types, those that involve only the superficial epidermis of the hoof and those that extend into the dermis. These cracks may be located anywhere on the hoof wall and may originate at the coronary band or at the ground surface. Hoof cracks result from a number of factors, the most important of which appears to be imbalance of the hoof either as a result of natural hoof growth or from trimming. Other factors include trauma, abscesses, environment, nutrition, and conformation.

THERAPY

Treatment is directed toward correcting any underlying disease state and proper balance of the foot. An unbalanced foot results in uneven distribution of pressure and stress cracks. Superficial cracks benefit from balancing alone; however, those that extend into the dermis require additional therapy. If infection is present, astringents or antibiotics are applied following curettage of the crack and removal of necrotic debris. Once the infection is eliminated, stabilization of the crack is of paramount importance. Stabilization is achieved by shoes with clips. Additional stabilization across the crack may be achieved with suturing or lacing, or applying fiberglass, acrylics, metal plates, clamps, or a combination of these devices.

NECROTIC PODODERMATITIS

Necrotic pododermatitis (canker) is a proliferative infectious condition involving the frog and adjacent sole. It is most commonly seen in the rear feet and frequently results from unhygienic conditions and lack of foot care. Canker has also been observed in horses that are pastured continuously on wetlands and is characterized by infection of the stratum germinativum and proliferation of the horn layer. A characteristic foul odor and a caseous exudate are usually present. Lameness is mild during the early stages, but with progression the lameness may become severe.

THERAPY

Therapy is prolonged and must be aggressive. All necrotic and proliferative tissues must be removed. This is best accomplished under general anesthesia, but in mild cases removal may be performed with regional anesthesia. A tourniquet facilitates debridement by reducing hemorrhage that obscures the surgical field. Following debridement the sole defect is packed with gauze soaked with povidone iodine° and a wa-

---

°E-Z Prep, Becton Dickinson, Franklin Lakes, NJ

terproof bandage applied. The horse is placed in a clean, dry environment and the bandage changed daily. Once the infection is controlled, antiseptic drying agents such as tincture of thimerosol† are used and a pressure bandage applied. In lieu of bandages a shoe with a steel plate that can be removed may be used. Strictly hygienic conditions must be maintained during treatment, which may take 6 to 8 weeks before healing is complete. Even under optimum conditions the prognosis for future soundness is guarded.

UPWARD FIXATION OF THE PATELLA

Upward fixation results from locking of the medial patellar ligament over the medial trochlea of the femur. When the patella is fixed in this position the horse is unable to flex the limb. Draft horses frequently have an abnormally straight hind limb or a long tibia that predisposes to this condition. Lack of muscle tone and poor conditioning are also contributing factors. The condition may appear to be unilateral; however, close observation will often show bilateral involvement.

Signs observed may range from a momentary catching of the patella to complete locking of the stifle. When only momentary catching occurs the horse may exhibit an abrupt anterior phase that may be confused with stringhalt. Signs are often exaggerated when the horse is circled with the affected limb to the inside. Walking uphill induces a crouched position in some horses and walking downhill may cause a jerky gait with slight dragging of the toe.

Signs observed with complete locking are obvious as the leg is extended with dragging of the toe. The patella may unlock after a few steps or it may remain locked for an extended period. Gonitis may be observed in those cases of long duration. Affected young animals should be examined closely for underlying osteochondrosis.

Therapy

In acute upward fixation, backing the horse will sometimes unlock the patella. Placing an inward and downward pressure on the patella while backing the horse will also help to free the patella. Cases that repeatedly lock or remain fixed will require a medial patellar desmotomy.

Momentary upward fixation of the patella is best treated initially by conditioning. Working the horse daily on both flat ground and inclines will strengthen the muscles, ligaments, and tendons. The condition is likely to return if work is interrupted.

When conditioning alone fails, a counterirritant° may be injected into the medial and middle patellar ligament. The goal of this therapy is to cause fibrosis and subsequent tightening of the ligaments, thus preventing the patella from catching. A total of 6 to 12 ml is divided into smaller amounts and injected at several sites in the medial patellar ligament. An additional 6 ml is similarly divided and injected into several sites in the middle patellar ligament. Care must be taken not to enter the joint. Mild lameness and swelling may be observed for a few days after injection. Light exercise should be continued and full work can be resumed in 7 to 10 days. Some individuals require repeat injections. Horses that do not respond favorably to this treatment will require a medial patellar desmotomy.

OSTEOCHONDROSIS

Osteochondrosis is part of a multifactorial orthopedic disease complex that includes angular limb deformities, flexor tendon anomalies, physitis, osteochondrosis, and osteochondritis dissecans. It most commonly involves the tibiotarsal and femorotibial/patellar joints of young, rapidly growing draft horses. Factors associated with the disease include trauma, genetics, conformation, calcium or phosphorus imbalances, and deficiencies in trace minerals (see p. 105 and p. 720). Since mare's milk is almost devoid of trace minerals, foals must rely on liver stores acquired during gestation. Commonly observed signs include lameness and joint effusion. The condition may be unilateral or bilateral and may be found in joints other than those mentioned.

Therapy

Prevention of the disease complex should be started during the last trimester of gestation. The mare should be fed a balanced ration, including a trace mineral supplement that contains copper, zinc, and magnesium. This diet provides the foal with adequate liver stores of trace minerals until it can consume adequate supplement. When the foal is weaned it should be fed a 14 to 16 per cent protein ration based on body weight and age, with good-quality grass or legume hay and free choice trace minerals. It is important that the foal not be overfed during the period of growth.

---

†Merthiolate, Eli Lilly and Co., Indianapolis, IN

°Maxlin Injection, Maxilin Medicines, Hudson, MA

When the disease is present, conservative therapy, including dietary adjustments, stall rest, and administration of polysulfated glycosaminoglycans,* may be attempted. Conservative therapy is recommended only for horses that are mildly affected or early in the disease process. Horses that do not respond to conservative therapy or are severely affected are surgical candidates. Arthroscopy is the surgical method of choice. The prognosis after surgical intervention is directly related to the severity and duration of the lesion. The postoperative use of hyaluronic acid† or polysulfated glycosaminoglycans will retard the inflammatory process and aid in healing. Conservative or surgical therapy is generally unrewarding in severely affected joints, multiple joint involvement, and long-standing disease.

DEGENERATIVE JOINT DISEASE
(Osteoarthrosis)

Degenerative joint disease is commonly observed in the draft horse. The two most common sites are the interphalangeal joints (ringbone) and the tarsal joints (spavin). Factors influencing the development of degenerative joint disease include trauma, weight, conformation, unbalanced feet, and use of the horse. Clinical lameness varies depending on the joint involved and the severity of pathological changes in the affected joint or joints.

Ringbone may be classified as high (proximal interphalangeal area) or low (distal interphalangeal area) and as articular or nonarticular. Nonarticular high ringbone is the type most commonly observed in the draft horse. It generally results from tearing of the ligamentous or joint capsular attachments surrounding the proximal interphalangeal joint. This tearing may result from direct trauma, poor conformation, or unbalanced feet. New bone deposition at the site of tearing causes irritation of the soft tissues surrounding the proximal interphalangeal joint and subsequent lameness. It is most commonly observed in the forelimbs and less frequently in the hind limbs. Horses with a base-narrow and toe-in or toe-out conformation are predisposed to development of high nonarticular ringbone on the lateral aspect of the pastern, whereas in a horse with a base-wide and toe-in or toe-out conformation the disease develops on the medial aspect of the pastern. The articular type is primarily found in young individuals and may be either high or low. The etiology appears to be related to undetected osteochondrosis or direct trauma.

Lameness related to ringbone varies from mild to severe. The more severe the condition, the greater the possibility that the articular surfaces are involved. Flexion and rotation of the pastern will usually elicit pain. Diagnosis is based on regional anesthesia and radiographs. Radionuclide scintigraphy may aid in the diagnosis of early cases not detected from radiographs.

Degenerative joint disease of the tarsocrural joint most commonly develops in the distal intertarsal and tarsometatarsal joints. It is most commonly observed in horses with poor conformation. Cow- or sickle-hocked individuals are predisposed to the development of degenerative joint disease as a result of abnormal stresses placed on the medial aspect of the tarsus. Additionally, undetected osteochondrosis may lead to tarsitis and degenerative joint disease later in life.

Signs are generally related to reduced flexion of the tarsocrural joint. The lameness tends to worsen with work and improves with rest. An asynchronous gluteal rise with the affected limb rising higher than the contralateral limb will be noted. A reduced arc of foot flight and shortened anterior phase of the stride may also be observed. The horse tends to land on the toe of the affected limb, thus wearing the toe excessively. An upper limb flexion test (spavin test) will generally worsen the lameness.

Diagnosis is based on clinical signs, positive flexion test, and improvement of the lameness after intra-articular anesthesia. Radiographic evidence of disease may not be seen in early cases with only articular surface involvement. In these cases radionuclide scintigraphy may provide imaging confirmation of disease.

THERAPY

Instability of the pastern area prior to the development of exostosis is best treated by stall confinement and external coaptation of the distal limb. This treatment should be maintained for 6 to 8 weeks to allow complete soft tissue healing. After this the horse should be placed in a small pasture for an additional 3 to 4 months before work is resumed. Work should gradually be increased over a 6- to 8-week period.

High nonarticular ringbone is best treated with nonsteroidal anti-inflammatory drugs and corrective shoeing. The toe of the foot and shoe should be rolled to decrease the work required to flex the pastern. Additionally, the shoe should be made as light as possible. Chronic cases and those that do not respond to conservative therapy may benefit from counterirritation therapy.

---

*Adequan, Luitpold Pharmaceuticals, Inc., Shirley, NY
†Equron, Solvay Animal Health Inc., Mendota Heights, MN.

Cases involving the articular surface of the proximal interphalangeal joint are best managed by arthrodesis of the joint. Arthrodesis has been quite successful in the lighter breeds; however, the potential complications of postanesthetic myositis, implant failure, and breakdown of the contralateral leg are quite high in the draft horse. Treatment of degenerative joint disease of the distal interphalangeal joint is often unrewarding. Conservative therapy, including corrective trimming, the use of nonsteroidal anti-inflammatory drugs, and injection of hyaluronic acid into the distal interphalangeal joint, is the most common mode of therapy. Often these horses must be retired, or occasionally euthanized if severe chronic lameness persists.

Therapy for degenerative joint disease of the tarsocrural joint is directed toward relief of pain and fusion of the distal tarsal joints. Shoes should be made of lightweight stock and the medial toe of the shoe should be rolled. Additionally, the hoof angle should be raised if clinically practical. These corrective measures ease flexion of the limb. The injection of 80 to 100 mg of methylprednisolone* per joint and 10 mg of hyaluronic acid into the distal intertarsal and tarsometatarsal joints may allow the horse to be used without the use of nonsteroidal anti-inflammatory drugs. Caution must be used with intra-articular injections because of the potential complication of joint infections or steroid arthropathy. With time and continued exercise the distal tarsal joints often fuse and the lameness will improve.

SHIVERS

Shivers is a progressive neuromuscular disease that is occasionally observed in the draft breeds. The disease primarily affects the hind limbs; however, it may also be observed in the forelimbs. It has been observed in Belgians and Clydesdales, but other breeds may be affected. The exact etiology is unknown but the disease often follows a viral infection or other systemic disease.

Mild cases may be difficult to detect. The signs occur at irregular intervals and may be stimulated by backing, turning, or making the individual step over an object. The affected limb is held off the ground in a flexed and abducted manner. The muscles of the upper limb, tail, or eyelids may quiver. After a short time the limb relaxes and the horse appears normal. Shivering should be distinguished from stringhalt or intermittent upward fixation of the patella.

THERAPY

No effective treatment is presently available. Improvement occurs with rest, but the condition returns when work is resumed. The prognosis for affected individuals is poor, since the disease is usually slowly progressive. Mildly affected individuals may be able to work provided the signs are not exacerbated by the work.

RHABDOMYOLYSIS (Azoturia, Tying Up, Monday Morning Sickness)

Rhabdomyolysis can be a severe, life-threatening condition. The disease is of particular importance in draft breeds because of their size and muscle mass. Rhabdomyolysis may occur as a result of prolonged anesthesia (postanesthetic myositis) or during work (exertional myopathy). The pathophysiology of postanesthetic myositis is discussed in the anesthesia section related to draft horses (see p. 100).

Exertional myopathy is most commonly observed in the fit individual that is not exercised for a period of time, continued on the same level of concentrate, and then returned to work. The pathophysiology is poorly defined but appears to be related to glycogen deposition in the muscle, lactic acid build-up, and a vascular response resulting in muscle ischemia.

Diagnosis is based on clinical signs and elevated muscle enzyme levels. It is important not to confuse rhabdomyolysis with other diseases, such as colic or laminitis. The creatine phosphokinase level rises (by 6 hours) and declines (by 36 to 72 hours) rapidly after the onset of the disease. The aspartate aminotransferase level rises (by 24 to 48 hours) and declines (by 2 to 3 weeks) more slowly than the creatine phosphokinase level. Both of these enzymes may be serially monitored to check the rate of recovery. Creatine phosphokinase levels of 30,000 to 40,000 IU and aspartate aminotransferase levels of 2000 to 4000 IU are not unusual.

THERAPY

Prevention is the most effective treatment of rhabdomyolysis. Animals whose work schedule is interrupted should have their grain ration reduced or stopped and be fed a good-quality grass hay. Work is resumed at light levels and gradually increased over a period of 10 to 14 days, with grain levels increased as work increases. Affected individuals may be susceptible to recurrence, and in these instances the addition of a

---

*Depo-Medrol, Upjohn Co., Kalamazoo, MI

commercial electrolyte mix and sodium bicarbonate (30 gm b.i.d.; ⅔ tablespoon) to the ration may be of benefit.

When rhabdomyolysis occurs, immediate therapy to restore tissue perfusion and prevent renal damage due to myoglobin infiltration should be instituted. The horse should be placed on an IV infusion of a balanced electrolyte solution° to promote tissue perfusion and diuresis. Furosemide† (1 mg per kg IV) may be utilized to initiate diuresis, provided hydration is adequate. Nonsteroidal anti-inflammatory drugs such as phenylbutazone, flunixin, and naproxen‡ (10 mg per kg PO or IV daily) should be utilized to reduce inflammation. Methocarbamol§ (15 to 25 mg per kg IV q.i.d.) may be given to aid muscle relaxation. Acepromazine maleate (0.05 mg per kg IM t.i.d.) may be administered to calm the animal and for its vasodilator effects. In severely affected individuals guaifenesin‖ (5 to 10 per cent, by IV infusion given to affect) may be needed for muscle relaxation and sedation. Hypocalcemia has been noted in some horses, so the administration of calcium gluconate¶ (500 ml diluted in 5 liters of lactated Ringer's solution and given IV over a 2- to 3-hour period) may be indicated. Medical grade dimethyl sulfoxide (1 gm per kg as a 20 per cent solution IV every 12 hours) may be given for its diuretic and analgesic properties. Dantrolene sodium# (loading dose of 10 mg per kg given PO, followed by 2.5 mg per kg PO every 2 hours) may be beneficial; however, it is primarily used for prevention and may be prohibitively costly. Supportive care such as soft bedding, frequent rolling, and muscle massage should be provided. The use of a full body sling may be beneficial but should only be utilized if adequate facilities, equipment, and personnel are available. Many horses will not tolerate the sling, and struggling may induce further damage.

Serial monitoring of creatine phosphokinase and aspartate aminotransferase levels to check the rate of recovery aids in prognosis. Clinical chemistries should return to normal levels before exercise is resumed. Horses with creatine phosphokinase levels higher than 100,000 IU, prolonged elevations in aspartate aminotransferase levels, and recumbency for longer than 48 to 72 hours have a poor prognosis. Serum electrolytes should be monitored daily and appropriate corrections made. Serum creatinine assays, urinalysis, and urinary fractional electrolyte excretions should be done to evaluate kidney function. Horses that develop signs of acute renal failure have a grave prognosis. Additional complications such as laminitis, diarrhea, and pneumonia may occur and further worsen the prognosis.

Supplemental Readings

Geiser, D. R.: Chemical restraint and general anesthesia in the draft horse. In Proceedings of the 35th Annual Meeting of the American Association of Equine Practitioners, December 1989, pp. 461–472.

Goble, D. O.: Selected problems in the draft horse. In Proceedings of the 34th Annual Convention of the American Association of Equine Practitioners, December 1988, pp. 607–610.

Goble, D. O.: Solutions to selected draft horse problems. In Proceedings of the 35th Annual Convention of the American Association of Equine Practitioners, December 1989, pp. 473–477.

Jones, R. D.: Management and care of common musculoskeletal problems of the draft horse. In Proceedings of the 35th Annual Convention of the American Association of Equine Practitioners, December 1989, pp. 487–493.

Mansmann, R. A.: Skeletal System. In Mansmann, R.A., McAllister, E.S., and Pratt, P.W. (eds.): Equine Medicine and Surgery, 3rd ed. Santa Barbara, Calif. American Veterinary Publications, 1982, pp. 944–1158.

Stashak, T. S.: Adams' Lameness of Horses, 4th ed. Philadelphia, Lea & Febiger, 1987.

Youvich, J. V.: The Equine Foot. Vet. Clin. North Am. (Equine Pract.) 5(1):1989.

°Lactated Ringer's Solution, Abbott Labs., North Chicago, IL
†Furosemide 5% Injection, Burns Vet Supply, Oakland, CA
‡Equiproxen, Syntex, West Des Moines, IA
§Robaxin, A. H. Robins, Richmond, VA
‖Guaifenesin, A. H. Robins, Richmond, VA
¶CalDex No. 2, Fort Dodge Labs., Fort Dodge, IA
#Dantrium, Eaton Pharmaceuticals, Norwich, NY

Upper Respiratory Problems of the Draft Horse

Dallas O. Goble, KNOXVILLE, TENNESSEE

Although draft horses suffer the multitude of upper respiratory problems that affect the light horse, the frequency of certain problems is markedly different in the two groups. Two problems that occur frequently in draft horses, laryngeal hemiplegia and guttural pouch empyema, produce special clinical problems and require special therapeutic considerations.

LARYNGEAL HEMIPLEGIA

Laryngeal hemiplegia is the most frequent upper respiratory problem causing respiratory dysfunction in the draft horse. Although there is evidence that this condition is inherited in light horses and draft horses, it is doubtful that horses will be selectively mated to eliminate this trait. Suggesting to breeders that heritability could be a factor in the frequency of occurrence may, however, influence breeding selection, which in time could reduce the frequency of the problem.

HISTORY AND CLINICAL SIGNS

Clinical signs of respiratory dysfunction due to laryngeal hemiplegia frequently follow viral respiratory infections and especially strangles. In some horses, signs may develop acutely: the horse starts making noise over a 1- to 3-week period of time. In others increased respiratory sounds develop over months to years. Increased sounds are not always found in horses with laryngeal hemiplegia; for example, one horse that did not make noise would occasionally choke down and become unconscious while in harness. Some physically fit horses with laryngeal hemiplegia that has not produced signs will show respiratory dysfunction when put back to work after being rested for several months. Occasionally the dysfunction improves or even disappears as the horse regains physical fitness.

Some affected horses may never have a detectable clinical problem because they are not asked to perform at a work load that demands high rates of air flow. This is especially true with some draft horses that pull light wagons or perform other low-intensity work. Laryngeal hemiplegia is not difficult to diagnose, but determining if it is producing work intolerance may be more challenging. Increased noise during exercise does not mean that hemiplegia is affecting performance. Careful questioning of the owner, a thorough physical examination, and observation of the horse being exercised at its intended work level are essential prior to initiation of therapy.

The methods for diagnosing laryngeal hemiplegia in the light horse apply to the draft horse. These include auscultation, the "grunt test," arytenoid depression, radiology, and endoscopy. Because it is difficult to palpate the muscular process and laryngeal structures in the draft horse, the arytenoid depression test is more difficult to perform in the draft horse than in the light horse.

The final diagnosis is dependent on endoscopic examination. A thorough examination of all pharyngeal and laryngeal structures should be performed to avoid omission of other concurrent problems. A hurried examination may lead to confusion of chondritis of the arytenoid cartilage with laryngeal hemiplegia, or a hypoplastic epiglottis may go unobserved. Obstructing nostril air flow for a few inspiratory efforts will aid in evaluation of pharyngeal lumen collapse, a not uncommon condition of draft horses. The arytenoid abduction resulting from the slap test (see *Current Therapy in Equine Medicine 1,* p. 497) can be more difficult to elicit and less reliable in the evaluation of laryngeal function in the draft horse than in the light horse.

THERAPY

Treatment of laryngeal hemiplegia is surgical. Until 1970, the standard treatment was laryngeal sacculectomy, accomplished through a ventral laryngotomy. This was frequently done with the horse standing, under local anesthesia and tranquilization. The procedure was reported to be 50 to 60 per cent effective in improving the clinical problem.

In 1970, laryngoplasty (laryngeal prosthesis, "tie back") was described. This surgical procedure is suggested to improve respiratory function in approximately 90 per cent of cases. The procedure is performed under general anesthesia and require an experienced surgeon. Postsurgical complications include chronic coughing, implant failure, and suture fistula that requires additional surgical intervention. Laryngoplasty has become the standard for optimal treatment.

It is vital that an experienced surgeon perform

laryngoplasty in the draft horse. Most surgery tables will not accommodate a horse weighing 2000 to 2500 lb and the surgery must be done on the floor. The short neck and heavy musculature at the surgical site make the surgical approach difficult, and anesthesia is associated with more frequent postsurgical complications such as myositis and neuromuscular weakness than in light horses.

In consideration of these factors I carefully evaluate the horse and the expectation of the horse's performance level. I specifically attempt to determine the degree of exercise intolerance at the time of examination in relation to the severity of respiratory sounds. The owner must be carefully questioned as to the importance of increased respiratory sounds as compared to work intolerance. Some owners are more concerned about respiratory sounds than about work intolerance. This is especially true of the owners of some show hitches. If work intolerance is present and is a major concern to the owner, I suggest an initial sacculectomy and then evaluation of the results after the horse has regained good physical fitness.

With the recent introduction of the neodymium:yttrium-aluminum-garnet (Nd-YAG) surgical laser (see p. 294), sacculectomy in the standing horse has become a simple procedure with minimal risk to the patient and minimal cost to the owner, compared with the traditional surgical procedure. The laser cable can be passed through the instrument channel of the fiberoptic endoscope and the saccule obliterated. The procedure is easily done on an outpatient basis, with sedation and application of a topical anesthetic to the saccule area. Additional benefits include reduced cost of hospitalization and elimination of the aftercare associated with sacculectomy performed via a laryngotomy. Phenylbutazone is usually administered before and for 3 to 5 days after surgery.

Endoscopy should be performed 30 to 45 days after surgery to evaluate healing and to determine if the horse should return to work. Healing is usually adequate 50 to 60 days after surgery and work may be resumed. The horse is slowly conditioned over a 60- to 120-day period. If there is no improvement after conditioning is complete, or if the signs worsen, the option of a surgical laryngoplasty is offered to the owner.

If the absence of respiratory sounds is critical to the horse's use, then laryngoplasty is the best option. This procedure offers better opportunity for reducing undesirable sounds to an acceptable level than any other procedure presently available. The risk of surgical and postsurgical complications should be explained fully to the owners. If the practitioner is not highly proficient at laryngoplasty, the horse should be referred to a surgical center.

GUTTURAL POUCH EMPYEMA

It is questionable whether the draft horse is more susceptible to this condition than the light horse, but in our practice it occurs more frequently in draft than in light horses. The greater frequency may be due to the less intensive management provided for draft horses than light horses. The duration of antibiotic therapy and the antibiotic dose are often inadequate in the draft horse, resulting in a higher frequency of complications associated with secondary infections. Since guttural pouch empyema is generally an extension of another infectious process, usually strangles, it follows that guttural pouch empyema occurs more frequently with a lower level of care.

CLINICAL SIGNS AND DIAGNOSIS

The clinical history frequently includes a previous respiratory infection, most commonly strangles *(Streptococcus equi)*. Several horses may have been affected initially and all may have recovered except for one or two individuals that continue to have an intermittent mucopurulent nasal discharge.

The classic clinical signs associated with guttural pouch empyema are swelling caudad to the mandible, a mucopurulent nasal discharge, and pain or swelling of the parotid gland area. Unfortunately, this combination of clinical signs is lacking in many cases, and correct diagnosis requires more involved examination techniques. This is especially true once the acute stage has passed and the condition is chronic.

Owing to the short, heavily muscled neck of the draft horse, palpation for swelling of lymph nodes, parotid glands, and structures behind the mandible is more difficult than in the light horse. Many draft horses are stoic and it is difficult to elicit a painful response. It is also difficult to apply digital pressure to the guttural pouch area in an effort to increase the volume of nasal exudate. The nasal exudate may be more profuse when the horse lowers its head, but this is not pathognomonic. The classic signs are more frequently present in acute than chronic disease.

The two most useful diagnostic aids are endoscopy and radiography. Although endoscopic observation of exudate from the pharyngeal openings of the guttural pouches is diagnostically significant, I prefer direct viewing of both pouches when possible. The flexible endoscope can usually be passed into the pouch with minimal restraint or sedation, depending on the horse's temperament. A biopsy cable is passed through the instrument channel of the endoscope and is used as a guide to direct the endoscope into the pouch. The type of exudate, the presence of chondroids, and the presence of mycotic lesions should be noted.

Radiographic evaluation is benefited by sedation of the horse so that the neck can be extended. This improves the visualization of the guttural pouches by reducing mandible juxtaposition. Even in a draft horse, a portable x-ray unit can provide good-quality radiographs of the guttural pouches. Fluid lines in the pouches will be observed with empyema. Radiographs will also aid in the diagnosis of chondroids. Radiographic visualization of chondroids is improved by infusion of a small amount of contrast material into the pouch. Caution must be observed when doing any of these procedures in animals with marginal airway patency. The stress of examination or respiratory compromise from tranquilization may induce total respiratory obstruction.

When there is palpable swelling of the caudal mandibular region, the hair may be clipped, a surgical preparation performed, and needle aspiration attempted. This procedure is not without risk of injury to nerves and vessels in the area. Also, one is not absolutely sure if the exudate obtained is from the guttural pouch or abscessed lymph node. A 16- to 18-gauge, 5- to 7.5-cm (2- to 3-inch) needle is usually of adequate length, but on occasion a longer needle is required.

THERAPY

In horses with compromised respiratory function due to intraluminal pharyngeal compression, a tracheostomy should be performed prior to other therapy. This reduces the stress of compromised respiratory function and eliminates the concern of total obstruction during treatment. Horses with empyema of the guttural pouches are frequently dehydrated from inability to drink, especially during hot weather. Rehydration with a balanced intravenous electrolyte solution should begin immediately.

Successful treatment requires systemic antibiotics and lavage of the affected guttural pouch or pouches. Local treatment of the guttural pouch entails either catheter placement and lavage or surgical drainage and lavage. If chondroids or inspissated exudate are present, surgical drainage is necessary. If the exudate is fluid, I prefer an indwelling catheter and daily flushing.

Systemic treatment with the appropriate antibiotic or combination of antibiotics will depend on the causative agent. A sample of the exudate should be taken prior to the initial antibiotic treatment to determine the organism or organisms present and their antibiotic sensitivity. Most of the infections involve *Streptococcus* spp. and therefore intramuscular procaine penicillin G (20,000 IU per kg b.i.d.) alone or in combination with trimethoprim-sulfa (15 mg per kg b.i.d.) per os is well advised until culture results are available. Regardless of the antibiotics or their sequence of administration, long-term treatment is generally necessary for success. In many cases, 2 to 4 weeks of continuous treatment will be required, and occasionally even longer periods may be necessary.

Lavage through a nasopharyngeal catheter in the guttural pouch is a vital part of treatment. Owing to the size of many draft horses, the catheters used in light horses are frequently of inadequate length. I use a 5.5-mm internal diameter Silastic endotracheal tube, 60 to 65 cm long, with an inflatable cuff 2.54 cm from the distal end.* The catheter can be placed into the affected pouch using a copper wire stylet for rigidity and endoscopic viewing through the opposite nostril. With practice, the catheter may be passed blindly. To facilitate placement, the distal 2 to 3 cm of the catheter is bent to approximately 30 degrees after the stylet has been inserted. It is preferable to inflate the cuff with tap water rather than air. The tube can then be sutured or taped at the external nares to maintain position.

The guttural pouch can be lavaged once or twice daily as the case dictates. I usually lavage the pouch twice a day for the first 3 to 5 days. As the volume of exudate decreases, I infuse once a day until exudate is no longer in the flush solution for at least 3 consecutive days. A low-cost, warm, nonirritating solution is used because the physical cleansing and dilution of the exudate is more important than the antibiotic or antiseptic that is added. I prefer a solution with a pH near 7.0. This requires buffering some of the commercial solutions with sodium bicarbonate, because their pH of 5.5 to 5.8 irritates the mucosa. Increasing irritation within the pouch may induce a neuritis and subsequent dysphagia. I do not use antibiotics in the solution, primarily to reduce cost. Warm physiologic saline with a pH near 7.0 is my solution of choice.

Tranquilization (usually with xylazine at 0.25 mg per kg) to lower the head and reduce the op-

---

*Bivona Inc., 5700 West 23rd Ave., Gary, IN

portunity for aspiration during lavage is recommended. About 500 to 1000 ml of solution per pouch is usually an adequate volume for each treatment.

Because of the frequency of postsurgical recovery problems in the draft horse, surgical intervention is best reserved for cases that do not respond to medical therapy alone.

Supplemental Readings

Cook, W. R.: Recent observations on recurrent laryngeal neuropathy in the horse: Application to practice. *In* Proceedings of the 34th Annual Convention of the American Association of Equine Practitioners, 1988, pp. 427–478.

Haynes, P. F.: Surgery of the equine respiratory tract. *In* Jennings, P.B. (ed.): The Practice of Large Animal Surgery, vol. 1. Philadelphia, W. B. Saunders, 1984, pp. 388–487.

Chemical Restraint and Anesthesia of the Draft Horse

Dennis R. Geiser, KNOXVILLE, TENNESSEE

Manual and chemical restraint and general anesthesia of large horses often present a challenge to the veterinary practitioner. Characteristics of draft breeds that may affect the response to chemical sedation and general anesthesia include height, weight, muscle mass, disposition, metabolic rate, and the relatively large amount of body mass in relation to the amount of nerve tissue.

The low metabolic rate, stoic attitude, and large body mass in relation to the amount of nervous tissue may potentiate the physiologic effects of drugs used for chemical restraint and general anesthesia. These characteristics affect the dose, duration of action, and rate of metabolism and elimination of anesthetic drugs. It is the clinical impression that draft breeds respond more profoundly to neurosuppressor drugs than do light breed horses. The use of drug dosages per kilogram of body weight that are based on the doses administered to light breed horses is not without risk. The size of the draft horse also contributes significantly to postanesthetic complications, prompting many veterinarians to attempt most surgical and diagnostic procedures with only chemical restraint and regional or local anesthesia.

CHEMICAL RESTRAINT OF THE STANDING HORSE

Investigation of drugs for chemical restraint has been carried out almost exclusively in light breed horses. Dosages for draft breeds are based on clinical experience and anecdotal exchanges between veterinarians. Draft breeds frequently respond more intensely to sedatives and tranquilizers than do light breeds, and severe ataxia is an undesirable side effect of some drugs or drug combinations. Careful selection of drugs and doses is necessary before restraint is undertaken. The administration of drugs by titration or to effect, although not always practical, is a good practice whenever possible, for example when using drugs with a short onset of action. The ideal drug or drug combination for restraint of the standing draft horse has yet to be discovered, but careful dosing of tranquilizers, sedative hypnotics, or drug combinations can result in acceptable restraint. Table 1 summarizes commonly used drugs and drug combinations. Dosages listed for the draft horse are based on clinical experience. These doses are compared to doses recommended in the literature for light breed horses.

ACETYLPROMAZINE

Acetylpromazine* produces mild sedation and dose-dependent hypotension in the horse. At therapeutic doses, it produces only minimal outward sedation with dulling of reflexes and slowing of avoidance responses. Most horses respond more consistently to acetylpromazine if placed in a quiet area for 10 to 15 minutes with minimal external stimulation. In draft horses, the recommended dosage varies between 0.033 and 0.066 mg per kg (0.015 to 0.03 mg per lb), given intravenously (IV). As a preanesthetic to general anesthesia, acetylpromazine is effective at 0.033 mg per kg (0.015 mg per lb) IV, given 15 to 20 minutes prior to induction. Low-dose preanes-

---

*PromAce, Fort Dodge Labs., Fort Dodge, IA

TABLE 1. INTRAVENOUS DOSES OF DRUGS FOR CHEMICAL RESTRAINT OF LIGHT AND DRAFT HORSES

Drug(s)	Sedation		Preanesthetic
	Light Horse (mg/kg)	Draft Horse (mg/kg)	Draft Horse (mg/kg)
Acepromazine	0.044–0.088	0.033–0.066	0.033
Xylazine	0.55	0.33–0.44	0.22–0.33
Xylazine as premed. to ketamine	1.1	—	0.88–1.1
Detomidine	0.02–0.04	0.01–0.03	0.005–0.01
Chloral hydrate	22–110	2.0–33.0	—
Xylazine	0.22–0.66	0.33–0.44	0.22–0.33
+ butorphanol	0.022–0.11	0.033–0.066	0.033–0.044
Acepromazine	0.055–0.066	0.033–0.055	0.033
+ butorphanol	0.066–0.11	0.055–0.066	0.055–0.066
Xylazine	0.48–0.99	0.44–0.55	—
+ morphine	0.44–0.66	0.33 (max)	—
Xylazine	0.66	0.33–0.44	—
+ meperidine	1.1	0.31–0.40	—
Acepromazine	0.044	0.033–0.44	—
+ meperidine	0.055	0.40–0.48	—
Acepromazine	0.044–0.066	0.033–0.044	—
+ chloral hydrate	13.2–33.0	22.0–33.0	—
Detomidine	0.011	—	—
+ morphine	0.099	—	—
Detomidine	0.022	0.01–0.02	—
+ butorphanol	0.044	0.044–0.066	—

thetic administration minimizes both the severity of hypotension and potentiation of other hypotensive anesthetic agents.

XYLAZINE

The imidazole derivative xylazine is a potent sedative-hypnotic and analgesic with some muscle-relaxing properties. Xylazine predominantly stimulates the α_2-adrenergic receptors, producing a dose-dependent systemic hypertension followed by hypotension, bradycardia due to second-degree heart block, and respiratory depression. Since the onset of sedation is rapid (3 to 5 minutes), additional increments of xylazine can be administered if lower doses do not produce the desired level of sedation. Xylazine produces more ataxia than acetylpromazine; therefore, xylazine must be used cautiously for procedures involving distal extremeties or for standing castration, especially at higher doses (0.55 to 1.1 mg per kg IV). Xylazine is useful for lowering the head for procedures in that area.

Draft horses are more sensitive to xylazine than light breeds. Doses between 0.33 and 0.44 mg per kg IV may be sufficient for most minor procedures in standing draft breeds. Xylazine may be associated with periodic awakening following external stimuation, which is a problem when working around the distal limb area. Xylazine sedation can be reversed with yohimbine† at 0.125 mg per kg IV, and this is particularly valuable if an overdose occurs or if it is necessary to move a heavily sedated draft horse, especially on slippery surfaces.

DETOMIDINE

Detomidine‡ is a sedative-hypnotic with physiologic effects similar to those of xylazine except that detomidine is more potent. The cardiopulmonary effects of detomidine are dose dependent, with doses higher than 0.04 mg per kg producing severe bradycardia and respiratory depression. Heart rate may decrease to less than 30 and respiration may be characterized by periods of closely spaced breaths followed by an apneic period. Detomidine may potentiate other respiratory depressants. Detomidine administered at suggested doses usually produces a short period of pronounced ataxia followed by a pe-

---

†Yohimbine hydrochloride, Sigma F and D Division, Ltd., St. Louis, MO
‡Dormosedan, Norden Labs., Lincoln, NE

riod in which the animal maintains a relatively stable, planted stance. The rear legs may be less stable than the forelegs and appear to be more sensitive to stimuli. The ataxia and periodic awakening seen with xylazine sedation occur less frequently with detomidine. The recommended dosage of detomidine in draft horses ranges between 0.01 and 0.02 mg per kg IV. Clinical sedation occurs within 5 minutes of administration, and peak effects occur in 15 minutes. Additional amounts may be administered if necessary. The duration of sedation is dose dependent and may be as long as 1.5 hours. One disadvantage of detomidine may be the reluctance of the patient to move after completion of a procedure; therefore, reversal with yohimbine at 0.125 mg per kg IV may be beneficial. In some horses, one-half the calculated dose of yohimbine may be sufficient after 1.5 hours of detomidine sedation.

Drug Combinations

In an attempt to decrease untoward effects, improve sedation, analgesia, and predictability, numerous drug combinations have been used in the horse (see Table 1). The combination of a tranquilizer or sedative-hypnotic with an opiate is termed *neuroleptanalgesia*. Many of the serious central nervous system (CNS) excitatory effects of opiates can be obviated by combining them with tranquilizers or hypnotics. One popular neuroleptanalgesic combination is xylazine and butorphanol.* Butorphanol is an opiate agonist-antagonist possessing minimal cardiopulmonary effects. When butorphanol is administered to a patient, some CNS stimulation may be observed, such as muscle tremors, head jerking, and lip and facial twitching. When butorphanol is combined with xylazine, these signs are greatly reduced. Butorphanol also exhibits a ceiling effect, a dose above which no increase in analgesia or side effects occurs. The ceiling dose of butorphanol reported for light breeds is 0.11 mg per kg IV or intramuscularly (IM). The dose of butorphanol used in combination ranges up to the ceiling dose, depending on the amount of analgesia desired. In draft breeds xylazine and butorphanol may be used at doses ranging from 0.33 to 0.44 mg per kg IV and 0.033 to 0.066 mg per kg IV, respectively. Administration of butorphanol 3 to 5 minutes after xylazine is preferred. The duration of good somatic analgesia with this combination is approximately 30 minutes.

Butorphanol may also be combined with detomidine to produce neuroleptanalgesia. Detomidine alone is a potent analgesic, and the increased analgesia achieved with this combination has not been fully investigated. Recommended dosages for the draft horse are detomidine, 0.01 to 0.02 mg per kg IV, followed in 10 to 15 minutes by butorphanol, 0.044 to 0.066 mg per kg IV.

Acetylpromazine and butorphanol combinations are widely used in light breed horses. Acetylpromazine alone produces mild sedation with little analgesia. The combination of acetylpromazine with butorphanol produces increased analgesia with minor ataxia and less of the forward pressing tendency that occurs in some patients after xylazine and butorphanol administration. In draft horses, acetylpromazine is used at 0.033 to 0.055 mg per kg IV, followed in 10 to 15 minutes by butorphanol, 0.055 to 0.066 mg per kg IV.

Many other drug combinations can be used for chemical restraint of standing draft horses. The sensitivity of the draft horse to tranquilizers and sedatives should always be considered when one is using these drugs, new drugs, or drug combinations. Whenever possible, it is prudent to begin with a low dose and titrate drugs to the desired effect.

GENERAL ANESTHESIA

Preanesthetic preparation for short procedures in normal draft horses under field conditions may only involve a complete physical examination. When the anticipated anesthetic time is longer than 30 minutes, whether injectable or inhalant methods are used, additional screening is indicated. The following should be considered in a preanesthetic evaluation: the signalment (weight, sex, age, etc.), the patient's primary problem, type of surgical procedure, body position required, the concurrent medical therapy, training or exercise program, feeding program, demeanor, and physical examination findings. Routine laboratory screening includes a complete blood cell count and blood urea nitrogen, creatinine, creatine phosphokinase, and aspartate aminotransferase determinations. Although a preanesthetic evaluation will not eliminate anesthetic or postanesthetic complications, it may identify horses that are high risks and in which elective procedures should be delayed or reevaluated. Hay and grain are withheld for 24 to 36 hours prior to anesthesia induction, but water is not generally withheld. For patients on high concentrate diets, the concentrate should be markedly reduced or eliminated several days before anesthesia induction. Horses must be placed in a nonbedded stall for 24 hours to prevent con-

---

*Torbugesic, Fort Dodge Labs, Fort Dodge, IA

sumption of bedding. Immediately prior to induction, the mouth is thoroughly flushed with water to reduce the chance of introducing foreign material into the trachea during respiration or intubation.

INDUCTION PHASE

Problems encountered during induction of general anesthesia in the draft horse include ataxia, physical control of the patient, excessive hypotension, and hypoventilation produced by the induction agents. A rapid, smooth induction with minimal ataxia and minimal cardiopulmonary depression is ideal. Preanesthetic tranquilization will aid induction by decreasing anxiety and potentiating the effects of the induction agents (see Table 1). The dosages of injectable anesthetics for draft breeds are listed in Table 2.

BARBITURATES

Ultrashort-acting barbiturates are frequently used alone or in combination with other drugs to induce general anesthesia in the horse. The administration of a precalculated bolus dose is necessary to produce a smooth induction. After bolus administration some horses collapse in the rear and tend to fall backward. Control of the head is vital to prevent trauma to the head and neck but is difficult to achieve in the draft horse. Repeated administration of barbiturates often results in prolonged, violent recoveries with severe hypotension and respiratory depression; consequently, ultrashort-acting barbiturates are not recommended for maintenance anesthesia in draft breeds. The dosage of ultrashort-acting barbiturates for anesthetic induction in draft horses ranges from 5.5 to 6.6 mg per kg given as an IV bolus following preanesthetic sedation.

TABLE 2. DOSES OF INJECTABLE AGENTS FOR ANESTHESIA OR INDUCTION OF INHALATION ANESTHESIA IN DRAFT HORSES

Anesthetic	Dosages for IV Route
Thiamylal sodium	5.5–6.6 mg/kg by IV bolus°
Guaifenesin	5%: 2.2 ml/kg°
	10%: 1.1 ml/kg
Guaifenesin	5%: 1 liter°,†
+	10%: ½ liter°,†
Thiamylal sodium	3.3–4.4 mg/kg
Xylazine	1.1 mg/kg
Ketamine	2.2 mg/kg
Guaifenesin	5% or 10% to effect
Ketamine	2.2 mg/kg by IV bolus
Detomidine	0.02–0.04 mg/kg
Ketamine	2.2 mg/kg

°After premedication.
†The average 1900-lb (850-kg) draft horse may require more than 1 liter of 5 per cent guaifenesin plus thiamylal or more than 500 ml of a 10 per cent solution plus thiamylal.

GUAIFENESIN

Guaifenesin is a muscle relaxant that acts at internuncial neurons of the spinal cord. Guaifenesin does not produce CNS depression or analgesia. There is a 4 to 5-minute lag between guaifenesin administration and effect. At concentrations greater than 10 per cent, guaifenesin produces significant intravascular hemolysis. This drug should be administered rapidly to produce smooth induction. When administered by gravity flow a minimum of a 12-gauge needle or catheter is recommended. When administered under pressure a 14-gauge catheter is sufficient. A calculated dose of 110 mg per kg IV as a 5 or 10 per cent solution can be used for induction. However, the amount necessary to produce recumbency will vary and the drug should be given to effect. A long period of ataxia may precede recumbency, which is dangerous to the horse and the personnel administering anesthesia. Another disadvantage of using guaifenesin alone in draft horses is that a large quantity is necessary to produce recumbency. At the above dose a 900-kg draft horse requires approximately 74 gm for induction. If a liter of 5 per cent guaifenesin is used (50 gm), two 1-liter bottles may be necessary. A liter of 10 per cent guaifenesin may be adequate. Although guaifenesin alone may be safe for induction of very debilitated patients, it is not recommended for induction in healthy patients scheduled for elective procedures, owing to the excessive ataxia prior to recumbency. Because guaifenesin alone lacks significant analgesic properties, its use as a singular anesthetic agent is questionable. Following administration of large quantities, long recovery periods and increased risk of toxicity should be expected.

Guaifenesin is most valuable when combined with other agents for induction and maintenance of anesthesia in healthy horses. Combining ultrashort-acting barbiturates with guaifenesin allows reduction of the barbiturate dose, but provides analgesia and CNS depression. Inductions are generally improved, although a period of ataxia still occurs during the induction phase. Premedication is recommended with low-dose acetylpromazine, xylazine, or detomidine. Usually 2 gm of ultrashort-acting barbiturate (4.4 mg per kg) is added to 1 liter of 5 per cent or 500 ml of 10 per cent guaifenesin. This combination can be used to induce anesthesia in draft horses. The use of 5 per cent guaifenesin and thiamylal° (3.3 mg per kg) has been recommended for induction prior to inhalation anesthesia. Additional guaifenesin and barbiturate should be available for horses weighing more than 1800 lb (800 kg)

°Bio-tal, Bio-Ceutic, Boehringer Ingelheim Animal Health, Inc., St. Joseph, MO

in case the initial dose is inadequate for induction or if the anesthesia is to be maintained by injectable methods. This combination has the disadvantage of prerecumbency ataxia, but less than that produced by guaifenesin alone. Induction is improved by administering guaifenesin until the patient is slightly ataxic or buckling of the limbs is noted, and then administering the barbiturate as a bolus. This combination is not recommended for long-term maintenance of anesthesia as prolonged recoveries may occur. Additional doses of barbiturate-guaifenesin combinations require a sequential reduction in the amount of barbiturate.

XYLAZINE AND KETAMINE

The combination of xylazine and ketamine[†] usually produces smoother inductions than guaifenesin-barbiturate combinations. Anesthesia with a xylazine-ketamine combination is characterized by short duration, poor muscle relaxation, good somatic analgesia, and active ocular and upper airway reflexes. The dose used in the draft horse is essentially that used in light breeds (xylazine, 1.1 mg per kg IV; ketamine, 1.76 to 2.2 mg per kg IV). Because xylazine-induced ataxia may make draft horses difficult to control, ketamine should be administered as soon as adequate xylazine sedation is noted. Ketamine given prior to adequate xylazine sedation often results in a violent recovery. Three regimens may be considered for maintaining anesthesia for *short* periods with xylazine and ketamine: (1) repetition of xylazine and ketamine at one half of the original dose, (2) administration of ketamine alone at one half of the original dose, with readministration of xylazine at one half of the original dose after the second ketamine supplementation, (3) administration of 200-mg increments of ketamine with the repetition of xylazine only after the third or fourth increment. The repeated administration of ketamine without repetition of xylazine may result in a difficult recovery.

Detomidine may be combined with ketamine for short-term anesthesia. Although adequate field experience is lacking at present, the suggested dose in the light horse is detomidine at 0.02 to 0.04 mg per kg IV, followed in 15 minutes by ketamine at 2.2 mg per kg IV. Because of the long duration of detomidine sedation and short duration of ketamine anesthesia, excessive ataxia may be noted upon recovery.

Several other induction protocols may be used in the draft horse. One protocol includes preanesthetic sedation with acetylpromazine (0.33 mg per kg IV), followed in 15 minutes by guaifenesin (5 to 10 per cent) until ataxia is noted. Ketamine is then given as a bolus (2.2 mg per kg IV).

Anesthesia can be induced or maintained for short periods by a mixture of guaifenesin and ketamine (ketamine, 2.2 mg per kg in 5 to 10 per cent guaifenesin). Another combination used for anesthetic induction and maintenance in light breeds is a mixture of xylazine (1.1 mg per kg) and ketamine (2.2 mg per kg) in 5 to 10 per cent guaifenesin. This combination has been reported for use in ponies and foals, but not reported specifically in draft breeds.

INHALATION ANESTHESIA

Inhalation anesthesia provides greater control of anesthetic depth and less opportunity for toxicity, and allows surgical procedures of longer duration to be undertaken with less frequent recovery problems. Inhalation anesthesia does, however, necessitate more sophisticated equipment and experienced personnel for patient monitoring.

The general principles of inhalation anesthesia are similar in all horses regardless of size. Following induction, the largest endotracheal tube that will comfortably fit the patient (20 to 40 mm) should be placed and the cuff inflated. Oxygen or oxygen-anesthetic mixtures are delivered following intubation. The administration of an oxygen-enriched mixture may reduce positional hypoxemia common in recumbent horses. Initial oxygen flow rates using a semiclosed, large animal circle system vary between 15.5 and 17.5 ml per kg per min. Four to 5 per cent halothane or isoflurane is administered initially and is reduced as physical monitoring of neural reflexes and cardiopulmonary parameters indicates. The goal is the lowest inhalant concentration that will provide adequate surgical analgesia and restraint. High anesthetic inhalant concentration is the greatest contributor to hypotension in the early anesthetic period. Most draft horses can be maintained on 2.5 to 3.0 per cent halothane.[°] Once an adequate anesthetic plane is reached the oxygen flow rate may be reduced to 8.8 to 11.0 ml per kg per min. Heart rates of 30 to 40 beats per minute and respiratory rates of 6 to 12 per minute are ideal. Monitoring mean arterial blood pressure is valuable; the pressure should be maintained above 65 mm Hg. Premature reduction of the inhalant anesthetic concentration may result in a "seesaw" anesthesia (frequent, alternating periods of light and deep anesthesia). It is a clinical impression that draft horses maintained on a high inhalant concentration or in "see-saw" fashion tend to have more postanesthetic complications. When isoflurane is

---

[†]Ketaset, Fort Dodge, IA

[°]Fluothane, Ford Dodge, IA

used, surgical anesthesia and recovery may occur more rapidly than with halothane.

During recovery the airway should be maintained after the anesthetic has been discontinued to facilitate supplementation of inspired air with 100 per cent oxygen. Oxygen can be administered via the anesthetic system, demand valve, or by insufflation at more than 15 L per minute until the orotracheal tube is removed.

POSTANESTHETIC COMPLICATIONS

Complications common with anesthesia of the draft horse are similar to those that occur in light breed horses and include myopathies, neuropathies, and edema plaques. Transient soft palate and pharyngeal paresis or turbinate congestion may occur following removal of the endotracheal tube. Close observation is required following extubation, and should these complications occur, reintubation may be necessary. A nasotracheal tube can also be passed and supplemental oxygen administered by insufflation if reintubation is difficult. Alternatively, the orotracheal tube can be taped in place and not removed until the patient is standing. Most patients recover well in a quiet, darkened recovery area.

The most common complication in draft horses is postanesthetic myopathy. Clinical signs of postoperative myopathy vary from mild lameness to inability to stand. The basic metabolic alterations are similar to those occurring in exertional myopathy or rhabdomyolysis. Predisposing factors include genetic predispostion, diet, level of exercise, endocrine alterations, size, and weight. These factors, plus the duration of anesthesia, the depth of anesthesia as it affects blood pressure and tissue perfusion, positioning as related to compartmental muscle pressure, and ventilation, determine the frequency of occurrence. Draft breeds exhibit an obvious predisposition to postanesthetic myopathy. Arterial hypotension, increased compartmental muscle pressure due to body weight, and hypoxemia related to inadequate pulmonary ventilation are critical contributory factors. Halothane-induced hypotension (mean arterial pressure less than 65 mm Hg) produces a dramatic decrease in muscle blood flow. This is exacerbated by the increase in intracompartmental muscle pressure which results from the weight of the horse and certain positions of the limbs. Loss of adequate muscle perfusion produces an anaerobic environment, localized lactic acidosis, and myodegeneration. There is also some evidence that halothane may directly affect calcium release in some tissues (as in malignant hyperthermia), triggering excessive muscle contraction or spasms.

Signs of muscle disease may be noted immediately when the horse attempts to stand or may not be evident for several hours after recovery. Signs vary from gait abnormalities in one or more limbs to inability to rise. Draft horses that are unable to stand after 48 to 72 hours have a poor prognosis, particularly if they have made frequent unsuccessful attempts to rise. These patients often exhaust themselves and tend to perpetuate the syndrome despite therapy.

Adductor myopathy has been reported in horses anesthetized for long periods of time in dorsal recumbency. This syndrome occurs when the rear limbs are passively flexed and can also be associated with pressure on the rear limbs during the surgical procedure.

Postanesthetic hemorrhagic myelopathy, reported in young, light breed horses, may occur in draft breeds anesthetized in dorsal recumbency. This syndrome is characterized by hemorrhage in the subarachnoid space at the thoracolumbar area of the spinal cord. Signs include inability to move the pelvic limbs, exaggerated extensor tone in the forelimbs, rigid extension of the hind limbs, and intercostal paralysis. Proper padding and avoidance of positional or surgical pressure may reduce the occurrence.

Postoperative neuropathies are usually associated with positioning and inadequate padding. These include transient or permanent paralysis of the facial, radial, or peroneal nerve.

Edema plaques occur as a result of improper padding of pressure point areas or localized hyperthermia at points of contact with the padding. These are most commonly found on the lateral shoulder, ilium, and masseter muscle areas. Plaques generally resolve without treatment. If they do not, hydrotherapy and nonsteroidal anti-inflammatory drugs can be used to assist resolution.

DANTROLENE

Dantrolene sodium* has been suggested for the prevention and treatment of myopathy in the horse. Dantrolene slows the release of calcium ions from the muscle sarcoplasmic reticulum, thereby decreasing the muscle cells' ability to contract. Recent investigations have indicated that dantrolene is rapidly redistributed and eliminated from the horse's body. After IV and PO administration the elimination half-lives are 129 and 136 minutes, respectively. The peak plasma concentration after oral administration occurs in 1.5 hours. As a possible preventative for postanesthetic myopathy, a preanesthetic loading dose of 10 mg per kg PO, followed in 1.5 to 2 hours by 2.5 mg per kg every 60 minutes, will maintain adequate plasma levels. For the treat-

---

*Dantrium, Norwich Eaton, Norwich, NY

ment of acute myopathy 1.9 mg per kg IV in physiologic saline over 10 minutes may be beneficial. The efficacy of dantrolene in the prevention of exertional or postanesthetic myopathy has not been proven in controlled studies.

Supplemental Readings

Court, M. H., Engelking, L. R., Dodman, N. H., et al.: Pharmacokinetics of dantrolene sodium in horses. J. Vet Pharmacol. Ther., 10:218–226, 1987.

Gleed R., Short, C. E.: A retrospective study of the anesthetic management of adult draft horses. Vet. Med. Small Anim. Clin., 75:1409–1414, 1990.

Grandy, J. L., Steffey, E. P., Hodgson, D. S., et al.: Arterial hypotension and the development of postanesthetic myopathy in halothane-anesthetized horses. Am. J. Vet. Res., 48:192–197, 1987.

Lindsay, W. A., Robinson, G. M., Brunson, D. B., et al.: Induction of equine postanesthetic myositis after halothane-induced hypotension. Am. J. Vet. Res., 50:404–410, 1989.

Muir, W. W.: Drugs used to produce standing chemical restraint in horses. Vet. Clin. North Am. (Equine Pract.), 3:17–44, 1981.

Thurmon, J. C., Benson, G.J: Injectable anesthetics and anesthetic adjuncts. Vet. Clin. North Am. (Equine Pract.), 3:15–36, 1987.

Sedation and Anesthesia of Mules and Donkeys

Nora S. Matthews and Tex Taylor, COLLEGE STATION, TEXAS

Mules and donkeys have been used by man for thousands of years. Although not nearly as numerous in the United States as in the past (their population peaked in 1920 at over 5 million) they are still raised as a labor source, as guard animals for the sheep industry, and for export to developing nations. As with other species, the worth of certain individuals is considerable (for example, imported miniature donkeys and Mammoth jacks), so the practitioner is more likely to see them when surgery is required. In the absence of specific information about anesthesia of mules and donkeys, veterinarians have generally assumed that they respond to the same methods and dosages as horses. This assumption sometimes leads to a frustrating and perhaps dangerous experience. This discussion presents specific information about mules and donkeys with respect to anesthetic drugs and techniques.

PREOPERATIVE ASSESSMENT

The preoperative assessment and preparation of mules, donkeys, and horses should be similar. A good history and physical examination may be all that is necessary, although it is helpful to have basic blood work, for example, packed cell volume and total protein measurements. More extensive biochemical or hematologic evaluations may be performed as indicated by the history and physical examination results. Normal values for mules and donkeys have been investigated and appear to be almost identical to normal values for the horse. Values for resting heart and respiratory rates, systolic blood pressure, and arterial blood gas values also appear to be similar to those values in the horse.

Although we have only limited data, weights obtained with an equine weight tape are within 5 to 8 per cent of actual values, so we use the weight tape for calculation of drug dosages when it is not possible to actually weigh the mule or donkey. As with the horse, we withhold grain for 12 hours before surgery.

RESTRAINT

Restraint of the mule or donkey is essential to preparation for anesthesia. A stout halter, a strong leadshank, and an immovable object are required. Catheter placement or intravenous (IV) injections can be accomplished with less difficulty *after* the mule or donkey has had an opportunity to test the strength of the tie. Unlike the horse, the mule or donkey, after sitting back and trying the rope, will generally stop fighting and stand quietly, if the rope has held securely. A nose twitch can be used but is less effective than in horses, and it is not as effective as solidly anchoring the mule to a post.

Mules in particular, and donkeys to a lesser extent, seem to object less to injections if the needle is laid against the skin and firmly pressed through into the vein. This is in contrast to the practice of rapidly inserting the needle ("popping") through the skin, as is done in most horses.

LOCAL/REGIONAL ANESTHESIA

Epidural anesthesia has been investigated in donkeys and it was reported that 8 to 10 ml (the weights of the donkeys were not reported) of 1 per cent procaine hydrochloride injected into the epidural space at the second intercoccygeal space produced sensory block while the animals remained standing. The injections were made with the needle at an angle of 30 degrees from horizontal (in contrast to insertion at 45 degrees preferred in the horse).

IV regional anesthesia of the thoracic limb has been used in the donkey. Physical restraint was used with the animal in lateral recumbency (the method of restraint was not reported), and 20 ml of 2 per cent lidocaine was injected into the radial vein following tourniquet application above the elbow. Tourniquet application for more than 90 minutes was associated with persistent lameness and edema. As in horses, other local nerve blocks or local infiltration have been used with or without tranquilization. Although there are very few reports of comparative anatomy, anatomical landmarks appear to be the same as in the horse.

TRANQUILIZATION AND SEDATION

Tranquilizers and sedatives that have been used in the mule and donkey include:

1. Propionyl-phenothiazine° (0.023 mg per kg IV).
2. Acetylpromazine† (0.1 mg per kg IM or IV).
3. Acetylpromazine (0.1 mg per kg) can be combined with etorphine‡ (0.0225 mg per kg) IV or IM to produce neuroleptanalgesia and as premedication before general anesthesia. The narcotic portion of this mixture can be reversed using the antagonist, diprenorphine.§ However, there have been reports of renarcotization after reversal when IV and subcutaneous doses of diprenorphine were used. It has been theorized that donkeys may metabolize the N-alkyl substituent of the diprenorphine molecule, thus converting the antagonist into an agonist. This "relapse" may produce a mild excitement. When this combination is used, the following guidelines are recommended: use equivalent doses of agonist and antagonist, keep the donkey under observation for 3 hours after remobilization, and protect the animal from extremes of temperature. A further half dose of diprenorphine may be given if incoordination occurs. However, this combination is not practical for routine use since it requires extensive paperwork to obtain and use the drug, and appropriate precautions in handling the drug must be observed, owing to its great potency and transdermal absorption.

4. Xylazine.∥ In the mule high doses of xylazine appear to be needed to produce good sedation reliably. A reasonable rule is to use the horse dose plus 50 per cent more (i.e., 1.65 mg per kg IV, 3.3 mg per kg IM). Generally, donkeys are effectively sedated with the horse dose (1.1 mg per kg IV, 2.2 mg per kg IM) or less.

5. Xylazine (1.1 per kg IV) and butorphanol¶ (0.044 mg per kg IV) are combined for neuroleptanalgesia or as a premedicant combination for ketamine anesthesia. When these drugs are used at these doses, mules are well sedated, and some donkeys are sedated enough to lie down. This combination is our preference for standing sedation.

6. Detomidine.# Since detomidine has been available in the United States only since January 1990, we have not used it in mules or donkeys. However, reports indicate that it is effective when used IV or IM at the horse dose plus 50 per cent (0.030 to 0.060 mg per kg).

While it may be possible to complete many procedures with tranquilization or sedation with or without a local anesthesia, practitioners should be especially cautious about procedures involving the hind legs in mules. They have always been known for the accurate aim of their kicks. Additional restraint, such as hobbles, tying up a leg, and so forth, should be considered in mules but are probably not necessary in donkeys. General anesthesia is often the safest choice.

INJECTABLE ANESTHESIA

Various combinations of injectable anesthetics have been used in mules and donkeys, with vary-

---

°Combelen, Bayer AG, Leverkusen, Germany
†PromAce, Fort Dodge Labs., Fort Dodge, IA
‡Large Animal Immobilon, Reckitt and Colman Pharmaceutical Division, Hull, MA
§Large Animal Revivon, Reckitt and Colman Pharmaceutical Division, Hull, MA

∥Rompun, Mobay Corp., Animal Health Division, Shawnee, KS
¶Torbugesic, Fort Dodge Labs., Fort Dodge, IA
#Dormosedan, Norden Labs., Lincoln, NE

ing advantages, disadvantages, and durations of recumbency.

1. Acetylpromazine and etorphine premedication (see previous section for doses), followed by ketamine (2.0 to 2.5 mg per kg IV). This combination is reported to produce an average of 13 minutes of recumbency.

2. Propionyl-phenothiazine (0.023 mg per kg IV) premedication followed by chloral hydrate (80 mg per kg IV). In donkeys the duration of anesthesia is 1.5 hours, and the donkeys recover after 3 hours. Recovery is smooth, but muscle relaxation is incomplete. Although this combination has probably been used in mules, we were not able to find any reports of its use.

3. Chloral hydrate (80 mg per kg IV) with thiopental sodium° (10 mg per kg IV). The duration of anesthesia is about 45 minutes, but muscle relaxation is incomplete. Although chloral hydrate is still used in some countries, its use in the United States has declined with the development of better, safer anesthetics. Chloral hydrate is a good hypnotic sedative, but the dose needed to produce anesthesia approaches the minimal lethal dose. It is no longer commercially available.

4. Thiopental or thiamylal† (4.4 to 8.8 mg per kg IV) may be given, with or without tranquilization, to produce anesthesia of approximately 20 minutes' duration. The dosage used, premedications, and precautions are the same as for the horse. Induction is very rapid, and a dose-dependent period of apnea may be seen. It is safer to administer the thiobarbiturates in combination with guaifenesin‡ (see below), so that the effects may be carefully titrated.

5. Thiamylal (4.4 mg per kg) mixed with guaifenesin, generally 1 liter of 5 per cent, may be administered rapidly IV for induction of anesthesia, following premedication with xylazine (0.4 mg per kg IV). Based on a small number of clinical cases, we believe that mules and donkeys may require approximately one-third less of this combination than a horse of comparable size, so administration should be accompanied by careful monitoring of heart rate, palpable pulse, and respiration.

6. Xylazine (1.1 mg per kg IV) followed by ketamine§ (2.2 mg per kg IV) produces an average recumbency time of 14 minutes in mules and 20 minutes in donkeys. This is less than the average recumbency time of 23 minutes in horses, and muscle relaxation is often incomplete, especially in mules in which this dose of xylazine does not always produce adequate sedation.

7. Xylazine (1.1 mg per kg IV) and butorphanol (0.04 mg per kg IV) followed by ketamine (2.2 mg per kg IV) produces longer recumbency times (25 minutes in mules, 24 minutes in horses, and 35 minutes in donkeys) with improved muscle relaxation. This combination is our preference of injectable anesthetics for short-term anesthesia since it consistently produces good sedation, a smooth induction, adequate muscle relaxation with analgesia, and a smooth, coordinated recovery.

8. Xylazine (1.1 mg per kg IV) followed by tiletamine-zolazepam‖ (a 1:1 mixture combined and dosed at 1.1 mg per kg IV) produces rapid recumbency with very good muscle relaxation. Recumbency times are fairly long, averaging 21 minutes in mules, 31 minutes in horses, and 43 minutes in donkeys. Several attempts are required for the animal to stand successfully. Because mules and horses may fall again after standing, we consider the recoveries unsafe in these animals unless they are assisted by the use of head and tail ropes. After standing, the animals are very ataxic and unsteady, especially in the hind limbs. Although donkeys require several attempts to stand, recoveries are not unsafe, probably because of the calmer disposition of donkeys. When they cannot coordinate their hind limbs, they resume recumbency quietly for several minutes before making another attempt to stand. The rapid onset of effects should make this combination useful for "darting" wild burros. Tiletamine-zolazepam can be reconstituted with xylazine instead of sterile water and IM dosages (2.2 mg per kg of xylazine with 2.2 mg per kg of tiletamine-zolazepam) used.

9. A combination of 1000 mg ketamine, and 500 mg xylazine mixed into 1 liter of 5 per cent guaifenesin, may be used for induction by bolus administration of 1.1 ml per kg IV, and for maintenance (2.2 ml per kg per hour IV) of anesthesia in mules and donkeys. This combination has been used very successfully in horses. Although we have used it in mules and donkeys, we feel that decreasing to 2.5 per cent guaifenesin makes it more useful and safer. In miniature donkeys, the small size necessitates careful calculation of the drug dose. A small animal administration set or buretrol is valuable to accurately measure the small volume required.

°Pentothal, Abbott Labs., North Chicago, IL
†Biotal, Bio-Ceutic Division, Boehringer Ingelheim Animal Health, St. Joseph, MO
‡Guaifenesin USP, Chemical Products Manufacturing Corp., St. Joseph, MO
§Ketaset, Fort Dodge Labs., Fort Dodge, IA

‖Telazol, A. H. Robins Co., Richmond, VA

INHALANT ANESTHESIA

When procedures lasting longer than one hour are planned, inhalant anesthesia is our preference. Mules and donkeys may be maintained in a manner similar to that for the horse. In our clinical experience mules and donkeys require essentially the same concentrations of halothane* or isoflurane,† although studies determining the minimum alveolar concentrations are lacking for these species. Induction can be accomplished using the injectable drug combinations outlined earlier under Injectable Anesthesia; endotracheal intubation is performed in the same manner and with the same size of endotracheal tube as for horses of comparable size. When animals are allowed to breathe spontaneously during anesthesia, respiratory rates appear to be higher (20 to 30 breaths per minute) with less chest excursion and more abdominal excursion than in the horse. Blood pressure may be monitored indirectly (using a Doppler or Dinamap unit) or directly by means of an anaeroid manometer or transducer and physiograph. Few data are available on "normal" blood pressure values for awake or anesthetized mules and donkeys. Our records indicate that mean blood pressure may be slightly lower than in the horse. We maintain a mean blood pressure of 50 to 55 mm Hg with no adverse consequences such as myositis. However, these data are from a very small number of cases; until more is known, one should probably plan to treat hypotension aggressively by lightening the plane of anesthesia and administering fluids and inotropic drugs.

Mules and donkeys appear to have a higher response threshold than horses, which makes them slightly more difficult to monitor. They will appear nonresponsive with no palpebral reflex, nystagmus, tearing, or blinking during minor stimuli, then be wide awake and move with a surgical stimulus.

Recovery is usually smooth; they will usually lie quietly without thrashing, until capable of standing. Complications such as myositis and leg fractures are much less common than in the horse.

Supplemental Readings

Al-Badrany, M. S., Abid, T. A., Singh, A. P., and Soliman, A. S.: Intravenous retrograde regional anaesthesia of thoracic limb in donkey. Indian J. Vet. Surg., *10*:5, 1989.

Dobbs, H. E., and Ling, C. M.: The use of etorphine/acepromazine in the horse and donkey. Vet. Rec., *91*:40, 1972.

Kinabo, L. D. B., and Bogan, J. A.: Disposition of triclabendazole in horses, ponies and donkeys. Equine Vet. J., *21*:305, 1989.

Samy, M. T., El-Sabaie, A., and Aly, M. A.: Blood gases and acid-base balance under the influences of different anaesthetic combinations in donkeys. Assiut Vet. Med. J., *17*:147, 1986.

Shoukry, M., Saleh, M., and Fouad, K.: Epidural anaesthesia in donkeys. Vet. Rec., *97*:450, 1975.

---

*Halothane, Halocarbon Labs, Inc., North Augusta, SC
†Aerrane, Anaquest, Madison, WI

Section 4

MUSCULOSKELETAL DISEASES

Edited by Alicia Bertone

Developmental Orthopedic Disease

Warren L. Beard, COLUMBUS, OHIO
Debra A. Knight, COLUMBUS, OHIO

Developmental orthopedic disease encompasses a complex of disease entities in the growing horse that are interrelated by a common pathophysiologic mechanism. Endochondral ossification, the process by which cartilage is converted to bone, occurs in the diaphysis, physis, and epiphysis of the long and cuboidal bones of the appendicular and axial skeletons. Genetic predisposition, nutrition, and physical factors, including trauma, may all play a role in the pathogenesis of developmental orthopedic disease, because all have the ability to disrupt the endochondral ossification process.

Endochondral ossification is a sequential process of replication, growth, and degeneration of chondrocytes; calcification and vascular invasion of the cartilage matrix; and finally differentiation of chondrocytes into osteoblasts with formation of lamellar bone. Disruption of this process leads to retention of cartilage that may form fissures in articular cartilage, result in osteochondral fragments, invaginate to form subchondral cysts, cause delayed ossification of the carpal or tarsal bones, or result in growth disparity and angular limb deformity. Skeletal lesions may manifest at any site where this process is perturbed. It should be recognized that the resulting condition is the local manifestation of a systemic process that may precede clinical recognition by months to years.

CLINICAL SYNDROMES

ANGULAR LIMB DEFORMITIES

Angular limb deformities develop in young foals. The deformity is named according to the joint involved and the direction of deviation of the limb distal to the affected area. Axial and abaxial deviation of the distal limb are termed *varus* and *valgus*, respectively. Carpal deformities are most frequently encountered, followed by deformities in the tarsus and fetlock. Bilateral involvement is common. The deviation may arise in the diaphysis of the long bone but more frequently occurs in the metaphysis, the epiphysis, or the cuboidal bones. The diagnosis may be made visually; however, radiographs are essential to determine the origin of the defect and to assess bone and joint configuration. Radiographs are usually taken on long cassettes. On the dorsopalmar view, lines drawn through the center of the long axis of the long bones on either side of the angulation will intersect at the origin of the deformity.

Therapy

Treatment and prognosis vary with the joint involved, the severity of the deformity, and the age of the foal at recognition of the condition. Discussion will be limited to irreducible acquired deformities. The degree of straightening that can be achieved is determined by the amount of residual growth at the involved physis. Carpus valgus is the most common deformity seen, and the site of the growth disparity is usually the distal radial physis. The carpal bones and the diaphysis of the radius and third metacarpal may contribute. Angulations of less than 5 degrees are considered to be mild deformities, those of 5 to 15 degrees are considered moderate deformities, and those of 15 to 30 degrees are considered severe deformities. Mild deformities in young foals can be successfully treated with controlled, light exercise in the hope of stimulating bone growth and limb straightening. Exercise may retard growth and exacerbate the deformity if compression exceeds the physiologic range. This is more likely to occur if the foal is of large body size, exercise is excessive, or the angulation is severe. Therefore, foals with moderate to severe deformities should be confined. Abnormal angulation causes uneven hoof wear, so the feet should be rasped as necessary.

Surgical treatment should be chosen if the deformity worsens or if no improvement is observed within 2 weeks. Hemicircumferential periosteal transection and stripping is the treatment of choice for moderate to severe deformities and for mild deformities that have not responded to conservative treatment. Moderate and severe deformities are usually surgically treated early to try to achieve correction when there is significant growth potential remaining in the physis. The surgery may be repeated in 1 to 2 months if correction is incomplete. Transphyseal bridging is commonly performed in conjunction with hemicircumferential periosteal transection and stripping in severe cases. For irreducible deformities, casts, splints, and limb braces may not provide additional benefit and may cause ulceration of the skin over bony prominences. Tarsal deformity may be treated in a manner similar to that for a carpal deformity, because the physes are physiologically similar in growth rate and closure. Tarsal valgus in one limb and varus in the contralateral limb ("windswept") is a congenital condition that may correct with time. Treatment of this congenital condition may be more difficult than treatment of the acquired condition because of abnormal formation of the associated soft tissues, such as the joint capsule.

Angular deformities of the fetlock differ from carpal and tarsal deformities in that early recognition is paramount to their correction. The physes of the distal metacarpus and tarsus cease growth by approximately 3 months even though they are radiographically apparent for 6 months. Radiographs are taken to ensure that the first phalanx and metacarpal or metatarsal bones are of normal shape. Conservative treatment consists of trimming the feet level and confinement, and is recommended only for mild cases and for foals less than 3 weeks old. Failure to achieve correction with conservative therapy leaves little opportunity for correction by other means, owing to the rapid growth plate closure. Surgical correction is by hemicircumferential periosteal transection and stripping plus, in most cases, transphyseal bridging.

PHYSEAL DYSPLASIA

Physeal dysplasia (physitis) usually is recognized in young horses from 6 to 18 months of age. The metaphyses are usually warm, painful, and enlarged. Lameness may be mild with stiffness, or severe. Affected locations are often multiple and include the distal physes of the radius, tibia, third metacarpus, and third metatarsus. Radiographic lesions consist of widened irregular physes, lysis and sclerosis, and occasionally cystic lesions. Physeal dysplasia tends to resolve more quickly in foals and weanlings than in yearlings. It is generally self-limiting unless cystic lesions are present in the bone.

Therapy

Treatment consists of dietary evaluation and correction if needed and phenylbutazone for horses exhibiting pain. In many cases, physeal dysplasia in the early phases responds favorably to correction of nutrient balance in the diet. The traditional treatment of reductions in feed intake and protein content is of questioned efficacy and, if severe, may restrict skeletal and muscular growth and reduce bone mineralization. A thorough evaluation of the feeding program for both adequacy and balance is essential before any changes are instituted. Samples of the hay, grain, and supplements making up the ration should be shipped to a qualified laboratory for nutrient analysis. Pasture analysis should be included if it is the predominant source of forage. The practitioner should request analyses for dry matter, crude protein, energy, total digestible nutrients (TDN), crude fiber, calcium, phosphorus, magnesium, potassium, sodium, sulfur, iron, copper,

TABLE 1. SUGGESTED DAILY NUTRIENT CONTENT OF THE TOTAL DIET FOR FOALS, WEANLINGS, AND YEARLINGS

Nutrient	Amount per Day		
	Foals*	Weanlings	Yearlings
Digestible energy, Mcal	13–15	15–18	18–20
Crude protein, gm	650–800	700–850	850–1000
Calcium, gm	35–45	40–50	40–50
Phosphorus, gm	25–35	30–40	30–40
Magnesium, gm	4–5	5–6	6–7
Potassium, gm	10–15	15–20	20–25
Copper, mg	120–160	150–180	175–200
Iron, mg	300–350	350–450	350–450
Manganese, mg	250–300	300–350	350–400
Zinc, mg	350–450	400–475	475–500
Iodine, mg	0.5–1	0.5–1	1–2
Selenium, mg	1–1.5	1–2	1–2

*For foals from 4 to 6 months of age.

manganese, and zinc. The weight per volume of each feed fed should be determined to calculate the nutrient content of the total ration. The suggested energy, protein, and mineral content of the total ration for young horses is given in Table 1. The recommended ratio of calcium to phosphorus is between 1.5:1 and 2:1. Higher levels of calcium are not likely to be a problem as long as adequate phosphorus is present. Decreases in energy intake are recommended if moderate to excessive condition (fat) is evident, or if the horse is confined to a stall for more than 7 days. When reductions in grain intake are indicated, the effect of this decrease on the protein and mineral content of the diet must be assessed and supplementation instituted where needed. The assistance of a reputable nutritionist can facilitate the evaluation and help with recommendations.

OSTEOCHONDROSIS
(Osteochondritis Dissecans)

Osteochondrosis lesions result from a defect in endochondral ossification in articular cartilage. Cartilage becomes thicker than is biomechanically ideal and cannot be nutritionally supported by the synovial fluid. This results in clefts, free cartilage flaps, osteochondral fragments, and misshapen joint surfaces. The first clinical sign is usually synovial effusion and may go unnoticed. Lameness is variable, reflecting the severity of the lesion and the joint involved. Lameness may not become apparent until after the horses are put into training. Degenerative arthritis is often the end result in untreated horses.

Osteochondrosis lesions have been described in almost every joint. Clinically the condition is usually noted in the hock, stifle, fetlock, shoulder, and cervical vertebrae. Bilateral lesions are common. Osteochondrosis should be a primary consideration in the differential diagnosis when synovial effusion is observed in young horses. The diagnosis is established by radiography; however, some lesions are inapparent radiographically and diagnostic arthroscopy may be indicated.

Therapy

Surgical removal is the treatment of choice if loose cartilage and bone fragments are present, especially if the horse is to be an athlete. Conservative therapy may be attempted in cases where surgery is not economically feasible, often with success. Prolonged stall rest (until lameness and effusion resolve) may result in resolution of some cystic lesions and healing of detached fragments. The goal of conservative therapy is to decrease the synovitis that results from the free fragments or exposure of subchondral bone. Intra-articular medication with hyaluronic acid is usually efficacious. Intra-articular corticosteroid administration will cause temporary resolution of the synovitis, but because use of these drugs may accelerate the degenerative process, they are contraindicated for long-term treatment.

The prognosis depends on the number of joints involved, the number and size of the lesions, the use of the horse, and the progression of articular cartilage damage. Lesions in the hock usually have a good prognosis following surgical treatment and often respond favorably to conservative management. Stifle lesions are often more extensive and the prognosis depends on the size and location within the joint. Osteochondrosis of the shoulder carries a fair to poor prognosis because the lesions involve a weight-bearing area.

There is no evidence that dietary changes have any effect on developing osteochondrotic lesions. The diagnosis of osteochondrosis in one or two weanlings or yearlings is generally followed by additional cases despite dietary intervention. Correcting the diet at this stage, however, may help to prevent the initiation of additional lesions and is therefore advised.

NUTRITIONAL GUIDELINES FOR PREVENTION OF DEVELOPMENTAL ORTHOPEDIC DISEASE

Attempts to reduce both the number of horses affected and the severity of the manifestations of developmental orthopedic disease in subsequent foal crops involve identification and evaluation of all factors currently believed to contribute to the disease process. A successful approach to prevention of these diseases through dietary means involves thorough evaluation of the nutrition program for brood mares, foals, and weanlings by a qualified nutritionist, farm veterinarian, and farm manager, and a strong commitment by the farm manager and his staff to comply with the recommendations. If nutrition is a major factor, failure at any of these levels will not satisfactorily reduce the number of horses affected. Empirical supplementation or restriction of the diet without nutrient analysis of the rations or evaluation of the feeding management is not advised.

Brood Mares

Prevention of developmental orthopedic disease in foals begins by providing the brood mare with a diet that is properly balanced and fortified. The energy, protein, and mineral content of a recommended ration for the last 4 months of gestation and lactation is given in Table 2. Commonly, mares are kept at pasture during the fall and early winter. Many mares are in their last trimester in these months and are not likely to receive sufficient quantities of some nutrients from pasture alone. Calcium and phosphorus supplementation may be necessary to meet increased needs. Recent research has also demonstrated that provision of supplemental trace minerals to mares has reduced the frequency of cartilage abnormalities in their foals. As a result, many commercial feeds have recently been reformulated. Several feed companies manufacture pelleted protein-vitamin-mineral supplements* that have been useful in providing the additional nutrients for gestating mares, particularly those that are fed little grain when pasture is plentiful. If additional grain is needed to meet the mare's en-

---

*Gro'N Win, Buckeye Feeds Mills, Inc., Dalton, OH; Spur and Foal-Prep, Manna Pro Corp., Los Angeles, CA; Tizwhiz Broodmare Ration and Tizwhiz 30 Plus, Tizwhiz Distributors, Delaware, OH

TABLE 2. RECOMMENDED DAILY ALLOWANCE OF NUTRIENTS IN THE TOTAL DIET OF MARES DURING LATE GESTATION AND EARLY LACTATION

Nutrient	Amount per Day	
	Late Gestation	Lactation
Digestible energy, Mcal*	18–22	25–30
Crude protein, gm	800–1000	1200–1500
Calcium, gm	35–45	50–60
Phosphorus, gm	25–35	30–40
Magnesium, gm	8–10	10–15
Potassium, gm	30–40	40–50
Copper, mg	250–300	250–300
Iron, mg	400–500	600–700
Manganese, mg	600–700	600–700
Zinc, mg	700–800	700–800
Iodine, mg	1–2	1–2
Selenium, mg	2–3	2–3

*Energy need may vary with age, desired body condition, and milk production.

ergy needs, these pellets can also be used in combination with commercial feeds to provide the necessary fortification. During lactation, the increase in fortified grain needed to supply additional energy usually provides the extra protein and minerals, eliminating the need for supplementation. The feeds should be used in accordance with the feeding guidelines suggested by the manufacturer.

Foals

The low concentrations of trace minerals in mare's milk and the presence of cartilage lesions in foals under 3 months of age suggest that mineral supplementation of the foal should begin early. Though many commercial feeds designed for foals are well-balanced and fortified, field experience indicates that most young foals rarely consume the amount of feed needed (5 lb or more) to provide them with the quantity of trace elements that has been shown to significantly reduce the occurrence of cartilage defects. For this reason, individual feeding of foals beginning at 2 to 3 weeks of age is recommended on farms where developmental orthopedic disease has become a problem. The protein-vitamin-mineral pellets discussed in the previous section have been useful for providing the necessary concentration of minerals in the small quantity that most foals are able to consume. The feed for the foal should be placed in a small box near the mare's feedtub. Tethering the mare prevents her from consuming the foal's feed. A small handful of grain may be added to enhance acceptability. The amount of pellet should be increased gradually. Foals should be eating 1 to 1½ lb of the pel-

lets by 4 months of age and 2 lb by 5 months.*
Once these goals have been reached, the grain mix selected for weanlings should be added. As grain intake increases, the pelleted supplement is decreased by 1 lb of pellets for each 3 lbs of grain mix. If oats are the grain of choice, the pellets should be used as the sole means of dietary fortification at 2 to 2½ lb per head per day. Providing the pelleted supplement in a creep feeder to a group of foals is not advised. Table 1 shows the recommended nutrient content for the diet of foals from 4 to 6 months of age.

WEANLINGS

Most weanlings will consume between 2 and 2.3 per cent of their body weight in feed per day. The diet should consist of 30 to 40 per cent hay and 60 to 70 per cent grain by weight. Older weanlings should receive the larger proportion of their diet as hay. Daily exercise is important for appetite stimulation, skeletal growth, and muscle development. Overfeeding is a major problem in the management of growing horses. Excessive weight gain may cause or exacerbate the development of physeal dysplasia, osteochondrosis, or angular limb deformities. Individual feeding, rather than group or creep feeding, provides greater control over nutrient intake, making special needs easier to address. Grain feeding in excess of 8 or 9 lbs per day is not necessary or recommended, unless hay quality is poor or horses are young and very active. Reexamination of the feeding program should be undertaken before reducing feed intake or initiating any supplementation when developmental orthopedic disease becomes evident. The reader is referred to the section on physeal dysplasia for a discussion of ration evaluation and Table 1 for the suggested nutrient content of weanling diets.

YEARLINGS

Diets for yearlings should maintain the balance and fortification previously established in weanling programs. The suggested nutrient content differs little from that of feeds for weanlings, except for a slight increase in energy needs (see Table 1). Most diets for yearlings should consist of 50 per cent hay and 50 per cent grain by weight. Overfeeding in preparation for sale or show can have the same adverse effects as described for weanlings, although at this stage, aggravation of existing, underlying disease is more likely than causation. For developmental orthopedic disease in yearlings, the nutritional treatment for weanlings applies. A storm of osteochondrosis in a crop of yearlings should be followed by a dietary evaluation of the brood mare, foal, and weanling programs rather than that of the yearlings alone, with the emphasis on prevention for the coming year.

Supplemental Readings

Auer, J. A., Martens, R. J., and Morris, E. L.: Angular limb deformities in foals. Part 1. Congenital factors. Compend. Cont. Ed. Pract. Vet., 4:S330–S339, 1982.
Auer, J. A., Martens, R. J., and Morris, E. L.: Angular limb deformities in foals. Part 2. Developmental factors. Compend. Cont. Ed. Pract. Vet., 5:S27–S35, 1983.
Fischer, A. T., and Barclay, W. P.: Osteochondrosis dissecans in the horse. Compend. Cont. Ed. Pract. Vet., 6:S123–S131, 1984.
National Research Council: Nutrient Requirements of Horses. Washington, D.C., National Academy Press, 1989.
Turner, A. S.: Diseases of bones and related structures. In Stashak, T. S. (ed.): Adams' Lameness in Horses, 4th ed. Philadelphia, Lea & Febiger, 1987.

---

*Feed one-fourth of the quantities listed when using Manna Pro Foal-Prep.

Diseases of the Spine

Mark D. Markel, MADISON, WISCONSIN

Horses with diseases of the spine can present with varied clinical signs, including lameness, localized pain, neurologic disorders, and alterations in appearance, attitude, and performance. For horses with neurologic signs, localization of the lesion may be possible based on a thorough neurologic examination. Most horses with diseases of the spine present with vague signs such as fever, lethargy, anorexia, diminished performance, and altered gait, making early diagnosis and localization of the lesion difficult. This chapter discusses infectious, mechanical/inflammatory, and traumatic conditions of the spine not normally associated with primary neurologic signs. These conditions include vertebral osteomyelitis, diskospondylitis, fistulous withers, crowding and overriding of dorsal spinous processes, ossifying spondylosis, and sacroiliac subluxation.

HISTORY

The clinical signs associated with diseases of the spine are highly variable. One relatively constant feature is a change in the horse's behavior or ability to perform. The onset of this change is usually insidious, but there may be a history of an acutely sore back associated with a traumatic episode. The horse may resent grooming, placing the saddle, tightening the girth, or picking up one or both hind limbs. Occasionally the horse may be reluctant to eat from the floor or may not lie down. If lameness is present, the hind limbs are the most frequently affected if there is a thoracolumbar spine lesion, and either the front or hind limbs may be affected if the cervical or cranial thoracic spine is involved.

PHYSICAL EXAMINATION

A thorough lameness, neurologic, and hematologic examination is essential in all horses with suspected spinal disease. With the horse standing squarely on all four limbs, conformation, symmetry of muscle groups, and deep or superficial swellings should be evaluated. The cervical vertebrae are palpated and the horse's neck manipulated dorsally, ventrally, and in both lateral directions to detect any localized pain or guarding of movement in the cervical region. The horse is observed when eating from the ground for abnormalities in head or neck motion. Beginning at the withers, the examiner palpates the dorsal spinous processes for the entire length of the back. The longissimus dorsi muscles should be pinched on either side of midline in the caudal thoracic, lumbar, and sacral regions to detect local regions of pain. The horse should dorsiflex and ventroflex the spine with these maneuvers and if reluctant to do so may be guarding motion of the spine, indicating a lesion in this region. The dorsal spinous processes are palpated to detect crepitus or pain. A rectal examination may elicit pain in the sublumbar group of muscles or detect swelling ventrad to the veterbral bodies if lesions of the lumbar or sacral regions are present.

The horse must be assessed at a walk, trot, and canter in a straight line and in large and small circles. Horses with spinal disease may have restricted forelimb or hind limb motion. With thoracolumbar disease, there may be restricted hind limb action accompanied by dragging of one or both toes. The horse may resent lateral motion of the affected spinal segment when circled. The horse should be worked on a longe line and then under saddle if it warms out of the abnormal gait. The clinician should observe the horse's response to saddling, tightening the girth, or mounting.

A thorough neurologic examination is necessary (see page 521) to help localize the lesion. A complete blood count (CBC) with measurement of fibrinogen will identify inflammatory lesions. If an infectious disorder such as fistulous withers, vertebral osteomyelitis, or diskospondylitis is suspected, a *Brucella abortus* titer should be determined. In addition, blood must be drawn for aerobic, anaerobic, and fungal culture, and if a potential site of infection is discovered, the region must be aspirated under diligent aseptic conditions and the fluid submitted for bacteriologic and fungal culture and cytologic examination.

If the lesion cannot be localized after a complete examination, radionuclide scintigraphy (bone scan) or a radiolabeled white blood cell scan can be very useful in localizing the lesion, particularly in difficult regions such as the thoracolumbar spine. After localization of the lesion, radiography of the suspected site is performed. With lesions such as cervical diskospondylitis and dorsal spinous process crowding and overriding, radiography should confirm the diagnosis. With lesions of the thoracolumbar spine, a radiographic diagnosis may be more difficult to establish, because the scatter reduces the quality of the image.

Radiographic examination of the spine, particularly of the thoracolumbar region, requires a 150 kVp, 1000 mA tube mounted on a three-dimensional overhead suspension. Rare earth intensifying screens with high-speed x-ray film will minimize both exposure and scatter. A parallel 12:1 grid with 43 lines per mm is used. Exposures vary from 20 to 200 mA and from 75 to 140 kVp, depending on the region of interest. If necessary, motion can be minimized by tranquilizing the horse with xylazine (0.5 to 1.1 mg per kg IV).

VERTEBRAL OSTEOMYELITIS

Vertebral body osteomyelitis is a rare but life-threatening condition in horses. Early signs are often limited to fever and back pain. The diagnosis may not be made until there are signs of spinal cord compression. If the infection has extended into the epidural space or paraspinal region, the prognosis is guarded (Fig.1).

Successful treatment of vertebral body osteo-

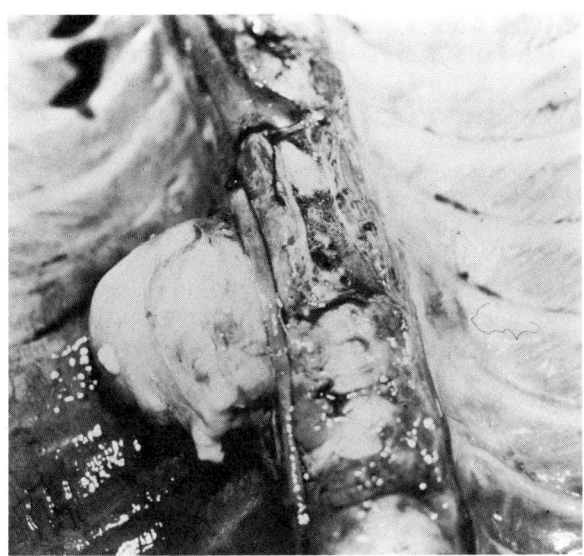

Figure 1. The ventral surface of the thoracic vertebrae at necropsy. A paravertebral abscess is ventrolateral to T12 and associated with vertebral body osteomyelitis.

myelitis depends on early detection, isolation of the causative organism, and appropriate antimicrobial agents. In all species, vertebral body osteomyelitis occurs most frequently in the young. Primary sites of infection should always be sought during clinical evaluation, because vertebral body osteomyelitis frequently represents secondary spread from another site of infection. In foals, umbilical abscess, patent urachus, and pneumonia have been primary infections. *Streptococcus zooepidemicus*, *Escherichia coli*, *Salmonella typhimurium*, *Rhodococcus equi*, and *Staphylococcus* spp., have been isolated from foals with vertebral body osteomyelitis. In adult horses, *Brucella abortus*, *Mycobacterium bovis*, *Streptococcus* spp. and *Aspergillus* spp. have caused the condition. Because of the wide variety of offending organisms, broad-spectrum antibiotics should be selected if an organism cannot be isolated. Long-term therapy of 2 to 6 months should be expected. Despite early and appropriate therapy, horses with vertebral body osteomyelitis have a guarded prognosis for survival because of the difficulty in eliminating the infection and frequent recurrences after cessation of antimicrobial therapy.

DISKOSPONDYLITIS

Diskospondylitis, inflammation of the vertebral bodies and the associated intervertebral disk, is rare in horses. Adults are affected more frequently than young animals. Diskospondylitis most frequently involves the cervical or upper thoracic vertebrae. Clinical signs include neck pain and ataxia, affecting the forelimbs to a greater degree than the hind limbs. Radiography frequently reveals a combination of destructive and productive lesions involving the affected vertebrae and disk space. Diskospondylitis is usually a septic condition and has been caused by *Brucella abortus* and *Streptococcus* spp. in horses. Since the lesion most frequently affects the cervical vertebrae, vertebral curettage combined with appropriate antimicrobial therapy may provide the best treatment. Horses with this condition have a guarded prognosis, and, despite debridement and appropriate antimicrobial therapy, the condition frequently progresses to cervical cord compression or meningitis, or both.

FISTULOUS WITHERS

"Fistulous withers" is inflammation of the bursa between the primary thoracic spines and the nuchal ligament. Fistulas extend to the skin with occasional migration ventrad to the associated vertebrae. In chronic cases the inflammation is suppurative and granulomatous. The primary lesion is either traumatic or inflammatory, initiated by *Onchocerca cervicalis*. Progression to a suppurative and granulomatous process is usually due to infection with *Brucella abortus* or *Actinomyces bovis*. Swelling of the bursae causes considerable pain and results in reluctance to move the head and neck. The swelling will ultimately fistulate with a typically copious and purulent exudate. Without treatment, lesions tend to be progressive with multiple draining tracts at the affected site. Because the location of the bursa provides poor natural drainage, lesions may extend ventrad to the dorsal spinous processes of the associated vertebrae.

When the clinical signs are consistent with fistulous withers, an aspirate of the site should be placed in blood culture bottles to ensure maximal isolation rates and submitted for culture and antimicrobial sensitivity testing. A diagnosis of *Brucella*-induced fistulous withers should be suspected with a history of association with cattle and the presence of the associated clinical signs. The diagnosis is confirmed by evidence of rising titers of antibodies to *Brucella abortus* or isolation of the organism.

Treatment of fistulous withers can be difficult and lengthy. Horses should be given ivermectin to limit or eliminate *Onchocerca cervicalis* infection. Because the condition is often due to intracellular organisms, treatment with trimethoprim-sulfa drugs is recommended. If the lesion becomes chronic, infected and necrotic material must be debrided and ventral drainage established.

In a case of proven *Brucella abortus* infection, the horse should be quarantined to prevent contact with other animals and human beings. Vaccination with three doses of live strain 19 *Brucella* vaccine may cause resolution of the disease and should be performed. If the lesion does not resolve with antimicrobial therapy or vaccination and becomes chronic, ventral drainage should be established and infected and necrotic material debrided. The prognosis for complete resolution of the lesion, whether or not it is caused by *Brucella abortus*, is guarded.

CROWDING AND OVERRIDING OF DORSAL SPINOUS PROCESSES

Impingement of the dorsal spinous processes occurs most frequently beneath the saddle area, at T12 to T17. The onset of the condition is often insidious and most prevalent in young, heavy Thoroughbreds used for jumping or dressage. Owners may report decreased performance, a change in attitude toward exercise, and a reluctance to lie down. Poor hind limb action at the trot or at fast exercise and poor jumping performance are nearly always features. Affected horses hold the thoracolumbar spine rigid and will not dorsiflex or ventroflex the spine normally, specifically when the longissimus dorsi muscles are pinched during physical examination. Radiography reveals overriding of adjacent spines, local periosteal reaction, small bony cysts, and false joint formation. The tips of the summits may overlap one another and often become abnormally shaped, presumably due to pressure from the adjacent spines. Injection of a local anesthetic at the affected spaces confirms the diagnosis.

Horses often respond to rest, but clinical signs frequently recur when exercise is resumed. Injection of corticosteroids into the affected area has been suggested as a palliative measure. Surgical removal of the summit of the affected spinous processes results in clinical improvement if the condition has responded to local peripheral nerve blocks.

OSSIFYING SPONDYLOSIS

Spondylosis, degeneration of the intervertebral disks with narrowing of the space and the development of ventral osteophytes, is seen in mature horses that have a history of marked rigidity of the spine associated with poor performance. There is usually no difficulty taking the weight of a rider, but there may be transient resentment to tightening the girth and mounting. Palpation of the spine is strongly resented, and forced ventroflexion or dorsiflexion may result in a violent reaction with kicking and efforts to prevent further palpation or manipulation. Bacterial or fungal infections apparently are not causative factors in this condition. The thoracic vertebrae (T9 to T16) are most commonly affected and the diagnosis can be confirmed by radiography. Radiography reveals flange or spurlike osteophytes arising from the ventral and ventrolateral borders of the vertebral bodies. At some sites, the osteophytes fuse to form a bridge of new bone across the intervertebral joint space. Ossifying spondylosis does not appear to be associated with diet. There is no specific treatment for this condition other than nonsteroidal anti-inflammatory therapy and limitation of exercise. Clinical signs usually persist until complete fusion occurs, a process that can take years.

SACROILIAC SUBLUXATION

The sacroiliac joint is crossed by many fibrous bands and the ventral sacroiliac ligament, which provides stability and immobility to the joint. The dorsal sacroiliac ligament coursing from the tuber sacrale to the dorsal spines of the sacral vertebrae also helps stabilize the joint. Signs of subluxation include prominence of the tuber sacrale, stiffness and shortening of hind limb stride with dragging of one or both toes, unilateral or bilateral hind limb lameness, and rolling motions of the hip. Manipulation of the ilium by palpation of the tuber coxae or sacroiliac joint elicits a painful response in acute cases. Often, there is history of a fall or slip, although subluxation may not be recognized for a period of time after the injury. Rectal palpation is usually not rewarding but may reveal motion or crepitation of the sacroiliac joint when performed with the horse walking. Radiography of the region may demonstrate only increased joint space of the sacroiliac articulation and slight rotation of the pelvis or sacrum; therefore, radiographic examination is usually not performed.

With acute sacroiliac subluxation, the horse should be stall rested for at least 1 month. If damage is severe, ankylosis of the joint may necessitate up to 6 months of rest. In horses that are unresponsive to stall rest or that have a chronic condition, injection of sclerosing agents into the damaged ligament may speed scar formation and resolution of the problem. The prognosis for return to performance is fair. Many horses demonstrate improvement in clinical signs after stall rest or treatment with sclerosing agents, but continue to have residual motion at the sacroiliac joint, although to a lesser degree than at the time of the initial injury.

Supplemental Readings

Adams, S. B., Steckel, R., Blevins, W.: Diskospondylitis in five horses. J. Am. Vet. Med. Assoc., *186*:270, 1985.

Jeffcott, L. B.: The diagnosis of diseases of the horse's back. Equine Vet. J., 7:69, 1975.

Jeffcott, L. B.: Disorders of the thoracolumbar spine of the horse—a survey of 443 cases. Equine Vet. J., 12:197, 1980.

Markel, M. D., Madigan, J. E., Lichtensteiger, C. A., Large, S. M., Hornof, W. J.: Vertebral body osteomyelitis in the horse. J. Am. Vet. Med. Assoc., *188*:632, 1986.

Wagner, P. C.: Diseases of the spine. In Mansmann, R. A., McAllister, E. S., and Pratt, P. W. (eds.): Equine Medicine and Surgery, 3rd ed. Santa Barbara, Calif., American Veterinary Publishing, 1982, pp. 1145–1158.

Muscular Disorders

Tracy A. Turner, ROCHESTER, NEW HAMPSHIRE

Muscular disorders of the performance horse are probably more prevalent than recognized. These disorders are usually expressed either as an exertional myopathy or as a muscle strain. Exertional myopathies may manifest as stress tetany, synchronous diaphragmatic flutter, exhaustion, postexercise fatigue, or exertional rhabdomyolysis. Exertional myopathies have in common loss of muscle function induced by some type of exertion.

EXERTIONAL MYOPATHIES

ETIOLOGY

The factors that predispose to exertional myopathy are varied. Diet, electrolyte balance, hormones, genetics, viremia, bacteremia, and exercise all play a role in the expression of the myopathy.

Diet:

Carbohydrates were the first dietary factors recognized as contributing to myopathies. A correlation exists among carbohydrate intake, exercise inconsistency, and myopathy. The exact reason why relative carbohydrate overload leads to a myopathy is not understood, but it is thought to be related to rapid glycogen breakdown, local lactic acidosis, and muscular vasoconstriction, which leads to muscle cramping.

Selenium deficiency is another dietary factor that may contribute to the development of myopathy. White muscle disease in foals can be initiated by sudden stress or muscular exertion in foals with selenium deficiency. The exact mechanism of action is not understood, but a similar muscle problem might be expected in adults fed selenium-deficient diets.

Electrolyte Imbalance:

Electrolyte balance affects neuromuscular irritability. Hypernatremia, hyperkalemia, hypocalcemia, hypomagnesemia, and acidosis increase neuromuscular irritability, which can lead to nervousness and muscular twitching. Conversely, hyponatremia, hypokalemia, hypercalcemia, hypermagnesemia, and alkalosis decrease neuromuscular irritability and, hence, performance. Hypokalemia also reduces the dilating ability of premuscular small arteries, thus leading to muscle hypoxia.

Hormones:

Hypothyroidism has been associated with myopathies. Thyroxine is involved in muscle oxidative metabolism, and low thyroxine levels would be expected to affect muscle function. Estrogen and progesterone may also be implicated in the development of myopathy. Although the relationship is not fully understood, fillies may be more prone to "tying-up" than colts.

Genetics:

Faulty calcium metabolism within the muscle cell is the basis of malignant hyperthermia, a genetic condition recognized in humans, pigs, and horses. The faulty calcium metabolism leads to excess calcium at the contractile unit. This leads to overcontraction of the muscle fiber, which manifests as cramping. This problem has been associated most commonly with halothane anesthesia. However, the effects of stimulants other than halothane and caffeine are unknown.

Infection:

Viral and bacterial infections can cause muscle damage that could lead to myopathies. For example, the influenza virus, which usually invades the respiratory tract, can invade the muscle if muscular stress occurs during the course of the disease. The virus then damages the muscle, potentially leading to a myopathy. *Acinetobacter calcoaceticus* infection has caused myositis in the horse, producing necrosis, scarring, and edema of skeletal muscle. This type of damage could predispose the horse to a later myopathy after successful recovery from the infection.

Exercise:

Exercise is the initiating cause of most types of myopathies. The amount of exercise needed to initiate a myopathy varies with the individual but is directly related to the training status of the animal. Most myopathies are associated with sudden increases or changes in exercise patterns in a horse that is not fit. Exertional rhabdomyolysis principally affects type II muscle fibers. This would indicate that rhabdomyolysis most commonly occurs as a result of high-speed exercise, generally above 600 m per minute (2:42 mile, 22 miles per hour).

DIAGNOSIS

The signs of the different exertional myopathies are varied but can be used to help determine the type of myopathy. Stress tetany usually produces muscle twitching and spasms: the horse appears jumpy and nervous. Synchronous diaphragmatic flutter presents as diaphragmatic contractions, seen as bilateral flank twitches, in synchrony with the heartbeat. The exhausted horse will be severely depressed with little interest in food or water. Pulse and respiratory rate will be elevated and will remain so despite adequate rest. Skeletal muscle cramps and spasms are often evident. Intestinal sounds are usually diminished in intensity and frequency or absent, with an accompanying loss of anal tone. In contrast, the horse with postexercise fatigue simply appears excessively tired for several days after exercise. The horse stands quietly with its head held low. Exertional rhabdomyolysis, also known as tying up, Monday morning sickness, or azoturia, presents as a stiff or stilted gait. The hind limbs and back are usually the most severely affected. Deep palpation of these muscles will usually elicit a pain response. Marked muscle dysfunction, characterized by reluctance or inability to move, is a hallmark of this condition. The affected horse will usually be anxious and sweating. Tachycardia, tachypnea, and hyperthermia are usually associated with the pain.

Laboratory Data:

Serum enzyme and electrolyte determinations are important elements in the diagnosis of exertional myopathy. Assessment of the degree of muscle damage is important. Creatine kinase (CK) is the most sensitive and specific indicator. This enzyme peaks within 6 hours after damage and declines within 2 to 3 days. Aspartate aminotransferase (AST), formerly called serum glutamic oxaloacetic transaminase (SGOT), reaches peak levels in 24 hours and declines in 7 to 14 days. Lactate dehydrogenase (LDH) peaks within 12 hours and remains elevated for 7 to 10 days. The type and level of muscle enzyme elevation can sometimes be used to determine the length of time since the muscle was damaged. Increased CK values without an increase in AST or LDH values indicate myodegeneration within the past 6 to 12 hours. Increased CK and LDH levels without an increase in AST levels indicate muscle damage within the past 24 hours. Increased AST and LDH levels without an increase in CK levels indicates damage sustained 3 to 4 days earlier.

Serum electrolyte determinations aid in evaluating the role of electrolyte imbalance in the myopathy. These values must be obtained so that any imbalances may be corrected. However, they do not reflect whole-body electrolyte status, specifically potassium. Serum potassium is a poor reflection of a whole-body electrolyte depletion, but serum electrolyte values do give a baseline to determine appropriate supplementation.

Urinalysis is also important. The identification of myoglobinuria is necessary in order to treat or prevent renal damage from myoglobin. If myoglobin has caused damage, casts in the urine and proteinuria will occur.

THERAPY

The first aim of treatment is to limit the muscle damage. In most cases, further exercise is contraindicated; however, this is dependent on the severity of the myopathy. If cramping is slight and fluids and electrolytes have been replaced, light walking may be helpful in restoring strength.

In horses suffering from dehydration or electrolyte imbalance, the administration of fluids and electrolytes is of first-order priority. Severe hypokalemia cannot be entirely corrected by intravenous (IV) fluid therapy, and oral (PO) supplementation should be administered as well. Since most of these horses are alkalotic, bicarbonate therapy would be inappropriate. If myoglobinuria has developed, fluid therapy should continue until the urine is clear.

Anti-inflammatory therapy is indicated to alleviate pain. The nonsteroidal agents are most commonly used. Administered at relatively high doses, all yield adequate results. Dimethyl sulfoxide administered IV at a dose of 1.0 gm per kg as a 10 to 20 per cent solution in saline or 5 per cent dextrose can also be beneficial as an anti-inflammatory agent. Corticosteroids, in addition to having potent anti-inflammatory action, reportedly cause relaxation of capillary sphincters and stabilize cellular membranes. If corticosteroids are used they should be administered within the first hours of illness. α-Adrenergic tranquilizers such as acetylpromazine have also been recommended to improve peripheral blood flow. In addition, these drugs also relieve anxiety. It is important that the horse be normovolemic prior to administration of alpha blockers. Administration of these drugs to the hypovolemic animal could result in catastrophic hypotension.

Severe pain may not be sufficiently relieved by anti-inflammatory agents, and narcotic derivatives such as meperidine hydrochloride or butorphanol tartrate may be indicated to relieve the pain. Combinations of these drugs with xylazine are also very useful and may help avoid the excitation occasionally noted in horses after narcotic administration. Detomidine may also be useful.

Two specific muscle relaxant drugs are dantrolene sodium and methocarbamol. Methocarbamol is administered slowly by IV injection at a dose of 15 to 25 mg per kg. The drug is reputed to reduce pain and relieve muscle spasms. Horses may become ataxic and depressed after methocarbamol administration. The efficacy of the drug in horses is not known. Dantrolene sodium may be the best agent for muscle problems. Administered at a dose of 2 mg per kg PO, the drug can prevent further muscle damage.

Prophylaxis

Dietary and exercise management are the two most important factors to consider in the prevention of exertional myopathies. The horse needs to be on a well-balanced ration that does not exceed its nutritional requirements. The ration must be varied according to the horse's exercise program. The horse's exercise program should be regular and consistent. Vitamin E and selenium have also been recommended to help prevention. Selenium should be supplemented up to five times the recommended requirements (see *Current Therapy in Equine Medicine* 2, p. 487). Dimethylglycine is a compound common to many foodstuffs. The drug is reputed to increase oxygen utilization and decrease lactic acid production. The recommended daily dosage is 1 to 1.6 mg per kg.

Dantrolene sodium has also been recommended as a preventative. Prophylactically, the drug is administered at 2 mg per kg PO once daily for 3 to 5 days, followed by 2 mg per kg PO every third day for 30 days. Caution must be maintained: this drug may be hepatotoxic, and its use over an extended period of time is questionable.

MUSCLE STRAIN

Muscle strains are classified according to severity from first to third degree. A first-degree muscle strain occurs when the limits of muscle elasticity have been reached. This is commonly referred to as a pulled muscle. A second-degree muscle strain or partial muscle tear occurs when the limits of muscle elasticity are exceeded. Tearing of connective tissue and muscle fibers occurs, but the continuity of the muscle is maintained. A third-degree muscle strain or complete muscle tear results in complete loss of muscle continuity.

Etiology

Numerous factors predispose to muscle strains. Among these factors are cold temperature, fatigue, insufficient training, and insufficient warm-up. Cold increases muscle tension and decreases circulation. This will lead to early muscle fatigue, which can lead to incoordinated muscle movement and strain. Fatigue, both muscular and general, predisposes the horse to muscle strain. As muscles fatigue they decrease not only in performance but also in elasticity, thus enhancing the likelihood of strain. General fatigue causes central nervous system incoordination of movement, which predisposes to strain. Proper training is designed to progressively increase the workload to develop muscle groups and increase stamina and recuperative properties. If training is insufficient, the horse is more prone to fatigue. Warm-up is necessary to increase circulation and capacity to eliminate muscle waste products. If this is not achieved, the muscle cannot sustain maximal performance.

Diagnosis

Muscle strain in the horse has been reported most commonly in the hind limb. Muscle strains of the longissimus and gluteal muscles have been termed *croup myopathy*, whereas muscle strains of the biceps femoris, semitendinosus, and semimembranosus have been termed *caudal thigh myopathy*. Muscle strains of other muscle groups most likely occur but have not been completely described.

Muscle strains can occur in any horse used for athletic endeavors. Lameness associated with these strains is variable. Croup myopathies usually cause less than a grade III (of V) lameness, whereas caudal thigh myopathies are usually associated with a lameness that is grade III or worse. Horses with croup myopathy usually exhibit stiffness, toe dragging, or short striding. This lameness may easily be confused with a stifle problem. Caudal thigh myopathy will most likely cause a hip hike or hoof slap gait. Hoof slap is the recognized characteristic sign of fibrotic myopathy.

Flexion tests will rarely exacerbate the lameness. Pain can usually be elicited over the corresponding area of muscle that has been strained. Unfortunately, the nature of these injuries is such that pain can usually be elicited on palpation of more than one area of muscle. Pain on palpation should always be reproducible. Firm pressure is generally more reliable than squeezing muscle masses when determining pain. Croup myopathy pain has been most commonly identified in three areas: the loin region, between the tuber sacrale and tuber coxae, and over the greater trochanter. Pain of the caudal thigh is most consistently identified over the caudal sacrum, caudad to the third trochanter of the femur, and at the musculotendinous junction of the semitendinosus muscle.

Thermography has been the most helpful diagnostic tool. There is a strong correlation between sites of pain and thermographic appearance. Thermographic cameras using infrared detectors are the most accurate but are expensive. Contact thermography or the use of hand-held infrared thermometers are two good alternatives. Contact thermography gives a visual display of temperature patterns, while infrared thermometers can be used to detect side-to-side temperature differences. Side-to-side temperature differences of 1° C are considered significant.

THERAPY

No specific treatment is available. Like a bowed tendon, a pulled muscle needs time to heal and regain its strength. Anti-inflammatory drugs and changes in work routine are of prime importance. Any of the nonsteroidal anti-inflammatories are suitable. In addition, the feed additive methylsulfmethoxine at 1 oz daily is useful in the treatment of muscle inflammation. Work routines are usually reduced, but stall rest may be contraindicated. Although the intensity of work is reduced, the length of workouts is increased. This is to increase warm-up and cool-down periods. The remainder of the exercise period should concentrate on light conditioning. In addition, many horses may benefit from massage, therapeutic ultrasound, or acupuncture. Strains of the musculotendinous junction of the semitendinosus muscle can be treated successfully by tenectomy of the tibial tendon at the insertion of the semitendinosus. Shoeing should be altered in some cases. Borium calks, stickers, and grabs can adversely affect the muscles. In cases that need more traction, the use of a shoe with in-line calks can be useful.

PROGNOSIS

Horses with croup myopathy tend to improve rapidly. The muscle strain usually resolves completely within 60 to 90 days. Caudal thigh myopathies are slower to resolve. Although horses may stay in work, the condition may take as long as a year to resolve. Healing in many of these cases, in particular the semitendinosus strain, may result in fibrous shortening of the musculotendinous junction, producing fibrotic myopathy and a permanent shortening of the horse's gait on the affected side. In such cases a semitendinosus tenectomy may be needed to restore the gait to normal.

Supplemental Readings

Hodgson, D. R.: Myopathies in the athletic horse. Compend. Cont. Ed. Pract. Vet., 7:S551, 1985.
Jeffcott, L. B.: Diagnosis of back problems in the horse. Compend. Cont. Ed. Pract. Vet., 3:S134, 1981.
Jones, W. E.: Equine Sports Medicine. Philadelphia, Lea & Febiger, 1989, p. 262.
Turner, A. S., and Trotter, G. W.: Fibrotic myopathy in the horse. J. Am. Vet. Med. Assoc., 184:338, 1984.
Turner, T. A.: Hindlimb muscle strain as a cause of lameness in horses. In: Proceedings of the 35th Annual Convention of the American Association of Equine Practitioners, 1989, p. 281.

Hyperkalemic Periodic Paralysis

Sharon J. Spier, DAVIS, CALIFORNIA

In recent years, a syndrome has been recognized in certain registered Quarter Horses that is characterized by intermittent episodes of muscle tremors and weakness, often resulting in collapse. These episodes or attacks are associated with severe hyperkalemia, while acid–base balance and renal function are normal. The condition in horses is nearly identical to a heritable condition in man known as hyperkalemic periodic paralysis. In man, hyperkalemic periodic paralysis is inherited as an autosomal dominant trait; the condition in horses appears heritable, but the mode of inheritance is currently under investigation. The pathogenesis of the condition is not entirely clear, but evidence suggests that a defect in muscle membrane transport is present.

CLINICAL AND LABORATORY FINDINGS

An accurate and detailed medical history must be obtained. Horses often have a history of recurrent episodes of weakness, muscle tremors, or collapse that may last for periods of a few minutes to hours. The frequency of observed episodes is highly variable, ranging from daily attacks to a single episode. Horses are usually 2 to 4 years old when episodes are initially noted, but the syndrome may be observed in foals as young as 2 months of age. Some affected horses may not exhibit signs until over 15 years. Affected horses are most commonly heavily muscled Quarter Horses in training for halter or performance use. Males have a higher prevalence of the condition, but mares and geldings are also affected.

The clinical manifestations can be confused with seizures, tying-up, or colic. Episodes typically begin with several minutes of muscle fasciculations or tremors of the neck and trunk muscles. These fasciculations usually become more diffuse, involving many muscle groups, and eventually proceed to involuntary recumbency. In horses that do not collapse, profound muscle weakness manifested as gait deficits, swaying, or staggering may be observed. If the horse is down, it may display hindquarter paresis ("dog-sitting") or be unable to stand when attempting to rise. During an episode, horses remain fully conscious and do not appear to be in pain. Generalized sweating is usually observed, but body temperature remains normal. Pulse and respiratory rates are variable, although modest increases are usually observed. Other clinical signs that may or may not be observed during an episode include prolapse of the third eyelid, anxious or nervous attitude, inspiratory stridor, darkened mucous membranes, and loose feces. Muscle tone during attacks is normal or increased. Usually the horses appear completely normal upon recovery with no indication of muscle stiffness or alteration in gait. These remarkable episodes of weakness and paresis usually resolve spontaneously.

Laboratory parameters during episodes include hyperkalemia (K^+ = 5.0 to 12.3 mEq/L) and increases in packed cell volume and total plasma protein. Blood gas values, renal function tests, and plasma glucose and calcium concentrations remain within normal limits. Muscle-derived serum enzyme activities are normal or only modestly increased. Resolution of clinical signs is accompanied by a rapid return of laboratory parameters toward normal. Physical examination findings and laboratory parameters between episodes are within normal limits.

ELECTROMYOGRAPHY AND MUSCLE HISTOPATHOLOGY

Electromyography (EMG) of affected horses invariably reveals numerous abnormalities, even between episodes when horses appear normal. The EMG abnormalities have a diffuse distribution. Increased insertion activity is indicated by bursts of activity with increased amplitude and prolonged duration following electrode insertion. There is also increased spontaneous activity not associated with movement of the electrode. The most consistent EMG abnormalities are complex repetitive discharges, although myotonic potentials, fibrillation potentials, and positive sharp waves are also observed. These EMG abnormalities are not specific to hyperkalemic periodic paralysis but are consistent with membrane irritability.

Gluteal muscle histopathology has not revealed consistent abnormalities, and only mild changes have been noted in some horses. These changes consist of intracellular vacuolation in type IIB fibers or nonspecific degenerative changes. At present, muscle biopsy is not a useful diagnostic tool for this condition, but could be helpful to distinguish hyperkalemic periodic paralysis from other myopathies.

DIAGNOSIS

The diagnosis is established by exclusion of secondary causes of electrolyte disorders such as chronic renal failure, drug therapy, or rhabdomyolysis. The episodes must be distinguished from seizure disorders or syncope. EMG abnormalities are not specific for hyperkalemic periodic paralysis but may be suggestive in combination with other physical and laboratory findings.

The condition is confirmed by documentation of hyperkalemia during an episode associated with typical clinical signs. Alternatively, an episode may be induced by provocative testing with oral potassium chloride.

POTASSIUM CHLORIDE CHALLENGE TEST

Horses must be fasted for 12 hours prior to administration of 88 to 160 mg per kg potassium chloride as an isotonic solution in water through a nasogastric tube. It is recommended to start with the lower dose of approximately 40 gm of KCl in 6 liters of warm water for a 450-kg horse and increase the dose by 20 gm per day if test results are negative. Because false negative tests can occur, known affected horses will not always exhibit abnormal clinical signs with this test at lower dosages of potassium chloride. Normal horses receiving 180 mg per kg have a modest increase in plasma potassium, but no abnormal clinical signs are observed.

Horses undergoing provocative testing must not be left unattended. Within 2 to 4 hours following administration of potassium chloride, typical clinical signs as described above are observed. Blood should be obtained to document hyperkalemia associated with signs of muscular weakness or tremors. Owners should be aware that provocative testing is not without risk to affected horses. Horses should be placed in a safe and well-cushioned area, and once the diagnosis is established, intravenous (IV) therapy should be administered without delay to alleviate the signs.

THERAPY AND CONTROL

Treatment of acute episodes with 23 per cent calcium gluconate (0.2 to 0.4 ml per kg diluted in 1 to 2 liters of 5 per cent dextrose given IV) usually results in rapid recovery. Alternatively, 5 per cent dextrose (4.4 to 6.6 ml per kg) or sodium bicarbonate (1 mEq per kg) administered rapidly IV are effective treatments for hyperkalemia.

Once a diagnosis of hyperkalemic periodic paralysis is made, the owners must be informed that the horse is at risk for future attacks. Many horses can be managed by dietary and stabling modifications. The dietary recommendations include decreasing the potassium content of the diet by changing from alfalfa hay (2.5 per cent K^+) to oat hay (1.5 per cent K^+) or by decreasing the proportion of alfalfa hay in the diet. The National Research Council estimate for potassium requirements for maintenance is 0.05 to 0.06 gm per kg, or approximately 0.4 per cent of the diet. The requirements for working horses are 1.1, 1.4, and 1.8 times the maintenance requirements for light, medium, and heavy work, respectively. When forages constitute the major portion of the diet, the potassium requirements are easily met. If oat hay is unavailable, then other forages can be provided as directed by potassium analysis of feed. Feeding equal portions of grain (oats contain 0.5 per cent K^+) two to three times daily and free access to salt is also beneficial. Avoid any rapid changes in diet, as these may induce an episode of hyperkalemic periodic paralysis. Access to a paddock or pasture is preferable to a stall to provide regular exercise. If the problem cannot be controlled by these measures, then acetazolamide, a carbonic anhydrase inhibitor diuretic, is very effective at preventing future episodes. Episodes can be controlled by daily administration of acetazolamide (2.2 mg per kg orally every 8 to 12 hours).

Hyperkalemic periodic paralysis in horses appears to have a genetic basis, although insufficient families have been studied to establish the mode of inheritance, degree of penetrance, or expressivity. Breeding of affected horses is not recommended, and prospective buyers of affected horses should be warned of the management constraints these horses require.

Supplemental Readings

Cox, J. H.: An episodic weakness in four horses associated with intermittent serum hyperkalemia and the similarity of the disease to hyperkalemic periodic paralysis in man. In: Proceedings of the Annual Convention of the American Association of Equine Practitioners, 1985, pp. 383–391.

Naylor, J. M., Robinson, J., Steiss, J. E., and Crichlow, E. C.: Hyperkalemic periodic paresis may be inherited as an autosomal dominant trait with incomplete penetrance [abstr. 12]. In: Proceedings of the 7th American College of Veterinary Internal Medicine Forum, 1989, p. 1027.

Robinson, J. A., Naylor, J. M., and Crichlow, E. C.: Electromyography in diagnosis of equine hyperkalemic periodic paresis [abstr. 14]. *In:* Proceedings of the 7th American College of Veterinary Internal Medicine Forum, 1989, p. 1028.

Rudel, R.: The pathophysiologic basis of the myotonias and the periodic paralyses. *In:* Engel, A. G., and Banker, B. Q. (eds.): Myology: Basic and Clinical. New York, McGraw-Hill Book Co., 1986, pp. 1287–1311.

Spier, S. J., Carlson, G. P., Holliday, T. A., et al.: Hyperkalemic periodic paralysis in horses. J. Am. Vet. Med. Assoc., 197:1009–1017, 1990.

Spier, S. J., Carlson, G. P., Pickar, J, et al.: Hyperkalemic periodic paralysis in horses. *In:* Proceedings of the 7th American College of Veterinary Internal Medicine Forum, 1989, pp. 499–500.

Nutritional Secondary Hyperparathyroidism

Joseph J. Bertone, COLUMBUS, OHIO

Nutritional secondary hyperparathyroidism (osteodystrophia fibrosa) was one of the first abnormal conditions of horses to be described. It has been called miller's disease and bran disease, because of its dietary associations, and bighead, because of the clinical sign. In this condition, calcium deficiency or malabsorption generates compensatory mechanisms that lead to bony deformation and dysfunction.

CALCIUM HOMEOSTASIS

Plasma ionized calcium concentration is regulated to precise limits despite wide, daily variations of intake and excretion. The mechanisms designed to regulate plasma calcium concentration rely on the interactions of parathyroid hormome, calcitonin, and vitamin D. However, many other factors, such as other hormones, acid–base status, plasma phosphorus and magnesium concentration, other electrolytes, and plasma proteins, contribute to the net plasma ionized and unionized calcium concentration.

Chief cells within the parathyroid gland synthesize and secrete parathyroid hormone. The stimulus for secretion is primarily decreased plasma ionized calcium and, to a lesser degree, magnesium concentration. This hormone directly influences target cells, primarily in bone, renal parenchyma, and the gastrointestinal (GI) tract, especially the ileum (Fig. 1).

Nutritional secondary hyperparathyroidism occurs as a consequence of the extreme biologic priority assigned to maintenance of plasma ionized calcium concentration. The compensatory mechanisms that develop in association with nutritional imbalances maintain mineral homeostasis. In short, chronic nutritional phosphorus excess and calcium shortage generate a need to extract calcium from other reserves, namely bone.

A relative decrease in plasma calcium concentration, and subsequent stimulation of parathyroid hormone secretion, may be accomplished by one or more of the five mechanisms in nutritional secondary hyperparathyroidism. First, decreased dietary calcium generates a mild reduction in plasma calcium concentration, which directly increases secretion of parathyroid hormone. Second, increased ingestion and absorption of excessive phosphorus yields a relative hyperphosphatemia. The hyperphosphatemia generates a mass action effect that drives the following reaction to the right:

$$Ca + HPO_4 \leftrightarrow CaHPO_4.$$

The generation of calcium phosphate reduces plasma ionized calcium concentration, which stimulates parathyroid hormone secretion. Third, hyperphosphatemia may also hinder the conversion of 25-hydroxycholecalciferol to 1,25-dihydroxycholecalciferol (Fig. 2), decreasing calcium resorption from the GI tract. Fourth, excess dietary phosphorus directly hinders small intestinal calcium absorption. Fifth, and less common, chronic ingestion of oxalate-containing plants may stimulate parathyroid secretion by binding GI calcium and decreasing the plasma-ionized calcium concentration. Regardless of the mechanism, hypocalcemia leads to stimulation of parathyroid secretory function and the associated morphological changes.

Hypocalcemia results in parathyroid gland cellular hypertrophy and hyperplasia. The increased parathyroid hormone activity increases the conversion of relatively inactive vitamin D

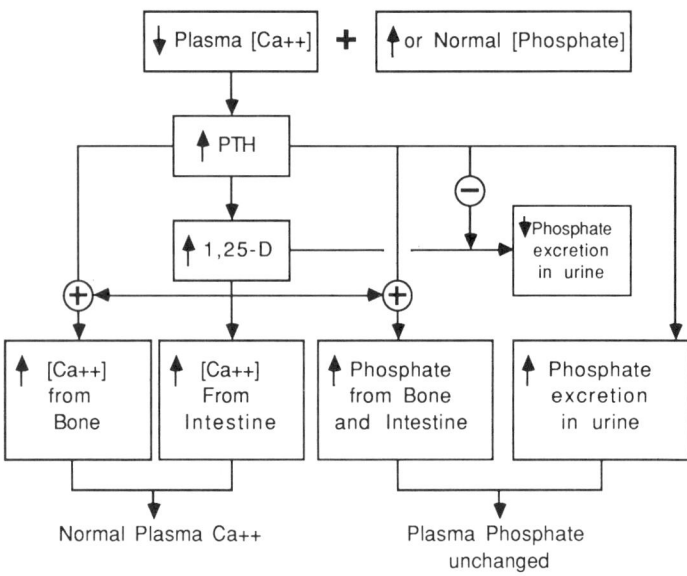

Figure 1. Parathyroid hormone and Vitamin D interaction when the plasma calcium concentration is decreased. The symbol ⊕ indicates a positive effect of parathyroid hormone and ⊖ indicates an antagonistic effect of hyperphosphatemia. (Adapted from Rose, B. D.: Clinical Physiology of Acid-Base and Electrolyte Disorders, 3rd ed. New York, McGraw-Hill Book Co., Inc., 1989.)

(25-hydroxycholecalciferol) to highly active vitamin D (1,25-dihydroxycholecalciferol), rather than the inactive product (24,25-dihydroxycholecalciferol) (see Fig. 2). Vitamin D alone results in decreased tubular excretion of phosphate. However, when plasma phosphate is normal or increased, the net result of vitamin D and parathyroid hormone effects is increased renal tubular excretion of phosphate and increased absorption of calcium (see Fig. 1). Bone resorption of calcium is accelerated, which increases the plasma ionized calcium concentration to tolerable levels. Continued ingestion of the unbalanced diet sustains the compensatory hyperparathyroidism and subsequently increases bone resorption. These phenomena generate the histologic and clinical manifestations of this disease.

The end result of bone resorption is dependent on many factors, including the rapidity and degree of bone resorption and the age and species of the animal. In general, young horses develop hyperostotic bone disease, or the classic clinical signs, facial bone enlargement. Older horses more commonly have little or no facial bone enlargement; they are iso-ostotic. Either scenario may occur. Therefore, this disease can present with a spectrum of bony responses dependent on the metabolic characteristics and demands of the animal and the mineral characteristics of its ration.

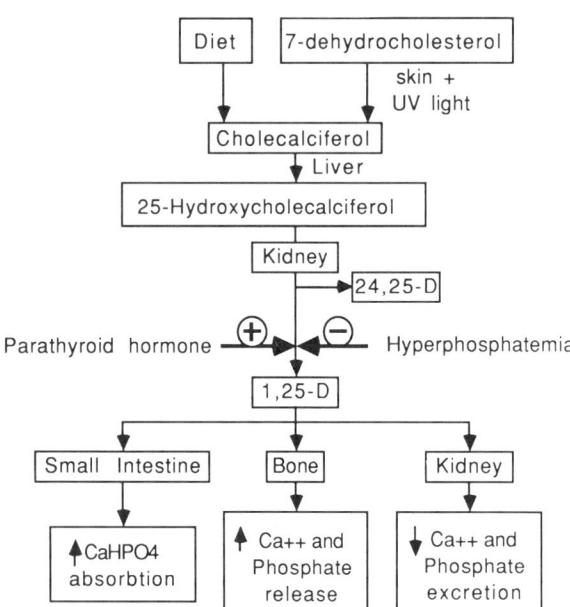

Figure 2. Vitamin D metabolism and target tissue effects. The symbol ⊕ indicates a positive effect on conversion of 25-hydroxycholecalciferol to 1,25-D and ⊖ indicates inhibition of conversion. (Adapted from Rose, B. D.: Clinical Physiology of Acid-Base and Electrolyte Disorders, 3rd ed. New York, McGraw-Hill Book Co., Inc., 1989.)

DIET

Commonly, horses that develop nutritional secondary hyperparathyroidism have been chronically fed grains with a high phosphorus content and poor to average hays with a decreased calcium content. Typically, these diets include oats (Ca, 0.07 per cent; P, 0.37 per cent) and poor-quality, mixed grass hay (Ca, 0.3 per cent; P, 0.3 per cent). Often the diets have increased grain to roughage ratios. Rice (Ca, 0.04 per cent; P, 1.8 per cent) or wheat bran (Ca, 0.12 per cent; P, 1.43 per cent) supplementation is also commonly associated with this condition.

In feeding programs that appear to be balanced, one should suspect pastures or hays with calcium to oxalate ratios that exceed 0.5 per cent. Oxalate chelates calcium in the GI tract, leading to calcium malabsorption. Some examples of oxalate-rich grasses include setaria *(Setaria sphacelata)*, green or blue panic *(Panicum* spp.), argentine or dallas grass *(Paspalum* spp.), and buffel grass *(Cenchrus ciliaris)*. The quantity of oxalates in these grasses is not great enough to lead to other signs of oxalate toxicity but is high enough to generate calcium malabsorption.

Young, growing, or hard-working horses of any sex or breed are particularly sensitive to this condition, because requirements for calcium and phosphorus of yearlings and lactating mares are greater than maintenance requirements for mature adult horses (Table 1). However, this condition may occur in any horse if the dietary imbalance is sufficient and the duration of exposure is sufficiently prolonged.

CLINICAL SIGNS

Although skeletal involvement is generalized with nutritional secondary hyperparathyroidism, abnormalities do not appear uniformly or consistently in any region. Early signs are often associated with the appendicular skeleton and include lameness in one or more limbs, painful joints, and stiff gait. Lameness is associated with increased osteoclastic resorption of circumferential lamellar bone. This process leads to weakened bone trabeculae and decreased support of articular cartilage. The cartilage is then easily disrupted during weight-bearing. Tendinous insertions become weakened and easily disrupted, adding to pain. Rarely, fractures may occur in advanced cases. The resorption of dental alveoli may lead to loose teeth and abnormal mastication.

As the disease progresses, demineralization of the skull, with or without fibrous proliferation, becomes more prominent. If conditions allow for the development of hyperostotic fibrous osteodystrophy, bilateral firm enlargements of the facial bones occur dorsocaudad to the facial crests. The horizontal rami of the mandibles are irregularly thickened. The nasal passages may become obstructed, resulting in upper airway noise. Cases have been observed in which the upper airway noise at exercise was the only presenting complaint, and lameness or other abnormal physical findings were not evident. In these cases, dietary, radiographic, and clinicopathologic findings corroborated the diagnosis.

DIAGNOSIS

The dietary history is integral to the diagnosis of this condition. In suspected cases, dietary indiscretions may be corrected prior to presentation and clinicopathologic data collection. If the disease has not progressed to a degree where conclusive radiographic changes are evident, a history that identifies the abnormal diet may be the only means of diagnosis.

Serum concentrations of calcium, phosphorus, and the activity of alkaline phosphatase often are within the normal reference range due to mechanisms that compensate for the mineral imbalance. Serum alkaline phosphatase may be mildly increased in horses with substantial disease.

Fractional excretion of phosphorus (FEP) appears to be the most useful means of diagnosing the disease and is calculated as follows:

$$\frac{\text{Serum creatinine}}{\text{Urine creatinine}} \times \frac{\text{Urine phosphate}}{\text{Serum phosphate}} = \frac{\text{FEP}}{100}$$

The increased secretion of parathyroid hormone and subsequent bone resorption is associated with increased urinary phosphate excretion (see Fig. 1). The disease should be suspected when other corroborating findings are present and FEP is greater than 0.5 per cent. If other urinary parameters are abnormal in the setting of increased phosphate excretion, then primary renal disease should be suspected. In my experience, FEP may return to normal within 24 hours of feeding a balanced diet. Therefore, if possible, blood and urine samples should be collected before dietary supplementation is initiated.

Intuitively, it would appear that fractional excretion of calcium values would be helpful. How-

TABLE 1. APPROXIMATE CALCIUM AND PHOSPHORUS REQUIREMENTS FOR HORSES*

	Percentage in Diet		Daily Dietary Content† (gm)	
	Ca	P	Ca	P
Foals < 6 mo	0.80	0.55	33	20
Weanlings	0.60	0.45	34	25
Yearlings	0.50	0.35	31	22
Two-year-olds	0.40	0.30	25	17
Mare, late pregnancy	0.45	0.30	34	23
Mare, lactation	0.45	0.30	50	34
Mature horses, maintenance	0.30	0.20	23	14

*From Schryver, H. F., and Hintz, H. F.: Minerals. *In* Robinson, N. E. (ed.): Current Therapy in Equine Medicine 2. Philadelphia, W. B. Saunders, 1987.
†Assumes 500 kg mature weight.

ever, calcium excretion values are often difficult to interpret because of the wide normal range and normal calcium crystalluria.

Bone density must be reduced by a minimum of 30 per cent to be evident radiographically. This limits the use of radiography in the identification of early cases of nutritional secondary hyperparathyroidism. Decreased density of the laminae durae dentes is often the earliest radiographic evidence of disease and may occur before the appearance of other abnormalities. The early appearance in this location is most likely associated with the thinness of cortices and the forces that increase bone turnover in this area. Later, facial bone density is lost. Only in advanced cases is there radiographic evidence of long bone cortical thinning and demineralization.

When there is evidence of the disease but the diet appears adequate, forages rich in oxalate should be suspected. Fecal calcium to phosphorus ratios greater than 2.35:1 would be indicative of this situation.

THERAPY

The primary goal of treatment is to decrease parathyroid hormone secretion by correcting the dietary mineral imbalance. All facets of the diet, including supplements, should be reviewed. Calcium intake should be supplemented to two to three times the daily requirement. It is important to note that horses at varying stages of development and performing different types of work have different calcium and phosphorus requirements (see Table 1).

Limestone (calcium carbonate) is a good source of calcium (35 per cent calcium) because it contains no phosphorus. If it is the sole calcium source, an unaffected yearling requires approximately 100 gm of limestone per day and an affected animal requires 300 gm. For therapeutic purposes, the diet should yield a calcium to phosphorus ratio of 3 or 4 to 1. Other sources of calcium in the diet should be included in these calculations. Bone meal contains a great deal of phosphorus and should be avoided. Excessive calcium supplementation (greater than five times maintenance requirements) in the recovery phase of this condition may result in greater bone density and decreased bone remodeling. This could result in decreased bone strength. Therefore, initial treatment should be aggressive, but the chronic treatment of the condition should not be overzealous. Affected animals should be confined early in the disease, until radiographic density of the affected areas has returned to normal. It should be remembered that return of radiographic density does not indicate full recovery. A judicious approach would be 1 year of supplemented dietary intake prior to return of the horse to strenuous exercise.

Anti-inflammatory therapy may be recommended if pain is excessive but should be used with caution. Reduced pain may increase activity, leading to pathologic fractures or more subtle complications. Horses with nutritional secondary hyperparathyroidism on a high oxalate content pasture should be removed from that pasture and treated as described.

The outcome of this condition is difficult to predict. Lameness may or may not resolve, depending on the severity and duration of the condition. Facial swelling, which most often does not resolve, requires months for recovery.

Supplemental Readings

Argenzio, R. A., Lowe, J. E., Hintz, H. F., and Schryver, H. F.: Calcium and phosphorus homeostasis in horses. J. Nutr., 104:18, 1974.

Capen, C. C.: Nutritional secondary hyperparathyroidism. In Robinson, N. E. (ed.): Current Therapy in Equine Medicine. Philadelphia, W. B. Saunders Co., 1983, p. 160.

Joyce, J. R., Pierce, K. R., Romane, W. M., and Baker, J. M. Clinical study of nutritional secondary hyperparathyroidism in horses. J. Am. Vet. Med. Assoc., 158:2033, 1971.

Krook, L., and Lowe, J. E.: Nutritional secondary hyperparathyroidism in the horse. Pathol. Vet., Suppl. 1:1, 1964.

Rose, B. D.: Clinical Physiology of Acid-Base and Electrolyte disorders, 3rd ed. New York, McGraw-Hill Book Co., Inc., 1989.

Swartzmann, J. A., Hintz, H. F., and Schryver, H. F.: Inhibition of calcium absorption in ponies fed diets containing oxalic acid. Am. J. Vet. Res., 39:1621, 1978.

Walthall, J. C., and McKenzie, R. A.: Osteodystrophia fibrosa in horses at pasture in Queensland: Field and laboratory observations. Aust. Vet. J., 52:11, 1976.

Differential Diagnoses of Medical Lameness: Nutritional, Toxic, Metabolic, and Other Conditions

Joseph J. Bertone, COLUMBUS, OHIO

Lameness is often associated with medical disturbances that are not traumatic or degenerative in origin. The association of musculoskeletal impairment and other diseases may range from lameness as the prominent sign of acute disease to lameness as the residual effect of a chronic disorder. This chapter reviews medical diseases, primarily nutritional, that have been associated with lameness as a clinical sign or presenting complaint. Table 1 lists medical diseases associated with lameness in North America. Several of the diseases, especially gastrointestinal (GI) and protozoal disorders, are associated with laminitis. Detailed discussions of these diseases may be found in other chapters.

VITAMIN E AND SELENIUM

Vitamin E and selenium (Se) function as antioxidants. Vitamin E prevents oxidation of membranes, while Se functions at the intracellular level in the glutathione peroxidase system. Se-dependent glutathione peroxidase activity occurs in striated and cardiac muscle, while liver and lung glutathione peroxidase activity is Se independent. This would explain why the signs associated with Se deficiency are most often affiliated with these Se-dependent tissues.

SELENIUM DEFICIENCY (WHITE MUSCLE DISEASE)

Decreased Se content in soils in the Great Lakes region and the Eastern, Gulf and Northwestern coasts places at risk horses located in or fed feeds from these areas. Deficiency is associated with chronic consumption of milk, forage, and grain containing less than 0.1 parts per million (ppm) Se. Foals 1 to 30 days of age are most often affected, but cases occur in foals up to 10 months of age. Se deficiency in foals may be associated with inadequate Se intake by pregnant or lactating mares. Mature horses are rarely affected. Muscular exertion may initiate the onset of signs. Severe deficiency is associated with oxidant-induced necrosis of both skeletal and myocardial muscle.

The most prominent clinical sign is muscular weakness. Muscle stiffness, myalgia, dysphagia, and terminal listlessness are often apparent. Young foals may exhibit severe myocardial, diaphragmatic, and respiratory muscle involvement. Increased plasma activity of muscle-related enzymes, such as aspartate aminotransferase, creatine kinase, and lactate dehydrogenase, with decreased glutathione peroxidase activity is diagnostic. When Se deficiency is the sole problem, hyponatremia, hypochloremia, hyperkalemia, and metabolic alkalosis are often evident. In severe cases, protein, blood, and myoglobin are identified in the urine. If the condition is severe, foals may develop cardiac failure, dyspnea, and pulmonary edema and frequently die within hours to 2 days after the onset of clinical signs.

Se deficiency in mature horses may affect muscles of mastication or the appendicular skeleton. Clinical signs often include a stiff gait. Se deficiency has also been implicated in exertional rhabdomyolysis.

Necropsy findings include steatitis and coagulative necrosis of muscles, particularly those of the hind limbs, neck, intercostal space, base of the tongue, and heart. Histologically, there is widespread coagulative necrosis, disruption, and calcification of muscle.

The response to treatment depends on the severity of the lesions at the time of diagnosis. Se deficiency may be treated by administering vitamin E and Se injection intramuscularly (IM) as directed by the manufacturer. Other required supportive care will be dictated by the condition at presentation and the severity of other organ system dysfunction.

Deficiency may be prevented by providing access to trace mineralized salt containing 15 to 30 ppm Se, or feeding a ration containing 0.5 ppm Se in dry matter content. Supplementation that increases the ration to above 0.5 ppm Se should be avoided. Some foals may be born or aborted with evidence of Se deficiency. Therefore, in deficient areas, the diets of pregnant mares should

TABLE 1. DISEASES THAT CAN CAUSE LAMENESS

Bacteria-Associated Disease	Dermatologic Disease	Gastrointestinal Disease	Neurologic Disease	Skeletal Disease	Toxin-Associated Disorders (Cont.)
Malignant edema (*Clostridium septicum*)	Cutaneous vasculitis	Abdominal abscess	Atlantoaxial, occipital malformation	Diskospondylitis	Snake bite
Rhodococcus equi infection	Dermatomycosis	Duodenitis-jejunitis	Bacterial, fungal, parasitic, protozoal, and viral meningitis	Immune-mediated polysynovitis	Strychnine toxicity
Septicemia	Equine monocytic ehrlichiosis	Ehrlichial enterocolitis	Botulism	Vertebral abscess or neoplasia	*Swainsonia* spp. poisoning
Sporadic abscesses	Fistulous withers (brucellosis)	Grain overload	Equine degenerative myeloencephalopathy	**Toxin-Associated Disorders**	Vitamin D toxicity
Tularemia	Idiopathic systemic gangrene of foals	Idiopathic enterocolitis	Equine protozoal myeloencephalitis	Arsenic toxicity	Vitamin K3 toxicity
Tuberculosis	Lymphangitis	Peritonitis	Femoral nerve disease	Bermuda grass poisoning	White snakeroot poisoning
Cancers	Mechanobullous disease	Salmonellosis	Herpesvirus myeloencephalitis	Black walnut (*Juglans nigra*) poisoning	**Urogenital Disease**
Angiosarcoma	Pastern dermatitis ("grease heel")	**Hemolymphatic Disease**	Lumbosacral plexus trauma	Blister beetle (cantharidin) toxicity	Bladder rupture
Associated hypercalcemia and dystrophic mineralization	Pemphigus foliaceous	Idiopathic equine aplastic anemia, bone marrow aplasia	Myotonia congenita	Chocolate, theobromine, cocoa toxicity	Interstitial nephritis
Extraskeletal bone and cartilage tumors	Phycomycosis, pythiosis	**Mammary Disease**	Neuroaxonal dystrophy	Fluorosis	Lower urinary tract obstruction
Fibroma	Purpura hemorrhagica	Mastitis	Obturator nerve disease	Larkspur poisoning	Pyelonephritis
Fibrosarcoma	Steatitis	**Metabolic Disease**	Peroneal nerve disease	Lead toxicity	Renal, ureteral, urethral calculi
Giant cell tumor	Sterile nodular panniculitis	Exhaustion	Rabies (peripheral and central)	Locoweed, astragalus, oxytropis poisoning	**Vascular Disease**
Hemangioma	Thrush	Hepatic lipidosis	Radial nerve disease	Mercury toxicity	Acute necrotizing vasculitis and thrombocytopenia
Hemangiosarcoma	**Diet-Associated Disorders**	Hyperlipemia	Spinal cord neoplasia	Moldy corn poisoning	Arterial, aortic, iliac, femoral thrombosis
Lymphoma	Copper deficiency	Lactation tetany, hypocalcemia, eclampsia, transit tetany	Spinal cord, or vertebral trauma	Moldy sweet clover, dicumarol toxicity	Peripheral arteriovenous fistula or aneurysm
Lymphosarcoma	Nutritional myodegeneration (white muscle disease)	**Muscular Disease**	Tetanus	Nonsteroidal anti-inflammatory toxicity	Spermatic cord thrombosis
Malignant and benign melanoma	Nutritional secondary hyperparathyroidism	Dystrophic myodegeneration	Tibial nerve disease	Organochlorine, chlorinated hydrocarbon toxicity	**Viral Disease**
Mastocytoma	Phosphorus deficiency	Exertional rhabdomyolysis	Togavirus encephalitis	Organophosphate, carbamate toxicity	Equine viral arteritis
Cardiac Disorders	Vitamin A deficiency	Gluteal paresis	**Protozoan-Associated Disease**	Potato dermatitis	Vesicular stomatitis
Atrial fibrillation	Zinc toxicity	Hyperkalemic periodic paresis	Borreliosis, Lyme disease	Psychogenic, excessive salt consumption	
Endocarditis	**Endocrine Disorders**	Polymyositis	Coccidioidomycosis	Reserpine toxicity	
Ventricular tachycardia	Hypothyroidism	Postanesthetic myonecrosis	Cryptococcal meningitis	Ryegrass poisoning	
Coagulatory Disorders	Pituitary adenoma	Shivering	**Respiratory Disease**	Selenium toxicity	
Factor VIII deficiency, hemophilia A			Hypertrophic osteopathy	Slaframine toxicity	
			Pleuritis, pleural effusion		
			Pneumonia		

Source: White, M. E., Lewkowicz, J., and Mohammed, H. O.: Consultant (online computerized database). Ithaca, New York: New York State College of Veterinary Medicine, 1990.

be adjusted, or they should receive parenteral Se formulations 3 to 4 weeks prior to foaling. Se injections are teratogenic in sows. Therefore, it would be judicious to avoid parenteral Se formulations early in pregnancy. In severe Se deficient areas, where Se deficiency has been documented, parenteral vitamin E and Se administration may be warranted shortly after birth and every 1 to 3 months during the first 6 months of life.

Selenium Toxicity

Acute, chronic, and neonatal Se toxicosis have been identified. Blind staggers, or what was once thought to be subacute Se toxicity, is more likely associated with plant-related hepatic toxins. In the acute form of the disease, often associated with excessive Se administration, neurologic and GI signs are more prominent than musculoskeletal dysfunction. The neonatal form results in hoof deformities in foals at birth and is associated with high concentration, chronic Se ingestion by pregnant mares.

Lameness is a prominent sign of chronic Se toxicity (alkali disease; bobtail disease). Most commonly chronic Se toxicity affects adult horses. Chronic Se toxicity is associated with the ingestion of plants containing greater than 5 ppm Se in dry matter content that yields a Se intake of 0.5 to 2 mg per kg of body weight. In the Rocky Mountains and Great Plains, soil Se levels are sufficient to result in toxic accumulation of Se in plants that do not readily do so. Some plants (e.g., *Grindelia squarrosa*) readily accumulate Se when grown in high Se concentration soils. Obligate or indicator plants are dependent on Se for growth (e.g., *Aster xylorrhiza*). Long-term elevations of blood Se concentrations lead to Se replacement of amino acid sulfhydryl groups and improper keratinization. Sulfhydryl groups are also replaced in oxidative enzyme pathways.

Clinical signs of chronic Se toxicity are often referable to keratinized tissues. The hair of the mane and tail (bobtail disease) becomes rough, coarse, and brittle. The coronary band swells and transverse grooves appear on the hoof. Often these signs are mistaken as evidence of laminitis. The hoof horn may separate from the underlying laminae. Extensive soft tissue calcification may occur. Affected animals have a stiff, stilted gait.

Chronic Se toxicity may be diagnosed if there is greater than a total ration Se content of 5 ppm of dry matter, 10 ppm in drinking water, 0.3 ppm in blood, 5 ppm in hair or hoof, or 2 ppm in liver or kidney. Hoof wall samples appear to be the most useful for diagnosis.

Treatment entails supportive hoof care and removal of horses from the Se source. Provision of high protein rations (20 per cent crude protein) may be useful in treatment and prevention. When the horse cannot be removed from high Se content pastures, supplementation with low Se concentration feeds may be somewhat preventative. Other treatments, such as arsenilic acid supplementation, are variably successful.

TRACE MINERAL IMBALANCES

Trace mineral balance, especially of zinc and copper, is important in normal endochondral ossification. Imbalances in these minerals have been associated with musculoskeletal disease.

Copper

Copper deficiency is rare, since dietary requirements of adult horses are small. Relative copper deficiency or malabsorption has been implicated in the pathogensis of osteochondrosis (see p. 722). Copper-responsive osteodystrophy is rare. In the few described cases, affected foals develop progressive lameness and reluctance to move. All limbs are affected to various degrees. Signs disappear after 100 mg copper IM and may be prevented by adding 20 mg of copper to the daily ration.

Zinc

Natural zinc deficiency has not been identified in horses. Experimental deficiency can be generated when zinc content is reduced to 4 ppm. Zinc content in natural feeds usually exceeds 20 to 50 ppm. Zinc-responsive osteodystrophy has been identified.

Zinc toxicity is most often associated with intake of excessive zinc supplement (greater than 200 ppm) or water with greater than 15 ppm zinc. When galvanized pipes come in contact with pipes made of copper or other metals, electrolysis may lead to excessive zinc release into drinking water. Pastures contaminated by smelters with a high zinc content effluent have also been implicated. Excessive zinc intake decreases calcium and copper absorption, which may lead to secondary deficiencies in these minerals and altered endochondral ossification. Bone and joint disorders have been consistently identified with zinc toxicity in horses. Clinical signs often include joint effusion, lameness, and stiffness. Radiographic lesions similar to those of osteochondrosis are described. Physitis, articular cartilage detachment, and flexor tendon contracture are seen.

Zinc toxicity or deficiency may be diagnosed if plasma levels fall out of the normal reference range of 0.8 to 2 ppm in plasma, 0 to 50 ppm in hepatic or renal tissue, or 5 to 10 ppm in pancreatic tissue. Pancreatic zinc content is the most diagnostic for zinc toxicity.

VITAMIN D

Vitamin D is required for intestinal calcium and phosphorus absorption, and parathyroid hormone function. These actions are essential for normal calcium and phosphorus homeostasis and ossification of endochondral cartilage. Toxic and deficient states can result in bone abnormalities.

VITAMIN D DEFICIENCY

Naturally occurring cases of vitamin D deficiency are rare. Deficiency is characterized by decreased bone calcification, osteosclerosis, osteomalacia, and osteitis fibrosa. Abnormal cartilage matrix is produced. Horses severely or chronically affected have tarsocrural joint effusion and are reluctant to stand or walk, doing so with difficulty and pain.

VITAMIN D TOXICITY

Rations that have been supplemented to contain greater than 25,000 to 50,000 IU of vitamin D fed daily for prolonged periods, or greater concentrations fed for shorter periods, may result in vitamin D toxicity. Iatrogenic toxicity has also been described. Most commonly, toxicity in horses is associated with ingestion of *Cestrum diurnum* (wild jasmine), which contains an active vitamin D analogue. Excessive vitamin D stimulates intestinal calcium absorption resulting in hypercalcemia, hypophosphatemia, soft tissue calcification, inhibited osteocytic osteolysis, osteopetrosis, osteonecrosis, and osteopenia. Growth is obstructed by inhibited cartilage maturation and cell proliferation in articular cartilage and metaphyseal growth.

Clinical signs of vitamin D toxicity include generalized stiffness, reluctance to move, decreased growth, partial to complete anorexia, and weight loss. Renal parenchymal calcification with polyuria and polydypsia are common. Tendons and suspensory ligaments are often sensitive to palpation. The diagnosis is based on evidence of excessive vitamin D intake through natural sources or administration/supplementation and the presence of clinical signs. Hypercalcemia is variably present, depending on the proximity of Vitamin D intake to initial examination. Treatment entails removal of the vitamin D or analogue source and supportive care. Often by the time diagnosis is made the prognosis is unfavorable.

FLUOROSIS

Requirements for fluoride are extremely small, and therefore deficiencies do not occur. Ingestion of fluoride at greater than 30 ppm of diet dry matter is toxic during growth and lactation. Fluoride at greater than 50 ppm is toxic during maintenance. Fluoride does cross the placental barrier. Therefore, excessive intake by pregnant mares may result in foals with mottled deciduous teeth and decreased birth weight. Little fluoride is secreted in milk.

Common toxic sources of fluoride are rock phosphates, phosphatic limestone, or fertilizer grade phosphates that have not been defluoridated. Industries that process minerals containing fluoride may release large amounts of fluoride into the air, with subsequent contamination of forage, soil, and water. Contaminated forage is most commonly associated with fluorosis. Grains do not readily accumulate fluoride. Wells located near phosphate rock may contain toxic concentrations.

Fluorosis is characterized almost entirely by signs involving bone. Dental abnormalities occur if horses are exposed to fluoride during development. Moderate exposure in young horses is associated with brown and black mottled dental enamel. More severe toxicity is indicated by pitted and eroded teeth. Mastication may be extremely painful and feed intake decreased by the exposure of sensitive dental tissue. Weight loss is often prominent. There may be increased bone thickness (periosteal hyperostosis) initially evident on the medial surface of the metacarpal and metatarsal bones. Later, mandibular and costal bones are affected. As the disease progresses, stiffness and lameness become prominent. Radiographically, there is thickening and increased density of bone. Bones fracture easily.

The diagnosis of fluorosis is based on signs, increased feed or water fluoride concentrations, and greater than 1300 ppm fluoride in ribs and vertebrae. Fluoride content of the ribs and vertebrae is more indicative of disease than other bones.

No treatment is effective in reversing clinical signs. Successful prevention requires removal of horses from the source.

Supplemental Readings

Hintz, H. F.: Nutrition. *In*: Robinson, N. E. (ed.): Current Therapy in Equine Medicine, 2nd ed. Philadelphia, W.B. Saunders Co., 1987, pp. 387–426.

Lewis, L. D.: The role of nutrition in musculoskeletal development. *In*: Stashak, T. S. (ed.): Adams' Lameness in

Horses, 4th ed. Philadelphia, Lea & Febiger, 1987, pp. 271–292.
Moore, R. A., Kohn, C. W.: Nutritional muscular dystrophy in foals. Compend. Contin. Educ. Pract. Veter., 13:476, 1991.

Schryver, H. F.: Mineral and vitamin intoxication in horses. Veter. Clin. North. Am. [Eq. Pract.] 6:295–318, 1990.
Traub-Dargatz, J. L., Knight, A. P., Hamar, D. W.: Selenium toxicity in horses. Compend. Contin. Educ. Pract. Veter., 8:771–776, 1986.

Intra-Articular Medication

Alan J. Nixon, ITHACA, NEW YORK

Intra-articular medication is directed toward diminishing the inflammatory response in both the synovium and cartilage, halting progressive cartilage degradation, restoring the normal joint environment, and alleviating pain. The commonly used medications perform these functions through differing mechanisms and to a variable degree.

CORTICOSTEROIDS

Although intra-articular corticosteroid use preceded the use of chondroprotective agents such as sodium hyaluronate and polysulfated glycosaminoglycan by several decades, controversy still surrounds the application and efficacy of steroids. Chondroprotective agents not only suppress inflammation within the joint but also maintain or enhance the metabolic activity of chondrocytes, synovial lining cells, and cells in the subchondral bone. Corticosteroids in recommended dosages suppress chondrocyte synthesis of matrix compounds such as collagen, proteoglycan, and hyaluronic acid, and may result in chondrocyte necrosis and cartilage hypocellularity. Steroids also reduce the synthesis of hyaluronic acid by synovial living cells but conversely may diminish hyaluronic acid depolymerization and dilution by virtue of their anti-inflammatory effects.

Nevertheless, corticosteroids are potent anti-inflammatory and analgesic agents and are often the only medication that will satisfactorily control recalcitrant synovitis. Experimental studies show that corticosteroids are extraordinarily effective in limiting cartilage proteolysis and inhibiting interleukin-1 (IL-1) production by the synovium. Recent evidence also indicates that dose rates lower than those currently recommended may provide anti-inflammatory effects that are beneficial to cartilage integrity by reducing degradatory enzyme activity, while not having the deleterious effects on chondrocyte morphology and synthetic activity seen at recommended dosages.

Corticosteroids provide an anti-inflammatory effect through stabilization of cellular lysosomal membranes, reduction of vascular permeability, decreasing leukocyte adherence to vessel walls, and inhibiting platelet aggregation and leukocyte diapedesis. Corticosteroids also reduce the inflammatory vasodilation associated with the acute phases of synovitis, reduce prostaglandin production, and diminish the production of superoxide radicals, although they have little radical scavenging action. Modulation of IL-1 production by corticosteroids has other beneficial effects, since IL-1 stimulates chondrocyte production of catabolic enzymes such as proteoglycanase (stromelysin), collagenase, and prostaglandins.

Corticosteroid preparations available for intra-articular use in horses include hydrocortisone acetate, methylprednisolone acetate, flumethasone, betamethasone acetate, and triamcinolone acetonide. Preparations and suggested dosages are listed in Table 1. The optimal dose varies with the potency of the steroid, its concentration, whether it is esterified or nonesterified, and the size of the joint cavity. A common misconception, however, is that poorly water-soluble esters are long-acting when given intra-articularly. The water solubility is generally irrelevant when the steroid is given directly at the site of action rather than systemically; the rate of hydrolysis of the ester within the joint is the critical feature. Short-acting corticosteroids include isoflupredone, flumethasone, and hydrocortisone, while triamcinolone acetonide, methylprednisolone acetate, and betamethasone acetate are medium- and longer acting steroids. The relative potency of these formulations varies, with betamethasone and flumethasone being the most potent (Table 2). Recent pharmacokinetic studies demonstrated detectable levels of methylprednisolone acetate in equine synovial fluid for only 2 to 6 days after injection; however, there were

TABLE 1. COMMONLY USED INTRA-ARTICULAR CORTICOSTEROIDS

Drug	Trade Name	Drug Concen.	Dose	Duration of Action
Triamcinolone acetonide	Vetalog°	6 mg/ml	1–3 ml	Medium
Flumethasone	Flucort†	0.5 mg/ml	1–3 ml	Short to medium
Isoflupredone	Predef 2x‡	2 mg/ml	3–10 ml	Short to medium
Betamethasone acetate	Betavet§	15 mg/ml	1.5–2.5 ml	Medium to long
Methylprednisolone acetate	Depomedrol#	40 mg/ml	2–3 ml	Long

°Vetalog, Solvay, Mendota Heights, MN.
†Flucort, Syntex Animal Health, Des Moines, IA.
‡Predef 2x, Upjohn, Kalamazoo, MI.
§Betavet, Schering-Plough Animal Health, Kenilworth, NJ.
#Depomedrol, Upjohn, Kalamazoo, MI.

TABLE 2. POTENCY OF ACTIVE MOIETY OF CORTICOSTEROID PREPARATIONS

Betamethasone	Most potent
Dexamethasone	↑
Flumethasone	
Triamcinolone	
Isoflupredone	
Methylprednisolone	
Prednisolone	↓
Hydrocortisone	Least potent

detectable levels of methylprednisolone, hydrolyzed from methylprednisolone acetate, for 5 to 39 days. Clearly, there is considerable individual variation in the rate of methylprednisolone acetate hydrolysis and loss from horses' joints. Clinical response generally lasts 3 to 4 weeks following intra-articular injection of 100 to 120 mg of methylprednisolone acetate; however, a shorter duration of action can be explained by the variation in the rate of methylprednisolone acetate hydrolysis and absorption from equine joints.

Triamcinolone acetonide, although classically regarded as a long-acting intra-articular steroid, has recently been shown to be relatively short-acting, the drug being cleared from carpal and tarsal joint fluid in approximately 3 days, and having effective tissue levels for only 4 to 5 days. However, the potency of triamcinolone acetonide remains high and total horse dosages need to be limited to 18 mg. Larger dosages have resulted in severe laminitis. Laminitis is most prevalent with the human formulation of triamcinolone known as Kenalog° (40 mg per ml). Other commonly used intra-articular steroids include betamethasone (Betavet†) and flumethasone (Flucort‡), in the dosages listed in Table 1.

Numerous references to adverse consequences following intra-articular steroid administration have tempered their use. Postinjection steroid flare, an acute inflammatory response resulting in increased heat, pain, swelling, and lameness, may occur up to 24 hours following injection. The synovitis dissipates rapidly, varies with the steroid product injected, and is reportedly due to the microcrystalline vehicle used in the preparation. The incidence approaches 2 per cent. Laminitis is a concern with any intra-articular steroid, especially triamcinolone and dexamethasone at high dosages.

Corticosteroid-induced arthropathy results from acceleration of preexisting degenerative joint disease. The potent anti-inflammatory and analgesic effects of steroids, their adverse effect on chondrocyte metabolism, and increased wear on a susceptible articular surface rapidly exacerbate preexisting joint degeneration. Resultant joint space narrowing, osteophyte formation, periarticular fibrosis, and calcification increase lameness. Steroid-induced arthropathy can be avoided by rest after injection and is rare when there are minimal radiographic changes prior to injection. However, recovery of chondrocyte metabolic activity after steroid administration, even in previously normal cartilage, may be delayed by as much as 16 weeks.

SODIUM HYALURONATE

Sodium hyaluronate products (Table 3) were initially used in combination with corticosteroids to compensate for some of the deleterious effects of steroids alone. Although numerous clinical papers attest to the benefit of sodium hyaluronate products in animals, they are still not approved for human use.

The initial reports of sodium hyaluronate use in horses made little attempt to categorize the type of joint disease being treated. Consequently, sodium hyaluronate developed a reputation as a cure-all that eventually disillusioned horse owners and veterinarians. Sodium hyaluronate has a profound beneficial effect on the soft tissues of the joint, including improved lubrication of the synovial membrane (which contributes upward of 50 per cent to the resistance of

°Kenalog: Westwood Squibb Pharmaceuticals, Buffalo, N.Y.
†Betavel: Schering-Plough Animal Health, Kenilworth, NJ.
‡Flucort: Syntex Animal Health, Des Moines, IA.

TABLE 3. SODIUM HYALURONATE PREPARATIONS AVAILABLE FOR INTRA-ARTICULAR USE IN THE HORSE

Trade name	Manufacturer	Concentration	Molecular weight, daltons (manufacturer's specs)	Molecular weight, daltons (measured)*	Vehicle	Recommended Dose
Hylartin V (Hylartil Vet) (Healon)	American Equine Prod., S. Norwalk CT Pharmacia, Sweden Pharmacia, Australia	10 mg/ml	3.5×10^6	2.88×10^6	NaCl–phosphate buffer and sterile water	20 mg
Hyvisc	Med. Chem. Products, Acton, MA Norden Labs Lincoln, NE	10 mg/ml	2.1×10^6	1.73×10^6	NaCl and sterile water	20 mg
Equron	Solvay Animal Health, Inc., Mendota Hts., MN	5 mg/ml	$1.5–2.0 \times 10^6$	0.9×10^6	NaCl	10 mg
Equiflex	Chesapeake Biological Laboratories, Baltimore, MD	5 mg/ml	1×10^6	N/A	NaCl	10 mg
Synacid	Schering-Plough Animal Health, Kenilworth, NJ	10 mg/ml	$0.15–0.20 \times 10^6$	0.13×10^6	Sterile water with preservatives	50 mg
Remobilase	Arnolds, Australia	10 mg/ml	7.5×10^4	N/A	Sterile water with preservatives	50 mg
Hyalovet 20	FIDIA, Abano Terme, Italy	10 mg/ml	$0.75–1.0 \times 10^6$	0.415×10^6	NaCl–phosphate buffer	20 mg
Connettivina II	FIDIA, Italy	2 mg/ml	7.5×10^4	N/A	5% glucose with preservative	20 mg

*Data from Loftus, S.A., et al.: Comparison of the properties of hyaluronate products used in treatment of joint dysfunction in horses. J. Eq. Vet. Sci., 8:117–120, 1988.

joint motion), return of steric hindrance at the synovium–blood barrier, which reduces protein and cellular influx to the joint, and additional direct anti-inflammatory effects through scavenging of oxygen-derived free radicals and suppression of prostaglandins. For these reasons it can exert a positive and at times permanent response when used to treat synovitis without serious degenerative joint disease. There are few beneficial effects of sodium hyaluronate on established full-thickness cartilage erosions, osteophytes, or joint ankylosis, and the drug will not dissolve chip fractures. The only benefit of sodium hyaluronate in situations of full-thickness cartilage loss is amelioration of the secondary synovitis.

The early literature attributes most of the beneficial effects of exogenous sodium hyaluronate to its viscoelastic properties and the restoration of endogenous hyaluronic acid layers at the synovial and cartilage surfaces. Since the rheological properties of sodium hyaluronate are largely related to the molecular weight and the concentration of sodium hyaluronate in the preparation, the larger molecular weight compounds (see Table 3) such as Hylartin and Hyvisc are frequently recommended over sodium hyaluronate preparations with molecular weight below 1×10^6 daltons. From a purely clinical standpoint, low molecular weight products (which tend to be less expensive) can be equally efficacious in ameliorating signs of joint disease. When synovial adhesions and pannus are to be avoided (as in most surgeries for carpal and fetlock fracture fragment removal), higher molecular weight preparations are recommended, because they inhibit proliferation of synovial fibroblasts.

Data support the use of repeated sodium hyaluronate dosages, usually at 2- to 3-week intervals. Depending on the inciting cause of synovitis, the effect may be permanent or transitory. Unlike repeated corticosteroid injections, extensive use of hyaluronate does not result in progressive joint deterioration and does not require rest from athletic activity. The ideal candidate for hyaluronate therapy has painful synovitis of recent onset, without radiographic evidence of degenerative joint disease or intra-articular fracture. Recalcitrant synovitis cases respond well to a combination of short-acting corticosteroids and sodium hyaluronate. Consideration of the compatibility of these agents within the joint or in the same syringe is important. Postinjection flares following use of sodium hyaluronate alone occur in up to 10 per cent of horses; a combination of drugs may increase the incidence.

POLYSULFATED GLYCOSAMINOGLYCAN

Polysulfated glycosaminoglycan (PSGAG), distributed under the trade names of Adequan° or Arteparon†, is one of the newer pharmaceuticals

---

°Adequan, Luitpold Pharmaceuticals, Shirley, NY
†Areteparon, Luitpold-Werk, Munich, Germany

marketed for equine intra-articular medication. This product is not new and has been used for several decades in people and in experimental animals in Europe. PSGAG is a mixture of low molecular weight (approximately 10,000 daltons) glycosaminoglycan (GAG) very similar in structure to chondroitin sulfate, the major GAG in normal cartilage. The product is derived from bovine lung and tracheal cartilage.

PSGAG is the most promising of a group of oversulfated heparinoids that have been tested for intra-articular use in recent years. Its mechanisms of action include a potent ability to competitively inhibit cartilage-degrading enzymes. In so doing, PSGAG preserves cartilage integrity by reducing breakdown and loss of cartilage components. Prostaglandin levels are reduced in culture conditions and this may have significant effects in reducing joint pain. PSGAG also stimulates chondrocyte synthesis of matrix components, especially in degenerate cartilage, and increases the synovial cell production of hyaluronic acid.

PSGAG has been evaluated in vivo in many types of experimental joint disease in different species. Almost without exception, it exerts a positive response by having both a chondroprotective role and the ability to stimulate chondrocytes and synoviocytes. Progression of degenerative joint disease has been attenuated with the use of PSGAG. Administered intra-articularly at a dose of 250 mg weekly for a minimum of 3 weeks, PSGAG has a clinical benefit in joint diseases characterized by mild to moderate cartilage damage. Most of these cases also have significant synovial effusion. Joints with severe cartilage damage, usually associated with moderate to severe radiographic evidence of degenerative joint disease, rarely respond for more than a few weeks to a course of PSGAG. While such a response may be sufficient in some circumstances, the cost–benefit analysis usually makes PSGAG an unsatisfactory choice in advanced degenerative joint disease cases.

PSGAG is frequently administered following chip fracture removal and cartilage debridement to assist in early return of normal synovial fluid parameters, to reduce elevated enzyme levels, to stabilize or improve the adjacent cartilage matrix proteoglycan and collagen levels, and to stimulate endogenous hyaluronate synthesis. The healing of the actual cartilage defect may be inevitably poor; however, the remaining articular cartilage and synovial environment should benefit.

In North America, Adequan has recently been approved for intramuscular (IM) administration in horses. The recommended dose of 500 mg should be administered every 3 to 4 days for a minimum of four and preferably seven injections. Systemic injection of PSGAG has been used for decades in people. PSGAG administered IM readily accumulates in articular cartilage, in apparently effective levels (greater than 1 μg per gm), and remains for at least 2 days. In horses, the IM route generally results in a clinical response, albeit of smaller magnitude than that accompanying intra-articular injection. Treatment of multiple joints in an individual horse probably will be effectively accomplished using IM PSGAG; however, additional controlled studies on increased dosages and frequencies are needed.

Because intra-articular injection of PSGAG at recommended dosages can potentiate infection, IM administration may be safer, although less efficacious. Where the intra-articular route is desired, a combination of PSGAG with 125 mg amikacin, an aminoglycoside antibiotic, has been recommended. Other side effects in horses include a nonspecific synovitis with lameness, which under most circumstances is self-limiting. Some difficulty can be encountered in differentiating a noninfectious severe synovitis from a low-grade septic arthritis. Under such circumstances, treatment for an infected joint, until proven otherwise, is prudent, since established infections following PSGAG have been extraordinarily difficult to resolve and the incidence of degenerative joint disease high. There are no published reports of anaphylactic reaction to systemic use of PSGAG in horses; however, acute anaphylaxis and death in two people have been reported.

SUPEROXIDE DISMUTASE (Orgotein)

Superoxide dismutase (SOD) is available commercially as a copper–zinc–metalloprotein of bovine liver origin, the drug version of which has been given the generic name of orgotein. It is marketed for systemic use in horses as Palosein.° The drug is available in single-dose vials of freeze-dried orgotein in sucrose. This product scavenges superoxide radicals and has general anti-inflammatory effects. Initial clinical studies suggested that Palosein administered intra-articularly had reasonable efficacy in the treatment of equine nonseptic joint diseases, was effective in treating navicular disease by juxtabursal injection, and had a profound anti-inflammatory effect when administered systemically. However,

---

°Palosein, Diagnostic Data Inc., Mountain View, CA

since then orgotein has not found widespread use. Orgotein can induce an intense synovitis. A more purified form of orgotein† incites minimal lameness and synovial reaction. Palosein apparently has acidic carbohydrate polymers present as impurities, which were removed from the Ontosein† product. The duration of action of these products is unknown.

OTHER INTRA-ARTICULAR MEDICATIONS

Rumalon‡ is a glycosaminoglycan–peptide complex from bovine cartilage and bone marrow that has shown promise in experimental and clinical trials in Europe and is under evaluation for use in horses. In people, it is injected IM in a series of 25 to 40 injections, 2 to 3 days apart, primarily to treat osteoarthritis. The series is often repeated every 6 months. Although Rumalon has been used in other countries for many years, it is not licensed for human or veterinary use in North America. Experimental studies in dogs suggest that Rumalon has marked chondroprotective effects, with reduced cartilage erosion, but has little stimulatory effect on proteoglycan synthesis or cell division.

Pentosan polysulfate (PPS) is a newer semisynthetic heparinoid similar in structure and function to Adequan and Arteparon and marketed under the trade name of Cartrophen.§ There is little published information concerning its use in animals and its advantages over Arteparon. Treatment of experimental animals, using 10 mg per kg administered IM every 2 days for 4 weeks, had a cartilage protective effect in a degenerative joint disease model. Information on the use of PPS in horses is not currently available.

Supplemental Readings

Balazs, E. A., and Denlinger, J. L.: Sodium hyaluronate and joint function. J. Equine Vet. Sci., 5:217–228, 1985.

Chunekamrai, S., Krook, L. P., Lust, G., and Maylin, G. A.: Changes in articular cartilage after intra-articular injections of methylprednisolone acetate in horses. Am. J. Vet. Res., 50:1733–1741, 1989.

Gustafson, S. B., McIlwraith, C. W., Jones, R. L., and Dixon-White, H. E.: Further investigations into the potentiation of infection by intra-articular injection of polysulfated glycosaminoglycan and the effect of filtration and intra-articular injection of amikacin. Am. J. Vet. Res., 50:2018–2022, 1989.

Loftus, S. A., Montplaisir, J. M., Kuo, J., and DeVore, D. P.: Comparison of the properties of hyaluronate products used in treatment of joint dysfunction in horses. J. Equine Vet. Sci., 8:117–120, 1988.

McIlwraith, C. W., Vachon, A.: Review of pathogenesis and treatment of degenerative joint disease. Equine Vet. J. Suppl, 6:3–11, 1988.

Tew, W. P.: Sodium hyaluronate and the treatment of equine joint disorders. In: Proceedings of the 30th Annual Meeting of the American Association of Equine Practitioners, 1984, p. 67.

Trotter, G. W., Yovich, J. V., McIlwraith, C. W., and Norrdin, R. W.: Effects of intramuscular polysulfated glycosaminoglycan on chemical and physical defects in equine articular cartilage. Can. J. Vet. Res., 53:224–230, 1989.

Yovich, J. V., Trotter, G. W., McIlwraith, C. W., and Norrdin, R. W.: Effects of polysulfated glycosaminoglycan on chemical and physical defects in equine articular cartilage. Am. J. Vet. Res., 48:1407–1414, 1987.

---

†Ontosein, Diagnostic Data Inc., Mountain View, CA
‡Rumalon, Robapharm, Munich, Germany
§Cartrophen, Arthropharm Pty-Ltd, Sydney, Australia

Infectious Synovitis

Alicia L. Bertone, COLUMBUS, OHIO

In the adult horse, infectious synovitis is most commonly caused by direct inoculation of bacteria into a joint from a puncture wound, laceration, or a needle. The bacterial virulence and number, joint environment, and immunologic status of the host determine if infection is established after joint contamination. Inoculation of as few as 100 virulent organisms can induce joint infection in normal horses. Hematogenous joint infection is more common in foals and is often accompanied by systemic illness, abscesses, or septicemia. Systemic treatment of such foals, other than treatment for the infectious arthritis, will not be addressed in this chapter. Polyarthritis is common when infection is of hematogenous origin, and therefore is more common in foals. Lyme disease, a hematogenous arthritis caused by the spirochete *Borrelia burgdorferi*, can, however, occur in horses of any age and should be considered as an infectious cause of polyarthritis of adult horses.

Inoculated bacteria localize in the synovial cells and synovia and multiply rapidly. During bacteremia, capillary loops with low blood flow (such as in the synovial capillaries) are sites of predilection for infection, presumably because of easier endothelial attachment and tissue invasion. The bacterial antigen attracts inflammatory cells to the synovium. The synovial and inflammatory cells release enzymes, prostaglandins, and free radicals that can amplify joint inflammation and articular cartilage destruction. Proteoglycan matrix loss can occur in less than 48 hours after infection. Collagen destruction and chondrocyte necrosis quickly ensue. Articular cartilage is slow to repair, and degenerative joint disease may result in permanent lameness. Because of the potential for rapid joint destruction, infectious synovitis should be regarded as a diagnostic and therapeutic emergency.

CLINICAL SIGNS AND DIAGNOSIS

The clinical signs of severe lameness, joint effusion, joint heat, and periarticular swelling warrant further diagnostic tests for joint infection. Lameness may not be severe early after joint inoculation with bacteria, after phenylbutazone administration, or if the joint is draining; therefore, any joint that has the cardinal signs of inflammation (especially with evidence of a puncture wound or a history of joint injection) should undergo further diagnostic testing.

The earliest and most reliable joint changes can be detected by analysis of the synovial fluid for total and differential white blood cell (WBC) number, and pH. More than 90 per cent neutrophils and a pH less than 7.1 are early, persistent, and consistent findings in infected synovia. The total WBC count is variable but usually greater than 30,000 cells per μl. Joints should be treated as if infected when appropriate clinical signs are present, the synovial fluid contains more than 30,000 cells per μl with more than 90 per cent neutrophils, or the joint has been punctured and is obviously contaminated.

Other confirmatory synovial fluid observations include reduced clarity, reduced viscosity, discoloration, increased total protein content, increased lactate levels, increased serum to synovial glucose difference, organisms demonstrable on Gram stain, and isolation of organisms from culture of the synovial fluid. Adjunct blood tests may reveal increased plasma fibrinogen, leukocytosis and neutrophilia, increased serum globulin, and decreased packed cell volume. An increased immunofluorescent antibody titer (above 1:250) for *Borrelia burgdorferi* is highly suggestive of Lyme disease.

Joint radiographs, synovial culture, bacterial sensitivity testing (for both aerobic and anaerobic organisms), and synovial biopsy are additional tests that are recommended for therapeutic and prognostic purposes. Radiographs may reveal foreign bodies, fractures, or osteomyelitis. Isolation of the organism and definition of its antibiotic sensitivity will direct antimicrobial therapy. Use of blood culture media will enhance isolation rates from synovial fluid and is recommended. Synovial biopsy may reveal organisms, provide another source of material for culture, reveal histologic changes that support the diagnosis, and suggest the duration of infection. A histologic diagnosis of suppurative synovitis (more than 70 per cent neutrophils) suggests acute, active bacterial infection. A chronic active bacterial infection lasting more than 2 to 3 weeks may contain up to 50 per cent mononuclear cells in the synovium. A lymphocytic, proliferative synovitis is compatible with borreliosis or immune-mediated synovitis (see p. 135).

THERAPY

Treatment ideally consists of systemic antimicrobial administration augmented with daily intra-articular administration in some instances; joint drainage, debridement, and lavage; anti-inflammatory medication; and joint physiotherapy.

Systemic Antimicrobial Therapy

Systemic antimicrobial therapy can eliminate clinical signs of septicemia and can help eliminate joint infection when combined with joint drainage. Most antimicrobial agents given systemically adequately penetrate normal synovial fluid, where their concentrations are identical to plasma concentrations. In inflamed but not infected equine joints, ampicillin and kanamycin achieve higher maximal concentrations than in corresponding serum. Infection in synovia may alter drug concentrations or effectiveness by affecting drug diffusion, drug solubility, protein binding, pKa (pH), and many other factors. Trimethoprim-sulfadiazine (TMP-SDZ) combination given to horses with joint infection at a dosage of 60 mg per kg per day (30 mg per kg orally q. 12 h.) is effective in maintaining greater than minimum inhibitory concentrations (MICs) for most isolates in the infected synovia. Gentamicin (2.2 mg per kg IV, t.i.d.) is active in equine infected synovia, but levels are below MIC for most isolates at the end of the interdosing interval. Because of toxicity, the systemic dose of gentamicin cannot be safely increased, but intra-articular administration can augment synovial fluid concentrations. Other systemic antimicrobial therapy that has not been evaluated experimentally in horses but seems clinically effective includes penicillin and cephalosporins (cephalothin, ceftiofur).

INTRA-ARTICULAR ANTIMICROBIAL THERAPY

Systemic gentamicin is expensive, potentially toxic, and unable to maintain MIC in infected synovia. Intra-articular administration provides the highest synovial concentrations (approximately 5000 µg per ml) with a minimum of chemically induced synovitis. Intra-articular gentamicin can augment, and in some instances possibly replace, systemic use of the drug. Intra-articular administration of 150 mg of unbuffered gentamicin eliminates joint infection sooner than systemic gentamicin, attains peak concentrations 1000 times higher than with systemic administration, and maintains synovial concentrations above MIC for more than 24 hours. Intra-articular amikacin (125 mg) is also effective. If gentamicin or amikacin therapy is selected, systemic therapy should supplement intra-articular administration.

JOINT DRAINAGE

Joint drainage as an accompaniment to antimicrobial therapy aids in the elimination of infection, reduces signs of sepsis, and allows removal of inflammatory debris. Three joint drainage techniques have been experimentally evaluated in horses with infectious arthritis: through-and-through lavage, arthrotomy and lavage, and arthroscopy with partial synovectomy and lavage. Arthrotomy provides continual joint drainage, less fibrin accumulation, and less synovitis than single, double, or triple through-and-through joint lavage. Delayed healing, exuberant granulation tissue, and fibrosis complicate healing of the arthrotomy by second intention. Tertiary closure of the arthrotomy after elimination of the infection provides a cosmetic alternative. Arthroscopy allows more thorough joint inspection and fibrin debridement, but in experimental studies arthroscopic debridement, partial synovectomy, and lavage provide less joint drainage, slower elimination of joint infection, more lameness, and more joint swelling than arthrotomy.

A logical joint drainage plan is to initially explore and debride the joint with the arthroscope. Synovium can be obtained for culture and histology. At the termination of the surgery, one of the joint portals is enlarged to a 2-cm arthrotomy for continued drainage. A sterile bandage is maintained and changed at least once daily. Once lameness has resolved and joint cultures are negative, the arthrotomy incision is closed for easier care and improved cosmesis. This approach has been successful in clinical cases.

ANTI-INFLAMMATORY THERAPY

In models of arthritis in other species, nonsteroidal anti-inflammatory drugs (NSAIDs) reduce joint destruction. Based on the contribution of inflammation to articular cartilage damage, and the risk of supporting limb laminitis in horses with infectious synovitis, NSAIDs should be given for their anti-inflammatory and analgesic effects. Corticosteroids delay the onset of clinical signs of joint infection in horses and may be immunosuppressive to the local joint environment. However, in two equine experimental studies, intra-articular corticosteroids did not potentiate or aggravate joint infection. Corticosteroid use early in infectious synovitis is not recommended, but its potent anti-inflammatory effects may be beneficial in postinfectious arthritis. This remains to be evaluated.

Intra-articular sodium hyaluronate (10 mg) given immediately following joint lavage reduces lameness and synovitis. Hyaluronate can provide anti-inflammatory properties, increase synovial viscosity, and improve joint soft tissue lubrication and, hopefully, joint flexibility.

Many other medications may be beneficial in the treatment of infectious synovitis, such as dimethyl sulfoxide, hyperimmune serum, and orgotein. Further investigation is necessary before promoting their use.

PHYSICAL THERAPY

Joint rest (stall rest) is recommended during the acute phases of synovitis to reduce joint injury and pain. Support bandages may immobilize and protect the joint. Passive flexion or swimming should be initiated after joint infection is eliminated and incisions are healed. Passive motion may improve joint flexibility, remodel fibrosis, prevent or stretch synovial adhesions, and improve cartilage nutrition. Other modes of physical therapy, such as cold laser treatment and ultrasound applications, have had some success.

Supplemental Readings

Bertone, A. L., Davis, D. M., Cox, H. C., Roberts, R. C., Kamerling, S., and Caprile, K: Arthrotomy versus arthroscopy and partial synovectomy for the treatment of experimentally induced equine infectious arthritis. Am. J. Vet. Res., 1991 (in press).

Bertone, A. L., Jones, R. L., and McIlwraith, C. W.: Serum and synovial fluid steady-state concentrations of trimethoprim and sulfadiazine in horses with experimentally induced infectious arthritis. Am. J. Vet. Res., 49:1681, 1988.

Bertone, A. L., McIlwraith, C. W.: A review of current concepts in the therapy of infectious arthritis in the horse. In: Proceedings of the 32nd Annual Convention of the American Association of Equine Practitioners, 1986, pp. 323–339.

Bertone, A. L., McIlwraith, C. W., Jones, R. L., Norrdin, R. W., Radin, M. J., and Lebel, J. L.: Comparison of various treatments for experimentally induced equine infectious arthritis. Am. J. Vet. Res., 48:519, 1987.

Burgess, E. C., Gillette, D., and Pickett, J. P.: Arthritis and panuveitis as manifestations of Borrelia burgdorferi infection in a Wisconsin pony. J. Am. Vet. Med. Assoc., 189:1340, 1986.

Gustafson, S. B., McIlwraith, C. W., and Jones, R. L.: Comparison of the effect of polysulfated glycosaminoglycan, corticosteroids, and sodium hyaluronate in the potentiation of a subinfective dose of Staphylococcus aureus in the midcarpal joint in horses. Am. J. Vet. Res., 50:2014, 1989.

Lloyd, K. C. K., Stover, S. M., Pascoe, J. R., and Adams, P.: Synovial fluid pH, cytologic characteristics, and gentamicin concentration after intra-articular administration of the drug in an experimental model of infectious arthritis in horses. Am. J. Vet. Res., 51:1363, 1990.

Martens, R. J., Auer, J. A., and Carter, G. K.: Equine pediatrics: Septic arthritis and osteomyelitis. J. Am. Vet. Med. Assoc., 188:582, 1986.

Tulamo, R. M., Bramlage, L. R., and Gabel, A. A.: Sequential clinical and synovial fluid changes associated with acute infectious arthritis in the horse. Equine Vet. J., 21:325, 1989.

Noninfectious Synovitis

Alicia L. Bertone, COLUMBUS, OHIO

Inflammation of the noninfected synovium can occur in association with joint trauma, degeneration, or immune-mediated disease. In traumatic synovitis, joint concussion and motion can disrupt synovium and articular cartilage. Inflammation associated with synovial healing and a reaction to cartilage breakdown products occurs. Proliferative synovitis can result from chronic trauma to synovial pads and is accompanied by hemorrhage and fibrosis. The dorsal pad of the metacarpophalangeal joint is particularly likely to be damaged. In degenerative joint disease, synovitis may be the inciting cause of degeneration and may be of traumatic, infectious, or immune-mediated etiology. Synovitis may also occur secondarily in progressive, spontaneous degenerative joint disease owing to the release of antigenic articular cartilage components, particularly polysulfated glycosaminoglycans and collagen. Eosinophilic synovitis has been reported in the horse in association with an intra-articular injection of methylprednisolone acetate.

Immune-mediated synovitis is associated with immunoglobulin G deposition in the synovium and usually a nonarticular focus of infection. Deposition of immunoglobulin in the synovium may be induced by an increased blood flow and filtration of immune complexes formed as a result of the primary infection. It is also possible that immunogenic bacterial byproducts may localize in the synovium and attract immunoglobulin. Immune complexes stimulate complement fixation and chemotaxis of lymphocytes and plasma cells, a type III Arthus-like reaction. A lymphocytic, plasmacytic synovitis results.

Systemic lupus erythematosus (SLE) is a specific immune-mediated systemic disorder in which antibodies develop against the animal's nuclear material. Clinical signs may involve many organ systems and include a nonerosive lymphocytic, plasmacytic arthritis. Two cases of a lupus-like syndrome have been reported in horses.

The interaction between synovium and articular cartilage in synovitis is complex. In infectious synovitis, the disease is initiated by the reaction of the synovium to the organism. In other forms of synovitis, the inflammation may be incited by trauma or an immune reaction. Once inflammation starts, it is perpetuated by inflammatory mediators such as interleukins and prostaglandins released by synovial or inflammatory cells. The synovial inflammation may not be as severe in noninfectious as in infectious forms of synovitis, but if chronic can produce articular cartilage changes by enzymatic degradation and alteration in synovial lubrication and nutrition.

Noninfectious synovitis is usually associated with less severe lameness and joint pain (arthralgia) and a milder, less fibrinous reaction than is infectious synovitis. Because the cause is joint concussion or systemic disease, multiple joints are often affected.

TRAUMATIC SYNOVITIS

Athletic horses, particularly racehorses, may exercise beyond the physiologic limits of concussive loading and joint excursion. Joints with a lot of motion, such as the fetlock, are particularly susceptible to direct trauma to the synovium or articular cartilage. Joint inflammation may be induced by the release of articular cartilage fragments into the synovia or as a direct response to the synovial trauma.

Diagnosis is usually based on the history and the presence of joint effusion, lameness, and resentment of joint flexion. Synovial fluid analysis in acute cases may reveal reduced viscosity and mild increases in white blood cell count (less than 10,000 cells per μl) and total protein content (less than 3.5 gm per dl). In chronic cases the synovial fluid cell count may be normal, but mild increases in protein content usually persist. Hemarthrosis, detected as bloody synovial fluid, may indicate articular cartilage damage. Radiographs are usually normal, but signs of degenerative joint disease such as osteophyte production, enthesiophytes, and joint narrowing develop in chronic cases of traumatic synovitis.

Treatment is joint rest. Anti-inflammatory medication such as phenylbutazone, 4 to 8 mg per kg per day given orally, hydrotherapy, and support bandages may speed resolution of clinical signs. Exercise can usually be resumed within 2 weeks, but recurrence is common if similar levels of exercise are expected as before injury. Intra-articular medication with drugs such as sodium hyaluronate is probably therapeutic for the joint and may prevent recurrence on resumption of exercise (see p. 128). Sodium hyaluronate is probably most beneficial for cases of acute traumatic synovitis. If cartilage damage is suspected, intra-articular or systemic administration of polysulfated glycosaminoglycans has been advocated. The anti-inflammatory potency of corticosteroids is often greater than necessary for the treatment of acute traumatic synovitis. Joint lavage is not usually necessary, owing to the low synovial fluid cell counts and the rapid response to rest.

OSTEOARTHRITIS

Osteoarthritis is the progressive degeneration of the articular cartilage. Pathologic changes include cartilage fibrillation and cracking, altered density of subchondral bone, and stiffening and thickening of joint soft tissues. Initiating factors may not be known. A slow process of release of proteins and enzymes from the degenerating cartilage stimulates release of substances from the synovium and incites inflammation. The process perpetuates itself, and ultimately mechanical strength of the joint is reduced and pain persists. Synovitis may initiate the degeneration and then resolve, but altered synovial physiology (and in some cases synovitis) persists throughout the disease process.

Clinical signs include joint stiffness, resentment of joint flexion, lameness, and radiographic signs consistent with degenerative joint disease. Bony and soft tissue proliferation may be palpable and visible at joint capsule insertions. Intra-articular anesthesia may improve but not eliminate the lameness. Joint effusion may be present if an active synovitis is present at the time of examination. Synovial fluid may be normal or have a slight increase in total protein content.

Alleviation of signs may necessitate reduction in expectations for athletic performance. Therapy is palliative. Initially, rest for 2 to 4 weeks is recommended to reduce any concomitant synovitis. Analgesics such as nonsteroidal anti-inflammatory drugs may be used as needed to maintain soundness. Shoeing with a half-round, light shoe and pad will ease breakover and concussion. Intra-articular medication with drugs such as sodium hyaluronate and polysulfated glycosaminoglycans may provide some relief, but as the disease progresses, these medications may not control the pain. Intra-articular corticosteroids provide the most pain relief for the longest duration. The effects on cartilage metabolism are of long duration and may be detrimental to the ultimate joint life span. Corticosteroids are often used in this disease, with understanding of their limitations, because they allow continued athletic use of the horse.

PROLIFERATIVE (VILLONODULAR) SYNOVITIS

The dorsal synovial pad of the fetlock joint is prone to traumatic injury when excessively dorsiflexed. Repeated trauma results in nodular fibrosis and enlargement of the pad. Joint capsule and metacarpal bone changes occur secondarily. Clinical signs suggestive of proliferative synovitis of the pad include excessive joint effusion and a palpable mass. The diagnosis can be confirmed with contrast arthrography or ultrasonography. If degenerative joint disease is not present, arthroscopic surgical removal of the mass can result in athletic soundness. Intra-articular steroids will shrink the mass and possibly prevent additional fibrosis when the horse is returned to exercise. Intra-articular steroids should be reserved for horses with evidence of degenerative joint disease and can be used alone or in conjunction with surgery.

NONEROSIVE IMMUNE-MEDIATED SYNOVITIS

IMMUNE-MEDIATED POLYSYNOVITIS

Multiple synovial effusions and a stiff gait affecting all four limbs has been described in foals with infection at sites other than the joints. Peripheral leukocytosis with neutrophilia, fever, and hyperfibrinogenemia is consistent with the systemic infection. Synovial fluid typically contains 500 to 10,000 cells per μl, mostly nondegenerated neutrophils and macrophages. Histologic examination of the synovium reveals lymphocytic, plasmacytic synovitis. Synovial culture and Gram stain are negative for aerobic and anaerobic bacteria or *Mycoplasma*. Rheumatoid factor titers, fluorescent antinuclear antibody titers, and lupus erythematosus (LE) cell preparations are negative. A Coombs test is positive in some cases.

The diagnosis is confirmed by demonstrating immune complexes in the synovium. Immunofluorescence staining of the synovium with fluorescein-labeled anti-equine IgG documents the presence and exact location of the immunoglobulin in the synovium.

Treatment is primarily directed at the focus of infection, as it may be life-threatening. Joint lavage may provide some temporary relief of arthralgia and, if performed with the arthroscope, can allow simultaneous synovial biopsy. A nonsteroidal anti-inflammatory medication such as phenylbutazone may provide some analgesic and anti-inflammatory benefit. If the infection resolves and the synovitis remains or recrudesces, treatment with oral prednisolone (1 to 4 mg per kg q. 48 h.) may relieve arthralgia and effusion. Clinical signs may recur upon discontinuation of the steroids. Intra-articular steroid administration may provide longer relief but has not been reported in the literature.

Systemic Lupus-Like Polysynovitis

A confirmed diagnosis of this condition requires fulfilling many clinicopathologic criteria and a confirmed case of lupus-like arthritis has not been reported in the horse. SLE-like syndrome should be considered in horses with the clinical signs described above for immune-mediated arthritis and in which a focus of infection cannot be located. Additionally, horses with lupus-like syndrome have positive SLE tests and fluorescent antinuclear antibody titers. Even with these criteria, however, the diagnosis of SLE-like syndrome should be reserved, because infection may be occult, and it is not currently known how many normal or ill horses have positive responses to LE tests or fluorescent antinuclear antibody titers. Other organ systems should be evaluated for immune-mediated disease, particularly the kidney for glomerulonephritis and the skin for dermatitis.

If SLE-like syndrome is the tentative diagnosis and the primary disease process is immune mediated, therapy should consist of anti-inflammatory medication such as oral prednisolone. Practically, however, a course of antibiotic therapy often precedes the use of oral prednisolone, since ruling out a focus of infection can be difficult. Recommendations for adjunct therapy, such as joint lavage and nonsteroidal anti-inflammatory medication, are the same as for other immune-mediated arthritides.

EOSINOPHILIC SYNOVITIS

Eosinophilic synovitis is rare in any species but has been reported in the horse following intra-articular injection of methylprednisolone acetate in the carpal joints. Clinical signs include joint effusion, resistance to joint flexion, joint heat, and lameness. Synovial fluid contained approximately 9,000 cells per μl, mostly mononuclear cells and 20 per cent eosinophils. Fifteen per cent of the macrophages had phagocytosed eosinophilic granules. Histopathologic evaluation of the synovium revealed an eosinophilic, plasmacytic synovitis compatible with a hypersensitivity reaction. Acute crystalline-induced synovitis (postinjection flare) occurs following intra-articular steroid injection but is usually self-limiting in 48 hours and has not been documented to produce an eosinophilic reaction. Joint lavage to remove remaining methylprednisolone acetate, associated vehicles, and inflammatory cells may reduce the inflammatory response and corresponding clinical signs.

Supplemental Readings

Byars, T. D., Tyler, D. E., Whitlock, R. H., George, J. W., and DeBuysscher, E. V.: Non-erosive polysynovitis in a horse. Equine Vet. J., 16:141, 1984.

Madison, J. B., and Scarratt, W. K.: Immune-mediated polysynovitis in four foals. J. Am. Vet. Med. Assoc., 192:1581, 1988.

McIlwraith, C. W.: Current concepts in equine degenerative joint disease. J. Am. Vet. Med. Assoc., 180:239, 1982.

Todhunter, R. J., and Lust, G.: Pathophysiology of synovitis: Clinical signs and examination in horses. Compend. Cont. Ed. Pract. Vet., 12:980, 1990.

Turner, A. S., Gustafson, S. B., Zeidner, N. S., McIlwraith, C. W., and Thrall, M. A.: Acute eosinophilic synovitis in a horse. Equine Vet. J., 22:215, 1990.

Vrins, A., and Feldman, B. F.: Lupus erythematosus-like syndrome in a horse. Equine Pract., 5:18, 1983.

White, N. A.: Synovial pad proliferation in the metacarpophalangeal joint. *In* White, N. A., and Moore, J. N. (eds.): Current Practice of Equine Surgery. Philadelphia, J. B. Lippincott Co., 1990, pp. 555–558.

Degenerative Joint Disease

Dean W. Richardson, KENNETT SQUARE, PENNSYLVANIA

Degenerative joint disease is a problem of overwhelming economic importance in the horse industry. Although many of the basic mechanisms of joint deterioration have been extensively investigated and defined, the complexity of the interactions of these mechanisms suggests that degenerative joint disease results from a number of processes leading to a final common pathway of disease. The joint as a whole can be considered as an organ comprised of multiple parts: articular cartilage, synovial lining, synovial fluid, joint capsule, articular ligaments, menisci, and subchondral bone. As in other body organs, failure of any component may lead to organ failure and clinical disease.

Although degenerative joint disease is clearly a consequence of both biological and mechanical factors, the initiating injury to one or more components of the equine joint is usually mechanical in nature. The underlying concept is that there is an imbalance between the load applied to some portion of the joint and that tissue's capacity to withstand that load. For example, overloading of the dorsal margin of the distal radial carpal bone in a racehorse may lead to mechanical failure of the bone and cartilage and an osteochondral fracture. The fracture in turn stimulates a series of biological and mechanical events that *may* lead to deterioration of the joint. The specific events occurring within each component vary because of the specific responses of the tissue. The combination of these responses is the disease we recognize clinically.

Articular cartilage is an extraordinary tissue, uniquely adapted to its mechanical function as the bearing surface of joints subjected to millions of loading cycles during an animal's life. Its mechanical function is directly related to its structure, and even subtle alterations in its structure or chemical composition can compromise its mechanical integrity and the continued function of the joint. Cartilage is a tissue without blood vessels, nerves, or lymphatic supply. Its living elements, the chondrocytes, live isolated lives within the cartilage, surrounded by a matrix of collagen and ground substance and nutritionally supported by diffusion from the synovial fluid and capillaries in the subchondral bone. The chondrocytes synthesize the collagen and ground substance components. Near the surface, chondrocytes are more closely packed and flattened in a tangential plane. Similarly, the collagen fiber network near the surface is tangentially arranged in an intertwined mat that is resistant to surface shearing loads. The chondrocytes in the deeper layers are surrounded by more matrix and are irregularly arranged until they reach the deepest layers, where they are radially aligned in columns perpendicular to the subchondral bony plate. The collagen network follows the same basic arrangement. Within the collagen framework, the ground substance is composed of enormous molecular aggregates, each comprised of a long backbone of hyaluronic acid to which side chains of proteoglycans are attached with a link protein. The proteoglycans have a protein core with varying side chains of glycosaminoglycans, including chondroitin-4 sulfate, chondroitin-6 sulfate, and keratan sulfate. The proteoglycan side chains are negatively charged and hydrophilic so that each side chain tends to repel another and bind a large volume of water. Water makes up 60 to 80 per cent of the wet weight of articular cartilage. The consequence of this construction is that cartilage functions like an elastic sponge with the water-expanded supramolecular aggregates holding the collagen meshwork in tension.

ETIOLOGY

Both biochemical and mechanical events can lead to alterations in the proteoglycan aggregates and/or collagen meshwork and subsequent loss of normal mechanical function of the cartilage (Fig. 1). In the horse, trauma due to acute or repetitive overload is the most important identifiable cause of cartilage damage. Direct trauma due to overload of a joint surface can affect cartilage in three basic ways. High shear forces on the surface of the cartilage can disrupt the normal tangential mat of collagen and expose the less shear-resistant radial zone of cartilage. Fibrillation or vertical clefting of the cartilage ensues, and there may be continued loss of ground substance from the deeper cartilage and progressive loss of mechanical function. A second mechanism of trauma results from remodeling of the subchondral bone in response to that trauma. Repetitively stressed bone inevitably stiffens. As the subchondral bone becomes stiffer, the internal stresses sustained by the overlying cartilage may increase and result in failure of its structure. Finally, trauma may cause an acute intra-articular event such as an osteochon-

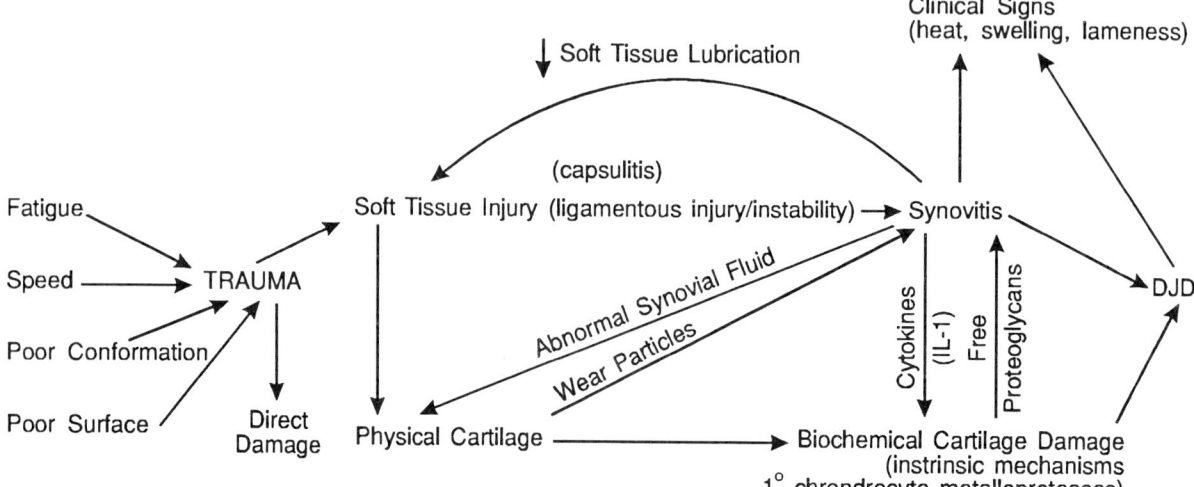

Figure 1. Destructive and reparative factors involved in degenerative joint disease. Reparative factors include decreasing joint trauma by increasing musculoskeletal and cardiopulmonary fitness, increasing proteoglycan synthesis by the stressed chondrocytes, and decreasing joint use with increasing pain, a protective mechanism that owners, trainers, and veterinarians continually abrogate. DJD, Degenerative joint disease.

dral fracture, ligamentous instability, or capsular tearing, any of which may lead to synovitis.

Synovitis in turn may lead to further changes in the joint through several mechanisms. The lubricating quality of the synovial fluid may be impaired as the normal balance of synovial lining cell synthesis and dialysis is altered. Enzymes capable of destroying cartilage, such as neutral metalloproteases, may be directly released into the synovial fluid by synovial mononuclear cells. Probably more importantly, cytokines such as interleukin-1 are released into the synovial fluid and activate proteoglycan-degrading enzymes within the cartilage. With severe synovitis, where activated neutrophils are present, lysozyme and free radicals may play a role in degradation of synovial fluid hyaluronic acid as well as cartilage matrix. Wear particles, cartilage debris, and proteoglycans leaching from physically or enzymatically damaged cartilage can in turn stimulate further synovitis and a vicious cycle can ensue, especially if the joint is subjected to continued trauma.

Cartilage was traditionally considered an inert tissue completely incapable of repair once injured, but it is now realized that chondrocytes are very active metabolically and do respond to injury. It is generally accepted that chondrocytes in the early, potentially reparable stages of osteoarthritis increase their synthesis of matrix components. Degenerative joint disease progresses when the joint's reparative responses are outpaced by the destructive influences. If cartilage deterioration progresses to the point of overt structural damage, its feeble repair mechanisms are overwhelmed, particularly if the joint continues to be traumatized. The goal of improving our understanding of the basic mechanisms of joint disease is to allow investigation of the destructive processes and promotion of the repair processes before widespread structural damage occurs in the joint.

CLINICAL SIGNS

There is an inconsistent correlation between the clinical signs of degenerative joint disease and the degree of morphological change. Much depends on the specific joint involved and the type and level of activity of the horse. Lameness as a clinical sign obviously invokes the stimulation of pain fibers. Most nociceptors are located in the joint capsule, so that capsulitis due to direct injury such as stretching or tearing of the capsule results in intense pain. Stretching of the capsule in the course of an inflammatory effusion can also induce pain. Inflammatory mediators released in response to wear debris, fracture particles, or even leached proteoglycans can directly affect pain receptors. A less well-defined mechanism of joint pain involves the juxta-articular bone. The presence of pain receptors in the subchondral bone is generally unproved, but it is known that there is a correlation between pain and intraosseous pressures. Changes in pressures within some bones may play a role in the pain and lameness seen with some degenerative joints.

Persistent inflammation in and around a joint

may lead not only to degenerative changes in the cartilage but also to changes in the periarticular connective tissue. Edema is succeeded by fibroblastic infiltration and fibroplasia. The joint becomes stiffer, and clinical signs may manifest when normal activity is constrained by the joint's decreased range of motion. In some cases, such as the old racehorse with "locked" fetlocks, the joint can become so constrained that clinical signs are minimized.

DIAGNOSTIC TESTS

In early degenerative joint disease, there are no radiographic changes and there is poor correlation between radiographic change and more advanced degenerative joint disease. Enthesiophytes, or dystrophic calcifications of capsular, ligamentous, or tendinous attachments, may be evident without significant change within the joint. Marginal or "true" osteophytes are proliferations of bone and cartilage at articular margins that are nonspecific responses to articular disease. They can develop in horses without causing clinical signs or necessarily progressing to clinically apparent disease.

Radiographic changes consistently associated with significant degenerative change include loss of radiographically demonstrable joint space caused by structural loss of cartilage and subchondral bone lysis. Subchondral sclerosis such as is seen on the radial facet of the third carpal bone in the tangential view has been proposed to be consistently associated with overlying cartilage change, but this association has not been proved.

There are no specific tests for degenerative joint disease. The diagnosis is based on localized clinical signs and typical radiographic changes. Because the initiating cause of the pathway to degenerative joint disease can be acute or insidious, the diagnosis is often made at varying stages of the disease. Early biochemical changes in cartilage cannot yet be identified in a clinical setting, and synovial fluid and serum markers of cartilage matrix loss have been disappointing to date. Similarly, synovial fluid analysis, while quite helpful in assessing the health and function of the synovial lining, is not a reliable means of measuring cartilage deterioration. Continued investigation in these areas may lead to more specific tests.

THERAPY

The most important therapy for any injured joint is rest. Continued hard use of a joint containing cartilage that is mechanically inferior due to matrix loss is likely to lead to structural failure of the cartilage and its eventual loss. Resting the joint when the cartilage has lost proteoglycans may allow replenishment of the ground substance before structural integrity is compromised. The amount of time required for equine cartilage to turn over or replace its ground substance is unknown but probably is a matter of several weeks to months.

Intra-articular therapy (see page 127) plays a major role in the management of degenerative joints, and the clinician must be aware of both the beneficial and detrimental effects of each medication. Nonsteroidal anti-inflammatory drugs (NSAIDs) are useful in the early treatment of an injured joint since they can suppress the inflammatory response of the soft tissues surrounding the joint. Their use can help decrease pain, edema, and swelling in and around the joint and thereby help minimize joint fibrosis and loss of normal range of motion of the joint. The chronic use of most NSAIDs in other species has been linked to decreased proteoglycan synthesis by chondrocytes. Further work in this area needs to be done in the horse, specifically identifying NSAIDs with minimal adverse effects on cartilage. Both NSAIDs and corticosteroids can be used with less concern and maximal benefit in joints such as the tarsometatarsal and distal intertarsal joints, where ankylosis is an acceptable end result.

Counterirritation in the form of rubefacients (liniments and paints), vesicants (blisters), and therapeutic ultrasound can be clinically helpful in managing the periarticular soft tissues but have little effect on the intra-articular degenerative processes. The benefit of more severe counterirritation such as thermocautery (firing) remains controversial, and most clinicians believe that the primary benefit to the joint is the enforced rest. "Freeze-firing" with liquid nitrogen, although not directly therapeutic, also may result in quick clinical improvement when done over nerves leading to the affected joint.

Cold, in the form of icing the joint, is very important in any acutely injured joint but is also valuable in managing the degenerative joint. Icing degenerative joints following exercise helps to limit the inflammation that inevitably occurs following hard use of a degenerative joint.

Surgical treatment of the degenerative joint is usually limited to the removal of overtly loose cartilage and bone serving as a source of continued synovitis. Resurfacing of damaged joint surfaces by means of abrasion arthroplasty (arthroscopic burning of damaged cartilage through the tidemark) or forage (drilling small holes through the damaged surface into vascular subchondral bone) is somewhat useful but limited by surgical accessibility and the surface area involved. Resurfacing with substances such as periosteum, perichondrium, or osteochondral grafts has limited applicability, but grafting of defects with cultured chondrocytes may be a practical alternative in the future.

Supplemental Readings

Gardner, D. L.: The nature and causes of osteoarthrosis. Br. Med. J., 286:418–424, 1983.
Hamerman, D.: The biology of osteoarthritis. N. Engl. J. Med., 320:1322–1330, 1989.
McIlwraith, C. W., and Vachon, A.: Review of pathogenesis and treatment of degenerative joint disease. Equine Vet. J., Suppl. 6:3–11, 1988.
Radin, E. L., and Rose, R. M.: Role of subchondral bone in the initiation and progression of cartilage damage. Clin. Orthop. Rel. Res., 213:34–40, 1986.

Sesamoiditis and Suspensory Desmitis

Joanne Hardy, COLUMBUS, OHIO

The proximal sesamoid bones and the suspensory ligament are components of the suspensory apparatus of the horse. Sesamoiditis and suspensory desmitis are common injuries of race and performance horses. Assessment of suspensory apparatus injury should include the sesamoid bones, the suspensory ligament, and the associated splint bones. Distal splint bone fractures are often associated with suspensory desmitis.

SESAMOIDITIS

CLINICAL SIGNS

Sesamoid fractures are more prevalent in the early stages of speed training, and suspensory ligament problems occur more commonly in the fit racehorse. This may be due to a differential rate in strength gain that occurs with training.

Both the sesamoid bones and the suspensory ligament have a limited blood supply. Additionally, the sesamoid bones lack an endosteal cavity and a periosteal covering. Therefore, both structures heal slowly. Healing is associated with scar tissue formation, which differs biochemically and mechanically from the original tissue and is functionally weaker.

Sesamoiditis is a performance-limiting injury. Lameness is most evident during periods of hard training or racing, and subsides with rest. The lameness is mild (grade 1 to 2 on a scale of 4) but may be more severe the day after training and is accentuated by fetlock flexion. Affected horses may show thickening of the soft tissue around the fetlock and tend to hold their fetlock in an upright position. Fetlock joint effusion is absent.

Intra-articular anesthesia of the fetlock joint will not improve the lameness. However, local anesthesia of the medial and lateral palmar nerves will markedly improve the lameness.

Radiographic lesions seen with sesamoiditis include lytic and proliferative changes on the abaxial surface of the sesamoid bones at the suspensory ligament insertion. Osteoarthritis of the fetlock joint may result in osteophyte formation at the apical and basilar aspects of the sesamoid bones, which should not be confused with sesamoiditis. The primary radiographic lesion of sesamoiditis is enlarged linear defects, sometimes referred to as vascular channels, measuring 2 mm or more in diameter, ill-defined, and often with a club-shaped appearance (Fig. 1). These findings have consistently been associated with lameness in the horse in training. Extensive osseous proliferation may also be observed in the chronic stage and is associated with healing.

In normal horses in training, one or two lytic linear defects less than 1 mm wide are often observed on the abaxial surface of the sesamoid bones without clinical signs. The number of these linear defects may increase with increased bone remodeling in response to training. Horses that have sustained other suspensory apparatus injuries including suspensory desmitis and flexor tendonitis and sesamoid fractures, may also have secondary changes in their sesamoid bones. The presence of three or more well-defined linear defects measuring 1 mm or less in diameter should be considered a reflection of increased bone metabolism resulting from training or inflammatory changes in adjacent structures, and not diagnostic of sesamoid disease. When these changes are present, soft tissue structures of the suspensory apparatus should be examined if lameness is present.

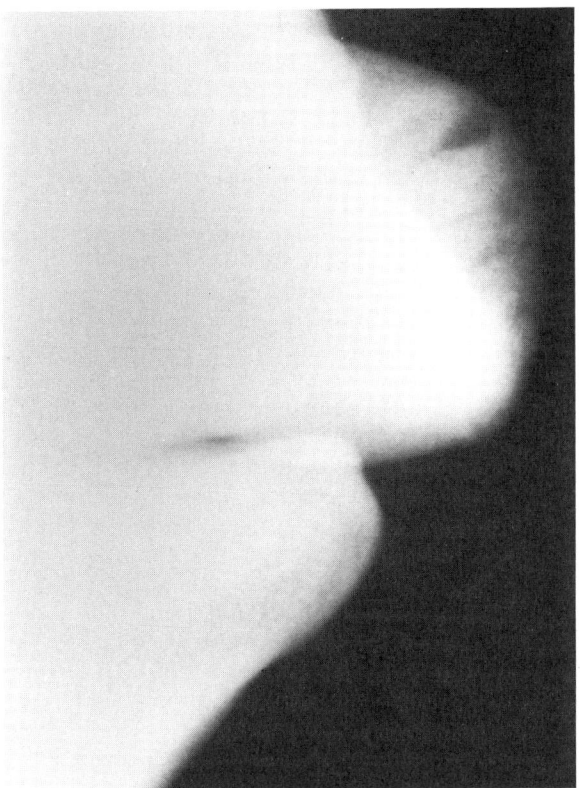

Figure 1. Radiographic findings of sesamoiditis in a 2-year-old Standardbred horse. Note the enlarged lytic areas on the abaxial surface of the proximal sesamoid bone.

THERAPY

Therapy for sesamoiditis is not rewarding. Most horses become sound with rest, only to show recurrence of lameness at speed. Extended rest periods of 6 to 12 months are advocated. Careful trimming and shoeing should provide adequate medial to lateral hoof balance and minimize stress on the suspensory apparatus. A shorter toe and removal of toe grabs will ease breakover. The angle of the hoof wall should be parallel to the pastern axis. Excessive heel height will increase strain on the suspensory apparatus, but an excessively short heel will have the same effect during the breakover phase of the stride at speed. Adjustments in the training schedule to emphasize extended work periods at lower speeds may be helpful. Some horses may be able to perform satisfactorily at lower performance levels, given adequate management.

SUSPENSORY DESMITIS

Injuries to the suspensory ligament can occur at the origin, body, medial and lateral branches, or insertion into the proximal sesamoid bone. The extensor branches of the suspensory ligament are rarely associated with disease. Clinical signs and prognosis will differ with the site of injury.

Injuries of the origin of the suspensory ligament are characterized by an acute, severe lameness that improves with a few days of rest. Usually there is no palpable swelling, and pain can be elicited by deep digital pressure over the origin of the suspensory ligament. Digital pressure maintained for 30 seconds over the affected area may exacerbate the lameness. Local infiltration of the origin of the suspensory ligament will relieve the lameness and is more specific than regional anesthesia of the palmar nerves. Because of the proximity of the lateral and medial palmar or plantar nerves, diffusion of the anesthetic may also result in regional anesthesia of the lower limb. Therefore, the lower limb should be eliminated as the source of lameness prior to local infiltration of the origin of the suspensory ligament. Additionally, the palmar outpouching of the carpometacarpal joint may extend as far distally as 4.5 cm; therefore, diffusion of the anesthetic into the carpometacarpal joint is possible. The carpus should be ruled out as a source of the lameness.

The differential diagnosis of pain originating at the proximal metacarpus or metatarsus includes proximal splint bone periostitis, distal accessory ligament desmitis in the front limbs, and incomplete palmar sagittal metacarpal fracture. Radiographic examination may reveal an avulsion fracture at the origin of the suspensory ligament (Fig. 2) and is useful to rule out other causes of lameness. Ultrasonographic examination of the suspensory ligament provides the most accurate assessment of the severity of the proximal suspensory injury. Therapy for injury to the origin of the suspensory is complete rest, generally for 3 to 6 months, until evidence of healing can be demonstrated ultrasonographically. Lameness will often recur if inadequate rest is provided. Nonsteroidal anti-inflammatory drugs such as phenylbutazone may be used in the acute stage. The prognosis for return to full athletic use is generally good if adequate rest is provided.

Injury to the ligamentous fibers of the body or branches of the suspensory ligament manifests with a moderate to severe lameness in the acute stage. Standardbreds are often affected in both front limbs and hind limbs, whereas Thoroughbreds are more commonly affected in the front limbs. A painful swelling may be apparent over the affected area; however, this will subside with a few days of local therapy, making palpation an unreliable tool for diagnosis. Small tears may not be associated with local swelling, but continued training will result in worsening of the tear and produce acute clinical signs. Damage of the sus-

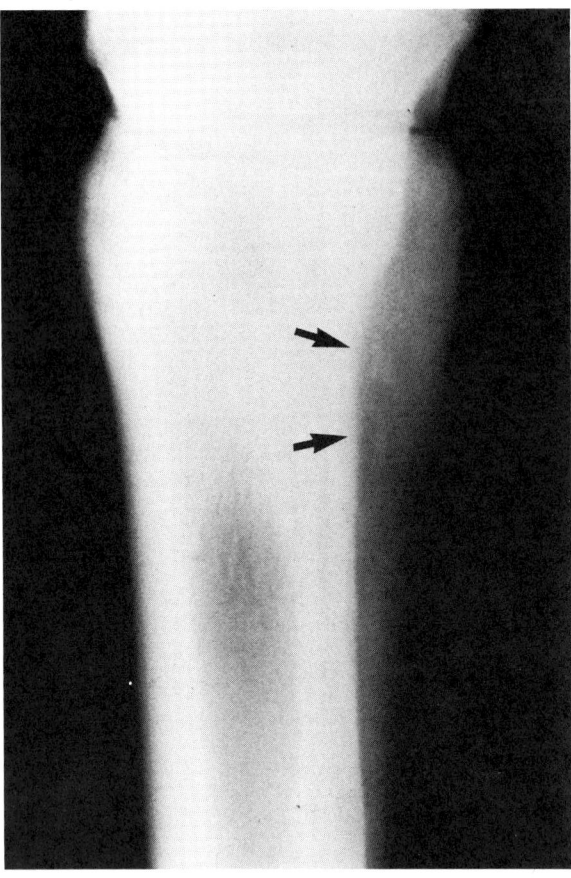

Figure 2. Radiograph of the proximal metacarpus in a horse with a suspensory avulsion fracture associated with a proximal suspensory desmitis.

Figure 3. (A) Cross-sectional ultrasonographic appearance of a normal suspensory branch (*arrows*). (B) Cross-sectional ultrasonographic appearance of the medial branch of the suspensory ligament demonstrating a grade 3 lesion.

pensory insertion into the sesamoid bones may result in periarticular edema and pain on fetlock flexion. Cytology of the joint fluid may show traumatic inflammation. However, intra-articular fetlock joint anesthesia will not relieve the lameness. Radiographs should be obtained to assess the integrity of the sesamoid and splint bones. Ultrasound examination of the suspensory ligament is the most useful technique to assess the presence and severity of suspensory damage and provides a basis for monitoring healing. A 7.5-MHz scan head without a standoff is used. Imaging of the entire suspensory ligament should be done. The origin of the suspensory ligament, the junction of the body and branches, and the suspensory insertion into the proximal sesamoid bones are more difficult locations to image. Accurate assessment of the injury entails measurement of the area of affected suspensory ligament in cross-section, length of damaged fibers and axial fiber alignment in longitudinal section, grading of the lesion's severity, and description of the lesion location (Fig. 3). Lesions are graded on a scale of 1 to 4: type 1 lesions are mostly echogenic; type 2 lesions are half echogenic and half anechoic; type 3 lesions are

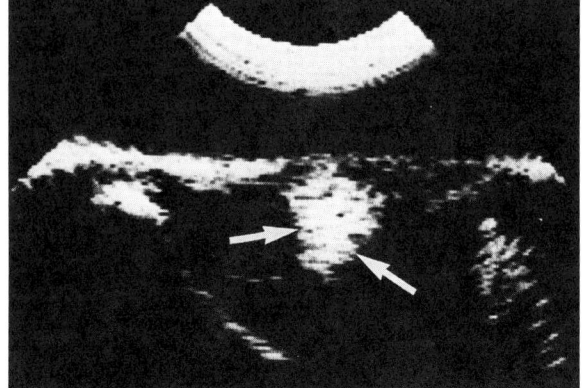

A

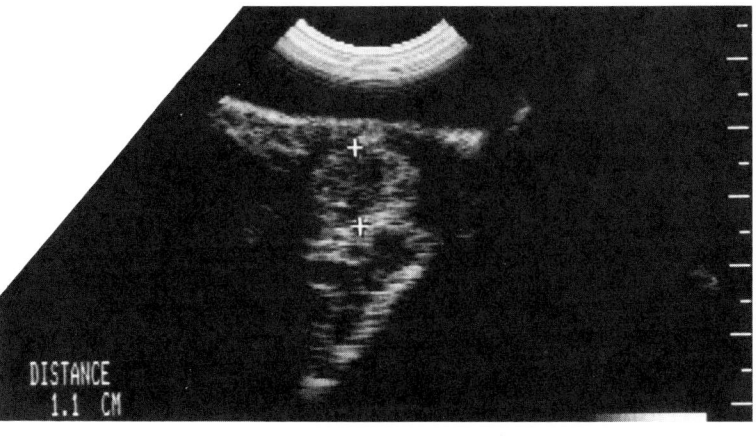

B

mostly anechoic; type 4 lesions are totally anechoic and represent the most pathologic state.

Therapy

The initial goal of therapy is to decrease the inflammatory reaction. Systemic anti-inflammatory agents such as phenylbutazone and or flunixin meglumine may be used. Local therapy may include ice packs and bandaging. If traumatic disruption of the suspensory apparatus is present, resulting in loss of support of the fetlock joint, it is essential to provide weight-bearing support to prevent stretching and thrombosis of the palmar arteries. Damage to these structures may result in temporary loss of blood supply to the hoof, with possible loss of the hoof wall. Fetlock joint support may be provided by means of a board splint or a Kimsey apparatus. Surgical therapy of suspensory desmitis includes ligament splitting and removal of the distal segment of fractured splints in selected cases. Ligament splitting has been used with success when a core lesion can be demonstrated in the body of the suspensory ligament, and may help vascularize the damaged area. In horses with distal splint fractures, surgical removal is suggested if the suspensory ligament injury is resolving with therapy and is not expected to severely limit the horse's performance. If severe damage had resulted in loss of fetlock joint support, long-term splinting (6 to 8 months), until scar tissue is strong enough to support the fetlock, has been used. Alternatively, fetlock joint arthrodesis has been used successfully. Laminitis of the opposing limb is a frequent complication in these cases, so functional weight-bearing should be provided as soon as possible.

In all cases, ultrasonographic reevaluation is an important aspect of therapy, as it provides an informed measurement of the degree and quality of healing prior to return to exercise. Resolution of lameness and improved external appearance of the suspensory ligament may give a false impression of adequate healing. Early return to work will often result in recurrence of the injury, often with additional damage.

Supplemental Readings

Bramlage, L., Gabel, A., and Hackett, R.: Avulsion fractures of the origin of the suspensory ligament in the horse. J. Am. Vet. Med. Assoc., 176:1004, 1980.
Ford, T. S., Ross, M. W., and Orsini, P. G.: A comparison of methods for proximal palmar metacarpal analgesia in horses. Vet. Surg., 18:146, 1989.
Genovese, R., Rantanen, R., Hauser, M., and Simpson, B.: Diagnostic ultrasonography of equine limbs. Vet. Clin. North Am. (Equine Pract.), 1:145, 1986.
Genovese, R. L., Rantanen, N. W., and Sherman, S. B.: The use of ultrasonography in the diagnosis and management of injuries to the equine limb. Compend. Cont. Ed. Pract. Vet., 9:945, 1987.
Hardy, J., Marcoux, M., and Breton, L.: Clinical significance of radiographic findings in the proximal sesamoid bones of two year old Standardbreds in training. J. Am. Vet. Med. Assoc. (in press).
O'Brien, T., Morgan, J., Wheat, J., and Suter, P.: Sesamoiditis in the Thoroughbred: A radiographic study. J. Am. Vet. Radiol. Soc. 12:75, 1971.
Ross, M., Ford, T., and Orsini, P.: Incomplete longitudinal fracture of the proximal palmar cortex of the third metacarpal bone in horses. Vet. Surg., 17:82, 1988.

Dorsal Metacarpal Disease

Susan M. Stover, DAVIS, CALIFORNIA

Dorsal metacarpal disease occurs in young horses galloping at racing speeds. The disease encompasses two disorders of the dorsal cortex of the third metacarpal bone, "bucked shins" and stress fractures. Bucked shins is an inflammation of the dorsal cortex. Stress fractures are incomplete fractures of the dorsal cortex.

BUCKED SHINS

Characteristically, bucked shins occur after a horse has first galloped several times at racing speeds, usually during the first year of race training. During this time the third metacarpal bones are subjected to a new and different pattern of loading than experienced earlier during training at the trot and slow gallop. These increased cyclical loads on the dorsal cortex result in inflammation. The ensuing deposition of new bone on the affected periosteal cortical surface results in a thickening of the dorsal cortex. When this adaptive process is completed, the third metacarpal bone is resistant to further damage and inflammation during subsequent training and racing.

DIAGNOSIS

At least 70 per cent of young horses in race training incur bucked shins. Thus, the disease should be suspected when horses exhibit decreased performance or forelimb lameness after they have begun to gallop at racing speeds. Most horses are affected bilaterally and consequently are unwilling to work at speed, but occasionally there is a distinct unilateral lameness. Bucked shins primarily affects the middle third of the dorsal cortex of the third metacarpal bone. The diagnosis is based on elicitation of a painful response to palpation of the dorsal and dorsomedial surfaces of the third metacarpal bones. Palpation should be performed with the limb bearing weight by quickly running the side of a finger over the dorsal and dorsomedial surfaces of the third metacarpal bone from proximal to distal with mild pressure, and then with the limb elevated by sequentially applying firm pressure with the fingertips to discrete regions to assess the entire dorsal and dorsomedial surfaces. Visible and palpable evidence of edema and inflammation of the overlying soft tissues is often detected, but the appearance of these signs may be delayed for up to 7 to 10 days following the first evidence of metacarpal pain. Initial signs are often diffuse, with localization of edema and harder soft tissue swelling occurring after 1 week following onset of the disease.

In the early stages of inflammation no abnormalities are observed on radiographs. High-quality radiographs or xeroradiographs may allow detection of active periosteal bony proliferation or subperiosteal cortical lucencies in the first weeks of the disease. Radiographs are also useful for eliminating other possible diagnoses, including incomplete stress fracture. Bone scintigraphy is a sensitive method for detecting metacarpal inflammation but is rarely necessary for the diagnosis of bucked shins in practice. Increased radiopharmaceutical uptake is apparent in a diffuse region of the midportion of the dorsal metacarpal cortex.

THERAPY

The dorsal cortex of the third metacarpi must be stimulated to thicken sufficiently so that the horse will no longer be susceptible to recurrence of bucked shins. Therefore, the ideal treatment includes continued training to stimulate adaptation of the dorsal cortex. However, the feasibility of continued training depends on the severity of disease and the degree of associated pain. In general, training can be continued in horses with mild to moderate pain that resolves after 2 to 4 days of rest. The intensity of training should be lessened—to trotting, for example—to prevent severe damage to the cortex, and then gradually intensified as resolution of the disorder allows. Horses that remain in moderate to severe pain after 1 week of rest usually need to be withdrawn from training for up to 3 months.

A multitude of adjunctive therapies such as icing, blistering, and pin firing are employed in the treatment of bucked shins. However, exercise modification and rest are considered the most beneficial therapies. Anti-inflammatory medication and physical therapy may allow continuation of a modified training program, as well as aid in the alleviation of pain and lessening of inflammation.

PROGNOSIS

Bucked shins delays the training of most horses. However, disease resolution is usually complete and the prognosis for return to training and racing is good. Bucked shins may recur in horses with severe disease that were not rested sufficiently prior to return to training, and in horses that were not trained adequately to stimulate adaptation of the third metacarpal bones for sustaining the stresses of racing.

PREVENTION

Traditionally, racing horses in the United States have been trained by a regimen that conditions horses with several months of trotting and slow galloping before galloping at racing speeds. A method that promotes adaptation of the third metacarpal bone and results in a thickened dorsomedial cortex earlier in the training regimen should enhance the resistance of this bone to bucked shins. Evidence suggests that horses must attain racing speeds in order to stimulate bone formation in the required dorsomedial location. Therefore, it has been hypothesized that beginning fast gallops over a short distance several times a week earlier in the training period will promote appropriate adaptation of the dorsal cortex and may reduce the incidence of bucked shins.

STRESS FRACTURES

Stress fractures of the third metacarpal bone are incomplete cortical fractures that most frequently occur in 3- and 4-year-old racing horses (i.e., later in the career of racing horses than bucked shins). Although stress fractures may occur in the same location on the third metacarpal bone as bucked shins, an association between bucked shins and stress fractures has not been clearly demonstrated.

Fractures characteristically occur in the middle or distal portions of the dorsal or dorsolateral aspects of the third metacarpal cortex. Most fractures course obliquely from the periosteal surface in a proximopalmar direction toward the endosteal surface of the dorsal cortex, but are rarely seen on radiographs to penetrate to the endosteal surface. Although fractures are most commonly unilateral and single, multiple fractures and bilateral fractures are occasionally found.

Stress fractures are also known as fatigue fractures because they are thought to result from the accretion of cortical microdamage incurred over months of repetitive metacarpal loading during training and racing. A fracture results when the accumulation of microdamage exceeds resolution by normal repair mechanisms.

Diagnosis

In contrast to horses with bucked shins, horses with a stress fracture usually exhibit a distinct forelimb lameness. Pain can usually be elicited from a discrete location by careful palpation of the third metacarpal dorsal cortex. With chronicity, a distinct firm enlargement, 2 to 3 cm in diameter, often overlies the fracture site.

Although radiographs are useful for the identification of incomplete cortical fractures, not all fractures can be observed on radiographs. Multiple oblique projections of the dorsal cortex may be necessary to highlight the fracture line. Xeroradiography may enhance the fracture line. Focal periosteal or endosteal bony proliferations often accompany a chronic incomplete cortical fracture and may be diagnostic for a fracture despite an inability to detect a fracture line on radiographs. Because periosteal and endosteal bony proliferation may persist for an indefinite time following resolution of a fracture, it may be necessary to perform a regional anesthetic block to determine the clinical significance of these radiographic abnormalities.

Bone scintigraphy is useful for the identification of acute fractures that are not visible on radiographs. A focal area of intense radiopharmaceutical uptake is considered diagnostic for a fracture. Scintigraphy may be indicated in horses with persistent fractures to help distinguish delayed or nonunion fractures from healing fractures. Delayed or nonunion fractures are associated with lesser degrees of radiopharmaceutical uptake than a healing fracture.

Therapy

Conservative and surgical therapies have been successfully used in the treatment of incomplete cortical fractures. Because conservative therapy necessitates a delay of several months in a horse's career and some fractures do not heal with conservative therapy, the practitioner is confronted with the dilemma of deciding whether to recommend conservative or surgical therapy at the initial time of diagnosis. Although surgical treatment has attendant anesthetic, surgical, and anesthetic recovery risks, economic and race scheduling pressures often dictate that initial treatment be surgical.

The majority of acute incomplete cortical fractures will heal with rest. Horses with these fractures should be removed from training and re-evaluated clinically and radiographically after 3 months. If the fracture is no longer evident radiographically, the horse is gradually returned to training. If the fracture line is less distinct, additional rest should be considered. If the fracture line is unchanged and the surrounding tissues are quiescent, a light exercise program of walking, trotting, or swimming is instituted in an attempt to stimulate fracture repair. If this regimen is unsuccessful after 2 to 3 months, surgical therapy is considered. Chronic fractures that result from continued training on a stress fracture are most refractory to conservative treatment and initial surgical therapy is recommended.

Interfragmentary drilling (osteostixis) has largely supplanted lag screw fixation for the surgical treatment of incomplete cortical fractures. Several holes are drilled transversely through the fracture line and into the medullary cavity. This procedure is believed to stimulate healing by (1) providing access for medullary vascular and mesenchymal elements necessary for repair to the fracture site, and (2) stimulating repair through controlled surgical trauma. At least 3 to 5 months of rest is required following surgical therapy before horses are returned to training. Clinical and radiographic reevaluation should be performed prior to recommending return to training.

Prognosis

The majority of acute stress fractures respond to rest alone. Unfortunately, it is difficult to predict which fractures will not respond to conservative treatment. Mild controlled exercise is beneficial for many horses with fractures refractory to rest alone. A good prognosis for repair and return to racing is also obtained with surgical treatment. The mean time for return to a race following osteostixis is reported to be approximately 9 months. Recurrence of fracture may occur following conservative and surgical treatments.

Supplemental Readings

Nunamaker, D. M.: Stress fractures of the third metacarpal bone. *In* White N. A. II, and Moore, J. N. (eds.): Current Practice of Equine Surgery. Philadelphia, J. B. Lippincott Co., 1990, pp. 622–626.

Specht, T. E., and Colahan, P. T.: Osteostixis for incomplete cortical fracture of the third metacarpal bone: Results in 11 horses. Vet. Surg., 19:34, 1990.

Medical Treatment of Tendinitis

Lawrence R. Bramlage, LEXINGTON, KENTUCKY

Tendinitis is one of the most frustrating musculoskeletal diseases to treat. The per centage of affected horses that return to previous level of performance is low. A rational approach to therapy, however, may make the difference between success and failure. The prognosis is poorer for maximal effort activities such as racing than for less demanding activities such as pleasure riding. The prognosis varies for different tendons and limbs. Because extensor tendons are able to heal from nearly any injury, treatment will not be discussed in this chapter. Hind limb flexor tendon injuries carry a more favorable prognosis than forelimb tendon injuries, and the deep digital flexor tendon tolerates injury better than the superficial digital flexor tendon. Injury to the superficial digital flexor tendon of the forelimb carries the worst prognosis for return to unimpaired function.

CLINICAL SIGNS AND DIAGNOSIS

Inflammation indicates damage, and therefore any heat, swelling, or pain on palpation of the tendons should be noted and followed for progression. Although persistence or recurrence of inflammation are key indicators of tendon damage, the amount of inflammation is not always a measure of the amount of tendon damage. The swelling may subside with therapy and tendon damage may still be present. If inflammation recurs or persists after the initial episode, diagnostic ultrasound examination is warranted to establish the degree of damage. It is as important to know when there is no injury as it is to know when the tendon is injured. Ultrasound examination aids in the determination of the presence and progression of an injury to a tendon. It may not be necessary for making a diagnosis of tendonitis, but it is important in defining the lesion and, therefore, in selection of treatment.

The goal in the medical treatment of tendinitis is to keep the inflammatory response to the minimum necessary to repair the injury, and to prevent it from affecting the remaining normal tendon. The inflammatory response results in edema and subsequently fibrous tissue deposition, which is detrimental to the elastic function of tendon. Fibrous tissue deposition is, however, the only means of repair available in the adult, and therefore necessary for healing. The therapeutic goal is to allow repair to proceed, but to modulate the response, and not let it become excessive and inflame the adjacent normal tendon.

THERAPY

ACUTE STAGE (0 to 48 hours)

The goal in the acutely injured tendon is to control the inflammatory response.

Physical Therapy

Ice is an effective inhibitor of inflammation. It constricts blood vessels, slows hemorrhage, reduces the amount of inflammatory mediators released into the injured tissue, slows the activity of the mediators of inflammation, and reduces the perception of pain. Cold application should be in 30-minute to 1-hour sessions at least three to four times a day.

Bandaging provides counter pressure against tissue swelling. Constant, firm, uniform pressure will keep tissue planes collapsed and reduce the quantity of tissue fluid that escapes from the vascular system into the tissues. Fluid within the tendon will lead to fibrosis and is not desirable.

Rest is essential during the 48-hour acute inflammatory phase of injury, because exercise may worsen the injury. In most instances, shoes should be removed. Since the superficial digital flexor tendon, which attaches to the pastern area, is most often injured, the heel should be lowered to straighten the fetlock angle and decrease the excursion of the superficial digital flexor tendon. It should not be elevated.

Pharmacologic Therapy

Nonsteroidal anti-inflammatory drugs (NSAIDs) are always indicated as part of the initial treatment of tendon inflammation. Interruption of the prostaglandin cascade, initiated by tissue injury, controls the inflammatory process. Flunixin meglumine (1.1 mg per kg) should be included in the initial treatment regimen because of its rapid onset of activity. Phenylbutazone (4.4 to 8.8 mg per kg) is preferable for long-term maintenance, owing to its longer half-life. Both drugs are often given simultaneously initially to get the fastest and most complete therapy. Other NSAIDs are available. Their use is a matter of personal preference and appropriate pharmacologic application.

Corticosteroids provide the most powerful anti-inflammatory therapy; however, they also have the undesirable effect of delaying healing and reducing repair strength for up to 1 year after administration. Some long-acting corticosteroids may also contribute to soft tissue calcification. Long-acting corticosteroid therapy is undesirable, but the use of an ultra-short-acting corticosteroid during the acute inflammatory phase can stop the inflammatory process and protect the remaining normal tissue. However, because there are other, safer means of accomplishing the same end, corticosteroids should be avoided in most instances.

Dimethyl sulfoxide (DMSO) is of benefit in the treatment of acute tendon inflammation. It is a free radical scavenger and may therefore prevent some of the detrimental effects of inflammation. Clinically, however, tendon inflammation is often discovered after free radicals would have been released in greatest amounts. The generally recommended systemic anti-inflammatory dose of DMSO is 2.2 mg per kg given intravenously (IV) and diluted in large volumes of fluid, although as little as 0.5 mg per kg given IV or orally by stomach tube has been described as being useful. There are few instances in which DMSO would be detrimental in the treatment of acute tendinitis.

Hyaluronic acid deposited around the tendon at the site of inflammation has proved beneficial in the treatment of tendon injuries in human hands. The goal is to prevent adhesions and maintain gliding function to preserve fine motor activity. Although adhesions are of concern in the horse, the main goal is to preserve weight-bearing function. Therefore, hyaluronic acid therapy must be weighed as to its cost-benefit ratio in the treatment of flexor tendon injuries in the horse. Injuries to tendons within tendon sheaths may benefit from hyaluronic acid administration into the tendon sheath to preserve the lubrication function of the sheath around the tendon and to prevent the development of adhesions between the sheath and tendon. The recommended dose of hyaluronic acid varies from 20 to 120 mg per treatment. The necessary minimum dose for efficacious coating of a digital tendon sheath probably is near the low end of this range, and the expense of treatment encourages a low dose.

Polysulfated glycosaminoglycans (PSGAGS) may have some use in the early treatment of tendon inflammation. They must be administered into the lesion to be effective. The efficacy of PSGAG remains speculative. Scientific documentation and the test of time are necessary.

Surgical Therapy

Surgical treatment is not recommended during the 48-hour acute inflammatory phase.

Monitoring

Monitoring the success of treatment in the first 48 hours of tendinitis is by physical examination. The goal is to arrest the progression of the disease.

SUBACUTE STAGE (2 to 21 days)

The goals of treatment in the subacute stage are to prevent the spread of inflammation into normal tendon, to reverse the acute inflammation to minimize permanent damage to the injured tendon, and to initiate the repair process for an orderly and functional reestablishment of the flexor tendon. In the subacute stage, fibrous tissue deposition necessary for repair begins and must be confined to the areas needing repair. Since coagulated tissue fluids and fibrin form the scaffold for fibrosis, the rapid removal of tissue fluids from tendon adjacent to the injury minimizes fibrosis in the normal tissue.

The signs of subacute tendinitis include heat, pain on tendon palpation, swelling, and, depending on the degree of damage, possibly lameness. Three courses of treatment are available: (1) removal from training and rest for an extended period to allow natural repair, (2) disregarding the inflammation, providing symptomatic treatment, and allowing continuation of exercise, or (3) accurate assessment of the damage with ultrasound examination and initiation of appropriate treatment.

Physical Therapy

Cold therapy should be alternated with warm temperatures for 4 to 6 days to help in removal of tissue fluid. Warm intervals should be three times as long as cold intervals, and the cycle can be repeated as many times as possible each day until the desired result is obtained. Four to 6 days after injury, fibroproliferation begins and fluid removal is no longer easily accomplished. Cold therapy can be stopped and warm temperatures are used to improve circulation and speed repair. Prolonged warm temperatures can be achieved by stimulating circulation through the use of topical medications, such as rubrifacients, and the use of an occlusive bandage (a "sweat bandage"). Pressure bandaging is useful to counteract swelling.

Hydromassage is a beneficial treatment that entails use of pressurized water from a hose, a "turbolator boot," a water treadmill, or a whirlpool. The water massages the injured tissue, aids in removal of stagnant tissue fluids, and speeds repair.

Exercise must be limited until tissue fluid accumulation is halted. At that point, unless complete structural integrity is lost, controlled mild exercise such as walking can begin, but free exercise is not advised. Mild, noninjuring exercise stimulates tissue fluid movement from areas of poor perfusion and stimulates improved perfusion throughout the entire tendon.

Pharmacologic Therapy

Nonsteroidal anti-inflammatory drugs should be continued through this stage. Corticosteroids are contraindicated, because their anti-inflammatory properties prevent repair. Topical DMSO can be applied until the tissue fluid has been evacuated. Once the fibroproliferative phase begins, DMSO should be discontinued, because it has a detrimental effect on the amount and quality of collagen formation within a scar. Hyaluronic acid therapy in the subacute period requires the same considerations as in the acute inflammation period. PSGAG therapy needs to be administered early in the acute phase to neutralize the damaging enzymes. Methysulfmethoxine has anti-inflammatory properties and may be a very rich source of available sulfur for tissue repair. The recommended dosage for treatment of injured tendons is 1 to 2 oz of methysulfmethoxine-containing feed supplement daily.

Surgical Treatment

Surgeries undertaken during the subacute phase include tendon transplantation, carbon fiber tow implantation and fragment injection, tendon splitting, and superior check ligament desmotomy. None is universally accepted as the treatment of choice. I prefer superior check ligament desmotomy and tendon splitting in selected cases.

Monitoring

Monitoring the response to treatment is primarily by observation of the clinical signs and repeat ultrasound evaluations. Surgical intervention alters the expected course of healing and appearance of the tendon.

REMODELING STAGE (21 to 60 days)

During this stage, treatment guides the repair process and produces a functional tendon or tendon substitute. Repair mechanisms should have started in the vascularized areas of the injured tendon. Medical or surgical steps should have been taken in the subacute period to ensure that the injured area of tendon revascularizes as completely as possible. During the remodeling stage, fibroblasts remodel and replace collagen according to the needs dictated by the local biomechanical forces. The fibroblasts produce as much collagen as is needed, and therefore as much scar as is necessary to accommodate the load on the tissues. It is difficult, however, for the fibroblasts to reproduce the elasticity of the stroma necessary for the repairing tendon to function as the original tissue.

Physical Therapy

Temperature-altering methods of therapy lose their efficacy during this healing period. Small recurrences of inflammation can and should accompany proper aggressive rehabilitation programs. Electronic aids, such as electromagnetic fields, direct electrical stimulation, and many others, have been advocated to assist tendon remodeling. Their benefit is questionable and their use may be detrimental, so it is recommended that they be avoided. Therapeutic laser treatment is losing popularity. Anecdotal success has been derived from treatment with "cold" lasers. The ability of the cold laser to penetrate to the tendon is questionable, though evidence does not indicate any detrimental effect of laser treatment.

Irritants were formerly used in this stage of healing in draft horses. These beasts of burden needed strong tendons, and therefore the production of fibrous tissue was encouraged. In the performance horse, however, preservation of a functional tendon is a more desirable end. Firing has been used in varying patterns to reinforce the injured tendon. Though still used in certain locales, firing has lost its popularity. Blistering as a means of stimulating an increased circulation makes sense theoretically and has been used for years. Stimulating remodeling, without the danger of stimulating more fibrosis, is the goal. Mild rubrifacients are safer than aggressive counterirritants. Any topical medication that is injurious to normal tissues is too strong to be useful in minimizing permanent tendon damage. Only mild circulatory stimulants are indicated. Injectable irritants carry the danger of stimulating an increase in unwanted fibrosis.

Bandaging in this phase is not likely to alter the size or character of the healing area. If inflammation reappears, bandaging should be used.

Controlled exercise is indicated during the remodeling stage. If exercise is excessive, fibrous tissue is produced rather than remodeled. If no stress is applied during the remodeling phase, the end result may resemble a tendon more adapted to pasture exercise than performance. The exercise regimen is an art and must be done according to the individual patient's needs. It is assumed that, like other tissues, tendon scars reach one half of their eventual strength in 6 to 8 weeks. Therefore, only very light exercise should be allowed for this stage. At 60 days, gradually increasing loads should be applied. Exercise aids such as underwater treadmills can assist in this process by requiring work against resistance and some weight-bearing while still avoiding strenuous loading. Swimming produces no weight-bearing load on the injured tendon and therefore does not create work-specific remodeling. This disadvantage can be overcome by combining some form of weight-bearing exercise in addition to or alternating with swimming. In most instances, however, special facilities are not available and are unnecessary. Four weeks of walking followed by 2 to 4 weeks of pasture exercise and then 4 weeks of jogging during or after the pasture exercise is a good start. Jogging keeps the rear quarter weight on the rear limbs and therefore lightly loads the tendon, stimulating remodeling but staying below the reinjury threshold.

There are sources of minor inflammation that must be overcome in the rehabilitation of a tendon. As a tendon is stretched after healing, adhesions must be stretched and in some instances torn in order to reestablish a full range of motion. Small sites of inflammation within the tendon, which may then spread to other parts of the tendon, appear and can recreate tendinitis. This problem can be overcome with careful retraining. Recognition of the minor inflammation caused by the breakdown of intratendinous and peritendinous adhesions and curtailment of strenous exercise until the inflammation subsides (generally a matter of days) eliminates the danger created by breaking down the adhesions and prevents the spread of inflammation into the recovering tendon. Adhesion problems are most likely to occur at each major increase in exercise level, for example, from trotting to galloping and from training to racing.

Supplemental Readings

Bramlage, L. R.: Superior check ligament desmotomy as a treatment for superficial digital flexor tendinitis: initial report. Proc. 32nd Ann. Conv. Am. Assoc. Equine Pract., 1986, pp. 365–370.

McIlwraith, C. W.: Diseases of joints, tendons, ligaments, and related structures. Adams' Lameness in Horses, 4th Ed. Philadelphia, Lea & Febinger, 1987, p. 447.

Navicular Syndrome

Tracy A. Turner, ROCHESTER, NEW HAMPSHIRE

Navicular syndrome is a complex of diseases or injuries involving the caudal aspect of the horse's foot. The pathogenesis of navicular syndrome is not known but is likely multifactorial, involving the navicular bone, its suspending ligaments, its blood supply, the coffin joint, navicular bursa, and deep digital flexor tendon. Navicular syndrome is the most common cause of chronic forelimb lameness in the horse.

The prevalence of navicular syndrome is highest among performance horses. Although the syndrome affects all types of equine athletes, there is a breed predisposition. Quarter horses, Thoroughbreds, and warmbloods have a higher frequency of navicular syndrome than other breeds. Navicular syndrome is most commonly diagnosed in horses 7 to 14 years old. Horses less than 3 or older than 15 years are three to five times less likely to develop navicular syndrome.

Hoof abnormalities predispose to the development of navicular syndrome. Broken hoof axis, underrun heels, shear heels, contracted heels, mismatched hoof angles, and small feet have been associated with the lameness. Each of these imbalances concentrates stress in the foot, particularly stress to the caudal aspect of the foot.

CLINICAL SIGNS AND DIAGNOSIS

The diagnosis of navicular syndrome is based on history and clinical signs. Historically, the lameness is characterized as chronic and intermittent in nature but it may be seen in its acute stages. Lameness is usually more noticeable after heavy work and improves with rest. Working the horse on a rough or hard surface and turning it in tight circles will exacerbate the lameness.

The diagnosis of navicular syndrome can be divided into gait changes, response to diagnostic tests, and response to local anesthesia. Navicular syndrome is usually characterized by a bilateral forelimb lameness. The horse tends to land on its toe, making its gait short and choppy. The lameness is accentuated by lunging at the trot. The inside limb is usually more lame than the outside limb. Lameness may be imperceptible on the straight because of the bilateral nature of the syndrome.

Diagnostic tests for navicular disease include hoof tester examination, wedge test, and flexion tests. Pain caused by application of hoof testers from the central sulcus to toe, from the collateral sulci to the contralateral hoof wall, and across the heels is consistent with navicular syndrome. The response should be consistent and uniform if it is due to navicular syndrome. Careful examination of the remaining portion of the foot with hoof testers must be made and evaluated relative to the pain in the navicular area. This is to make sure the pain elicited from the navicular area is not from another area of the foot. A negative response to hoof testers is still compatible with navicular syndrome.

Two types of wedge tests may aid in the diagnosis of navicular syndrome. In the hyperextension test, the horse's foot is placed on one end of a board and the opposite end of the board is raised (Fig. 1). This maneuver increases tension on the deep flexor tendon and navicular sup-

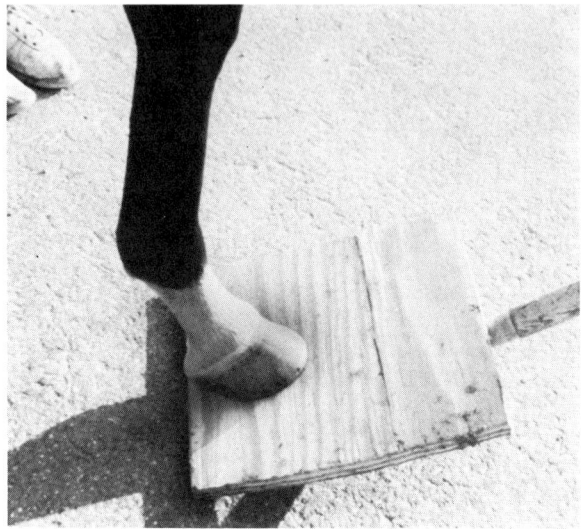

Figure 1. Hyperextension test for the diagnosis of navicular syndrome. Gradually elevating the board increases the tension on the deep digital flexor tendon and the navicular suspensory ligament. A positive response is indicated by the horse jumping off the board or by an exacerbation of lameness.

porting mechanism. A positive response is recorded if the horse jumps off the board or if the lameness is exacerbated when the horse is trotted off. The frog pressure test is performed by placing a block of wood directly under the caudal two thirds of the frog (Fig. 2). The opposite limb is held off the ground, forcing the horse to stand on the block. The wood exerts pressure directly on the navicular bone, bursa, and deep flexor tendon. A positive response is characterized by exacerbation of the lameness when the

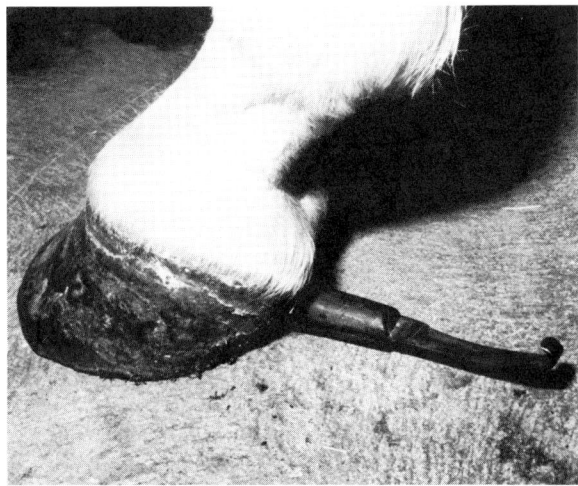

Figure 2. Frog pressure test for the diagnosis of navicular syndrome. The test places pressure on the middle and caudal thirds of the frog. An exacerbation of lameness denotes a positive result.

horse is trotted. Although positive responses to these tests are consistent with navicular syndrome and provide valuable information as to the possible sources of pain, negative responses do not rule out navicular syndrome.

Distal limb flexion, flexion of the metacarpophalangeal and proximal and distal interphalangeal joints, also provides useful additional information regarding navicular syndrome. A positive response is noted if the lameness is exacerbated when the horse is trotted after flexion. Because a positive response could be expected for many conditions involving the distal limb, this test is not pathognomonic for navicular syndrome. This test must be evaluated relative to the horse's response to regional anesthesia.

Regional anesthesia is invaluable in determining the location of lameness. The horse with navicular syndrome should improve at least 90 per cent following medial and lateral palmar digital nerve block. Horses with other lamenesses secondary to navicular syndrome, such as pedal osteitis and suspensory desmitis, are important exceptions. In addition to palmar digital nerve blocks, findings on distal interphalangeal and navicular bursa anesthesia add useful information relative to the diagnosis. These must be performed either prior to palmar digital anesthesia or after sensation has returned to the foot. Distal interphalangeal anesthesia should alleviate pain associated with conditions involving the distal interphalangeal joint cavity, including the areas of the navicular bone in communication with the joint. Anatomical studies indicate that such areas do not include the navicular bursa. Navicular bursa anesthesia could be expected to desensitize structures in direct contact with the bursa, but complete block of sensation in those structures may not be achieved.

Once the clinical diagnosis of navicular syndrome is made, imaging of the bone and adjacent structures should be performed. Imaging information suggests the possible cause of pain and therefore will aid in the selection of treatment. Radionuclide scintigraphy, thermography, and radiography each provide valuable information regarding the presence of navicular syndrome. Scintigraphy provides information regarding rate of bone turnover, and thermography provides information regarding the circulation to the navicular area. However, scintigraphy and thermography are not techniques available to the average practitioner. Radiography remains the best means of assessing changes in the navicular bone.

There are five radiographic changes associated with navicular syndrome: marginal osteophytes, bone remodeling, enlarged synovial fossae, cysts, and flexor cortex changes (Fig. 3). Although none of these changes is pathognomonic, all provide insight into the possible inciting injury. Three radiographic projections are needed to completely assess the navicular bone: a 60-degree dorsopalmar (DP) projection, lateral projections, and palmaroproximal palmarodistal (PP-PD) projections. The DP projections provide the most useful information regarding the presence of marginal osteophyte formation, remodeling of the proximal and distal borders of the navicular bone, cyst formation, and enlarged synovial fossae. The PP-PD view is most useful for evaluating the flexor cortex. A lateral view is helpful in confirming the presence of any of these changes.

Marginal osteophyte formation ("spurs") is calcification of the abaxial collateral sesamoidean ligaments along the wings of the navicular bone; remodeling is calcification of either the axial portions of the collateral sesamoidean ligament or the impar ligament. Occasionally, changes along the impar ligament may be seen as chip fractures. Radiographic demonstration of these changes may indicate a primary injury to one of the ligaments of the navicular bone. Enlarged synovial fossae ("lollipops") may indicate an inflammatory process in the distal interphalangeal joint. The presence of cysts tends to indicate a primary navicular bone lesion, and flexor changes may indicate an injury to the deep flexor tendon.

THERAPY

Treatments for navicular syndrome are varied but can be divided into three categories: shoeing, medicinal, and surgical. Shoeing for navicular syndrome has been approached from three methods. The classic method is to raise the heels of the shoe or foot and roll the toe. This is thought to reduce strain on the deep flexor tendon. The second method is to use an egg bar shoe to increase caudal support and help stabilize the foot. This approach has not met with uniform success. The most successful type of shoeing is to approach each case individually. The first goal of shoeing is to correct any preexisting hoof problems. Hoof problems such as broken-hoof axis, underrun heels, shear heels, contracted heels, and small feet are common problems associated with navicular syndrome and must be corrected. The second goal is to enhance the normal physiologic functions of the foot. These functions are to bear weight and absorb concussion. All weight-bearing structures of the foot (hoof wall, bars, frog) should be utilized. The shoe should

152 / NAVICULAR SYNDROME—continued

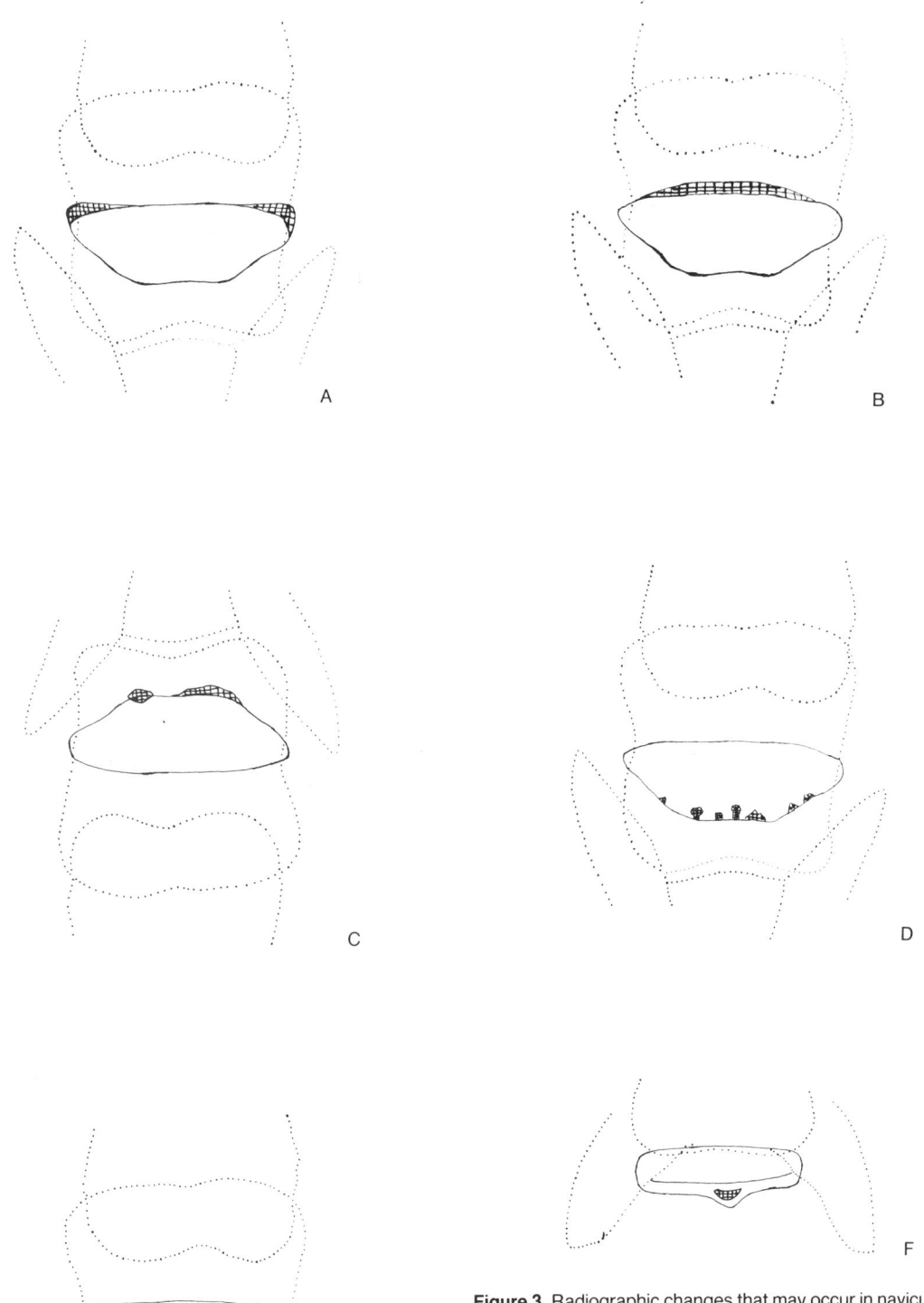

Figure 3. Radiographic changes that may occur in navicular syndrome. (*A*) Marginal osteophyte formation, spur formation, calcification of the margins of the navicular suspensory ligament. (*B*) Bone remodeling change consisting of calcification of the central portions of the navicular suspensory ligament. (*C*) Bone remodeling change consisting of calcification of the impar ligament. Remodeling along the impar ligament may also appear as a chip fracture. (*D*) Enlarged synovial fossae. Variations include the classic "lollipop" appearance or pyramid along the wings, or coalesced pyramids along the distal border. (*E*) Navicular cyst-like lesion. (*F*) Flexor cortical lesions, which usually occur along the median ridge.

be fitted full, that is, fitted so that it is larger than the hoof, thus allowing for hoof expansion. Along those same lines, it is important to maintain an adequate cup in the sole. This is absolutely necessary if the hoof is to expand. Two other aids to hoof expansion are placement of nails forward to the bend in the quarters and slippering the heels of the pad or shoe. Ease of breakover through the use of a roller, square, or rocker toe should help the foot travel better and therefore improve function. This may also reduce some strain on the caudal hoof.

Medicinal therapy involves anti-inflammatory, analgesic drugs and vasoactive drugs. The use of anti-inflammatory, analgesic drugs such as phenylbutazone is the most common treatment. The analgesic effect can be extremely useful when managing navicular syndrome, not only by reducing pain but also by allowing the horse to use its foot more normally, thereby promoting the beneficial effect of the shoeing. These drugs may also aid circulation via antiplatelet activity. The importance of this fact has not yet been investigated with regard to navicular syndrome.

Vasoactive drugs are the newest innovation in medicinal therapy. Warfarin and isoxsuprine hydrochloride were the first two drugs suggested as treatment for navicular syndrome. Warfarin is administered to slow thrombosis. Before administration of warfarin begins, the horse's one-stage prothrombin time must be measured. Dosage begins at 0.018 mg per kg per day and may be increased by 20 per cent weekly until the one-stage prothrombin time is increased by 2 to 4 seconds. The efficacy of this therapy has been reported to be between 40 and 80 per cent. A serious disadvantage of this treatment is hemorrhage, which can occur almost anywhere. Also, warfarin interacts with protein-bound drugs (Table 1). This interaction can lead to increased plasma concentrations of warfarin and fatal hemorrhage. Vitamin K_1 should always be readily available when this drug is used. Because of these problems this treatment has not found wide acceptance.

Isoxsuprine hydrochloride has been reported to increase distal limb circulation. Effective doses range between 0.6 and 1.8 mg per kg administered orally (PO). Initially, the drug should be administered at 0.6 mg per kg twice daily until the horse becomes sound. If soundness is not reached within 2 weeks, the dosage is increased to 1.2 mg per kg. The dosage can be increased to as high as 1.8 mg per kg if soundness is not reached within an additional 2 weeks. Once the horse has been sound for 2 weeks, the dosage interval can be reduced to a daily dosage. Long-term efficacy has varied between 40 and 87 per cent. Disadvantages of this treatment are that isoxsuprine is considered a forbidden substance by the American Horse Shows Association and that vascular resistance does not change at these dose levels.

Two new drugs that may be used more in the future are metrenperone and pentoxyllin. Mentrenperone is a serotonin antagonist and reduces the vascular contractile response to serotonin. Experimental dosages are 0.1 mg per kg PO twice daily. The efficacy of the drug has been reported to be similar to that of isoxsuprine hydrochloride. Pentoxylline increases red blood cell deformability and reduces the risk of thrombosis. The clinical dose that has been used is 7 mg per kg per day PO. The efficacy of this drug has not been reported. One disadvantage of medicinal therapy is that most equine associations and competitive groups regulate medication. It is imperative that the veterinarian be familiar with these rules prior to prescribing medication.

If shoeing and medication fail to control the lameness, there are surgical alternatives. One procedure, the collateral sesamoidean desmotomy, has recently shown promise. Initial studies indicated 70 per cent efficacy. However, these results have not been repeated, and others have not had as encouraging results. The procedure appears to be most efficacious when performed on horses with a broken back hoof axis. Palmar digital neurectomy remains the most reliable surgical procedure for navicular syndrome. The surgery does not alter the disease, it only alleviates the pain. Neurectomy will be no more pain alleviating than a palmar digital nerve block. Long-term studies have shown that 60 per cent of horses that undergo neurectomy remain sound for more than 1 year.

Treatment of navicular syndrome is difficult because there is more than one cause and form of the disease process. Diagnostic improvements may allow a more specific description of the navicular syndrome, which may better focus our therapy. Therapy will vary according to the cause and may use one or all of the treatment modalities: shoeing, medicinal, or surgical. When specific treatments can be matched to the

TABLE 1. DRUGS THAT INTERACT WITH WARFARIN

Protein-bound antibiotics
Antihistamines
Barbiturates
Chloral hydrate
Corticosteroids
Griseofulvin
Aspirin
Phenylbutazone

specific disease process, there will be an improvement in the consistency of therapeutic success rates.

Supplemental Readings

Colles, C. M.: Concepts of blood flow in the etiology and treatment of navicular disease. *In:* Proceedings of the 29th Annual Meeting of the American Association of Equine Practitioners, 1983, p. 265.

Rose, R. J., Allen, J. R., Hodgson, D. R., et al.: Studies on isoxsuprine hydrochloride for the treatment of navicular disease. Eq. Vet. J., *15*:238, 1983.

Turner, T. A.: Shoeing principles for the management of navicular disease in horses. J. Am. Vet. Med. Assoc., *189*:298,1986.

Turner, T. A., and Fessler, J. F.: The anatomic, pathologic, and radiographic aspects of navicular disease. Compend. Cont. Ed. Pract. Vet., *4*:S350, 1982.

Wright, I. M.: Navicular suspensory desmotomy in the treatment of navicular disease: Technique and preliminary results. Equine Vet. J., *18*:443, 1986.

Laminitis

Gary M. Baxter, ATHENS, GEORGIA

Laminitis or acute laminar degeneration is an inflammation of the laminae within the hoof. The complex interdigitating system of primary and secondary laminae provides a firm bond between the hoof wall and the laminar corium. Damage to the laminae results in breakdown of this interdigitation and the underlying distal phalanx separates from the hoof wall. Vasoconstriction within the digit, microthrombosis, perivascular edema, arteriovenous shunting of blood at the level of the coronary band, and venoconstriction are all pathophysiologic mechanisms proposed to cause laminitis. All produce hypoperfusion of the digit, leading to ischemia, necrosis, and edema of the laminae. In particular, the venoconstriction is thought to increase capillary pressure and hydrostatic movement of fluid into the interstitial space. Numerous secondary inflammatory and systemic alterations occur with laminitis, making differentiation between the initiating cause(s) and secondary manifestations extremely difficult.

There are numerous predisposing factors for laminitis in horses (Table 1). Excessive carbohydrate intake is the classic cause of laminitis and has been used to reproduce the syndrome experimentally. However, any systemically ill and potentially endotoxemic horse is at risk for developing laminitis. The risk is even more pronounced if the horse is overweight or has been treated with systemic corticosteroids. Sudden diet changes or overeating of highly digestible high-energy feed such as lush pasture or alfalfa may also induce laminitis. Horses worked excessively on a hard surface may exhibit signs of laminitis from traumatic tearing of the laminae. Support laminitis occurs when one limb has to bear an excessive amount of weight because of severe lameness in the contralateral limb. Direct exposure of the feet to or ingestion of black walnut wood shavings can lead to laminitis, which is usually transient once contact is eliminated.

CLINICAL SIGNS

Laminitis can be broadly classified into acute, subacute, refractory, and chronic stages. The condition is more commonly seen in the front feet but may involve all four feet or a single digit. Lameness associated with laminitis can range from very slight to failure to bear weight to refusal to stand. The gradations of lameness associated with laminitis as described by Obel are as follows: grade 1—the horse lifts its feet repeatedly, often every few seconds; grade 2—the horse moves willingly at a walk, but the gait is characteristic of laminitis; the horse does not resist lifting of a forefoot; grade 3—the horse moves reluctantly and vigorously resists attempts to lift a forefoot because of pain in the contralateral digit; grade 4—the horse must be forced to move and may be recumbent.

The higher the Obel grade of lameness, the greater the likelihood of permanent damage to the laminae. Unfortunately, acute laminitis in most horses is not recognized by the owners until the disease has reached grade 3. By this time significant laminar degeneration may have already occurred, thus reducing the chances of a complete recovery.

ACUTE LAMINITIS

The acute form of laminitis should be considered a medical emergency and aggressive treatment must be initiated promptly. Severe lameness can develop rapidly and is obvious when the

TABLE 1. PRECIPITATING FACTORS IN EQUINE LAMINITIS

Carbohydrate overload
   Excess grain intake
   Lush pasture (grass laminitis)
   Feed change to high-energy legume
Endotoxemia, sepsis, shock
   Colitis
   Proximal enteritis
   Small intestinal strangulation/obstructions
   Retained placenta, metritis, abortion
   Septicemia or toxemia from any cause
Excessive unilateral weight-bearing (support laminitis)
   Severe lameness
   Rehabilitation of fracture repair
Management
   Ingestion of cold water by overheated horse
   Unconditioned horse worked on hard surface (concussion or road laminitis)
   Overweight horses or ponies
   Trimming hooves too short
   Black walnut wood shavings used for bedding
Miscellaneous
   Treatment with corticosteroids
   Hypothyroidism
   Diet of plants containing estrogens
   Continuous estrus in mares
   Allergic-type reactions to certain medications

horse walks on a hard surface or is forced to turn in a circle. Increased digital pulses and heat over the hoof wall are nearly always present and pain is elicited when the toe is compressed with hoof testers. Strides are shortened, with each foot placed quickly back on the ground. If the pain is very severe, or if all four feet are affected, the horse may be recumbent.

Large, overweight horses with primary septic, endotoxemic, or metabolic conditions are prime candidates for distal displacement (sinking) of the distal phalanx. The entire laminar interdigitation becomes detached from the hoof wall, permitting the distal phalanx to drop within the hoof wall. These horses often have involvement of all four feet and are severely lame. Cavitation or depression along the coronary band is often the first clinical sign of sinking. With time, blood or serum may ooze from the coronary band. Sinking may occur alone or in combination with rotation of the distal phalanx. Sinking of the distal phalanx in a single digit secondary to severe lameness in the contralateral limb has occurred. These horses were not systemically ill but were overweight and presumably overloaded the affected digit.

Subacute Laminitis

Subacute laminitis is a milder degree of acute laminitis. The same clinical signs may be present but often are less pronounced (Obel grades 1 and 2). Horses that have been worked on hard surfaces, have had the hooves trimmed too short, or have been exposed to black walnut wood shavings often exhibit subacute laminitis. Clinical signs often resolve quickly, and permanent laminar damage usually does not occur.

Refractory Laminitis

All too frequently, acute laminitis does not respond to aggressive medical therapy. If no improvement is seen within 7 to 10 days, or if an acute exacerbation of the disease occurs after an initial improvement, the laminitis should be considered refractory. Refractory laminitis suggests continued laminar degeneration, severe inflammation and edema within the digit, and a poor prognosis. Rotation or distal displacement of the distal phalanx is inevitable if signs of laminitis cannot be controlled within 10 to 14 days. Severe refractory laminitis can result in complete hoof wall detachment or penetration of the sole by the tip of the distal phalanx.

Chronic Laminitis

Chronic laminitis occurs when rotation or distal displacement of the distal phalanx has occurred and there is no active laminar necrosis or inflammation. Laminar damage results in abnormal hoof growth, seen as diverging rings around the hoof wall; these rings are wider at the heel than at the toe. Classically, the toes are long, the heels are overgrown, and the sole has dropped, resulting in a flat or convex appearance to the bottom of the foot. Because of the abnormal horn growth and changes in the digital vasculature of horses with chronic laminitis, subsolar abscesses are very common. In addition, the dorsal hoof wall may become detached from the underlying laminae, widening of the white line predisposes to "seedy toe," and recurrent attacks of acute laminitis are likely.

DIAGNOSIS

Any horse with increased pulse amplitude in the digital arteries, increased heat within the foot, pain over the toe elicited with hoof testers, and lameness should be suspected of having laminitis. Horses with chronic laminitis will often travel using a heel–toe placement of their feet to avoid concussion of their toes. Acute laminitis requires an abaxial sesamoid or low palmar–plantar nerve block to alleviate the pain, whereas horses with chronic laminitis may improve significantly with a palmar digital nerve block because of the dropped, bruised sole and secondary abscessation. In some horses with severe acute laminitis it may be very difficult to completely desensitize the digit. Lateral radiographs of the affected digit(s) should be taken immediately to serve as a baseline for subsequent radiographic comparison and to determine if the horse has had laminitis previously. Serial radiographs are often essential to monitor progression of the disease. Radiographically, laminitis can be divided into five categories: (1) no observable abnormalities, (2) distal displacement of the distal phalanx (Fig. 1), (3) rotation of the distal phalanx, (4) rotation and sinking of the distal phalanx, and (5) rotation of the distal phalanx with secondary chronic changes. Very early radiographic signs suggestive of laminitis include widening of the area between the distal phalanx and the dorsal hoof wall and roughening along the dorsal aspect of the distal phalanx. The degree of rotation of the distal phalanx can be determined. The greater the rotation, the poorer the prognosis for return to athletic function (Fig. 2).

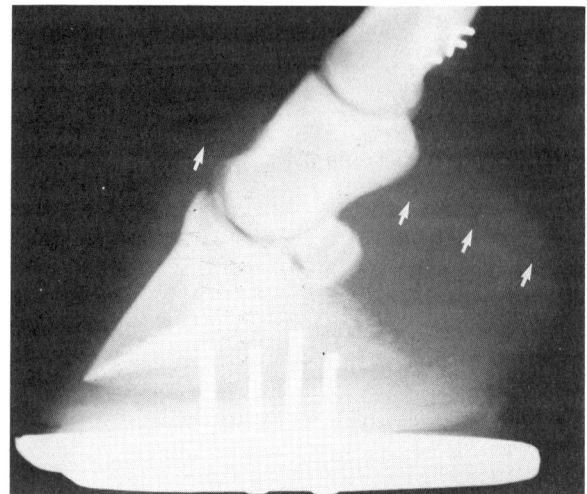

Figure 1. Lateral radiograph of a front foot of a horse with severe laminitis. A sinker line *(arrows)* suggests distal displacement of the distal phalanx.

THERAPY

In most situations it is more rewarding and effective to prevent laminitis than to treat the disease once it has occurred. Preventative measures should be taken with horses "at risk" for the development of laminitis. Laminitis has been associated with endotoxemia and therefore the systemic effects of endotoxemia should be minimized. Other therapy includes maintaining hydration, treating septicemia, maintaining frog pressure, proper feeding and management, and administration of anti-inflammatories and anticoagulants such as acetylsalicylic acid (aspirin)° or heparin.† Presently, the use of heparin in horses with laminitis is controversial since it causes red cell agglutination in vitro. Clinical problems associated with agglutination have not

---

°Acetylsalicylic acid, Butler Co., Columbus, OH
†Heparin sodium, Elkins Sinn, Inc., Cherry Hill, NJ

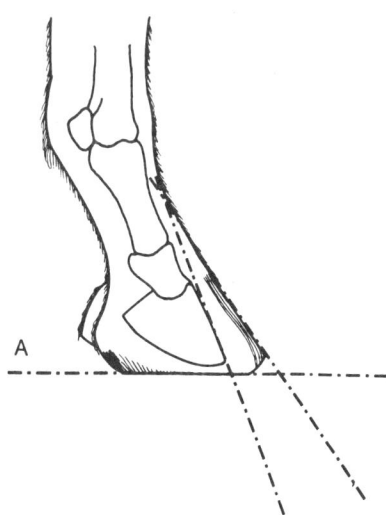 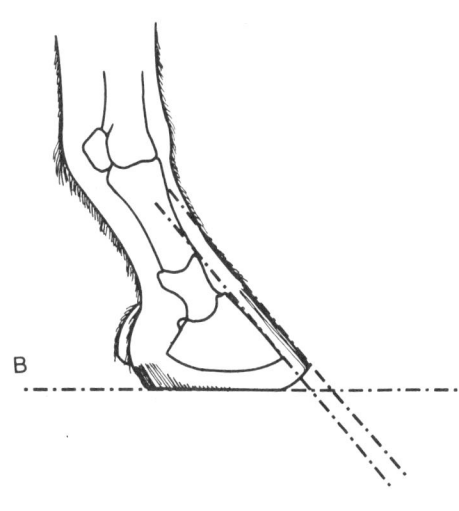

Figure 2. Diagrams of the distal equine limb, demonstrating the measurement of distal phalanx rotation. When distal phalanx rotation has occurred (*A*), the angle of the hoof wall (formed by the line drawn parallel to the dorsum of the hoof wall and the horizontal line) subtracted from the angle of the distal phalanx (formed by the line drawn parallel to the dorsum of the distal phalanx and the horizontal) equals the degree of distal phalanx rotation. In a foot unaffected by laminitis (*B*), the amount of rotation is zero. (From Stick, J. A.: Laminitis. *In* Robinson, N. E. (ed.): Current Therapy in Equine Medicine 2. Philadelphia, W. B. Saunders Co., 1984, p. 280. Reproduced by permission.)

been seen. Although heparin has been shown to prevent experimentally induced laminitis in horses, a recent retrospective study failed to demonstrate a significant benefit of heparin prophylaxis.

Despite recent advances in identifying the cause of laminitis, most treatment regimens remain empirical. Because extensive laminar damage can occur within 24 hours of the onset of acute laminitis, aggressive therapy must be given at the first suspicion of the disease. The goals of treatment include (1) correcting the primary illness or removing the causative factor, (2) blocking the pain–hypertension cycle, (3) improving digital blood flow and laminar perfusion, (4) preventing or correcting rotation or sinking of the distal phalanx, and (5) promoting keratinization and healing of sole and hoof defects (Table 2).

When a precipitating factor for laminitis is known, such as lush pasture, excessive grain feeding, or exposure to walnut wood shavings, the horse should be promptly removed from the environment. Mineral oil should be given via nasogastric tube to horses with alimentary disease to minimize further absorption of endotoxins. Grain and legume hay should be eliminated from the diet and the horse fed only grass hay until the signs of acute laminitis have resolved. If the horse or pony is overweight, a weight-reducing diet should be instituted.

In most cases, the primary illness must be treated concurrently with the laminitis. This usually includes intravenous (IV) fluids, parenteral antimicrobials, flunixin meglumine°, and possibly plasma. Therapy specifically directed at laminitis includes dimethyl sulfoxide (DMSO),† phenylbutazone, and aspirin. DMSO (0.1 mg per kg IV) is a free radical scavenger and potent anti-inflammatory agent directed primarily at preventing the cellular reperfusion injury that occurs in ischemic tissue. No studies have docu-

---

°Banamine, Schering Corp., Kenilworth, NJ
†Domoso, Syntex Animal Health Inc., West Des Moines, IA

TABLE 2. SUMMARY OF TREATMENT OF LAMINITIS

GOAL 1: REMOVE CAUSATIVE FACTOR OR CORRECT PRIMARY ILLNESS
Techniques
1. Determine potential cause(s) and remove from environment.
2. Combat endotoxemia, septicemia, and hemoconcentration.
   a. Systemic antimicrobials
   b. Flunixin meglumine
   c. Intravenous fluids
   d. Mineral oil PO
   e. Hyperimmune plasma

TABLE 2. SUMMARY OF TREATMENT OF LAMINITIS (*Continued*)

3. Preventive care.
   a. Frog support or pressure
   b. Well-bedded stall
   c. Periodic hand walking

GOAL 2: BLOCK PAIN–HYPERTENSION CYCLE
Techniques
1. Local anesthesia of digit: Reserved for animals in severe pain. Not recommended more than once daily. Do not walk horse excessively after desensitization.
2. Analgesics.
   a. Phenylbutazone: 4.4 mg/kg b.i.d. IV or PO for 3–5 days, then decrease dose gradually
   b. DMSO: 0.1 g/kg diluted to 10% solution IV b.i.d. for 3–5 days
3. Sand stall or deep bedding; padding of sole and frog.

GOAL 3: IMPROVE DIGITAL BLOOD FLOW AND LAMINAR PERFUSION
Techniques
1. Vasodilators.
   a. Acetylpromazine: 0.02 mg/kg IV or IM 3–6 times daily
   b. Isoxsuprine hydrochloride: 1.2 mg/kg PO b.i.d.
2. Anticoagulants.
   a. Aspirin: 10–20 mg/kg PO every other day
   b. Heparin (?): 40–80 IU/kg IV or SC 2–3 times daily
3. Maintain frog pressure and support of sole.

GOAL 4: PREVENT FURTHER ROTATION OR SINKING OF DISTAL PHALANX
Techniques
1. Maintain frog pressure with padding or shoes.
2. Deep digital flexor tenotomy.
3. Inferior check ligament desmotomy?
4. Elevated-heel shoes?
5. Foot casts?
6. Hoof trimming: Remove excess toe and heel in chronic laminitis.
7. Hoof wall resection?
8. No known method to prevent sinking of the distal phalanx.

GOAL 5: PROMOTE KERATINIZATION AND HEALING OF HOOF AND SOLE DEFECTS
Techniques
1. Proper trimming of underrun sole and detached hoof wall.
2. Foot soaking and local antiseptics.
3. Systemic antimicrobials?
4. Shoeing: Must provide support to frog and sole; variety of methods available.
5. Methionine:° 10 gm/day.
6. Methylsulphonylmethan (MSM)† 0.5–1.0 gm/day.
7. Commercially available supplements for hoof growth:‡ Use as directed.
8. Topical hoof dressings.

GOAL 6: MAINTAIN SYSTEMIC HEALTH IN HORSES WITH CHRONIC LAMINITIS
Techniques
1. Prevent and treat pressure sores.
2. Ensure adequate feed and water intake, especially if horse is recumbent.
3. Prevent impactions of the bowel by use of bran mashes, good quality feed, and fluids.
4. Thyroid replacement?

°D-L-methionine powder, Butler Co., Columbus, OH.
†MSM, Vitality Systems, Inc., Gaston, OR.
‡Horse sho-hoof, Manna Pro Corp., Los Angeles, CA.

mented the efficacy of DMSO in laminitis, but clinical impressions dictate its continued use. Likewise, phenylbutazone (4.4 mg per kg) is essential for treating any form of laminitis because it reduces the inflammation, edema, and pain within the digit, thus promoting return of normal foot function and preventing progressive laminar damage. Aspirin (10 to 20 mg per kg) is used to inhibit platelet aggregation by decreasing thromboxane synthesis, which could predispose to microthrombus formation within the laminae when perfusion is sluggish. This dosage of aspirin has minimal anti-inflammatory properties, and the drug can be safely combined with other nonsteroidal anti-inflammatory drugs.

Peripheral vasodilator therapy should only be used in horses with a stable cardiovascular system. The goal is to improve laminar perfusion and to counteract the increased sympathetic tone that often accompanies laminitis. The most commonly used agents include acetylpromazine* and isoxsuprine hydrochloride.† Phenoxybenzamine‡ is less available and therefore less commonly used (Table 2). It is unknown if these drugs actually improve circulation to the microvasculature of the laminae. Additionally, oral isoxsuprine at 0.6 mg per kg does not cause systemic vasodilation in normal horses. However, acute and refractory cases of laminitis appear to benefit from acetylpromazine therapy.

Radical trimming of the feet of horses with acute laminitis should be avoided. Shoes should be pulled and if the toes are long, they should be shortened. Counterpressure on the frog should be maintained using compressible gauze, cotton, or commercially available frog pads§ to promote digital circulation and to counteract downward rotation of the distal phalanx. Some horses with distal displacement may become more lame when pressure is applied to the frog and sole. Presumably this occurs because the digital cushion and vascular system are compressed between the solar aspect of the distal phalanx and the horny sole. Therefore, prevention of sinking is difficult since support of the frog and sole by any means may further compress the solar vasculature. Padding and support of the feet can also be achieved by placing the horse on sand, soft ground, or on deep bedding. Walking should be avoided in horses with acute laminitis because of the potential to further damage the already compromised laminae. Routine local anesthesia of the digit with subsequent forced exercise is contraindicated. However, periodic desensitization of the affected digit(s) stops the pain–hypertension cycle temporarily and can greatly improve the patient's attitude. Local anesthesia may also cause dilation of the digital vasculature. Warm or cold hydrotherapy or foot soaks can be used but probably do little to alter the course of the disease.

CORRECTIVE TRIMMING AND SHOEING

Treatment of chronic laminitis primarily involves corrective trimming and shoeing and preventing recurrent acute flare-ups. Permanent laminar damage has already occurred and epidermal hyperplasia results in a wedge of epithelium between the dorsal hoof wall and distal phalanx. Initial therapy for chronic laminitis often entails removing underrun sole and debriding abscesses. Foot soaking in a dilute povidone–iodine* and magnesium sulfate† solution will speed resolution of the infection. Systemic antimicrobials may also be used. Corrective trimming should attempt to return the distal phalanx to its normal anatomical position and provide a nonpainful weight-bearing surface. This usually involves shortening the toes, lowering the heels, and protecting the sole (Fig. 3). Several trimmings at 4 to 6-week intervals are often required to obtain normal alignment in horses with severe distal phalangeal rotation.

Hoof wall resection has become more commonplace in treating both acute and chronic laminitis (Fig. 4). Resection is mostly used for chronic laminitis where the hoof wall is unattached, as demonstrated by a gas line on radiographs or with subsolar abscessation. However, it may also be used in acute or refractory cases of laminitis to relieve the pressure from fluid accumulation within the edematous laminae. In addition, hoof wall resection or stripping has been advocated for horses with sinking of the distal phalanx to remove the pressure-induced ischemia and pain that occurs at the dorsal coronary corium. The hoof wall can be removed with a circular sander, electric drill with a bur-tipped drill bit, or hoof rasp. Hoof wall resection can be combined with corrective shoeing to protect the exposed sensitive tissue.

The goals of shoeing horses with laminitis are (1) to protect the painful area of the sole and

---

*Acepromazine, Butler Co., Columbus, OH
†Isoxsuprine, Chelsea Labs., Division of Rugby Labs., Rockville Centre, Long Island, NY
‡Dibenzyline, Smith Kline & French Labs., Philadelphia, PA
§Lilly Pads, Therapeutic Equine Products, Inc., Indianapolis, IN

*Betadine, Purdue Frederick Co., Norwalk, CT
†Epsom salt, Humco Lab., Texarkana, TX

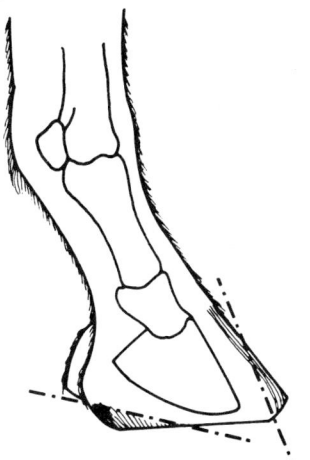

Figure 3. Areas of hoof to be removed during corrective trimming in a horse with chronic laminitis. *Vertical line* shows the amount of hoof wall to be removed so that it parallels the dorsum of the distal phalanx. *Horizontal line* shows the amount of heel areas of hoof to be removed so that the weight-bearing surface of the distal phalanx is parallel to the ground. (From Stick, J. A.: Laminitis. *In* Robinson, N. E. (ed.): Current Therapy in Equine Medicine 2. Philadelphia, W. B. Saunders Co., 1987, p. 281. Reproduced by permission.)

hoof wall from ground contact, (2) to prevent further tissue destruction or rotation of the distal phalanx, (3) to provide support to the foot, and (4) to enhance healing of the digit. The shoe with or without a pad can be used to lower or elevate the heel, depending on the situation, but should not apply direct pressure to the solar surface or exposed sensitive tissue. Farriers and veterinarians alike have claimed success with nonadjustable heart bar shoes, adjustable heart bar shoes, reverse shoes and pads, wide-web shoes, regular shoes and pads, egg-bar shoes, wide-bar shoes, boiler-plate shoes, and most recently the Thera-Flex shoe inserts.* Silicone rubber is often used between the pad and sole to further decrease concussion on the sole. Recently, an elevated heel shoe has been used to treat acute laminitis. The shoe is designed to reduce the pull of the deep digital flexor tendon, thus preventing rotation of the distal phalanx. The ideal shoe has not been developed and the type of shoe used often depends on personal preference and the expertise of the farrier. However, using shoes that do not provide frog or sole support to the feet is thought to increase the likelihood of further rotation or sinking of the distal phalanx. Regardless of the type of shoe used, it is very important that the farrier work with the practitioner and understand the principles of shoeing horses with laminitis.

SURGICAL THERAPY

It has been hypothesized that the pull of the deep digital flexor tendon is important in promoting rotation of the distal phalanx (Fig. 5). Tenotomies of the deep digital flexor tendon can be performed in the palmar–plantar aspect of the pastern or in the mid-metacarpal–metatarsal regions to counteract this rotating force (Fig. 6). Good success has been reported with tenotony at the midpastern region for treating chronic refractory laminitis with severe rotation of the distal phalanx. Tenotomy at the midcannon bone appears to relieve the pain associated with laminitis but may not alter the ultimate outcome. Only 5 of 20 horses with acute or chronic lamin-

---

*Thera-Flex shoe inserts, Thera-Flex Inc., Lawrenceburg, KY

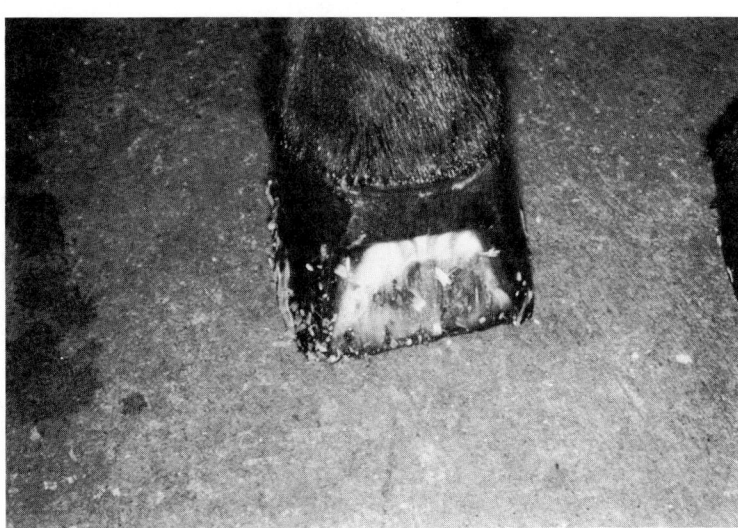

Figure 4. Dorsal hoof wall resection has been performed on a horse with chronic laminitis. The dorsal hoof wall was detached from the underlying laminae and was removed with a sander.

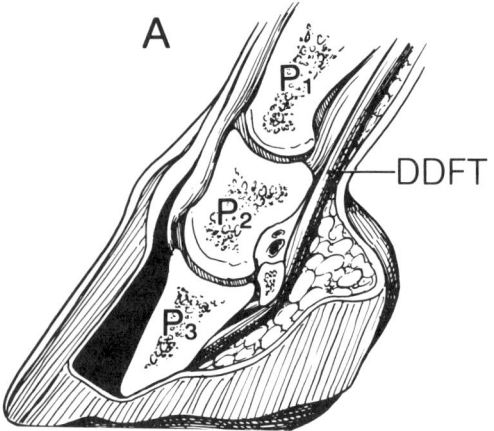

Figure 5. Pull of the deep digital flexor tendon *(DDFT)* on the palmar–plantar aspect of the distal phalanx. Transection of the tendon may prevent further rotation of the distal phalanx. P_1 = proximal phalanx, P_2 = middle phalanx, P_3 = distal phalanx. (Courtesy of Dr. Douglas Allen, University of Georgia.)

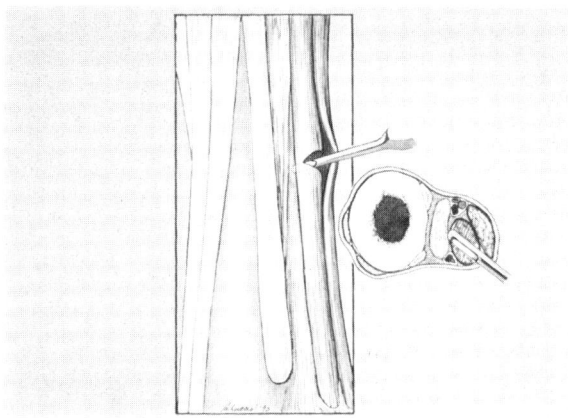

Figure 6. Transection of the deep digital flexor tendon in the midmetacarpus. A guarded bistoury is used to prevent trauma to the palmar vessels and nerves. (Courtesy of Dr. Robert Hunt, University of Georgia.)

itis that underwent a tenotomy at the midcannon bone at our hospital survived longer than one year. Only one of these horses was completely sound. This most likely reflects the severity of the laminitis and does not mean that tenotomies should not be performed. The location of the tenotomy depends on the health of the horse, the degree of rotation of the distal phalanx, financial constraints of the owner, and personal preference. Tenotomy at the midpastern requires general anesthesia, whereas tenotomy at the midmetacarpus–metatarsus can be performed in the standing animal following a high palmar nerve block and sedation. Either technique should be seriously considered as a salvage procedure in the treatment of refractory or severe chronic laminitis, especially if conventional therapy is failing.

PROGNOSIS

The prognosis of any horse with laminitis is guarded. Factors determining the prognosis include (1) the duration of acute laminitis, (2) the number of feet affected, (3) the amount of distal phalanx rotation, (4) whether sinking has occurred, (5) whether secondary abscessation and osteomyelitis of the distal phalanx occurs, and (6) the aftercare provided by the owners. Horses with less than 5.5 degrees rotation of the distal phalanx can return to performance. Horses with subacute or acute laminitis that responds to therapy within 7 to 10 days may also recover completely. Horses with refractory and severe chronic laminitis are unlikely to perform again, and many of these horses will be euthanized because of the continued pain, lack of response to therapy, and severe permanent laminar and hoof wall changes. In addition, horses in which the distal phalanx sinks or sinks and rotates have an extremely guarded prognosis. If they recover, they are likely to be pasture sound at best.

Supplemental Readings

Allen, D., White, N. A., Foerner, J. F., et al.: Surgical management of chronic laminitis in horses: 13 cases (1983–1985). J. Am. Vet. Med. Assoc., 189:1604–1606, 1986.

Baxter, G. M.: Equine laminitis caused by distal displacement of the distal phalanx: 12 cases (1976–1985). J. Am. Vet. Med. Assoc., 189:326–329, 1986.

Belknap, J. K., and Moore, J. N.: Evaluation of heparin for prophylaxis of equine laminitis: 71 cases (1980–1986). J. Am. Vet. Med. Assoc., 195:505–507, 1989.

Colles, C. M., and Jeffcott, L. B.: Laminitis in the horse. Vet. Rec., 100:262–264, 1977.

Goetz, T. E.: Anatomic, hoof, and shoeing considerations for the treatment of laminitis in horses. J. Am. Vet. Med. Assoc., 190:1323–1332, 1987.

Hunt, R. J., Allen, D., Baxter, G. M., et al.: Mid-metacarpal deep digital flexor tenotomy in the management of refractory laminitis in horses. Vet. Surg. 20:15–20, 1991.

Moore, J. N., Allen D., Clark, E. S.: Pathophysiology of acute laminitis. Vet. Clin. North Am. (Equine Pract.), 5:67–72, 1989.

Stick, J. A., Jann, H. W., Scott, E. A., Robinson, N. E.: Pedal bone rotation as a prognostic sign in laminitis of horses. J. Am. Vet. Med. Assoc., 180:251–253, 1982.

Yelle, M.: Clinicians' guide to equine laminitis. Equine Vet. J., 18:156–158, 1986.

Appendicular Inflammatory Disorders

Valerie A. Fadok, DENVER, COLORADO

Several disparate etiologic agents can cause inflammation with significant swelling in the limbs of horses; these include infectious, parasitic, immunologic, and environmental insults (Table 1). It is vital to determine the cause in order to treat the inflammation rationally and effectively. This discussion reviews the causes of appendicular inflammation in the horse, diagnostic techniques, and therapeutic options.

INFECTIOUS CAUSES

BACTERIAL INFECTIONS

Infectious causes of appendicular inflammation include a variety of bacterial and fungal agents. Ulcerative lymphangitis, a bacterial infection of the cutaneous lymphatics, is a sporadic disease that is classically and most commonly caused by *Corynebacterium pseudotuberculosis*. Other organisms isolated from similar clinical lesions include *Rhodococcus* (formerly *Corynebacterium*) *equi* and *Pasteurella hemolytica*. The disease usually follows contamination of a wound, particularly in horses subjected to poor general hygiene and management. This disease appears more commonly in the rear limbs and is characterized by multiple nodules that ulcerate and drain. Edema and fibrosis are particularly prominent in infections caused by *C. pseudotuberculosis*. Sporotrichosis is the major differential diagnosis; the infection also can present as nodular dermatitis of the limbs (see below). The diagnosis of ulcerative lymphangitis can be confirmed by biopsy and culture. Early diagnosis and therapy is vital, because progressive fibrosis associated with chronicity can be permanently disabling. Systemic treatment with penicillin, 40,000 to 80,000 IU per kg b.i.d., is recommended, accompanied by surgical drainage and warm soaks. Antibiotic therapy should be continued for a minimum of 4 to 6 weeks.

Bacterial cellulitis and abscessation of the proximal limbs of horses, without the nodular appearance of ulcerative lymphangitis, has also been attributed to infections with *Corynebacterium pseudotuberculosis* and *Rhodococcus equi*. These infections can be associated with considerable lameness, pitting edema, fever, and depression, prior to the development of ulceration and draining tracts. *C. pseudotuberculosis* infections have been reported with increasing frequency from the western states, particularly California, where it is known to cause inguinal and pectoral abscesses, or "pigeon chest." The pathogenesis of these lesions is not known. Suggested vectors for the bacteria include hornflies, ticks, and *Habronema* larvae. It has been suggested that *Strongyloides westeri* larvae can carry *R. equi* into the skin.

Infections with these organisms can be difficult to treat. Topical therapy with hot packs or warm soaks and surgical drainage of abscesses are important. Care should be taken when draining these abscesses to dispose of the exudate carefully, to avoid contamination of the environment. The exudate should be cultured to determine the bacteria causing the disease, and sensitivity testing performed to select an appropriate systemic antibiotic. *C. pseudotuberculosis* is usually sensitive to penicillin; however, high dosages, such as those recommended above, should be used. *R. equi* may be resistant to penicillin, requiring the use of an alternative antibiotic. Erythromycin (10 to 15 mg per kg three to four times a day), given orally in combination with rifampin (5 mg per kg twice a day), is often effective against this organism. Protection against insect attack by the use of topical insecticides or repellents is advisable to prevent spread of these infectious organisms.

Bacterial cellulitis caused by microbes such as *Staphylococcus* spp., β-hemolytic streptococci, and, rarely, *Clostridium* spp. can also occur in the limbs of horses. Again, these diseases usually occur as a result of wound infection; poor wound management and a dirty environment probably also contribute. Most clostridial infections are associated with injection sites; subcutaneous gas production is often a feature. Clostridial infections may be fatal unless treatment is begun immediately. Diagnosis should be made by culture as soon as possible, particularly if there is a history of nonresponsiveness to routinely used antibiotics. Systemic antibiotic therapy should be based on sensitivity results, and treatment should continue for several weeks. Clostridial infections usually respond well to penicillin therapy, and this antibiotic should be administered immediately if this organism is suspected. Sur-

TABLE 1. POTENTIAL ETIOLOGIC FACTORS ASSOCIATED WITH INFLAMMATORY DISEASE IN THE LIMBS OF HORSES

Infectious
  Bacterial
    Corynebacterium pseudotuberculosis
    Rhodococcus equi
    Pasteurella hemolytica
    Staphylococcus spp.
    Streptococcus spp.
    Clostridium spp.
    Dermatophilus congolensis
    Pseudomonas mallei (glanders; restricted to Eastern Europe, North Africa, and Asia [see p. 761])
  Fungal
    Sporothrix schenkii
    Pythium spp. (Protista rather than true fungal organism)
    Eumycotic mycetoma *(Curvularia geniculata)*
    Deep mycoses (blastomycosis, histoplasmosis)
  Parasitic
    Habronema spp.
Immunologic
  Purpura hemorrhagica (strangles, viral infections, idiopathic)
  Vasculitis, nonpurpuric (bacterial and viral infections, idiopathic)
  Systemic lupus erythematosus
Environmental
  Photoactivated vasculitis
  Venomous insect and snake bites

gical opening of abscesses and draining tracts will facilitate healing. Clostridial infections in particular should be lanced to oxygenate the tissues. Nonspecific topical therapy such as warm water soaks or hot packs applied two to three times a day are also very helpful.

Staphylococcal spp. can also cause granulomatous nodular lesions (botryomycosis) on the limbs of horses; these lesions also usually result from wound or surgical contamination. Diagnosis is made by biopsy of the lesion. Best results are obtained by completely excising the lesions and administering systemic antibiotics, based on culture and sensitivity results, for several weeks.

Dermatophilus congolensis is an opportunistic bacterium that invades skin that has been macerated by continual moisture and traumatized by minor cuts and insect bites. In areas where the disease is prevalent, severe dermatophilosis can cause significant swelling and pain in the lower limbs, accompanied by lameness. Horses that develop this syndrome have usually been kept on poorly drained pasture, especially during heavy rains. The classic cuplike crusts are diagnostic; however, the lesions can coalesce into firm, adherent plaques of crust overlying exudative, painful, ulcerative lesions. These infections can be associated with other bacteria, such as the pathogenic staphylococcal species. The *Dermatophilus* component can be easily diagnosed by mincing the crusts in saline on a glass slide, allowing it to dry, and using a simple stain such as Diff-Quik. The organisms appear in chains with the typical "railroad track" appearance. Systemic antibiotic therapy with penicillin should be instituted, along with topical therapy aimed at drying the skin. Warm water soaks or hot packs, with povidone iodine washes twice a day, will facilitate healing. If staphylococcal involvement is suspected, culture and sensitivity testing should be performed, as pathogenic staphylococcal species can be resistant to penicillin. It is important to keep the horse in dry conditions, that is, off pasture and in a clean, dry stall, if possible.

FUNGAL INFECTIONS

Several fungal organisms have the potential to invade the skin as opportunists through wounds; these usually cause localized granulomatous lesions. Two diseases can cause extensive limb involvement: sporotrichosis and pythiosis (phycomycosis).

Sporotrichosis

Sporotrichosis is a subcutaneous mycotic infection caused by the dimorphic fungus *Sporothrix schenckii*, an organism found in soil and vegetation. It usually gains entrance into the skin through wounds. The organism in the horse seems to spread most commonly through the lymphatics, causing cording and nodular lesions resembling beads on a chain. The nodules can ulcerate and drain a serosanguinous or blood-tinged purulent exudate. Abscesses may also form. Diagnosis is confirmed by biopsy and culture. Biopsies show a pyogranulomatous dermatitis; special stains may or may not show the organism. Exudate or a biopsy specimen should be submitted to a mycology laboratory for culture confirmation of the diagnosis.

The classic treatment for sporotrichosis is iodide therapy. Sodium iodide can be given orally at a dosage of 20 to 40 mg per kg daily for several weeks. Therapy with hot packs or warm to hot hydrotherapy is especially important in this disease, as the organisms seem particularly sensitive to heat. Experience suggests that iodide therapy is helpful in many cases; however, some horses either fail to respond completely, relapse after treatment is stopped, or cannot tolerate the side effects, which can include loss of appetite, depression, fever, and serous nasal and ocular discharges. Iodides can also cause alopecia and scaling skin in some horses. Proven alternatives to iodide therapy for sporotrichosis have not been developed specifically for the horse. Griseofulvin at a dosage of 10 gm daily for 2 weeks, then 5 gm daily for another 7 weeks, has been reported to be effective in one horse that was not cured with iodides. In human patients with sporotrichosis, alternative therapy with amphotericin B, ketoconazole, or more recently itraconazole has been suggested. The toxicity of amphotericin B and the problems associated with its intravenous administration make it an undesirable drug to use in horses. The use of ketoconazole in man has shown that some patients with sporotrichosis do not respond to this drug. The use of ketoconazole in horses with sporotrichosis has not been reported; however, the pharmacokinetics of this drug used orally in the horse have been studied. Ketoconazole for oral administration should be dissolved in acid (0.2N HCl) to promote absorption from the gastrointestinal tract. It can be given at a dosage of 30 mg per kg one to two times a day; it is very expensive. Itraconazole (1 to 2 mg per kg) has become the drug of choice for the treatment of sporotrichosis in man. It has also been used successfully in dogs and cats at a dosage of 5 to 10 mg per kg, although the lower end of the dosage range seems effective. One equine clinician (M. Levy, pers. commun., 1990) has used itraconazole in the treatment of a horse with sporotrichosis of greater than 1 year's duration. The drug was given at 3 mg per kg twice a day in the grain; after 2 months of therapy, the swelling of the affected limb was decreased, and the lesions had stopped oozing and begun to dry. Itraconazole, therefore, would appear to have great potential in the treatment of iodide-resistant equine sporotrichosis; its expense would necessarily restrict its use.

Pythiosis

Pythiosis, or phycomycosis, is actually not a fungal disease. It is caused by the Protista organism *Pythium*, formerly called *Hyphomyces destruens*. This disease occurs primarily in the Gulf Coast states. The organism lives in water or in moist, decaying vegetation and gains entrance to the subcutaneous tissues through wounds. The motile zoospores actually show chemotaxis toward damaged plant or animal tissue. The organism induces a severe pyogranulomatous reaction as it spreads through the tissues. The growth of the lesions is extremely rapid, suggesting the more colorful colloquial name of "swamp cancer." The organism has a tropism for blood vessels, and hemorrhage is frequently associated with these lesions. Anemia, therefore, can complicate the clinical picture. Pruritis, lameness, and edema are also seen. The characteristic "leeches" or "kunkers" found in the multiple draining tracts represent cores of necrotic tissue and *Pythium* organisms. This disease can only be successfully treated if it is diagnosed early. Like a malignancy, the lesions rapidly destroy surrounding tissue and can metastasize to local lymph nodes and occasionally into the abdominal cavity. Diagnosis should be made as soon as possible by biopsy of the lesions.

Experience suggests that the most successful treatment combines complete surgical excision with immunotherapy, using a vaccine made from the *Pythium* organism. The vaccine is made from *Pythium* cultured in vitro, homogenized in saline, and adjusted to 5 mg per ml. Two ml is administered once weekly in the pectoral muscles for at least three injections. A common side effect is localized swelling at the site of injection; the severity of this swelling has correlated positively with response to therapy, so it is not an indication to stop the vaccine. In some horses, sterile abscesses may develop; these may be treated with hot packs. The vaccine can be given initially, and the horse observed over 10 to 14 days for beginning resolution of the lesion. During this time, the lesions can be treated nonspecifically with povidone–iodine washes and soaks to decrease bacterial contamination. Once the lesion has begun to resolve, surgical excision can be performed. Experience suggests that vaccine alone will only cure very small lesions. It is not uncommon for lesions to recur, so that multiple surgeries may be required. The expense of this type of treatment, combined with the fact that diagnosis is often made after extensive spread of the organism has taken place, results in many owners deciding to euthanize their horses.

Parasitic Infections

The major parasitic disorder causing localized or multifocal granulomatous lesions on the limbs of horses is cutaneous habronemiasis. The eosinophilic granulomas, which develop at the site of wounds in which the vector fly *Stomoxys calcitrans* deposits the larvae, are believed to be a hypersensitivity response. This disease seems to have declined in prevalence greatly with the use of ivermectin for horses. Habronemiasis is the major differential diagnosis for pythiosis in horses in the Gulf Coast states. Diagnosis of this disease can be made by biopsy, which should always be performed on granulomatous diseases of the limbs. Habronemiasis may complicate other lesions, such as sarcoid, squamous cell carcinoma, and exuberant granulation tissue.

If habronemiasis is diagnosed, the granulomas will respond to corticosteroid therapy. Prednisone can be given at a dosage of 1.0 mg per kg daily for 1 to 2 weeks, then tapered. The deworming program should be evaluated. Ivermectin could be included in the program to decrease the likelihood of developing this disease. Ivermectin has also been reported to cause resolution of habronemiasis lesions; however, it may not be important to kill the larvae at the lesion site, as they will probably die from the inflammation they have induced.

IMMUNOLOGIC CAUSES

Immunologic causes of inflammatory limb disease in horses include purpura hemorrhagica, the other cutaneous vasculitides that do not resemble purpura, and systemic lupus erythematosus (SLE).

Purpura hemorrhagica is a cutaneous vasculitis seen in some horses with a recent history of *Streptococcus equi* infection (strangles) or equine influenza. Some cases are idiopathic. The syndrome is characterized by severe and often sharply demarcated edema of the head and limbs and petechial hemorrhages of the mucous membranes. Diagnosis can be confirmed by biopsy, which shows a neutrophilic, nectrotizing vasculitis associated with hemorrhage and edema. Treatment should be instituted as soon as possible to decrease the necrosis that will develop and to avoid sequelae such as infection and myositis. If a bacterial infection is found as the underlying cause, systemic antibiotic therapy should be instituted. Usually streptococcal infections can be treated successfully with penicillin. Antibiotic therapy is also indicated if secondary pyoderma is present in the vasculitic skin lesions. Corticosteroids can be given to alleviate the inflammation associated with the vasculitis. Prednisone or prednisolone should be given at 1 to 2 mg per kg daily and continued until the disease begins to remit; the dosage can then be lowered *slowly* to 0.25 to 0.5 mg per kg every other day, or to a dosage that will control the disease. Several weeks of therapy may be required. Diuretics have been recommended by some clinicians to reduce edema; furosemide can be used for the first few days at a dosage of 1 mg per kg b.i.d. Other palliative treatments such as hydrotherapy and mild exercise will assist recovery.

Cutaneous vasculitis may also present without the signs of petechial hemorrhage and severe edema seen with purpura hemorrhagica. Early lesions may resemble papular urticaria; crusting, alopecia, and erythema develop as the disease progresses. Shaving the urticarial lesions may reveal papules and plaques with a necrotic center. These lesions are ideal for punch biopsy. The vasculitis may be eosinophilic, neutrophilic, or have mixed inflammatory infiltrates; fibrinoid degeneration may also be noticed.

Making a diagnosis of vasculitis obligates the veterinarian to search for an underlying cause, which can include bacterial or viral infections, drug reactions, or possibly lupus-like disorders; many cases have no known cause (see p. 510). The treatment of vasculitis is the same as for purpura hemorrhagica. Some equine patients do not seem to respond to prednisone therapy very well; i.e., the drug does not control the lesions except at very high dosages, or frequent relapses occur. Sometimes changing the steroid to dexamethasone, used at 0.1 to 0.2 mg per kg daily, will improve response to therapy. Dexamethasone, a longer acting steroid, is not ideal for alternate-day therapy; however, it may be possible to treat initially with this drug, and then switch to prednisone when the disease is well under control.

A disease syndrome resembling SLE has been diagnosed rarely in horses. It has a variable clinical presentation; however, one of the presentations has included edema of the extremities. The diagnosis is made by finding a positive antinuclear antibody titer in association with appropriate clinical signs. Other signs associated with lupus in the horse have included panniculitis, alopecia, leukoderma, and scaling, as well as thrombocytopenia, proteinuria, fever, polyarthritis, depression, and weight loss. If skin lesions are present, they should be biopsied to assist in confirmation of the diagnosis. Experience with treating lupus-like disorders in the horse is limited; however, glucocorticoids would be the drug of choice. Prognosis is unpredictable; however, it seems likely that treatment should continue for life. Glucocorticoids should be given at the lowest possible alternate-day dosage that controls the disease.

ENVIRONMENTAL CAUSES

A fascinating form of photosensitization in the horse, termed *photoactivated vasculitis*, causes significant painful edema restricted to nonpigmented lower limbs. Associated skin changes may include erythema, scaling, and crusting. Unlike the more conventional photosensitivity disorders, this disease does not affect nonpigmented skin on other parts of the body. It occurs during the summer months in geographic areas with plenty of sunlight. The etiology and pathogenesis of this disorder have not been determined; however, known photosensitizing agents or liver disease have not been found. The diagnosis can be made by skin biopsy, which shows vasculitis in the superficial dermis; thrombosis may also be seen. Treatment requires that the horse be stalled during the day to reduce exposure to sunlight; corticosteroids such as prednisone (1 to 2 mg per kg) should be given daily for at least 10 days to 2 weeks. The dosage can then be reduced gradually over the next 4 to 6 weeks. Warm water soaks may be helpful to remove crusts and exudate. Most horses with this disorder recover without incident; a few may relapse when reintroduced to sunlight. Until the etiologic agent is identified, no specific therapy can be recommended. It may be helpful to determine whether the horse has been exposed to the known photosensitizing plants, or if relapse occurs while the horse is on a particular pasture or feed.

Supplemental Readings

Miers, K. C., and Ley, W. B.: Corynebacterium pseudotuberculosis infection in the horse: Study of 117 clinical cases and consideration of etiopathogenesis. J. Am. Vet. Med. Assoc., 177:250–253, 1980.

Miller, R. I.: Equine phycomycosis. Compend. Cont. Ed. Pract. Vet., 5:S472–S479, 1983.

Prades, M., Brown, M. P., Gronwall, R., and Houston, A. E.: Body fluid and endometrial concentrations of ketoconazole in mares after intravenous injection or repeated gavage. Equine Vet. J., 21:211–214, 1989.

Rebhun, W. C., Shin, S. J., Ing, J. M., Baum, K., Pattern, V.: Malignant edema in horses. J. Am. Vet. Med. Assoc., 187:732–736, 1985.

Scott, D. W.: Large Animal Dermatology. Philadelphia, W. B. Saunders Co., 1988.

Stannard, A. A.: Photoactivated vasculitis. In Robinson, N. E. (ed.): Current Therapy in Equine Medicine 2. Philadelphia, W. B. Saunders Co., 1987, pp. 646–647.

Section 5

ALIMENTARY TRACT DISEASE

Edited by Michael J. Murray

Diagnostic Procedures for Evaluation of the Alimentary System

Michael J. Murray, LEESBURG, VIRGINIA

In addition to a thorough physical examination, rectal examination, and routine laboratory tests, several diagnostic procedures may be selected to enhance the evaluation of a horse with a known or suspected disorder involving the alimentary system. Each procedure is limited in the type and extent of information it yields, and thus the clinician should select the complement of procedures that is most likely to provide the information necessary to make a proper diagnosis and determine the appropriate therapy.

ENDOSCOPY

The availability of specialized endoscopy equipment has expanded the use of this procedure in evaluating the equine alimentary tract. In order to select the equipment that will be most applicable to the practice situation, the practitioner must determine what examinations will need to be performed.

The typical endoscope used in equine practice consists of an insertion tube that is 70 cm to 100 cm long and 10 to 14.5 mm in outer diameter, dimensions that restrict use of the endoscope for many gastrointestinal (GI) examinations. A diameter of 10 mm will allow passage through the turbinates of young foals, whereas the larger diameter tube can only be inserted through the nasal passages of adults.

In an adult horse, the proximal esophagus can be examined with an endoscope that has a 110-cm-long insertion tube. A 180-cm-long endoscope is usually necessary to view the entire length of the esophagus. A length of 110 cm is sufficient to reach the stomach of foals up to 30 to 40 days old, but a length of 150 to 180 cm is necessary for weanlings, and 200 cm is needed to examine the stomach of yearlings and adults. An insertion tube length of 200 cm is sufficient to examine the duodenum of foals up to approximately 6 months of age, while a length of 275 cm to 300 cm is required to examine the duodenum of adult horses.

Endoscopy of the rectum and distal small colon

can be performed with most flexible endoscopes in use in equine practice. It should be preceded, as much as possible, by careful evacuation and saline lavage of the rectum and distal small colon. The mucosal surface should appear pink to pale red and should have a smooth, velvety appearance. Mucosal edema or thickening, hyperemia, irregularities, defects, tears, and intraluminal masses are abnormal findings that may be encountered. Because of the concern for trauma to the rectum and small colon, the horse should be adequately sedated and restrained prior to preparation and examination of the distal alimentary tract.

The practitioner has several options when selecting endoscopic equipment. There are two basic types available: equipment based entirely on a fiber optic system, and equipment based on an electronic, video chip system. Both fiber optic and video systems are available from several manufacturers, with costs and availability of endoscopes suitable for examination of the equine alimentary system varying by manufacturer. Currently, companies that stock or will make endoscopes to the specifications required for examination of the equine alimentary system include Fujinon, Olympus, Pentax, and Schott. In 1987 Welch Allyn introduced an electronic endoscope designed for use in the horse. Unfortunately, the company no longer offers this equipment.

RADIOGRAPHY

Radiography of the alimentary tract can be a useful diagnostic tool in the evaluation of the oral, esophageal, and abdominal portions of the alimentary system. The size of the patient and the capabilities of radiographic equipment available will determine which procedures can be performed. As with all radiographic procedures, safety must be the primary consideration in the development and performance of a radiographic technique. Radiography of the abdomen of weanlings, yearlings, and adult horses requires a high-exposure technique and is accompanied by significant scatter radiation. Nonetheless, radiography often provides the most valuable information in the evaluation of certain cases.

Many portable units, with settings ranging from 60 kV and 30 mA to 90 kV and 15 mA, are suitable for making good-quality radiographs of the teeth, pharynx, and esophagus in adults and the entire alimentary tract in young foals. The use of rare earth screens with high-latitude film, in conjunction with a focused grid, will enhance the capabilities and quality of films made with a portable radiography unit. Also, techniques that take advantage of air–tissue interfaces, such as an oblique view of the teeth with the paranasal sinuses superimposed on the dorsal arcade of teeth, or the use of positive contrast media will yield diagnostic films at lower exposures.

Radiography is particularly useful in the evaluation of disorders of the thoracic esophagus and abdominal viscera in foals. In young foals, obstructions caused by meconium impactions, fecal impactions, displacements, volvulus, stricture, and congenital malformations can be deduced from the appearance of visceral distention and accumulation of gas. The presence of peritonitis or abscessation also may be determined in some cases. The use of barium contrast medium is useful in evaluating the esophagus, stomach, and proximal small intestine, and intestinal transit. With the aid of barium contrast enema, the distal colon and rectum can be outlined. Suspensions of 20 to 40 per cent barium sulfate, at 10 to 20 ml per kg, can be used to evaluate the esophagus, stomach, and small intestine. Disorders such as megaesophagus, cardia stricture, severe gastric ulceration, pyloric stricture, duodenal stricture, and cholangitis secondary to duodenitis can be diagnosed with contrast radiography.

ULTRASONOGRAPHY

Ultrasonography images certain soft tissue structures associated with the alimentary system and often is complementary to radiography. Limited penetration, 20 to 25 cm, and the loss of resolution at increased depth of penetration restrict the use of ultrasonography in the abdominal viscera. Thus, the technique is often limited to evaluating structures within 1 to 25 cm, and optimally 1 to 15 cm, of the body wall. Nonetheless, in many cases ultrasonography provides information not obtainable by other techniques.

It is preferable to clip the site to be examined, although in young foals and horses with a short hair coat this may not be necessary. Liberal application of ultrasound couplant gel to the site prior to the examination often yields satisfactory results without clipping. A sector scan head is preferable to a linear scan head, although use of the latter provides more information than not using it at all. The scan head frequency used depends on the size of the animal and the depth of the structure to be examined. Increasing the scan head frequency improves the resolution but decreases the depth of penetration. Thus, a scan head frequency of 5.0 to 7.5 MHz may be sufficient for examination of the foal abdomen or cervical esophagus in adult horses, whereas a scan head frequency of 2.0 to 5.0 MHz will usually be required to examine abdominal viscera in adults.

It is important to recognize that gas within the bowel stops the penetration of the sound waves, and thus no structures deep to the gas–bowel wall interface can be examined. This fact can be used to the practitioner's advantage, since clear visualization of proximal and distal bowel walls suggests that fluid, not gas, is present within the bowel lumen. Although this may be a normal finding, distention with fluid, or adynamic ileus, suggests an abnormality.

Ultrasonography of the abdomen should be performed in a standard manner, so that pertinent structures are examined each time. A protocol for examining the abdomen has been described by Rantanen.

Several abnormalities may be detected with ultrasonography, including peritoneal effusion, adhesions, abscesses, neoplasms, duodenal dilation or ileus, increased bowel wall thickness, dorsal displacement of the colon over the nephrosplenic ligament, and cecal impaction. The keys to an effective examination are good knowledge of the anatomy of the abdominal viscera, particularly within 20 cm of the body wall, and frequent use of this diagnostic tool. As with any procedure, the quality of the information obtained increases with the experience of the individual performing the procedure.

PARACENTESIS

Abdominal paracentesis is performed routinely in patients with suspected disorders of the abdominal viscera. The technique and sample evaluation are described elsewhere in this section (see page 238). Several slides should be prepared and air dried at the time the sample is collected, for several reasons. Cells can degenerate within the collection tube. Bacteria, which may have contaminated the sample during collection, can be phagocytosed within a few minutes, and thus on cytologic examination give the impression that intracellular bacteria are present within the peritoneal fluid. Also, it is useful to save unstained slides, which can be sent to a veterinary pathologist for further evaluation.

LAPAROSCOPY

Laparoscopy can offer important diagnostic information regarding the abdominal cavity while being little more invasive than percutaneous biopsy. The procedure does not entail general anesthesia or a prolonged recovery period but does require specialized, relatively expensive equipment. Required equipment includes a laparoscopic telescope, laparascopic cannula with trocar and obturator, fiber optic light source and cable, insufflator, and biopsy or manipulation instruments.

Laparoscopy has many indications but should always be preceded by a careful physical examination and abdominal palpation per rectum. Negative findings are common if one is merely exploring the abdomen for some suspected abnormality. If abdominocentesis is to be part of the diagnostic workup, it should be performed prior to laparoscopy, because of laparoscopy's effect on abdominal fluid values. A primary indication for laparoscopy is a palpable abdominal mass that requires further characterization. Biopsy or aspiration of these masses is readily accomplished with the proper instrumentation. Contraindications to laparoscopy include acute colic with distended viscus, adhesions to the area where the laparoscopic instruments are inserted, and diaphragmatic hernias.

Structures and landmarks that may be examined include the dorsal abdominal cavity (for the presence of metastatic lesions or adhesions), the serosal surfaces of the colon, small intestine and stomach, the urogenital tract, and the spleen and liver.

BIOPSY

The value of alimentary tract biopsy will depend on the site and method of biopsy, the amount of tissue obtained, and the completeness of the history and request provided to the pathologist who will examine the biopsy specimen. Because small biopsy samples are often submitted, it is essential that a thorough history and an indication of what disorder is suspected be provided. In addition to histologic evaluation, bacteriologic culture, electron microscopy, and direct and indirect fluorescent antibody staining can be performed.

The decision to perform a biopsy is often based on the ease of obtaining a sample and the relative value of the evaluation that can be made. Very small samples, such as those obtained with an endoscope biopsy instrument, provide limited information, although they are relatively easy to obtain. Full-thickness bowel specimens obtained via a ventral midline or flank laparotomy provide much more information but are more difficult to obtain.

The choice of tissue to biopsy is often difficult. Performing a biopsy through the endoscope allows the practitioner to choose the biopsy site based on the appearance of the mucosal surface, which is frequently the most reflective of an inflammatory disorder. When a biopsy specimen is obtained through a laparotomy, the serosal surface of the bowel may not reflect a disorder within the bowel wall, and thus the decision as to which portion of the bowel to biopsy may be random. In this case, several biopsy specimens should be obtained. The practitioner should determine the likely site of the alimentary tract disorder prior to biopsy, so that the site selected is most representative.

Rectal mucosal biopsy specimens are easily obtained. Many instruments can be used for this purpose; a uterine biopsy forceps works well. A fold of mucosa can readily be pinched between two fingers, and a sample of this tissue is obtained. The size of the sample is adequate for histologic and bacteriologic examination.

Full-thickness bowel specimens obtained at surgery are most valuable in evaluating the morphology of the bowel. Bacteriologic culture of a tissue sample should be performed when an inflammatory disorder is suspected.

FECAL EXAMINATION

Cytologic, biochemical, bacteriologic, immunologic, and electron microscopic evaluations can be performed on fecal samples. Additionally, observation of the consistency, color, the presence of foreign material such as sand or gravel, and the presence of parasites should be included in the examination of the alimentary system. In addition to fecal consistency, fecal particle size can be used to evaluate the efficiency of mastication, or colonic transit time. Increased particle size with loose or watery stool is suggestive of decreased colonic transit time.

Cytologic examinations are primarily used to evaluate the parasite burden of the animal. Ova of large and small strongyles, tapeworms, roundworms, and *Strongyloides westeri* are most common. Coccidia are occasionally observed. Examination of fecal white blood cells has been advocated in the evaluation of horses and foals with enterocolitis; however, these cells are very labile. Their presence in large numbers indicates that an inflammatory process is present and that the inflammation is in the distal colon or associated with decreased transit time.

Fecal occult blood testing has been recommended to diagnose gastric ulcers, duodenal ulcers, and other potentially hemorrhagic disorders of the alimentary tract. However, the test is of limited diagnostic value in the adult horse, since negative results can be obtained when a large amount of blood is present in the proximal portion of the GI tract. The sensitivity of most commercially available tests is poor, and negative results can occur in the setting of severe gastric bleeding.

Fecal culture is an essential component in the evaluation of many patients. Bacteriologic culture techniques for fecal samples routinely employ selective media that are designed to isolate *Salmonella*. These media include selenite broth, tetrathionate broth, brilliant green agar, and *Salmonella–Shigella* agar. Less selective media, McConkey's and eosin methylene blue agars, are desirable to culture other potential gram-negative bacterial pathogens such as *Escherichia coli*. The presence alone of *E. coli* in the feces does not determine its pathogenicity. Enterotoxigenic *E. coli* have been isolated from foals with diarrhea, but special tests must be performed to determine whether an isolate produces enterotoxin.

The presence of rotavirus in a fecal sample can be determined by use of an enzyme-linked immunosorbent assay (ELISA)[*] or an agglutination test.[†] Both assays test for the presence of viral particles in the feces. The ELISA is more sensitive than the agglutination test but less specific. Thus, the agglutination test is likely to give more false negative results, and the ELISA is likely to give more false positive results. The ELISA is more time-consuming and less convenient to perform than the agglutination test. When rotavirus is a concern, particularly as a farm problem, a reasonable approach is to screen fecal samples with the agglutination test, and repeat samples that are negative with the ELISA test.

ABSORPTION/DIGESTION TESTS

Tests that evaluate the ability of the equine intestinal tract to digest and absorb nutrients have a more limited clinical application than in human or small animal medicine but can be useful in the evaluation of horses with chronic weight loss, suspected small intestinal inflammation or neoplasia, gastric and small intestinal partial obstruction, and postoperative malabsorptive disorders. To date, the available, effective absorption tests that can be routinely performed in a clinical setting are limited to evaluation of the small intestine. For absorption tests to be diagnostic, the intestinal disorder either must be diffuse or must affect the delivery to and transit through the small intestine.

---

[*]Rotazyme II, Abbott Labs., North Chicago, IL
[†]Rotalex, Medical Technologies Corp., Somerset, NJ

Maldigestion tests are performed to evaluate exocrine pancreatic function and small intestinal mucosal brush border disaccharidase activity. Pancreatic exocrine deficiencies have not been described in the horse, probably because equine pancreatic secretions consist primarily of water and bicarbonate and have less enzymatic activity than in monogastric species. Mucosal brush border disaccharidase-related maldigestion is relevant in viral and bacterial enteridites of foals, particularly rotavirus and coronavirus enteritides. Lactose tolerance can be tested by administering a 20 per cent solution of D-lactose at a dosage of 0.5 to 1 gm per kg. This dosage should result in an approximate doubling of the serum glucose level within 60 minutes of administration.

Clinically applicable absorption tests include the D-glucose and D-xylose absorption tests. The glucose absorption test is relatively easy and inexpensive to perform. However, cellular uptake and metabolism of glucose, as well as intestinal absorption, influence the results and thus are undesirable variables. The D-xylose absorption test measures intestinal absorptive capacity more directly. The results of both tests, though, are affected by gastric emptying rate and small intestinal transit time. Absorption and digestion tests should be performed following an 18- to 24-hour fast, and should be interpreted as reflecting GI transit as well as intestinal digestion and absorption.

The D-glucose and D-xylose tests are performed similarly. Following an 18- to 24-hour fast, a 10 per cent solution of D-glucose or D-xylose, 0.5 to 1 gm per kg, is administered via nasogastric tube. For the measurement of glucose, blood is collected in sodium fluoride tubes, and for the measurement of D-xylose, blood is collected in heparinized tubes. Samples are taken at 0, 30, 60, 90, 120, 150, 180, 210, and 240 minutes following administration.

Blood glucose levels should peak at twice the resting values within 120 minutes and return to baseline by 6 hours. Peak levels of D-xylose normally range from 20 to 25 mg per dl and occur 60 to 120 minutes following administration. The normal curve resembles an inverted V. Delay or flattening of this curve may reflect delayed gastric emptying, increased intestinal transit time, or impaired intestinal absorption. Accurate interpretation of the results of these tests will depend on the results of other diagnostic evaluations. Additionally, different types of diet have been shown to significantly affect the height, although not the shape, of the absorption curves. In general, diets that have a higher digestible energy content result in a lower peak in the curve.

Other absorption and intestinal function tests can be performed but require the use of radioisotopes. Thus, their use is restricted to facilities that can measure and safely handle the disposal of these isotopes. Intestinal fat absorption has been evaluated in the horse by administering ^{3}H-oleic acid by nasogastric tube and measuring plasma ^{3}H by liquid scintillation. The injection of $^{51}CrCl_3$, which binds to serum albumin, and measurement of fecal ^{51}Cr has been performed to document enteric protein loss.

Supplemental Readings

Fischer, A. T., Lloyd, K., Carlson, G. P., et al.: Diagnostic laparoscopy in the horse. J. Am. Vet. Med. Assoc., 189:289–292, 1986.

Fischer, A. T., Kerr, L. Y., O'Brien, T. R.: Radiographic diagnosis of gastrointestinal disorders in the foal. Vet. Radiol., 28:42–48, 1987.

Merritt, A. M., Kohn, C. W., Ramberg, C. F., et al.: Plasma clearance of ^{51}Cr albumin into the intestinal tract of normal and chronically diarrheal horses. Am. J. Vet. Res., 38:1769, 1977.

Pearson, E. G., Smith, B. B., McKim, J. M.: Fecal blood determinations and interpretations. In: Proceedings of the 33rd Annual Meeting of the American Association of Equine Practitioners, 1987, pp. 77–83.

Rantanen, N. W.: Diseases of the abdomen. Vet. Clin. North Am. (Equine Pract. Diagn. Ultrasound), 2:67–88, 1986.

Roberts, M. C., Norman, P.: A re-evaluation of the D$^+$-xylose absorption test in the horse. Equine Vet. J., 11:239–243, 1979.

Dysphagia

Christopher M. Brown, EAST LANSING, MICHIGAN

Strictly defined, dysphagia means inability to swallow. However, the term is often applied to disorders in which the horse experiences difficulty or inability to eat. As such, problems with prehension and chewing as well as swallowing are considered. For clinical practice this broader usage is more appropriate as many of these horses present with "trouble eating" rather than an owner's complaint of "trouble swallowing." In this chapter the broad consideration will be used. A detailed consideration of specific dental and related problems is not included (see *Current Therapy in Equine Medicine 2*, p. 6, for dental problems).

EVALUATION

Difficulty in eating can be caused by a wide range of diseases. The final diagnosis depends on an accurate data base, generated from the history, observation, physical findings, and the results of special tests and ancillary investigations.

HISTORY

Particular attention should be paid to the duration of onset of the problem and the rate, sudden or gradual. Most problems arising from trauma are sudden in onset and often improve initially. On the other hand, many neurologic problems are gradual in onset and worsen with time. Concurrent problems in other horses should be determined. Similar signs in others suggest common causes, such as infectious agents or exposure to toxic substances, such as moldy corn or lead.

OBSERVATION

Observation is an invaluable and essential aspect of the evaluation of any horse with dysphagia. It is important to determine if the horse actually wants to eat and drink or is simply disinterested. Many ill horses are inappetent; on the other hand, many dysphagic horses are hungry but cannot eat. Watching the horse attempting to eat will give valuable clues to the causes. Can the horse grasp the food and move it around in its mouth? Can the horse chew? Does food come down the nose? Does the horse cough when eating? In addition, the stall should be examined for chewed and unchewed food. In the stalls of dysphagic horses that aspirate food into the larynx and then cough, there is often food splattered around the walls near the manger and food trough. Water buckets are also worth examining: unchewed or partially chewed food may be floating in the water.

PHYSICAL EXAMINATION

In addition to a general physical examination, particular attention should be paid to the head and neck, including an evaluation of the cranial nerves. Rabies is a potential cause of dysphagia, and therefore, in cases of recent onset, the examination may be postponed or performed with the examiner wearing protective clothing and gloves. The examiner must have an adequate titer of rabies antibodies. This is important, because a detailed oral examination, including visual and manual evaluation, is vital.

ADDITIONAL TESTS

If the history and physical examination have not revealed the cause of the problem, then endoscopic and radiographic evaluation of the pharynx, larynx, guttural pouches, and upper esophagus may be helpful. Barium swallow examination is a simple and useful technique that may be used to outline anatomical abnormalities radiographically, or to demonstrate pharyngeal dysfunction when there are no apparent anatomical lesions. In addition, laboratory evaluations, including hematology, serum biochemistries, aspiration, and cytology or culture of lesions, and in a few cases cerebrospinal fluid analysis, may be helpful.

CAUSES AND THERAPY

Eating is a complex integrated function that can be divided into three phases: prehension, chewing, and swallowing. Damage to the sensory, motor, or mechanical components of this process may lead to difficulty in eating.

PREHENSION

Horses have a profuse sensory innervation of the muzzle and well-developed facial muscles, enabling excellent grasping ability with the lips. Prehension depends on good motor control of the tongue and facial muscles integrated by sensory input from the oral mucosa, lips, and by sight. Damage to one or more of the neurological or muscular components or damage to the mechanical components (i.e., incisor teeth and jaws) may cause prehension problems. Facial paralysis, usually unilateral, is fairly common in horses. The nerves are vulnerable as they pass over the body of the masseter muscle. In addition, infections of the guttural pouch may lead to facial nerve paralysis. Occasionally horses with polyneuritis equi (neuritis of the cauda equina) may have cranial nerve lesions. Any lesion of the central nervous system could potentially damage the sensory or motor component of prehension, but one would expect additional signs referrable to these lesions, not merely prehension abnormalities.

In unilateral facial paralysis the muscles of the lips, nostrils, and cheek are flacid on the affected side. If the nerve damage is close to the origin of the nerve, the muscles moving the ear and facial muscles of the eye may be affected. The muzzle deviates away from the affected side and the lip droops on the affected side. Food accumulates between the cheek teeth and cheek, forming an obvious bulge. Food drops from the mouth from this area. If only unilaterally affected, these horses manage to eat adequately to maintain body weight. Bilateral cases of facial paralysis are rare, but affected horses may have more difficulty eating and may lose weight.

Tongue dysfunction due to trauma or following damage to cranial nerve XII could also cause problems with prehension, chewing, and swallowing. Tongue paralysis is rare. Tongue lacerations are frequent, but even very severe ones heal well, and although there may be a period of difficulty in eating, the problem usually resolves in 1 or 2 weeks. Mandibular or maxillary fractures are fairly uncommon but may lead to difficulty in prehension, particularly if the incisor teeth are involved. The diagnosis is based on clinical, physical, and radiographic findings.

Basal ganglial lesions may develop in horses exposed to yellow star thistles or Russian knapweed (see *Current Therapy in Equine Medicine 2*, p. 675). These horses are unable to prehend food and unable to move the bolus to the pharynx. They can, however, swallow. There is no specific therapy.

Most horses with the above problems are interested in eating and make frequent but frustrated attempts to do so. They may bury their muzzles in hay or grain, attempting to drive food into the pharynx. When drinking they may immerse their heads in water to the level of the eyes.

Management of horses with prehension problems depends on the cause and how much food they can eat. Fractures or severe lacerations may require surgical correction. Some traumatic lesions may resolve with time, perhaps with concomitant anti-inflammatory medication. Problems secondary to neurologic abnormalities may be untreatable. Often the only course of action is to provide supportive therapy and see if the problem resolves with time. If the animal is suspected of having a specific disease, such as protozoal myeloencephalitis, then specific therapy may be indicated. In all cases, nutritional support may be needed if intake is inadequate. This is best achieved by means of an indwelling stomach tube (see p. 724). The food should be a slurry made from commercial complete horse food pellets. This will provide adequate calories, and additional water can be given down the tube.

Chewing

Difficulty in chewing is usually due to dental disease. This can range from retained deciduous premolars in young horses to marked chronic gingival and buccal erosions resulting from abnormal tooth wear in older horses. A detailed oral examination is usually enough to diagnose the problem. Therapy for these problems was described in previous editions of this book (see *Current Therapy in Equine Medicine 2*, p. 6).

Occasional causes of difficulty in chewing include fracture of the mandible, lesions of the temporomandibular joint, and atrophy of the masseter muscles.

Horses with severe problems with chewing, in which the lesions may resolve, may benefit from supportive nutritional care as outlined earlier for horses with prehension problems.

Swallowing

Swallowing is a complex integrated activity. A bolus is initially formed at the back of the tongue and is pressed against the hard palate. It is forced caudally, the oropharynx relaxes, and the soft palate elevates, sealing the palatopharyngeal arch. The tongue moves caudally, pushing the bolus into the oropharynx. The hyoid swings rostrodorsally and the larynx and common pharynx are drawn forward. The epiglottis flips back to help seal the glottis. The bolus enters the common pharynx and the constrictor muscles of the pharynx squeeze it caudally through the relaxed cranial esophageal sphincter into the esophagus.

This sequence of events relies on motor and sensory components of cranial nerves V, IX, X, XI, and XII, together with their central integration and coordination. Abnormalities of the nerves of this area or structural alterations of adjacent tissues can lead to varying degrees of dysfunction and dysphagia.

Problems with swallowing can be divided in three broad groups based on cause: neurologic, muscular, and mechanical. Each is described below.

NEUROLOGIC CAUSES

Neurologic causes can be roughly divided into central and peripheral lesions. Central lesions causing abnormal swallowing can occur almost anywhere along the integrating pathways and from the cerebral cortex to the cranial nerve nuclei of the brain stem. Thus, swallowing problems may occur with cerebral trauma; viral encephalitides such as rabies and equine encephalitis; protozoal myeloencephalitis; toxic neuropathies such as leukoencephalomalacia (moldy corn poisoning) and lead poisoning; brain abscesses; and occasionally migrating helminth parasites. Although dysphagia may be a significant clinical sign in these settings, often other signs predominate. Depending on the cause, other signs may include altered mental status, ataxia and weakness, and additional cranial nerve signs such as head tilt, facial paralysis, and blindness. A thorough neurological evaluation will alert the clinician to the possible cause. Again, the examiner should take precautions against the possibility of rabies.

Damage to the peripheral nerves involved in swallowing most commonly occurs as they pass adjacent to the guttural pouch. Most frequently such nerve damage results from extension of fungal and bacterial infections into tissues around the pouches. Several cases of dysphagia have also resulted following the use of irritating irrigation solutions for the treatment of guttural pouch infections. Most typically iodine–hydrogen peroxide solutions have been implicated.

The diagnosis of dysphagia of neural origin is based on endoscopic examination of the pharynx and the guttural pouch. Radiographic evaluation may be of some help if involvement of the bones of the skull base is suspected.

Therapy for neurological causes of swallowing problems is often unrewarding. Some problems, such as leukoencephalomalacia, are refractory or untreatable. Others, such as guttural pouch infections, may be treatable, but often significant dysfunction persists following resolution of the inciting cause. Generally speaking, if the neurological problem has been present for 2 to 3 weeks without signs of improvement, the prognosis is poor.

MUSCULAR PROBLEMS

Myopathies and muscular dysfunctions are rare causes of dysphagia in horses. Occasional foals with nutritional myopathy secondary to vitamin E and selenium deficiency may experience problems suckling and swallowing. However, they also usually show signs of generalized myopathy, with weakness and dyspnea. In these cases evaluation of serum levels of vitamin E, selenium, and creatinine kinase are valuable diagnostic aids. Therapy with vitamin E and selenium may be helpful, but aspiration pneumonia may be a significant limiting problem.

In some areas of the United States botulism is a fairly common cause of muscular dysfunction in horses. In addition to exhibiting some degree of dysphagia, these animals often are weak or become very weak with minimal exercise. Clinical signs are suspicious and EMG evaluation may be a valuable diagnostic aid. In some locales where the disease is frequent, specific antisera are available. Therapy is expensive. Nutritional supportive therapy administered through a stomach tube is also indicated.

MECHANICAL FACTORS

Mechanical causes of dysphagia relate to abnormalities of structures involved in swallowing, such as the soft palate and hyoid apparatus, or of structures around the pharynx, such as the retropharyngeal lymph nodes.

Disorders of the soft palate are uncommon. Occasionally foals are born with a cleft soft palate and are unable to seal the palatopharyngeal arch. They have difficulty suckling, and when they swallow, milk escapes down their nostrils. The diagnosis is based on clinical signs and is confirmed endoscopically. The cleft is not easily visualized on oral examination. Successful surgical corrections have been reported, but many attempts are not successful. These foals are frequently euthanized. In adult horses, occasional thickening of the soft palate occurs leading to dysphagia. The cause is not known, and biopsies of the affected palate indicate chronic inflammation. The condition is suspected when endoscopy reveals the soft palate bulging up into the nasal pharynx. However, a barium swallow examination is invaluable, as the ventral surface of the soft palate will be outlined, allowing assessment of its thickness. For those unfamiliar with the technique and interpretation of pharyngeal radiographs with barium swallow, it is suggested that a normal horse be studied at the same time as the patient.

Because the cause of the soft palate thickening is unknown, specific therapy is not available. Experience with many of these horses suggests that the problem resolves with time. Affected horses rarely develop malnutrition, and therefore supportive therapy is not usually needed.

Pharyngeal neoplasia is uncommon in horses and is a very rare cause of dysphagia. Occasionally horses with cutaneous lymphoproliferative diseases develop multiple large (1 to 2 cm) masses in the pharynx and may be dysphagic. Endoscopic biopsy and radiology will assist in the diagnosis.

Pharyngeal trauma, usually following vigorous unsuccessful attempts at stomach intubation or aggressive use of the balling gun, may cause severe pharyngeal edema and swelling, leading to dysphagia. Endoscopic evaluation is usually enough for diagnosis. Therapy is empirical. Nutritional support administered through a stomach tube may be needed if the horse cannot eat; often nonsteroidal anti-inflammatory agents are used as well. The prognosis is usually good unless the pharynx has ruptured and a local infection has resulted.

An occasional cause of dysphagia in young horses is a subepiglottic cyst. These cysts are probably congenital, but the cause is unknown. Large cysts may interfere with normal swallowing. The diagnosis is based on endoscopic and radiographic findings and treatment is surgical (see p. 281).

Infection and abscessation of retropharyngeal lymph nodes may cause sufficient swelling to occlude the pharyngeal lumen and cause problems in swallowing. The most common cause in young horses is *Streptococcus equi* infection (strangles). Thus, the disease is often present in many young horses on affected premises, although only a few will develop retropharyngeal abscessation and dysphagia. The diagnosis is based on the history, clinical signs, epidemiologic evidence, endoscopic findings, radiography, and culture results. Therapy depends on the severity of the problem. Some animals may be dyspneic as well as dysphagic and a tracheostomy may be needed to relieve the dyspnea. Some may require anesthesia and surgical drainage of the retropharyngeal area. Drainage is not easy and should only be attempted in severe, life-threatening situations. Most horses will improve with antibiotic therapy. It may be useful to begin with intravenous penicillin, 20,000 IU per kg four times daily. After 4 to 6 days therapy can be changed to procaine penicillin G given intramuscularly twice daily at 20,000 IU per kg per day. These animals may need therapy for 3 to 4 weeks. In addition, nutritional support may be necessary.

A similar problem may result if guttural pouch empyema develops and the drainage from the pouch is poor or nonexistent. In these cases the pouch fills with purulent material, which again leads to pharyngeal occlusion. Dysphagia may result not only from the physical pressure but also from cranial nerve involvement. Surgical drainage of the pouch and appropriate antibiotics are indicated.

Chronic otitis media in horses may lead to osteoproliferation at the articulation of the stylohyoid and the base of the skull. Over time ankylosis occurs, which may limit the movement of the hyoid apparatus and cause some problems in swallowing. More often these horses develop problems when the ankylosis fractures and acute signs develop, probably due to a combination of mechanical and neurologic causes. The diagnosis is based on endoscopic examination of the pouch and radiography. Therapy at this stage is unrewarding.

Supplemental Readings

Baum, K. H., Modransky, P. D., Halpern, N. E., and Banish, L. D.: Dysphagia in horses: The differential diagnosis. Part I. Compend. Cont. Ed. Pract. Vet., *10*:1301, 1988.

Freeman, D. E.: Diagnosis and treatment of diseases of the guttural pouch: Parts I and II. Compend. Cont. Ed. Pract. Vet., 2:S3, S25, 1980.

Wagner, P. C., Rantanen, N. W., and Grant, B. D.: Differential diagnosis of dysphagia in the horse. Mod. Vet. Pract., 60:1029, 1979.

Esophageal Obstruction

Eleanor M. Green, COLUMBIA, MISSOURI

The primary function of the esophagus is transport of a food bolus and secretions from the pharynx to the stomach, and prevention of retrograde movement of both esophageal and gastrointestinal (GI) contents. Esophageal dysfunctions include abnormalities of esophageal transit of materials aborally and failure to retard retrogression of esophageal contents in an oral direction. Esophageal disorders are categorized as obstructive, inflammatory, traumatic, neoplastic, congenital, and motility disturbances. Virtually all esophageal disorders are associated with some degree of esophageal obstruction, which can be divided into intraluminal obstruction, intrinsic narrowing (stricture), extraluminal compression, and diverticula.

CLINICAL SIGNS

The clinical manifestations of esophageal disease range from subtle to obvious, depending on the anatomical site affected, the severity and duration of the condition, and coexisting secondary problems (Table 1). The classic clinical manifestation of esophageal obstruction is dysphagia (Table 2). Feed material mixed with saliva is regurgitated through the nares during, shortly after, or hours after feeding. The relationship between a swallow and regurgitation is diagnostically significant (see Table 1). At the onset, mechanical obstructions may allow passage of liquids but not solid materials, while abnormal transport of both solid and liquid substances oc-

TABLE 1. CLINICAL SIGNS OF ESOPHAGEAL DISEASE

Sign	Definition	Clinical Implication
Dysphagia	Difficult swallowing	Relentless, progressive: Anatomic disorder
		Episodic, nonprogressive: Motility disorder
Obstruction	Inability to transport a bolus (food or liquid) past an affected esophageal segment	Intrinsic obstruction
		Extrinsic compression
Inability to initiate swallows	Inability to form and transport a bolus	Central nervous system disease
Regurgitation	Retrograde flow of swallowed food or liquid into the nasopharynx or oropharynx	Anatomic disorder
		Motility disorder
		Timing in relation to the swallow is important to indicate the level of the esophageal lesion
Aspiration	Contamination of tracheobronchial tree and lungs by esophageal or gastric contents	Secondary to many esophageal disorders
Melena	Gastrointestinal bleeding	Esophagitis
		Esophageal ulcer
		Neoplasia

TABLE 2. DISORDERS OF THE SWALLOWING MECHANISM

Dysfunction	Definition	Clinical Implication

Pharyngeal dysphagia	Difficulty moving food bolus from pharynx to cervical esophagus
	Feed and water exit through nasal cavity immediately following each swallow
		Intrinsic obstruction:
		  Proximal esophageal obstruction
		  Proximal neoplasia
		  Pharyngitis
		Extrinsic compression:
		  Lymphadenopathy—retropharyngeal or cranial cervical lymph node
		  Proximal neoplasia
		  Guttural pouch distention
		UES motility disorder:
		  Failure to open during a swallow
		  Failure to close following a swallow

Esophageal dysphagia	Difficulty moving food bolus from UES to LES
	Feed or feed and water exit through the nasal cavity
	Unless the esophagus is fully impacted with material, there is delay in regurgitation for variable periods following a swallow
		Intrinsic obstruction:
		  Feed impaction
		  Foreign body
		  Stricture
		  Diverticulum
		  Neoplasia
		Extrinsic compression:
		  Lymphadenopathy—caudal deep cervical or mediastinal lymph node
		  Neoplasia
		  Vascular ring anomaly
		Motility disorder:
		  Esophagitis
		  Megaesophagus
		  Achalasia
		  UES dysfunction
		  Neuromuscular disorders
		  Myopathy
		  Vagus neuropathy

Esophagogastric dysphagia	Difficulty moving food bolus from distal esophagus to stomach
	Feed or feed and water exit through the nasal cavity
	Unless the esophagus is fully impacted, there is a considerable delay in regurgitation after swallows
		Intrinsic obstruction:
		  Distal feed impaction
		  Distal foreign body
		  Distal neoplasia
		Motility disorder:
		  LES hypotension
		  Esophageal spasm
		  Achalasia

Abbreviations: UES, upper esophageal sphincter; LES, lower esophageal sphincter.

curs early in the course of esophageal motility disorders. Bile-stained regurgitated material, as opposed to gastric fluid alone, indicates a small intestinal origin.

Other clinical signs of esophageal obstruction are relatively nonspecific, such as ptyalism and halitosis. Esophageal pain is suggested by repeated deglutition and retching. Intermittent extension or flexion of the neck is also characteristic. Focal cervical swelling may be indicative of an obstruction of the cervical esophagus. More extensive swelling can indicate dilation of the entire cervical esophagus. Warm and painful swelling indicates cervical cellulitis, while esophageal perforation is accompanied by subcutaneous emphysema or a draining fistulous tract.

Abrupt onset implies an acute impaction, such as a feed or foreign body obstruction. An insidious onset is more compatible with a developing esophageal stricture, megaesophagus, or an expanding neoplasm or lymph node. Weight loss indicates chronicity.

DIAGNOSTIC PROCEDURES

Nasogastric Intubation

Passage of a nasogastric tube is an inexpensive field technique that provides immediate evidence of an esophageal obstruction and suggests its approximate location. The procedure is not without danger, as a compromised esophagus can be readily perforated. Advancement of a nasogastric tube to the stomach does not preclude the possibility of an obstruction. In some cases the tube may be diverted beyond partial obstructions, strictures, or diverticula, or even through an esophageal tear.

Esophageal Radiography

Radiographic evaluation of the esophagus verifies and further defines esophageal obstruction. Portable radiographic equipment can often generate a diagnostic study of the cervical region in most adult horses and a complete study in foals. Tranquilizers are used only when essential and for specific indications, for example, to eliminate esophageal spasm.

Lateral projections of the pharynx, cervical, thoracic, and, rarely, the abdominal esophagus make up the survey radiographs. The normal resting esophagus is collapsed, empty, and radiographically indistinct. Small amounts of intraluminal air may be transiently present. The esophageal silhouette may be outlined by pathologic accumulations of air, fluid, and feed material. Impacted feed material appears as a dense granular pattern, while radiodense foreign objects may be clearly visualized. Luminal obstructions and motility disorders result in intraluminal collection of air. Esophageal perforation leads to subcutaneous emphysema, apparent as extraluminal radiolucency. Thoracic structures may be displaced by an enlarged esophagus.

Although some esophageal obstructions can be fully defined on survey radiographs, contrast esophagography often provides greater clarification. The most useful contrast agent is barium sulfate,* which can be administered per os (PO) or through a nasogastric tube. Barium paste† offers the advantage of better adherence to, and therefore better depiction of, the esophageal mucosa. The dose of either form of barium varies widely according to the disorder, degree of esophageal dilation, and site of obstruction; however, 60 to 180 ml is generally adequate. With a normal contrast esophagram, the esophagus is collapsed and the longitudinal folds are outlined. An obstruction may disrupt the flow of contrast material, and radiolucent foreign bodies may be outlined. Esophagitis is recognized by thickening of the longitudinal folds, pooling of contrast material commensurate with the degree of motility disturbance, and filling defects where contrast material adheres to ulcerated areas. A narrowing of the contrast column is compatible with stricture, extrinsic compression, or neoplasia. Dilated areas adjacent to narrowed areas indicate pre- and poststenotic dilation, while extensive dilation signifies megaesophagus. Diverticula usually appear as eccentric, contrast agent–filled spaces, although contrast material may readily flow past a feed-filled diverticulum. Radiographic evidence of dysphagia is provided by the presence of contrast material within the tracheal lumen (Figs. 1A, B). Circumferential lesions such as strictures and eccentric lesions such as diverticula, large ulcers, and extrinsic compression are better demonstrated after administration of up to 500 ml of contrast material through a cuffed nasogastric tube, under pressure. Feeding contrast agent mixed with grain offers a superior method to evaluate esophageal transit of a food bolus. The normal esophageal transit time for solid substances is a matter of seconds. If repeated radiographs show that the contrast-accentuated food bolus has moved only minimally, impaired esophageal transit is confirmed. Common causes of delayed transit in-

---

*Redi-Paque, Burns-Biotec Labs., Inc., Oakland, CA
†Esophotrast, Armour Pharmaceutical Co., Kankakee, IL

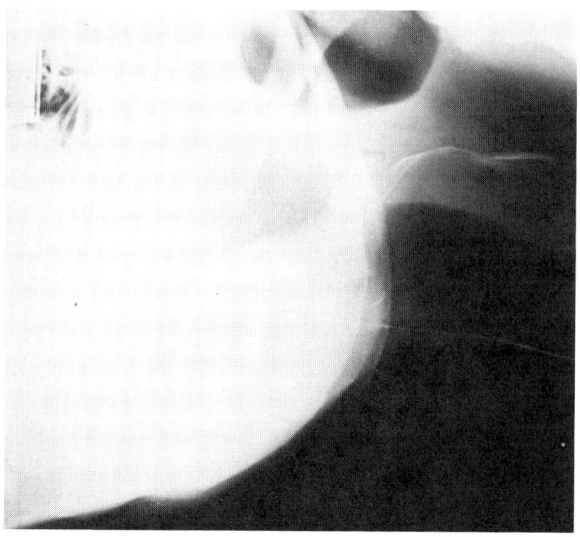
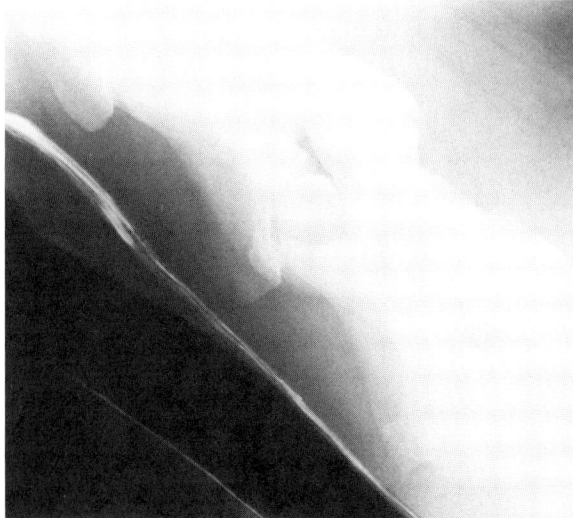

Figure 1. (*A*) Contrast esophagogram of the upper esophagus and pharynx of an adult horse with a history of chronic dysphagia and clinical evidence of aspiration pneumonia. The esophagogram demonstrates a normal outline of the esophagus; however, excessive contrast material has gained access to the trachea, the ventral aspect of which is well outlined. In the absence of a mechanical obstruction, a functional obstruction was suspected. With normal esophageal peristalsis, normal laryngeal function, and radiographic evidence of closure of the upper esophageal sphincter, the diagnostic entities to be ruled out included a glossopharyngeal nerve lesion, a brain stem lesion, or failure of the upper esophageal sphincter to open adequately during the pharyngeal stage of swallowing. (*B*) Contrast esophagogram of the midcervical esophagus of the same horse as in *A*. Contrast material is present throughout the entire length of the cervical esophagus. The cervical esophagus is of a normal diameter, and normal longitudinal folds are outlined by contrast material.

clude postobstructive focal esophagitis, stricture, and motility disorders.

Double-contrast esophagography entails insufflation of the esophagus with contrast agent and air. Focal narrowing, pre- and poststenotic dilation, mucosal lesions, and small neoplasms are accentuated.

Suspicion of esophageal perforation warrants the use of a water-soluble contrast agent.*,† Periesophageal contrast material supports the tentative diagnosis (Fig. 2). If perforation is not observed, the study should be repeated with barium.

Esophagoscopy

Esophageal endoscopy demonstrates lesions not defined by esophagography. At the same time, diagnostic samples such as biopsy specimens, mucosal scrapings, or refluxed gastric fluid can be collected for laboratory analysis. Transendoscopic treatment procedures include foreign body retrieval and neodymium:yttrium-aluminum-garnet (Nd-YAG) laser surgery.

Physical restraint alone is optimal for esopha-

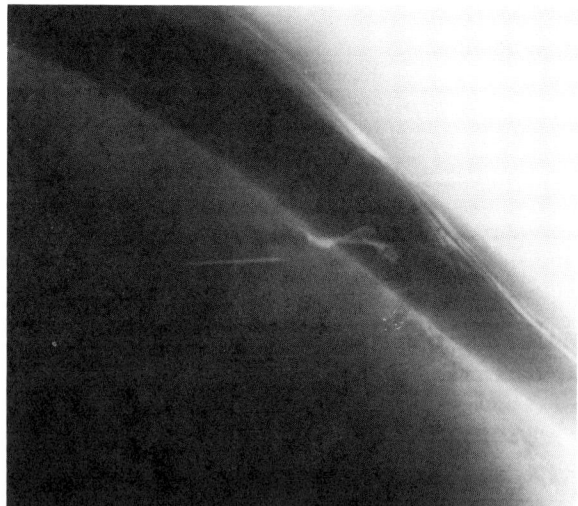

Figure 2. Contrast esophagogram of an adult horse with a perforated midcervical esophagus. Contrast material has gained access to the periesophageal tissues through the esophageal perforation. The penetrating foreign object can be visualized, associated with subcutaneous emphysema. The contrast study was necessary to confirm that the esophagus was involved, because all other radiographic findings on the survey film could have been explained by a foreign object penetrating only the overlying skin.

---

*Gastrograffin, E. R. Squibb & Sons, Inc., Princeton, NJ
†Oral Hypaque Solution, Winthrop Labs., New York, NY

goscopy so that esophageal motility is preserved. For less tractable horses and during more prolonged procedures, xylazine hydrochloride,* detomidine hydrochloride,† or various drug combinations may be advantageous. The esophagus should be examined as the endoscope is advanced and withdrawn.

The whitish pink esophageal mucosa typically forms longitudinal folds that become more prominent distal to the upper (cranial) esophageal sphincter. Progression of the endoscope through the normally collapsed, elastic esophagus causes the mucosa to form multiple transverse folds that, along with the normal longitudinal folds, disappear with insufflation. Normal luminal narrowing of the esophagus may be appreciated at several levels, including the postpharyngeal area, thoracic inlet, heart base, and terminal esophagus. Visible peristalsis, which routinely succeeds swallows and distention, is more evident in the distal esophagus. The lower (caudal) esophageal sphincter is usually closed, but opens in response to a peristaltic wave. For completeness, gastroscopic examination accompanies esophagoscopy, because gastric lesions accompany many esophageal disorders.

An esophageal obstruction can be accurately localized endoscopically and the obstructing substance discerned. Fluid that has collected proximal to the obstruction may require removal by suction to improve visibility. Extreme dilation and poor motility suggest chronicity. After the obstruction has been alleviated the esophageal mucosa can be evaluated. Circumferential, deep mucosal ulceration characteristically leads to stricture formation. Once formed, a stricture appears endoscopically as a narrowed site that cannot be distended with insufflation. Longitudinal or transverse folds (or both) likewise persist when the esophagus is distended. The mucosa may or may not be disrupted. Significant quantities of feed and fluid material can be accommodated by the proximally enlarged esophagus.

Other obstructive disorders have distinctive endoscopic features. Luminal stenosis without mucosal lesions is typical of extrinsic compression. With diverticula, the intact mucosa forms a saclike evagination from the lumen. The extent of injury or esophageal perforation can be determined endoscopically. Esophagitis may be identified by reddened areas resulting from inflammation and by thickened longitudinal folds. Linear mucosal ulcers that progressively worsen toward the cardia and visible retrograde movement of gastric fluid through the cardia into the distal esophagus verify a reflux esophagitis. White or green-tinged elevated mucosal plaques and nodular ulcerated mucosa are features of fungal esophagitis. A motility disorder is suggested by extreme distention before and after insufflation, absence of peristalsis, and impaired clearance of swallowed materials. With megaesophagus and other motility disorders, it is common to find impacted feed recurrently in an esophagus in which the obstruction is easily resolved. Neoplasms may be characterized by visible mucosal ulcers or nodular masses. Transendoscopically applied Lugol's solution (3 per cent) can be used to differentiate between normal mucosa, which stains brown, and inflamed or neoplastic mucosa, which does not stain. Toluidine blue (1 per cent) will stain early lesions of squamous cell carcinoma.

CLINICAL PATHOLOGY

Esophageal obstruction is associated with excessive loss of salivary secretions. Hyponatremic, hypochloremic, metabolic alkalosis may develop. The acid-base disturbance induced by diminished feed and water intake somewhat offsets this alkalosis. Consequently, the acid–base status accompanying esophageal obstruction can be highly variable, though rarely severe. Blood volume and electrolyte homeostasis are maintained initially by decreased urine volume, decreased fecal volume, and transcellular ion and fluid shifts. Hemoconcentration and severe electrolyte and acid–base imbalances signify a chronic state in which compensatory mechanisms are overwhelmed.

THERAPY

Acquired intraluminal obstruction is the most commonly diagnosed esophageal disorder in the horse. Although a diversity of substances has been recognized, impacted feed material is found most frequently. Esophageal obstructions are not immediately life-threatening and may even resolve without treatment. Many more cases are likely undetected, even by the owner, than require veterinary attention; nevertheless, prompt and effective treatment of the clinical case is vital to thwart complications. Esophageal obstructions should be handled initially as emergencies in order to limit esophageal spasm at the site of the mass, gradual drying of the impaction, resultant esophageal inflammation, receptive relaxation distal to the mass, progressive dilation of the proximal esophagus to accommodate increas-

---

*Rompun, Mobay Corp., Shaunee, KS
†Dormosedan, SmithKline Beecham, Animal Health, Exton, PA

ing quantities of ingested and secreted materials, eventual loss of esophageal motor function, and aspiration associated with dysphagia. The major treatment goals are resolution of the obstruction, maintenance of homeostasis, and prevention of secondary complications (Table 3).

REMOVAL OF THE OBSTRUCTION

The basic approach to removal of the obstruction is gentle esophageal lavage in conjunction with restriction of ingestion. To facilitate patient acceptance of treatment, to encourage lavage fluid to flow rostrally, and to promote relaxation of esophageal musculature, horses should be sedated with xylazine hydrochloride, detomidine hydrochloride, or either agent combined with butorphanol tartrate.°

Lavage of a feed impaction entails passage of a nasogastric tube to the site of obstruction, where small increments of warm water are repetitively pumped against the impaction with either a stomach pump or dose syringe. The lavaged fluid either egresses through the nares of the lowered head or it can be removed by suction through an independently placed suction tube. Patience and gentleness are usually rewarding. If immediate success is not achieved, the horse can be intermittently placed into a stall with no access to feed, water, or bedding. Because the desire to eat customarily persists, a muzzle may be required. Esophageal peristalsis may be capable of propelling the softened mass through the esophagus, so that alternate lavage and rest ordinarily lead to resolution of the impaction.

Numerous modifications of the lavage technique can be employed. A cuffed nasogastric tube° will facilitate lavage under increased pressure, which should be applied cautiously. The inflated cuff also promotes the flow of lavaged material through the tube, bypassing the pharynx and discouraging aspiration. Continuous lavage is achievable by means of a smaller tube inserted through the larger, cuffed tube. A small-bore, cuffed endotracheal tube may be used in lieu of the cuffed nasogastric tube as a guide for the smaller lavage tube. Without the use of cuffed tubes, increased lavage pressure can also be achieved by applying external pressure to the cervical esophagus above the obstructed site. Impactions of the cervical esophagus may be amenable to external massage.

Before surgery is undertaken in the refractory case, the conservative approach could be continued with the patient anesthetized. Placement of an endotracheal tube and positioning of the patient with the head lowered negate the risk of aspiration. More vigorous lavage in a more relaxed esophagus with an immobile animal can be very productive.

Theoretically, lubricating agents like mineral oil or softening agents like dioctyl sodium sulfosuccinate (DSS) could be beneficial in the refrac-

---

°Torbugesic, Bristol Labs., Syracuse, NY

°Bivona, Inc., Gary, IN

TABLE 3. TREATMENT OF ACQUIRED ESOPHAGEAL OBSTRUCTION

Problem	Treatment
RESOLUTION OF THE OBSTRUCTION	
Esophageal spasm	Sedation with xylazine, detomidine, acepromazine, or drug combinations.
Esophageal pain	Analgesia with NSAID, xylazine, detomidine, torbugesic, or drug combinations.
Esophageal feed impaction	*Esophageal lavage:* Nasogastric tube—pass tube to affected site and gently lavage with warm water. Cuffed nasogastric tube—pass tube to affected site, inflate cuff, gently lavage. Endotracheal tube—pass tube into esophagus, inflate cuff, pass smaller bore tube through endotracheal tube, gently lavage. Lavage under moderate pressure—pass cuffed nasogastric tube to obstructed site and lavage with greater pressure; or pass nasogastric tube to obstructed site, apply pressure externally above obstruction, and lavage with greater pressure. Under anesthesia—position with head lowered; pass endotracheal tube into trachea and inflate cuff; pass nasogastric tube to affected site and gently lavage; lavage with mineral oil or dioctyl sodium sulfosuccinate (DSS).
Esophageal foreign body	*Transoral manual removal:* For objects lodged within the postpharyngeal esophagus. *Transendoscopic retrieval:* Pass endoscope to obstruction and retrieve with grasping forceps or snare. Break larger objects into pieces and remove individually. *Esophagotomy:* For objects with sharp surfaces, caustic agents, and objects buried within the esophageal mucosa.

TABLE 3. TREATMENT OF ACQUIRED ESOPHAGEAL OBSTRUCTION *Continued*

Problem	Treatment
MAINTENANCE OF HOMEOSTASIS	
Dehydration without hemoconcentration	Oral fluids
Dehydration with hemococentration	Intravenous fluids: Balanced polyionic solution. Replacement of deficit: (% dehydration) × (body weight in kg) = deficit in 1. Maintenance: 2 to 3 ml/kg/hr.
Metabolic alkalosis	Normal isotonic saline
Metabolic acidosis	Acetate polyionic solution
Electrolyte imbalances	Specific replacement as determined by measured alterations. Hyponatremia/hypochloremia—oral electrolyte solution or IV isotonic saline. Hypokalemia—dietary roughage or oral electrolyte solution or IV potassium at 0.25 mEq/kg/hour.
PREVENTION OF COMPLICATIONS	
Tracheobronchial aspiration	Alleviate obstruction as soon as possible. Prevent access to feed, water, and bedding until obstruction is alleviated and esophageal function has returned. Use of cuffed tubes, either within esophagus or within trachea.
Aspiration pneumonia	*Broad spectrum antimicrobial therapy (Example):* *Gram positive:* Procaine penicillin G—22,000 IU/kg IM b.i.d. *Gram negative:* Gentamicin sulfate—2.2 mg/kg IM or IV t.i.d. Amikacin sulfate—6.6 mg/kg IM or IV b.i.d or t.i.d. *Anaerobic bacteria:* Metronidazole—15 mg/kg PO t.i.d.
Esophageal inflammation	*NSAID (Cyclo-oxygenase inhibitors):* Flunixin meglumine—1.1 mg/kg IV b.i.d. Phenylbutazone—1 to 2 g/500 kg IV or PO b.i.d.
Esophageal stricture	*Control inflammation:* NSAID. NPO except liquids (rest affected part). *Inhibit fibrous tissue synthesis:* Corticosteroids (inhibit procollagen synthesis). Colchicine—1 mg/100 kg PO s.i.d. (inhibits procollagen secretion). *Esophageal dilation:* Bougienage SID for 2 weeks. Re-evaluate prior to cessation of bougienage.
Recurrence of obstruction	*Dietary management:* Normal diet, if minimal esophageal trauma and normal esophageal function. Slurry of pelleted feed and small quantities of moistened, nonirritating roughage, if moderate trauma and minimal alteration of esophageal transit. NPO except liquids, if severe trauma and significantly altered function.
Esophageal diverticulum	Prompt relief of the obstruction. Gentle techniques during examination and treatment.
Weight loss to starvation	Adequate nutrition, selection of which depends upon the individual circumstances (Normal diet to pellet slurry, enteral feeding, or total parenteral nutrition).

NSAID = nonsteroidal anti-inflammatory drugs; NPO = nothing per os.

tory case. Aspiration of these substances poses a significant risk, so they should be used only with some device or set of circumstances to prevent aspiration. Agents that digest starch might assist in the dispersion of a persistent feed impaction.

If the obstruction is caused by a foreign object, lavage will be ineffectual. A proximal foreign body might be reached by hand through the mouth. Some objects can be retrieved with grasping forceps and various snares passed through the endoscope. Swallowed nasogastric tubes can be recovered in this fashion. Some large objects can be broken with forceps into smaller, removable pieces. Care should be taken in retracting a foreign body through the pharynx, as dislodging can occlude the airway. If numerous intubations are necessary to extract multiple pieces, a large-bore tube should be used as a guide for the endoscope to protect the esophageal mucosa from undue trauma. Transendoscopic retrieval should not be attempted for objects that have rough surfaces, are caustic, or are embedded within the mucosa.

Although extrinsic compression of the esophagus can be caused by the thyroid gland, thymus, abscess, diaphragmatic hernia, and persistent right aortic arch, most commonly lymphadenopathy accounts for compression. Lymph nodes in close proximity to the esophagus include the medial and lateral retropharyngeal, cranial, middle and caudal deep cervical nodes, and the mediastinal nodes. Alleviation of the resulting esophageal compression depends on treatment of the primary condition. Lymphadenopathy is usually related to neoplasia or inflammation, either septic or nonseptic.

Esophageal surgery is a last resort for the alleviation of esophageal obstructions, unless an irretrievable foreign object, esophageal stricture, chronically obstructing diverticulum, or neoplasia is confirmed. Detailed descriptions of esophageal surgical techniques and indications for each are found elsewhere. The Nd-YAG laser offers a modern, relatively noninvasive approach to conditions previously considered impossible or very difficult to treat. In the future, diseases such as squamous cell carcinoma may be diagnosed in earlier stages with the more frequent use of endoscopy, and subsequently treated surgically in the standing horse with the laser unit.

MAINTENANCE OF HOMEOSTASIS

Maintenance of homeostasis in the patient with an esophageal obstruction is aimed primarily at fluid, electrolyte, and acid–base status. The majority of cases of esophageal feed impaction are relatively normal in this respect and require no specific treatment. If the horse is clinically dehydrated but not hemoconcentrated and if the obstruction is incomplete, oral fluids will suffice. Intravenous (IV) fluids are indicated if hemoconcentration ensues, signified by elevated packed cell volume and plasma protein concentrations. Specific electrolyte replacement hinges on individual imbalances. Acid–base derangements rarely warrant specific correction. Isotonic saline solution is effective in reversing a mild metabolic alkalosis, as is a balanced polyionic solution for a metabolic acidosis. Sodium bicarbonate is seldom indicated.

TREATMENT OF COMPLICATIONS

Complications secondary to esophageal obstruction include aspiration pneumonia, temporary or prolonged esophageal dysfunction mediated by trauma and inflammation, esophageal stricture, diverticulum formation, and esophageal perforation. Dysphagia is invariably associated with tracheal contamination by feed material and salivary secretions. Intact defense mechanisms effectively prevent the development of clinical pneumonia unless they are deficient or overwhelmed by excessive of aspiration. If aspiration pneumonia is suspected from the clinical course or confirmed by physical, radiographic, and laboratory findings, antimicrobial therapy should be instituted. Ideally, the selection of the antimicrobial regimen hinges on culture and sensitivity testing of a transtracheal wash specimen. Rational drug selection, before or in lieu of laboratory confirmation, is based on the prediction of a mixed bacterial population comprised of gram-positive aerobic, gram-negative aerobic, and anaerobic bacteria. Penicillin (e.g., procaine penicillin G,* 22,000 IU per kg intramuscularly [IM] b.i.d.), an aminoglycoside (e.g., gentamicin sulfate,† 2.2 mg per kg IM or IV t.i.d., or amikacin sulfate,‡ 6.6 mg per kg IM or IV b.i.d.), and metronidazole§ (15 mg per kg PO t.i.d.) provide broad-spectrum coverage. Clinical impression suggests that most cases of aspiration pneumonia associated with esophageal obstruction resolve without significant impairment of function.

Esophageal inflammation at the obstructed site can be diminished by the use of anti-inflammatory drugs such as flunixin meglumine‖ (1.1 mg per kg IV b.i.d.) and phenylbutazone¶ (1 to 2 gm per 500 kg IV or PO b.i.d.). These drugs are especially warranted in the setting of mucosal trauma. Adequate hydration is imperative during the administration of these potentially toxic drugs. If deep, circumferential mucosal ulceration is detected endoscopically, corticosteroids are theoretically of benefit to minimize scarring and stricture, by inhibition of procollagen synthesis; however, a recent double-blind study in human patients with severe esophageal trauma showed no benefit of corticosteroids in preventing esophageal stricture. With particularly se-

---

*Procaine penicillin G, Pfizer, New York, NY
†Gentocin, Schering Corp., Kenilworth, NJ
‡Amikin, Bristol Labs., Evansville, IN
§Flagyl, Schiapparelli Searle, Skokie, IL
‖Banamine, Schering Corp., Kenilworth, NJ
¶Butazolidin, Cooper's Animal Health, Inc., Kansas City, MO

vere trauma, colchicine (1 mg per 100 kg body weight PO s.i.d.) offers another rational choice, by inhibition of procollagen secretion. The efficacy of colchicine has not been documented in horses.

NUTRITION

Dietary management following relief of an esophageal obstruction relates to the degree of esophageal injury incurred. For transient obstructions accompanied by minimal, superficial esophageal mucosal trauma with no functional alteration, the normal diet can be resumed immediately. When moderate mucosal damage occurs with minimal changes in esophageal transit of a food bolus, a slurry of pelleted feed, either without roughage or with a nonirritating roughage such as lush grass, can be offered immediately. If the esophageal damage is severe, the esophagus remains dilated, and esophageal transit is significantly impaired, voluntary intake should be limited to liquids and all solid material should be withheld for approximately 72 hours. Feed materially can be gradually reintroduced coincident with mucosal healing and return of esophageal tone and peristalsis. Initially, small amounts of a pelleted slurry can be offered frequently, followed by a soft, moistened roughage such as grass. If esophageal flaccidity and dysfunction are persistent and the value of the horse warrants the expense, parenteral or enteral nutrition may be considered as temporary measures to provide adequate nutrition (see p. 724–36). Unfortunately, in some cases, prolonged esophageal dilation (acquired megaesophagus) is irreversible. If a stricture forms despite preventive measures, a slurry of a complete pelleted feed, containing both grain and roughage, can be offered indefinitely. Some patients will also tolerate small quantities of fine, moistened roughage, which is more desirable than pelleted feed alone, because of the association of impaction colic with insufficient dietary roughage.

Esophageal bougienage is a mechanical dilating technique that is well established in human medicine and occasionally used in companion animal medicine, but is currently experimental in the horse. Most effective for acute, postobstructive stenosis, bougienage entails daily passage of a mechanical dilator beyond a stenotic region. Commercial dilators available in human medicine are insufficient in length and diameter for direct application in the horse. A specially designed nasogastric tube° fitted with a double-thickness rubber cuff has been used successfully to prevent stricture formation in cases of deep, circumferential esophageal ulceration and stenosis following chronic feed impaction. The tube is passed beyond the stenotic area, the cuff is filled with water, and the distended tube is slowly withdrawn through the stenotic area. The procedure is repeated daily for approximately 2 weeks, the period during which stricture formation is most aggressive.

Treatment of reflux esophagitis is aimed at the inciting cause, such as enteritis, gastric outflow obstruction, or gastroparesis. Metoclopramide† can be used to treat small intestinal ileus, to coordinate gastric and upper small intestinal motility, and to increase lower esophageal sphincter tone. Neurologic side effects of metoclopramide are not infrequent. Bethanechol‡ (0.4 mg per kg t.i.d.) is warranted in the treatment of gastric disease to stimulate gastric emptying, increase esophageal contractions in the lower esophagus, and increase lower esophageal sphincter pressure. The H_2-receptor antagonists cimetidine§ (8.8 to 16 mg per kg PO t.i.d.), ranitidine‖ (2.2 to 5.0 mg per kg PO t.i.d.), or famotidine¶ increase lower esophageal sphincter tone directly and reduce acid secretion.

Esophageal perforation may occur from the lumen or as a complication of a cervical laceration or penetrating foreign object (see Fig. 2). Although primary surgical closure may be attempted, most cases are allowed to heal by secondary intention. Initially the horse may be fed through an esophagotomy tube, which enters the esophageal lumen through the perforated site. As the esophageal wound heals, the esophagotomy tube is replaced with a nasogastric tube, fixed in place temporarily. The variety of enteral formulations that can be administered through these tubes is discussed elsewhere. A small esophagocutaneous fistula may heal uneventfully. More aggressive therapy is indicated if cellulitis, mediastinitis, pleuritis, and toxemia result.

Supplemental Readings

Brook, G., and Schmidt, G. R.: Prerenal azotemia in a pony with an esophageal obstruction. Equine Vet. J., 11:53, 1979.

°Bivona Inc., Gary, IN

†Reglan, A. H. Robins Co., Richmond, VA
‡Urecholine, Merck Sharp & Dohme Labs., West Point, PA
§Tagamet, Smith Kline & French Labs., Philadelphia, PA
‖Zantac, Glaxo, Inc., Research Triangle Park, NC
¶Pepcid, Merck Sharp & Dohme Labs., West Point, PA

Green, E. M., Roth, J. E., and McClure, R. C.: Recurrent esophageal obstruction in the horse: Neurologic considerations. Proc. Ann. Conv. Am. Assoc. Equine Pract., 1986, p. 423.

Green, S., Green, E. M., and Aronson, E.: Squamous cell carcinoma: An unusual cause of choke in a horse. Mod. Vet. Pract., 67:870, 1986.

Greet, T. R. C.: Observations on the potential role of esophageal radiography in the horse. Equine Vet. J., 14:73, 1982.

Heffron, C. J., and Baker, G. J.: Endoscopic observations on the deglutition reflex in the horse. Equine Vet. J., 11:137, 1979.

Murray, M. J., Ball M. M., and Parker, G. A.: Megaesophagus and aspiration pneumonia secondary to gastric ulceration in a foal. J. Am. Vet. Med. Assoc., 192:381, 1988.

Stick, J. A., Robinson, N. E., and Krehbiel, J. D.: Acid-base and electrolyte alterations associated with salivary loss in the pony. Am. J. Vet. Res., 42:733, 1981.

Tasker, J. B.: Fluid and electrolyte studies in the horse: IV. The effects of fasting and thirsting. Cornell Vet., 57:658, 1967.

Todhunter, R. J., Stick, J. A., Trotter, G. W., et al.: Medical management of esophageal stricture in seven horses. J. Am. Vet. Med. Assoc., 185:784, 1984.

Gastroduodenal Ulceration

Michael J. Murray, LEESBURG, VIRGINIA

Just as the term *colic* describes a clinical presentation and encompasses a large number of disorders, gastroduodenal ulceration describes a clinical finding the cause of which is likely to be multifactorial and different from case to case. Within the umbrella term *gastroduodenal ulceration* are included symptomatic and asymptomatic cases, focal or multifocal ulceration involving the squamous or glandular mucosal linings of the stomach, gastritis, gastric emptying disorders, duodenitis, duodenal ulceration, and complications resulting from these disorders.

Gastric ulceration affects large numbers of foals, yearlings, and adult horses, and different clinical syndromes and lesion distribution occur in each group. Gastric ulceration may occur as a primary problem or may occur secondary to another intestinal disorder. Duodenal ulceration occurs primarily in foals, although it has been diagnosed in yearlings. It is a rare finding in adult horses.

PATHOGENESIS

In consideration of possible pathogenic mechanisms, the anatomical location of the ulcer must be taken into account. In general, ulceration is considered to result from an imbalance of aggressive and protective factors. The principal aggressive factors are hydrochloric acid and pepsin, while protective factors include the mucus–bicarbonate barrier, prostaglandin E_2 (PGE_2), mucosal blood flow, cellular restitution, and growth factors such as epidermal growth factor. The relevance of any protective factor depends on whether the squamous or glandular mucosal surface is considered. Gastric motility also is important, since delayed gastric emptying and prolonged gastric contractions have been implicated in the pathogenesis of ulcers. Mucosal protection of the duodenum relies on an alkaline or neutral pH, with factors such as PGE_2 and mucosal blood flow of probable relevance. It is noteworthy that many ulcerating disorders in man are considered to result from mucosal protective deficiencies rather than from acid hypersecretion.

The squamous mucosa of the equine stomach lacks a mucus–bicarbonate layer, and the relevance of other mucosal protective factors for this tissue is undetermined. Thus, ulceration of the gastric squamous epithelial mucosa may result primarily from excessive exposure to hydrochloric acid and possibly pepsin. Excessive exposure to acid results from increased acid secretion or delayed gastric emptying, or both. One apparent protective mechanism of the gastric squamous mucosa is hyperkeratosis, a thickening of the keratinized layer of the squamous muscosa. This occurs in the healing phase of squamous ulceration as well as with active ulceration.

Foals are capable of gastric acid secretion by 2 days of age, if not earlier, and in one study the pH of some sites of the gastric mucosal lining was lower in foals than in adult horses. Immature regulation of acid secretion and incompletely developed mucosal protective processes in young foals could contribute to ulcer development, particularly in the gastric glandular and duodenal mucosa.

Currently, specific pathogenic mechanisms of gastric and duodenal ulceration in foals and horses remain unknown, and in consideration of the different ulcer syndromes that occur, there are likely to be several different mechanisms. Stress is frequently cited as a contributing factor to gastroduodenal ulceration in foals. In two recent reports, foals with a variety of clinical disorders had a prevalence of glandular mucosal lesions of 23 to 40 per cent, compared to 5 to 10 per cent in normal foals. Studies including large numbers of foals will need to be performed before specific foals at risk of developing gastroduodenal ulceration can be identified.

CLINICAL SYNDROMES

Foals

Gastric Ulceration

The clinical signs that typically are associated with gastric ulcers in foals include bruxism, dorsal recumbency, salivation, interrupted nursing, and colic. These signs, though, are observed in the minority of foals with ulcers and usually reflect the presence of lesions in the gastric glandular mucosa or duodenum, or both. Signs of salivation or esophageal reflux are indicative of gastric outlet obstruction or pseudo-obstruction, reflecting significant ulceration associated with the pylorus or duodenum, or both.

The majority of foals with gastric ulcers do not have lesions in the glandular mucosa or duodenum but have lesions distributed in the nonglandular, or squamous mucosa. Most lesions occur adjacent to the margo plicatus along the greater curvature. Such foals usually are not symptomatic, although this seems to depend on lesion location and severity. Typical signs in symptomatic foals with squamous mucosal lesions include diarrhea, poor growth, rough hair coat, and a "pot belly" appearance. In cases with severe or diffuse squamous ulceration, bruxism or colic may be present.

The distribution of lesions in the squamous mucosa varies with the age of the foal. In foals less than 1 month old, lesions typically originate in the squamous mucosa adjacent to the margo plicatus along the greater curvature. These lesions are frequently associated with desquamation of the squamous epithelium (Fig. 1). Desquamation, the shedding of surface epithelial layers, appears as flakes or sheets of epithelium. Desquamation occurs in the majority of foals up to 35 days of age. In most foals, lesions in the squamous mucosa adjacent to the margo plicatus along the greater curvature resolve without treatment and without causing a clinical problem.

In some young foals, erosive, ulcerative lesions adjacent to the margo plicatus coalesce into larger or deeper areas of ulceration. At this point, there may be hemorrhage associated with

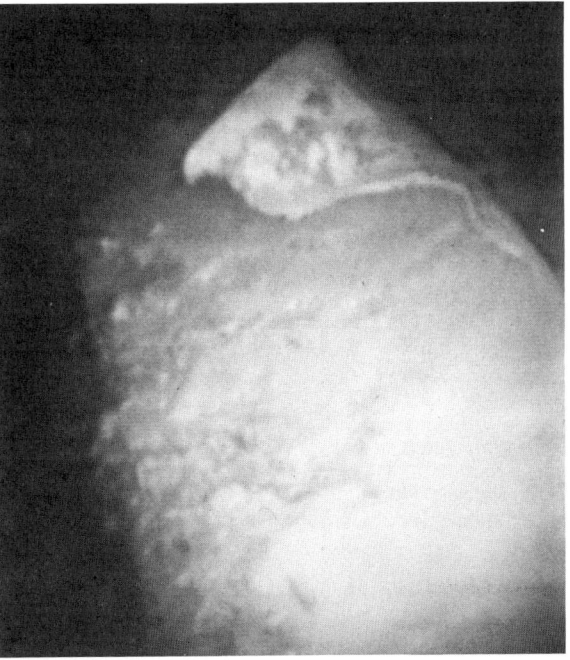

Figure 1. Endoscopic view of the stomach of a clinically normal 14-day-old Thoroughbred foal. There is a large sheet of desquamating squamous epithelium along the greater curvature.

the lesions. Clinical signs may occur, with diarrhea the most frequently observed sign.

In foals older than 3 months, lesions become more prevalent in the squamous mucosa surrounding the cardia and along the lesser curvature between the cardia and pylorus. Lesions also are found in the squamous mucosa of the fundus and adjacent to the margo plicatus. These lesions can be very severe and often are associated with clinical signs such as diarrhea, poor appetite, poor growth, and poor bodily condition.

Gastric ulcers in foals may result in significant blood loss, resulting in anemia and hypoproteinemia, but this is usually the case only in young foals. Perforation is a dramatic, although infrequent, sequela to gastric ulceration. In many cases, perforation is not preceded by signs typical of gastric ulceration, and foals are found acutely depressed or dead. Theoretically, a small perforation along the greater curvature could be sealed by the greater omentum. In fact, most foals presenting with perforation have significant peritonitis, and many perforations occur along the lesser curvature of the stomach. Peritonitis secondary to perforation can have a tremendous fibrinous component, and it is possible for peritoneal fluid cell count and protein content to be normal, because of sequestration of cells and protein in fibrin clots within the omentum (Fig. 2). Careful inspection of a Wright- or Gram-

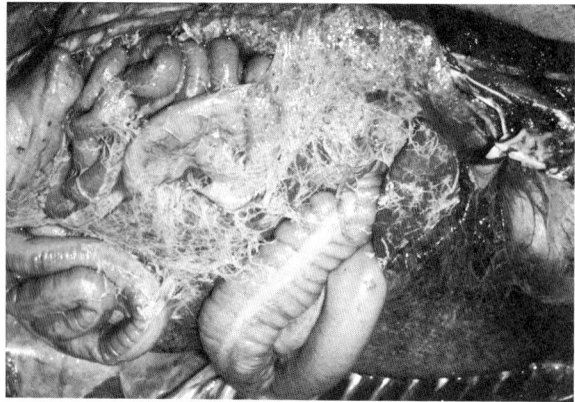

Figure 2. Fibrinous peritonitis in a 6-week-old foal that presented with fever, depression, and intermittent bruxism. There was a focal perforation of the proximal duodenum. Analysis of peritoneal fluid revealed a low nucleated cell count and protein concentration, but mixed types of bacteria were seen.

stained slide for bacteria may confirm a perforated viscus.

Duodenal Ulceration

Duodenal ulceration occurs in foals of all ages, and was found in 28 of 511 foals necropsied at the University of Florida. The signs of duodenal ulceration are the same as for some cases of gastric ulceration and include bruxism, colic, and diarrhea. In many cases duodenal and gastric ulcers occur concurrently. Gastric ulceration that is secondary to duodenal ulceration tends to be severe and is frequently associated with gastroesophageal reflux and esophagitis.

In general, the sequelae of duodenal ulceration are more severe than gastric ulceration. These include duodenal perforation with peritonitis or adhesions, duodenal stricture with complete or partial obstruction, and ascending cholangitis and hepatitis. Lesions occur primarily in the proximal duodenum and range from diffuse inflammation to focal bleeding ulcers.

Duodenal ulceration can be difficult to confirm ante mortem. Duodenoscopy is the most specific means of diagnosis. Excessive enterogastric reflux of bile through the pylorus suggests duodenal dysfunction. If gastroendoscopy, but not duodenoscopy, can be performed, gastric lesions, particularly in the squamous mucosa of the lesser curvature dorsal to the pyloric antrum, will often be very severe when duodenal ulcers are present. In such cases, histamine H_2 antagonist therapy may be less effective in resolving gastric lesions than in cases of primary gastric ulceration.

Other useful diagnostic procedures include radiography, evaluation of peritoneal fluid, serum liver enzymes, particularly biliary-associated enzymes (γ-glutamyl transpeptidase, alkaline phosphatase), and serum bile acids. With severe duodenal ulceration, survey radiographs of the cranial abdomen may reveal accumulation of fluid within the stomach, and gas ascending the biliary ducts. If barium contrast is placed in the stomach, complete emptying is usually delayed more than 2 hours, and an irregular mucosal border may be noted in the descending duodenum. If stricture has occurred, this may be noted. If the descending duodenum is to be imaged, the volume of contrast material placed in the stomach should not exceed 0.5 to 1 liter in a foal and 1 to 2 liters in a weanling or yearling, or the proximal descending duodenum will be obscured by contrast material within the stomach.

Yearlings

In yearlings most lesions are confined to the squamous mucosa, particularly adjacent to the margo plicatus. Normal yearlings do not have gastric ulcers, although mild erosions of the squamous mucosa have been noted. Ulcers have been associated with recurrent colic, poor bodily condition, poor appetite, and intermittent diarrhea. Recently, yearlings have been diagnosed with delayed gastric emptying, resulting in severe, often bleeding, gastric ulceration. The cause of the delayed emptying was not determined, and although duodenal ulceration or partial pyloric outflow obstruction could not be ruled out, the typical signs expected with duodenal ulceration were absent. Affected animals had poor bodily condition, poor appetite, and intermittent diarrhea. One animal was observed to belch. Diagnosis was confirmed by barium contrast upper gastrointestinal (GI) radiography, failure to empty stomach contents following withholding of feed for more than 16 hours, or response to prokinetic drugs.

Adult Horses

Gastric ulceration affects a large number of adult horses. Clinical signs include poor appetite, poor condition, mild to severe colic, attitude changes, and poor racing performance. The association of these signs, some of which are obscure or subjective, with gastric ulcers has been confirmed based on the results of endoscopic examinations and effective treatment with histamine H_2 antagonists. In one study gastric lesions were significantly more prevalent and more severe in symptomatic horses than in normal horses. Horses in active training for racing were at great risk (greater than 80 per cent) of having gastric ulcers. The cause of the high rate of gastric ulceration in such horses was not determined, but in the majority of horses examined, nonsteroidal anti-inflammatory drugs (NSAIDs) were not a factor. Administration of NSAIDs can initiate and exacerbate gastric ulceration. In addition to racing horses, horses of several breeds and in a variety of uses have had clinically relevant gastric ulceration.

In adult horses, spontaneous gastric lesions occur most frequently in the squamous mucosa, and uncommonly in the glandular mucosa. Glandular ulceration is observed with greater frequency after the administration of NSAIDs. Lesions usually occur adjacent to the margo plicatus along the greater or lesser curvatures. In several cases, lesions have been associated with hemorrhage, appearing as either active bleeding or darkened, coagulated blood. However, bleeding from ulcers in the gastric squamous mucosa is *not* usually associated with anemia or hypoproteinemia, and if these abnormalities are present another cause must be determined.

DIAGNOSIS

The diagnosis of gastric ulceration is based on the presence of age-related characteristic clinical signs, endoscopic findings, and response to treatment. Gastric ulceration in the majority of foals and horses is definitively diagnosed with gastroendoscopy. Endoscopy demonstrates the location of gastric ulcers and can be used to assess the severity of the lesions and response to therapy. Expected clinical signs and the results of diagnostic tests such as fecal occult blood and contrast radiography can be unreliable indicators of gastric ulcers.

Before gastroendoscopy is performed, suckling foals up to 20 days old should be allowed to nurse, but not to consume solid feed for 8 to 10 hours. Older foals and mature horses should not have solid feed for 10 hours. This time period is required to ensure complete emptying of ingesta from the stomach. Most young foals do not require sedation for the gastroendoscopic examination to be performed, although sedation with xylazine, 0.6 mg per kg, can facilitate the examination. Minimal restraint is usually satisfactory during the procedure. The most objectionable part of the examination is the initial insertion of the endoscope through the nasal turbinates. Chemical sedation is required if the foal is to be placed in a recumbent position so that the entire glandular mucosa can be examined. Combinations of xylazine (0.6 mg per kg) and butorphanol (0.01 to 0.02 mg per kg) or xylazine and diazepam (0.05 to 0.10 mg per kg) are useful for this procedure.

Sedation of older foals and horses is necessary. Passage of the endoscope into the esophagus is facilitated by injecting water through the biopsy channel and inducing a swallow. The stomach is distended by insufflation of air through the endoscope and until the nonglandular and glandular regions of the gastric surface can be observed. Distention with air is tolerated by foals and horses, and has been associated with signs of abdominal discomfort only rarely in the patients examined by the author.

As the examiner views along the greater curvature of the stomach, the squamous mucosa of the nonglandular fundus, the margo plicatus, and glandular fundus are observed (Fig. 3). The squamous mucosa appears as a pale to white tissue. In foals the squamous mucosa is very thin in the first several days of life and appears pale pink to white. From the endoscopist's perspective the margo plicatus, the junction between the squamous and glandular gastric mucosal epithelium, is seen to proceed dorsally, then ventrally along the greater curvature. The glandular mucosa appears as dark pink to red, with a smooth, glistening texture.

The endoscope is then advanced along the longitudinal curvature of the stomach until the lesser curvature and cardia can be observed (see Fig. 4). At this location the squamous mucosa surrounding the cardia, lesser curvature, and, in foals with an empty stomach, the pyloric antrum and pylorus can be observed. With a 200-cm-long endoscope, the duodenum can be entered

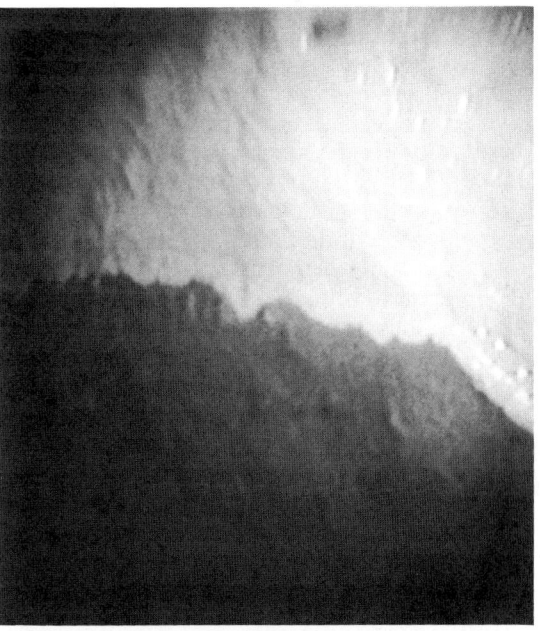

Figure 3. Endoscopic view along the greater curvature of the stomach, showing the squamous mucosa of the nonglandular fundus, the margo plicatus, and the glandular fundus.

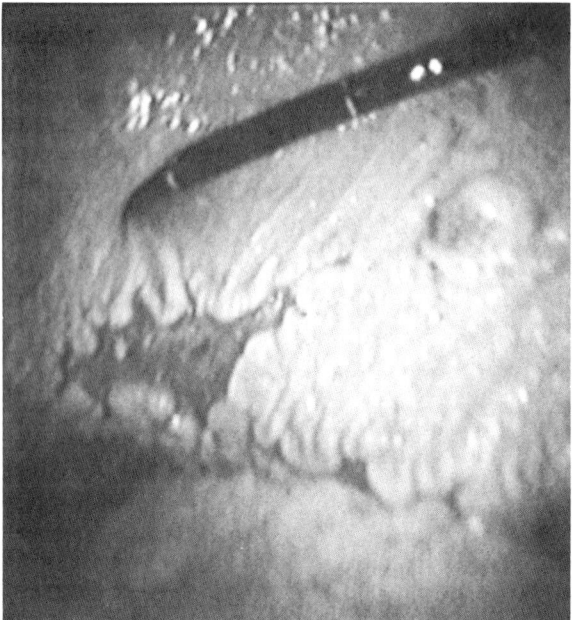

Figure 4. Ulceration of the squamous mucosa along the lesser curvature. Notice the endoscope insertion tube through the cardia.

TABLE 1. THERAPEUTIC AGENTS FOR USE IN TREATING GASTRIC OR DUODENAL ULCERS IN FOALS AND HORSES°

Agent	Dosage, Route, and Timing
Histamine type 2 receptor antagonists	
Cimetidine (Tagamet)	6.6 mg/kg PO, IV, 4–6 times daily
Ranitidine (Zantac)	6.6 mg/kg PO, IV, 3 times daily
Famotidine (Pepsid)	3.3 mg/kg PO, 3 times daily†
Nizatidine (Axid)	6.6 mg/kg PO, 3 times daily‡
Proton pump inhibitor	
Omeprazole (Losec)	1.0–2.0 mg/kg PO, 1–2 times daily
Antacids	
Mylanta II	124 mEq/oz§
Maalox	78 mEq/oz
Riopan	66 mEq/oz
Amphogel	58 mEq/oz
Mucosal protectants	
Sucralfate (Carafate)	2–4 gms PO, 2–4 times daily
Prostaglandin E_2 analogue	
Misoprostil (Cytotec)	200 μg, 4 times daily with food‖

°Only the dosage for ranitidine has been tested for clinical efficacy in horses.
†Dosage based on unpublished data comparing effect of 3.3 mg/kg famotidine with effect of 6.6 mg/kg ranitidine on equine gastric fluid pH.
‡Dosage based on equivalent potency with ranitidine in man. Data on effect in horses not available.
§Acid neutralization capacity, in mEq/oz of selected antacids. See text for dosage.
‖Human adult dose.

in foals up to 6 months of age. In horses, an insertion tube length of 275 to 300 cm is required.

The pylorus is observed ventral and to the left of the cardia. In foals, reflux of bile-tinged fluid from the duodenum into the stomach is occasionally observed and is considered normal. Frequent bile reflux is abnormal, reflective of small intestinal obstruction or adynamic ileus. When observing the cardia and pylorus it is important to recognize that the endoscope is pointing cranially, so that the left side of the animal appears on the left side of the endoscopist's field of view. The endoscope is advanced to the pylorus, and from this point the normal contractions of the stomach, with some guidance by the endoscopist, are usually sufficient to advance the endoscope into the duodenum. The duodenal mucosa should have a uniform pink, velvety appearance. The common duodenal papilla may be observed, with bile emptying from the common bile duct.

THERAPY

Currently, the primary objective in the treatment of gastric ulcers in foals and horses is to reduce or neutralize acid secretion so that the gastric mucosal epithelium can heal (see Table 1). Gastric acid secretion can be temporarily attenuated with the use of histamine type 2 receptor (H_2) antagonists. Cimetidine° and ranitidine† are

---

°Tagamet, Smith Kline & French Labs., Inc., Carolina, PR
†Zantac, Glaxo Inc., Research Triangle Park, NC

the most frequently used; both inhibit gastric acid secretion in the horse.

The preferred dosage of cimetidine or ranitidine is 6.6 mg per kg. Cimetidine should be administered four to six times daily and ranitidine three times daily to be effective. There is tremendous individual variability in horses' responses to H_2 antagonists, with suppression of acid secretion and increased gastric pH lasting from 1 to 20 hours following a single dose of 6.6 mg per kg of ranitidine. Interestingly, lower dosages, from 1.1 to 2.2 mg per kg, have been effective in alleviating clinical signs of gastric ulcers (diarrhea, inappetance, etc.), but gastroendoscopic examination has revealed that significant ulceration was still present. Thus, a dosage of 6.6 mg per kg administered three times daily (ranitidine) or four to six times daily (cimetidine) currently is recommended to achieve complete healing of the ulcers.

The H_2 antagonist therapy should continue for 10 to 20 days to ensure complete healing. In most cases, 3 weeks of treatment is required to achieve complete healing. Eighty to ninety per cent of adult horses treated with ranitidine, 6.6

mg per kg administered every 8 hours for 3 weeks, had complete healing of gastric ulcers, whereas at 2 weeks complete healing had occurred in only 15 to 40 per cent. It has become apparent from treating horses in training for racing that if the horse is kept in training while being treated, clinical signs resolve but the lesions do not. Once the medication is discontinued, clinical signs often return. Thus, for healing of the ulcers to be achieved, treatment with an H_2 antagonist should be accompanied by refraining from training.

Other H_2 antagonists, famotidine* and nizatidine,† are available for use in humans, but an effective dosage in the horse has not been established at this time. Omeprazole,‡ a drug that completely blocks gastric acid secretion by inhibiting the hydrogen ion pump, is approved for use in humans and blocks gastric acid secretion in horses. The product is available as enteric-coated granules in capsules, and the integrity of the enteric coating cannot be disrupted, since acidity destroys the drug's activity. This may make effective administration of the drug difficult in foals and horses. An effective dosage in the horse has not been established but may be in the 1.0 to 2.0 mg per kg range.

The use of antacids in the treatment of gastric ulcers has not been critically examined in horses. In people, antacids must be taken frequently, six to ten times daily, to have a significant effect on the healing of peptic ulcers. There also may be a rebound secretion of acid in response to the increase in gastric pH following antacid administration. Thus, antacids may be effective in treating equine gastric ulcers, but the dosage and frequency of administration necessary to achieve healing are undetermined.

Antacids have been used to resolve clinical signs of gastric ulcers, particularly poor appetite, in mature horses. Additionally, I have recommended the use of antacids in horses that were successfully treated with an H_2 antagonist, in an attempt to prevent or minimize recurrence of gastric ulcers. Administration of 200 to 250 ml of an aluminum hydroxide or magnesium hydroxide antacid (such as Mylanta II§), three times daily, has apparently been effective in preventing recurrence of *clinical signs* in horses in which ulcers had healed with H_2 antagonist therapy.

Sucralfate,‖ a sulfated polysaccharide, is effective in the treatment of peptic ulcers in humans. The mechanism of action may involve adherence to ulcerated mucosa, stimulation of mucus secretion, and enhanced PGE synthesis. These are all factors relevant to glandular mucosa, and the efficacy of sucralfate in treating ulcers in the equine gastric squamous mucosa remains undetermined. Sucralfate may bind to ulcers in the squamous mucosa, and thus have some protective effect, but the efficacy of sucralfate in treating squamous ulceration of the equine stomach remains doubtful. Sucralfate should have greatest efficacy for ulcers in the gastric glandular mucosa and duodenum, and even in this context its efficacy in horses has not been tested. Currently, it is advisable to use sucralfate as an adjunct to H_2 antagonist therapy, and not alone.

The use of the synthetic PGE_2 analogue misoprostil* has been effective in the treatment of duodenal ulcers in humans, and the mechanism of action is proposed to be both inhibition of gastric acid secretion and mucosal cytoprotection. However, side effects that include abdominal discomfort (cramping) and diarrhea frequently occur in people taking misoprostil.

Prokinetic drugs stimulate GI motility and enhance gastric emptying. They are used in cases in which delayed gastric emptying is suspected or confirmed. Metoclopramide† has been used in selected cases to prevent gastroesophageal reflux and enhance gastric emptying. An effective dosage is approximately 0.25 mg per kg, given by IV drip or subcutaneously, three to four times daily. Several adverse effects occur with metoclopramide in the horse, and the drug appears to have a very narrow margin of safety. Consequently, bethanecol,‡ a cholinergic agonist, is preferred. In cases of acute gastric atony, 0.025 to 0.030 mg per kg given, subcutaneously, every 3 to 4 hours has been effective in promoting gastric motility and emptying. Oral maintenance dosages of 0.30 to 0.45 mg per kg given three or four times daily are effective. Diarrhea has been observed with the higher dosages, but resolved when the dosage was decreased.

If medical therapy is ineffective, or if sequelae of duodenal ulceration cause complications, surgical intervention may be required. Gastroenterostomy has been reported to be effective in some cases, through bypassing the affected portion of duodenum and allowing for gastric emptying. However, the reported survival rates in such cases are poor, due primarily to the severity of the disorder when surgery has been attempted.

---

*Pepcid, Merck Sharp & Dohme Labs., Rahway, NJ
†Axid, Eli Lilly Inc., Indianapolis, IN
‡Prilosec, Merck Sharp & Dohme Labs., Rahway, NJ
§Mylanta II, Stuart Pharmaceuticals, Wilmington, DE.
‖Carafate, Marion Labs., Kansas City, MO

*Cytotec, Searle Labs., Inc., Skokie, IL
†Reglan, A. H. Robbins, Richmond, VA
‡Urecholine, Merck, Sharp & Dohne Labs, Rahway, NJ

Supplemental Readings

Campbell-Thompson, M. L., and Merritt, A. M.: Effect of ranitidine on gastric acid secretion in young male horses. Am. J. Vet. Res., 48:1511–1515, 1987.
Furr, M. O., and Murray, M. J.: Treatment of gastric ulcers in horses with histamine type 2 receptor antagonists. Equine Vet. J., Suppl. 7:77–79, 1989.
Hammond, C. J., Mason, D. K., and Watkins, K. L.: Gastric ulceration in mature Thoroughbred horses. Equine Vet. J., 18:284, 1986.
Murray, M. J.: Endoscopic appearance of gastric lesions in foals: 94 cases (1987–1988). J. Am. Vet. Med. Assoc., 195:1135–1141, 1989.
Murray, M. J., Grodinsky, C., Anderson, C. W., Radue, P. F., and Schmidt, G. R.: Gastric ulcers in horses: A comparison of endoscopic findings in horses with and without clinical signs. Equine Vet. J., Suppl. 7:68–72, 1989.
Murray, M. J., Hart, J., and Parker, G. A.: Equine gastric ulcer syndrome: Endoscopic survey of asymptomatic foals. In: Proceedings of the 33rd Annual Convention of the American Association of Equine Practitioners, 1987, pp. 769–776.
Wilson, J. H.: Gastric and duodenal ulcers in foals: A retrospective study. In: Proceedings of the 2nd Equine Colic Research Symposium, 1986, p. 126.

Physical and Laboratory Evaluation of the Horse with Colic

Sharon J. Spier, DAVIS, CALIFORNIA
Jack R. Snyder, DAVIS, CALIFORNIA

Acute abdominal pain (colic) in the horse is one of the most frequent emergency conditions encountered in practice. Because there are numerous causes for abdominal pain, or colic, including intestinal and nonintestinal disorders, a complete and systematic physical examination should be performed in each case. The approach to diagnosis should be uniform and should be based on findings on the medical history, physical examination, rectal examination, and a few laboratory aids. The location and severity of the lesion causing the pain should be determined. In most cases with intestinal disorders, the cause of abdominal pain can be attributed to one or another of the following conditions: nonstrangulating obstructions (e.g., impaction), strangulating obstructions (e.g., volvulus or torsion), nonstrangulating infarctions (e.g., verminous arteritis), duodenitis–proximal jejunitis or colitis, or peritonitis. If the horse does not respond to conservative therapy with analgesics, stomach decompression, or laxatives, or if its physical status deteriorates, referral to a surgical facility for further evaluation should be pursued.

APPROACH TO DIAGNOSIS

Although acute abdominal pain is a relatively frequent occurrence, the majority of cases, probably greater than 90 per cent, respond readily to analgesic therapy. The primary aim of the initial examination is to distinguish horses with a mild or uncomplicated disease process from those with a potentially life-threatening disorder requiring further monitoring, surgery, or intensive care. The earlier these serious disorders are recognized and specific therapy instituted, the better is the prognosis for recovery.

SIGNALMENT

The age of the horse with colic should signal the veterinarian to consider specific conditions, for example, meconium impaction in a foal 1 to 2 days old, strangulating umbilical hernia or ascarid impaction in weanlings (6 to 12 months), or strangulating lipoma in a horse older than 14 years. Some conditions have a sex predisposition; for example, uterine torsion or large colon volvulus typically affects broodmares and inguinal hernia affects stallions. The breed of horse may occasionally suggest certain disorders: large-bodied horses such as the European breeds appear to have a higher prevalence of nephrosplenic entrapment of the left colon, and Miniature Horses have a predisposition to small colon impaction.

HISTORY

The nature and duration of abnormal clinical signs are very important. Horses with mild or intermittent pain of more than 24 hours' duration and minimal physiologic abnormalities are less likely to have a life-threatening disorder than a horse in continuous pain for more than 2 to 4 hours with deterioration in physical parameters. It is important to determine if any medications that could mask pain have been administered by the owner or another veterinarian. If the horse is exhibiting moderate to severe signs of pain, such as rolling or continuous pawing, a short-acting analgesic such as xylazine can be administered to calm the horse and relieve the owner's anxiety before further questioning. Assessment of the patient's cardiovascular status should, however, precede administration of any drug.

Information should be obtained regarding housing and feed, any changes in diet, anthelmintic therapy, previous medical history, any past history of abdominal pain or surgery, and whether any other horses are affected. Often, changes in diet, weather, or exercise will trigger intestinal upsets. However, it is also common to find no apparent initiating factors for an abdominal crisis.

The medical history of the affected horse and other horses on the farm can be helpful in detecting some types of disorders, such as parasitism, salmonellosis, enterolithiasis, equine monocytic ehrlichiosis (Potomac horse fever), and intra-abdominal abscesses due to streptococci. The owner should be asked when defecation was last observed and what the fecal consistency was. Were the feces hard and dry, or did the horse have diarrhea?

The breeding history and pregnancy status should be documented. Uterine torsions in late gestation will cause acute abdominal pain. Colonic impactions and 360-degree large colon volvulus are observed in postparturient mares. Scrotal or inguinal hernias in stallions are often associated with breeding.

The nature and progression of clinical signs and the response to therapy are often the most useful factors in determining the need for surgical intervention. It is vital to determine the value of the horse to the owner, especially if surgery or intensive therapy is anticipated. The insurance status should be reviewed by the owner, and the insurance carrier notified if surgery or euthanasia is being considered.

PHYSICAL EXAMINATION

Examination of a horse with abdominal pain should begin with a routine physical examination. Initially, general observations should ascertain the attitude of the horse, the degree of abdominal distention, and any signs of self-induced trauma. With few exceptions, horses with fever or signs of depression rather than overt pain will have a disorder requiring medical rather than surgical therapy. Exceptions include horses with severe shock resulting from strangulating obstructions of more than 4 hours' duration. Rectal findings in these horses are, however, often indicative of a surgical lesion. Close monitoring of all horses with colic is essential.

Adult horses with distention in the flank region usually have a large intestinal disorder causing obstruction and gas trapping proximal to the obstruction. Foals, however, may have abdominal distention with either large or small intestinal lesions.

During the initial examination it is important to record vital signs, including pulse rate and quality (strong, fair, or poor), respiratory rate and quality (e.g., eupnea, tachypnea, or dyspnea), rectal temperature, mucous membrane moistness and color, capillary refill time, skin turgor, temperature of the extremities, digital pulses, and abdominal borborygmi. A rapid pulse rate (greater than 52 beats per minute) of fair or poor quality, a capillary refill time greater than 2 seconds, poor skin turgor, and cool extremities are indicative of hypovolemia or poor perfusion. These signs reflect the effects of a severe gastrointestinal (GI) disorder on the cardiovascular system and signify the need for fluid therapy.

Digital pulses and evidence of lameness should be closely monitored, because of the association of abdominal disorders and laminitis. Laminitis can be mistaken for colic if there are similar clinical signs, such as an elevated heart rate, refusal to rise, and sweating.

Borborygmi, audible with a stethoscope, do not indicate normal bowel motility. However, an absence of borborygmi suggests an absence of motility. Presence of low-pitched, progressive sounds in all four quadrants of the abdomen is a favorable sign.

Passage of a nasogastric tube into the stomach is indicated for most if not all cases of colic. If the pulse rate is greater than 60 beats per minute, a tube should be passed without delay. Removal of enterogastric reflux can relieve pain and prevent gastric rupture. Once the tube is in the stomach, gastric reflux should be checked by siphoning. Water is introduced by dose syringe and negative pressure applied. If only gas is obtained, the tube should be inserted further and attempts repeated.

If gastric reflux is obtained, the volume should be recorded. The pH can be easily checked with pH paper strips. The pH of stomach contents should be less than 5; a higher pH implies that alkaline small intestinal contents are present. The odor and color of the reflux are also informative. Foul odor accompanies the presence of blood and bile, or indicates prolonged bowel stasis. Dark brown reflux or the appearance of precipitate resembling coffee grounds suggests that gastric or duodenal hemorrhage is present. Reflux in cases of proximal enteritis (duodenitis, jejunitis) is often brown and foul-smelling.

The teeth should be inspected for enamel points, as poor mastication may predispose to intestinal impaction. The odor of the breath should be noted. A foul odor implies that the horse has been anorectic or has had spontaneous reflux of gastric contents, and a serious disorder should be suspected.

RECTAL EXAMINATION

A complete rectal examination is essential for evaluation of a horse with colic. However, the benefits and risks must be understood by the owner. Proper restraint, and tranquilization if necessary, should be practiced. Adequate sedation can usually be achieved with xylazine (0.3 to 0.5 mg per kg IV) alone or in combination with butorphanol (0.012 to 0.02 mg per kg IV). Generous amounts of lubrication should be used, as many horses will be dehydrated. If straining is excessive, it may be beneficial to infuse a topical anesthetic into the rectum (20 to 50 ml of lidocaine diluted 1:1 with water) or to perform epidural anesthesia (see p. 27).

Feces in the rectum should be evaluated for consistency, blood or melena, foul odor, and mucus. In cases of heavy parasitism, ascarids or small strongyles may be observed in the feces or on the rectal sleeve. Examination for sand is done by mixing feces with water in a plastic palpation sleeve and allowing the sand to settle in the fingers of the sleeve. If significant amounts of sand are present, a sand impaction should be suspected. If no feces are present and large amounts of mucus are observed, a prolonged duration of the condition is suggested.

In the normal horse, the left side of the abdomen should contain the small colon, left ventral colon, pelvic flexure, and left dorsal colon. By moving the hand cranially, the examiner should be able to palpate the spleen adjacent to the body wall, with the nephrosplenic ligament and left kidney located dorsally. The cranial mesenteric artery may be palpated on midline if the horse is not straining. On the right side of the abdomen, the cecum may be identified as a soft structure containing gas and ingesta, a prominent ventral band, and sacculations. The small intestine usually cannot be identified in the normal horse. The ovaries, uterus, bladder, and inguinal rings are palpable in the caudal abdomen.

In a horse with intestinal obstruction, positive anatomical identification of structures may be difficult. However, even without identification, a great deal can be gained from a few observations. If the distended bowel is palpable, is it large bowel or small intestine? Is there one loop or several loops? If the distended bowel is large bowel, is it in its normal anatomical orientation or displaced? Is a feed impaction or foreign body impaction present?

The small colon can be easily identified by the presence of fecal balls, its mobility in the abdomen, wide bands, and sacculations. An impacted small colon impaction feels like a tortuous tubular structure, distended with digesta, with distinct taeniae. If the distended bowel has taeniae and sacculations and is not small colon, it can only be cecum or ventral colon.

Determine if the bowel is distended with gas or ingesta. Bowel with gaseous distention springs back to shape immediately after pressure is released. Bowel filled with ingesta feels doughy, and an impression remains in the bowel after the palpator releases pressure. Bowel with fluid contents feels similar to gas-filled bowel. In many cases of colic the contents of the large colon are dry secondary to dehydration. This should not be mistaken for an intestinal impaction, in which the colon is distended, heavy, and difficult to move in the abdomen. The distention can be so great that the sacculations may not be readily palpable. The dehydrated colon is contracted and sacculations are palpably distinct. The distended bowel should also be palpated for increased tissue thickness indicative of intestinal edema. If intestinal tissue edema is palpable, a strangulating obstruction should be considered, and surgery may be indicated.

If palpation or traction on any structures elicits a painful response, this may aid in locating a lesion. For instance, traction on the ventral band of the cecum induces pain when the ileum is incarcerated, implying that surgery may be required.

Certain specific disorders such as pelvic flexure impaction and nephrosplenic entrapment of the large colon may be diagnosed from rectal examination findings (see p. 196). In many cases, however, rectal examination findings must be combined with other physical laboratory parameters to make a presumptive diagnosis. It should be remembered that only the caudal abdomen is accessible for palpation; approximately 60 per cent of the abdomen is beyond reach of the examiner.

ABDOMINAL PARACENTESIS

Evaluation of peritoneal fluid is easy, rapid, and informative. Changes in peritoneal fluid occur rapidly in response to inflammatory changes involving the peritoneum or intestinal tissues. Fluid transudation occurs from lymphatic or venous obstruction or increased capillary permeability. The nature and composition of the fluid depend on the extent of vascular occlusion or the severity of inflammatory changes. Notable exceptions, in which peritoneal fluid remains normal despite devitalized bowel, do occur. Intussusceptions, or entrapment of small bowel in the epiploic foramen, are examples where the exudate from compromised bowel may not be reflected by a single abdominal paracentesis.

Normal peritoneal fluid is clear, straw colored, serous, and does not coagulate. It has a protein content of less than 2.5 gm per dl and less than 5,000 nucleated cells per ml. Peritoneal fluid becomes turbid when increased numbers of leukocytes and increased protein are present. Pink or red fluid is indicative of free hemoglobin or hemorrhage. Large volumes of dark brown or green fluid with a fetid odor obtained from several sites suggests bowel rupture, but cytology should be performed for confirmation. The cellular populations vary widely, and there is considerable overlap among abdominal disorders. The results should be interpreted as supporting a number of disorders rather than a specific diagnosis.

The initial response to inflammation or vascular occlusion is an increase in the amount of fluid and leakage of vascular proteins. Because the increase in fluid volume is difficult to monitor, the first sign of an abnormality is usually a peritoneal fluid protein content greater than 2.5 gm per dl. Fibrinogen content increases, and levels greater than 10 mg per dl in the peritoneal fluid suggest an acute inflammatory process. Fibrinogen content also increases as a result of blood contamination. Progressive vascular damage causes diapedesis of red blood cells (RBCs) into the abdominal cavity. Migration of white blood cells (WBCs) follows the increase in RBCs. The WBC count and protein content may be elevated without a concurrent rise in RBCs in cases of abdominal abscesses or peritonitis.

The differential WBC count may be used to determine if the disorder is acute, as indicated by an increased granulocytic component, or chronic, as indicated by an increased total cell count with high numbers of large mononuclear cells.

In the presence of extensive bowel ischemia, bacteria and endotoxins escape into the abdominal cavity. Bacteria present within WBCs or free in the peritoneal cavity indicate a poor prognosis. Numerous bacteria of mixed types or plant material free in the peritoneal fluid indicate massive bacterial contamination of the abdomen following bowel rupture. To distinguish peritoneal fluid from intestinal contents, the examiner should look for phagocytized bacteria within neutrophils, which should be numerous in peritoneal fluid. Intestinal contents contain numerous mixed types of bacteria, plant material, and very few WBCs.

ADDITIONAL LABORATORY TESTS

In the evaluation of a horse with acute abdominal pain, measurement of packed cell volume (PCV), total plasma protein (PP), and total WBC count is essential. The PCV and PP are useful indicators of hydration, and the total WBC count helps detect conditions that will respond to medical therapy. For further evaluation, serum electrolyte determinations, renal function tests, blood gas analysis, and liver enzyme assays are useful in assisting diagnosis and therapy.

Interpretation of the PCV is affected by breed, excitement, age, training, and general health. "Hot-blooded" horses—Arabians, Thoroughbreds, Quarter Horses, and Standardbreds—have PCV values several per centage units higher than "cold-blooded" horses (European breeds and draft horses). Stress or excitement increases PCV through splenic contraction. Horses in strenuous training have a higher PCV than horses at rest, while aged horses often have a resting PCV within low normal limits. Horses with chronic disease or endoparasitism have a low hematocrit. Despite these variations, elevations in PCV have been found to be a significant prognostic indicator in cases of colic. In one report, horses with PCV values up to 45 per cent had a greater than 80 per cent chance of survival, whereas PCV values above 60 per cent were associated with only a 25 per cent chance of survival.

Plasma protein does not vary with breed, training, or changes in sympathetic tone. Hemoconcentration, indicated by increases in PCV and PP, develops slowly over 24 to 48 hours when there is no water intake. In contrast, severe hemoconcentration develops within hours when strangulating obstruction occurs. Hemoconcentration is secondary to extracellular fluid shifts from the plasma water compartment into obstructed bowel. Serial measurement of PCV and PP, along with physical parameters, is useful for assessing response to fluid therapy.

The total WBC count may be useful in detecting early cases of colitis, in which a decreased WBC count is observed. Neutropenia in the presence of fever with mild to moderate abdominal pain and severe depression is commonly seen in the early cases of enteritis. However, neutropenia reflects systemic endotoxemia and is not specific for enteritis. The leukogram in most cases of intestinal obstruction reveals a stress response, with modest elevations in mature neutrophils. Total WBC counts are elevated or within the upper normal range. In the presence of endotoxemia and sepsis, the leukogram is characterized by a decreased total WBC count with a degenerative leftward shift to immature granulocytes. Changes in polymorphonuclear morphology, such as Doehle bodies, foamy cytoplasm, and "toxic" granulation, are frequently seen. Leukopenia due to neutropenia, accompanied by a leftward shift on the leukogram and lymphopenia, calls for a guarded prognosis.

Serum electrolyte levels will vary with the severity and duration of illness, fluid and acid–base balance, intake, and renal function. Serial measurements of serum sodium, potassium, and chloride levels are valuable for providing appropriate fluid therapy.

ACID–BASE STATUS

The acid–base status depends on the nature and duration of the disorder and the level of obstruction. In most cases of intestinal obstruction, the acid–base status is within normal limits. Metabolic alkalosis may occur following loss of hydrogen and chloride ions when gastric reflux is evacuated. If hypovolemia occurs, it will be accompanied by lactic acidosis. Acid–base disorders occurring with GI disease are frequently difficult to predict. Most acid–base imbalances will correct following fluid volume replacement, so that routine treatment with bicarbonate should be avoided unless base deficit has been measured. Base deficits greater than 10 mMol/L should be treated with sodium bicarbonate.

RENAL AND LIVER FUNCTION TESTS

Laboratory tests that are indicative of renal function, such as blood urea nitrogen (BUN), serum creatinine, and urinalysis, are useful. Many cases of acute abdominal pain have a reduced plasma volume, resulting in prerenal azotemia, and in many cases of colic some degree of renal dysfunction is also present. This may be an important consideration if the use of potentially nephrotoxic nonsteroidal anti-inflammatory agents or aminoglycoside antimicrobials is considered. Liver function tests, such as sorbitol dehydrogenase (SDH), γ-glutamyltransferase (GGT), alkaline phosphatase (AP), fractionated bilirubin, and serum bile acid concentrations, may be useful in the differential diagnosis of mild abdominal pain or anorexia. Cholelithiasis should be considered when recurrent episodes of abdominal pain and clinical or pathologic evidence of obstructive liver disease are present. Increasing levels of GGT, AP and bilirubin, increased serum bile acids, and bilirubin are suggestive of cholelithiasis.

HEMOSTASIS

Hemostatic abnormalities associated with acute abdominal disorders have gained increased attention in recent years because of the clinical association of colic with thrombotic disease. Horses with severe abdominal conditions such as colitis or volvulus of the large colon appear to have an increased prevalence of jugular and mesenteric thrombosis; and laminitis, a condition that may be due to coagulation abnormalities, is a common complication of these disorders. Abnormalities in coagulation parameters are frequently reported in clinical cases of colic. The development of local and disseminated intravascular coagulation (DIC) occurs subsequent to endotoxemia and is an important factor in the pathogenesis of intestinal ischemia. Endotoxin can initiate the intrinsic clotting cascade by direct activation of factor XII. Endotoxin-activated neutrophils, ruptured endothelial cells, and other damaged tissue exudes tissue thromboplastin (factor III or tissue factor), initiating the extrinsic pathway.

Numerous tests of the intrinsic and extrinsic coagulation pathways are available. A suitable assessment of hemostasis can be made by measurement of platelet count, plasma fibrinogen, prothrombin time (PT), partial thromboplastin time (PTT), and fibrin degradation products (FDP). Plasma antithrombin III (AT-III) may be a useful prognostic indicator but is not readily available to date. The laboratory diagnosis of DIC is based on finding at least three of the following abnormalities: prolonged PT, prolonged PTT, elevated FDP, and thrombocytopenia. In the horse, hypofibrinogenemia does not frequently accompany DIC.

Hemostatic abnormalities are commonly detected in equine colic. Prolonged PTT and elevated fibrinogen levels are frequently observed, while thrombocytopenia, elevated FDP levels, and prolonged PT are indicative of a serious systemic disorder and a more guarded prognosis. A coagulation profile does not assist in diagnosis or in making the decision for surgery, but may aid in establishing the prognosis and suggesting the need for transfusion of blood components.

ANCILLARY DIAGNOSTIC AIDS

In select cases, abdominal radiography, including contrast-enhanced studies, or laparoscopy may be used to establish diagnosis. It should be recognized, however, that in many cases a definitive diagnosis is not established until an exploratory laparotomy is performed. The main emphasis for diagnosis should be to determine whether the abdominal pain can be treated medically or is amenable to surgical treatment.

THE DECISION FOR SURGERY AND PROGNOSTIC INDICATORS

In general, the cardinal signs of intestinal displacement requiring surgical correction are the following: severe abdominal pain that responds poorly or not at all to analgesic therapy; discolored peritoneal fluid containing increased protein, erythrocytes, and nucleated WBCs; and indications of obstruction or displacement of intestinal viscera on rectal examination. Not all of these signs need be present in a patient requiring abdominal surgery. For best chances for recovery, the decision for surgery should be made as early as possible. At the same time, unnecessary laparotomies should be avoided.

Therefore, the decision for referral to a surgical center or to perform surgery must be based on a combination of factors rather than waiting for all of the cardinal signs to become apparent (see *Current Therapy in Equine Medicine 2*, p. 30). History and signalment are important, with particular attention to the duration and severity of abdominal pain and findings on rectal examination. Horses with intestinal tympany, spasmodic colic, or gastric dilation may show signs of severe abdominal pain or sweating, but there is usually improvement in 2 to 4 hours.

During the physical examination, assessment of the cardiovascular status is critical. Alterations in vital signs, such as an elevated heart rate, prolonged capillary refill time, and mucous membrane discoloration, often reflect hypovolemia or endotoxemia from ischemic bowel. An uncertain diagnosis, progressive deterioration in cardiovascular status, and signs of unremitting abdominal pain are indications for exploratory laparotomy. Horses that continue to exhibit pain following administration of medications such as flunixin meglumine or xylazine, horses that require repeated doses of analgesics, horses with significant amounts of gastric reflux, or horses with distended small bowel on rectal examination may benefit from early referral.

Laboratory data generally do not assist in determining the need for surgical intervention. However, many of the laboratory tests mentioned earlier will help in assessing the degree of cardiovascular compromise to organ systems, determining therapy, and estimating prognosis.

If surgery is anticipated, it should be performed before bowel necrosis occurs and before severe changes in peritoneal fluid are observed. This is most important when the large bowel is involved. Changes in peritoneal fluid occur later in the course of large bowel disease as compared to small intestinal disease, and resection of large bowel is more difficult. When the decision for surgery is not clear, serial changes in peritoneal fluid may be used as a diagnostic aid.

In summary, the degree of pain, findings on rectal examination, the presence of gastric reflux, and peritoneal fluid analysis offer the best indications of the need for surgery. The decision to refer a case to a surgical facility should be made as early as possible. It is often best to refer the horse for further monitoring and evaluation rather than wait until surgery is essential. The importance of supportive therapy by the referring veterinarian cannot be overstated. This includes the use of IV fluid therapy prior to and during transport, and transporting the horse with a nasogastric tube in place. A brief history and record of therapy, such as the dosage and type of analgesics, antimicrobials, or laxatives, administered by the referring veterinarian should accompany the horse to the referral center.

Supplemental Readings

Bramlage, L. R.: Examination in acute abdominal crisis. *In* Mansmann, R. A., McAllister, E. S., Pratt, P. W. (eds.): Equine Medicine & Surgery. Santa Barbara, Calif., American Veterinary Publications, 1982, pp. 548–559.

Colahan, P. T.: Evaluation of horses with colic and the selection of surgical treatment. Compend. Cont. Ed. Pract. Vet. 7:S141–152, 1985.

Johnstone, I. B., and Crane, S.: Haemostatic abnormalities in horses with colic: Their prognostic value. Equine Vet. J., 18:271–274, 1986.

Morris, D. D., and Beech, J.: Disseminated intravascular coagulation in six horses. J. Am. Vet. Med. Assoc., 183:1067–1072, 1983.

Nelson, A. W.: Analysis of equine peritoneal fluid. Vet. Clin. North Am. (Large An. Pract.), 1:267–274, 1979.

Parry, B. W., Gay, C. C., and Anderson, G. A.: Assessment of the necessity for surgical intervention in cases of equine colic: A retrospective study. Eq. Vet. J. 15:216–221, 1983.

Traub, J. L., Rantanan, N., Reed, S., Schecter, L.: Cholelithiasis in four horses. J. Am. Vet. Med. Assoc., 181:59–62, 1982.

Rectal Examination of the Colic Patient

Norbert Kopf, VIENNA, AUSTRIA

Rectal examination is essential in each case of colic. Findings should always be considered in conjunction with the results of physical examination, nasogastric intubation, abdominocentesis, and laboratory data. Rectal exploration should always be performed before paracentesis in order to recognize extremely enlarged portions of bowel and to prevent accidental penetration of distended loops of intestine. To determine the type of intestinal obstruction, internal palpation is the most useful technique. Palpation findings usually give an indication of the need for surgical intervention or conservative treatment. The value of rectal examination depends on the experience of the examiner and cooperation of the patient. It is impossible to survey the peritoneal cavity completely by internal palpation, because only the pelvic cavity and the caudal portion, or approximately 40 per cent, of the abdominal cavity can be explored.

Frequently, rather subtle signs or hints found during examination yield information pointing to conditions in deeper abdominal regions. In other cases, the location and the type of the obstruction can be identified precisely—for example, incarcerated inguinal hernia and left dorsal displacement of the large colon.

TECHNIQUE

To minimize the risk of damage to the rectum, horses with unrelenting pain should be treated with analgesics or sedatives such as xylazine° (0.1 to 0.2 mg per kg). Use of a twitch is almost always necessary to prevent straining. An alternative method of restraint is the simple fixation of a hindleg with a rope attached to the pastern and led between the forelegs to the neck. If the veterinarian examines with the right arm the left hindleg is fixed, and vice versa. The anus of the horse and the gloved hand should be lubricated sufficiently to reduce resistance and mucosal irritation when the hand is inserted. First, the mucosa of the ampulla should be examined for any lesions, and blood or clots on the withdrawn arm. Rectal mucus and the contents of the rectal ampulla are noted and fecal balls are eliminated. The next reinsertion of the arm should be as deep as possible when the rectum is flaccid to facilitate examination of deep regions. The size of the rectal tube in relation to the palpator's hand is assessed from the tension of the rectal wall over the examiner's wrist, hand, and forearm. Limitation by a short mesorectum also will be identified. Often the lumen travels ventrally. The examiner should follow this ventral deviation and then raise the arm dorsally to straighten the rectum. Figure 1 shows the stressed areas, which are usually predisposed to iatrogenic lesions. Initial manipulation of tissues with a half-inserted arm, and examination of the pelvic cavity first, usually causes tenesmus and propulsive contractions of the rectum. Consequently, thorough investigation of more cranial structures is prevented.

EXAMINATION FINDINGS

NORMAL RECTAL FINDINGS

Rectal findings in the healthy animal (Fig. 2) include well-formed, soft fecal balls in the rectal ampulla that have an aromatic odor. The rectal mucosa is finely folded. The small colon is identified by fecal balls, which can be moved in all directions. At the right side, the cecum often can be recognized as a soft viscus containing some gas. The only portion of the cecum that can always be identified is the ventral taenia. In small horses ventral and medial taeniae can be palpated. If the cecum contains some gas or ingesta, its dorsal adhesion to the abdominal wall can be touched going from the aorta to the right side. At the left flank the caudal edge of the spleen can be found. Usually the caudal pole of the left kidney and the suspensory ligament of the spleen or nephrosplenic ligament can be identified. Two or three fingers can be inserted into the nephrosplenic space between the dorsal part of the spleen and the left kidney. In small horses the cranial mesenteric root can be investigated by fingertips as a flaccid folded band running in a ventral direction. Parts of the large colon frequently cannot be identified. By passing the hand along the ventral abdominal wall, it is often possible to feel some bands or the pelvic flexure if it contains ingesta. The caudal part of the abdominal cavity can normally be reached in all directions without any resistance.

°Rompun, Haver-Lockhart, Shawnee, KS

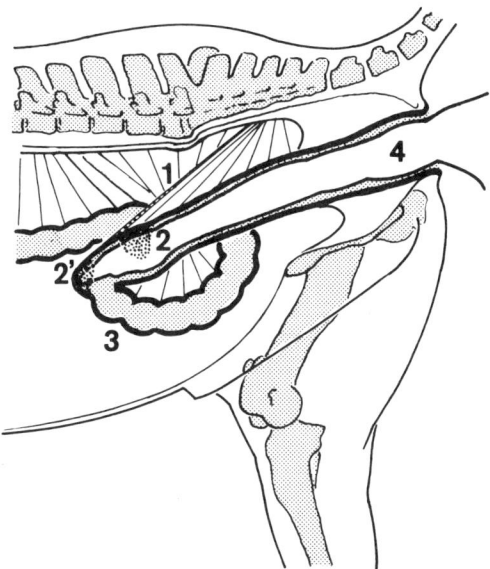

Figure 1. Technique of deep rectal examination. 1, Stretched mesorectum; 2, 2′, Areas of increased extension of the rectal wall; 3, Ventral deviation of the small colon; 4, Position of the arm in relation to the abdominal and pelvic cavity.

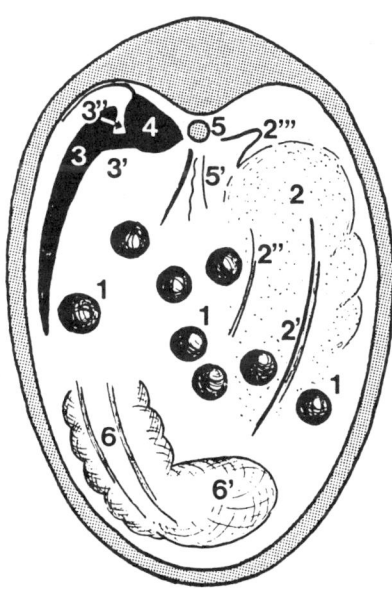

Figure 2. Normal rectal findings. 1, Fecal balls marking the small colon; 2, Cecal base containing some gas; 2′, Its ventral taenia; 2″, Its medial taenia; 2‴, Its adhesion to the dorsal abdominal wall; 3, Spleen; 3′, Its suspensory ligament; 3″, Nephrosplenic space; 4, Kidney; 5, Aorta; 5′, Cranial mesenteric root; 6, Large colon, bands of the ventral portion; 6′, Pelvic flexure.

PATHOLOGICAL FINDINGS

The common location of rectal tears is in the dorsal bowel wall at the cranial limitation of the rectal ampulla (see p. 232). Lubricant on the glove with a sanguinous tinge after the first inspection of this area requires careful investigation. Bloody and malodorous brownish fluid is also found in all conditions that compromise the vascular supply of the small colon with or without compromise of its lumen. Injuries of the rectum are best explored by the more sensitive bare hand. The smooth mucosa disappears and the surface is rough.

In cases of intestinal obstruction the rectum frequently contains no fecal material and the rectal mucus is inspissated. Small dry fecal balls coated with pasty mucus signify delayed transport of the feces. By contrast, chronic impaction of the cecum often causes a diarrhealike stool. To interpret the findings of rectal examination correctly, one must pay particular attention to the consistency, form, position, location, or tenseness of both the intestine and mesentery. The taeniae are important structures for identification of specific segments of the large bowel. Intestinal impactions cause enlargement of the constipated parts of the bowel and have a pasty or doughy consistency. Digital impressions remain for some time.

In dilations of the intestine caused by gas accumulation, impressions disappear at once. By pressing the bowels against the abdominal wall or pelvis, the examiner can identify lesions such as edema and infarction that increase the thickness of the bowel wall. Localized intestinal pain can also be reproduced in this manner. In stallions and geldings, palpation of the vaginal ring should be a routine part of the examination.

Intravaginal inguinal herniation of the small intestine occurs if the peritoneal ring is large. Rectal findings in this condition are an enlarged loop of the small intestine with abnormal fixation at the abdominal wall in the inguinal region, acute pain, and a taut mesentery. External palpation of the scrotum completes this diagnosis.

Obstructions of the small bowel are characterized by distended loops of small intestine that are compressible to varying degrees. The diameter may vary from 5 to 12 cm, depending on the duration of the condition. In cases of high obstruction or in late cases, the dilated second flexure of the duodenum surrounding the dorsal adhesion of the cecum can be recognized. The strangulated part of the small bowel can be identified by the thickening of its wall. In all cases of small bowel obstruction the ingesta inside the large colon becomes more solid because of dehydration. Dehydration also reduces the size of the large colon, making the constrictions and sacculations of the ventral part of the large colon palpably more distinct (Fig. 3). Touching the strangulated intestinal or mesenteric parts may cause pain. In a high obstruction of the small in-

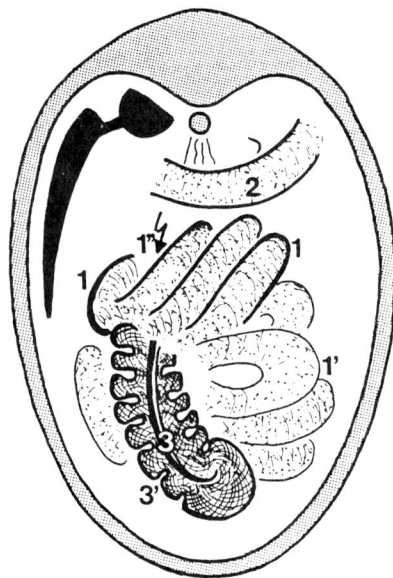

Figure 3. Rectal findings in small bowel obstruction. 1, Strangulated parts of small intestine, distended loops with thickened wall; 1', Prestenotic loops of small bowel, tympanic without thickening of the wall; 1" (⚡), Painful area; 2, Caudal flexure of the distended duodenum; 3, Large colon containing solid ingesta; 3', Its contracted sacculations.

testine, distended loops may not be within reach. In this situation, however, gentle traction on the ventral taenia of the cecum in a caudal direction is very painful. *Ileal impaction* can be diagnosed by rectal examination in early cases only. The obstipated ileum feels like a large sausage, the end of which is fixed in the right dorsal region at the base of the cecum; the cecum itself is poststenotic and therefore empty and not palpable. Tension on the taut mesentery of the ileum produces pain. In late cases the constipated ileum cannot be palpated because the distended loops of the caudal portion of the prestenotic jejunum fill the caudal part of the abdominal cavity and the ileum may be dislocated in a cranial direction.

In cases of *ileocecal intussusception* a blunt mass can be felt in the right dorsal region. The mass is fixed at its dorsomedial pole and can be moved like a pendulum in transverse and sagittal directions. Touching the point of fixation often elicits pain. In all cases of small bowel obstruction *gastric dilation* occurs. A dislocation of the spleen in the ventromedial and caudal direction is an indication of tremendous gastric dilation.

Acute dilation of the cecum produces obvious rectal findings as the form of the organ can be recognized very clearly. The ventral taenia, the large-caliber sacculations, and the deep constrictions can be felt. Impactions of the cecum can be diagnosed because of the typical form of this bowel, its dorsal junction to the abdominal wall, and the doughy consistency. Sometimes a relapsing spastic impaction of the overhanging part of the cecal base occurs. It can only be reached in medium-sized horses, is recognized because of its oval form, and can be moved like a pendulum in a transverse direction. In severe cases of recurrent *impaction of the cecum* hypertrophy of the circular layer of the smooth muscles of the base and the body of the cecum can be recognized even if the cecum is not well filled. In all cases of *strangulation of the large colon* there is a large amount of gas distention of the cecum proximal to the obstruction. When the cecum is distended with gas, its apex tends to "float up" and the ventral taenia becomes positioned in an oblique or transverse direction.

One of the most common findings in horses with colic is *impaction of the left ventral portion of the large colon*. The colon is enlarged and the obstipation has a cone-formed end at the pelvic flexure (Fig. 4). The two free taeniae of the ventral large colon can be felt as longitudinal grooves, separated by 90 degrees in relation to the circumference of the intestinal tube. The consistency of the obstipated ingesta depends on the tone of the intestinal wall and can change suddenly during the manual investigation. Because of the enlargement, the sacculations and constrictions are not recognizable. This is a very significant difference from cases of *pseudoimpac-*

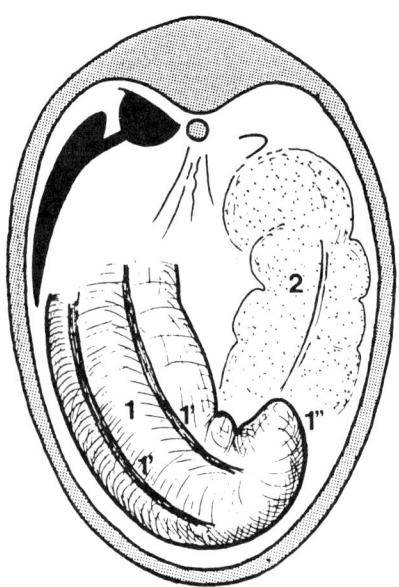

Figure 4. Rectal findings in impaction of the left ventral colon. 1, Enlarged large colon containing doughy ingesta; 1', Its two free taenia (Distanced 90 degrees in relation to the circumference of the intestinal tube); 1", Cone-formed end of the obstipation at the pelvic flexure; 2, Tympanic cecum.

tion of the large bowels caused by the dehydration in cases of small bowel obstruction. This difference must be noted to prevent improper interpretation of cases in which the firmness of the contents of the large colon is increased.

Impaction of the ampulla of the right dorsal portion of the large colon has the shape and dimensions of a soccer ball, approximately 30 cm in diameter. Often it will not be within reach. Only in medium-sized horses in which the cranial mesenteric root can be investigated easily can the caudal part of the constipated ampulla coli be reached. The cranial mesenteric root can be pressed against the background of the dome-like protrusion of the constipated dorsal colon and serves as a helpful guide in identifying the location of the obstipated ingesta.

Occlusion of the large colon by enteroliths also occurs at the junction of the right dorsal and transverse colon. If the occluding stone can be touched, there is no question about the type of obstruction. The prestenotic parts of the large colon are greatly distended by gas, as in all cases of strangulation and volvulus of the large colon in which the occlusion is total.

Extreme distention of the large colon with gas and tremendous tension on its taeniae are the cornerstones in rectal identification of *torsion or flexion* of this intestinal part. After a few hours, the twisted bowels become edematous, and the thickened intestinal wall, haustra, and longitudinal bands are readily palpated. In some cases the ventral colon can be located dorsal to the dorsal colon. Because of the distention, the large bowel cannot be moved. In some cases it is positioned in a transverse direction, with the curvature of the pelvic flexure dislocated either toward the right flank or in a cranial direction. In dramatic cases of *torsion of the entire large colon* tympany may be so severe that it is impossible to explore the cranial regions of the abdominal cavity (Fig. 5).

A frequently observed condition is the *strangulation of the large colon by the suspensory ligament of the spleen*—the so-called left dorsal displacement of the large colon (Fig. 6). The location of the strangulation can be investigated by rectal palpation. If the dislocated portion of the colon is large, the bands (taeniae) run diagonally to converge at the nephrosplenic space on the left dorsal quadrant of the abdomen. By palpating from the caudal pole of the left kidney toward the left abdominal wall, the examiner can feel the taeniae of the large colon crossing dorsally to the nephrosplenic ligament. The spleen is almost always situated in its normal position but may be hidden by tympanic parts of the dislocated colon. In a few cases of left dorsal dis-

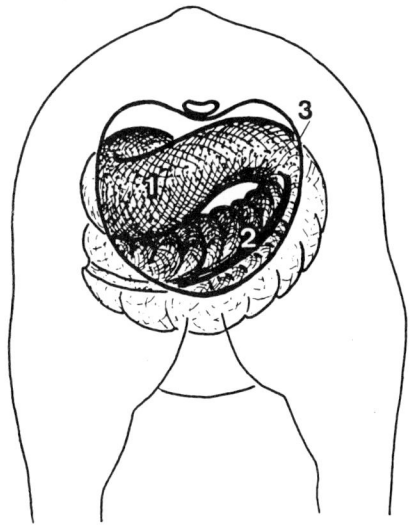

Figure 5. Rectal findings in torsion of the whole large colon. 1, Tympanic dorsal portion; 2, Edemous and gaseous distended ventral part of the large colon in transverse position with clearly contoured sacculations and constrictions; 3, Limitation of pelvic cavity (deeper regions cannot be explored).

placement of the large colon, only the impacted pelvic flexure is strangulated over the suspensory ligament of the spleen. This condition is easily recognized from the wheel-like form of this intestinal part, with a diameter of the intestinal tube of 15 to 20 cm.

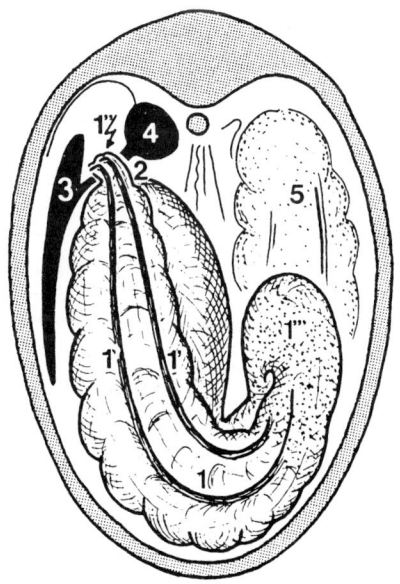

Figure 6. Rectal findings in left dorsal displacement of the large colon. 1, Enlarged large colon with accumulation of gas and ingesta: 1', Tensed oblique sinistrodorsocranial converging taenia; 1" ($\frac{1}{2}$), Location of strangulation with pain on palpation; 1''', Dislocated tympanic pelvic flexure; 2, Suspensory ligament of the spleen (covered by the large colon); 3, Spleen; 4, Kidney; 5, Prestenotic tympany of the cecum.

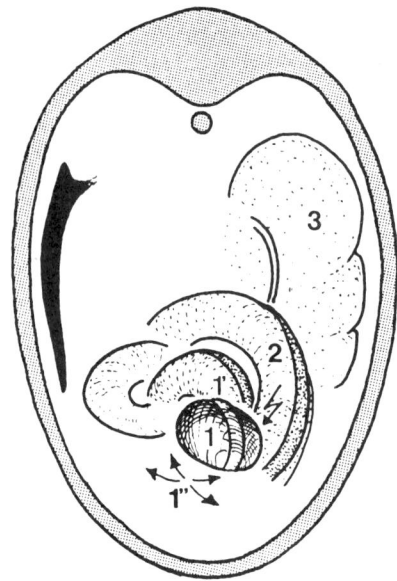

Figure 7. Rectal findings in occlusion of the small colon by an enterolith. 1, Obstructed bowel part with local pain on palpation (↯); 1', prominent free taenia; 1" Possible directions of manual displacement; 2, Tympany of the prestenotic part of the small colon; 3, Cecum.

A similar condition is *right dorsal displacement of the large colon* between the tympanic cecum and the right abdominal wall. The large colon is flexed in a rightward and caudal direction and covers the cecum. The edematous fat of the mesentery containing the large blood vessels between the ventral and the dorsal colon has a jellylike consistency.

Obstruction of the small colon by foreign bodies or fecal concretions can be diagnosed accurately on rectal examination (Fig. 7). The occluding body is usually situated at the ventral abdominal wall near the pelvic inlet and can be moved in all directions. The broad and prominent antimesenteric band of the small colon can be palpated and helps to identify this bowel section. The tympanic prestenotic loops of the small colon have a diameter of approximately 6 to 10 cm and are curved like wheels.

In cases of impaction or volvulus of the small colon, deep rectal examination often is not possible. Only the forearm can be inserted to touch the distended loops of the small colon. In such cases the caudal mesenteric root can be felt because it is tense. This is not found in any other condition, because the free-floating mesentery of the small colon normally is not noticeable.

Pain elicited on palpation of the visceral surface of the abdominal wall is an indication of acute *diffuse peritonitis*. In cases in which rupture of an abdominal viscus has occurred the dorsal part of the abdominal cavity feels empty and there are floating flaccid intestinal loops in the ventral part. The peritoneum may feel rough because of adherent fecal particles, and in cases of gastric or cecal rupture there is evidence of emphysema in the supraperitoneal space.

To completely assess intestinal or intraperitoneal injury, rectal examination should always be complemented by abdominocentesis. In an analysis of 150 cases at our university, a definitive diagnosis was obtained in 75 patients by rectal palpation alone. In an additional 27 per cent an indication for surgical treatment was obtained by rectal exploration. Only in 6 per cent of these cases was a false diagnosis caused by errors in interpretation of rectal findings. In 9 per cent of the horses rectal examination was not practicable because the horses were too small.

Supplemental Readings

Huskamp, B., Daniels, H., and Kopf, N.: Magen- und Darmkrankheiten. In Dietz, O., and Wiesner, E. (eds.): Handbuch der Pferdekrankheiten für Wissenschaft und Praxis, Vol. 2, VEB. Jena, Gustav Fischer Verlag, 1982.

Huskamp, B., and Kopf, N.: Die Verlagerung des Colon ascendens in den Milznierenraum beim Pferd (Hernia spatii lienorenalis coli ascendentis). Tierarztl. Prax., 8:327, 495, 1980.

Huskamp, B., and Kopf, N.: Right dorsal displacement of the large colon in the horse. Equine Pract., 5:20, 1983.

Kopf, N.: Rectal findings in horses with intestinal obstruction. *In:* Proceedings of the 1st Colic Research Symposium, University of Georgia, Athens, 1982.

Kopf, N., and Huskamp, B.: Die rektale Untersuchung beim Kolikpferd. Prakt. Tierarzt, 59:259, 1978.

Pharmacologic Management of Colic

E. Susan Clark, ATHENS, GEORGIA

Gastrointestinal (GI) lesions can cause important changes in intestinal motility, absorption, and secretion, thereby resulting in an accumulation of fluid and electrolytes in the intestinal lumen at the expense of both intestinal distention and depletion of the intravascular fluid compartment. Hypovolemia can compromise cardiovascular stability and tissue perfusion. Intestinal distention due to mechanical obstruction or motility disorders causes abdominal pain. Physical examination findings associated with these conditions include tachycardia, dry mucous membranes, altered mucous membrane color, prolonged capillary refill time, cold extremities, nasogastric reflux, and the rectal examination finding of intestinal distention.

GI diseases that disrupt either the intraluminal contents or the blood supply to the intestinal lamina propria can initiate a progression of mucosal degeneration. Subsequent to this destruction of the mucosal epithelial barrier, bacterial endotoxin gains access to the peritoneal cavity and the systemic circulation. Once in the general circulation, endotoxin causes a progressive syndrome of multisystemic disturbances. Clinical signs typically exhibited by horses with endotoxemia are tachypnea, alterations in mucous membrane color and moistness, pyrexia, and abdominal pain (see page 225).

Although disruption of both intestinal function and the mucosal epithelial barrier during GI disease processes initiates these numerous adverse effects on the GI, cardiovascular, and other body systems, only certain of these effects are amenable to pharmacologic therapy. Therapeutic agents include analgesics to control visceral pain, agents to normalize intestinal contractions during adynamic ileus, anti-inflammatory drugs to reduce the adverse effects of endotoxin, and drugs to improve cardiovascular function during endotoxic and hypovolemic shock.

ANALGESICS

Relief of visceral pain in horses with severe colic is important to minimize injury to personnel attending the patient during evaluation and therapy. Owner distress over animal pain is a consideration even in mild cases. Unfortunately, analgesics may mask clinical signs that must be monitored for proper case management. Therefore, analgesic therapy (Table 1) must be tailored to the case, based on knowledge of the potency, mechanism of action, and side effects of analgesic drugs and a current assessment of the patient's condition.

NONSTEROIDAL ANTI-INFLAMMATORY DRUGS

Dipyrone, phenylbutazone, and flunixin meglumine are the nonsteroidal anti-inflammatory drugs (NSAIDs) used for analgesia in horses with abdominal pain. The therapeutic and adverse effects of these drugs result from inhibition of cyclooxygenase enzyme-mediated biosynthesis of prostaglandins. Because prostaglandins are directly responsible for provoking pain only when present in large concentrations, it may be assumed that NSAIDs only provide analgesia for pain elicited by intestinal inflammation or ischemia. Of more relevance to pain, prostaglandins increase both sensitivity to other painful stimuli and pain perception in the central nervous system (CNS). Antagonism to the increased CNS perception of pain probably accounts for the pain relief provided by administration of NSAIDs to horses with abdominal pain caused by increased mesenteric tension.

Dipyrone, phenylbutazone, and flunixin meglumine differ greatly in efficacy in the treatment of visceral pain in horses. Dipyrone is a very weak analgesic drug that provides only short-term relief in a few cases of very mild abdominal pain. When it does relieve pain it is very useful, because several doses can be safely administered over a few hours. In general, phenylbutazone provides no more relief from visceral pain than does dipyrone. However, the toxic side effects of phenylbutazone are numerous and include GI ulceration and nephrotoxicity. For this reason, the dosage of phenylbutazone should not exceed 4.4 mg per kg every 12 hours.

Flunixin meglumine is the most effective NSAID for control of visceral pain in horses. The duration of analgesia produced by flunixin varies from less than 1 hour to more than 24 hours, depending on the cause and severity of the pain. Administration of flunixin meglumine is sometimes necessary for control of severe abdominal pain in horses needing transport to a referral center. Although this drug has toxic side effects similar to phenylbutazone, the greater risk asso-

TABLE 1. ANALGESICS USED FOR TREATMENT OF VISCERAL PAIN IN HORSES

Analgesic	Trade Name	Manufacturer	Dosage
Dipyrone	Novin	Mobay Animal Health	11 mg/kg IV
			11 mg/kg IM
Phenylbutazone	Phenylbutazone	Butler	2.2–4.4 mg/kg IV
Flunixin meglumine	Banamine	Schering	0.25–1.1 mg/kg IV or IM
Xylazine	Rompun	Mobay Animal Health	0.2–0.4 mg/kg IV
			0.5–1 mg/kg IM
Detomidine	Domosedan	Norden	10–30 µg/kg IV
Choral hydrate			20–50 mg/kg IV°
			40–100 mg/kg PO
Pentazocine lactate	Talwin-V	Winthrop	0.8 mg/kg IV
Butorphanol tartrate	Torbugesic	Bristol	0.05–0.1 mg/kg IV or IM

°Recommended dosage when chloral hydrate (12%) is combined with magnesium sulfate (6%).

ciated with the use of flunixin meglumine devolves from its ability to mask clinical signs of intestinal strangulation or obstruction. Flunixin meglumine may reduce heart rate, provide comfort, and improve mucous membrane color. It is important, therefore, to monitor rectal examination findings, nasogastric reflux, heart rate, and respiratory rate after administration of flunixin meglumine. Severe small intestinal or large colon distention discerned on rectal examination may be consistent with small intestinal volvulus or large colon torsion, respectively. Recurrence of abdominal pain after administration of flunixin meglumine in horses with moderate, mild, or no intestinal distention may suggest nonstrangulating obstruction, inflammatory disease of the intestine, or inflammatory disease of the peritoneum. Reduced dosages of flunixin meglumine (0.25 to 0.75 mg per kg given intravenously [IV] or intramuscularly [IM] may provide sufficient analgesia in some cases.

SEDATIVES

Sedatives decrease CNS awareness of pain. Xylazine, the sedative most commonly used for colic in horses, produces both sedation and analgesia by stimulating α_2-adrenoceptors in the CNS, thereby decreasing neurotransmission. At dosages of 1.1 mg per kg IV, the visceral analgesia provided by xylazine is similar to that of the narcotics and flunixin. The duration of effect of xylazine is much shorter (usually 10 to 40 minutes) than that of flunixin, making xylazine more useful for controlling pain during evaluation of the cause of colic and of the need for specific therapy. Potentially detrimental side effects of xylazine include bradycardia, decreased cardiac output, transient hypertension followed by hypotension, ileus, and decreased intestinal blood flow. The bradycardia, hypertension, and intestinal hypoperfusion last only a few minutes. In contrast, the ileus and hypotension can be prolonged. A reduced dosage of xylazine (0.2 to 0.4 mg per kg IV) can be administered in an attempt to reduce the severity and duration of the side effects. In addition, administration of lower dosages of xylazine with narcotic agonists may produce superior analgesia with fewer side effects.

Detomidine is a new α_2-adrenoceptor agonist that is a more potent sedative and analgesic agent than xylazine. Administration of dosages of detomidine that cause bradycardia and hypertension similar in degree and duration to that caused by xylazine produces significantly more intense and more prolonged analgesia and sedation than xylazine. The analgesia is superior to that achieved with flunixin and can mask abdominal pain and changes in heart rate and respiratory rate for up to 90 minutes. Although the potent effects of detomidine will mask pain, the sedation provided may allow examination and transportation of those horses with severe abdominal pain nonresponsive to other analgesics.

Although chloral hydrate effectively reduces the response to painful stimuli, it does not provide analgesia. Therefore, this drug is not routinely used in horses with colic. On the other hand, this hypnotic sedative produces minimal cardiovascular, respiratory, or GI side effects. Therefore, chloral hydrate is sometimes useful for controlling pain in some colic patients. Although the duration of effect of chloral hydrate after IV administration is short (15 to 60 minutes), a more prolonged duration of action can be obtained with oral administration.

NARCOTIC ANALGESICS

Morphine sulfate, meperidine hydrochloride, oxymorphone, butorphanol tartrate, and pentazocine lactate have been used as visceral analgesics in horses. The analgesic and sedative effects of these drugs result from interaction with central and/or peripheral opioid receptors. Morphine, meperidine, and oxymorphone are opioid receptor agonists. The narcotics increase regional intestinal contractions, thereby causing intestinal transit to be prolonged and sometimes causing abdominal pain. In addition, opiate agonists may reduce intestinal secretions and thus predispose to impactions. Cardiovascular changes and respiratory depression are usually minimal. However, morphine, meperidine, and oxymorphone tend to increase locomotor activity and cause behavioral side effects. Although these drugs are occasionally used to increase the analgesic effect of xylazine in intractable patients, their clinical use is generally precluded by those excitatory effects.

In contrast, pentazocine lactate and butorphanol tartrate both stimulate opioid receptors and oppose the action of the agonists of opioid receptors. Therefore, these opiate agonist–antagonists are infrequently excitatory and have fewer GI side effects than the pure opiate agonists. Excitement and behavioral alterations rarely occur at recommended dosages. Butorphanol tartrate may cause excitement when administered IV at dosages exceeding 0.2 mg per kg. Pentazocine is more effective than dipyrone but less effective than xylazine and flunixin in relieving visceral pain. The degree of analgesia produced by butorphanol is superior to that achieved with pentazocine and flunixin, and is similar to that produced by xylazine. The duration (15 to 90 minutes) of the analgesic effect of butorphanol is shorter than that of flunixin, thereby reducing the risk associated with masking signs of pain. The combination of xylazine and butorphanol (0.01 to 0.075 mg per kg) can be used for analgesia in horses with moderate to severe abdominal pain.

PHARMACOLOGIC AGENTS THAT ALTER MOTILITY

Intestinal distention due to hypomotility is a complication of many GI diseases that result in colic. Postoperative ileus is the most common indication for pharmacologic manipulation of intestinal contractile activity. There are two general methods by which drugs may correct ileus caused by any disease. First, drugs may directly stimulate contraction of the intestinal smooth muscle. Second, certain agents block the mechanism by which the disease inhibits motility, thereby restoring normal contractions. By nonspecifically stimulating motility, drugs acting by the first mechanism usually induce spasmodic contractions. This undesirable effect results in intermittent abdominal pain and increased regional contractions, resulting in slowed intestinal transit. Therefore, the preferred method of correcting postoperative ileus is to specifically antagonize the inhibiting neurogenic or hormonal processes.

The specific mechanism by which stimulation of the visceral and parietal peritoneum during surgical manipulation reflexly inhibits motility is unknown. There is evidence from studies in other species that postoperative ileus involves hyperactivity of sympathetic reflexes. β-Adrenoceptor blockade with propranolol significantly reduces the duration of postoperative ileus in humans. In an experimental model of postoperative ileus in ponies, however, propranolol was not effective in improving intestinal transit. α_2-Adrenergic inhibition with yohimbine blocks colonic ileus created by peritonitis in some laboratory animals and is effective in correcting experimental postoperative ileus in horses.

Some studies of experimentally induced postoperative ileus in ponies have implicated dopaminergic hyperactivity as an important factor in the pathogenesis of postoperative ileus. Unfortunately, in the author's experience, clinical use of metoclopramide, a nonspecific dopaminergic antagonist, in the treatment of equine postoperative ileus has been variably effective. Furthermore, metoclopramide is unsuitable for use clinically as it produces severe CNS side effects. Because metoclopramide nonspecifically stimulates intestinal contractions by facilitating the release and action of acetylcholine, abdominal pain has occurred as a frequent side effect of treatment. In contrast, domperidone, a newer dopaminergic antagonist, does not cross the blood–brain barrier or interact with cholinergic mechanisms in the GI tract. Like metoclopramide, domperidone (0.2 mg per kg IV) does, however, block dopaminergic receptors and prevent postoperative ileus induced experimentally in ponies. Domperidone deserves attention as a potential therapeutic agent for treatment of postoperative ileus in horses.

Endotoxemia may also play a role in the pathogenesis of postoperative ileus. Many GI diseases causing colic damage the intestinal mucosal epithelium, thereby allowing absorption of endotoxin into the systemic circulation. Even very mild endotoxemia results in profound inhibition of motility of the stomach, jejunum, ileum, cecum, and large colon. Quiescence of GI contractile activity during endotoxemia results from both a prostaglandin-dependent mechanism and a prostaglandin-independent mechanism. It appears that the prostaglandin-independent mechanism involves α_2-adrenoceptors. Flunixin meglumine (1.1 mg per kg IV), phenylbutazone (2.2 mg per kg IV), and yohimbine (0.075 mg per kg IV), an α_2-adrenoceptor agonist, have been effective in restoring intestinal motility during ileus induced by experimental endotoxemia. The role of these mechanisms in induction of ileus in clinical cases has not been investigated.

Of the drugs that directly stimulate intestinal contractions, neostigmine has been used clinically. Disorganized, segmental contractile activity caused by nonspecific agents does not improve aboral progression of ingesta. The resulting contractions increase intestinal wall tension, thereby causing pain and impeding intestinal blood flow. Neostigmine methylsulfate (0.02 mg per kg given subcutaneously [SC]), a drug that reversibly inactivates the enzyme acetylcholine esterase that degrades acetylcholine, has been administered to stimulate intestinal contractions in horses. The duration of effect is very short (15 to 30 minutes) and the contractile activity may not correspond to propulsive motility. In some studies this drug decreased propulsive motility of the jejunum and delayed gastric emptying in horses. Neostigmine can cause abdominal pain when administered to healthy horses and patients with colic. This pain could be a result of spasmodic regional contractions. Metoclopramide may increase contractions by facilitating the action of normally released acetylcholine, thereby being less likely to induce painful spasmodic contractions.

Bethanecol, a cholinomimetic agent, has been used to stimulate motility, especially in the most proximal portion of the intestinal tract. The drug has been administered at 0.025 mg per kg SC every 6 to 8 hours, followed by maintenance dosages of 0.3 to 0.4 mg per kg orally every 6 to 8 hours to stimulate gastric motility in patients with delayed gastric emptying due to gastric ulceration. Potential side effects include salivation and stimulation of gastric acid secretion.

Cisapride is a prokinetic agent under investigation for treatment of ileus in horses. Its mechanism of action appears to be through facilitating release of acetylcholine. Although the drug presently is not for clinical use in horses, both experimentally induced ileus in horses and postoperative ileus have been successfully treated with cisapride. Further investigation of the clinical safety and efficacy of cisapride is warranted.

Anti-Inflammatory Agents

The primary indication for use of anti-inflammatory agents in treatment of colic patients is to block production of the mediators of the metabolic and hemodynamic alterations seen in endotoxemia. Although accumulating evidence indicates that endotoxemia adversely alters the function of most tissues, few if any of these pathophysiologic consequences result from direct effects of the endotoxin molecule. In contrast, it is known that the pathophysiology of endotoxemia revolves around the ability of the endotoxin molecule to elicit the formation and release of vasoactive and pro-inflammatory substances. In this light, it is currently believed that anti-inflammatory agents are beneficial to the treatment of endotoxemia.

Nonsteroidal Anti-Inflammatory Agents

By inhibiting cyclooxygenase-mediated production of the arachidonic metabolites responsible for some of the vasoactive effects of endotoxin, NSAIDs are currently believed to be of benefit in endotoxemia. Flunixin appears to be more effective than phenylbutazone or dipyrone at suppressing prostaglandin-mediated effects of endotoxemia in the horse. Consequently, flunixin is frequently administered to patients with intestinal ischemia and endotoxemia.

Because certain end products of cyclooxygenase enzyme are necessary for maintenance of local blood flow and integrity of renal tubular and GI epithelial cells, toxicity is a potential problem with therapy with NSAIDs. In addition, concern has been expressed regarding possible potentiation of NSAID toxicity by endotoxemia and hypovolemia. Furthermore, because administration of flunixin at a dosage of 1.1 mg per kg can mask clinical signs of intestinal strangulation, treatment of endotoxemia with this dosage of flunixin before obtaining a definitive diagnosis for the cause of endotoxemia and abdominal pain may be contraindicated. Reduced dosages of flunixin (0.25 mg per kg every 8 hours) decrease thromboxane production during experimental endotoxemia with a lower potential for causing toxic side effects and masking pain and therefore are recommended for treatment of endotoxemia.

Dimethyl Sulfoxide

Dimethyl sulfoxide (DMSO) is a hygroscopic solvent that has been used therapeutically for its anti-inflammatory properties. Although the mechanisms of its anti-inflammatory effects are not entirely known, many attribute these to its ability to detoxify hydroxyl radicals generated by neutrophils as part of the inflammatory process and by enzymatic processes in reperfused ischemic tissue. Therefore, there is a theoretical basis for using DMSO to help prevent endotoxin-mediated sequelae and damage to reperfused ischemic tissue. A low dosage of DMSO (0.1 gm per kg IV as a 10 per cent solution every 6 to 12 hours) has been used in patients with endotoxemia and strangulating obstruction; however, there have been no controlled studies of its efficacy. Rapid administration of more concentrated solutions (≥20 per cent) often results in hemolysis.

It is believed that surgery can induce peritoneal inflammation leading to formation of peritoneal adhesions. Therefore, anti-inflammatory drug therapy is also indicated in patients requiring abdominal surgery. In contrast to dosages used for therapy of endotoxemia, high dosages of NSAIDs are recommended for treating peritonitis. Flunixin (1.1 mg per kg) should be administered before and every 12 hours for 36 hours after surgery.

DRUGS USED TO IMPROVE CARDIOVASCULAR FUNCTION

Because the venous return to the heart is decreased, both endotoxic and hypovolemic shock result in decreased cardiac output. The usual method of restoring venous return and therefore cardiac output is IV administration of large volumes of fluids. Furthermore, endotoxin directly affects the myocardium to decrease contractility, thereby further reducing tissue perfusion. Clinically, this becomes most important during anesthesia with cardiodepressant drugs. Dopamine stimulates α- and β-adrenoceptors and dopaminergic receptors. Administration of dopamine at 2.5 to 5 μg per kg per minute increases cardiac output in conscious horses, anesthetized horses, and endotoxemic ponies. By increasing cardiac output and dilating local vascular beds, these dosages of dopamine may improve perfusion of the kidney and visceral organs. As the dosage of dopamine increases, however, excessive stimulation of α- and β-adrenoceptors may result in tachycardia, arrhythmias, and constriction of local vascular beds. Because these adverse effects of higher dosages of dopamine are affected by sympathetic nervous system activity, dosages at which these effects are noted in diseased animals are variable. Therefore careful monitoring of the patient's status must accompany use of this drug. Dopamine hydrochloride (200 mg) dissolved in 500 ml of either 0.9 per cent sodium chloride or 5 per cent dextrose solution and administered at 3 ml per minute provides a dosage of 2.5 μg per kg per minute in a 450-kg horse. The dosage may be increased to not greater than 5 μg per kg per minute to achieve the desired effect. However, if either tachycardia, arrhythmias, or excitation develop, dopamine infusion should be discontinued. Dopamine is rapidly metabolized, and therefore the duration of affect after cessation of dopamine infusion is only several minutes. Dobutamine is a more specific agonist of β-adrenergic receptors. This drug can be used to improve cardiac output; however, its vasodilator properties are not as potent as those of dopamine.

LAXATIVES

Laxatives (Table 2) are commonly used in the treatment of colic to increase the water content and softness of ingesta, thereby facilitating intestinal transit. Laxatives are usually used for treating impactions of the large colon in adult horses and foals. The most effective therapy for these conditions is hydration of the impacted ingesta with fluids administered orally (PO) and IV. Laxatives used in conjunction with fluids aid this process. Medication should not be administered PO to animals with nasogastric reflux. Laxatives that may worsen pain and intestinal distention by stimulating intestinal motility and secretion are contraindicated in horses with surgically correctable diseases.

MINERAL OIL

Mineral oil is the most commonly used laxative in equine practice. Its effects are considered mild and probably result from lubrication of ingesta and interference with water absorption. Because oil penetrates ingesta poorly, softening of the impacted mass by oil probably contributes little to its action. Therefore, mineral oil is most effective in facilitating passage of ingesta already dislodged from the impacted mass.

PSYLLIUM HYDROPHILIC MUCILLOID

Psyllium hydrophilic mucilloid is the most common bulk-forming laxative used in equine

TABLE 2. LAXATIVES USED IN TREATMENT OF COLIC IN HORSES

Laxative	Dosage	Maximum Frequency of Administration	Maximum Duration of Treatment
Mineral oil	10 ml/kg	q. 24 h.	Safe for prolonged use
Psyllium hydrophilic mucilloid	1 gm/kg	q. 6–24 h.	Safe for prolonged use
Magnesium sulfate	0.4 gm/kg, diluted	q. 24 h.	3 days
Dioctyl sodium sulfosuccinate	10–20 mg/kg, diluted	q. 48 h.	2 days

practice. This agent absorbs water, causing the fluid and ion content of feces to increase. Because psyllium is effective and safe it is useful for treating simple impactions of ingesta. In addition, psyllium-derived products seem to be particularly useful for treating impactions caused by sand ingestion. After the sand obstruction has resolved, 2 to 3 weeks of therapy may be necessary to rid the colon of the sand. Psyllium is sometimes used as a preventative to sand accumulation. However, after continuous administration for several weeks, the colonic bacteria may develop the ability to metabolize psyllium, thereby reducing its efficacy. Therefore, in horses grazing in sandy environments, daily administration for 3 weeks every 4 to 6 months may be preferable to continuous administration.

Magnesium Sulfate

Magnesium sulfate is used as an osmotic laxative in horses. Because undiluted magnesium sulfate causes enteritis via osmotic damage to the mucosal cells, each dosage (0.2 gm per kg) should be diluted in 4 liters of warm water and administered by nasogastric tube. Administration of magnesium sulfate once daily may be necessary for treating severe impactions; however, therapy should be discontinued after 3 days to avoid enteritis and magnesium intoxication.

Dioctyl Sodium Sulfosuccinate

Dioctyl sodium sulfosuccinate (DSS) is a stimulant laxative that reduces surface tension to allow water to penetrate a mass of ingesta. In addition, DSS increases fluid and electrolyte secretion by enterocytes. For treatment of persistent impactions, the recommended dose of DSS may be repeated in 48 hours.

Supplemental Readings

Clark, E. S., and Becht, J. L.: Clinical pharmacology of the gastrointestinal tract. Vet. Clin. North Am. (Equine Pract.), 3:101, 1987.

Muir, W. W.: Analgesics in the treatment of colic. *In* Robinson, N. E. (ed.): Current Therapy in Equine Medicine 2. Philadelphia, W. B. Saunders, 1987, pp. 27–29.

Semrad, S. D., and Moore, J. N.: Endotoxemia. *In* Robinson, N. E. (ed.): Current Therapy in Equine Medicine 2. Philadelphia, W. B. Saunders, 1987, pp. 81–87.

Risk and Prognostic Factors in Colic

Mathew Reeves, KENNETT SQUARE, PENNSYLVANIA

RISK FACTORS

A risk factor is any characteristic that is associated with disease occurrence. Age, gender, breed, occupation, previous health history, environmental exposure, geographic location, diet, and life-style are all potential risk factors for disease. Identification of risk factors is important, because high-risk populations can be identified as target groups for preventive interventions and more frequent health examinations. If risk factors for a disease are defined, prevention of the disease by controlling the exposure to the risk factors may be feasible. Risk factors are usually identified using epidemiologic study designs such as cross-sectional, case–control, or cohort studies. The first two designs are particularly efficient in identifying risk factors when relatively little is known about the causes of a disease, such as colic, whereas the cohort design is better for defining cause-and-effect relationships once tentative risk factors have been defined by previous studies.

There is limited published material concerning potential risk factors for equine colic. A small number of published hospital-based case–control studies limited themselves to age, sex, and breed relationships, because such data are readily available for the control population (all other horses treated at the hospital). Although some useful information has been generated by these studies, there are potentially major biases that could adversely affect these results. Of particular concern are differential referral or admission rates that can create or mask significant associations. Age, sex, and breed differences between colic and noncolic control populations seen at university hospitals appear to be relatively minor. With regard to total colic admissions to university hospitals there are conflicting reports concerning age-associated risk. It seems, however, that horses less than 2 years old or more than 11 years old may be at higher risk of referral with colic. Horses over 15 years old appear to be at greater risk of requiring surgery to correct a colic problem. This seems to be related, in part, to the higher frequency of strangulation obstruction of the small intestine due to pedunculated lipoma or epiploic foramen entrapment in older horses. Horses less than 3 years old are at greater risk of small intestinal and ileocecal intussusception, small intestinal volvulus, and incarcerated umbilical hernia. Horses less than 6 months old may be at increased risk of small colon disease requiring surgery.

There appears to be little risk associated with gender when total colic admissions are compared to the total hospital control populations. One study did find mares to be at a greater risk for admission with colic and to have a higher prevalence of small intestinal intussusception, intra-abdominal abscess, and adhesions. Such associations have not been repeated elsewhere, however. Obviously, conditions such as scrotal hernia, uterine torsion, and broad ligament hematomas are gender-related conditions. It is well recognized that large colon torsions and displacements are an occupational hazard of the brood mare; however, the strength of this association has yet to be quantified by any scientific studies.

Breed differences in the proportion of colic cases seen at university hospitals are probably most likely to show bias in differential referral rates, and any reported associations should be viewed with extreme caution. Arabian horses are overrepresented among the colic population in some studies, Standardbred horses and ponies were overrepresented in one report, and three other reports did not show any breed-associated risk when assessing total colic admissions. Standardbred horses appear to have a higher prevalence of scrotal hernias than other breeds, while Shetland ponies may have a higher prevalence of small colon impactions. In one study, Thoroughbreds were overrepresented among cases of epiploic foramen entrapment.

Several case series reports from different geographic areas have served to identify regional differences in the type of colic conditions observed. In general, large colon conditions appear to be more common in the western United States and small intestinal problems more common in the eastern United States. However, in recent years conditions of the large colon have also been more frequently observed in the eastern United States. Cases of enteroliths have a well-defined geographic distribution. Specific loci include southern California, Indiana, and Florida.

Apart from age, sex, breed, and geographic factors, there are, to the author's knowledge, no reports that have assessed any other potential risk factors. There is a desperate need for epidemiologic studies to define potential risk factors. Obvious targets for investigation include diet, feeding practices, housing, exercise, transport history, parasite control measures, occupation, breeding history, genetic influences, previous health history (especially previous colic history), and meteorological influences. There are many anecdotal reports of weather changes inducing colic, although the one study that addressed this complex issue failed to find any association between weather changes and colic incidence. However, it may be that weather changes act as an intervening factor or trigger for colic.

Several well-recognized risk factors for colic have been identified anecdotally over the years. These factors include an imbalance of roughage to concentrate feeding, which leads to a relative overfeeding of concentrates; inadequate water supply; moldy hay or grain; poor parasite control; and previous colic episodes in certain horses. The relative significance and interrelationship of these factors to other risk factors needs to be defined. Several recent articles described potential physiological mechanisms that could induce colic and identified management practices, such as intermittent feeding, that could induce GI tract disturbances. Such findings are very intriguing but should be viewed with caution until epidemiological studies have identified that certain feeding practices are true risk factors for colic.

The problem of obtaining accurate information from horse owners and trainers about the intensity, duration, time of onset, and discontinuation of the many different potential exposures is enormous. The increasing use of horse health records on farms can greatly help investigators. Such record keeping should be actively encouraged by the equine industry. Accurate details of management and feeding practices are probably best obtained by farm visits.

PROGNOSTIC FACTORS

An essential part of the clinical evaluation of the colic patient involves the estimation of the prognosis. An accurate estimate is important, because economic factors often play an integral role in the owner's decision to continue therapy. Even without financial concerns, owners are naturally interested in the likely outcome of their horse, especially if surgery is performed. The veterinarian is required to make an estimate based on relatively limited information derived from the physical examination and any available laboratory tests. Often the approach taken by the clinician is one of educated guess work, which often lacks objectivity. Estimates are usually phrased in terms such as "poor," "guarded," "fair," or "good," but the exact meaning and implication of these terms vary considerably among clinicians, let alone horse owners and trainers. The use of such terms exemplifies our inability as clinicians to accurately determine the likelihood of survival based on purely subjective means.

Most published studies agree that parameters that reflect the degree of cardiovascular compromise are the most useful prognostic guides. This is not surprising, as the leading cause of death in colic patients is acute circulatory failure (shock) secondary to intestinal infarction. Useful parameters include arterial blood pressure, pulse amplitude, heart rate, capillary refill time, oral mucous membrane color, packed cell volume, mental depression, hemostatic abnormalities, blood pH, blood bicarbonate, blood lactate, blood glucose, anion gap, and blood urinary nitrogen. All of these parameters simply reflect the degree of shock in the patient. Other parameters such as abdominal sounds, intestinal hydrostatic pressure, abdominal pain, nasogastric reflux, rectal examination findings, and peritoneal fluid parameters have also been shown to be prognostically useful. In general, these parameters correlate with the degree of intestinal pathology. Obviously, the more extreme the intestinal damage, the greater the degree of shock, the poorer the prognosis.

Most of the previous literature has evaluated the usefulness of single parameters. The method of evaluation and the form by which this assessment is made depend on the type of data. The effects of categorical variables—that is, variables that have no meaningful scale of measure, such as abdominal sounds, sex, and degree of abdominal pain—can be measured by calculating odds ratios (OR). Odds ratios are quantifiable measures of association or risk. An example of such data is shown in Table 1. For each parameter there is a null value (OR = 1) to which all the other OR values are compared. For example, horses that have a depressed attitude are 8.4 times more likely to die than colic-affected horses with a normal attitude. For continuous variables—that is, variables that have a meaningful scale of measure, such as heart rate (beats per minute) or packed cell volume (per cent)—probabilities of survival can be calculated for given values of a variable. This approach is illustrated

TABLE 1. ODDS RATIOS FOR DEATH FROM COLIC FOR SINGLE CATEGORICAL VARIABLES

Variable	No.	No. That Died	Odds Ratio
Pain controllability			
Controllable without analgesics	215	17	1.0
Controllable with analgesics	763	116	2.1°
Uncontrollable	137	80	16.4°
Self-inflicted trauma			
Absent	1227	124	1.0
Present	320	128	6.0°
Attitude			
Normal	149	5	1.0
Depressed (toxic)	1031	233	8.4°
Alert	369	26	2.2
Pulse character			
Normal	970	71	1.0
Weak	286	150	14.0°
Mucous membrane color			
Normal (pink)	919	52	1.0
Pale or pale pink	356	59	3.2°
Red	128	44	8.4°
Cyanotic	124	68	38.2°
Injected	22	6	6.7°
Icteric	33	8	5.2°
Abdominal sounds (frequency)			
Normal	301	16	1.0
Increased	145	5	0.6
Decreased	801	102	2.6°
Absent	286	119	12.7°
Rectal examination			
Normal	350	42	1.0
Abnormal	812	194	2.3°
Peritoneal fluid color			
Normal	371	32	1.0
Serosanguinous	74	34	9.0°
Cloudy	142	28	2.6°
Bloody	57	20	5.7°
Opaque	64	25	6.8°

Data obtained from The Morris Animal Foundation Colic Survey.
No., total number of horses in category; No. that died, number of horses that died in category.
°$P < 0.01$.

in Table 2. The problem with using only a single variable is that no one parameter can reliably discriminate between cases that will survive and those that will not. Therefore, an estimate based on an individual parameter is likely to be unreliable and should only be used as a rough prognostic guide.

An alternative method that can be used to determine prognosis is to combine the information of several individual parameters into one test statistic. This approach, called multivariable analysis, overcomes the problem of using only one variable at a time. Multivariable statistical analysis methods such as multiple logistic regression have several important advantages. They are especially useful when dealing with an event that has a dichotomous outcome, i.e., an outcome that has only two possible events, such as lived/died, surgical/medical. Multivariable analysis

TABLE 2. ESTIMATES OF PROGNOSIS USING SINGLE CONTINUOUS PARAMETERS

Parameter	Values			
Peritoneal fluid total protein, gm/dl	2.0	3.0	4.0	5.0
P(d)	0.23	0.44	0.67	0.84
Blood glucose, gm/dl	150	200	250	300
P(d)	0.42	0.64	0.8	0.9
Cap. refill time, sec	2.0	3.0	4.0	5.0
P(d)	0.39	0.67	0.87	0.95
Heart rate, bpm	40	60	80	100
P(d)	0.18	0.48	0.65	0.79
Packed cell vol, %	30	45	60	65
P(d)	0.17	0.46	0.78	0.85
Systolic arterial blood pressure, mm Hg	140	110	80	50
P(d)	0.06	0.31	0.76	0.95
Age, yr	5	10	15	20
P(d)	0.37	0.43	0.49	0.55
Anion gap, mEq/L	<20	20–25	>25	
P(d)	0.19	0.53	1.0	
Blood lactate, mg/dl	19	36	72	
P(d)	0.12	0.70	0.97	

P(d) = probability of death.

methods are used to combine information from several variables into one probability statistic (with a range of 0 to 1) that can be used to predict the likelihood of an event. Confounding variables and interactions between variables can also be evaluated using this method.

The first use of multivariable analysis in equine colic patients was by Parry in 1983. This study used discriminant analysis to formulate a model that used systolic blood pressure, blood lactate, blood urinary nitrogen, and packed cell volume to predict the outcome. Although the model was 93 per cent accurate in predicting the outcome of cases, there was no independent validation; that is, the assessment of accuracy was determined using the same cases from which the model was developed. Three other prognostic models using logistic regression have been subsequently developed.

Following are two examples illustrating the use of a multivariable prognostic model. The model was based on a retrospective study of colic cases admitted to the University of Minnesota veterinary hospital. The model requires the following data to be collected: age, sex, surgical or medical treatment, capillary refill time (CRT), packed cell volume (PCV), and heart rate (HR). From these data the probability of death $(P(d))$ for a colic case can be calculated.

EXAMPLE 1

A 26-year-old Quarterhorse gelding was evaluated for colic. The following parameters were determined: HR = 36 bpm, CRT = 2 sec, PCV = 42%. Only medical treatment was necessary. The logistic equation has the following general form:

$$P(d) = \frac{1}{1 + e^{-y}}$$

where y is equal to the log odds of death, which is calculated using the following equation:

$$\begin{aligned}y =\ & -6.873 + (0.02375 \times \text{Age [yr]}) \\ & + (-0.07433 \times \text{Sex}_1) + (0.6414 \times \text{Sex}_2) \\ & + (3.283 \times \text{Surg}) + (0.4184 \times \text{CRT}) \\ & + (0.03869 \times \text{PCV}) + (0.02183 \times \text{HR})\end{aligned}$$

where $\text{Sex}_1 = 1$, $\text{Sex}_2 = 0$ for stallions; $\text{Sex}_1 = 0$, $\text{Sex}_2 = 1$ for geldings; $\text{Sex}_1 = 0$, $\text{Sex}_2 = 0$ for females; Surg = 0 for medical treatment, Surg = 1 for surgical treatment.

Therefore, the log odds of death for this horse equals:

$$\begin{aligned}y =\ & -6.873 + (0.02375 \times 26) \\ & + (-0.07433 \times 0) + (0.6414 \times 1) \\ & + (3.283 \times 0) + (0.4184 \times 2) \\ & + (0.03869 \times 42) + (0.02183 \times 36) \\ =\ & 2.366.\end{aligned}$$

The probability of death $(P(d))$ is then calculated using the logistic regression equation:

$$P(d) = \frac{1}{1 + e^{-y}} = \frac{1}{1 + e^{-(2.366)}} = \frac{1}{11.66} = 0.08.$$

Therefore, the horse has a low probability of death of 0.08, which is to be expected, given the relatively normal parameters found on the physical examination.

EXAMPLE 2

A 12-year-old Thoroughbred mare was evaluated for colic. The following parameters were determined: HR = 66 bpm, CRT = 3 sec, PCV = 48%. The horse required surgical treatment. The $P(d)$ for this horse was calculated from the model as 0.78. A large colon torsion was found and corrected at surgery. The bowel was of questionable viability, but the position of the volvulus precluded colonic resection. The horse was euthanized 48 hours after surgery because of progressive endotoxemia and shock.

An advantage of this method is that the owner is given an actual numerical estimate of the prognosis, i.e., 0.08, rather than the subjective statement, "I believe the prognosis is good," or 0.78, rather than "the prognosis is fair to guarded." This information helps the owner become more actively involved in the decision-making process, especially if surgical intervention is advised.

To the author's knowledge, none of the predictive models mentioned above have gained acceptance in the clinical environment. There are several possible reasons for this. The first is the apparent complexity of the models. However, with the use of a computer or even a programmable calculator, use of these models is greatly simplified. Data entry can be made very simple and a probability of the event (with an associated confidence interval) generated in a few seconds.

The lack of independent validation, which involves evaluating the model's performance on a different population of cases from the one used to generate the model, has been one of the major limitations of these models so far.

The majority of these models have been developed from referral hospital cases, where the prevalence of surgical cases and associated case fatality rates are high. The performance of these models will be affected when used in a general practice environment, where the prevalence of serious colic cases is much lower. The estimate of the probability of death generated from the logistic regression model can, however, be readily adjusted for the influence of varying prevalence of disease by applying Bayes' theorem. For simplicity this will not be illustrated here, but it is important to note that a good estimate of the prevalence of death (i.e., case fatality rate of colic cases) in the population of colic cases being tested must be known before these models can be used effectively. Case fatality rates for colic can vary dramatically from less than 5 per cent in a general practice to 40 per cent or more in referral centers. Such changes in prevalence will dramatically affect the estimates of prognosis and must be accounted for.

Finally, it is important to recognize the limitations associated with all clinical predictions. Clinical predictions are never certain but are inherently probabilistic. A prognosis of 70 per cent means that a favorable outcome is most likely, but an unfavorable outcome cannot be ruled out completely. If the patient dies, the estimate can hardly be regarded as wrong, as it is simply a probabilistic statement. This obvious fact should always be stressed to the owner, especially before expensive treatment is undertaken. A 100 per cent guarantee of survival should never be given for any colic case.

Supplemental Readings

Martin, S. W., Meek, A. H., and Willeberg, P.: Veterinary Epidemiology: Principles and Methods. Ames, Iowa, Iowa State University Press, 1987.

Orsini, J. A., Elser, A. H., Galligan, D. T., Donawick, W. J., and Kronfeld, D. S.: Prognostic index for acute abdominal crisis (colic) in horses. Am. J. Vet. Res., 49:1969, 1988.

Parry, B. W., Anderson, G. A., and Gay, C. C.: Prognosis in equine colic: A comparative study of variables used to assess individual cases. Equine Vet. J., 15:211, 1983.

Parry, B. W., Anderson, G. A., and Gay, C. C.: Prognosis in equine colic: A study of individual variables used in case assessment. Equine Vet. J., 15:337, 1983.

Puotunen-Reinert, A.: Study of variables commonly used in examination of equine colic cases to assess prognostic value. Equine Vet. J., 18:275, 1986.

Reeves, M. J., Curtis, C. R., Salman, M. D., and Hilbert, B. J.: Prognosis in equine colic patients using multivariable analysis. Can. J. Vet. Res., 53:87, 1989.

Reeves, M. J., Curtis, C. R., Salman, M. D., Stashak, T. S., and Reif, J. S.: Descriptive epidemiology and risk factors indicating the need for surgery and the evaluation of prognosis: The Morris Animal Foundation colic study. In: Proceedings of the 33rd Annual Convention of the American Association of Equine Practitioners, 1987, p. 83.

Reeves, M. J., Gay, J. M., Hilbert, B. J., and Morris, R. S.: Association of age, sex, breed factors in acute equine colic: A retrospective study of 320 cases admitted to a veterinary teaching hospital in the USA. Prev. Vet. Med., 7:149, 1989.

Sackett, D. L., Haynes, R. B., and Tugwell, P.: Clinical Epidemiology: A Basic Science for Clinical Medicine. Boston, Little, Brown, 1985.

Sembrat, R. F.: The acute abdomen in the horse: Epidemiologic considerations. Arch. Amer. Coll. Vet. Surg., 4:34, 1975.

Tennant, B., Wheat, J. D., and Meagher, D. M.: Observations on the causes and incidence of acute intestinal obstruction in the horse. In: Proceedings of the 18th Annual Convention of the American Association of Equine Practitioners, 1972, p. 251.

White, N. A.: The epidemiology of the equine acute abdomen. In: Proceedings of the 30th Annual Convention of the American Association of Equine Practitioners, 1984, p. 291.

White, N. A., and Lessard, P.: 1986. Risk factors and clinical signs associated with cases of equine colic. In: Proceedings of the 32nd Annual Convention of the American Association of Equine Practitioners, 1986, p. 637.

Duodenitis–Proximal Jejunitis

Douglas Allen Jr., ATHENS, GEORGIA
E. Susan Clark, ATHENS, GEORGIA

Hemorrhagic-necrotic duodenitis–proximal jejunitis (DPJ), sometimes referred to as anterior enteritis or proximal enteritis, is a common disease of horses. When DPJ was first described in 1977, it was hypothesized that the disease was caused by thrombosis of the vasculature supplying the duodenum and proximal jejunum. Since that time, however, it has been determined that the clinical signs, clinicopathological findings, and gross and histopathological lesions in horses with DPJ are different from those in horses with thromboembolic colic. DPJ is now recognized as a distinct disease syndrome; however, the etiology and pathogenesis are unknown. Because the primary differential diagnosis is small intestinal obstruction with many signs in common with strangulation obstruction, prompt diagnosis of DPJ is important. Unfortunately, at present, a definitive diagnosis depends on identification of characteristic lesions at surgery or necropsy.

Damage to the mucosal epithelium and capillary endothelium in the proximal small intestine permits transmucosal secretion of fluid and electrolytes into the intestinal lumen. It has been hypothesized that enhanced secretion of fluid and electrolytes into the intestinal lumen also occurs, compounding the problem. In more severe cases, villous denuding and villous capillary endothelial damage contribute to the large volume of gastrointestinal (GI) reflux. The clinically relevant events that result from this intestinal damage are proximal small intestinal distention and nasogastric reflux, dehydration, and circulatory shock. In addition, hyponatremia, hypochloremia, hypokalemia, and acid–base alterations can develop secondarily. Although hypochloremia due to secretion of chloride ions into the stomach can result in metabolic alkalosis, poor tissue perfusion and bicarbonate loss in the small intestine ultimately lead to metabolic acidosis.

CLINICAL SIGNS

DPJ can occur in horses of any age but most commonly affects adult horses on adequate to high levels of nutrition. Frequently a history of a marked increase in dietary concentrates or a recent change in concentrate quality is obtained. The owner or handler will usually indicate that the horse was normal and ate well but was found with signs of acute colic without any apparent predisposing factors.

Although the clinical signs of DPJ usually follow a consistent pattern, the duration of illness and patient morbidity are variable and seem to increase with the severity of the small intestinal lesions. Most horses with DPJ present with a history of an acute onset of moderate to severe abdominal pain. Other clinical signs include copious amounts of nasogastric reflux that is occasionally orange-brown colored with a fetid odor, moderate to severe small intestinal distention, a mild fever, dehydration, injected mucous membranes, lack of intestinal sounds, prolonged capillary refill time, heart rate greater than 60 bpm, and tachypnea. The abdominal pain usually abates after gastric decompression, but the horse remains severely depressed, perhaps the most consistent and characteristic clinical sign of the disease. If the fluid that accumulates in the proximal intestinal tract is not removed periodically, signs of abdominal pain recur. The body temperature, volume of nasogastric reflux, and frequency of borborygmal sounds appear to be greater in horses with DPJ than in horses with small intestinal obstruction. On the other hand, horses with small intestinal obstruction have higher heart and respiratory rates and a more prolonged capillary refill time.

Clinical laboratory findings include an increased packed cell volume above that expected relative to the increase in plasma protein levels, a metabolic acidosis in longstanding or severe cases, markedly elevated peritoneal fluid protein concentration (often in excess of 3 gm per dl), and a mild to moderate elevation of the peritoneal white blood cell count (usually in excess of 10,000 cells per μl). The peritoneal fluid is usually yellow and turbid, but in severe cases diapedesis occurs, resulting in a serosanguinous color. The white blood cell count in the peripheral blood may be normal or increased (neutrophilia).

PATHOLOGY

A definitive diagnosis of DPJ can be made in most cases by gross examination of the duodenum and proximal jejunum at surgery or necropsy. In horses with DPJ, lesions are consistently found in the duodenum, but the severity and frequency of lesions in the jejunum are variable. Less commonly, lesions are found in the pyloric portion of the stomach; uncommonly, they are found in the ileum and large intestines. The lesions of DPJ are transmural, with the serosal surface appearing smooth and containing bright red to dark red petechial and ecchymotic hemorrhages. Inflammation and edema cause a palpable thickening of the wall of the affected intestine. The mucosa is a deep red color and, depending on the amount of mucosal damage and subsequent intraluminal hemorrhage, the proximal small intestinal contents may be similarly discolored, therefore explaining the orange-red tint frequently found in the initial gastric reflux. While the stomach and proximal small intestine are moderately distended with fluid, the distal jejunum and ileum, if unaffected, are usually flaccid.

The histological lesions in the duodenum and proximal jejunum vary in severity. Lesions include hyperemia and edema of the mucosa and submucosa progressing to villous epithelial degeneration, epithelial cell sloughing, marked neutrophil infiltration, hemorrhages in the muscular layers, and fibrinopurulent exudation on the serosa. Thus, the term hemorrhagic-necrotic duodenitis–proximal jejunitis has been used as a more descriptive name for this disease. The lesions described are very similar to those reported in humans and neonatal pigs with *Clostridium perfringens* infections.

DIAGNOSIS

The similarities of the various small intestinal diseases that manifest with colic pose a diagnostic and therapeutic challenge. Most conditions of the equine small intestine that cause distention, GI reflux, dehydration, and acute abdominal pain (i.e., strangulation obstructions, intraluminal obstructions, and intramural or extramural occlusion of the intestinal lumen) require surgical intervention. General anesthesia and surgery in a horse with a definitive diagnosis of DPJ is usually unnecessary and increases the morbidity in an already compromised patient. Unfortunately, it is rare that a clear-cut diagnosis of DPJ is made based on clinical and clinicopathological data. Table 1 provides guidelines for deciding whether a case should be medically or surgically managed.

THERAPY

The cause of DPJ is unknown, and treatment remains empirical, consisting of aggressive supportive therapy. Persistent GI reflux necessitates gastric decompression every 1 to 2 hours to relieve pain and prevent gastric rupture. Approximately 4 to 8 liters of gastric fluid can be collected during decompression. These horses should receive nothing per os until small intestinal function has returned. This is recognized clinically by cessation or reduction of nasogastric

TABLE 1. PHYSICAL AND LABORATORY EXAMINATION FINDINGS IN HORSES WITH DUODENITIS–PROXIMAL JEJUNITIS

Examination	Duodenitis-Proximal Jejunitis		Surgical Candidate
Attitude	Depressed/painful	Painful	Painful
Heart rate, bpm	40–80	≥80	40–80
Respiratory rate, breaths/min	16–28	24–40	15–35
Rectal temperature, °F	101.5–102.5	≤101	99–101
Capillary refill time, sec	>3	≥3	1.5–3
Auscultable intestinal sounds	Mildly to markedly depressed	Markedly depressed to absent	Mildly depressed to absent
Nasogastric reflux: volume (gal.) and character	3–4 gal, ± malodorous, orange-brown color	2–3 gal., ± malodorous	2–3 gal. with ingesta
Rectal examination	Dilated to moderately distended	Moderately to markedly distended	Mild to moderately distended; ± ileal impaction
Response to nasogastric decompression	Depressed and quiet	Temporary to no relief of pain	Temporary to no relief of pain
Complete blood count	±Leukocytosis with mature neutrophilia	±Leukocytosis with slight neutrophilia	Normal to elevated WBC
Peritoneal fluid protein, gm/dl	±3, but may be >4.5	2.5–4.5	2.5–3.5
Peritoneal fluid nucleated cell count, cells/μl	≤5000	Varies up to 20,000	3000–12,000

reflux to 1 to 2 liters over a 2-hour period. The duration of enhanced transmucosal fluid movement and intestinal ileus that results in GI reflux varies with the severity of the intestinal lesion. Thus the time necessary for gastric decompression is also variable but is usually 3 to 7 days. Some horses have reflux for up to 2 weeks. Rectal examinations after the first day of therapy may or may not reveal distended loops of small intestine, depending on the frequency of removal of the reflux and the severity of the initial lesion.

Intravenous (IV) administration of a balanced electrolyte solution is necessary initially to treat the shock, electrolyte imbalances, and prerenal azotemia, and later to maintain intravascular fluid volume. This may require continuous fluid therapy and in large horses may necessitate administration of fluid through both jugular veins or through 10-gauge catheters. The massive IV fluid therapy that is usually required in this disease will commonly accelerate the flux of fluid from the vasculature into the intestinal lumen because of a reduced intravascular osmotic pressure and an increased capillary perfusion pressure. This will initially result in an increased volume of GI reflux. Thus, during the initial hours of therapy, even aggressive IV fluid administration will result in only moderate clinical improvement.

The clinical responses, as evidenced by improved hydration status, decreased nasogastric reflux, improved attitude, and improvement in parameters reflecting kidney function (decreased blood urea nitrogen and creatinine levels), will usually correlate with improvement of the damaged intestine.

Nonsteroidal anti-inflammatory agents should be used judiciously to avoid masking the clinical signs of a potential surgical lesion. A reduced dosage of flunixin meglumine (0.25 mg per kg t.i.d. or q.i.d.) can be used. Because *Clostridium* spp. is one suspected etiological agent, penicillin is commonly used as the antimicrobial of choice. However, aminoglycosides may also be administered to horses with DPJ that demonstrate signs of endotoxemia and bacteremia.

Conservative therapy is sufficient in most cases of DPJ and it has been suggested that surgical intervention may add excessive stress to an already compromised animal. In cases with more than 7 days of nasogastric reflux, excessive fluid losses that cannot be corrected with conventional fluid therapy, or clinical and laboratory findings strongly suggestive of an intestinal obstruction, surgery should be considered as an option. When a clinical diagnosis of DPJ has been made and surgery is used to augment therapy, two approaches have been employed. A right flank laparotomy using a resection of the last rib has been performed in the standing horse to approach the duodenum and cecal base. A small stoma can be made between the duodenum and cecum using a hand-sewn 1-cm to 1.5-cm side-to-side anastomosis. This stoma decompresses the proximal small intestine by shunting the fluid to the cecum for reabsorption, and will later close. Perhaps a more effective method of evaluating and decompressing the small intestine in horses with DPJ is via a ventral midline celiotomy. Although more stressful on the patient than a standing flank laparotomy, this approach permits a more complete evaluation of the GI tract and facilitates development of a more physiological intestinal shunt. Upon entrance into the abdominal cavity, dilated small intestine is immediately apparent. After the extent of the diseased intestine is determined, a segment of normal distal jejunum is laid side-to-side to the proximal diseased intestine in an isoperistaltic fashion and as far proximal as possible without extending into the abdominal cavity. A small 1-cm to 1.5-cm hand-sewn anastomosis can then be made between the two segments of intestine. This provides an adequate stoma for direct intestinal decompression while minimally compromising the digestive and absorptive capacity of the small intestine. Potential complications of this procedure include the development of an intestinal incarceration through the loop that is formed and the development of small intestinal adhesions.

Complications of DPJ include adhesions of the proximal small intestine and laminitis. Approximately 95 per cent of horses with DPJ survive the primary intestinal insult with appropriate management. Losses from this disease are more commonly related to secondary complications such as laminitis, intra-abdominal adhesions, and vascular thrombosis. Because laminitis is commonly encountered as a result of DPJ, prophylaxis is routinely incorporated into the medical therapy and consists of analgesic doses of nonsteroidal anti-inflammatory drugs, and peripheral vasodilatory agents once cardiovascular stability is attained. Other therapeutic interventions that have been employed include dimethyl sulfoxide (DMSO) administered IV at a wide range of dosages (20 mg per kg two to three times daily, up to 1 gm per kg, diluted in isotonic electrolyte solution). Routine foot care is indicated, and where practical, horses should be stalled in deep wood shavings or sand to provide sole and frog support. Otherwise the sole and frog area can be supported somewhat with gauze sponges or rolled gauze held in place with an adhesive elastic bandage.

Intra-abdominal adhesions are much less frequently encountered after DPJ. Specific prophylaxis for this complication is not routinely used; however, the supportive measures and therapies used for the initial disease and the possible laminitis should be sufficient.

Supplemental Readings

Blackwell, R. B., and White, N. A.: Duodenitis proximal jejunitis in the horse. *In:* Proceedings of the Equine Colic Research Symposium, 1982, p. 106.

Johnson, J. K., and Morris, D. D.: Comparison of duodenitis proximal jejunitis and small intestinal obstruction in horses: 68 cases (1977–1985). J. Am. Vet. Med. Assoc., *191*:849–854, 1987.

Morris, D. D., and Johnston, J. K.: Peritoneal fluid constituents in horses with colic due to small intestinal disease. *In:* Proceedings of the 2nd Equine Colic Research Symposium, 1986, pp. 197–199.

Tyler D. G., White, N. A., Blackwell, R. B., and Allen, D.: Pathology of equine duodenitis proximal jejunitis (anterior enteritis). *In:* Proceedings of the 2nd Equine Colic Research Symposium, 1986, pp. 197–199.

Strangulating and Nonstrangulating Obstruction of the Small Intestine

Kenneth E. Sullins, LEESBURG, VIRGINIA

Acute abdominal disease is the leading cause of death in horses. Current statistics show that somewhat less than half of horses with surgical colic have small intestinal lesions and that small intestinal lesions requiring surgical correction are among the most serious forms of colic. Unexplained geographic differences exist with respect to the occurrence of colic of various etiologies. Reports from Germany, for example, indicate much higher rates of small bowel strangulation within the epiploic foramen than do reports from the United States. These differences could be due to the type and age of the horse population, feeding practices, or differences in the efficacy of parasite control programs.

Simple obstruction of the small intestine is most often due to ileal impaction, a condition largely localized to the southeastern United States. The exact cause is unknown, but type of hay is suspected to play a role. Other potential causes of simple obstruction or impaction usually reach the colon before lodging. Thickening or dysfunction of the ileocecal valve can contribute to intermittent or acute ileal obstruction. This type of distal obstruction results in accumulation of a great volume of fluid and gas before acute pain or nasogastric reflux occurs. Incomplete obstruction may or may not cause intermittent colic, but chronic small intestinal distention will result in gross luminal dilation and mural thickening, structural changes that alone cause no apparent dysfunction.

Strangulation obstruction of equine small intestine is common. Causes include incarceration in the epiploic foramen or some other internal defect such as a mesodiverticular band or mesenteric rent; inguinal, umbilical, diaphragmatic, or direct hernia; strangulation by a pedunculated lipoma or fibrous band; and volvulus. The incidence of such problems may be age related because of the type of structure causing the problem. Strangulation obstruction most often involves the more mobile distal jejunum or ileum where the mesentery is longer.

The sequence of events in strangulation of bowel begins with venous occlusion by the incarcerating structure. Intramural edema follows, eventually precluding reduction of the affected segment to the normal position. With time and hypoxia, the venous obstruction becomes more complete and capillaries become more incompetent. Intramural hemorrhage follows for as long as the arterioles are patent. Interstitial extravasation of blood causes the seromuscular surface to initially become blotchy, followed by the characteristic blackening of strangulated small intestine. In the later stages of strangulation, the vascular stasis progresses to total thrombosis.

When the ischemic bowel becomes reperfused, the transmural histologic appearance worsens. Two reasons for this phenomenon are biochemical reperfusion injury and mechanical disruption of tissue as edema and hemorrhage continue with the return of blood pressure.

Among the biochemical mediators of reperfusion injury are oxygen free radicals, which rapidly react to form reactive hydroxyl radicals. These oxygen-derived radicals degrade hyaluronic acid and collagen and cause peroxidation of the cellular lipid membranes; these changes account for disruption of every structural tissue component. The net effect on the intestine is biochemical disruption of the bowel wall, followed by structural collapse with mechanical stress of edema and hemorrhage that occurs because the capillaries are leaking. Last to be affected are the muscular layers because the metabolic rate is much lower than that of the mucosa.

CLINICAL SIGNS

The clinical signs suggesting small intestinal obstruction are summarized in Table 1. The only noninvasive method of definitively diagnosing small intestinal obstruction in adult horses is manual detection of distended loops of small intestine per rectum. When loops of tightly distended small intestine are palpable, exploratory surgery is usually indicated. The notable exception is proximal duodenitis–enteritis, in which multiple loops of small intestine and the duodenum caudal and medial to the cecum will be quite evident per rectum but generally are not tightly distended. This type of distention will reduce following reflux through a nasogastric tube. Outwardly visible abdominal distention is not a usual feature of small intestinal obstruction; however, an exception is distention of the entire small intestine due to volvulus or an extremely distal obstruction. Radiography may help with the diagnosis in some foals, but potentially correctable flatulence due to small intestinal ileus can appear similar to obstructed bowel. When the decision is unclear from the above, clinical signs, including the severity and duration of pain, metabolic status, amount of nasogastric reflux, and peritoneal fluid parameters, must be considered when making the decision for surgery (see Table 1).

THERAPY

Mild simple obstruction or flatulence may not require surgery if motility can be maintained with fluid and electrolyte therapy and suppression of the sympathetic response by control of pain. Small intestinal obstructions correctable with medical managment are, however, uncommon.

The management of pain and the maintenance of fluid balance in the horse with colic are described on pp. 201 and 18, respectively. The

TABLE 1. SUMMARY OF COMMON FINDINGS IN HORSES WITH SMALL INTESTINAL OBSTRUCTION*

Pain	Variable from simple depression to severe pain that does not respond to medication.
Metabolic status	Heart rate > 40 bpm (usually higher, but serious infarctive disease can be present with low heart rates for long periods of time).
	Peripheral pulse weakens as disease progresses.
	Mucous membranes pale, injected, muddy, or cyanotic.
	Capillary refill time 2 to 5 seconds, depending on severity.
	Hematocrit 45 to 60 or higher in severe cases.
	Plasma protein increases with dehydration (7.0 to 8.5 mg per dl). May decrease with prolonged leakage into lumen of bowel.
	Acid–base status normal to metabolic acidosis. Lactate concentration increased.
Peritoneal fluid	Normal if problem is short-lived, a very small segment of small intestine is strangulated, or with some intussusceptions.
	Mild increases in protein (>2.5 gm per dl) and variable cells in the presence of inflammatory disease or strangulations of intermediate duration. Color may be pink or light red.
	Significant increases in protein (>3.5 gm per dl) and cells (variable) with serosanguinous color in the presence of severely compromised bowel of some duration.
Rectal exam	Multiple loops of small intestine that rise dorsally as distention increases. Smaller diameter and softer palpable loops may not indicate true obstruction.
Nasogastric intubation	Reflux of several liters of fluid from stomach and small intestine often accompanies palpable small intestinal distention. Large-volume reflux may be present without significant findings on rectal examination.
Intestinal sounds	Increased with spasmodic colic or enteritis if horse is hydrated.
	Decreased with more serious obstruction producing transmural pathology.
Temperature per rectum	Normal to slightly elevated. Significant elevations are reason to suspect enteritis as the cause of pain, and surgery is seldom indicated.

*Modified from Robertson, J. T.: Small intestinal strangulation obstruction. *In* Robinson, N. E. (ed.): Current Therapy in Equine Medicine 2. Philadelphia, W. B. Saunders, 1987.

techniques of laparotomy are beyond the scope of this text. What follows is the approach to different types of lesions that may be encountered during surgery and techniques for the management of postoperative complications.

Intraluminal obstructions may be broken down manually in some cases, but removal of the mass through an enterotomy is often required. Ileocecostomy may be necessary to relieve or prevent recurrence of ileal impactions by tenacious masses of fine grass.

Resection of segments of small intestine located in accessible regions with an adequate length of distal healthy bowel is accomplished with an end-to-end anastomosis and closure of the mesenteric rent. I prefer the simple interrupted crushing suture method of end-to-end anastomosis because there is less luminal compromise and the bowel retains the ability to dilate as needed. It is important to exclude most of the mucosa from the suture path, because it tends to evert between sutures and cause inflammation. Some surgeons prefer a "functional end-to-end" stapled anastomosis; however, the everted end-to-end stapled anastomosis is to be avoided. When the distal stump of small intestine is inadequate, the only choice is a jejunocecal anastomosis. The preferred procedure is a side-to-side anastomosis that can be constructed with sutures or staples. Stapling is more efficient and much cleaner than suturing. When intestine is thickened, the staple rows must be oversewn to ensure a secure closure.

Determination of the limits of resections can be difficult. Clearly defined necrotic lines of demarcation may be present, but the bowel that was distended proximal to the obstruction can be significantly compromised. Surgical experience is invaluable in making the needed distinctions; however, intravenous sodium fluorescein and Doppler detection of intramural blood flow can be useful intraoperative adjuncts. The physiological limit of resection has been shown to be 40 per cent of the total length of the small intestine. This fact often causes the surgeon to give the benefit of the doubt to any bowel of questionable viability.

Luminal distention sufficient to make the bowel wall tense can cause intramural ischemia leading to either acute infarction of intestine or subacute to chronic postoperative complications. Because gas and fluid accumulate upstream, all small intestine proximal to an obstruction is at risk. The degree of bowel distention is difficult to assess intraoperatively. However, pressure measurements can be made, and horses with intraluminal pressures above 17 mm Hg rarely survive. In foals, small intestinal distention to a pressure of 25 mm Hg for 2 hours causes localized peritoneal adhesions. Foals have a greater propensity than adults for developing peritoneal adhesions. This is a trait of all young animals and people, and the reason has not been clearly defined.

Umbilical hernias may strangulate only one wall of small intestine (Richter's hernia). The signs may be subtler than those of complete obstruction, but the consequences for the involved segment are no less significant than more conventional stangulations. Edema surrounding the umbilicus may be the only early sign.

Postoperative complications are observed more commonly following small intestinal disease than after correction of large colon strangulations. For the most part, few long-term complications follow large colon conditions, as long as the horse survives the early postoperative period. One likely cause of the unpredictably poor outcomes of small intestinal surgery is inability to identify sublethal ischemic damage.

Postoperative peritoneal adhesions are the most significant complication following abdominal surgery, particularly when the primary problem has involved the small intestine. Decades of opinion and speculation have led surgeons to consider adhesions as "overhead" in the business of abdominal surgery: adhesions result from simply opening the abdomen and handling bowel. Definition of the pathophysiological role of ischemia and distention has allowed recognition that many postoperative sequelae in fact result from pathological processes present as part of the initial problem before surgery. Surgeons today have sufficient knowledge and experience to avoid most iatrogenic causes of adhesions such as excessive serosal abrasion, leaving exposed or contaminated intestinal tissue edges, or contaminating the abdomen with glove powder or ingesta. Unfortunately, specific locations of pathology or preexisting conditions may preclude application of the most desirable techniques.

Measures can be taken to enhance survival of ischemic bowel or minimize postoperative complications. Of primary concern is maintenance of blood flow and prevention of shock accompanying the often septic conditions. Fluid therapy is necessary to maintain fluid volume and stabilize electrolytes for normal myoelectric activity and intestinal motility. Broad-spectrum antibiotics minimize intestinal bacterial proliferation that worsens toxemia and decreases patient survival. Flunixin meglumine is the most effective nonsteroidal anti-inflammatory drug available for the treatment of horses with endotoxemia and is capable of ameliorating severe endotoxic metabolic compromise. The combination of antibiotics and flunixin meglumine has been shown to minimize or prevent local peritoneal adhesion formation following experimental intestinal ischemia in adult horses and foals. While the clinical case is much less controlled than research trials, these results indicate that these agents should be used whenever ischemia or other inflammatory processes have occurred.

There is reason to support the use of systemic free radical scavengers such as dimethyl sulfoxide (DMSO) to reduce the effects of ischemia and reperfusion injury. Experimental results have been variable, but recent work in the horse provided encouraging results. I continue to use DMSO (175 mg per kg, delivered as a 10 per cent solution) when ischemic intestine is anticipated. Research in other species has indicated that DMSO should be administered before the affected intestine is reperfused.

Heparin is another systemic medication that has been proposed for use in the prevention of ischemic complications by maintenance of microvascular patency and prevention of serosal fibrin accumulation. Experience has shown that for purely ischemic events, heparin in dosages exceeding clinical safety is required before any benefit is observed. However, for the surface phenomenon of septic peritonitis, heparin (20 to 90 IU per kg) has consistently been demonstrated to be beneficial through reduction of adhesions and serosal abscesses and increasing survival in laboratory animals. Anecdotally in the horse, I have observed adhesion-free resolution of confirmed fibrinopurulent peritonitis using heparin therapy. Although objective evidence of an effective dose is not available for horses, I have used 60 to 80 IU per kg SC b.i.d. Heparinized horses should be monitored clinically for bleeding and clinicopathologically for a reduction in hematocrit. Documentation of the effect of the heparin on the activated partial thromboplastin time (APTT) of the patient is advisable. Septic peritonitis resulting from continued leakage of ingesta probably is not a correctable condition.

When placed on serosal surfaces before trauma is induced, topically protective medications such as sodium hyaluronate have been beneficial in reducing adhesions due to excessive serosal trauma. Recent work has indicated that carboxymethylcellulose may incite a significant inflammatory reaction on its own. There is no evidence that topical agents can reduce adhesion formation in the presence of transmural pathology.

Return of small intestinal motility is another significant postobstruction consideration. Of primary concern is maintenance of hydration and electrolyte balance. Until the horse is able to remain hydrated on maintenance fluids or maintain its own hydration by oral water intake, solid food should not be allowed. In cases with severe small intestine distention or dysfunction, removal of large volumes of secretions by nasogastric tube may be necessary for several days before motility returns. Intraoperatively, the most significant procedure to facilitate return of motility is leaving the small intestine as empty as possible. Atraumatic manipulation of fluid and gas into the cecum has no adverse effect and significantly shortens postoperative ileus when no primary intestinal pathology is present. I have not found pharmacologic stimulation of intestinal motility useful, with the exception of agents that stimulate gastric emptying when that has been a primary problem. Older reports in the literature indicated that agents such as neostigmine were dangerous in the presence of a new intestinal anastomosis; the issue is controversial.

Supplemental Readings

Allen, D., and White, N. A.: Effect of small intestinal distention in the horse. Vet. Surg., 14:45, 1985.

Lundin, C. S., Sullins, K. E., White, N. A., Clem, M. F., DeBowes, R. M., and Pfeiffer, C. A.: Induction of peritoneal adhesions with small intestinal ischemia and distention in the foal. Equine Vet. J., 21:451, 1989.

McCord, J. M.: Oxygen-derived radicals: A link between reperfusion injury and inflammation. Fed. Proc., 46:2402, 1987.

Nonstrangulating and Strangulating Obstruction of the Ascending Colon

Jack R. Snyder, DAVIS, CALIFORNIA
Sharon J. Spier, DAVIS, CALIFORNIA

The ascending (large) colon is often the site of disorders leading to acute abdominal pain in horses. In some geographic areas such as California, veterinarians report that the majority of colic cases are associated with problems originating from the large colon.

Because the large colon is attached to the body wall by a single attachment at the most proximal and distal aspects of the colon, extensive movement within the abdominal cavity may occur. These movements within the abdominal cavity may lead to abnormal displacements, especially when combined with alterations in colonic weight and gas production. Since the large colon functions in water absorption and microbial digestion, conditions interfering with these processes may result in severe dehydration and luminal distention, with subsequent pain and shock.

Colonic obstruction can occur with or without vascular occlusion. Conditions that do not cause vascular obstruction are referred to as *nonstrangulating intestinal obstructions* and include intraluminal obstructions and simple displacements. Conditions associated with vascular obstruction are referred to as *strangulating obstructions* and in the large colon are most likely seen with colonic volvulus. In the following discussion, abnormalities of the large colon are classified as either nonstrangulating or strangulating intestinal obstruction. However, depending on the severity of the obstruction, conditions that are nonstrangulating may become strangulating.

NONSTRANGULATING OBSTRUCTIONS

LARGE COLON IMPACTION

Colonic impaction is one of the most common forms of colic. The causes of impaction remain unclear, but alterations in colonic motility due to a malfunction in the intrinsic or extrinsic nerve supply, or both, possibly associated with a stressful environmental change, may lead to impaction. Damage to intrinsic nerve function or blood supply from parasite migration may also play a role in the etiology of colonic impaction, although this is also difficult to confirm. Predisposing factors to ingesta impactions include coarse feed, poor dental maintenance or worn teeth, and dehydration.

CLINICAL SIGNS AND DIAGNOSIS

Horses with impactions caused by ingesta present with mild to moderate pain and decreased fecal output. Feces are often hard, dry, and mucus covered. Horses with impactions usually have a history of decreased food intake progressing to complete refusal to eat. If water intake is also decreased, signs of dehydration will develop.

The physical examination often reveals a normal rectal temperature and respiratory rate. Heart rate is variable; it may be normal or slightly elevated, depending on the severity of the impaction. Gastric reflux is usually absent. Unless vascular damage to the intestinal tissue has occurred, the results of peritoneal fluid analysis are normal. Intestinal sounds will vary according to the duration of the impaction. Initially, sounds may be variable and may with time continue to decrease until completely absent.

Rectal examination often reveals a large, firm, ingesta-filled colon. However, with some right dorsal and transverse colon impactions, rectal examinations are inconclusive. In such horses, the left colon and pelvic flexure may be distended with gas, although in the correct anatomical position. When confirmation cannot be made by rectal examination, diagnosis is based on the clincal signs and ruling out other possibilities. Radiographs may also be used for confirmation of impactions in foals, ponies, or American Miniature Horses.

THERAPY

Ingesta impactions are usually managed conservatively with mild analgesic agents, laxatives, and fluid therapy. Oral fluids may be used if gastric reflux is absent. Proper hydration must be maintained to allow the impaction to soften. If hydration is not maintained, fluid from the intestinal tract will be absorbed to maintain systemic hydration, thus worsening the impaction. Laxatives such as mineral oil are vital for relieving an impaction. Two to four liters of mineral oil per horse (450 kg) can be given per os (PO) by stomach tube every 12 to 24 hours. Other treatments that help soften impaction include the anionic surfactant dioctyl sodium sulfosuccinate (DSS) at a dosage of .01 to .06 gm (5% solution diluted in 2 to 4 liters water) per kg PO as needed. Higher dosages or prolonged administration may result in diarrhea and should be used with caution. DSS works as an emulsifying, wetting, and dispersing agent, functioning to soften the impaction. Other products that may be used in the conservative management of impactions include saline cathartics such as magnesium sulfate or Epsom salts. The saline cathartics retain water in the intestinal lumen by their osmotic properties, resulting in softening of the impaction. When this therapy is used, adequate systemic hydration is mandatory since significant amounts of body fluids are moving into the intestinal lumen. This is especially important if the impaction causes the Epsom salts to be maintained proximal to the mass, causing a continued influx of fluid.

The duration of conservative therapy before surgery is considered depends on each individual case. Indications for surgery include unrelenting pain, increased peritoneal nucleated cells or protein content, or colonic displacment. If the horse is alert, drinking water, and starting to pass feces, conservative therapy may be continued.

Sand Impactions

Horses that consume sand may develop an intraluminal obstruction. Sand may be present in the hay or may be ingested from the environment. Horses, especially young foals, may also deliberately eat sand. Coarse sand frequently accumulates in the right colon, transverse colon, and pelvic flexure, while fine sand may accumulate in the ventral colon. Because of the abrasiveness of the sand, colonic irritation may occur, causing mucosal damage leading to bacteria or toxin absorption. Additionally, long-standing sand impactions may result in a weakened colonic wall, predisposing to rupture.

CLINICAL SIGNS AND DIAGNOSIS

Horses with sand impactions present with the same signs as horses with ingesta impactions. Rectal examination often allows palpation of firm sand in the colon; however, sand that has accumulated in the distal right colon or transverse colon may be difficult to detect with palpation. Excessive sand accumulation can also be observed by taking four to six fecal balls, after rectal examination, inverting the glove over them, and filling the sleeve with water. The fecal balls are mixed, forming a slurry, and the sleeve is suspended for several minutes, allowing the sand to settle into the fingers. Frequently horses will have minor amounts of sand; however, if there is an excessive amount, a diagnosis of sand impaction can be made. It is important for the veterinarian to know the amount of sand observed in feces from normal horses in the practice region before determining the amount that is abnormal. As with other impactions, radiography or ultrasonography may be used to diagnose sand impaction in small horses. Recently, abdominal auscultation has been reported as being useful for detecting sand in the large colon. The movement of sand within the intestine can be ausculted from the ventral abdomen.

THERAPY

The same laxatives used for treating feed impaction may also be used for conservative therapy of sand impaction. The laxative of choice for sand impactions is Psyllium hydrophilic mucilloid° at a dose of 0.25 to 0.5 kg per 450 kg, placed in 4 to 8 liters of water and given PO through a stomach tube. Once in contact with water, the mucilloid forms a gel that is difficult to pump through the nasogastric tube. The gel lubricates and binds with the sand, moving it distally and clearing the impaction. After the initial doses the mucilloid can be given dry, mixed with sweet feed.

The amount given and the duration of therapy depends on the individual case. The veterinarian must closely monitor the feces for the clearance of sand. Prolonged therapy, even after clinical signs have been relieved, may be necessary for removal of the sand. In certain geographic areas it may be necessary to monitor farms very closely for prevention of sand impaction. Prevention requires feeding above the ground or away from sandy soil, and grazing in pastures where adequate growth prevents horses from picking up sand. Horses that seek out sand to eat are difficult to manage. Muzzles or stall confinement may be necessary.

As with other forms of impaction, surgery is indicated if there is unrelenting pain, alteration in the peritoneal fluid constituents, colonic displacement, or deterioration in the horse's condition.

Foreign Body Obstructions

Intraluminal obstruction by foreign bodies usually occurs in the small colon or transverse colon, but obstructing masses are often also

---

°Metamucil, Procter and Gamble, Cincinnati, OH

found in the large colon. Obstructions often occur in young horses and are formed by nondigestable materials. These include bedding materials, rope, fence materials with rubber, and other less common materials such as feed bags and plastic such as tarpaulins. The presenting signs are similar to those of any intraluminal obstruction and generally surgery is required for removal.

DISPLACEMENT OF THE ASCENDING COLON

The normal spatial arrangement of the colon is maintained by contact with the other abdominal organs and under normal circumstances is fairly constant. However, the position of the colon may be deranged by altered motility or altered digestive mechanisms. If a section of colon retains ingesta it may sink, whereas increased gas production will cause the colon to rise. These abnormal mechanisms may lead to various types of displacements, including right and left dorsal displacement [renosplenic (nephrosplenic) entrapment], volvulus of the colon less than 270 degrees (nonstrangulating), and colonic retroflexion.

Left Dorsal Displacement

Large horses such as the warm bloods or large Thoroughbreds appear to be prone to left dorsal displacement. In this condition the large colon becomes trapped within the nephrosplenic space, placing the colon between the left kidney medially, the nephrosplenic ligament ventrally, the spleen laterally and dorsally, and the dorsal body wall.

Entrapment of the colon may occur by two mechanisms. The pelvic flexure of the colon may travel through the nephrosplenic space dorsally, becoming entrapped. Alternatively, the colon may move up between the body wall and spleen until it is trapped in the nephrosplenic space. The latter may occur during splenic contraction when the colon, if gas-filled, can travel dorsally between the spleen and body wall. The colon becomes trapped once the spleen returns to normal size. Alternatively, during gastric distention the spleen may displace ventromedially, resulting in a space between the spleen and body wall, allowing the colon to travel through the gap and continue dorsally up to the nephrosplenic space.

In mild cases only the pelvic flexure becomes entrapped, but more often a significant portion of the colon becomes entrapped. In severe cases as much as two thirds of the ventral and dorsal colon may become entrapped. In these severe displacements the colon frequently moves cranially and the pelvic flexure positions itself next to the diaphragm. If the colon moves between the spleen and body wall and is entrapped, it will twist at least 180 degrees at the site of constriction. The twist occurs because the dorsal colon initially travels between the spleen and body wall in its normal relationship with the ventral colon, but ends up beneath the ventral colon in the nephrosplenic space. Because of the reduction in luminal space, gas and ingesta accumulate. Under most circumstances there is not enough distention to cause vascular compromise of the tissue; however, it is not uncommon to find congestion and edema at the site of entrapment.

CLINICAL SIGNS AND DIAGNOSIS

The horse with a nephrosplenic entrapment often presents in mild to moderate pain, depending on the extent of colonic displacement and distention. As greater lengths of colon become entrapped, increased tension on the mesentery and severe distention of the colon occur, leading to increased pain and systemic shock.

In most cases the temperature and respiratory rate are within normal limits. The heart rate is normal to slightly elevated, depending on the severity of the condition. Rectal examination may reveal a distended large colon, caudomedially displaced spleen, and, if the horse is amenable to palpation, the colon may be palpable traversing over the nephrosplenic ligament. Results of peritoneal fluid analysis are variable but frequently within normal limits.

THERAPY

Both conservative and surgical methods have been reported for correcting a nephrosplenic entrapment. If the colon is trapped between the spleen and body wall, surgical correction may not be necessary as the colon often will return spontaneously to a normal position. If only the pelvic flexure is entrapped and the horse is not in pain, conservative management and denying access to feed may allow spontaneous correction. However, if there is no response to conservative therapy, or if there are indications that a large portion of the colon is trapped, more active therapy is indicated. In nonsurgical treatment the horse is administered a short-acting anesthetic, such as xylazine and ketamine, and positioned into right lateral recumbency. The horse is lifted by the legs with a hoist, held for 1 minute, and returned to dorsal recumbency. The horse is slowly positioned into left lateral recumbency and the 360 degree rotation is completed as the horse stands.

If conservative methods are not effective, or if

the entrapment is severe and the horse's condition is deteriorating, then surgical correction must be employed. Surgical correction should be attempted through a ventral median celiotomy. This approach is preferred to a left flank approach because it allows better visualization and room for manipulation of the bowel.

Right Dorsal Displacement

This condition is characterized by two types of displacements. In the most common, the colon turns at the mesenteric attachment and passes between the cecum and body wall in a caudal direction. Once caudal to the cecum, the colon frequently turns 180 degrees around the cecum, thereby placing the pelvic flexure in the cranial part of the abdomen. Less frequently, the large colon turns cranially around the caudal aspect of the cecum, placing the colon between cecum and body wall, with the pelvic flexure lying adjacent to the diaphragm. Frequently, in either type of displacement, the colon twists 180 degrees to 360 degrees at the mesenteric root, although 180 degrees is the most common. The etiology of right dorsal displacements is unknown; however, the mechanisms are probably similar to those involved in other displacements. Feeding practices and alterations in colonic motility and function lead to changes in weight and gas formation within the various sections of colon.

CLINICAL SIGNS AND DIAGNOSIS

The clinical signs, which are similar to those of left dorsal colon displacement, vary according to the extent of distention and intestinal damage. Gastric reflux is usually absent and the abdominal fluid analysis is normal unless there has been vascular compromise causing damage to the colonic tissue. Rectal examination often reveals a large, gas-distended colon and absence of the pelvic flexure. The cecum is palpated medial to the colon.

THERAPY

Therapy usually entails surgical intervention, especially if displacement is severe or associated with volvulus. Conservative therapy by maintaining hydration and fasting may allow self-correction of a mild right dorsal displacement. The prognosis is good following surgical treatment.

Other Displacements

The pelvic flexure may displace cranially (retroflexion) in either a lateral, medial, dorsal, or ventral plane. The clinical signs, diagnosis, and therapy are similar to those of other colonic displacements.

STRANGULATING OBSTRUCTIONS

Colonic Volvulus

A volvulus greater than 270 degrees causes vascular obstruction, often resulting in severe colonic devitalization. Large colon volvulus has been identified in 11 per cent to 17 per cent of horses undergoing surgical intervention for colonic abnormalities. Despite improvements in surgical technique and postoperative care, the survival rate following correction of a large colon volvulus is low (21 per cent to 42 per cent). There appears to be no breed predilection for colonic volvulus, but adult horses and brood mares have the highest incidence. Volvulus is most common during the summer months, with a lesser incidence in spring. This relationship may result from the association between volvulus and parturition. However, in a recent study an equal number of volvulus cases occurred in females not associated with parturition, indicating that the pathogenesis and etiology are probably multifactorial.

During surgery, volvulus is most commonly observed at the base of the colon. However, the twist may occur at any point of the large colon. The sternal and diaphragmatic flexure is the second most common location. The twist is usually dorsomedial.

There appear to be at least two types of vascular insults to the colon during a volvulus. Venous obstruction has been reported as the initial insult because of the common clinical observation of extensive colonic edema, congestion, and hemorrhage. However, a volvulus may result in a pale gray serosa with minimal edema, congestion, and hemorrhage. This indicates that the initial vascular insult is both arterial and venous obstruction.

CLINICAL SIGNS AND DIAGNOSIS

The clinical signs of volvulus depend on the degree of volvulus, the duration of vascular occlusion, and the length of colon involved. The majority of horses with a volvulus exhibit signs of severe pain. The duration of colic most likely depends on a variety of factors; however, there is a correlation between the degree of volvulus and duration of clinical signs: horses with volvulus of more than 360 degrees present earlier than horses with volvulus of 270 degrees. Although there is overlap between these two groups, the time difference probably reflects the degree of vascular compromise in the two groups.

Horses with a large intestinal volvulus often present with severe abdominal distention and shock. Shock is indicated by cold extremities, weak pulse, dehydration, poor mucous membrane color, and increased capillary refill time. Usually tachycardia and tachypnea are present; however, some horses with a severe volvulus may not have a marked increase in heart rate.

The diagnosis of a colonic volvulus is usually not difficult to make because the history and clinical signs are often suggestive. Rectal examination often reveals a large, gas-distended colon, and with careful palpation an edematous colonic wall can be felt. The results of analysis of the peritoneal fluid are highly variable. In most cases this analysis is of little value in determining the severity of bowel damage, especially in comparison to the extreme changes that occur with strangulating obstructions of the small intestine.

THERAPY

Surgical intervention is necessary for correction of a volvulus and should be attempted as soon as the diagnosis is made and the horse is stabilized. Acid-base or electrolyte disturbances should be corrected and if hemoconcentration is present, fluids should be administered. Large volumes of fluids are often necessary and can be administered using two large-bore (10 to 14 gauge) catheters. Potent analgesic agents are necessary to control severe pain.

PROGNOSIS

The prognosis depends on the severity of the vascular compromise and the damage to the colon. In mild cases in which the return of colonic vascular circulation, color, and motility predicts bowel viability, the prognosis is good. In contrast, if there are severe, gross morphological alterations to the colon, colonic viability is less likely and the prognosis is guarded to poor. Colonic resection has been reported and in some cases may increase survival of horses with severe colonic damage. This procedure is most effective if the twist is located away from the colonic base.

COLONIC INTUSSUSCEPTION

Colonic intussusception is rare. The condition may be nonstrangulating or strangulating, depending on the duration and degree of pressure on the intussusceptum. Few cases have been reported; however, the most common site appears to be the left colon and the pelvic flexure.

Clinical signs accord with the degree of intraluminal obstruction and vascular compromise. Frequently, pain is mild to moderate and there is a gradual reduction of fecal output.

The results of abdominal fluid analysis vary depending on whether or not the intussusceptum is exposed to the abdominal cavity and the level of damage to the colonic tissue. Rectal examination often reveals gas distention within the ascending colon. The intussusception may be palpated as a thick colonic mass; however, this is usually the exception and most commonly, as with other intussusceptions, nothing diagnostic can be felt.

Surgical intervention is necessary for reduction or resection of the affected segment. Because of the severity of this condition and the potential for abdominal contamination, the prognosis is very poor.

Supplemental Readings

Barclay, W. P., Foerner, J. J., and Phillips, T. N.: Volvulus of the large colon in the horse. J. Am. Vet. Med. Assoc., 177:629–630, 1980.

Bertone, A. L., Stashak, T. S., Sullins, K. E., and Ralston, S. L.: Experimental large colon resection at the cecocolic ligament in the horse. Vet. Surg., 16:5–12, 1987.

Boening, K. J. and von Saldern, F.: Nonsurgical treatment of left dorsal displacement of the large colon of horses under anesthesia. In: Proceedings of the Second Equine Colic Research Symposium. Athens, GA, University of Georgia 1986, pp. 325–327.

Ducharme, N. G., Horney, D. F., Baird, J. D., Arighi M., and Burton J. H.: Extensive large colon resection in the pony: I. Surgical procedures and clinical results. Can. J. Vet. Res., 51:66–75, 1987.

Fisher, A. T., and Meagher, D. M.: Strangulating torsions of the large colon in the horse. Compend. Cont. Ed. Pract. Vet., 8:525–530, 1985.

Hackett, R. P.: Colonic volvulus and intussusception. In Robinson, N. E. (ed.): Current Therapy in Equine Medicine 2. Philadelphia, W. B. Saunders Co., 1987, pp 66–68.

Harrison, I. W.: Equine large intestinal volvulus: A review of 124 cases. Vet. Surg., 17:77–81, 1988.

Huskamp, B.: The diagnosis and treatment of acute abdominal conditions in the horse: The various types and frequency as seen at the animal hospital in Hoochmoor. In: Proceedings of the First Equine Colic Research Symposium. Athens, GA, University of Georgia 1982, pp. 261–272.

Huskamp, B.: Torsion of the large colon in the horse (torsio coli ascendentis). In Pfeiffer, C. J. (ed.): Animal Models for Intestinal Disease. Boca Raton, CRC Press, 1985.

Huskamp, B.: Displacement of the large colon. In Robinson, N. E. (ed.): Current Therapy in Equine Medicine 2. Philadelphia, W. B. Saunders Co., 1987, pp 60–65.

Koch, C.: The diagnosis and medical management of obstructive diseases of the large colon. In: Proceedings of the 26th Annual Convention of the American Association of Equine Practitioners, 1980, pp. 221–229.

McIlwraith, C. W.: Equine digestive system. In Jennings, P. B. (ed.): The Practice of Large Animal Surgery, Vol 1. Philadelphia, W. B. Saunders Co., 1984, pp 554–663.

Morris, D. D., and Johnston, J. K.: Peritoneal fluid constituents in horses with colic due to small intestinal disease. In: Proceedings of the Second Equine Colic Research Symposium. Athens, GA, University of Georgia 1986, pp. 134–142.

Sellers, A. F., and Lowe, J. E.: Review of large intestinal motility and mechanisms of impaction in the horse. Equine Vet. J., 18:261–263, 1986.

Snyder, J.R., Pascoe, J. R., Olander, H. J., Spier, S. J., Meagher, D. M., and Bleifer, D. R.: Strangulating volvulus of the ascending colon in horses. J. Am. Vet. Med. Assoc., 195:757–764, 1989.

Snyder, J. R. and Spier, S. J.: Diseases of the large intestine associated with acute abdominal pain. In Smith, B. P. (ed.): Large Animal Internal Medicine. St Louis, Mosby–Year Book, 1990, pp. 694–703.

Tennant, B. C.: Intestinal obstruction in the horse. In: Proceedings of the 21st Annual Convention of the American Association of Equine Practioners, 1975, pp. 426–439.

White, N. A., and Lessard, P.: Risk factors and clinical signs associated with cases of equine colic. In: Proceedings of the 32nd Annual Meeting of the American Association of Equine Practitioners, 1986, pp. 637–644.

Enteroliths

Harold F. Hintz, ITHACA, NEW YORK
Jack R. Snyder, DAVIS, CALIFORNIA

Enteroliths are mineral concretions that form in the large intestine. They are primarily composed of struvite (magnesium ammonium phosphate). The minerals precipitate around a nidus. Many different objects have been reported to constitute the nidus, including nails, pins, needles, coins, and buttons. The most common nidal objects are small stones such as chert (silicon dioxide). The rate of growth probably depends on several factors, but there is evidence that some enteroliths can grow to a size that can cause intestinal obstruction within a year.

EPIDEMIOLOGY

Enteroliths were frequently reported by veterinarians in the 1800s, particularly in England. The incidence of reported cases apparently decreased in the early 1900s, but in the late 1970s the number of reports of cases, particularly in California, started to increase. For example, during the period of 1970 to 1975 at the University of California, Davis, enteroliths were surgically removed from an average of two horses per year. By 1985 the number of surgical cases had increased to 43 annually. Data from the Veterinary Medical Data Program from 18 North American university veterinary medical teaching hospitals indicated that more than half of the reported cases were from the UC Davis clinic. The universities in states in the southern half of the United States were likely to have a higher rate of cases than universities in the northern half. Louisiana State University reported the highest rate per 10,000 patients at risk (48.2). UC Davis reported 42.2. However, UC Davis had the highest total of cases. Most northern veterinary colleges reported less than 8 cases of enteroliths per 10,000 patients. Illinois was an exception, with 27.6 cases per 10,000 patients at risk.

Arabians and Morgans had the highest relative risk of all breeds. Gender did not significantly influence risk.

ETIOLOGY

Diet has been frequently suggested as a factor in the etiology of enterolithiasis. In the late 1800s it was concluded that the concentration of nitrogen, magnesium, and phosphorus in the diet and hence in the large intestine influenced the incidence of enterolithiasis. Many of the enteroliths were found in horses fed wheat bran. Bran contains significant amounts of the above elements. Several studies indicated that when wheat bran was removed from the diet, the incidence of enteroliths decreased. Recently, alfalfa has been suggested as a possible factor, because alfalfa provides nitrogen and alfalfa raised in some parts of California is likely to be relatively high in magnesium. Furthermore, significant amounts of the nitrogen of the alfalfa is likely to reach the colon.

Another critical factor may be the pH of the large intestine. It has been suggested that when the pH is 6.5 or lower, the incidence of enteroliths is decreased. Alfalfa is an excellent buffer and is known to promote alkalinity in the rumen. Thus, alfalfa could promote an alkaline pH in the colon of the horse. Intestinal motility may also be a factor. A greater rate of motility could presumably increase the rate of excretion of the enteroliths when they are small. A decreased motility could lead to greater rate of formation.

DIAGNOSIS

The diagnosis is based on history, physical examination, and rectal examination findings. The degree of pain varies according to the extent of distention and the vascular compromise caused by the obstructing enterolith. With a partial intraluminal obstruction the horse will continue to pass scant amounts of liquid feces, gas, or mineral oil. In most patients the abdominal fluid remains normal until the calculus causes pressure necrosis of the surrounding intestinal tissue. In some cases it may be advantageous to perform rectal palpation with the horse on a slight incline, such as a hill or loading chute, thereby allowing the intestinal tract to move caudally and possibly allowing palpation of the enterolith. The calculi vary in location within the intestinal tract; however, the right dorsal colon is frequently the site for larger stones. Other locations include the transverse and small colon. Stones may develop singly, in which case they are round and smooth. Multiple stones are usually tetrahedral in shape, due to contact with apposing stone surfaces.

Abdominal radiographs may be valuable in cases where the diagnosis is uncertain; however, in large horses the technique is less rewarding.

THERAPY

Once a diagnosis has been confirmed, a surgical removal is the usual method of therapy. Because alkaline colonic pH may be a factor causing enteroliths, acidification of colonic contents is a possible treatment for small, nonobstructing stones. No controlled clinical studies have been conducted to determine the effectiveness of vinegar treatment for enterolithiasis. However, there have been anecdotal reports from farms that the incidence of enteroliths decreased when horses were fed 8 oz of vinegar twice daily. One farm reported that horses developed diarrhea when the vinegar was first added to the diet. Some owners report that some horses are initially reluctant to eat grain with vinegar. However, we have not experienced any difficulty in inducing horses to eat the grain plus vinegar. Further studies are needed to determine the effectiveness of vinegar and how frequently it must be used.

PREVENTION

Decreasing magnesium intake might be beneficial, not only because of the lowered magnesium concentration in the colon but because magnesium promotes an acid pH in the colon. However, the magnesium concentration in the diet should not be less than the NRC requirement of 0.1 per cent. Decreasing the hay to grain ratio can also decrease colonic pH. The colonic pH of ponies fed only hay is 6.9, but when the feed ratio is one third hay and two thirds grain, the pH is reduced to 6.4. Feeding grain alone is not practical, but when grain is the only feed the colonic pH decreases to 6.2. When the ratio of grain to hay is changed, energy intake may increase and lead to increased weight gains unless intake is controlled. Perhaps the higher incidence of enteroliths in warmer states is related to lower grain intake because of the greater availability of pasture and the lower energy requirements resulting from warmer weather. It is also possible that the higher incidence of enteroliths in Arabians and Morgans than in Thoroughbreds and Standardbreds might be a result of the higher level of grain fed to racing horses.

The feeding of vinegar may also decrease the colonic pH. When ponies receiving a diet of two thirds hay and one third grain are given 112 ml of apple cider vinegar twice per day, the colonic pH decreases from 6.5 to 6.0 after about 21 days. No adverse effects have been seen when vinegar is administered for as long as 90 days. Of course, rapid and severe changes in colonic pH to 5.0 or less could result in colic or laminitis. Vinegar need not be fed continuously. Six weeks on and 6 weeks off vinegar could possibly maintain a colonic pH that is not conducive to enterolith formation. Fecal pH may indicate the colonic pH, but the correlation between fecal pH and colonic pH is not tight.

Some horses are fed sodium bicarbonate in an attempt to promote athletic performance, because bicarbonate may decrease the build-up of lactate in the muscle. Vinegar should not be recommended if horses are receiving bicarbonate.

Supplemental Readings

Blue, M. G., and Wittkopp, R. W.: Clinical and structural features of equine enteroliths. J. Am. Vet. Med. Assoc., 179:79, 1981.

Evan, D. R. Trunk, D. A., Hibser, N. K., Everman, T., and London, C. A.: Diagnosis and treatment of enterolithiasis in equidae. Compend. Cont. Ed. Pract. Vet., 3:S383–S391, 1981.

Hintz, H. F., Lowe, J. E., Livesay-Wilkens, P., Schryver, H. F., Soderholm, L. V., Tennant, B. C., Hayes, H. M., Lloyd, K., Buechner, V., Liskey, C., and Wheat J. D.: Studies on equine enterolithiasis. In: Proceedings of the 34th Annual Convention of the American Association of Equine Practitioners, 1988, p. 53.

Hintz, H. F., Hernandez, T. M., Soderholm, L. V., Evans D. R., and Schryver, H. F.: Effect of vinegar supplementation on pH of colonic fluid. *In:* Proceedings of the Equine Nutrition and Physiology Society, Stillwater, OK, May 18–20, 1989, 1989, p. 116.

Hintz, H. F., Lim, M. C., Soderholm, L. V., Schryver, H. F., and Lowe, J. E.: Enteroliths in horses. *In:* Proceedings of the Cornell Nutrition Conference, 1987, p. 95.

Lawrence, L., Kline, K., Miller-Graber, P., Siegel, A., Kurcz, E., Fisher, M., and Bump, K.: Effect of sodium bicarbonate on racing thoroughbreds. J. Anim. Sci. 68:673–677, 1990.

Lloyd, K., Hintz, H. F., Wheat, J. D., and Schryver, H. F.: Enteroliths in horses. Cornell Vet., 77:172, 1987.

Endotoxemia

Robert J. MacKay, GAINESVILLE, FLORIDA

Endotoxins are large aggregates of lipopolysaccharide (LPS) and protein that are derived from the outer wall of gram-negative bacteria. Lipid A and the core polysaccharide segment to which it is linked comprise the more constant or core glycolipid region of the LPS molecule. Most, but not all, of the adverse biological effects of endotoxin are associated with the lipid A portion of the core glycolipid. The O-region of lipopolysaccharide is a highly variable array of polysaccharide chains that contain the antigenic determinants that define serologically the LPS molecule (and the bacterial species from which it is derived).

Endotoxemia is the presence of endotoxin in the blood. When the term is used clinically, it additionally implies the presence of clinical signs due to circulating endotoxin. This term should not be confused with either bacteremia, which refers only to the presence of viable bacteria in the blood, or septicemia, which is defined here as systemic disease caused by the multiplication of microorganisms in the blood.

Although endotoxin is ubiquitous in the environment, it normally is effectively excluded from the body by the skin and the mucous membranes of the respiratory, urogenital, and gastrointestinal tracts. Because of the presence in the intestine of resident large populations of gram-negative bacteria, the gut wall is particularly challenged to contain high concentrations of endotoxin. At least 2.25 gm of free endotoxin is safely sequestered in the ventral colons and cecum of an average adult horse. Passage of only 1 μg of this material into the systemic circulation may cause fever and leukopenia. Small amounts of endotoxin probably do escape from the intestine into the portal and systemic circulations and are removed by the liver, primarily by binding to Kupffer cells.

Any condition that compromises the integrity of the gut wall could result in clinical endotoxemia. Intestinal damage caused by invasive microbial or parasitic organisms, chronic inflammatory disease, edema, physical and chemical causes of ulceration or perforation, or vascular compromise could all allow the transmural passage of free endotoxin or endotoxin-containing gram-negative bacteria. When an invasive organism is itself a source of endotoxin (e.g., *Salmonella* spp.), the likelihood of endotoxemia is much greater. If sufficient endotoxin escapes into the portal circulation, the ability of the liver to remove it may be overwhelmed and systemic endotoxemia ensues. When hepatic function is impaired, the endotoxin-binding capacity of the liver is compromised and the likelihood of endotoxemia is increased proportionately. In cases of portal hypertension and inflammatory bowel disease in humans, endotoxin may gain access to the systemic circulation by passage through lymphatics. Even in the absence of structural changes to mucosal walls, the permeability of these barriers to endotoxin can be increased by the local actions of vasoactive substances such as histamine, bradykinin, and some eicosanoids. Such a mechanism may be involved in the endotoxemia reportedly associated with carbohydrate overload of horses.

Infection of any tissue by gram-negative bacteria theoretically can cause endotoxemia. For example, septic postpartum metritis is thought frequently to cause endotoxemia in mares. Although it has been shown that circulating endotoxin facilitates the passage of bacteria across the gut wall, it is widely assumed that most cases of endotoxemia in the adult horse occur without associated bacteremia. In neonatal foals, however, endotoxemia in association with gram-negative bacteremia likely is relatively common.

When endotoxin contacts blood, the resulting events are so widespread and complex that it is difficult to sort out the changes that are critical to the clinical outcome from those that can be considered epiphenomena. Figure 1 shows these initial events. The interaction of endotoxin with

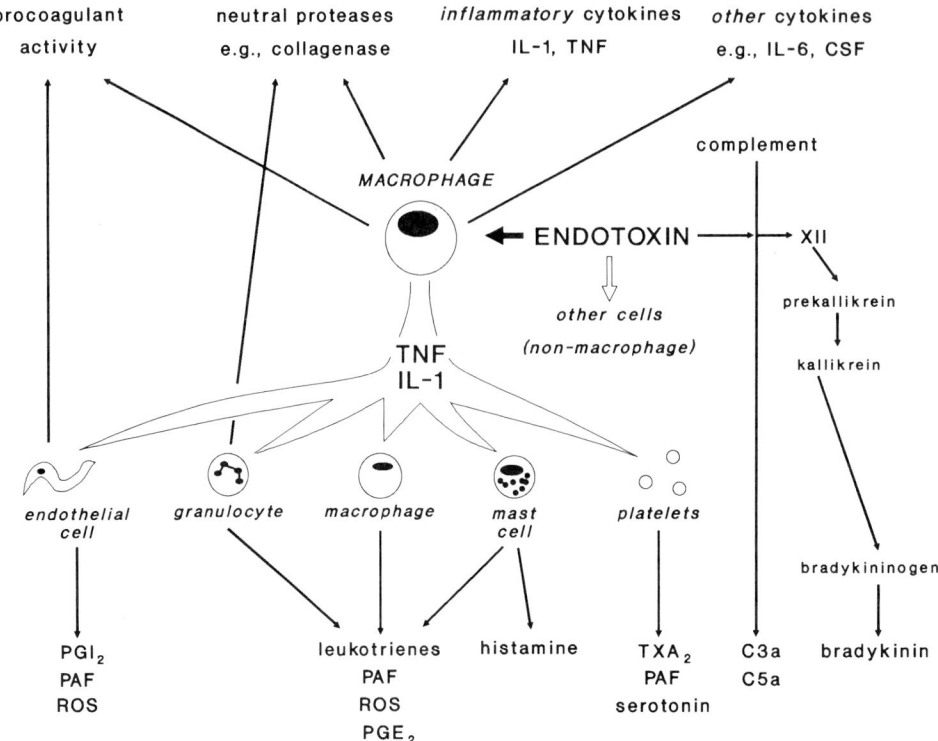

Figure 1. The mediators of endotoxemia. The critical and central role of the macrophage/monocyte is emphasized in this diagram; however, it is important to note that the direct interaction of endotoxin with other cells, such as platelets, also contributes to the clinical signs of endotoxemia. (C = complement, IL = interleukin, TNF = tumor necrosis factor, PGI_2 = prostacyclin, PGE_2 = prostaglandin E_2, TXA_2 = thromboxane A_2, PAF = platelet-activating factor, ROS = reactive oxygen species.)

cells of the mononuclear phagocytic system, such as monocytes and macrophages, sets in motion most of the changes of endotoxemia. Binding to macrophages is followed within 30 minutes by the secretion into the circulation of a small number of extremely potent proteins termed cytokines, the most important of which are tumor necrosis factor (TNF) and interleukin-1 (IL-1). When injected experimentally into animals, TNF and, to a lesser extent, IL-1 can reproduce virtually all of the signs of endotoxemia. Interleukin-6, colony-stimulating factors, macrophage inflammatory peptides, and interferons also are secreted cytokines that contribute to the clinical signs of endotoxemia.

The inflammatory cytokines (IL-1 and TNF) are potent mediators with direct actions on many cells and soluble systems and also induce the production of other mediators that amplify the process. One important mediator that is liberated is the phospholipid platelet-activating factor (PAF), a potent inflammatory substance with activity in many tissues. Also outlined in Figure 1 are the important direct interactions of endotoxin with the complement proteins and factor XII, each of which yields active peptide products of potential importance in endotoxemia. The final events in the inflammatory pathways include a number of mediators such as eicosanoids (thromboxanes, prostaglandins, leukotrienes), vasoactive and chemotactic peptides (histamine, serotonin, bradykinin, C3a, C5a), secreted proteases (collagenase, elastase) and reactive oxygen species (particularly hydroxyl radical).

In addition to the development of circulatory shock, other changes are induced whose clinical relevance is either less important or unclear. These include elevations in blood levels of the stress hormones glucagon, cortisol, and epinephrine, induction of the acute phase protein response, elevations in the levels of endogenous opioids, alterations in carbohydrate, amino acid and lipid homeostasis, and changes in the circulating concentrations of certain metal ions.

PATHOPHYSIOLOGY

The principal responses of the horse to circulating endotoxin are fever, leukopenia, and alterations in blood pressure, hemostasis, and glucose metabolism.

FEVER

Elevation in rectal temperature and a decline in the number of circulating neutrophils are the two most sensitive indicators of endotoxemia. The intravenous (IV) injection of less than 1 ng

LPS per kg body weight is sufficient to evoke a febrile response within 2 hours. The magnitude and duration of fever are dose dependent but quite variable among individual horses. Endotoxin fever is induced primarily by the central actions of IL-1 and TNF (the two principal endogenous pyrogens) and is mediated by prostaglandin E_2 (PGE_2). The secretion of macrophage inflammatory peptides contributes to fever via a prostglandin-independent mechanism.

Neutropenia

Endotoxemia causes endothelial cells to express receptors for neutrophils. Once bound to the epithelium, the marginated neutrophils are "activated" by exposure to inflammatory mediators (e.g., TNF, leukotriene B_4). Activated marginated neutrophils damage vessels and render them leaky by discharging their granule contents and toxic reactive oxygen species onto the adjacent endothelium and basement membranes. Neutrophils that have been activated by exposure to the mediators of endotoxemia are usually described as "toxic" in appearance.

Under the influence of colony-stimulating factors and other mediators, immature neutrophils are released into the circulation and neutrophil production by the bone marrow is stimulated. Thus, the net effect of endotoxin on circulating neutrophils is an initial neutropenia with a left shift, followed by a mature neutrophilia.

Hemodynamic Effects

The pulmonary and systemic circulations respond differently to endotoxemia. In the lungs there is increased vascular resistance and pulmonary hypertension followed by pulmonary capillary congestion. These changes stem from the action of endotoxin on intravascular pulmonary platelets and macrophages, leading to the preponderant activity of mediators with vasoconstrictor activity, such as thromboxane A_2 from platelets. Although these changes are associated with a reduction in Pa_{O_2}, only rarely does this progress to a syndrome resembling adult respiratory distress syndrome.

In adult horses treated with a moderate sublethal dose of LPS, there may be an initial period of systemic hypertension followed by a more sustained fall in blood pressure. The early pressor effects of platelet-derived mediators and catecholamines likely mediate the initial rise in blood pressure. A combination of decreased peripheral vascular resistance, myocardial depression, and reduced plasma volume contributes to the subsequent hypotensive phase. Following the interaction of activated neutrophils and endothelial cells, the influence of vasoconstrictors is greatly outweighed by the combined action of vasodilators such as endothelial prostacyclin (PGI_2) and PGE_2 from leukocytes. Plasma-derived peptides such as C3a and bradykinin contribute an additional vasodilatory influence. Marginated neutrophils damage the endothelium and basement membrane of capillary beds, allowing plasma to leak into the interstitium. Leukotrienes, PAF, and C5a appear to have important mediator roles in this process. TNF shifts water into myocytes and other cells, thus causing a further contraction in circulating blood volume without changing total body water. The ability of the heart to respond to falling blood pressure is impaired by the actions of endotoxin-induced circulating myocardial depressant factor, which reduces cardiac myocontractility. It has been suggested that inflammatory cytokines also directly interfere with myocardial function.

Hemostasis

The net early effect of endotoxin on the hemostatic system increases coagulability. There is widespread platelet aggregation due to the effects of released thromboxane A_2 and exposure of damaged endothelium. Activation of the intrinsic pathway of coagulation is initiated via direct effects of endotoxin on factor XII (Hageman factor); more important, the increased expression of procoagulant activity (tissue factor) by endothelial cells and macrophages causes intensive activation of the extrinsic clotting cascade. At the same time, the anticoagulant influence of thrombomodulin, an endothelial protein, is downregulated by TNF. During this hypercoagulable phase, there may be spontaneous thrombosis of major as well as minor vessels. As a consequence of fibrinolytic pathway activation, which occurs secondary to coagulation, there is increased production and impaired degradation of fibrinopeptides, which themselves cause vasoconstriction of small vessels. With widespread coagulation, severe consumption of platelets and clotting factors combined with intense fibrinolysis may induce a hemorrhagic diathesis. Thus, states of hypercoagulability and hemorrhage may coexist in the same animal. Clinically significant hemorrhage as a result of endotoxemia is very rare in the horse.

Glucose Homeostasis

Within 30 minutes of the injection of a sublethal amount of endotoxin, there is a rise in blood glucose due to enhanced glycogenolysis stimulated by elevated circulating catecholamines. Once glycogen stores have been depleted, blood glucose levels decline to normal or subnormal levels. This tendency toward hypoglycemia is most pronounced in neonatal foals with gram-negative bacterial infections. Hypoglycemia occurs as a result of greatly increased glucose utilization by tissues, particularly by inflammatory leukocytes and skeletal muscle. Because much of the glucose utilization by leukocytes is via anaerobic glycolysis, lactic acidosis develops. The increased availability of lactic acid along with increases in the plasma concentrations of the stress hormones (glucagon, catecholamines, and glucocorticoids) stimulates gluconeogenesis and actually tends to increase glucose availability. The resulting plasma concentration of glucose depends on the balance between glucose production and utilization.

REDUCED EFFECTIVE BLOOD FLOW TO CRITICAL TISSUES

During severe endotoxemia, systemic hypotension, vasoconstriction, capillary congestion, extravasation of plasma, plugging of capillaries by platelets, and intravascular coagulation compromise blood flow to vital organs. Erythrocytes and leukocytes become more rigid and lose their normal ability to deform and squeeze through small capillaries. The resultant cellular plugging of small vessels is considered an important phenomenon in endotoxemia of humans and dogs; the significance in horses is unknown.

Low Pa_{O_2}, defective oxygen extraction by tissues, and hypoglycemia may all compound the deleterious effects of inadequate blood flow during endotoxemia. Hypoxic conditions prevailing in endothelial cells favor the formation of xanthine oxidase, an enzyme that catalyzes the formation of locally toxic, reactive oxygen species such as hydroxyl radical. The systemic manifestations of nutrient and oxygen starvation of tissues may include renal failure (ischemic tubular necrosis), depression and stupor (cerebral hypoxia/hypoglycemia), laminitis (pedal laminar ischemia), ileus, or colic (intestinal ischemia). Compromised blood flow to vital organs may become so severe that the condition becomes irreversible. This vaguely defined condition is known as multiple organ failure and is the usual cause of death due to endotoxemia.

CLINICAL SIGNS

Depending on the LPS dose, the clinical signs of experimental endotoxemia may range from fever without obvious malaise to multiple organ failure and death. It is assumed but not proved that a similar spectrum of signs can be attributed to the endotoxemia that complicates some natural diseases of horses. Obviously, the signs of these diseases that are not exclusively due to endotoxin (e.g., severe pain due to bowel strangulation or diarrhea in horses with *Salmonella* colitis) may greatly influence the overall clinical presentation.

Typically, in an adult horse exposed to a moderate sublethal IV bolus injection of LPS (e.g., 1 μg per kg body weight), there is an immediate period of mild tachypnea. This early sign usually is so mild as to easily be missed by the untrained observer. Beginning within an hour of injection, however, depression, restlessness, and inappetence gradually are manifest. Within 2 hours of injection, body temperature increases progressively. Auscultable intestinal sounds usually cease abruptly during this period and remain depressed for several hours. Intermittent signs of colic usually are seen and may cause the horse to go down, usually without rolling. Small amounts of loose feces may be passed but this would not usually be described as diarrhea. Heart and respiratory rates increase steadily for the first 4 to 6 hours after LPS injection and may peak at about 50 per cent above normal rates before beginning to decline. During the first hour, the visible mucous membranes are pale and peripheral pulses are strong (phase of peripheral vasoconstriction). As the horse enters the hypotensive phase of endotoxemia (beginning about an hour after receiving a moderate dose of LPS), mucous membranes become progressively more congested, the capillary refill time is prolonged, and a dark "toxic" line may become apparent around the gingival margins of the teeth. Clinical evidence of dehydration such as reduced skin turgor and sunken dull eyes likely will become apparent at this stage. These signs of circulatory insufficiency as well as signs of depression and malaise persist for several hours after injection, while the rectal temperature may remain elevated for up to 18 hours.

At lethal LPS doses (e.g., 100 μg per kg) in experimental animals or in clinical patients with severe endotoxemia, signs of circulatory failure and disordered hemostasis dominate the clinical picture. Usually these horses are stuporous and totally anorectic. As systemic blood flow becomes more compromised, rectal temperature may drop into or below the normal range. Urine output is reduced or nonexistent. In addition to dark, congested mucous membranes, other signs include rapid, weak peripheral pulses, cold extremities, sweating, and occasionally muscle tremors and recumbency.

Petechial and ecchymotic hemorrhages may be seen on mucous membranes. A poor prognostic sign is the development of a hypercoagulation syndrome, during which routine venipuncture or catheter placement may result in thrombosis along the entire visible length of the jugular veins (or other superficial veins). If both jugular veins are thus occluded, there often is massive swelling of the soft tissues of the head, and associated laryngeal edema may cause signs of upper respiratory tract obstruction. Infarcts of bowel segments may cause severe colic signs unresponsive to treatment. In those rare cases with a severe pulmonary component, there may be hemorrhage into the respiratory tract with progressive tachypnea and dyspnea.

If moderately to severely affected animals survive for more than 24 hours, there usually is visible edema of the ventral abdomen and limbs. Signs of laminitis may first become apparent at this stage and may progress in severity even as the other systemic signs of endotoxemia improve.

LABORATORY DIAGNOSIS

With the exception of the early and profound neutropenia (usually accompanied by a left shift and a toxic appearance of stained cells) and the dose-dependent hypoglycemia described above, the clinicopathological signs of endotoxemia are nonspecific and reflect altered tissue perfusion or disordered hemostasis. There is a dose-dependent lactic acidosis, increased anion gap, and a reduction in Pa_{O_2}. Elevations in serum activities of lactate dehydrogenase, alkaline phosphatase, and creatine kinase reflect damage to organs such as the liver, muscle, intestine, and brain. Increased blood urea nitrogen and serum creatinine concentrations occur secondary to reduced renal perfusion (prerenal azotemia), and in severe cases, there is also a component of uremia secondary to ischemic renal damage. In the latter circumstance, dipstick examination of urine should reveal abnormal amounts of protein and blood. In moderate and severe cases of endotoxemia, there is a dose-dependent reduction in the circulating platelet count to less than 100,000 per μl, and moderate prolongation of the prothrombin and/or activated partial thromboplastin times. Titers of fibrin degradation products of greater than 1:5 indicate uncompensated fibrinolysis occurring as part of a widespread coagulopathy.

THERAPY

The strategy for management of horses with endotoxemia has two components: provision of circulatory support and specific inhibition of endotoxin-mediated processes. In cases in which an intestinal "accident" is the cause of endotoxemia, medical support is secondary to the paramount issue of surgical correction of the problem.

SUPPORTIVE THERAPY

Blood volume expansion is the cornerstone of treatment for moderate and severe acute endotoxemia. Many of the signs of acute endotoxemia relate to leakage of plasma into the interstitial spaces and movement of water into cells. A balanced polyionic solution should be used in an attempt to restore plasma volume by expanding extracellular fluid volume (ECF). The ECF deficit should be estimated by reference both to clinical parameters of dehydration (see p. 18) and by measurement of the hematocrit and plasma protein concentration. In early endotoxemia, plasma protein concentration is a more useful indicator of ECF than is the hematocrit, as the latter is greatly influenced by catecholamine release and splenic contraction.

Fluids should be infused through an indwelling IV catheter, inserted under aseptic conditions. The initial fluid deficit can be roughly estimated as follows:

$$\text{ECF deficit (liters)} = \frac{(PP-7)}{PP} \times (0.22)BW,$$

where PP = plasma protein concentration (gm per dl) and BW = body weight (kg).

For example, for an endotoxemic 450-kg horse with a plasma protein concentration of 8.5 gm per dl, the estimated deficit would be 17.5 liters. This equation assumes that the plasma protein concentration of the horse prior to disease onset was 7.0 gm per dl and that the ECF volume of a healthy horse is 22 per cent of body weight. This is a conservative estimate, as even early in the course of endotoxemia there is likely some loss of plasma protein into the interstitium. The estimated deficit should be given rapidly at 10 to 20 ml per kg per hour (5 to 10 L per hour for a 450-kg horse) and then continued at a rate at least 50 per cent above maintenance (i.e., at 1.5 L per hour or more in a 450-kg horse). Urination should begin during the rapid replacement of estimated losses. Ideally, the fine control of fluid replacement should be based on serial measurements of plasma protein concentration.

Some clinicians prefer the early use of crossmatched plasma transfusions (5 liters for a 450-kg horse, 1 to 2 liters for a neonate) to replace the extravasated colloid. In septic neonatal foals, plasma has the additional advantage of providing immunoglobulin.

Unless the initial blood pH is less than 7.2, or the bicarbonate or total CO_2 concentration is less than 15 mEq per L_{ECF}, sodium bicarbonate probably does not need to be given initially. Improvements in peripheral perfusion and renal function caused by volume expansion likely will improve acid–base balance in these less severe cases. If the pH is below 7.2, 50 to 100 per cent of the estimated deficit (see p. 18) should be provided during the period in which the initial fluid deficit is being replaced. Acid–base balance should then be reevaluated and additional bicarbonate provided if the pH is still less than 7.2. For this purpose, a 5 per cent solution of sodium bicarbonate can simply be added to or "piggybacked" onto a bag of physiologic saline. Bicarbonate-containing solutions should not be used with fluids containing calcium salts, as the calcium carbonate will precipitate. IV fluids should be supplemented with potassium (10 to 20 mEq per L) regardless of whether or not there is measured hypokalemia, as serum potassium levels will decline as acidosis is corrected. All fluids given initially to septic neonates or to hypoglycemic adult horses should be supplemented to 5 or 10 per cent glucose and glucose levels should be closely monitored in the blood and urine.

There currently is much interest in the use of hypertonic saline for rapid volume expansion in horses with septic shock. This appears to be an attractive therapy as small volumes of fluids can be used and the experimental results have been promising. Hypertonic saline is thought to act by shifting water from the intracellular to the extracellular space, by stimulating autonomic reflexes, and by directly stimulating myocardial contractility. A current recommendation is to administer 4 ml per kg of 7.5 per cent NaCl IV over 20 minutes. The use of hypertonic saline is in its infancy and further work needs to be done before its routine use can be recommended.

If, once blood volume has been adequately replaced, anuria or hypotension (mean arterial pressure less than 60 mm Hg as measured by tail cuff manometer) persists, the selective use of catecholamines should be considered. Dobutamine (2 to 15 µg per kg per minute) may be used in an effort to increase systemic blood pressure by improving cardiac myocontractility. Low-dose dopamine (1 to 3 µg per kg per minute) improves renal and brain perfusion by causing selective peripheral vasodilation. A useful protocol that should improve renal perfusion while maintaining or improving systemic blood pressure is as follows: dilute 1 vial each of dobutamine° (250 mg) and dopamine† (200 mg) into 500 ml of saline or 5 per cent dextrose and infuse the mixture at 0.45 ml per kg per hour (200 ml per hour in a 450-kg horse). This will provide 3 µg per kg per minute of dopamine and 3.6 µg per kg per minute of dobutamine. Blood pressure and heart rate should be monitored (e.g., by tail cuff manometer) frequently during the infusion, especially in neonates.

ANTIBIOTICS

There is no universally accepted practice as to the use of antibiotics in horses with endotoxemia. I use antibiotics in the following situations in which a horse is suspected of having endotoxemia: (1) in all foals less than 3 months of age; (2) where there is a known or suspected extraintestinal gram-negative infection; (3) in horses with a degenerative left shift or total neutrophil count of less than 1000 per µl; and (4) where there is clinical evidence of dyshemostasis, such as jugular thrombosis or mucosal petechial hemorrhages. It should be noted that effective antibiotic therapy can theoretically cause a transient worsening of clinical signs by causing the release of a pulse of endotoxin from killed bacteria. This possibility should be anticipated and minimized by the timely use of anti-inflammatory drugs.

ANTIENDOTOXIN ANTISERUM

There is evidence in horses and other animals that serum containing antibodies against the core glycolipid of LPS can protect against the effects of injected endotoxin. In prospective studies in humans and in horses, the use of antiserum early in the course of disease also improved survival in gram-negative sepsis. Although other studies in horses failed to demonstrate a beneficial effect of antiendotoxin serotherapy, its use seems well justified in cases of moderate to severe endotoxemia. The product that is available commercially° is a serum from horses hyperimmunized with a bacterin-toxoid prepared from a mutant *Salmonella typhimurium* strain. The suggested regimen is 1.5 ml per kg body weight diluted at least twofold in IV fluids. A hyperimmune plasma produced in horses against an *E. coli* J5 mutant† is being marketed for use in foals but is not yet licensed by the U.S. Department of Agriculture or marketed for use in adult horses. Obviously, serotherapy is most likely to be useful if used early in the course of disease.

NONSTEROIDAL ANTI-INFLAMMATORY DRUGS (NSAID)

Through their inhibition of cyclooxygenase activity (Fig. 2), NSAIDs reduce the formation of

---

°Dobutrex, Eli Lilly Industries, San Juan, Puerto Rico
†Dopamine hydrochloride, Abbott Labs., North Chicago, IL

°Endoserum, Immvac Inc., Columbia, MO
†Polymune-J, Veterinary Dynamics Inc., Chino, CA

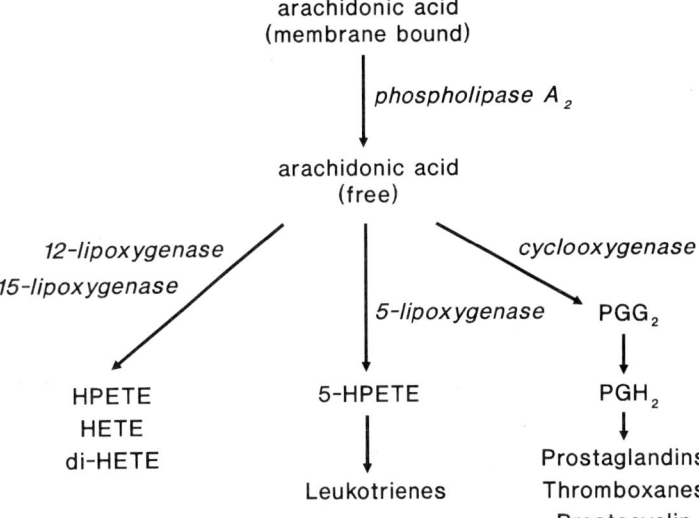

Figure 2. Possible routes of arachidonate metabolism. (From Hansen, B.: Leukotrienes: Biology and role in disease. J. Vet. Intern. Med., 33:59, 1989. Reproduced by permission.)

prostanoid metabolites (thromboxanes, leukotrienes, and prostaglandins) from arachidonic acid and thereby attenuate most of the adverse effects of endotoxin. Phenylbutazone, aspirin, and flunixin meglumine are examples of this class of drugs that are commonly used in horses. Flunixin has proved particularly effective in experimental endotoxemia in the horse. When used at 0.25 mg per kg every 6 hours, maximal antiendotoxic effects are produced without obscuring the signs of colic or risking toxic side effects of the drug. It should be noted that flunixin does not significantly affect endotoxin-induced leukopenia. Because it is a potent inhibitor of platelet aggregation, aspirin often is used in an attempt to prevent or treat the disorders of coagulation seen during endotoxemia. A safe dose for an adult horse is one 60-grain aspirin tablet given orally every other day. This dose can be used concurrently with low-dose flunixin.

GLUCOCORTICOIDS

This class of drugs potentially has many useful actions in combatting the effects of endotoxemia. These include reduced production of eicosanoids (inhibition of phospholipase A2), inhibition of TNF production by macrophages, stabilization of cell membranes, and prevention of neutrophil activation. Unfortunately, these beneficial effects are minimal unless the drug is given at or before the first contact of endotoxin with blood. On the negative side, glucocorticoids depress the phagocytic activity of macrophages and neutrophils, inhibit immune responses, delay wound repair, and, most important, greatly increase the likelihood of laminitis. Therefore, corticosteroids should not be given routinely to horses with endotoxemia. Their use might be considered (1) in horses in the very early stages of severe endotoxemia or (2) if they can be given in advance of the anticipated release of endotoxin into the circulation—for example, prior to the initiation of antimicrobial therapy in a foal with septicemia, or possibly before the surgical correction of a large colon torsion in an adult horse. For the treatment of septic shock, the recommended dosage of dexamethasone is 0.5 to 2 mg per kg; for prednisolone sodium succinate it is 2 to 5 mg per kg.

HEPARIN

The use of heparin in endotoxemia is highly controversial. It prevents microvascular thrombosis by promoting the anticoagulant activity of antithrombin III. Unfortunately, antithrombin III is rapidly consumed during systemic coagulopathies, and it is therefore unlikely that heparin would be helpful in reversing serious intravascular coagulation syndromes in horses.

Depending on the experimental setting, there is evidence both for and against the efficacy of heparin in preventing laminitis in horses that may have endotoxemia. When given at the recommended IV or subcutaneous (SC) dose of 40 to 100 units per kg b.i.d. or t.i.d., heparin markedly increases intravascular agglutination of red blood cells. Thus, it could be argued that the use of heparin might actually exacerbate the degree of cellular plugging due to endotoxemia. Until more evidence for its efficacy is available, the use of heparin probably should be restricted to horses that (1) have had abdominal surgery or (2) are at high risk for the development of laminitis (especially after overeating of grain).

Scavengers of Reactive Oxygen Species

There is little doubt that toxic reactive oxygen species play a role in the pathophysiology of equine endotoxemia, yet only minimal efforts have been made to intervene therapeutically at this level. There is some evidence that allopurinol, an inhibitor of xanthine oxidase activity, may be useful in preventing ischemic damage during endotoxemia. It may be especially useful for preventing the reperfusion injury that is thought to occur after the correction of bowel strangulations. A recommended dosage of allopurinol is 5 mg per kg given IV. Because dimethyl sulfoxide (DMSO) has been shown to be a potent scavenger of hydroxyl radicals, it seems reasonable to use this agent in the treatment of equine endotoxemia. DMSO can be given IV as a 20 per cent solution in saline at dosages of 0.2 to 1 gm per kg every 6 to 12 hours. Because of concerns about renal toxicity, it is important that adequate blood volume and renal function be established before DMSO therapy is begun.

Current research in experimental animals and the horse indicates additional ways in which to inhibit the multiple pathways of endotoxin action. A partial list of promising areas now being investigated includes the following: (1) inhibition of PAF action by PAF receptor antagonists, (2) inhibition of leukotriene synthesis or action by 5-lipoxygenase inhibitors and leukotriene receptor blockers, (3) prevention of endotoxin-induced changes in erythrocyte deformability by hemorrheologic agents such as pentoxifylline, (4) direct binding of endotoxin by nontoxic antibiotics such as taurolin, (5) neutralization of TNF by specific antibodies, (6) use of potent antiproteases to combat widespread release and activation of serine proteases, and (7) inhibition of reactive oxygen species formation by the use of combinations of superoxide dismutase and catalase.

Supplemental Readings

Beutler, B., and Cerami, A.: Cachectin: More than a tumor necrosis factor. N. Engl. J. Med., 316:379, 1987.
Hansen, B.: Leukotrienes: Biology and role in disease. J. Vet. Intern. Med., 3:59, 1989.
Mahaffey, E. A., and Moore, J. N.: Erythrocyte agglutination associated with heparin treatment in three horses. J. Am. Vet. Med. Assoc., 189:1478, 1986.
Moore, J. N., Hardee, M. M., and Hardee, G. E.: Modulation of arachidonic acid metabolism in endotoxic horses: Comparison of flunixin meglumine, phenylbutazone, and a selective thromboxane synthetase inhibitor. Am. J. Vet. Res., 47:110, 1986.
Spier, S. J., Lavoie, J.-P., Cullor, J. S., Smith, B. P., Snyder, J. R., and Sischo, W. M.: Protection against clinical endotoxemia in horses by using plasma containing antibody to an Rc mutant E. coli (J5). Circ. Shock, 28:235, 1989.
Ward, P. A., Warren, J. S., and Johnson, K. J.: Oxygen radicals, inflammation, and tissue injury. Free Radical Biol. Med., 5:403, 1988.

Rectal Tears

Aubrey N. Baird, COLLEGE STATION, TEXAS

Practitioners are not commonly faced with disruption of the rectum or distal small colon; however, when a rectal tear occurs, it can be a life-threatening situation for the horse as well as a serious medicolegal problem for the practitioner. Noniatrogenic rectal tears have been reported, but rectal tears usually are a sequel to rectal palpation of the genitourinary or gastrointestinal (GI) tract.

Contrary to some published opinions, inexperience of the examiner does not always contribute to a rectal tear. More important factors are the care and patience of the palpator, restraint of the horse, and the predisposition of the horse to tearing. Arabian horses appear predisposed to rectal tears, possibly because of their smaller rectum or a natural resistance to palpation by excessive straining. Male horses of all breeds seem more likely to suffer rectal tears than females. This may be because females are palpated more and become accustomed to the procedure. Also, males are usually palpated for GI lesions, which may be accompanied by dehydration, thus making the rectal mucosa more friable. In addition, the rectal tube may be smaller in the male due to the presence of accessory sex glands and the absence of the vagina ventrally.

Most rectal tears occur in the dorsal aspect of the rectum (between 10 and 2 o'clock; 1000 and 1400 hours) approximately 25 to 30 cm from the anus. These tears are usually cranial to the peritoneal reflection and have the potential to communicate directly with the abdominal cavity. Rectal tears that occur caudal to the peritoneal reflection may lead to retroperitoneal abscesses that may extend into the abdominal cavity or require draining into the rectum or vagina.

Rectal tears are classified according to severity and tissue layers disrupted. Grade 1 rectal tears disrupt only the mucosa and leave all other layers intact. Grade 2 rectal tears disrupt only the muscularis layer of the rectal wall, leaving the mucosa and serosa intact. Grade 3 rectal tears disrupt the mucosa, submucosa, and muscularis and are subdivided according to location. Grade 3A rectal tears leave only the serosal layer of the rectal wall intact. Grade 3B rectal tears occur in the dorsalmost part of the rectal wall and therefore enter the fat-filled space between the two leaves of serosa that make up the mesocolon. The mesocolon prevents direct exposure to the abdominal cavity but is susceptible to abscessation when contaminated with feces and often ruptures, creating a grade 4 tear. Grade 4 rectal tears disrupt all layers of the rectal wall, allowing direct communication with the abdominal cavity and potential gross fecal contamination. It is important to determine the severity of the rectal tear because the treatment and prognosis vary with severity.

Once a grade 3 or 4 rectal tear has occurred, immediate diagnosis and treatment is imperative to enhance the probability of the horse's survival. When a rectal tear happens, the practitioner will usually detect a sudden release of tension from the rectum associated with a peristaltic wave or will directly palpate abdominal organs. Occasionally the palpator may not be aware that the rectum has torn until removing the gloved hand from the rectum and seeing blood, while others may not suspect a rectal tear until the horse passes blood in the feces following palpation. Any horse that exhibits signs of abdominal pain, such as sweating, pawing, and increased heart rate, within 2 hours of rectal palpation or breeding should be examined for the presence of a rectal tear.

DIAGNOSIS

If a rectal tear is suspected, the horse should be sedated immediately to facilitate further examination and relieve anxiety. Next, mepivacaine hydrochloride (100 mg for a 450-kg horse) should be administered between the first and second coccygeal vertebra with a 1.5- to 2-inch (3- to 5-cm) 20-gauge needle for caudal epidural anesthesia. This should prevent the horse from straining, slow the passage of ingesta, and again facilitate further examination. The rectal tear may be seen and evaluated with the use of a speculum. However, many tears occur too far proximal to the anus for speculum observation. The rectum often contracts immediately caudal to the tear, again making speculum examination impossible. Therefore, bare-handed palpation with the horse restrained, sedated, and under epidural anesthesia is the best method for locating and evaluating a rectal tear. Bare-handed palpation is best; a surgical glove decreases sensitivity of palpation and is not recommended.

The well-lubricated bare hand should be carefully inserted into the rectum to remove all feces present and minimize fecal contamination of the wound. The tear can be located by circumferential palpation of the rectum from the anus cranially in 3- to 4-inch (7- to 10-cm) increments until the tear is detected. The size and severity of the tear can then be evaluated by careful palpation. It has been recommended that the tear be located by repeated insertions of the hand into the rectum, but that is not necessary. A grade 1 tear, which may be difficult to detect without experience, may be palpated as a defect in the mucosa with the muscularis intact and no other change in the rectal wall. Grade 2 rectal tears do not cause luminal bleeding and do not generally require treatment. These tears are felt as a dimple in the rectal wall lined with mucosa; the texture of the lining does not change. The rectal wall is compromised, which may be a problem on subsequent palpation. More serious tears should not be difficult to identify. Grade 3 rectal tears create an obvious void in the rectal wall and expose either the thin serosa in a grade 3A tear or the fat-filled mesorectum in a grade 3B tear. A diverticulum lined by these structures usually forms when the muscularis, submucosa, and mucosa are disrupted. This diverticulum tends to fill with feces if proper steps are not taken and may lead to abscessation or formation of a grade 4 tear. Direct communication with the abdominal cavity and easy palpation of abdominal organs signify the presence of a grade 4 rectal tear.

INITIAL MANAGEMENT

The initial management of a rectal tear is aimed at preventing fecal contamination of the injury. Particulate fecal matter filling the serosa-lined diverticulum of a grade 3 tear may not directly enter the abdominal cavity but does increase peritoneal inflammation owing to bacterial leakage and may contribute to progression of the tear by irritating the serosa. First-aid measures that prevent fecal contamination of the rectal tear have improved survival rates in a series of cases recently reviewed. The initial management of grade 3 tears is most crucial and will be described here. Suggestions for management of other rectal tears are discussed under Therapy.

If a grade 3 rectal tear is identified after sedation and epidural anesthesia, prevention of fecal contamination of the injury and timely referral of a good surgical candidate to a surgical facility are of the utmost importance. All the fecal material within reach should be gently removed from the rectum. A rectal pack has proved beneficial in preventing fecal contamination of a grade 3 rectal tear. This pack can be made of 3-inch stockinette filled with approximately 0.25 kg of moistened roll cotton. If stockinette is not available, the practitioner may elect to use ingenuity and available resources to construct a tubular structure of absorbant material that would serve as a suitable substitute. The pack may be sprayed with dilute povidone–iodine solution and should be well lubricated with surgical jelly (Fig. 1). The pack is carefully inserted until the cranialmost aspect of the pack is approximately 10 cm craniad to the tear and not within the tear (Fig. 2). The pack should fill but not distend the rectum. After the pack has been positioned, more cotton may be added to the stockinette to ensure adequate packing to the anus. The pack should then be secured by either towel clamps or purse-string suture closure of the anus. Maintaining epidural anesthesia is a necessity of rectal packing, because the presence of the pack will stimulate rectal straining if the epidural anesthesia wears off. The epidural anesthesia is usually effective for 3 to 4 hours and may need to be repeated to ensure safe arrival at a surgical facility.

Other aspects of the initial management include administration of mineral oil via nasogastric tube to help soften the feces, which will be important in the definitive treatment. Dioctyl sodium sulfosuccinate (DSS), up to 9 gm PO (6 to 8 oz of 5% solution), may also be used for this purpose. The animal should be started on a broad-spectrum antibiotic regimen (such as penicillin and gentamicin) to treat the peritonitis that is inevitable. The horse should not be fed between the time of the injury and evaluation at a surgical facility so as to decrease the amount of ingesta in the intestinal tract. Tetanus toxoid booster or antitoxin may be appropriate, as determined from the vaccination history. While preparing the horse for shipment to a surgical facility, the practitioner must remember that client communication is very important whenever a complication of treatment such as this occurs.

The laboratory evaluation of the rectal tear patient is in no way a minor concern. However, for the practitioner in the field, palpation of the tear, provision of first aid, and referral of a good surgical candidate are more important than establishing baseline data. Most horses with rectal

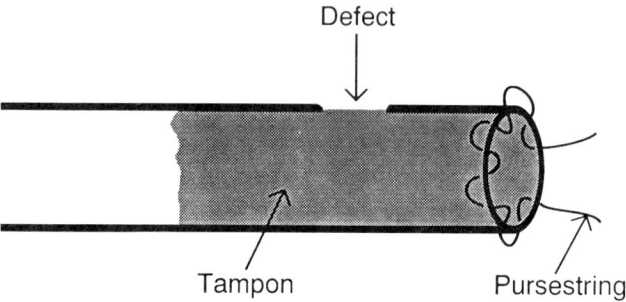

Figure 2. A pack (tampon) positioned in the rectum from the anus to cranial to the defect and secured with a purse-string suture.

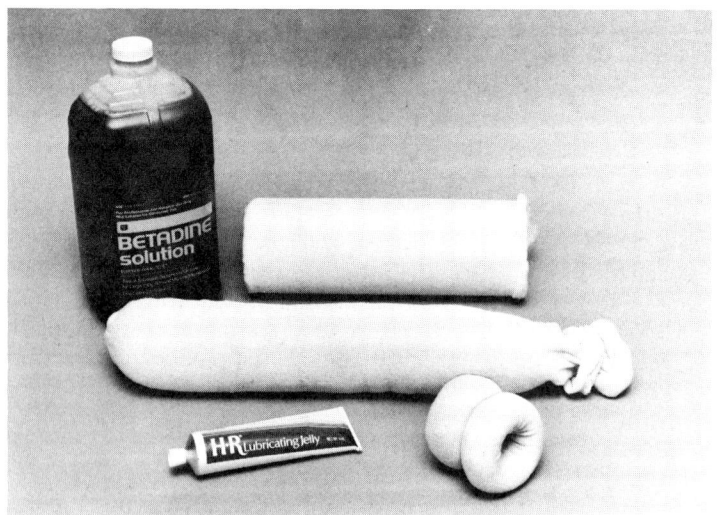

Figure 1. Materials used for rectal packing as a first-aid measure for initial management of rectal tears. A completed pack with the open (caudal) end to the right, to which more cotton can be added after placement, is surrounded by lubricating jelly, povidone–iodine solution, cotton, and stockinette.

tears will not require treatment for shock unless a grade 4 tear is present with gross fecal contamination of the abdominal cavity. This can be determined by palpation and usually necessitates euthanasia of the horse.

THERAPY

Grade 1 rectal tears do not require intensive therapy and usually have a good prognosis. Some surgeons may choose to suture the mucosal rent, but this is not routinely needed. The animal should be placed on antibiotics, because peritonitis usually accompanies rectal tears. A modified diet to soften the feces decreases the possibility of progression of the tear. Most grade 1 rectal tears will heal in 7 to 14 days.

Grade 2 rectal tears are seldom of clinical significance. Since the mucosa is not disrupted, these tears do not bleed into the rectal lumen. The practitioner may feel a sudden relief of tension during palpation, but these injuries are more likely to be an incidental finding on subsequent palpation. If the rent in the muscularis is large enough to create a mucosa-lined diverticulum, suturing per rectum may be indicated. However, this treatment is not routinely advised unless the tear is 4 cm in diameter or larger. In one case an ultrasound probe entered the mucosa-lined diverticulum of a large grade 2 tear, converting it to a grade 4 tear.

Grade 3 rectal tears require the initial treatment described above as well as surgical intervention to minimize peritonitis and prevent progression of the lesion to a grade 4 tear. Several surgical techniques can be used to treat grade 3 rectal tears. Most of these techniques divert the flow of feces away from the rectal tear to allow the injury time to heal. Some also entail suturing the tear to enhance healing and prevent the formation of a rectoperitoneal fistula. The technique used depends on the surgeon's preference and the individual case. A detailed description of these techniques is beyond the scope of this text. Techniques that have been described are placement of a temporary rectal liner with suture of the tear per rectum, suturing via rectum alone, creation of a temporary colostomy, creation of a temporary loop colostomy, and suturing via laparotomy (see *Current Therapy in Equine Medicine 2*, pp. 77–78).

A temporary indwelling rectal liner can be secured craniad to the rectal tear for the diversion of feces past the tear. The defect is sutured by a blind one-handed technique in the standing animal after the liner has been placed under general anesthesia. The liner is usually passed in the feces in 10 to 14 days, which allows time for the tear to heal.

The temporary colostomy technique divides the rectum cranial to the defect. The open distal end of the proximal segment exits the body wall. The proximal end of the distal segment is closed with a Parker–Kerr closure. After the defect heals, the two segments of the rectum are anastomosed to establish normal flow of ingesta.

The temporary loop colostomy technique does not divide the rectum but diverts the flow of feces away from a rectal defect by exteriorizing a loop of small colon craniad to the tear through the body wall. After the tear heals, this communication is closed to establish normal flow of ingesta.

At the Texas Veterinary Medical Center the temporary rectal liner with one-handed blind suture of the tear has yielded better results than those reported with other techniques. Although this repair is not easy, neither is it impossible. It has not caused trauma to the lesion or adjacent tissues and has not tended to break down, as reported by others. Peritoneal lavage is an essential part of therapy for these cases.

Grade 4 rectal tears communicate directly with the abdominal cavity and will result in gross fecal contamination if not treated promptly. The peritonitis and adhesions that accompany gross fecal contamination make the prognosis for these horses poor. Treatment of grade 4 rectal tears is a heroic measure, once there is gross fecal contamination of the abdomen. If discovered promptly and if appropriate first aid is provided to prevent spillage of feces into the abdomen, grade 4 rectal tears are treated similarly to grade 3 tears. A colostomy should be used for fecal diversion in these cases rather than the temporary indwelling liner to ensure adequate healing of the tear before termination of the fecal diversion. Suture of the grade 4 defect is imperative to prevent rectoperitoneal fistula formation. The peritonitis that accompanies grade 4 rectal tears will require aggressive treatment.

PREVENTION

Practitioners must take precautions when rectally palpating to prevent injury to the horse. The horse must be properly restrained. No single method of restraint is appropriate for all horses. Different methods include a twitch, lip chain, sedation, epidural anesthesia, and stock confinement. Attempting to palpate a horse without adequate lubrication may also contribute to the occurrence of rectal tears. Gentle examination will decrease the likelihood of rectal injury. In addition, the examiner should ascertain that the animal's rectum will accommodate the examiner's arm to reduce the possibility of rectal injury.

SUMMARY

Available evidence suggests that rectal tears are not always due to negligence if the horse is adequately restrained and the examiner patiently performs a careful examination. When a rectal tear does occur, the practitioner must be responsible for prompt recognition and first-aid treatment. Reported survival rates for horses with grade 3 rectal tears have varied from 20 to 60 per cent. This variability is largely due to differences in initial management and timely referral to a surgical facility.

Supplemental Readings

Arnold, J. S. and Meagher, D. M.: Management of rectal tears in the horse. J. Equine Med. Surg., 2:64, 1978.
Arnold, J. S., Meagher, D. M., and Lohse, C. L.: Rectal tears in the horse. J. Equine Med. Surg., 2:55, 1978.
Baird, A. N., Taylor, T. S., Watkins, J. P.: Rectal packing as initial management of grade 3 rectal tears. Equine Vet. J. Suppl. 7:121, 1989.
Taylor, T. S., Watkins, J. P., and Schumacher, J.: Temporary indwelling rectal liner for use in horses with rectal tears. J. Am. Vet. Med. Assoc., 191:677, 1987.
Watkins, J. P., Taylor, T. S., Schumacher, J., et al.: Rectal tears in the horse: An analysis of 35 cases. Equine Vet. J., 21:186, 1989.

Peritonitis

Susan D. Semrad, MADISON, WISCONSIN

The peritoneal cavity includes the abdominal cavity, pelvic cavity, and extra-abdominal extensions or vaginal processes. A single layer of mesothelial squamous cells with microvilli overlying loose areolar connective tissue and adipose tissue lines the peritoneal cavity and covers the intra-abdominal viscera. In health, the peritoneum secretes a serous fluid that lubricates the abdominal cavity, minimizes intra-abdominal adhesion formation, has minimal antibacterial properties, and acts as a bidirectional semipermeable barrier between the blood and the abdominal cavity.

Inflammation of the mesothelial lining of the peritoneal cavity is termed *peritonitis*. The inflammatory process is characterized by hyperemia, exudation, suppuration, chemotactic phagocytosis, increased peritoneal permeability to toxins (with subsequent absorption), peritoneal effusion, and fibrin deposits on the peritoneal surface.

Peritonitis may be classified according to origin (primary or secondary), onset (peracute, acute, chronic), region affected (diffuse, localized), and presence of bacteria (septic, nonseptic). In primary peritonitis the route of bacterial spread is not evident. Bacteria may enter the abdomen via the bloodstream or lymphatic system, or by transmigration through the bowel wall. Primary peritonitis is uncommon in horses but may be associated with impaired host defenses. In secondary peritonitis, bacteria enter the peritoneum or retroperitoneal space most commonly following disruption of the integrity of the gastrointestinal (GI) tract by disease, injury, or surgical contamination. In the horse, peritonitis is usually acute, diffuse, and secondary to traumatic or chemical insults or infectious disease processes. Localized peritonitis in the horse is most frequently associated with abdominal abscesses.

Any agent or disease process that causes irritation of the peritoneum or inflammation of abdominal viscera or that compromises the wall of hollow abdominal organs may foster the development of peritonitis (Table 1). The severity of the peritonitis is related to the initial underlying disease process, the nature of the infective agent, the natural host defenses, the extent of multiorgan involvement, the speed of early recognition and intervention, and the response to initial therapy. The severity of diffuse septic peritonitis is also related to the site of GI leakage and subsequent type of bacterial contamination. From the stomach distally along the GI tract, the absolute number of bacteria increases markedly, as does the ratio of anaerobic to aerobic organisms. Upper GI perforations may result in abdominal contamination with a relatively small bacterial load, whereas colonic leaks result in release of a large number of mixed organisms. In either case, the resulting peritonitis may be severe.

A variety of infectious agents has been isolated

TABLE 1. CONDITIONS ASSOCIATED WITH PERITONITIS

Infectious or Septic	Nonseptic	Traumatic	Parasitic	Iatrogenic
Intestinal accidents with perforation or transrenal movement of bacteria	Ruptured bladder, ureter, or kidney	Penetrating abdominal wound	Verminous arteritis	Intraperitoneal injections
	Hemoperitoneum	Blunt abdominal trauma	Parasitic larval migration (S. edentatus)	Cecal trocharization
Abdominal, renal, or retroperitoneal abscess	Chemical agents: bile, talc, barium, chyle, gastric or pancreatic juice	Breeding accident	Perforating lesions (ascarids, tapeworms)	Liver biopsy
		Foaling accident		Enterocentesis
Enteritis	Drugs	Esophageal injury		Rectal tear
Septicemia	Foreign body (sponges, drain)	Ruptured diaphragm		Peritoneal dialysis
Ascending urinary tract infection	Neoplasia—abdominal ovarian			Uterine perforation during biopsy, infusion, or artificial insemination
Urachal infection	Urinary tract obstruction			
Metritis, pyometra	Cholelithiasis			
Uterine rupture or perforation	Hepatitis			
Castration	Pancreatitis			
Surgical complications:	Urolithiasis			
Anastomosis failure	Splenitis			
Wound dehiscence	Gastric rupture			
Faulty asepsis				
Nonviable tissue				
Bowel trauma				
Equine influenza				
Equine viral arteritis				
Equine infectious anemia				
African horse sickness				
Streptococcus equi				
Chemical irritation with secondary infection				

From Smith, B.P. (ed): Large Animal Internal Medicine. Philadelphia, C.V. Mosby Co., p. 674. With permission.

from the abdominal fluid of horses with peritonitis. Fifty-six per cent of the positive samples yielded a single species and 26 per cent yielded two species. Anaerobic bacteria of the *Bacteroides* spp. (penicillin-resistant *B. fragilis* isolated from 10 to 20 per cent of positive cases) and members of the family Enterobacteriaceae (primarily *Escherichia coli*) are commonly isolated. Although many bacteria isolated in mixed infections are nonpathogenic by themselves, they may be essential for the pathogenicity of the bacterial mixture.

Contamination of the abdomen and injury to the mesothelial cells initiates an inflammatory response and a cascade of events that results in the release of histamine and vasoactive substances from peritoneal mast cells; vasodilation and hyperemia; an increase in peritoneal and vascular permeability; an influx of protein-rich fluid, macrophages, polymorphonuclear cells, humoral opsonins, natural antibodies, and serum complement into the peritoneal cavity; chemotactic phagocytosis; depression of the peritoneal fibrinolytic activity; fibrin deposits on the peritoneal surface; and reflex ileus of the GI tract. Although initially of benefit by confining the contamination and infection, these processes may become deleterious, resulting in hypovolemia, hypoproteinemia, dilution of opsonin concentrations, reduction in peritoneal oxygen tension, ileus with bowel distention, ischemia of the bowel wall and absorption of bacteria and toxins, and adhesion formation. The cardiovascular compromise, renal insufficiency, and endocrine and metabolic alterations observed reflect the degree of hypovolemia and endotoxic shock present.

CLINICAL SIGNS

Clinical signs of peritonitis depend on the primary disease process, infectious agents involved, and extent of disease when the animal is first examined. The spectrum of pathologic conditions ranges from localized peritonitis with little systemic involvement and minimal clinical signs to generalized peritonitis accompanied by severe toxemia or septicemia, or both. Most often the clinical signs are nonspecific but suggestive of GI dysfunction. Common presenting signs include colic, ileus, pyrexia, anorexia, weight loss, and diarrhea.

Horses with peracute peritonitis, such as occurs after rupture of the intestine, present with profound toxemia, weakness, depression, tachycardia, tachypnea, circulatory failure, and rapid deterioration. Death may occur within 4 to 24 hours. Fever and abdominal pain may or may not be evident, depending on the stage of shock and the mental status of the animal.

Signs associated with acute diffuse peritonitis include abdominal pain, sweating, pawing, muscle fasciculations, elevated heart and respiratory rates, thready peripheral pulses, red to purple mucous membranes, prolonged capillary refill time, dehydration, depression, and anorexia. Body temperature is variable. Abdominal pain, resulting from a combination of visceral and parietal pain, is most evident in the early stages of the disease. Parietal pain characterized by immobilization, reluctance to move, splinting of the abdominal wall, and sensitivity to external abdominal pressure predominates in most cases. GI motility and fecal output may be transiently increased early in the disease process, but ileus most frequently occurs. Resultant intestinal stasis may lead to intestinal distention, gastric reflux, and abdominal discomfort. Reluctance to perform an abdominal press because of pain and dehydration results in decreased fecal output, constipation, or impaction.

Horses with localized, subacute, or chronic peritonitis may present with signs of depression, anorexia, weight loss, intermittent fever, ventral edema, exercise intolerance, decreased or absent intestinal sounds, and mild dehydration. Abdominal pain may be chronic and low grade, intermittent, or absent. Heart rate and respiratory rate may be normal. Fecal output may be normal; however, cases with chronic diarrhea have been reported. Infrequently, pleural effusion, polyuria, and polydypsia have been noted.

Peritonitis can occur in the postpartum mare due to uterine perforation or uterine or intestinal bruising during foaling. The resultant peritonitis may be acute and generalized but often is low grade, diffuse or localized, and insidious in onset. Clinical signs in the latter case are vague but include depression, hypophagia, restlessness, and low-grade pain. Temperature, pulse, and respiratory rate may be normal or elevated. Vaginal or rectal examination may confirm a uterine perforation. On rectal palpation, a pain response may be elicited or fibrinous adhesions noted over the affected area of the uterus. Clinicopathological changes will reflect the degree of endotoxin absorption and systemic response.

DIAGNOSIS

Peritonitis is suspected based on a history of predisposing factors, clinical signs, and findings on physical examination. The stage of disease and the primary underlying disease process will determine the clinicopathological alterations present in the peripheral blood. Findings on rectal examination are variable. Abnormalities reported include a gritty feeling to the serosal and parietal surface of the peritoneum due to fibrin deposition, a dull, dry texture to the peritoneum, decreased fecal or dry fecal material in the intestine, pain on palpation of fibrous adhesions, mesenteric bands, or inflamed surfaces of the peritoneum, intestinal impaction or distention secondary to ileus, or an abdominal mass (abscess or neoplasia). In many cases no abnormalities can be detected on rectal examination.

In peracute or acute peritonitis with overwhelming toxemia, severe leukopenia with an absolute neutropenia and a degenerative left shift are commonly present. Protein sequestration and fluid exudation into the peritoneal cavity lead to hypoproteinemia and dehydration. An elevated packed cell volume (PCV) with a proportionate increase in total protein content may be seen early in the disease process, reflecting the degree of dehydration present. As protein loss into the abdomen continues, the PCV may increase while a normal or disproportionally low protein level is observed. Hyperfibrinogenemia may be present if the process has been ongoing for 48 hours or more.

In acute peritonitis of longer duration and in localized or chronic peritonitis, the changes in total white blood cell (WBC) count are often less dramatic. WBC counts may be normal or a neutrophilic leukocytosis may be seen. A small number of immature neutrophils, lymphopenia, lymphocytosis, or monocytosis may be present. A decrease in the albumin–globulin ratio is frequently present. A normocytic, normochromic anemia reflective of chronic disease may be observed.

Alterations in the blood chemistry parameters depend on the underlying cause of the peritonitis, organ compromise induced by toxemia, and the hydration status of the animal. In peracute and acute peritonitis, metabolic acidosis and losses of sodium, potassium, and chloride may be significant. Such alterations are uncommon in chronic peritonitis.

ABDOMINOCENTESIS

Abdominocentesis will confirm the presence of peritonitis but may not elucidate the primary pathological process. The preferred site for performing an abdominocentesis is on the midline or to the right of the midline in an area 4 to 6 inches caudad to the xiphoid process. In an obese or heavily pregnant mare it may be necessary to choose the most dependent portion of the abdomen. The left paramedian area should be avoided due to the possibility of splenic perforation.

The chosen area should be clipped and surgically scrubbed to allow better visualization of the vascular pattern on the skin and cleansing of the area. Sample contamination or development of cellulitis or a localized abscess is decreased by proper clipping and scrubbing of the area. To further decrease the possibility of contamination, sterile surgical gloves are worn. If an 18-gauge, 1½-inch disposable needle is used, no local anesthetic is required. The needle is placed through the skin with a quick movement of the hand and then slowly advanced until fluid is obtained. The needle may be rotated gently between the fingers to initiate fluid flow. In the absence of fluid, an additional needle may be placed 1 to 2 inches from the original site.

Preparation of the site for performing abdominocentesis using a blunt, 4-inch teat cannula or 6-inch female dog urinary catheter is as described above. Two to 3 ml of a local anesthetic is used to infiltrate the skin and subcutaneous tissues at the chosen site and followed by a final surgical scrub. A small incision is made through the skin and subcutaneous tissues and into the abdominal tunic or linea alba with a No. 15 scalpel blade. Sterile gauze sponges may be placed around the hub of the blunt instrument to prevent contamination of the sample from incisional bleeding. With firm, steady pressure, the blunt cannula is passed through the skin incision, subcutaneous tissue, and peritoneum. The catheter is slowly advanced until fluid is obtained. Gentle rotation or redirection of the catheter may be necessary to initiate fluid flow. If difficulty is encountered in passing the blunt instrument through the abdominal wall, the stab incision may be deepened, with care taken not to penetrate the peritoneum.

A fluid sample for cytology and total protein determination is collected in a tube containing EDTA. Samples for bacterial culture must be collected either in a sterile tube without additive, or with a culturette, or in transport media. Special biochemical tests, including electrolyte and creatinine concentration if uroperitoneum is suspected, are conducted on samples collected in a tube without additives. Once collected, the color, odor, turbidity, PCV, and protein content of the fluid can be determined rapidly. Blood-tinged fluid may be indicative of a splenic puncture, intra-abdominal or iatrogenic hemorrhage, or intestinal necrosis. A comparison of the PCV of the sample with that of the peripheral blood will help differentiate among splenic puncture, abdominal hemorrhage, and blood contamination during sample collection. Samples obtained by splenic puncture usually have a higher PCV than peripheral blood. A high number of small lymphocytes should be apparent on smears made from samples obtained after splenic puncture. Peritoneal fluid analysis associated with intraperitoneal hemorrhage commonly reveals a PCV lower than that in peripheral blood, erythrocytophagia, and few or no platelets (Table 3).

Peritoneal fluid varies in quantity, color, and character. It may be serosanguinous, turbid, flocculent, or purulent, the result of a transudate, an exudate, or modified transudate or exudate (Table 2). Normal peritoneal fluid is odorless, nonturbid, and clear to light yellow in color. Early in the inflammatory process the elevated WBC count is due primarily to an increase in polymorphonuclear cells (nondegenerative or degenerative). In chronic cases, mononuclear cells and macrophages increase in relation to the polymorphonuclear cells. Mesothelial cells may become hyperplastic and mimic neoplastic cells in chronic cases. The WBC count in acute peritonitis ($>100,000$ per mm^3) is higher than in chronic peritonitis (20,000 to 60,000 per mm^3); however, this is not always the case. Peritoneal protein levels are elevated. WBC count and protein level reflect the degree of peritoneal effusion and hydration status of the animal. Total WBC performed by automated methods may give falsely low readings if the cells within the peritoneal fluid are degenerate. Collection of only a small volume of peritoneal fluid into an EDTA tube may falsely elevate total protein values (see Table 2).

Cytological evaluation of the peritoneal fluid may reveal bacteria free or phagocytized in the leukocytes. Gram stain may be especially helpful if antimicrobial therapy has already been administered or if an anaerobic infection is present. Frequently, bacterial cultures are negative when cytological evaluation or Gram stain indicate the presence of bacteria. Failure to identify bacteria on cytological examination, however, does not rule out septic peritonitis.

Peritonitis is more difficult to diagnose after abdominal surgery because manipulation of the bowel causes an elevation in peritoneal WBC count and total protein content. Persistently high peritoneal WBC counts and protein concentrations in conjunction with systemic signs suggest peritonitis, especially if bacteria are observed within the WBCs or extracellularly in high numbers, or the WBCs appear degenerative.

Radiographs may reveal free fluid, ileus, or free gas (ruptured viscus) in the abdomen. Ab-

TABLE 2. PERITONEAL FLUID ANALYSIS

Condition	Color	Turbidity	Protein	Fibrinogen	RBC Count/μl	WBC Count/μl	WBC Type
Normal	Yellow to straw-colored	Clear	<2.5 gm/dl	<100 mg/dl, no clot	5000 ± 1000	<5000 (some sources <10,000)	Neutrophils + macrophages > mononuclear cells; ± eosinophils
Inflammation	Straw-colored to serosanguinous	Turbid	>2.5 gm/dl	>100 mg/dl ± clot	Normal or mildly elevated	5000–15,000	Acute ↑neutrophils, nontoxic; chronic ↑ macrophages, monocytes ± reactive mesothelial cells
Compromised bowel	Serosanguinous orange to red brown (late stage)	Turbid to flocculent	>2.5 gm/dl	>100 mg/dl ± clot	138,000 ± 50,000	15,000–60,000	↑Neutrophils with degenerative changes ± free or intracellular bacteria; ↑macrophages
Bowel content	Green to brown	Turbid to flocculent	>2.5 gm/dl	>100 mg/dl ± clot	Increased but variable	Above normal but total count variable	↑Neutrophils with toxic changes or degenerate neutrophils; ↑ macrophages ± bacteria ± plant material
Septic peritonitis	Serosanguinous to purulent	Turbid, opaque or flocculent	>2.5 gm/dl	>100 mg/dl ± clot	Variable	Variable—acute case often >100,000; chronic 20,000–60,000	Acute: ↑neutrophils with toxic changes or degenerate neutrophils ± bacteria Chronic: ↑macrophages, fewer degenerate or toxic neutrophils, ± reactive mesothelial cells
Neoplasia	Variable—yellow to orange-red	Clear to turbid	Variable, often ≥2.5 gm/dl	Variable ± clot	Often mildly elevated	Variable; normal to mild-moderate elevation	Similar to chronic inflammation ± degenerate neutrophils if tumor necrosis present; ± exfoliated neoplastic cells
Intra-abdominal hemorrhage, acute	Pink to red	Opaque	<Peripheral blood	Usually no clot	PCV < peripheral blood	<Peripheral blood	Morphology and distribution like peripheral blood, few platelets, ± erythrocytophagia
Chronic or previous hemorrhage	Pink to red-brown	Opaque	Variable		PCV < peripheral blood	Variable	↑Macrophages; neutrophils hypersegmented, pyknotic; no or few platelets; erythrocytophagia
Splenic tap	Red	Opaque	Similar to peripheral blood	>100 mg/dl, clot	PCV > peripheral blood	variable	↑Lymphocytes and platelets; little or no erythrocytophagia

TABLE 3. DIFFERENTIAL DIAGNOSIS OF PERITONITIS OR PERITONEAL EFFUSION

	Acute Peritonitis	← Chronic Peritonitis →	
Presenting signs:	Depression, anorexia, toxemia, ± abnormal stance, pain	Weight loss, anorexia, ± exercise intolerance	Weight loss, anorexia; chronic or intermittent abdominal discomfort ± exercise intolerance
Adult:	Salmonellosis Intestinal accident (intussusception volvulus, displacement) Septic metritis Pyelonephritis Acute pleuritis Rhabdomyositis Laminitis Potomac horse fever Nonstrangulating infarction Abdominal mass (abscess, tumor) Pancreatitis Ruptured uterine artery Abdominal trauma (blunt, perforating) Acute hepatic failure Diaphragmatic hernia	Malnutrition Parasitism Abdominal abscess Abdominal adhesions Cystitis Urolithiasis Phenylbutazone toxicosis Chronic pleuritis Chronic liver disease Neoplasia Protein-losing enteropathy Cardiac disease Histoplasmosis Gastric ulcer	Abdominal abscess Enterolithiasis Impaction (sand, ingesta foreign body) Abdominal adhesions Cholelithiasis Parasitism Chronic salmonellosis Nonstrangulating infarction Neoplasia Urolithiasis Gastric ulcer
Foal:	Ruptured bladder Septicemia Meconium impaction Gastroduodenal ulcer Acute enteritis Intestinal accident Foreign body impaction	Abdominal abscess Malnutrition Parasitism Pulmonary abscess Chronic pneumonia Neoplasia Chronic liver disease	Gastroduodenal ulcer and/or stricture Parasitism Abdominal abscess Neoplasia

dominal contrast studies may help to identify or confirm a site of leakage from the intestinal or urinary tract. Ultrasonography may show free fluid, fibrin, adhesions, or an abscess or mass in the abdomen.

THERAPY

Early and aggressive therapy is required if treatment of peritonitis is to be of benefit. In the acute phase primary consideration is given to stabilization of the animal, which includes arrest of endotoxic, septic, and hypovolemic shock; correction of metabolic and electrolyte abnormalities, dehydration, and hypoproteinemia; and management of pain. Antiendotoxin antiserum* (1.5 ml per kg) may be administered to neutralize circulating endotoxin and increase the protein concentration in hypoproteinemic horses. An alkalinizing fluid is recommended for the correction of mild to moderate metabolic acidosis. Specific electrolyte abnormalities, commonly hypokalemia and hypocalcemia, must be identified and corrected to help reestablish homeostasis and GI motility. In the absence of blood gas and electrolyte determinations, adequate volumes of a balanced electrolyte solution are required to correct hydration status and support the cardiovascular system. If total protein content is less than 4.5 gm per dl and the horse is dehydrated, administration of plasma must be considered before large volumes of fluid are given, owing to the risk of inducing pulmonary edema and further fluid loss into extravascular spaces. Surgical exploration after stabilization of the animal may be necessary to correct the primary problem, decrease peritoneal contamination, or remove a foreign body. Nonsteroidal anti-inflammatory drugs (NSAIDs) are of benefit because of their antiprostaglandin, anti-inflammatory, and analgesic effects. These agents should be used cautiously in hypovolemic, hypoproteinemic, or compromised horses, as toxicity may result. Restoration and maintenance of normal hydration will help to decrease the toxic potential of these agents. Flunixin meglumine† at reduced doses (0.25 to 0.5 mg per kg IV q. 8 h.) effectively suppresses eicosanoid production and provides mild analgesia. Relief of abdominal dis-

*Endoserum, Immvac, Columbia, MO

†Banamine, Schering Corp., Kenilworth, NJ

comfort may also improve water and food consumption. If gastric reflux is present, decompression by passage of a nasogastric tube is required and often aids in relief of pain and correction of ileus.

Administration of a mild laxative such as mineral oil or psyllium is indicated if constipation or intestinal impaction is present and gastric reflux is absent. Restoration of normal hydration will facilitate movement of water into the intestinal tract and the action of laxative agents, such as psyllium. Harsh or irritant laxatives, such as dioctyl sodium sulfosuccinate or hypertonic saline, should be avoided until the integrity of the bowel has been determined.

ANTIMICROBIALS

The mainstays of therapy in peritonitis are broad-spectrum antimicrobial agents and correction of the primary disease process. Antimicrobials are administered to control bacteremia and metastatic foci of infection, to reduce suppurative complications after bacterial contamination, and to prevent local spread of existing infection. Antimicrobial therapy should be initiated as soon as the diagnosis of peritonitis is made but after a sample of peritoneal fluid has been obtained for culture and sensitivity testing. Delay in the initiation of therapy until bacterial culture results are available will decrease the likelihood of a successful outcome. Antimicrobial therapy can later be adjusted as indicated by culture and sensitivity results. Intravenous administration of antimicrobials is preferred in hypovolemic and "shocky" animals, owing to unreliable perfusion of tissues and resultant delay in uptake and distribution following other routes of administration. Intra-abdominal infections are typically multimicrobial, involving both aerobes (*Escherichia coli, Streptococcus equi, Streptococcus zooepidemicus, Rhodococcus equi*) and anaerobes (*Bacteroides, Peptostreptococcus, Clostridium, Fusobacterium*).

Antimicrobial combinations are commonly used and have been shown to decrease mortality and abscess formation. Seventy per cent of cases of peritonitis are successfully treated with antibiotics and supportive therapy. Most antimicrobials reach more than 50 per cent of the serum level in the peritoneal fluid after systemic administration. In horses, concentrations of procaine penicillin in peritoneal fluid following intramuscular injection (22,000 IU per kg) are maintained in excess of the minimum inhibitory concentration (MIC) for *S. equi* and *S. zooepidemicus* for up to 12 hours. Gentamicin concentrations in peritoneal fluid after administration of 3.3 mg per kg exceed 4 μg per ml, thus exceeding the MIC for *E. coli* (1 to 4 μg per ml) and for *R. equi* (0.25 μg per ml) for at least 2 hours and 6 hours, respectively.

Bactericidal antimicrobials are preferred as the immune response and phagocytic cell activity may be decreased by the disease process. Aminoglycosides are effective against the majority of gram-negative aerobes but are ineffective against anaerobes. These agents, alone or in combination with NSAIDs, must be used cautiously in hypovolemic or marginally hydrated horses as drug-induced renal toxicity may develop. Although most gram-positive aerobes and anaerobes are sensitive to penicillin, *Bacteroides fragilis* is commonly resistant to penicillin and the cephalosporins. Metronidazole frequently is effective against the resistant anaerobes but is not effective against aerobes. Commonly used antibiotic combinations include penicillin or ampicillin and gentamicin; penicillin or ampicillin and amikacin; and trimethoprim–sulfadiazine and penicillin. Metronidazole (15 to 25 mg per kg q. 6–8 h., PO) is often added to these combinations for coverage against *B. fragilis*. Generally, the dosage used to treat intra-abdominal infections should be at the higher end of the recommended dosage range, at least until patient improvement is noted.

The duration of antimicrobial therapy depends on the severity of the peritonitis, primary etiology, response to therapy, and occurrence of complications. Response to therapy may be assessed by monitoring the horse's clinical status, complete blood cell (CBC) count and differential, plasma fibrinogen concentration and character of the peritoneal fluid. Improvement in vital signs, appetite, attitude, and weight gain may be noted before the clinicopathological abnormalities resolve. On this basis, therapy is often discontinued prematurely, resulting in incomplete resolution of the problem or relapse. As the peritoneal infection and inflammation resolve, the peripheral CBC, differential, and fibrinogen concentration return to their normal ranges. If previously present, toxic changes in the WBC profile disappear. Gradually the WBC count and protein concentration in the peritoneal fluid decline. Degenerative neutrophils are replaced by nondegenerative neutrophils and mononuclear phagocytic cells until a normal cell population within the peritoneal cavity is reestablished. Recognition of bacteria in the peritoneal fluid and obtaining a positive bacterial culture are often difficult following initiation of antimicrobial therapy and thus are not sensitive indicators of resolution. Generalized septic peritonitis requires 1 to 6 months of antimicrobial therapy. Longer therapy is necessary in cases complicated by cellulitis, abdominal abscess, and the development of septic foci in other organs.

ABDOMINAL DRAINAGE

Intermittent drainage of abdominal fluid through a teat cannula, female dog urinary catheter, Foley catheter, or indwelling drain is beneficial. Abdominal drainage is advocated to aid in removal of offending bacteria, toxins, and debris; to decrease adhesion formation and pain; to increase antimicrobial contact within the peritoneal surface; to foster return of intestinal motility; and to help relieve distress due to increased intra-abdominal pressure. Complications associated with use of abdominal drains or repeated abdominoparacentesis include retrograde infection; local irritation; pneumoperitoneum; subcutaneous seepage around drain and cellulitis; protein, electrolyte, and fluid volume loss; puncture of the bowel during drain placement; and plugging of the drain.

If the animal is hypovolemic and hypoproteinemic, volume replacement and administration of plasma should be considered before large quantities of fluid are removed from the abdomen. In foals and dehydrated horses, rapid removal of large quantities of abdominal fluid may precipitate a hypotensive, hypovolemic crisis. In such animals fluid volume replacement before or during abdominal drainage is required. Removal of fluid from the abdomen of a foal should be done gradually. In some foals, thoracocentesis may also be necessary to remove fluid that has accumulated in the pleural space following movement across the diaphragm. Respiratory compromise in the foal is often relieved by peritoneal drainage or thoracocentesis. Gastric ulceration and rupture should always be ruled out as a cause of peritonitis in foals. Stressed, ill foals should also be treated prophylactically for gastric ulcers (see p. 188).

PERITONEAL LAVAGE

The use of peritoneal lavage is controversial, especially in cases of localized or chronic peritonitis where there is the possibility of spreading infection. Lavage may be more beneficial in cases of generalized peritonitis in which little therapeutic response has been seen with antimicrobials, and fluid drainage. It should not, however, be used without caution or as the sole therapy. Two approaches to peritoneal lavage are commonly described: retrograde irrigation through a ventrally placed ingress–egress drain, and placement of ingress catheters in both paralumbar fossae for infusion of fluids, with placement of a drain along the ventral abdominal midline for removal of infused fluid and peritoneal exudate. Because of the anatomy and the massive amount of intestinal viscera and mesentery, effective abdominal lavage is difficult to achieve in the horse, and the efficacy of both methods has been questioned. Greater success may be achieved if peritoneal lavage is performed at the time of surgical exploration to identify and correct the underlying cause of the peritonitis.

PERITONEAL DIALYSIS

In certain instances, such as uroperitoneum or renal failure, where blood chemistry derangements are severe, peritoneal dialysis has been used successfully. Peritoneal dialysis reliably corrects electrolyte and metabolic disturbances without causing rapid electrolyte or volume changes. Dialysis catheters are best placed in a surgical setting but may be placed with sedation and local anesthetic. Although no universal protocol for peritoneal dialysis has been established in the horse, instillation of 2 liters of hypertonic dialysis solution° alternated with peritoneal drainage has proved effective in the foal. Serial electrolyte determinations should be made to monitor systemic response to dialysis.

Radical surgical debridement, open peritoneal drainage, or treatment of the peritoneal cavity as an open wound after exploration and debridement of the peritoneal cavity has been effective in treating humans and dogs with peritonitis. This procedure is less practical in horses due to their postoperative ambulatory state. A modified approach has been recommended in horses, which involves closure of the abdominal wall with stainless steel wire, leaving skin and the subcutaneous space unsutured, thus allowing peritoneal fluid to drain through the incision. The abdominal wall is bandaged to help support the abdomen and keep the wound clean.

OTHER THERAPY

Heparin given intraperitoneally, subcutaneously, or intravenously has been recommended to prevent the deposition of fibrin and to render bacteria more susceptible to cellular and noncellular clearing mechanisms. Studies on the effectiveness of heparin in preventing abdominal adhesions have yielded inconsistent results, and its use remains controversial. Neither the effectiveness of heparin in preventing abdominal adhesions nor the ideal dosage for use in the horse is known.

Treatment of ileus reduces pressure on the diaphragm, enhances respiratory efforts, venous return from abdomen, intestinal perfusion, and

---

°Dianeal, Travenol Labs., Deerfield, IL

transfer of phagocytes to the peritoneal cavity, and promotes return of appetite. Treatments may include nasogastric intubation and decompression; correction of electrolyte imbalances, especially K^+ and Ca^{++}; and removal of excess abdominal fluid and debris. Use of neostigmine, bethanecol, or metaclopromide to enhance GI motility has been recommended. The response of ileus in the horse to these pharmacological agents has been disappointing. With compromised or disturbed bowel, the possibility of inducing bowel rupture must also be considered.

Nutritional demands are increased during peritonitis owing to protein loss, an increased metabolic rate, and altered utilization of energy sources. Increased energy demands must be met through oral or parenteral supplementation with hypertonic alimentation solutions, but with caution so as not to induce laminitis.

Differentiation of septic peritonitis from abdominal disease secondary to verminous arteritis may be difficult. Peripheral blood and peritoneal fluid alterations may be similar, especially if verminous arteritis is complicated by intestinal ischemia or infarction. In horses with verminous arteritis and mild intestinal damage, the CBC count and peritoneal fluid character may be unremarkable. A peripheral eosinophilia or the presence of an increased number of eosinophils in the peritoneal fluid is suggestive of parasite-induced intestinal damage. When peritonitis secondary to verminous arteritis is suspected, larvicidal doses of anthelmintics should be administered after the horse is stabilized. Agents effective against verminous arteritis without intestinal infarction include thiabendazole (440 mg per kg for 2 consecutive days), fenbendazole (50 mg per kg for 3 consecutive days or 10 to 15 mg per kg for 5 consecutive days), and ivermectin (0.2 mg per kg).

PROGNOSIS

Prognosis depends on the severity and duration of the peritonitis, primary etiological insult, and occurrence of complications, including abdominal adhesions, abdominal abscesses, laminitis, and organ failure. Generally, if early, aggressive therapy and rapid correction of the primary lesion is achieved, prognosis is fair to good in localized and mild acute diffuse peritonitis. In chronic cases or cases complicated by severe abdominal contamination, intestinal penetration, or diarrhea, prognosis is poor.

Supplemental Readings

Bohnen, J. M. A., Matlow, A. G., Mustard, R. A., et al.: Antibiotic efficacy in intraabdominal sepsis: A clinically relevant model. Can. J. Microbiol., 34:323–326, 1988.

Dyson, S.: Review of 30 cases of peritonitis in the horse. Equine Vet. J., 15:25–30, 1983.

Hirsh, D. C., and Jang, S. S.: Antimicrobial susceptibility of bacterial pathogens from horses. Vet. Clin. North Am., 3:185–187, 1987.

Hosgood, G.: Peritonitis: Part I. A review of the pathophysiology and diagnosis. Aust. Vet. Pract., 16;184–190, 1986.

Hosgood, G.: Peritonitis: Part II. Principles of treatment. Aust. Vet. Pract., 17:3–9, 1987.

Hovda, L. R.: Abdominocentesis. In: Proceedings of the Annual Postgraduate Conference. Madison, Wis., 1987, vol. 3, pp. 33–37.

Markel, M. D.: Prevention and management of peritonitis in horses. Vet. Clin. North Am. (Equine Pract.), 4:145–156, 1988.

McIlwraith, C. W.: Equine digestive system. In Jennings, P. P. (ed.): The Practice of Large Animal Surgery, 1st ed. Philadelphia, W. B. Saunders, 1984, pp. 554–664.

Wilson, J., and Gordon, B. J.: Interpreting the diagnostic tests for colic. In Gordon, B. J., and Allen, D. (eds.): Colic Management in the Horse, 1st ed. Lenexa, Kan., Veterinary Medicine Publishing, 1988.

Acute Colitis

Michael J. Murray, LEESBURG, VIRGINIA

Colitis is inflammation of the cecum and large colon and can result in profuse diarrhea, severe fluid and electrolyte deficits, metabolic acidosis, endotoxemia, and septic shock. Several pathophysiological processes may occur simultaneously in horses with colitis, and metabolic parameters must be monitored frequently so that treatment can be directed to meet the current requirements of the patient and medication requirements can be anticipated.

PATHOGENESIS

The known causes of colitis in juvenile and adult horses are limited. Frequently the cause is not determined. The most frequently diagnosed infectious cause of diarrhea in horses is *Salmonella*. *Salmonella* is associated with several virulence factors that contribute to invasiveness, colonic fluid secretion, and local and systemic inflammatory responses. A large number of *Salmonella* serotypes have been associated with equine colitis, and overall more than 1700 serotypes of *Salmonella* have been described. *S. typhimurium*, *S. agona*, *S. krefeld*, and *S. st. paul* are serotypes frequently isolated in horses. Dozens of other serotypes are isolated sporadically. Salmonellae are ubiquitous in the environment, and from 1 to 10 per cent of asymptomatic horses tested shed *Salmonella* in the feces. Horses are not considered to be carriers, per se, of *Salmonella*, as there are apparently no host-adapted *Salmonella* species affecting the horse. Horses can shed *Salmonella* for several weeks to months and may serve as reservoirs of infection.

In acutely affected horses, large numbers of highly infective *Salmonella* bacteria can be shed in the diarrheic feces. Susceptible animals, such as young foals, hospitalized horses, and horses under stress, can be infected by doses of *Salmonella* that are 100 to 1000 times less than those required to infect immunocompetent normal horses. Thus, particular care should be taken in the management of horses and foals with diarrhea in environments in which animals are at risk—for example, in hospitals, on breeding farms, and at racetracks. Asymptomatic shedders generally pass a relatively small number of *Salmonella* bacteria in the feces and do not appear to pose an important threat to healthy horses, although asymptomatic shedders have been responsible for outbreaks of salmonellosis in hospitals and on breeding farms.

Salmonellosis typically is characterized by an acute, septic colitis resulting in profuse diarrhea. In most cases, with treatment, the severe diarrhea and associated metabolic disorders improve within 7 to 10 days of the onset of illness. Horses that have severe diarrhea and septicemia for 10 days or longer are unlikely to survive, even with intensive therapy, since these horses often have extensive loss of colonic mucosa and chronic colitis. Other clinical syndromes of salmonellosis include fever and leukopenia, colic, and proximal enteritis with gastric reflux.

A recently identified infectious agent causing acute diarrhea in the horse is *Ehrlichia risticii*, the causative agent of equine ehrlichial colitis (Potomac horse fever). This disorder is covered in another part of this section (see p. 250).

Clostridium perfringens type A has been described as a cause of peracute toxemic colitis (colitis X), but the role of this organism in the initiation of acute diarrhea in the horse has not been clearly defined. The clinical signs described for intestinal clostridiosis are similar to those of septic colitis caused by *Salmonella*, and the diagnosis has been determined based on increased fecal concentrations of *Clostridium perfringens* type A. More recently, another organism, resembling *Clostridium cadaveris*, has been implicated as the cause of experimentally induced colitis in horses and ponies. A definitive role for clostridial organisms in equine colitis remains to be determined.

Colitis has occurred secondary to the use of certain antibiotics, including oral and parenteral lincomycin and tetracycline, oral trimethoprim-sulfamethoxazole, oral erythromycin, and oral penicillin. The pathophysiology of the resulting colitis and diarrhea may involve altered volatile fatty acid synthesis, colonization and invasion of the colon by pathogenic bacteria, and the release of bacterial toxins. *Salmonella*, *Clostridium perfringens*, and *Clostridium difficile* have been implicated in such cases.

The administration of excessive dosages of nonsteroidal anti-inflammatory drugs (NSAIDs) (see p. 16) has been associated with the onset of diarrhea secondary to the development of hypoproteinemia and cecal and colonic mucosal edema. The inhibition of prostaglandin synthesis by these drugs disrupts mucosal blood flow and other mucosa-protective mechanisms in the bowel. In addition to hypoproteinemia, affected horses often have signs of severe septicemia. Horses with diarrhea and septicemia secondary to excessive administration of NSAIDs often are slow to respond to therapy, and may require a long duration of intensive care.

CLINICAL SIGNS

In many cases of colitis the etiology is not determined, even after exhaustive diagnostic procedures have been performed. However, the clinical features of colitis are similar, regardless of the cause. Most cases of equine colitis encountered by practitioners are typified by increased bowel secretion, hypoproteinemia, septicemia, and inflammation of the bowel.

A tremendous volume of fluid and electrolytes is lost through the inflamed colon, rapidly leading to severe dehydration, electrolyte disturbances, and metabolic acidosis. Several factors may contribute to active secretion, which occurs when mucosal cells are stimulated to pump fluid and electrolytes into the lumen, and passive fluid secretion, which results from increased capillary permeability and a breakdown in the ability of the colonic interstitium to counteract edema formation. Active secretory processes are generally characterized by a large volume of transmucosal fluid and electrolyte movement, with a negligible protein component in the secreted fluid. Passive secretory processes, however, usually involve alterations in the mucosal interstitium, and the secreted fluid may contain a significant amount of protein. Additionally, disruption of normal colonic function results in failure to absorb fluid and electrolytes entering the large intestine from the small bowel.

Protein exudation through the inflamed cecum and colon is common, leading to intra- and extravascular hypoproteinemia and edema formation. Additionally, in the septic, anorectic patient, plasma protein catabolism occurs. Catabolism of other proteins also occurs because of the hypermetabolic state of the septic patient. Hypoproteinemia can contribute to fluid losses, complicate therapeutic measures, and exacerbate pathological changes within the already damaged large intestine.

There is often severe inflammation of the large colon and cecum, as well as systemic manifestations of inflammation and septicemia. Within the umbrella of local and systemic inflammatory responses are a great number of mediators that produce a multitude of adverse effects. These include endotoxin, tumor necrosis factor, enterotoxin, complement, prostaglandins, leukotrienes, bradykinin, histamine, serotonin, oxygen radicals, collagenases, elastases, and many more.

Prostaglandins, leukotrienes, bradykinin, and serotonin enhance active fluid secretion; oxygen radicals and collagenases disrupt the interstitium of the lamina propria and submucosa; prostaglandins, leukotrienes, bradykinin, histamine, serotonin, and enterotoxin increase capillary perfusion and permeability; and leukotrienes and complement recruit neutrophils. Acute systemic effects occur secondary to the actions of endotoxin on macrophages and mesothelial cells, which release a multitude of mediators that affect homeostasis, coagulation factors, and the cellular arm of the immune system. Recently, tumor necrosis factor (cachexin) has been postulated to be the common macrophage-derived mediator of many of these effects.

DIAGNOSIS

The diagnostic evaluations performed on horses with diarrhea are intended to provide the veterinarian with information to accurately assess the horse's condition, and thus direct therapy toward specific requirements of the horse.

The first part of the evaluation is a thorough physical examination, with particular attention paid to (1) the horse's hydration status as judged from skin turgor, gum moisture, and capillary refill time; (2) evidence of septicemia, such as injected mucous membranes, mucous membrane color, and capillary refill time; (3) cardiovascular function, indicated by heart rate and rhythm, the character of the peripheral pulse, and capillary refill time; and (4) signs of laminitis such as lameness, digital pulse, and heat in the hoof walls. Horses with colitis often are moderately to severely dehydrated, with either purplish or brick-red mucous membranes. Purple mucous membranes reflect venous congestion and poor venous return, while a brick-red color reflects arteriole–venule shunting and poor tissue oxygen exchange.

Laboratory tests should include a complete blood cell count with white blood cell (WBC) differential count and morphology to assess the severity of toxemia, measurement of plasma protein and total solids to assess the horse's hydration status or protein loss, and measurement of fibrinogen to assess the severity of inflammation. The total WBC and neutrophil counts initially decrease in most cases of acute colitis regardless of the etiology.

The morphology of the WBCs reflects the severity of the inflammatory response and the degree of sepsis. "Toxic" changes, such as basophilia, granulation, and vacuolation of the cytoplasm and scalloped borders of the cell membrane, do not reflect injury to the neutrophils by toxins but reflect the cells' response to antigenic stimulation and the production of chemicals that are toxic to bacteria. The magnitude of these changes in circulating neutrophils reflects the severity of sepsis. Often the initial sign of the horse's recovery is an improvement in the toxic appearance to the neutrophils. The continued presence of neutrophils with a scalloped cell membrane adherent to red blood cells, cytoplasmic vacuolation, granulation, and basophilia for more than 10 days is indicative of chronic colitis that is unlikely to resolve.

Serum chemistry tests should include measurement of electrolytes (sodium, chloride, potassium, and calcium), blood urea nitrogen (BUN), and creatinine. Acid–base status is assessed by measurement of blood pH and either bicarbonate or total CO_2. Horses with diarrhea typically are hyponatremic, hypochloremic, and hypokalemic. With inappetence, hypocalcemia occurs. The severity of these electrolyte disturbances should be monitored, often daily, so that appropriate therapy may be undertaken. Parameters that assess renal function, BUN and creatinine, are frequently increased for several reasons. Prerenal azotemia due to dehydration and decreased glomerular filtration accounts for some of the increase. Horses that are adequately hydrated yet moderately hyponatremic (serum sodium 120 to 128 mEq per liter) may remain azotemic because of a decrease in glomerular filtration rate. Correction of hyponatremia in such cases corrects the azotemia. Azotemia may also reflect tubular dysfunction secondary to endotoxemia and septicemia. Urinalysis may reveal glucosuria and an increased γ-glutamyl transferase–creatinine ratio due to proximal tubular cell damage, and a specific gravity disproportionately low for the degree of dehydration present.

The acid–base status can be evaluated by estimating serum bicarbonate from the serum total CO_2, or directly from a venous or arterial blood gas analysis. Low pH, decreased HCO_3^-, and a reduced total CO_2 indicate metabolic acidosis. A venous oxygen partial pressure greater than 60 mm Hg indicates poor capillary perfusion and oxygen delivery to the tissues. Such horses usually have brick-red mucous membranes.

At least five fecal cultures for *Salmonella* should be performed on all horses with diarrhea to enhance the chances of isolating *Salmonella*. Samples with little solid matter often yield negative culture results, even when the horse is infected. Formed fecal samples are more likely to result in a positive culture from infected horses. Five to ten grams of feces should be submitted in selective media such as tetrathionate or selenite broth, and brilliant green or *Salmonella-Shigella* agar. Culture of a rectal mucosal biopsy specimen can identify some positive *Salmonella* cases that are negative on fecal culture.

In areas where equine ehrlichial colitis (Potomac horse fever) occurs, paired acute and convalescent blood samples should be submitted for indirect fluorescent antibody (IFA) testing for antibodies to *Ehrlichia risticii*. This is the current recommended test, although more sensitive tests, such as an enzyme-linked immunosorbent assay for serum antibody levels or DNA replication assays that detect ehrlichial antigen in blood, may be available for evaluation of clinical samples in the future (see p. 251).

THERAPY

Because the pathophysiology of equine colitis is complex, treatment often incorporates several medications. Many treatments provide well-documented benefit, while the efficacy of others is based on empirical judgment. In many cases the outcome is determined by a complication of colitis, and not by the colitis itself.

Fluid Therapy

Fluid administration is the treatment of primary importance and most cases will require intravenous (IV) administration in the early stages of colitis. With several commercially available IV fluid products that are sterile and packaged in volumes suitable for use in adult horses, IV fluid administration in the field is becoming more common. The fluids used must replace water, sodium, chloride, and potassium losses. Often, large volumes are required for several days.

Fluid requirements are based on the horse's fluid and electrolyte deficits and its anticipated losses. Parameters for estimating the degree of dehydration are listed in Table 1. Horses with ongoing protein losses may present with "normal" plasma protein levels when severely dehydrated. Hematocrit and physical examination findings are most useful for determining hydration status in such horses. For a 500-kg (1100-lb) horse that is 8 per cent dehydrated, 40 liters of fluid are required to correct dehydration, and maintenance fluid requirements may be as great as 120 ml per kg per day, or 60 liters in a 500-kg horse.

In a severely dehydrated horse (packed cell volume [PCV] >65 per cent, dry gums, tachycardia, poor skin turgor) fluids can be adminis-

TABLE 1. CLINICAL PARAMETERS FOR ASSESSING HYDRATION

Parameter	Degree of Dehydration		
	Mild (4%–6%)	*Moderate (7%–9%)*	*Severe (>9%)*
Skin turgor	Good to fair	Fair	Poor
Gum moisture	Good to fair	Sticky	Dry
Capillary refill time, sec	1–2	2–4	>4
Packed cell volume, %*	40–50	50–65	>65
Total protein, gm/dl†	6.5–7.5	7.5–8.5	>8.5

*Normal PCV is dependent on breed and level of athletic training. For example, Thoroughbred and Standardbred horses in training may have a normal PCV up to 45 per cent, whereas inactive horses will have a normal PCV of 32 to 38 per cent. Normal PCV of draft breeds is 25 to 30 per cent.

†In horses with significant enteric protein losses and dehydration, total plasma protein may be similar to normal values, even in severely dehydrated horses.

TABLE 2. INTRAVENOUS FLUID DELIVERY

Selection	Advantage	Disadvantage
Catheter		
Polypropylene: 10 or 12 ga.	Large volumes administered rapidly	Thrombophlebitis
Teflon: 14 or 16 ga.	Moderate volumes	Thrombophlebitis, kinks in catheter
Silicon elastomere: 16 ga.	Minimal thrombophlebitis, long-term placement	Limited rate of administration
Polyurethane: 16 ga.		
Vein		
Jugular	Ease of catheterization, ease of maintenance, ease of access	Sequellae of thrombophlebitis
Lateral thoracic	Relative ease of catheterization, relative ease of maintenance and access, minimal sequellae of thrombophlebitis	Usually restricted to 14 and 16 ga. catheters
Saphenous		Relative difficulty placing and maintaining catheter

tered IV at a rate of approximately 1 liter per minute, using two 5-liter bags of fluids administered simultaneously through a two-lead arthroscopic irrigation set, with 10-gauge catheters in place in each jugular vein.

The use of hypertonic saline in the treatment of severe hypovolemic shock has recently been advocated. Normal saline solution is 0.9 per cent (900 mg per 100 ml) sodium chloride, while hypertonic solutions are 7 to 8 per cent (7000 to 8000 mg per 100 ml) solidum chloride. Hypertonic saline has been reported to be of benefit in treatment of acute hemorrhagic shock and in a model of equine endotoxemia. Administration of 1 to 2 liters of hypertonic saline results in improved systemic blood pressure and cardiac output, and buys time until adequate fluid replacement can be administered. The mechanism of action is not completely understood but is not an osmotic effect whereby fluid is drawn into the vasculature. The effect appears to be vagally mediated and requires passage of the solution through the lungs. Hypertonic saline solution administration to horses has not been thoroughly evaluated in clinical settings, and thus specific indications and possible contraindications for its use remain to be determined.

The choice of IV catheter system and vein for fluid and medication delivery depends on several factors, including the volume, rate, and type of fluid to be administered, the potential for coagulopathies and venous thrombosis, and the duration of IV catheterization required (Table 2). Polypropylene catheters° are available in sizes (10 or 12 gauge) that permit rapid administration of large volumes of fluid, but are thrombogenic and unsuitable for long-term catheterization in colitis cases. Teflon catheters† (14 or 16 gauge) are less thrombogenic but can cause jugular thrombosis in septic patients. These catheters also are prone to kinking and cracking with continuous use. Silicone elastomer‡ and polyurethane§ catheters are the least thrombogenic and because they are quite flexible do not readily form permanent kinks. However, to date the largest size available is 16 gauge, limiting the rate of fluid administration. These latter catheters are most appropriate for long-term use in horses with colitis, and can be maintained in the jugular veins of septic patients, usually with minimal complications. Catheterization of the lateral thoracic vein is often preferable to the jugular vein, because thrombosis of the jugular vein can result in severe swelling of the head.

As horses begin to recover, they often will consume fluids orally, and frequently they will select solutions that contain electrolytes in which they are deficient. For example, horses with a mild to moderate bicarbonate deficit often will selectively consume water with added bicarbonate. Hypokalemic horses may prefer solutions containing potassium. Offering horses a variety of solutions for oral consumption allows the animal to select based on its requirements. We offer buckets containing water, water with baking soda (5 to 10 gm of baking soda per liter), water with potassium chloride (3 to 6 gm of "lite salt" per liter), and water containing a commercial balanced oral electrolyte replacement.

PLASMA THERAPY

Most horses with colitis become hypoproteinemic and may require plasma, because hypoproteinemia can compromise the clinician's ability to rehydrate the patient through fluid administration. Albumin is the principal plasma protein

---

°Medicut, Argyle, St. Louis, MO
†Abbott Cath-T, Abbott Labs., North Chicago, IL
‡Centrasil, Travenol Labs, Deerfield, IL
§L-Cath, Lutner Medical Products, Santa Ana, CA

that regulates plasma oncotic pressure. With colitis, albumin typically decreases to less than 2.0 gm per dl. Such horses will require 5 to 10 liters of plasma containing 3.0 gm of albumin per dl to significantly increase the plasma albumin concentration toward normal. Further plasma transfusions may be required if protein losses continue. Plasma also contains fibronectin, protease inhibitors, complement inhibitors, antithrombin III, and other inhibitors of hypercoagulability, and thus may be of benefit beyond improvement of plasma oncotic pressure. With the price of a 900-ml bag of commercial plasma ranging from $70 to $105, the cost of effective plasma therapy in adult horses is often prohibitive.

NUTRITIONAL THERAPY

The nutritional needs of the septic colitis patient were underemphasized in the past. Affected horses are frequently anorectic, and the disruption of normal physiological processes in the inflamed cecum and colon limits the effectiveness of these organs in the digestion and absorption of nutrients. Several mediators of inflammation and septicemia alter protein and calorie metabolism, resulting in a catabolic state. Thus, even if the horse eats, it is likely to be in a severe caloric deficit for some time. Normally, an average horse requires 10,000 to 15,000 kcal per day. A septic horse may require 25,000 kcal per day. In a catabolic patient, muscle and fat tissue are mobilized and used in lieu of ingested nutrients. The plasma protein pool, including albumin and immunoglobulins, also is catabolized. In many cases of colitis, the decrease in plasma protein may be due as much to catabolism as to leakage through the inflamed colon.

The nutritional requirements of the septic horse with colitis may be supplemented enterally or parenterally. The nutrients in these supplementations must be digestible and absorbable within the small intestine, since the inflamed colon has diminished ability to digest or absorb nutrients. Calories, digestible protein, fat, electrolytes, and vitamins should be provided (see p. 724). In most cases, the volume of a feed gruel that can be administered through a nasogastric tube to an anorectic horse is insufficient to supply the horse's nutritional needs. Commercial products are available for enteral nutritional supplementation of humans, but they need to be evaluated in the context of colitis and other disorders in horses.

Parenterally administered solutions containing glucose, balanced amino acid solutions, lipid emulsions, balanced electrolyte and trace minerals, and vitamins have been administered to adult horses with colitis. Based on a small number of cases, this therapy appears promising in terms of minimizing protein losses and decreasing the duration of illness. Providing for part of the horse's nutritional requirements (8,000 to 12,000 kcal per day) is possible with glucose–amino acid solutions that are of moderate cost (see p. 732). In some cases, administration of parenteral nutrition obviates the need for plasma transfusion. Thus, the overall cost of providing nutritional supplementation, enteral or parenteral, to horses with colitis may well be offset by quicker recoveries and diminished requirement for other costly treatments.

ENDOTOXIN ANTISERA

Because many of the clinical signs accompanying equine colitis appear to be attributable to the effects of endotoxin, the development of specific therapy to neutralize endotoxins has been a goal in the past few years. Commercially produced sera that contain antibody effective against the endotoxin produced by a variety of gram-negative organisms, including *Salmonella*, have recently become available for use in horses.[*,†] At this time the efficacy of these products in treating horses with colitis remains undetermined, but this type of therapy has a sound basis and should be considered.

ANTI-INFLAMMATORY AGENTS

The use of NSAIDs is a common practice in equine colitis patients. Flunixin meglumine[*] in particular is appropriate for treatment of equine endotoxemia because it prevents several of the pathophysiological changes induced by endotoxin.

A medication with potential anti-inflammatory benefit in colitis cases is dimethyl sulfoxide (DMSO). It scavenges hydroxyl radicals produced by metabolically activated neutrophils that have invaded the cecum and colon. The dosage is 100 to 200 mg per kg per day.

ANTIMICROBIAL THERAPY

The use of antimicrobials in the treatment of colitis is controversial. In cases of colitis caused by *Ehrlichia risticii*, tetracycline, 6.6 to 11 mg per kg (3 to 5 mg per lb) given IV twice daily is effective. In other cases of colitis, including *Salmonella* colitis in which specific antimicrobial sensitivities of the isolated organisms have been determined, the efficacy of antimicrobial administration is less well documented. Many clini-

---

[*]Polymune J, Veterinary Dynamics, Inc., Chino, CA
[†]Endoserum, Immvac, Columbia, MO
[*]Banamine, Schering Corp., Kenilworth, NJ

cians feel that the use of an antimicrobial for which the *Salmonella* has demonstrated sensitivity, such as chloramphenicol, trimethoprim-sulfa, gentamicin, amikacin, or a third-generation cephalosporin, does not significantly alter the course of the disease or hasten the elimination of the organism from the body. In septic, neutropenic patients, the use of broad-spectrum antibiotics is justified to prevent bacteremia or organ colonization by *Salmonella* and other enteric organisms.

Antisecretory Therapy

Medications that minimize or abolish colonic fluid secretion would be of tremendous benefit in the treatment of equine colitis. Medications such as kaolin, bismuth subsalicylate, and activated charcoal are frequently used, but their efficacy has not been established. These medications are more effective in foals with diarrhea, probably as a result of an effect on the small intestine rather than the colon.

Several medications that demonstrate antisecretory activity have been examined in non-equine species; these medications include NSAIDs, narcotic agonists, α_2-adrenergic agonists, and drugs that affect cellular calcium metabolism. The antisecretory effects of these drugs have been demonstrated more for the small intestine than the colon, and thus the clinical effectiveness of any of these agents in horses with colitis remains undetermined. Phenoxybenzamine, an α_1-adrenergic antagonist, has been used effectively in selected cases of equine colitis. However, the drug can cause severe hypotension.

PROGNOSIS

The prognosis for horses with acute colitis that receive appropriate fluids, electrolytes, and other supportive treatment is good, with the majority surviving without complications. The most frequent complications that occur are catheter site infection, thrombophlebitis, and laminitis. Horses that recover will usually show signs of improvement within 7 days of the onset of illness, and in the author's experience, invariably by 10 days. Horses that remain septic and have diarrhea for more than 10 days generally have a poor prognosis for survival.

Supplemental Readings

Allen, D., Kvietys, P. R., Granger, N.: Crystalloids versus colloids: Implications in fluid therapy of dogs with intestinal obstruction. Am. J. Vet. Res., 47:1751–1755, 1986.
Bertone, J. J.: Intravenous hypertonic saline solution and endotoxemia in horses. Proceedings of the 7th Annual Meeting of the American College of Veterinary Internal Medicine, 1989, pp. 476–479.
Carter, J. D., Hird, D. W., Farver, T. B., Hjerpe, C. A.: Salmonellosis in hospitalized horses: Seasonality and case fatality rates. J. Am. Vet. Med. Assoc., 188:163–167, 1986.
Ewert, K. M., Fessler, J. F., Templeton, C. B., et al.: Endotoxin-induced hematologic and blood chemical changes in ponies: Effects of flunixin meglumine, dexamethasone, and prednisolone. Am. J. Vet. Res., 46:24–30, 1985.
Kemp, D. T.: A comprehensive guide to intravenous fluid therapy in horses. Vet. Med., 83:193–212, 1988.
Prescott, J. F., Staempfli, H. R., Barker, I. K., Bottoms, G. D., Latshaw, H. S., Johnson, M. A.: A method of reproducing fatal idiopathic colitis (colitis X) in ponies and isolation of a *Clostridium* as a possible agent. Equine Vet. J., 20:417–420, 1988.
Spier, S. J., Lavoie J.-P., Cullor, J. S., Smith, B. P., Snyder, J. R., Sischo, W. M.: Protection against clinical endotoxemia in horses by using plasma containing antibody to an Rc mutant *E. coli* (J5). Circ. Shock, 28:235–248, 1989.

Potomac Horse Fever
Jonathan E. Palmer, KENNETT SQUARE, PENNSYLVANIA

Potamac horse fever is an ehrlichial typhlocolitis caused by *Ehrlichia risticii*. It is enzootic in many regions of the United States and Canada and has been reported in Europe. Although the disease appears to be more prevalent near large waterways, it is found in a variety of climatic settings. Horses under all management schemes are at risk. The disease occurs in two epidemiological patterns. In the most common pattern, horses may be affected anywhere within the enzootic area independent of local population densities.

Thus, most farms only experience one or two cases. Cases occur in isolated horses away from the major traffic patterns on the farm. Because cases are not clustered in areas of horse concentration, the disease is as likely to occur in pastured horses as it is in stabled horses. If more than one case occurs on a farm, the second and subsequent cases are likely to occur in horses grazed on different pastures or housed in different stables from the first. In the second epidemiological pattern, cases cluster on a farm or racetrack. A high percentage of horses on the farm may be affected, or the outbreak may be clustered in one area such as a certain group of barns on a racetrack. When tested, even asymptomatic horses have high antibody titers, indicating past subclinical infection. New horses introduced to the farm are at high risk of developing disease.

The disease is seasonal, occurring from late spring until early fall. The vast majority of cases occur in July, August, and September and can be clustered in time. Although cases may sporadically occur in the early summer, there may be a sudden onslaught of cases throughout the enzootic area with the onset of hot weather.

The method of transmission is unclear. Epidemiological evidence and controlled studies indicate that direct contact is not important in transmission. Vectors including blood-sucking arthropods such as ticks have been sought but none have been implicated. Oral transmission can occur, but direct horse-to-horse transmission does not occur. With oral transmission possible, and since *Ehrlichia* is shed in horse feces, transmission may involve a coprophagic insect. Horses may be a dead-end host, or concentration within a vector may be involved.

A reservoir for the causative *Ehrlichia* has not been identified. Recovered horses do not retain the organism in their blood or other tissues, although the possibility of an enteric carrier state has not been ruled out. Once Potomac horse fever has occurred in an area, recurrence in subsequent years is likely. The recurrence is independent of the horse population. Thus, even if an enzootic farm is depopulated for a year or more, Potomac horse fever is likely to recur with the introduction of new horses.

CLINICAL SIGNS

The clinical signs produced by *Ehrlichia risticii* infection vary greatly among individuals. The mildest and most common form of disease results in depression, partial to complete anorexia, and decreased borborygmi. Other horses may have a fever between 102° and 107° F (39° to 43° C) accompanying these signs. The fever is biphasic, but the initial fever spike is often missed since it occurs several days before other signs and may last only a few hours. Some affected horses develop diarrhea. The diarrhea is often low volume, cowlike in consistency, and short-lived (1 to 3 days). In other cases the diarrhea can be high volume, dehydrating, and watery. Watery diarrhea may be transient or may continue for 5 to 7 days. Colic may also occur. Most often the colic is mild, but occasionally horses with diarrhea will stop passing feces, develop complete ileus, and show signs of severe endotoxemia and profound depression or severe colic. These horses often die within hours.

The frequency with which laminitis develops varies between enzootic areas and years. It may be a rare clinical manifestation or it may be almost universally present. It may be mild and transient or severe and life-threatening. Laminitis may be an early sign, may occur during the acute stage of the disease, or may occur during convalescence.

In utero infection can occur. The only well-documented case occurred in a mare with experimentally induced disease when she was three months pregnant. There was no indication of disease in the fetus when the organism was isolated four months later. Antibodies have been detected in fetal blood after abortion, but the role of *E. risticii* in these abortions is unclear.

There are no unique laboratory findings in horses with Potomac horse fever. A mild to extreme leukopenia with neutropenia and lymphopenia may occur early in the disease. This may be followed by a leukocytosis that can range up to 30,000 cells per μl (an unusual finding in other enteric diseases). If the horse develops diarrhea, chemistry abnormalities typical of acute diarrhea will occur.

DIAGNOSIS

The diagnosis of Potomac horse fever cannot be based on clinical signs alone, because the clinical picture is not unique. A working diagnosis may be made when a horse develops typical clinical signs in a known endemic area. Confirmation of the working diagnosis is usually attempted with serology studies, but because of the typical serological response, only about one half of cases can be definitively diagnosed by this means. The diagnosis in the other half remains uncertain.

The most commonly used serological test is an indirect fluorescent antibody test. This test is plagued by nonspecific binding of sera, leading to false positive results, and poor antigen preparations, leading to false negative results. The experience of the laboratory personnel and the use of proper controls correlate with the accuracy of the results.

Even when the serological results are accurate, the test is often not diagnostic. Most horses develop antibody titers at the time signs are evident or even before clinical disease is noted. Titers are present within a day of development of signs and reach a peak within a week or less. Titers may then drop slightly or plateau. Titers may have already reached their plateau when the clinician is first asked to examine the animal. Thus, for serology to be diagnostic, the initial sample must be taken at the onset of signs and a second sample must be obtained for comparison (but can be drawn within a week of the first). A fourfold or greater increase or decrease in titer is diagnostic. Horses with Potomac horse fever almost always have titers of 1:160 or greater. Yet despite care in sampling time, approximately 50 per cent of horses with acute disease will have paired titers within 1 dilution of each other. Serologically, these cases cannot be distinguished from horses with past exposure that maintain titers over 1:5120 for more than a year. If a horse has had signs of disease for 4 or 5 days and has a negative titer, it is highly unlikely that it has Potomac horse fever. Use of oxytetracycline does not change the antibody response, but vaccination may further confuse the picture. Vaccination usually produces low to moderately high titers that wane in 6 to 9 months. Horses that develop Potomac horse fever after vaccination may have a tremendous anamnestic response with titers rising above 1:100,000 despite lack of protection from disease.

Although serology is often used as a diagnostic aid, it is more important as an epidemiological tool, identifying endemic areas. Practical diagnosis aimed at directing therapy is often based on identifying typical signs in a horse living in an endemic area. Serology remains a valuable tool in retrospective confirmation of the diagnosis but, being retrospective, can play little role in directing rational therapy.

THERAPY

Clinical signs present in individual cases dictate the degree of therapeutic intervention. Mild transient cases characterized by fever, depression, and anorexia may require only symptomatic analgesic or antipyretic therapy. Other cases with more severe disease, colic, ileus, diarrhea, or laminitis may require intensive therapy.

Ehrlichia risticii is very sensitive to the tetracycline antimicrobials. The antimicrobial of choice for Potomac horse fever is intravenous oxytetracycline at 6.6 mg per kg s.i.d. Once daily dosage is sufficient because of the high sensitivity of the pathogen to the drug. Response to therapy is often dramatic, with resolution of fever, improvement in attitude, and return of appetite within 12 hours of the first dose. Established enteritis may not improve as rapidly, and the course of laminitis may be independent of the therapy. If clinical recovery is complete after 5 days of therapy, the oxytetracycline may be stopped. Occasionally there are relapses requiring longer therapy for a total of 10 to 14 days. Because of the biology of the pathogen, resistance to the drug is highly unlikely. If the disease recurs, a second course of the antimicrobial should be as effective as the first. If improvement is not noted after initiation of therapy, reassessment of the diagnosis is in order. Although oxytetracycline therapy has been associated with adverse reactions, such as fatal enteritis, the benefits of the therapy far outweigh the risks in the treatment of Potomac horse fever. The dilemma facing the practitioner is the diagnosis, which, in the absence of a rapid diagnostic aid, is based on an educated guess.

If signs of acute enterocolitis are present, aggressive fluid therapy is of utmost importance. Although the diarrhea may be low volume and transient, dehydration and electrolyte imbalances may be severe. As in other diarrheal diseases, the horse is hyponatremic, hypochloremic, hypokalemic, and has a metabolic acidosis with azotemia, all of which should be treated accordingly (see p. 18).

PREVENTION

Once Potomac horse fever has occurred in an area it is likely to recur in future years. Even if a farm is depopulated for a period, when new horses are placed on the farm recurrence is likely. Attempts at insect control on the farm or in individual horses has not resulted in prevention of disease. Isolation of affected and recovered individuals is not rational because of lack of direct transmission, yet if other contagious enteric diseases are among the differential diagnoses, isolation may be wise. Without an understanding of the mode of transmission a rational plan to block transmission is impossible.

Resistance to reinfection after recovery from natural disease is solid and lasts 2 years or more. Killed bacterins have been developed, but the protection is incomplete and short-lived. At best, 80 per cent of vaccinates are protected from most clinical signs. Because of the short duration of protection, revaccination every 4 months may be needed to ensure a reasonable likelihood of protection. Because of the delay between vaccination and the development of immunity, vaccination during an outbreak is of little value. The use of prophylactic oxytetracycline during an outbreak is not recommended since it will only prolong the incubation period and may interfere with the host's response to the disease.

Supplemental Readings

Meinersmann, R. J., Palmer, J. E., Bullis, J. A., Ganser, R. D., Benson, C. E., and Whitlock, R. H.: Serology for diagnosis of equine ehrlichial colitis. In: Proceeedings of a Symposium on Potomac Horse Fever. Louisville, KY, Veterinary Learning Systems Co., 1988, pp. 33–36.

Palmer, J. E.: Prevention of Potomac horse fever. Cornell Vet., 79:201–205, 1989.

Palmer, J. E., Benson, C. E., and Lotz, G. W.: Serologic response of experimental ponies orally infected with *Ehrlichia risticii*. Equine Vet. J. Suppl., 7:19, 1989.

Palmer, J. E., Benson, C. E., and Whitlock, R. H.: Resistance to development of equine ehrlichial colitis in experimentally inoculated horses and ponies. Am. J. Vet. Res., 51:763, 1990.

Palmer, J. E., Whitlock, R. H., and Benson, C. E.: Clinical signs and treatment of equine ehrlichial colitis. In: Proceedings of a Symposium on Potomac Horse Fever. Louisville, KY, Veterinary Learning Systems Co., 1988, pp. 49–54.

Hepatic Disease

Thomas J. Divers, ITHACA, NEW YORK

Hepatic disease occurs frequently in horses, but the liver has a large functional reserve, and 60 per cent or more of normal liver function must be lost before clinical signs of hepatic failure occur. Only horses with obstruction of the biliary system or extensive hepatic parenchymal disease exhibit clinical signs of hepatic failure.

Equine hepatic diseases can be divided into three groups based on the frequency with which they cause hepatic failure: (1) hepatic disease that rarely, if ever, progresses to hepatic failure, (2) hepatic diseases that only sporadically cause hepatic failure, and (3) hepatic diseases that frequently cause hepatic failure.

ETIOLOGY

An elevation in serum hepatic enzyme levels is often found in association with multisystemic diseases or mild hepatotoxic insults. These conditions rarely progress to liver failure, and the clinical signs almost certainly result from disease in another organ system.

A number of hepatic diseases may sporadically progress to hepatic failure, including aflatoxicosis, leukoencephalomalacia (moldy corn poisoning, see p. 369), alsike clover or klein grass poisoning, portal vein thrombosis, obstruction of the bile duct, pancreatic disease, duodenal ulceration, displacement of the large colon, hepatic abscessation, hepatic neoplasia, perinatal herpes I infections, portocaval shunts, and congenital biliary atresia. Serum hepatic enzyme levels may be elevated in any of these diseases and the clinical signs could result from hepatic dysfunction.

Acute hepatic failure has been reported in horses that are fed mycotoxin-contaminated corn (see p. 369). Aflatoxin is the mycotoxin most likely to produce hepatic failure in the horse. In some parts of the world, horses grazing on alsike clover or klein grass may sporadically develop hepatic failure. Portal vein thrombosis and hepatic failure as part of a generalized thrombotic crisis have also been seen in a foal grazing on fescue pasture.

Primary pancreatic diseases such as eosinophilic inflammation or granulomatous or neoplastic processes can cause secondary hepatic failure by obstruction of the bile ducts with subsequent hepatic fibrosis in adult horses.

Hepatic diseases caused by neoplasia or abscess are sporadic and unique in that clinical signs may occur without extensive hepatic involvement. Three tumors cause hepatic parenchymal destruction or bile occlusion (or both) and result in hepatic failure: (1) hepatocellular carcinomas, which occur more frequently in yearlings and young adults; (2) biliary carcinomas, which are more common in older horses; and (3) a rare diffuse hepatic lymphosarcoma. Hepatic abscessation is most commonly caused by clostridial or enteric pathogens. Clostridial infections are often associated with infarction of a portion of the liver.

Biliary obstruction secondary to gastrointestinal (GI) disease may sporadically cause hepatic failure. Two horses have been observed in which displacement of the large colon obstructed the biliary system. Both horses had colic for periods of 1 to 3 days, severe icterus, high serum concentrations of direct bilirubin greater than 5.0 mg per dl, and elevated biliary enzyme levels. Enzyme levels quickly returned to normal after surgical correction of the displaced colon. Foals with duodenal ulceration can develop cicatrix of the duodenum, which may then obstruct the common bile duct.

Congenital diseases of the liver only occasionally cause liver failure in foals. Foals infected in utero with herpesvirus type I may be born with severe hepatic necrosis and may develop signs of hepatic failure if the animals survive for a day or more. Congenital biliary atresia was reported to cause hepatic failure in one foal. Congenital portovenous shunts should also be considered in young foals that develop neurological signs when dietary protein consumption is increased.

Only a few diseases of the equine liver frequently cause hepatic failure. One of the most common in the adult horse is Theiler's disease, an acute to subacute hepatitis of unknown etiology. Outbreaks of the disease occur frequently in the autumn in the northwestern United States, affecting one to several horses on a farm over a 2- to 3-month period. Because Theiler's disease has been associated with administration of a biological of equine origin, it is also called serum hepatitis. Although equine-origin biologicals are rarely used in adult horses, Theiler's disease remains a frequent cause of hepatic failure. Its association with serum administration, multiple affected horses on some farms, and the apparent seasonal incidence suggest an infectious blood-borne etiological agent. Although the liver lesions seen in Theiler's disease suggest that the disease has been present for a few days, the clinical onset is usually peracute. The course of the disease is rapid, with most horses either succumbing to the disease or recovering within 5 to 7 days. A few horses have malaise and fluctuating hepatic enzyme levels for several weeks or months. Other horses on affected farms may develop subclinical hepatic disease.

In certain areas of the world, the ingestion of plants containing pyrrolizine alkaloids, for example *Amsinckia*, *Senecio*, or *Crotolaria* spp., is the most common cause of hepatic failure. Consumption most commonly occurs through contaminated hay, especially spring-cut alfalfa and alfalfa cubes. The liver damage associated with pyrrolizidine alkaloid ingestion is often acute, occurring within a 6-month period after ingestion of the toxic plant. In a few cases there may be signs of chronic disease such as weight loss.

Cholelithiasis, the most frequent cause of obstructive hepatic failure in adult horses, is discussed on p. 259.

Tyzzer's disease, caused by *Bacillus piliformis*, is a highly fatal acute hepatitis and septicemia that occurs in foals 9 to 42 days of age. Some affected foals die peracutely of septicemia; others are depressed and severely hypoglycemic. If affected foals live for 24 hours, icterus and neurological signs become pronounced.

Hepatic failure occurred in several newborn foals in the United States in 1982 and 1983 as a result of oral administration of a microorganism inoculum containing the toxic agent ferrous fumarate. This syndrome has not been seen since the product was withdrawn.

Hyperlipemia and subsequent hepatic failure is most common in ponies and rare in warm-blooded horses. An acute onset of hepatic failure may be triggered by late pregnancy, lactation, or other stresses that cause rapid mobilization of free fatty acids from adipose tissue. In some cases, fatty infiltration makes the liver so friable that hepatic rupture occurs.

Chronic active hepatitis is the pathological diagnosis in several horses with hepatic failure. While no single cause is known, some cases may result from chronic cholangiohepatitis of predominantly periportal areas. A pony recovering from Theiler's disease also developed microscopic lesions classified as chronic active hepatitis. Hepatic cirrhosis occurs occasionally from one of the aforementioned causes or other toxic insults.

CLINICAL SIGNS

Except for liver abscess or neoplasia, equine hepatic disease without failure causes few clinical signs. If liver disease is secondary to disease of another organ system, clinical signs are associated with the primary disease site, for example, duodenal strictures that cause biliary obstruction.

Clinical signs resulting from hepatic failure usually involve the central nervous system. Depression, head pressing, uncontrolled circling, compulsive walking, seizure, and coma are the most common neurological signs. Ataxia and excessive yawning may be among the earliest clinical signs of hepatoencephalopathy, which is a result of increased blood ammonia, hypoglycemia, imbalance of the ratio of serum aromatic to branched-chain amino acids, or increases in other false neurotransmitters.

The clinical signs in horses with hepatic failure resulting from cholelithiasis or cholangiohepatitis are described on p. 259.

Although most horses with hepatic failure have a decrease in coagulation factors, spontaneous bleeding is not a common clinical sign. Severe hemorrhage into the GI tract and severe pulmonary hemorrhage have, however, been observed in horses with hepatic fibrosis. Excessive hemorrhage from self-inflicted wounds often occurs.

Weight loss may be noted in some chronic hepatic diseases, especially pyrrolizidine alkaloid toxicosis, chronic active hepatitis, neoplasia, hepatic cirrhosis, cholangiohepatitis, cholelithiasis, and hepatic abscessation.

Photosensitization is a not uncommon finding in white horses with liver failure. It may be the first clinical sign in cases of pyrrolizidine alkaloid toxicity or biliary obstruction. Although icterus is present in most horses with hepatic failure, it may not be seen in some cases of pyrrolizidine alkaloid toxicosis or chronic fibrosis, or in peracute hepatic disease and failure. Laminitis, ventral edema, and diarrhea occur in ponies with hyperlipemia and acute hepatic failure. Diarrhea is an uncommon finding in horses with liver disease, although it may be a major clinical sign associated with portal vein thrombosis. Discolored urine, either bilirubinuria or hemoglobinuria, may be observed in some horses with hepatic failure. An acute fulminant intravascular hemolytic syndrome is occasionally seen as a terminal event in equine liver failure.

DIAGNOSIS

LIVER ENZYMES

A tentative diagnosis of hepatic disease is usually made by finding abnormally elevated serum hepatic enzyme levels. The magnitude of the elevation does not always correlate with the degree of hepatic dysfunction. Acute, focal, or mild diffuse lesions may cause marked increases in serum hepatic enzyme levels, while chronic, diffuse, and severe diseases may cause only mild elevations. A large number of hepatic enzymes may be measured in the serum. The clinician should be familiar with specificity, serum half-life, the primary site of production (hepatocellular versus biliary) of the enzymes, and the stability of the collected sample. Measurement of hepatic enzyme levels can be useful in determining the presence or absence of active hepatic disease, the primary location of the hepatic disease (i.e., biliary versus hepatocellular), and the progression of acute cases of hepatic disease.

γ-Glutamyl transferase (transamino peptidase, GGT) is the most useful screening enzyme. Elevations in serum GGT levels are generally considered to be of hepatic origin. The enzyme is produced from the biliary epithelium and has its most dramatic elevations in the serum of horses with biliary disease. Biliary hyperplasia occurs rapidly in the diseased equine liver, and the serum GGT level rises quickly even in horses with primary hepatocellular disease. It is rare for horses to show clinical signs of hepatic failure without having an elevation in GGT. GGT levels may be normal or only mildly elevated in peracute hepatocellular necrosis or chronic hepatocellular cirrhosis. GGT is thought to have a moderately long half-life ($t\frac{1}{2}$) in the serum. Stored samples are stable for 36 hours at room temperature and 30 days if frozen. Serum GGT levels may remain elevated for several months in some liver diseases, particularly pyrrolizidine alkaloid toxicosis, cholangiohepatitis, obstructive biliary disease, or chronic active hepatitis. Horses with predominantly hepatocellular disease (for example, Theiler's disease) may have increasing concentrations of GGT in the serum despite showing clinical improvement. This should not be alarming if the hepatocellular enzyme levels are decreasing and probably represents a continued secondary biliary reaction. In evaluating horses with hepatic failure early in the course of the disease, comparison of serum GGT levels and the serum concentration of a hepatocellular enzyme can be useful in predicting the primary location of the disease. Cholelithiasis, septic cholangitis, biliary fibrosis, or neoplasia should be suspected in horses with marked serum GGT elevations but only mild to moderate elevation in hepatocellular enzymes.

Many clinically normal foals have elevations of GGT two to three times normal for the first 2 weeks of life. Some young performance horses examined because of decreased performance may have a threefold to fourfold elevation in GGT levels without any other laboratory evidence of hepatic disease. It is not known if this is a result of hepatic induction of the enzyme, pancreatic disease (for example, *Strongylus edentatus* migration), or secondary biliary reaction from a prior hepatocellular insult. Most horses return to normal within 30 to 60 days.

Aspartate aminotransferase (AST, SGOT) is the most commonly measured equine hepatocellular enzyme. It is very stable in serum, routinely assayed at most laboratories, and quite sensitive to liver damage; elevations usually occur even after minor hepatic insults. Without an elevation in AST there is a low probability that a horse has *active* hepatocellular disease. AST is not liver specific, however, and increased levels may be associated with muscle disease or hemolysis.

Sorbitol dehydrogenase (SDH) is a hepatocellular specific enzyme sometimes measured in equine practice. The short $t\frac{1}{2}$ makes it very useful in monitoring improvement in hepatic disease. The major disadvantage of SDH is that the laboratory measurement is not automated and many laboratories do not perform the test. If serum is separated from the blood soon after collection, the equine enzyme is 90 per cent stable at room temperature or with refrigeration for up to 48 hours. An alternative to measuring SDH is to measure isoenzyme 5 of lactic dehydrogenase (LDH⟨5⟩). Isoenzyme 5 of LDH has a t½ similar to that of SDH and therefore can be measured to assess resolution of hepatic disease. The LDH⟨5⟩ is 90 per cent stable in the serum at room temperature for 36 hours. Although the enzyme is occasionally called liver LDH, it is not specific for the liver but is also found in muscle. Differentiation of muscle versus liver LDH⟨5⟩ can be made by concurrently measuring muscle-specific creatine phosphokinase (CPK), which has a similar half-life. If the CPK is normal and the LDH⟨5⟩ is elevated, it can be assumed that the horse has liver disease.

BILE ACIDS

An increase in serum bile acids is an extremely sensitive indicator of equine hepatic disease. Bile acids are rapidly elevated (within to 1 to 2 days) after the onset of hepatic disease, but their use as a measure of dysfunction can be difficult, because increases may occur without extensive hepatic disease. Highest serum values occur with obstructive biliary diseases and portocaval shunts. Some laboratories measure only those bile acids conjugated with glycine, and 86 per cent of equine bile acids are conjugated with taurine. The measurement of total bile acids is preferred in the horse. Total bile acid concentrations of greater than 20 μM per L are highly suggestive of hepatic disease.

Horses with hepatic failure are unable to convert ammonia to urea and may have decreased blood urea nitrogen (BUN) and increased blood ammonia concentrations. Low BUN may also be noted in horses with anorexia and cachexia. Blood ammonia levels should be determined soon after the blood has been drawn, which limits the practicality of this function test.

Hypoglycemia is not common, but blood glucose values may be low and clinical response to glucose therapy can be dramatic. Ponies with hyperlipemia syndrome have a marked elevation in plasma triglyceride levels and the plasma is usually grossly discolored (milky).

FUNCTION TESTS

Exogenously administered substances that are metabolized by the liver may be useful as hepatic function tests. The sulfobromophthalein (BSP) clearance test is useful in evaluating hepatic function in horses suspected of having extensive liver dysfunction in the absence of elevations in serum bilirubin levels and icterus. In the adult horse, 1 gm of BSP is given intravenously (IV) in one jugular vein after a preinjection blood sample has been collected. Subsequent samples are taken from the opposite jugular vein at approximately 3 minutes, 5 minutes, 7 minutes, 9 minutes, and 11 minutes. It is not critical that the samples be collected at these exact times, but it is important that the exact time the sample is collected be recorded. BSP concentration is graphed as a function of time; a t½ greater than 4.5 minutes is highly suggestive of decreased hepatic function.

OTHER TESTS

Serum bilirubin concentrations, particularly the indirect or unconjugated fraction, are above the normal range in most cases of hepatic failure in the horse. In primary cholestatic disease, 50 per cent or more of the serum bilirubin may be conjugated. Serum bilirubin levels may also be mildly or moderately elevated in horses with anorexia, but serum liver enzyme levels usually remain normal.

Bilirubinuria is observed in many cases of liver failure. The determination of bilirubinuria can be made by simple urine dipstick evaluation, or a tentative determination can be made by shaking the urine in a test tube and observing a greenish discoloration of the urine foam. Bilirubinuria without evidence of hemolysis is highly suggestive of hepatic failure.

The prothrombin time is elevated in most cases of equine liver failure. Plasma fibrinogen concentration may be abnormally low as a result of decreased production. Albumin and globulin concentrations are usually not markedly decreased, and severe hypoproteinemia is rare.

The moderate elevation in packed cell volume (PCV) is often poorly amenable to fluid therapy. A more dramatic elevation in PCV (65 to 70 per cent) has been seen in horses with hepatocellular carcinomas. Plasma bicarbonate should be measured in order to provide proper fluid therapy.

Leukograms are not very helpful except in horses with suppurative cholangitis or biliary choleliths. Elevated white blood cell counts and plasma fibrinogen levels occur in spite of the chronic hepatic disease and failure.

MICROSCOPIC EXAMINATION

Antemortem microscopic examination of the liver may provide diagnostic or prognostic information in horses with pyrrolizidine alkaloid toxicosis, Theiler's disease, cholangiohepatitis, Tyzzer's disease, and hepatic masses but will not provide a definite diagnosis for most other vascular, toxic, infectious, or obstructive conditions involving the equine liver.

Microscopic examination of the liver may be performed on formalin-fixed tissues obtained with a Tru-Cut biopsy needle* or on cytological examination of a needle aspirate. The examination of fixed tissue is usually preferred, but the more rapid (hours vs. days) cytological examination may be of diagnostic or therapeutic benefit in some diseases (for example, Theiler's disease). A 4-inch, 18-gauge needle may be used for aspiration. A sample of liver for microscopic examination can usually be obtained under field conditions by percutaneous biopsy in the right 12th intercostal space just above a line drawn from the olecranon to the tuber coxae. The risks are minimal. Although prothrombin and partial thromboplastin times are usually elevated, clinical bleeding problems associated with the biopsy are rare. If bleeding tendencies are noted prior to attempting the biopsy, 4 to 6 liters of compatible fresh plasma from a normal horse may be given prior to the biopsy. Occasionally a piece of colon or lung may be obtained inadvertently during the procedure but this rarely causes a clinical problem. If colonic ingesta is noted on the biopsy instrument, antimicrobial therapy should be started.

ULTRASONOGRAPHY

Ultrasonography is a valuable noninvasive method of evaluating the hepatic parenchyma and selecting a site for biopsy. The liver can be imaged on the right side of the abdomen along the entire ventral lung field from the 6th to 15th intercostal spaces in young horses. In older horses with atrophy of the right liver lobe or in horses with decreased hepatic mass caused by Theiler's disease or cirrhosis, imaging of the liver on the right is difficult. However, the left portion of the liver can still be imaged from the 7th to 9th intercostal spaces ventral to the lung margin. A 3.0- or 5.0-MHz sector or linear scanner can be used to image the liver. The 5.0-MHz transducer improves resolution but provides less tissue penetration than the 3.0-MHz transducer.

The scan should be performed in the intercostal spaces after the hair has been clipped, the skin cleaned, and an ultrasound coupling gel applied. The liver should be scanned in at least two mutually perpendicular planes. The portal and hepatic vessels can be imaged coursing through the hepatic parenchyma (Fig. 1). The walls of the portal veins are more echogenic than the hepatic veins. The hepatic veins are often anechoic, and blood can be seen flowing toward the caudal vena cava, which usually cannot be imaged suc-

*Travenol Labs., Deerfield, IL

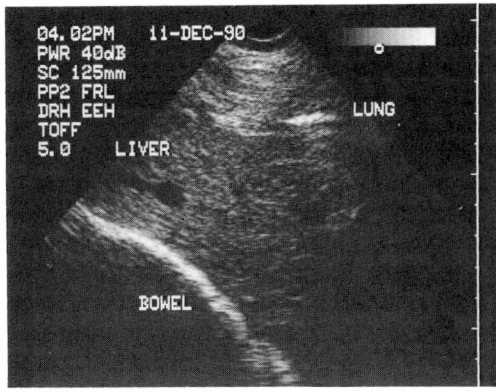

Figure 1. Ultrasonogram of the liver of a normal horse. The liver has a relatively uniform density, with anechoic areas representing blood vessels coursing through the liver parenchyma.

cessfully in the adult. The bile ducts are very small in the normal liver and have echogenic walls. The bile ducts are often not visible in the normal horse.

The detection of distended bile ducts with hepatomegaly suggests obstructive liver disease. Choleliths can be visualized within the biliary tree as echogenic masses, often casting an acoustic shadow (Fig. 2). Sonolucent choleliths have also been reported in the horse and contained bilirubin. The hepatic parenchyma in these horses is usually more echogenic than normal as a result of chronic hepatic fibrosis. Distention of the bile ducts has been seen with biliary obstruction in foals with duodenal ulceration. Thickening of the bile ducts and increased echogenicity of the bile and surrounding structures has been seen with suppurative cholangitis in a foal.

A widespread, relatively uniform increase in echogenicity of the hepatic parenchyma occurs

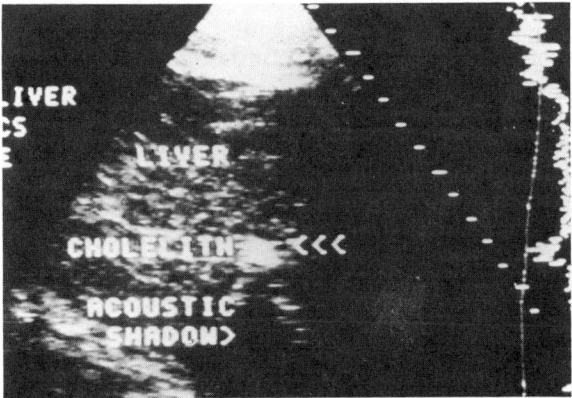

Figure 2. Ultrasonogram of the liver of a horse with a cholelith. The cholelith shows as an echogenic focus. The surrounding liver parenchyma is more echogenic than normal, probably as a result of hepatic fibrosis. Reproduced from J. Am. Vet. Med. Assoc. *194*:405, 1989.

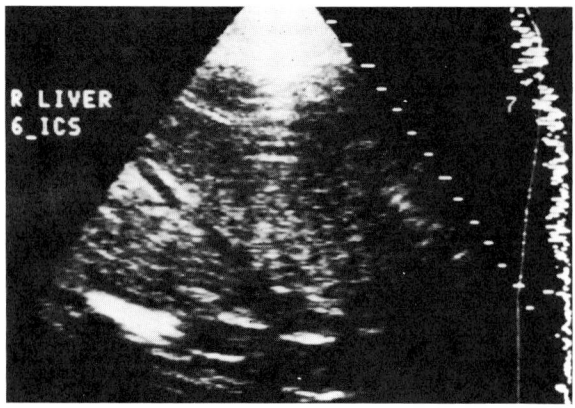

Figure 3. Ultrasonogram of the liver of a horse with hepatic fibrosis. The liver has a diffuse increase in echogenicity. The anechoic bile duct is surrounded by an increase in echogenicity. The focal areas of increased echodensity may represent choleliths.

with any disease resulting in diffuse cellular infiltration (for example, fatty liver, hepatic inflammation, fibrosis) (Fig. 3). Focal masses of increased echogenicity have been reported in association with primary hepatic neoplasia but can also occur with abscessation. Complex patterns of echogenicity (varying echogenicity and texture) suggest neoplasia.

Large fluid-filled structures in the liver or underneath the capsule may be imaged in horses with cysts, hematomas, or abscesses. Hematomas often are loculated, with some internal echoes representing clot formation, whereas abscesses usually contain more echogenic material. Rupture of the liver has been diagnosed in one horse by means of ultrasound.

THERAPY

The treatment of hepatic failure is usually medical and supportive, although in a few instances surgery may be indicated. The initial therapy for hepatic failure should be directed toward correction of any abnormal behavior (hepatoencephalopathy). If the horse is extremely restless or convulsing, it should be sedated before further therapy is attempted. Xylazine will sedate most horses. Most sedatives and tranquilizers are metabolized by the liver, and therefore their use should be kept to a minimum. Following chemical restraint of the affected horse, therapy can be directed at the cause of the hepatoencephalopathy. If the blood glucose concentration is low, a 10 per cent glucose solution should be administered IV. This may result in a dramatic alleviation of the clinical signs. Therapeutic measures directed toward decreasing the blood ammonia concentration are also indicated. These include nasogastric administration of a mild laxative such as mineral oil; oral administration of neomycin, 50 to 100 mg per kg four times daily; or oral administration of lactulose, 150 to 200 ml per adult horse, four times daily. Nasogastric intubation should be performed with care since excessive trauma to the nasal cavity, esophagus, or stomach may result in severe and prolonged hemorrhage. Prolonged neomycin administration may cause diarrhea.

Although acidosis may be severe, attempts at correction must be made slowly, as a rapid increase in pH exacerbates the hepatoencephalopathy. Persistent acidosis has a poor prognosis. Dehydration and polycythemia may also exacerbate acid–base imbalances and should be corrected with balanced electrolyte solutions. A nonresponsive polycythemia has a poor prognosis.

To somewhat decrease the hepatic work load, a continual 5 per cent dextrose drip may be administered IV. Too rapid or intermittent administration can acutely exacerbate the polycythemia and complicate carbohydrate metabolism. No more than 1 liter of 5 per cent dextrose per hour should be given IV to the adult horse unless hypoglycemia is documented. Ponies with hyperlipemia should be treated with glucose, galactose, and insulin. A 200-kg pony should receive 30 IU of Protamine Zinc Insulin intramuscularly (IM) and 100 gm of glucose orally twice daily on the first and succeeding odd days. On even days, 15 IU of Protamine Zinc Insulin is given IM twice daily and 100 gm of galactose is given PO once daily. Heparin, 40 IU per kg, may be given subcutaneously twice daily in hopes of enhancing lipase activity. Therapy for any initiating disease process, for example laminitis, should be provided. This routine should be continued until the serum is no longer grossly lipemic and the affected pony is eating. IV balanced electrolyte fluids are also important in azotemic ponies.

Horses with hepatic failure that maintain a fair appetite are often best treated by dietary management. Dietary management is important in the recovery of horses with acute hepatitis or hepatopathy and may prolong life in cases with chronic hepatic disease. Energy and protein (mostly as branched-chain amino acids) requirements should be met. A reasonable diet includes one part beet pulp with one-quarter to one-half part cracked corn mixed with molasses and provided four to six times daily, up to a total of 20 to 30 lb. for the adult horse. Small meals given frequently are ideal because of difficulties with gluconeogenesis. If this diet is unpalatable, sorgum may be substituted for beet pulp. If the affected horse will not eat, forced feeding should be considered. An oral paste with a high branched-chain to aromatic amino acid ratio can be formulated (8 parts L-leucine, 2 parts L-valine, 1 part L-isoleucine) for forced feeding. IV preparations with high concentrations of branched chain amino acids are available, but they are expensive and must be given slowly. Vitamin B_1, folic acid and vitamin K_1 should be given at least weekly. Grazing of mixed grasses is permitted and should be encouraged as long as affected horses can be protected from sunlight.

Bactericidal antibiotic therapy is indicated for horses with suppurative cholangitis. A diagnosis of suppurative cholangitis is usually made before the organism or its antibiotic sensitivity is known. Therefore, a broad-spectrum drug regimen such as a combination of ampicillin and gentamicin or trimethoprim-sulfa is preferred for the initial therapy. Antimicrobial therapy can be adjusted once the offending organism has been identified. High levels of IV penicillin and an aminoglycoside should be administered to foals with suspected Tyzzer's disease. Penicillin in high doses should also be used for treating suspected anaerobic abscesses of the liver.

Surgery may be indicated as part of the therapy for liver failure in foals with duodenal stricture or in horses with colonic displacements that result in biliary obstruction. Foals with portacaval shunts require surgical repair if desirable growth and performance are expected. Surgery for cholelithiasis is indicated unless diffuse fibrosis is already present.

Horses considered to have chronic active hepatitis may be given steroids or cholchicine, although the therapeutic benefit is questionable. If steroids are to be used, prednisolone, 200 mg per day for the adult horse, is recommended.

Supplemental Readings

Angsubhakorn, N. S., Poomvises, P., Romruen, K., and Newberne, P. M.: Aflatoxicosis in horses. J. Am. Vet. Med. Assoc., 178:274, 1981.

Church, S., West, H. J., and Baker, J. R.: Two cases of pancreatic adenocarcinoma in horses. Equine Vet. J., 19:77, 1987.

Cornick, J. L., Carter, R. G., and Bridges, C. H.: Klein grass associated with hepatotoxicity in the horse. In: Proceedings of the American College of Veterinary Internal Medicine. Washington, D.C., 1986, p. 14.

Gay, C. C.: Infectious necrotic hepatitis (black disease) in a horse. Equine Vet. J., 12:26, 1980.

Giles, C. J.: Outbreak of ragwort *(Senecio jacobea)* poisoning in horses. Equine Vet. J., 15:248, 1983.

Jeffcott, L. B., and Field, J. R.: Current concepts of hyperlipidemia in horses and ponies. Vet. Rec., 116:461, 1985.

Johnston, J. K., Divers, T. J., and Reef, V. B.: Cholelithiasis in horses: Ten cases (1982–1986). J. Am. Vet. Med. Assoc., 194:405, 1989.

Lessard, P., Wilson, W. D., Olander, H. J., Rogers, Q. R., and Mendel, V. E.: Clinicopathologic study of horses surviving pyrrlizidine alkaloid *(Senecio vulgaris)* toxicosis. Am. J. Vet. Res., 47:1776, 1986.

Naylor, J. M.: Hyperlipemia. In Robinson, N. E. (ed.): Current Therapy in Equine Medicine 2. Philadelphia, W. B. Saunders, 1987, pp. 114–116.

Biliary Disorders

Josie L. Traub-Dargatz, FORT COLLINS, COLORADO

CHOLELITHIASIS

Cholelithiasis is the presence of calculi in the common bile duct or gallbladder; choledocholithiasis is the presence of calculi in common bile duct. Since the horse has no gallbladder, choledocholithiasis is probably the preferable term. Calculi have been reported to occur singly or multiply and vary in diameter from a few millimeters to 12 cm in the horse. The calculi may be found incidentally at necropsy or may produce clinical signs.

The etiology of cholelithiasis in the horse is not definitively known. Ascending bacterial infection with subsequent biliary stasis is a possibility, because enteric organisms have been cultured from the liver of horses with cholelithiasis. Retrograde infection from the duodenum up the common bile duct apparently occurs antecedent to cholelith formation. Salmonellosis has been associated with cholelithiasis in horses and is one of the bacteria-associated biliary infections in humans. Hematogenous infection of the biliary system secondary to bacteremia may occur in the horse.

CLINICAL SIGNS

The clinical signs are most likely the result of cholestasis and inflammation or infection of the biliary system. The most consistent clinical presentation is mild colic with historical evidence that the horse has had repeated bouts of mild colic lasting for one to several days and recurring in some cases for over a year. In some horses, fever, icterus, and weight loss have been associated with colic. Dullness and dementia have been reported in a limited number of horses with cholelithiasis and are signs of hepatoencephalopathy. The mean age of horses with cholelithiasis is 11 years (range, 5 to 23 years). No breed or sex predilection has been reported.

LABORATORY FINDINGS

Clinicopathological findings include leukocytosis due to neutrophilia in several but not all reported cases. Hyperproteinemia and hyperfibrinogenemia are relatively consistent findings. The leukocytosis and hyperfibrinogenemia are thought to be the result of cholangitis. Serum chemistry abnormalities include markedly increased γ-glutamyl transferase (GGT) values (130 to 2920 IU per L) and alkaline phosphatase (AP) values (300 to 3550 IU per L), with a moderate increase in aspartate aminotransferase (AST) values (267 to 837 IU per L) and sorbitol dehydrogenase (SDH) values (40 IU per L). In the majority of horses with cholelithiasis, both total bilirubin (2.3 to 13.4 mg per dl) and direct bilirubin (0.5 to 8.54 mg per dl) values are increased. The ratio of direct to total bilirubin is greater than 0.25 in most horses with cholelithiasis. The marked increase in cholestatic enzymes such as GGT and AP in the setting of moderate elevation in hepatocellular enzymes such as AST, SDH and a direct bilirubin value exceeding 25 per cent of the total bilirubin value is the result of the cholestasis associated with cholelithiasis. Serum bile acid concentrations have been reported as 607 to 1387 μg per dl in two of three cases of cholelithiasis.

Horses with cholelithiasis may have an abnormal clotting profile and increased blood ammonia level. These findings indicate that the degree of hepatic insufficiency is severe. Prolongation of partial thromboplastin and prothrombin time in comparison to control values is due to reduced synthesis of coagulation factors in the liver and indicates marked hepatocellular damage. An increased blood ammonia level has been associated with marked hepatocellular damage and development of hepatoencephalopathy.

Abdominocentesis is indicated in horses with recurrent colic. In horses with cholelithiasis, peritoneal fluid is sometimes increased in volume and has an orange color; cytologically the fluid may be consistent with a chronic active inflammatory process.

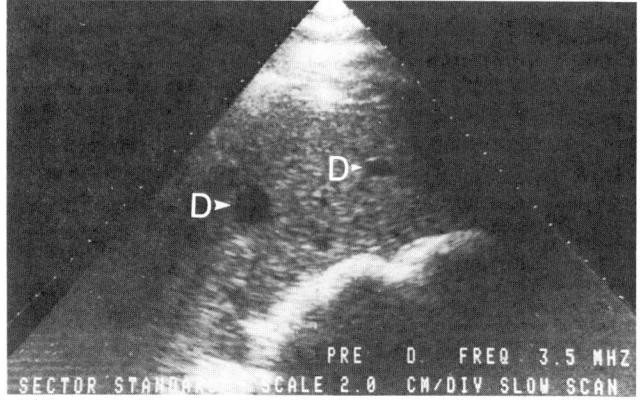
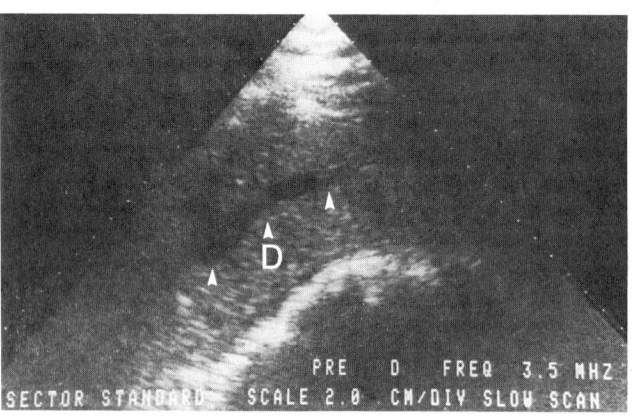

Figure 1. (*A*) Ultrasonographic image of horse with enlarged liver and dilated bile ducts imaged in cross-section. *Arrows D* are dilated ducts. (*B*) Ultrasonographic image of horse with enlarged liver and dilated bile duct imaged longitudinally. *Arrows D* are along dilated duct.

Bilirubinuria, due to clearance of direct (conjugated) bilirubin into the urine, may be recognized as a green-orange discoloration of the urine and detected as a positive bilirubin reaction on the urine dipstick. Since horses do not normally excrete bilirubin in the urine, the presence of bilirubin should alert the clinician to cholestasis.

Ultrasonography

Ultrasonography of the liver of horses with evidence of cholestasis can result in a preoperative or antemortem diagnosis of cholelithiasis. Ultrasonographic findings include visualization of a large area of liver from the right side, suggestive of hepatomegaly, dilation of the bile ducts (Figs. 1A, B), and hyperechoic areas that may result in acoustic shadowing (Fig. 2). The biliary system is not normally seen ultrasonographically. Distention of the biliary system detectable with ultrasonography is abnormal in the horse and indicates cholestasis, but this finding is not pathognomonic for cholelithiasis. It is important that the ultrasonographer attempt to differentiate vascular structures from ductile structures, but this is not always possible. A double parallel portal sign (i.e., visualization of the duct and vessel in same scan) has been considered definitive evidence of ductule dilation in man but rarely occurs in the horse. Evaluation of the tubular structure with a pulsed Doppler technique can differentiate a vessel with flow from a dilated duct, which would not have flow. Overall, it is difficult to be sure if tubular structures seen within the liver parenchyma ultrasonographically are vessels or dilated ducts. Vascular structures in the liver can become prominent in certain situations such as heart failure (Fig. 3) and be confused with dilated bile ducts. Only the demonstration of hyperechoic areas within distended ducts is diagnostic for cholelithiasis. The degree of echogenicity and acoustic shadowing will vary with the density and mineral content of the choleliths. Those containing calcium bilirubinate or calcium phosphate are most echodense. It is difficult to image single choleliths in the common bile duct because of the central location of the obstructing cholelith, often near the bile duct opening. The difficulty lies in finding a window to image this area of the horse's liver. Air-filled lung precludes imaging from the dorsum, gas-filled bowel precludes imaging from the ventrum, and if there is not a large area of liver on the right side to act as an imaging win-

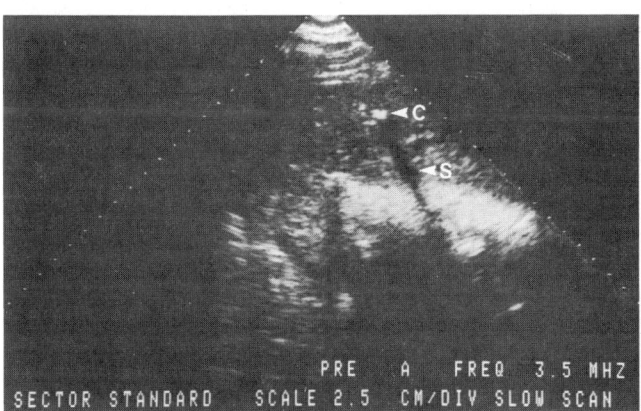

Figure 2. Ultrasonographic image of horse with choleliths *(arrow C)* in peripheral bile ducts. Note acoustic shadowing *(arrow S)* created by choleliths and hepatic fibrosis.

Figure 3. Ultrasonographic image of horse with congestive heart failure. Dilated tubular structures are hepatic vasculature. Note treelike branching pattern.

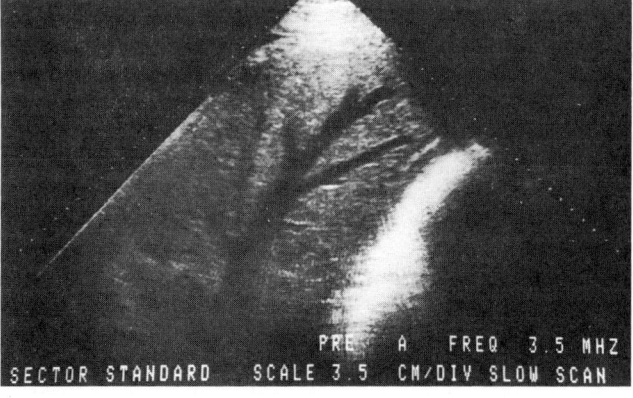

dow, the common bile duct cannot be examined completely. The depth from the body wall to the medial surface of the liver and the common bile duct is extremely variable and depends on the volume of the thorax, the amount of material in the large colon, and the presence of liver disease and other conditions that could cause visceral displacement, such as pregnancy and ascites. Older horses without a large area of liver on the right side should be imaged from the left side. If peripheral choleliths are present, they may be imaged from the left side.

LIVER BIOPSY

Liver biopsy is indicated if the clinical signs, hematology, serum chemistry, and ultrasonography of the liver indicate cholelithiasis. A coagulation profile should be determined before the biopsy is performed because prolongation of the activated partial thromboplastin time and thrombin time can occur in horses with liver disease. If clotting times are prolonged, a plasma transfusion may be beneficial. Clinically significant problems due to liver biopsy are uncommon, but precautions should be taken in horses with bleeding tendencies.

A Tru-Cut° or a Franklin-modified Vim Silverman† biopsy needle can be used to obtain the liver biopsy. The author prefers to utilize ultrasonography to guide the biopsy instrument into the liver. (The location of the biopsy site will vary among horses when ultrasonography is used to direct the biopsy.) The location for obtaining a liver biopsy without the aid of ultrasonography was described previously (see p. 257).

Histopathology as well as bacterial culture should be performed on liver tissue obtained by biopsy. Histopathological findings in horses with cholelithiasis are not specific for cholelithiasis but will provide prognostic information. Findings indicative of a poor prognosis include periportal fibrosis, bile duct proliferation, accumulation of bile pigment, and hepatocyte necrosis.

THERAPY

The prognosis for recovery and long-term survival of horses with cholelithiasis is guarded and depends on the degree of hepatic fibrosis occurring concurrently with the cholestasis. The prognosis for recovery should be discussed with the client before therapy is pursued.

Medical therapy consists of antimicrobial treatment to resolve biliary infection. Because enteric bacteria are often involved in the biliary infection, the antimicrobials used include penicillin in combination with an aminoglycoside such as gentamicin. Trimethoprim-sulfa may also be used, with or without concurrent penicillin therapy. It may be difficult to achieve adequate biliary concentrations of antibiotic if there is biliary obstruction, and therefore tissue and blood levels are of greater importance. In humans, ampicillin or a cephalosporin have been suggested for less severe cases, with the addition of an aminoglycoside or metronidazole in more seriously ill patients with cholangitis or cholestasis. Antimicrobial therapy for several weeks is indicated, and thus the horse needs to be monitored for potential adverse effects, such as gentamicin nephrotoxicity or trimethoprim-sulfa–associated diarrhea.

Cholelithotripsy and choledochotomy have been performed in horses with cholelithiasis. Surgical intervention may be performed in horses with recurrent colic and extremely high serum levels of biliary enzymes (GGT and AP) suggestive of obstructive cholestasis even in the absence of definitive ultrasonographic evidence of cholelithiasis. Liver biopsy is advocated before surgery to evaluate the degree of hepatocellular damage and fibrosis. The success of these operations has been limited by extensive hepatic fibrosis, multiple stones throughout the biliary tree that could not be removed, choleperitoneum in the setting of choledochotomy, and postoperative *Salmonella*-induced diarrhea. The source of *Salmonella* may have been the biliary system once the patency was reestablished. The prognosis for horses with cholelithiasis is extremely guarded even with surgical intervention.

Dissolution of choleliths with bile acid therapy has not been attempted in the horse and may be of limited benefit as therapy requires several months and is directed toward cholesterol calculi. Biliary calculi in the horse are brown-pigmented and contain principally calcium bilirubinates, sodium taurodeoxycholate and calcium phosphate, cholesterol esters, bile acids, and bilirubin.

Dietary recommendations include feeds such as timothy hay, milo, and corn that are rich in branched-chain amino acids, and a source of B vitamins such as brewers yeast. Depending on the horse's hydration and energy status, it may initially require intravenous polyionic fluids with dextrose and possibly B vitamins added. Branched-chain amino acids and lactulose therapy may be indicated if the horse has hepatoencephalopathy. Parenteral nutrition has been used in selected cases.

°Travenol Laboratories, Inc., Deerfield, IL
†Mueller and Company, Chicago, IL

CHOLANGITIS

Cholangitis or cholestasis without cholelith formation is a differential diagnosis in horses with clinical signs and laboratory evidence of cholestasis. Diagnostic ultrasonography of the liver could assist the clinician in ruling in cholelithiasis if calculi were seen but could not differentiate the condition if no choleliths were visualized. Possible causes of cholestasis in the horse include neoplasia, abscesses, and granulomas that obstruct bile flow. Cholangitis without cholelithiasis is difficult to differentiate from cholelithiasis without exploratory laparotomy or necropsy. The medical management of cholangitis without cholelithiasis is the same as for cholelithiasis, so the distinction between the two conditions is of concern only if surgical intervention is contemplated. The decision for surgical intervention can be a difficult, since the two conditions can be difficult to differentiate.

Supplemental Readings

Carlson, G. P.: The liver. *In* Mansmann, R. A., McAllister, E. S., Pratt, P. W. (eds.): Equine Medicine and Surgery, 3rd ed. Santa Barbara, Calif., American Veterinary Publications, 1982, p. 633–643.

Johnston, J. K., Divers, T. J., Reef, V. B., and Acland, H.: Cholelithiasis in horses: Ten cases (1982–1986). J. Am. Vet. Med. Assoc., 194:405, 1989.

Modransky, P. D.: Ultrasound-guided renal and hepatic biopsy technique. Vet. Clin. North Am. (Equine Pract.), 2:115, 1986.

Munro, R., and Sorrell, T. C.: Biliary sepsis: Reviewing treatment options. Drugs, 31:449, 1986.

Pearson, E. G.: Diseases of the hepatobiliary system: Diagnosis of liver disease. *In* Smith, B. P. (ed.): Large Animal Internal Medicine, 1st ed. St. Louis, MO, C. V. Mosby Co., 1990, p. 837.

Rantanen, N. W.: Diseases of the liver. Vet. Clin. North Am. (Equin Pract.), 2:105, 1986.

Roussel, A. J., Becht, J. L., and Adams, S. B.: Choledocholithiasis in a horse. Cornell Vet., 74:166, 1984.

Scarratt, W. K., Saunders, G. K., and Fessler, R. L.: Cholelithiasis and biliary obstruction in a horse. Compend. Cont. Ed. Pract. Vet., 7:S428, 1985.

Traub, J. L., Grant, B. D., Rantanen, N. W., McElwain, T., Wagner, P. C., and Bayly, W. M.: Surgical removal of choleliths in a horse. J. Am. Vet. Med. Assoc., 182:714, 1983.

Traub, J. L., Rantanen, N., Reed, S., and Schecter, L.: Cholelithiasis in four horses. J. Am. Vet. Med. Assoc., 181:59, 1982.

Tulleners, E. P., Becht, J. L., Richardson, D. W., and Divers, T. J.: Choledocholithotripsy in a mare. J. Am. Vet. Med. Assoc., 186:1317, 1985.

Van Der Luer, R. J. T., and Kroneman, J.: Three cases of cholelithiasis and biliary fibrosis in the horse. Equine Vet. J., 14:251, 1982.

Section 6

UPPER AIRWAY DISEASES

Edited by Richard P. Hackett and Normand G. Ducharme

Diseases of the Nasal Passages

James T. Robertson, COLUMBUS, OHIO
Clara K. Fenger, COLUMBUS, OHIO

The incidence of nasal cavity disease in the horse is low, but the diagnosis should be considered in any horse with nasal discharge, malodorous breath, facial swelling, respiratory stridor, and exercise intolerance. The specific clinical signs associated with nasal cavity diseases will vary according to the individual disease process.

Examination of the nares and nasal passages begins with a visual inspection of the head from the front and each side. Any nasal discharge, facial swelling, asymmetry, or conformational abnormalities should be noted. The nostrils, alar folds, and the rostral portion of the nasal septum and premaxillary region can be digitally palpated. The air flow through each nostril is evaluated by placing the palm of each hand in front of each nostril. Percussion of the paranasal sinuses for decreased resonance may reveal concurrent sinus involvement. If exercise intolerance and respiratory noise are part of the history, the horse should be observed at exercise. During exercise, the nostrils should be observed for maximal dilation and symmetry of movement. Any evident stridor should be characterized as to location (nasal vs. guttural) and phase of respiration (inspiratory, expiratory, or both).

The nasal passages can be further evaluated with endoscopy and radiography. Accurate radiographic assessment of the nasal septum and symmetry of the turbinates and nasal passages requires a perfect dorsoventral view of the skull. The overall width of the nasal passages may be difficult to assess endoscopically or radiographically unless there is marked narrowing or deformity. Space-occupying lesions of the nasal passages are usually easily identified and characterized with both techniques.

DISEASES OF THE NOSTRILS

ATHEROMA

Atheromas, or epidermal inclusion cysts, develop in the diverticulum of the nostril. It is a unilateral condition that most commonly becomes apparent in horses 1 to 3 years old. The etiology is unknown but is likely due to aberrant epithelial tissue remaining after embryogenesis. The skin overlying the atheroma is normal, but as the cyst enlarges a facial swelling becomes apparent at the caudal limit of the nasal diverticulum. The cyst contents are a sterile, thick, proteinaceous substance. Histopathological evaluation shows a lining of layered epidermis covering the inner surface of the cyst. Atheromas are principally a cosmetic problem, although they occasionally become large enough to obstruct air flow through the nostril.

Atheromas require surgical resection or drainage for resolution. There are three surgical approaches: drainage to the external surface, drainage through the false nostril, or surgical removal. After surgical drainage, the cavity should be packed with iodine-soaked gauze to cauterize the epithelial lining and minimize the chance of recurrence. This packing may be removed after 24 to 48 hours and the wound allowed to heal by second intention. If atheromas recur after drainage, surgical resection is indicated. The cyst is dissected through an incision over the lateral skin surface and the incision is closed primarily.

ALAR FOLD OBSTRUCTION

The alar fold or "false nostril" is a thick fold of skin and mucous membrane that lies in the dorsal part of the nostril and forms the floor of the nasal diverticulum. In normal horses, the alar fold is retracted from the airway when the nostril is dilated. In some horses with excessive alar fold tissue or congenitally narrow nasal passages, the alar folds are drawn into the nasal passage during inspiration, producing an obstruction. A loud, vibrating nasal noise is present during inspiration. Alar fold obstruction can be diagnosed by temporarily retracting both folds and observing the horse during exercise. This retraction can be achieved by three different techniques. The first involves passing a suture, under local anesthesia, through the free edge of each alar fold and tying it over the bridge of the nose. The second method entails placing a metal ring in the free edge of each fold, then passing a string through each ring and tying it over the bridge of the nose. A third alternative is to pass a mattress suture through the alar fold and the roof of the false nostril to fix the fold in a retracted position.

In horses in which temporary retraction of the alar folds results in partial or complete resolution of the nasal obstruction, bilateral alar fold resection is indicated. The wounds heal in approximately 10 days and exercise can be resumed at that time.

NOSTRIL LACERATION

Circumferential lacerations around the rim of the nostril require surgical repair. If the wound is allowed to heal by second intention, the free edges of the nostril may stricture, occluding the airway. The tissues should be carefully apposed in at least two layers with large vertical mattress sutures in the skin. Often the challenge is not so much in the wound repair, but in preventing wound dehiscence, caused by the horse rubbing its nose. If these wounds break down and are not resutured or are initially allowed to heal by second intention, the stricture will produce a result that is unacceptable both cosmetically and functionally.

FACIAL NERVE PARALYSIS

Trauma to the facial nerve often results in paralysis of the nostril and muzzle on the affected side. The muzzle is deviated away from the affected side and the nostril is unable to dilate. Any ability of the animal to dilate the nostril or to move the muzzle toward the affected side is a good prognostic sign and function will usually return, although it may take months. Severe injury leading to fibrosis of the endoneurium can result in permanent nostril paralysis, leading to nostril collapse during exercise. In order to salvage a racehorse, radical resection of the external nares may be attempted. The results are not cosmetic.

A horse with mild injury to both facial nerves may have subtle signs that go unnoticed on casual observation. The nostrils may be symmetrical and dilate at rest, but there may be a very slight deviation of the muzzle. As the horse begins to fatigue during exercise, however, the nostrils may collapse during inspiration, producing a severe obstruction. This type of facial nerve trauma may follow an accident with the horse in cross-ties. The resultant paresis usually resolves but may take 6 to 12 months for complete recovery.

DISEASES OF THE NASAL CAVITY

NASAL SEPTAL DISEASES

Congenital Deviation

Wry nose is a congenital deviation of the nasal septum and nasal and premaxillary bones. This condition can range from subtle to severe. The exact cause of wry nose is not known, although it has been anecdotally associated with the teratogenic effecs of the administration of some deworming compounds and with endotoxemia during early pregnancy. It is likely that an intrauterine disturbance in the development of the maxilla during embryogenesis produces the deformity. This condition probably is not heritable.

The clinical effects of a wry nose depend on its severity. A mild nasal and septal deviation constitutes no more than a cosmetic defect, while severe deviation of the septal premaxilla and nasal bones results in nasal obstruction, complete maxillomandibular malocclusion, and an unacceptable appearance. Severely affected foals have difficulty nursing from the mare and prehending solid food. These foals are usually euthanatized because they have little chance of becoming successful show or performance horses, even with surgery. With proper care, some of these foals can go on to be breeding animals.

If the foal is not suffering from an obstructed airway and is able to nurse and eat without difficulty, no immediate treatment is indicated. It is best to let the foal grow at least to yearling size and allow the head to mature before performing corrective surgery, which is usually a nasal septum resection. A major risk of nasal surgery in a foal, particularly removal of a portion of the nasal septum, is significant bony nasal deformation and retardation of growth of the upper jaw.

Horses with a mild septal deviation can be put into training and evaluated for evidence of obstruction. Some performance horses can tolerate a mild deviation. If the deviation causes exercise intolerance, the deviated portion of the nasal septum can be resected in an attempt to remove some of the obstruction.

If a foal with a severe deviation is to be kept alive, it is important to ensure that the foal ingests an adequate volume of colostrum. Many of these foals have failure of passive transfer because of inability to suckle successfully. If the nasal obstruction is not severe, these foals may survive and reach adulthood without surgical correction, but initially they must be bottle- and bucket-fed milk. Special feeding may be required because of their inability to prehend food owing to malocclusion. In foals in which the nasal obstruction causes an exaggerated respiratory effort at rest, surgical correction should be attempted immediately. Also, any foal with moderate to severe deviation that is intended as an athlete should undergo surgical correction within the first months of life.

The prognosis for athletic performance in a foal with a significant maxillomandibular malocclusion is guarded, even with surgical correction. The surgery entails a combination of premaxilla and nasal bone osteotomies and nasal septal resection with some form of internal or external fixation to stabilize the bones following osteotomy. Although there is a report of cosmetic success in one foal, in our experience these foals develop into adults with significant facial deformity, maxillary underbite, and some degree of persistent nasal obstruction.

Congenital Cyst

Cysts of the nasal septum are congenital and are usually discovered in weanling-age foals when the cyst expands to a size that produces airway obstruction. Temporary improvement can be achieved by draining the cyst, and a permanent cure can be effected by resecting that portion of the nasal septum containing the cyst. Cystic tissue may also be present in the adjacent turbinates. The prognosis following resection of a nasal septal cyst is good, although some facial deformity may result.

Acquired Septal Diseases

Trauma causing fracture of the nasal bones and injury to the nasal septum can result in septal thickening and distortion, particularly in foals. Septal thickening with cystic degeneration has been observed in horses following a respiratory infection. In some young horses, nasal septal thickening develops as a result of cartilage degeneration; the etiology is unknown. Neoplastic infiltration and amyloid deposition can occur in the nasal septum and nasal cavity, but both conditions are rare. The prognosis of infiltrative diseases is poor, but surgical therapy may afford temporary palliation. Nasal septal deviation may also occur as a result of pressure from expansion of space-occupying lesions of the paranasal sinuses.

Horses with an acquired thickening or deformity of the nasal septum usually have some degree of airway obstruction and make a nasal respiratory noise during exercise. A careful visual examination of the head may reveal a deviated premaxilla (wry nose) or a slight conformational change; flattening and widening over the nasal bones may be observed in some young horses with nasal septal thickening. Digital examination of the rostral portion of the septum usually reveals a palpable thickening or deformity. On endoscopic examination, the deformity of the nasal septum may be apparent and the nasal passage may appear narrow. The diagnosis is confirmed with a dorsoventral radiograph of the skull. The entire length of the septum, from the nostrils to the ethmoid bone, is visible on a dorsoventral radiograph. A near perfect dorsoventral view is necessary because obliquity of the skull will produce distortion of the septum and confound evaluation of its width and shape.

Occasionally, a horse with a septal thickening will present a diagnostic challenge if there is absence of facial deformity, no palpable abnormalities of the rostral septum, and lack of obvious narrowing on endoscopic examination. The loud nasal respiratory noise heard during training should, however, provide a hint of the problem. The diagnosis is then confirmed with radiographic evaluation.

The severity and extent of the septal disease must be assessed before surgery so that the appropriate technique for resection can be selected. The prognosis is better in horses with a septal lesion located rostral to the caudal limit of the hard palate (or rostral to the level of the fifth upper tooth). Removal of the caudalmost portion of the septum necessitates modifications in technique, which makes the procedure more difficult and increases the chance for serious complications. However, if the diseased portion of septum is not removed in its entirety, there is little likelihood of postoperative improvement in performance. If the abnormal portion of the septum is completely removed, the horse's performance should improve, although it is likely that some nasal respiratory noise will still be evident during exercise.

In preparation for surgery, the surgeon should evaluate the horse's hematocrit, platelet count, and hemostasis profile. A compatible blood donor should be identified and 4 liters of blood collected. An intraoperative transfusion may be necessary if blood loss becomes excessive. The owner must be made aware of the risk of fatal hemorrhage during the procedure. The surgical techniques for septal resection are described elsewhere.

Necrosis of a portion of the nasal septum can occur secondary to severe systemic disease. It is likely that this is related to disseminated intravascular coagulation or vasculitis. In most cases a foul-smelling bilateral nasal discharge develops suddenly as the affected tissue sloughs. Once the primary problem has resolved and the septum has healed, the animal may be asymptomatic or may exhibit stridor during exercise. Necrosis resulting in a communication between the nasal passages may be discovered incidentally during routine nasogastric intubation.

Intranasal Neoplasms

Intranasal neoplasms are relatively rare and generally occur in older horses. Neoplasms that originate in the nasal cavity reportedly occur with one-half the frequency of neoplasms originating in the paranasal sinuses. Large tumor masses occupying the nasal cavity frequently invade the adjacent paranasal sinuses. Various types of carcinomas, including squamous cell carcinoma and sarcomas such as osteogenic sarcoma and lymphosarcoma, have been reported to originate in the nasal passages. In our practice, the most frequently encountered nasal neoplasm is squamous cell carcinoma. This tumor type originates in the nasal epithelium and is usually very aggressive and invasive, frequently metastasizing to the retropharyngeal lymph nodes. Rarely, neoplasms of the nasal cavity such as nasal-maxillary fibrosarcoma or adenocarcinoma are encountered in the neonate.

In the early stages of nasal tumor development, the clinical signs include a unilateral reduction in nasal air flow and a mucopurulent or serosanguinous nasal discharge, depending on the degree of tissue destruction. As the neoplasm enlarges, nasal obstruction worsens and facial swelling develops over the nasal passages or sinuses of the affected side.

The obstructing tumor mass will be evident on endoscopy and may prevent passage of a small-diameter endoscope through the ventral meatus. Radiographs of the head will demonstrate the tumor density occupying the nasal cavity and, in more advanced cases, distortion and destruction of the surrounding bony structures. Frequently an expanding tumor causes nasal septal deviation and may cause dental distortion. If a neoplasm is suspected, a biopsy of the mass should be performed with a biopsy forceps passed through a flexible fiber-optic endoscope or a forceps passed up the nasal passage under endoscopic guidance. Alternatively, a biopsy specimen can be obtained surgically through a small trephine opening in the nasal or maxillary bones. The biopsy can result in considerable hemorrhage. Small tumor masses can be ablated with a neodymium:yttrium-aluminum-garnet (Nd:YAG) laser through an endoscope, treated with cryosurgery, or resected surgically. Treatment of a large malignant tumor is rarely attempted and euthanasia is the usual option. To date, very few horses with nasal cavity carcinoma or sarcoma have been treated with any kind of success, regardless of the treatment modality. Treatment is unlikely to accomplish any significant remission.

Granulomas

Fungal granulomas of the nasal passages of horses are rare, and occur most commonly in tropical and subtropical climates. Causative organisms include *Coccidiodes immitis, Cryptococcus neoformans, Histoplasma, Aspergillus* spp., *Pseudallescheria boydii, Rhinosporidium* spp., *Hyphomyces destruens,* and *Conidiobolus coronatus.* There does not appear to be an age predilection. Affected animals are usually seen for evaluation of respiratory stridor, exercise intolerance, chronic unilateral nasal discharge, or epistaxis. Clinical findings are variable. There may or may not be impedance to air flow through the affected side. The sinuses may have reduced resonance on percussion if the granuloma has penetrated the sinus cavities. Results of hematological and serum biochemical analyses are usually normal but may reflect an inflammatory response in cases with systemic or secondary bacterial involvement. Endoscopic evaluation of the nasal passages will usually reveal the granuloma. Radiography may delineate involvement of the sinuses or calcification within the granuloma.

Nasal granulomas may be treated by debulking, with or without antifungal therapy. Some cases have been successfully treated with surgical resection alone. Medical therapy alone is usually unsuccessful.

Nasal Polyps

Nasal polyps are fibrous masses of inflammatory tissue that can arise from the submucosal connective tissue of the nasal passages or from the alveolus of an upper second or third cheek tooth. Nasal polyps can be single or multiple but are usually unilateral. Polyps located in the nares or rostral portion of the nasal cavity and associated with an alveolus usually consist of a single mass attached by a stalk to the alveolus, and may be visible at the nostril. Polyps originating from the nasal mucosa in the more caudal portion of the nasal cavity are visible on endoscopic examination. No specific etiological agent has been identified.

As a nasal polyp enlarges, it produces airway obstruction detectable as decreased air flow through the nostril on the affected side. A respiratory noise will develop as the obstruction worsens. The diagnosis is straightforward if the polyp is visible and can be made easily with an endoscope if the polyp is located in the caudal portion of the nasal cavity. Radiographs of the skull will demonstrate the soft tissue mass in the nasal cavity and reveal any tooth root involvement.

A number of different techniques for polyp removal are available. The method chosen will depend on the size and location of the polyp. Generally, those originating in the rostral portion of the nasal cavity can be amputated at the base of the stalk with a snare passed through the nostril. The area of attachment can be curetted through a trephine opening in the nasal cavity. If the polyp originates in an alveolus, the affected tooth should be repelled and extracted. Polyps in the caudal aspect of the nasal cavity are best ablated with the Nd:YAG laser passed through an endoscope. Masses in the caudal nasal cavity are difficult to reach surgically through nasal or sinus flaps or trephinations. Some may be amenable to the application of a cryogen, such as liquid nitrogen, through a tube passed up the nostril, under endoscopic guidance.

Congenitally Narrow Nasal Passages

A horse with congenitally narrow nasal passages may have some respiratory noise at rest, particularly when relaxed in the stall. Some affected animals may demonstrate noise solely at exercise. This can be a difficult diagnosis because there is no pathology of the nasal septum or turbinates, only narrowing of the nasal meati throughout the length of the nasal passages. On physical examination, most horses with this condition have a refined head that is quite narrow over the nasal bones. They generally make a nasal inspiratory noise that varies in intensity with the degree of narrowing. Some noise may also be generated from the nostrils and alar folds. Sedation with xylazine will frequently produce a marked respiratory stertor in a horse with this condition. The ventral nasal meatus may be narrowed, making it difficult to pass a stomach tube or standard-sized endoscope. Radiography is of little value in making this diagnosis because nasal cavity width is difficult to estimate. However, radiographs of the head should be obtained to rule out nasal septal disease.

The prognosis associated with congenital narrowing of the nasal passages depends on the severity of the condition and the intended use of the horse. Horses that are mildly affected may benefit from an alar fold resection if there is a nostril component to the obstruction. More severely affected horses, particularly those in race training with associated exercise intolerance, have a poor prognosis. Alar fold resection and nasal septum removal can be attempted, but a poor prognosis should be given.

Choanal Atresia

A rare condition, choanal atresia results from failure of the bucconasal membrane to rupture during the early stages of development of the fetus. The result is a membranous or bony obstruction at the juncture of the nasal passages and nasopharynx. The atresia can be unilateral or bilateral, complete or incomplete. A complete bilateral obstruction will likely result in fatal asphyxia unless an emergency tracheostomy is performed.

Choanal atresia can be diagnosed on the basis of endoscopic and contrast-enhanced radiographic studies that demonstrate an obstruction of the choanae. Successful surgical correction of bilateral choanal atresia has been reported. The obstruction was approached through nasal bone flaps on each side of the nasal septum and the obstructive tissue was resected with a portion of the nasal septum. The authors recommended maintaining intranasal tubes for 6 to 8 weeks after surgery to prevent renewed obstruction. Some facial deformity developed as a result of the surgery. The bucconasal membrane can also be resected through a laryngotomy incision (Richard Hackett, D.V.M., Cornell University; pers. commun.). A flexible fiber endoscope should be passed through the nasal cavity. The light can be seen through the thin membrane, facilitating identification of its limits.

Laser ablation with the Nd:YAG laser passed through an endoscope may be an alternative approach to ablation of a membranous obstruction. This treatment modality would provide a noninvasive solution to the problem and could be repeated if a stricture developed after surgery.

Rhinitis

Inflammation of the mucosa of the nasal passages with accompanying nasal discharge can be associated with many infectious respiratory diseases. Common viral causes include rhinopneumonitis, influenza, and rhinovirus. In the early stages of viral infection, there is a proliferation of the virus particles in the nasal and pharyngeal mucosa with an associated serous nasal discharge. Bacterial rhinitis occurs secondary to mucosal disruption from the viral infection and is accompanied by a mucopurulent exudate. Bacterial rhinitis can also occur in conjunction with primary infection of other components of the respiratory system, such as in strangles and pneumonia. Further discussion of respiratory viruses is found on p. 316.

Other Conditions

Nutritional secondary hyperparathyroidism ("big head" or osteodystrophia fibrosa), a skeletal disease that develops in horses fed a ration containing an excess of phosphorus in relation to calcium, such as in high grain diets, may cause nasal obstruction due to excessive proliferation of fibrous tissue (see page 119). Horner's syndrome, caused by an injury to the sympathetic nerve supply to the head, can also cause nasal obstruction. Impaired vasoconstriction of the blood vessels in the mucous membranes of the nasal passages of the affected side allows persistent congestion. The clinical signs of Horner's syndrome include ptosis of the upper eyelid, miosis of the pupil, and facial sweating on the affected side. The skin over the head of the affected side is warmer than on the contralateral side. This syndrome is seen most frequently in conjunction with laryngeal hemiplegia as a result of perivascular injection around the jugular vein. In racehorses, Horner's syndrome results in a significant obstruction to air flow that produces exercise intolerance and some nasal respiratory noise.

Necrosis of the turbinates can result from direct trauma or may occur secondary to infection. This condition is characterized by a chronic fetid nasal discharge. The diagnosis is based on the history, clinical signs, endoscopic examination, and radiographs of the turbinates. The turbinates can be approached and curetted or resected through a nasal bone flap. Severe hemorrhage should be expected and nasal packing is necessary to stop bleeding. A tracheostomy is usually required for recovery from anesthesia.

Supplemental Readings

Aylor, M. K., Campbell, M. L., Goring, R. L., and Hillidge, C. J.: Congenital bilateral choanal atresia in a Standardbred foal. Equine Vet. J., 16:396–398, 1984.

Boulton, C. H.: Equine nasal cavity and paranasal sinus disease: A review of 85 cases. J. Equine Vet. Sci., 5:268–275, 1985.

Brearley, J. C., McCandlish, I. A. P., Sullivan, M., and Dawson, C. O.: Nasal granuloma caused by *Pseudallescheria boydii*. Equine Vet. J., 18:151–153, 1986.

Gordon, L.: The cytology and histology of epidermal inclusion cysts in the horse. J. Eq. Med. Surg. 2:371–374, 1978.

Hodgin, E. C., Conaway, D. H., and Ortenburger, A. I.: Recurrence of obstructive nasal coccidioidal granuloma in a horse. J. Am. Vet. Med. Assoc., 184:339–340, 1984.

Miller, R. I., and Campbell, R. S. F.: Clinical observations on equine phycomycosis. Aust. Vet. J., 58:221–226, 1982.

Schmotzer, W. B., Hultgren, B. D., Watrous, B. J., Wagner, P. C., and Kaneps, A. J.: Nasomaxillary fibrosarcomas in three young horses. J. Am. Vet. Med. Assoc., 191:437–439, 1987.

Tate, L. P.: Applications of lasers in equine upper respiratory surgery. Vet. Clin. N. Amer. (Equine Pract.) 7:165–199, 1991.

Tulleners, E. P., and Raker, C. W.: Nasal septum resection in the horse. Vet. Surg., 12:41–47, 1983.

Valdez, H., McMullan, W. C., Hobson, H. P., and Hanselka, D. V.: Surgical correction of deviated nasal septum and premaxilla in a colt. J. Am. Vet. Med. Assoc., 173:1001–1004, 1978.

van Andel, A. C. J., Gruys, E., Kroneman, J., and Vaerkamp, J.: Amyloid in the horse: A report of nine cases. Equine Vet. J., 20:277–285, 1988.

Diseases of Paranasal Sinuses

Victor C. Speirs, BERNE, SWITZERLAND

Diseases of the paranasal sinuses may be categorized by origin as traumatic, infectious, cystic, or neoplastic. The clinical signs are not always pathognomonic for a specific disease; those present depend not only on the primary condition but also on which of several adjacent structures are affected.

ANATOMY

There are six pairs of paranasal sinuses that communicate either directly or indirectly with the nasal cavity via the nasomaxillary apertures. These are the frontal, sphenopalatine and maxillary sinuses and the dorsal, middle, and ventral conchal sinuses. The maxillary sinus is divided into rostral and caudal compartments by a septum. The ventral conchal sinus communicates with the rostral maxillary sinus, the middle conchal sinus communicates with the caudal maxillary sinus, and the dorsal conchal sinus is continuous with the frontal sinus. When the septum between the maxillary sinuses is intact there are therefore just two sinus systems, each communicating separately with the nasal passage, i.e., the rostral maxillary sinus and the other sinuses. If the septum is naturally incomplete or has been perforated by disease there is communication between all sinuses. The roots of the last four cheek teeth (last premolar and three molars) usually lie partly or completely in the maxillary sinuses, the third and fourth in the rostral maxillary sinus and the fifth and sixth in the caudal maxillary sinus. In young horses the teeth occupy most of the maxillary sinus cavity, but with age they recede and the sinuses increase in size correspondingly.

CLINICAL SIGNS

The clinical signs of sinus disease include nasal discharge, facial deformity, halitosis, dyspnea, epiphora, difficult or painful mastication, a draining tract to the exterior, and, rarely, a full-thickness defect in the wall of a sinus.

Nasal discharge is usually present with sinusitis and is the product of inflammation of soft tissues and bone secondary to infection or necrosis. It may be serous, mucoid, purulent, blood-stained, or a mixture of these, depending on the type and stage of the disease. A fetid breath usually indicates an anaerobic infection due to dental disease, accompanied by communication between the mouth and the paranasal sinus.

A generalized enlargement of the facial regions overlying a sinus is likely to indicate expansion of a lesion within the sinus. The lesion may be neoplastic, cystic, or filled with fluid or exudate secondary to obstruction of sinus drainage. Osteodystrophia fibrosa also produces facial deformity, but the lesions are not restricted to the sinus regions. A localized swelling over a bone suture, especially the frontonasal suture, indicates periostitis with new bone production. Dental disease involving a tooth lying outside the maxillary sinuses will also produce a localized swelling. More extensive dental disease such as chronic ossifying alveolar periostitis also causes facial bulging that is bilateral. Distention of the ventral conchal sinus causes partial or complete obstruction of the nasal passage, and even deviation of the nasal septum with gradual occlusion of the contralateral nasal passage. The obstruction of the nasal passages can cause respiratory distress.

Partial or complete obstruction of the nasolacrimal duct will cause epiphora. Although trauma can damage the duct, outward displacement of the facial bones is the usual cause.

The presence of dental disease may cause pain while chewing, which may be manifested as head tilt, slow eating, or dropping of partially chewed food from the mouth ("quidding"). Relevant dental problems are fracture and infundibular necrosis with periapical abscessation.

A permanent opening to the exterior may be the result of trauma involving extensive loss of bone or may be an indication of previous surgery. Facial trauma or previous surgery may occasionally result in a residual septic focus with osteomyelitis or a sequestrum and a draining tract.

DIAGNOSIS

Useful diagnostic procedures include visual examination, percussion, radiology, rhinoendoscopy, passage of a nasal tube, sinusoscopy, sinocentesis, and oral examination. In most cases sinus disease is unilateral and the normal side can be used for comparison with the affected side. Visual examination will detect any facial deformity. Percussion with or without auscultation helps detect space-occupying fluid or tissue masses by virtue of loss of the normal resonance. Radiography is an indispensable diagnostic aid. The value of the technique is enhanced if lateral, oblique, and ventrodorsal projections are obtained to ensure visualization of teeth, medial expansion of the ventral conchal sinus, and the presence of fluid lines. Fluid lines are best identified when the horse is standing.

Rhinoendoscopy will demonstrate, in the middle nasal meatus, exudate that has come from the nasomaxillary apertures, and medial expansion of the ventral conchal sinus. Patency of a nasal passage is also tested by ease of passage of a tube into the pharynx. Sinusoscopy may occasionally be useful if the examiner's vision is not obscured by blood, exudate, or tissue masses. Sinocentesis reveals the presence of fluid and provides a sample for laboratory identification of organisms and their sensitivity to antimicrobial agents (see *Current Therapy in Equine Medicine 2*, p. 606). Oral examination is used to check dental abnormalities such as fractures, infundibular necrosis, or loose or missing teeth.

TRAUMATIC DISORDERS

Acute trauma is usually accompanied by hemorrhage into the sinus(es) with epistaxis and, depending on severity, fracture of the bones overlying the sinuses. Fractures may be open or closed and may involve localized penetrating wounds or depression of facial bones. Dyspnea may be present if the nasal passages have been injured. Management of the acute case will depend on the extent of the injury but may include the establishment of a patent airway by temporary tracheostomy or nasal intubation, restoration of facial contour by elevation of depressed bone fragments, removal of loose bone fragments, immobilization of loose fragments by interfragmentary wiring, catheterization of the nasolacrimal duct to ensure patency to the nasal cavity or drainage into the sinus, and antimicrobial therapy. Surgery may require local or general anesthesia.

The clinical signs of chronic trauma include facial deformity, a defect in the wall of the sinus, epiphora, and purulent nasal discharge from residual sinus infection, osteomyelitis, or bone sequestrae. Suture line periostitis usually regresses over a period of years as a result of remodeling and seldom requires removal of the exostosis. Depression fractures may be treated by refracture and elevation or, more easily, by augmentation with carbon fiber or silicone. Residual infection is managed by exploration (see below) and removal of septic foci. Defects in the wall of the sinus require primary closure, which may involve grafting and skin expansion techniques if the defect is large.

SINUSITIS

Sinusitis is usually unilateral and tends to occur in horses 4 to 10 years old. It has a dental origin in approximately 50 per cent of cases, most frequently involving the third or fourth cheek teeth. Sinusitis is usually accompanied by accumulation of exudate within the sinus system (empyema), because the slitlike nasomaxillary openings are not capable of draining thick or inspissated exudate.

CLINICAL SIGNS

The main clinical sign is a unilateral purulent exudate. Chronic cases may be accompanied by facial deformity and epiphora. Dental involvement may cause halitosis, painful mastication, and localized swelling.

DIAGNOSIS

The presence of fluid within the sinuses is confirmed by sinocentesis and radiography. Radiography also allows identification of dental involvement. Aspiration of fluid is necessary for identification of cellular contents, and microorganisms and their antibiotic sensitivity. Aspiration is best done through a small hole made with a bone drill or Steinman pin. Because of intersinus communication it is usual to drill first into the caudal maxillary sinus. Depending on the integrity of the septum between the maxillary sinuses, access to the rostral maxillary sinus may also be necessary (see *Current Therapy in Equine Medicine 1*, p. 483). Trephination provides larger access but is not necessary for diagnosis.

THERAPY

The two most important aspects of successful treatment are control of the primary cause and establishment of adequate drainage between the sinuses and the nasal passage. Use of antibiotics without surgical treatment is virtually useless, although temporary control of nasal discharge is usually achieved. Access to the sinuses for examination, debridement, lavage, or dental repulsion is achieved with trephination or bone flap elevation. The choice of technique depends on the necessary exposure; both can be used to access maxillary and frontal sinuses. Thickened mucosa containing microabscesses should be removed as completely as possible. If drainage into the nasal passage is inadequate, it should be improved by the creation of an opening in the medial wall of the ventral conchal sinus. This can be done from either the nasal or sinus side. Inspissated exudate can lodge in poorly drained parts of the sinus system, particularly the ventral conchal sinus, from which it should be removed, if necessary by penetrating the bone plate ventral to the infraorbital canal. Removal of one or more teeth leaves a patent alveolus, which should be plugged with gauze or an acrylic while granulation tissue forms.

Postoperative sinus care consists of twice daily lavage with a balanced electrolyte solution, mild antiseptic, or plain water if there is excessive exudate and debris. Lavage is continued until the discharge is clear. Antimicrobial therapy is indicated if there is infection of bone and soft tissues or dental involvement, otherwise lavage with adequate drainage is satisfactory.

The prognosis is always guarded, particularly for primary sinusitis and whenever chronic infection is present.

CYSTIC SINUS DISEASE

The etiology and pathogenesis of cystic sinus disease are not known with certainty. The condition is characterized by accumulation of fluid within one or more of the sinuses and gradual enlargment of the sinus system, resulting in facial distortion and dyspnea. Frequently an obvious cyst is present, but sometimes there is no evidence of a cystic membrane, thus indicating that the fluid may accumulate because of outflow obstruction. Cysts sometimes appear to originate in dental structures, but they may also originate in mucosal or submucosal sites in the sinuses, usually the maxillary sinus.

Clinical Signs

Facial deformity, dyspnea, and nasal discharge are the main signs. Most cases are unilateral, with the right and left sides affected in an equal number of cases. There is no sex predisposition. Horses of any age may be affected, from young foals suspected of having congenital cysts to aged horses. Epiphora is sometimes present.

Diagnosis

The diagnosis is based on clinical signs and findings on sinocentesis and radiography. Fluid obtained by sinocentesis is usually amber and relatively clear; in uninfected cases it has an unremarkable cellular population. Radiographic findings may include sinus opacification, fluid lines, thickening of sinus walls, deviation of the nasal septum and displacement of the ventral conchal sinus, flattening and distortion of affected teeth, and soft tissue mineralization.

Therapy

Treatment entails surgical exposure of the sinus cavity to allow thorough removal of the cyst and restoration of adequate nasomaxillary drainage. This is best done with a bone flap sinusotomy. Whenever possible, all remnants of the cyst and its capsule should be removed to minimize the possibility of recurrence. Postoperative management includes sinus lavage through a trephine hole or preferably through an indwelling system placed during surgery. Antibiotic use is indicated if preexisting infection is present. A favorable outcome can be expected if treatment is carried out before there has been extensive distortion of tissues and involvement of teeth.

NEOPLASIA

Neoplasia of the paranasal sinuses typically occurs in older horses. It is characterized by an insidious onset, a protracted clinical course, and a poor prognosis.

Clinical Signs

The first sign is usually a unilateral mucopurulent nasal discharge containing variable amounts of blood. Enlargement of the neoplasm may be accompanied by bulging of facial bones, encroachment on nasal passages with subsequent dyspnea, and obstruction of the nasolacrimal duct. If invasion occurs into adjacent structures there may also be ocular, dental, and neurological disturbances.

Diagnosis

A blood-stained nasal discharge with development of facial deformity and dyspnea is strongly suggestive of sinus neoplasia. Sinocentesis may allow identification of cell type. Radiography is useful in revealing tissue masses in the sinuses and destruction and displacement of bone. If obstruction is present there will be a fluid accumulation in the sinuses with opacification and fluid lines. Neoplasms likely to be encountered reflect the variety of tissues normally found in the sinuses and are most likely to be malignant, although metastasis is rare. Reported neoplasms originate from soft tissue, cartilage, and bone.

Therapy

Treatment is often palliative but is rarely successful because of the malignant nature of most of the lesions and because of the advanced stage of disease at the time of diagnosis. Successful therapy requires removal or destruction of the neoplasm, which is rarely possible. Cryosurgery and, where available, irradiation are useful methods of destroying residual neoplastic tissue. The prognosis is very poor.

Supplemental Readings

Boles, C.: Treatment of upper airway abnormalities. Vet. Clin. North Am. (Large Anim. Pract.), 1:127, 1979.
Boulton, C. H.: Equine nasal cavity and paranasal sinus disease. J. Equine Vet Sci., 5:268, 1985.
Lane, J. G., Gibbs, C., Meynink, S. E., and Steele, F. C.: Radiographic examination of the facial, nasal and paranasal sinus regions of the horse: I. Indications and procedures in 235 cases. Equine Vet. J., 19:466, 1987.
Lane, J. G., Longstaffe, J. A., and Gibbs, C.: Equine paranasal sinus cysts: A report of 15 cases. Equine Vet. J., 19:537, 1987.
Madewell, B. R., Priester, W. A., Gillette, E. L., and Snyder, S. P.: Neoplasms of the nasal passages and paranasal sinuses in domesticated animals as reported by 13 veterinary colleges. Am. J. Vet. Res., 37:851, 1976.
Mason, B. J. E.: Empyema of the equine paranasal sinuses. J. Am. Vet. Med. Assoc., 167:727, 1975.

Ethmoidal Hematoma

William A. Lindsay, MADISON, WISCONSIN

The ethmoid turbinates are paired structures located on the floor of each frontal sinus. For unknown reasons, encapsulated hematomas may arise from the area of the ethmoid labyrinth. These may be discrete polyps or large expansile masses that involve the frontal sinus, the sphenopalatine sinus, the maxillary sinuses, or the nasal cavity. This lesion has no counterpart in other species, and the etiology remains unknown. One hypothesis is that the hematoma may form following trauma inflicted by a nasogastric tube.

The most frequent initial sign is intermittent, unilateral epistaxis while the horse is at rest. The amount of blood present at the nostril is never life-threatening, usually just a trickle. With time, the unilateral epistaxis may become persistent, but the volume is never excessive. If the hematoma enlarges, there may be obstruction to air flow, facial distortion, coughing, and choking.

This condition does not occur frequently. In a survey of 235 horses referred for radiography of the facial area and paranasal sinuses, ethmoidal hematoma was diagnosed in 10 cases. There appears to be no predilection for the left or right side. Bilateral ethmoidal hematoma is rare.

CLINICAL SIGNS AND DIAGNOSIS

Ethmoidal hematoma is suspected in a horse with unilateral epistaxis and is confirmed by direct endoscopic observation. During endoscopy, it is advisable to observe the architecture of the normal ethmoidal labyrinth before examining the affected side. An abnormal mass of inconsistent size and shape is often seen when the endoscope is placed in the middle meatus. The mass is usually well encapsulated and characteristically a greenish to black color. The mucosa may be ulcerated in some areas, permitting the escape of blood.

Radiography is an important diagnostic aid, although in the early stages the abnormal roentgen signs may be subtle. A lateral projection with the beam centered at the medial canthus of the eye may be obtained using portable equipment. Radiography is extremely helpful in determining the extent of the ethmoidal hematoma and any involvement of adjacent paranasal sinuses. Abnormal roentgen signs have been observed in a significant number of affected horses. The hematoma will cause alterations in soft tissue densities of the ethmoid turbinate area.

A biopsy specimen may be obtained either transendoscopically or via a trephine hole made in the frontal sinus. Additionally, an arthroscope or flexible pediatric endoscope may be introduced into the frontal or caudal maxillary sinuses to assist the clinician in obtaining a biopsy specimen.

Conditions to be excluded when nasal hematoma is a consideration include nasal trauma or nasal foreign body, nasal polyps, ulcerative rhinitis, fungal infection of the nasal passages, necrosis of the turbinate bones, epistaxis originating from the lower respiratory tract, neoplasia of paranasal sinus, and mycotic infection of the guttural pouch.

THERAPY

Surgical removal of an ethmoidal hematoma is recommended. The use of a wire snare, passed through the ventral meatus, has been reported as a method of removing a discrete hematoma attached by a pedicle. Most frequently a bone flap must be created in the frontal or nasal bone. Preoperative radiographs are critical in determining both the location and dimensions of this flap. Because considerable blood loss is likely to occur during surgery, a preoperative hemogram and clotting profile are recommended. A suitable blood donor should be readily available.

After a bone flap of adequate size has been created, the margins of the ethmoidal hematoma are delineated. Placement of a gauze bandage through the flap, into the nasal cavity and exiting at the nostril, prior to dissection is advisable. The ensuing dissection of the hematoma is blunt and must be accomplished as completely and quickly as possible. The cavity is packed with gauze to control hemorrhage and the packing is removed gradually during the first postoperative week. Moderate bleeding following removal of the pack is common. Cryosurgery has been reported to be an effective method of reducing intraoperative blood loss. Small ethmoidal hematomas appear to be ideal candidates for laser therapy.

Complications during surgery are related to blood loss: systemic hypotension may predispose to cardiac arrhythmias and postanesthetic myopathy. A 40 per cent prevalence of hematoma recurrence following surgery has been reported. There are also reports of successful 2- and 3-year follow-ups. In two diagnosed cases the horses received no treatment and the clinical signs remained static over several years of follow-up.

Supplemental Readings

Cook, W. R., and Littlewort, M. C. G.: Progressive haematoma of the ethmoid region in the horse. Equine Vet. J., 6:101, 1974.

Etherington, W. G., Vasey, J. R., and Horney, F. D.: Ethmoid hematoma of the equine. Can. Vet. J., 23:231–234, 1982.

Hanselka, D. V., and Young, M. F.: Ethmoidal hematoma in the horse. Vet. Med. (Small Anim. Clin.), 70:1289, 1975.

McIlwraith, C. W., and Turner, A. S.: Equine Surgery: Advanced Techniques. Philadephia, Lea & Febiger, 1987, pp. 244–246.

Platt, H.: Haemorrhagic nasal polyps of the horse. J. Vet. Pathol., 115:51, 1975.

Specht, T. E., Colahan, P. T., Nixon, A. J., et al.: Ethmoidal hematoma in nine horses. J. Am. Vet. Med. Assoc. 197:613–616, 1990.

Diseases of the Guttural Pouches

Dan L. Hawkins, GAINESVILLE, FLORIDA

The guttural pouches are paired, ventral diverticula of the auditory tubes. They are thought to help in equalization of air pressure across the tympanic membrane. The pouches are located beneath the base of the cranium and atlas and oppose each other medially. They are dorsal to the nasopharynx and are bounded laterally by the vertical rami of the mandible and parotid salivary glands. The floor of each pouch is reflected over the stylohyoid bone, which serves to divide the pouch into medial and lateral compartments. The average volume of each pouch is about 300 ml, the lateral compartment representing about one-third the volume. The pouches are lined with ciliated epithelium that contains principally mucous glands. Contained within the wall of or in close apposition to the guttural pouch are the internal maxillary, external carotid, maxillary, and linguofacial arteries and various veins. In addition, there are cranial nerves VII and IX through XII, the cranial cervical ganglion, sympathetic and cranial laryngeal nerves as well as retropharyngeal lymph nodes. Each pouch communicates with the pharynx through a slitlike opening in the caudodorsal part of the lateral wall of the pharynx just below the level of the choanae. Internally, both sides of the opening are covered by folds of mucous membrane (medial and lateral laminae of the eustachian tubes) that aid the control of air flow in and out of the pouch. These membranous folds permit air to enter the guttural pouches during expiration and swallowing, with subsequent emptying during inspiration.

TYMPANY

CLINICAL SIGNS AND DIAGNOSIS

Tympany of the guttural pouches is generally diagnosed on the basis of the anamnesis and physical examination. Individuals with tympany may present from birth to approximately 18 months of age. Fillies are affected twice as frequently as colts. Nonpainful tympanic swelling of the parotid region that resonates on percussion is a conspicuous clinical sign. The problem is usually unilateral but can be bilateral. Most cases are characterized by stertorous breathing and dyspnea; in addition there may be milk in the nostrils, coughing, nasal discharge, aspiration pneumonia, or dysphagia. Mildly affected animals may be bright, alert, and afebrile, with normal pulse and respiratory rate; however, an increase in activity may elicit signs of upper airway obstruction.

Paracentesis by means of a needle and decompression can be used to determine whether the right, left, or both pouches are involved. If the parotid distention does not completely disappear after paracentesis of the affected side, then the problem is bilateral. Alternatively, catheterization through the nasopharyngeal orifice can be used diagnostically and to relieve the condition pending treatment if the catheter is secured in place. Endoscopy is used to evaluate upper airway distortion, to identify the origin of nasal discharge, and to guide catheter placement. Radiography will help verify the diagnosis, reveal the presence of a fluid line in the affected pouch and demonstrate any secondary pulmonary disease.

ETIOLOGY AND PATHOGENESIS

Tympany of the guttural pouches is thought to develop secondarily to a congenital defect in the lateral mucosal fold of the nasopharyngeal orifice. Functionally or structurally it acts as a one-way valve, permitting air to enter the pouch but not escape. Folds of restricting tissue, redundant plica salpingopharyngea, and excessive mucous membrane attached to the medial lamina of the auditory tube are some of the structural abnormalities that have been noted. Frequently there are no gross abnormalities present at the orifice. Empyema may be present in some cases, presumably due to impairment of normal clearance of pouch secretions.

THERAPY

Conservative management of tympany of the guttural pouches has been unsuccessful. A surgical approach through Viborg's triangle (outlined by the vertical ramus of the mandible, the sternocephalicus tendon, and the linguofacial vein) affords the best visualization of the laminae covering the pharyngeal orifice on the inside of the guttural pouch. Establishing communication between both pouches by fenestration of the medial septum and resection of the medial lamina are the two procedures that are done separately or in combination. For unilateral involvement, each procedure has worked when used alone; however, I prefer to use both procedures in combination. For bilateral tympany, a combination of the two should be used. With unilateral tympany, resection of the medial lamina should permit escape of air that enters the pouch, provided there is no postoperative scarring. Fenestration of the medial septum ensures equalization of air pressure in both pouches by allowing air to escape through the opposite, normal pharyngeal orifice. Use of both procedures improves the chances for a successful outcome in the event that either procedure fails. Even with these precautions, approximately one third of cases may recur, making a second surgery necessary.

The surgical wound may be left to heal by secondary intention, in which case the pouch is lavaged daily with an appropriate, nonirritating antibiotic solution until the wound has sealed, approximately 10 to 14 days later. If the pouch appears healthy at surgery, primary closure may be considered. If pulmonary disease is present, additional systemic antibiotic therapy should be administered after a tracheal wash sample has been obtained for culture and sensitivity testing.

The prognosis is usually good after surgical treatment of a unilateral problem. If resection of the membranous flap is performed or if the disease is bilateral, there is a greater chance for recurrence. The presence of pneumonia or other complications changes the prognosis to guarded or poor, depending on the severity.

EMPYEMA

CLINICAL SIGNS AND DIAGNOSIS

The diagnosis of guttural pouch empyema should be considered in any horse with a chronic mucopurulent nasal discharge. Although the discharge may be bilateral, it is generally more profuse on the affected side. Pharyngitis, a frequent sequela of guttural pouch empyema, may result in coughing, dorsal displacement of the soft palate, or decreased exercise tolerance. External swelling is generally not seen in mild cases. Protracted, severe cases may be accompanied by nontympanic, painful swelling in the throat latch, the head carried lower and more extended than normal, reluctance to turn the head, or dysphagia and pharyngeal paralysis.

The diagnosis of guttural pouch empyema may be confirmed with radiography, endoscopy, and catheterization. Lateral radiographs of the guttural pouches should show distention of the pouch, a fluid line in the pouch, or radiodense material in the case of inspissation or chondroids.

Pharyngeal endoscopy may demonstrate mucopurulent exudate coming from the pharyngeal opening of the guttural pouch, suggestive of guttural pouch empyema. This tentative diagnosis should be made with the understanding that both false negative and false positive results are possible. Exudate may not be seen at the pharyngeal orifice in some cases of inspissation. Conversely, cloudy mucus coming from the pharyngeal orifice in patients with pharyngitis may represent extension of the pharyngeal inflammation to the mucous membrane lining the guttural pouch, with no accumulation of fluid in the pouch (i.e., empyema). Passage of the endoscope through the pharyngeal orifice will permit visualization of the pouch and give the best assessment. One method of directing the endoscope into the pouch is to pass biopsy forceps through the channel of the endoscope and allow it to protrude several centimeters into the field of vision. The forceps is then introduced under the medial lamina of the orifice with endoscopic guidance and serves as a guide wire over which the endoscope can be threaded. Both pouches should be examined even if the disease appears to be unilateral.

Fluid is collected for culture and sensitivity testing by catheterization of the pouch or directing a needle through Viborg's triangle and aspirating a sample. If only a small amount of fluid is present, the pouch can be filled with a polyionic solution so that a lavage sample can be obtained. If the pouch is not distended, obtaining a sample percutaneously may be difficult.

Etiology and Pathogenesis

The mucous membrane lining the guttural pouches is probably involved in any viral or bacterial infection of the upper respiratory tract. Therefore, guttural pouch empyema is most frequently secondary to some other primary disease process. Generally, any accumulation of exudate during an acute infection is transient and resolves concurrently with resolution of the upper respiratory tract infection.

Chronic guttural pouch empyema is most frequently caused by β-haemolytic streptococcal infection of the upper respiratory tract. In the cases that become chronic, the inflammation is well established in the pouch mucous membranes, producing a persistent nasal discharge. Systemic antibiotics usually affect the discharge only temporarily. With streptococcal infections, adjacent retropharyngeal lymph nodes not uncommonly abscess and rupture into the pouch. Neoplasia, fungal granulomas, or any process that affects the natural outflow of the pouch may permit a secondary infection to become established as chronic empyema. The exudate in chronic cases that have not been treated will often become inspissated into the consistency of cottage cheese and will not drain. This material may change further into discrete concretions referred to as chondroids. It is the protracted, chronic cases that produce severe distention of the guttural pouches externally and collapse of the nasopharyngeal lumen, with attendant dyspnea and dysphagia.

Therapy

In acute, mild guttural pouch empyema, the upper respiratory tract disease and empyema may resolve in 7 to 14 days with systemic administration of appropriate antibiotics. If systemic therapy is inadequate or if the condition becomes chronic, repeated local irrigation is safe and effective, providing local treatment and drainage of exudate. Surgery is generally employed for the most severe cases, particularly when the consistency of the exudate hampers its removal by lavage.

Guttural pouches are treated locally by infusing solutions through indwelling catheters or catheters placed into the pouch intermittently. Each method has advantages and disadvantages. Both may traumatize the medial lamina of the orifice, and the use of indwelling catheters may induce tissue necrosis. The Chamber's mare catheter is commonly used for intermittent infusion. A No. 10 French polypropylene male canine urinary catheter can be made into an indwelling catheter by threading a stiff wire into it, bending the tip into a spiral, and heating it in boiling water for 5 minutes to reform the polypropylene. After cooling, the catheter with the wire inside is straightened and 3 to 4 cm of the tip is bent to a 30-degree angle to aid passage under the medial lamina of the orifice. Once in the pouch, the wire is removed and a small piece of tape is used as a butterfly on the flanged end to suture it to the nostril. Retaining intrauterine catheters with grapples that can be detached should be avoided for obvious reasons.

Infusion solutions and the treatment protocol used vary depending on the attending clinician's preference. Repeated irrigation helps evacuate exudate containing inflammatory cells, cellular debris, destructive enzymes, and inflammatory mediators that inhibit local defense mechanisms. However, irritating solutions should not be used, because they may induce further inflammation of the mucous membranes, resulting in increased production of exudate, which interferes with accurate evaluation of the clinical response. They may also cause pharyngeal dysfunction and other neurological complications by creating a local neuritis of cranial nerves associated with the pouches. If antibiotics or antiseptics are included in the solution, consideration should be given to their effectiveness in the prevailing pH of the medium and in the presence of exudate. Most treatment regimens call for either once or twice daily infusions of a 1-liter volume for approximately 7 days, followed by catheter removal and a rest period for evaluation of the clinical response. At the time of infusion the horse should keep its head down (sedation with xylazine may be necessary) to avoid aspiration of fluid into the trachea. Throughout the course of treatment and convalescence the horse should be fed off the ground to encourage drainage from the pouches.

The solution most commonly used to infuse guttural pouches has been 10 per cent (vol/vol) povidone-iodine in saline. Recent work demonstrated that this strength induced focal inflammatory infiltrates, hemorrhage, necrosis, and lymphoid reaction in normal guttural pouches. I prefer to use 5 per cent (vol/vol) povidone-iodine in saline, hypertonic saline, or buffered polyionic solution, depending on the severity of the case. I generally do not incorporate antibiotics into the solution because the added expense and short contact time make their use in this manner impractical. A more feasible approach is to either instill the appropriate antibiotic into the pouch after infusion and drainage or to use it systemically as adjunct therapy. Systemic use of the antibiotic results in higher tissue concentrations for longer time periods.

When medical and local treatment has not been successful, surgical drainage through Viborg's triangle or the Whitehouse (ventral) approach is indicated to ensure continued, complete drainage of exudate. The incision is allowed to heal by secondary intention and irrigation is directed through the external incision. Whenever the exudate is inspissated or chondroids have formed, surgery is indicated to remove the material and establish a means of irrigation and drainage. A distended pouch can be approached through Viborg's triangle in the standing horse. General anesthesia is necessary if the pouch is not distended or if the Whitehouse approach is elected. In horses with compression of the pharynx it is often necessary to maintain a Dyson tracheotomy tube in the trachea until the horse can safely breathe through the upper airway. If surgery under general anesthesia is elected, the anesthetic gas is administered via an endotracheal tube placed in the tracheotomy site. Although these approaches are straightforward, they should be done carefully and with proper respect for the important nerves and vessels in the guttural pouch walls. Treatment with systemic antibiotics should follow surgery for several days to control any infection that may have spread to the surrounding tissue during the surgery.

The prognosis following successful treatment of guttural pouch empyema is favorable if the condition is treated early and aggressively. Cases with inspissation also respond reasonably well to treatment unless there are complicating factors, such as permanent pharyngeal dysfunction or neoplasia. These changes then preclude a satisfactory outcome or may contribute to recurrence.

MYCOSIS

CLINICAL SIGNS AND DIAGNOSIS

The three most common signs of guttural pouch mycosis are epistaxis not induced by exercise, unilateral mucoid nasal discharge, and pharyngeal paresis (dysphagia). The condition usually affects mature horses but does occur in yearlings and has been seen in foals rarely. Epistaxis varies from a trickle of blood in one nostril to several liters during an episode. Typically a horse will have had one to several such episodes over a 2- or 3-week period before presentation or a fatal hemorrhage. Frequently a unilateral mucoid nasal discharge precedes the initial hemorrhage by several weeks. Approximately 50 per cent of horses with epistaxis due to guttural pouch mycosis will die if they are not treated.

Dysphagia is the second most common clinical sign noted with guttural pouch mycosis. It may develop before the initial epistaxis, acutely with an episode of epistaxis, gradually as the condition progresses, or during the healing phase of the disease. Some horses with dysphagia or other neurological signs may recover partially or entirely following treatment or spontaneous regression, depending on the extent of involvement of the affected nerve. Pulmonary disease secondary to pharyngeal dysfunction must be evaluated and considered in the overall prognosis.

Other secondary clinical signs have been reported less frequently as manifestations of guttural pouch mycosis. Some of these include parotid pain, abnormal head posture, head shyness or shaking, abnormal respiratory noise, Horner's syndrome, facial paralysis, and unilateral atrophy of the tongue muscles. The variety of these signs relates to invasion or scarring of important nerves in the affected guttural pouch.

Endoscopy of the pharynx and affected guttural pouch is the most important procedure used to diagnose and evaluate guttural pouch mycosis. The presence of food material on the mucous membranes of the pharynx, persistent dorsal displacement of the soft palate, and laryngeal hemiplegia generally indicate that pharyngeal paresis is present. Blood-tinged mucus may be seen exiting the pharyngeal orifice of the involved guttural pouch if a hemorrhagic episode has occurred recently. Although examination of the pouch may often be frustrating or unrewarding, due to the presence of clotted blood, extreme care should be exercised. Dislodging the clot by stressing the horse or trying to inspect the pouch may precipitate fatal hemorrhage. The fungal lesion itself may make the anatomy difficult to understand precisely in some cases. The dorsal roof of the medial compartment near the articulation of the stylohyoid bone with the petrous temporal bone is the most common location of the fungal lesion. In this location the lesion may overlie the internal carotid artery, the vagus (X) nerve, and the glossopharyngeal (IX) nerve. Another common site is the lateral wall of the lateral compartment in the area of the external carotid artery and its branches. Lesions may occur in more than one area within a pouch or may be bilateral. The size and color of the diphtheritic membrane may vary. It may appear as a black, yellow, brown, or white irregular mass firmly attached to the underlying tissue and covered with necrotic debris and clotted blood. These diphtheritic lesions have been noted as incidental findings on necropsy of horses not showing any clinical signs of guttural pouch mycosis. Pale scar tissue can be seen in the location of the previously diagnosed fungal lesion as early as 5 weeks following surgical treatment. Both guttural pouches should be examined even if the disease appears to be unilateral.

Other diagnostic procedures that can be done to further evaluate cases include radiography and angiography. Radiographs of the skull will reveal any secondary bony involvement. Angiography is used to identify specific arteries that are affected and to increase the examiner's confidence in the presurgical evaluation.

Etiology and Pathogenesis

Although a variety of fungal organisms have been isolated from diphtheritic lesions, *Aspergillus nidulans* has been incriminated most often. No bacterial species has been consistently isolated from the affected tissue. Organisms found associated with the lesions occur naturally in the environment of horses, and therefore the exact cause of the disease is not known. The lack of light, warmth, humidity, and poor ventilation of the guttural pouch interior are contributing factors promoting fungal growth. However, it is unknown what specific predisposing factors unite in individual cases to cause the development of guttural pouch mycosis with an opportunist organism like *Aspergillus nidulans*. Even more interesting is the reason why the mycelia invade such specific anatomical areas in the guttural pouches.

Histopathologic examination of the lesions has demonstrated fungal mycelia in highest density in the superficial layers and decreasing in numbers into the deeper parts of the lesion. Erosion of arterial walls results in aneurysm formation and rupture. The mycelia or the inflammatory response they evoke may also extend into the pharyngeal wall (creating a fistula) or into underlying bone, tendon tissue, or the median septum. Changes reported in affected cranial nerves range from slight swelling of the myelin sheaths and Schwann cells with dilation of intraneural vessels to penetration of nerve fibers with necrosis. It is presumed that horses with less severe neurological changes have the best chance of recovery from impaired neurological function. Nerves of the guttural pouch can be affected by mycelial invasion, submucosal extravasation associated with hemorrhagic episodes, or perineural fibrosis during the healing phase following treatment.

Therapy

Thrombosis of the involved arteries is probably the key to a successful outcome following surgical treatment, medical treatment, or spontaneous recovery. Treatment soley by local infusion or nebulization of antifungal agents is of questionable value and generally regarded as unsatisfactory. It is technically difficult to achieve significant contact time of the agent with the lesion on the roof of the medial compartment without endoscopic guidance at every treatment. It is unknown how well agents penetrate the superficial layer of mucus and necrotic tissue to affect underlying fungal growth. The response, if any, to medical treatment alone is viewed by many clinicians as too slow and uncertain to risk the possibility of a fatal hemorrhage. The fact that some horses do recover spontaneously without treatment makes evaluation of medical treatment difficult. In one study six horses with guttural pouch mycosis were treated surgically and received no medical therapy. All six recovered completely, and regression of the lesions was noted as early as 5 weeks after surgery. Generally, when local medical therapy is included in postoperative care, the consensus is that it may be beneficial and probably will not be harmful.

Transfusions of compatible whole blood and polyionic solutions should be used as supportive therapy as indicated in cases with recent hemorrhagic episodes. If daily local antifungal therapy is elected, it should be continued for 4 to 6 weeks, whether employed as the sole method of treatment or in conjunction with surgery. Several agents are active against mycelial fungi such as *Aspergillus nidulans*. Amphotericin B is only used systemically and is effective against *Aspergillus nidulans*. However, the expense and risks of serious toxic side effects make it unsuitable. Thiabendazole given orally twice daily at 10 to 20 mg per kg has been effective against *Aspergillus* in dogs. It has antifungal activity and is thought to stimulate the immune system.

The imidazole compounds have strong, broad-spectrum activity against mycelial fungi and other microbes. Ketoconazole is used orally at 10 mg per kg twice daily for *Aspergillus* infections in horses. This form of administration is expensive, but ketocanazole is the safest potent systemic antifungal agent available. Miconazole solutions (1 mg per ml) can be used to irrigate the pouch lining on a daily basis. Although econazole is more active against mycelial forms than miconazole and has good penetration, it is currently unavailable in a form suitable for infusion. Clotrimazole similarly cannot be formulated to be used topically in the guttural pouch.

Povidone–iodine in a 5 to 10 per cent solution (vol/vol) is fungicidal and has been used extensively in guttural pouch infusion. As an iodophor solution, there is minimal information about its efficacy against fungi growing in tissue, although it has good penetration. Natamycin is a good agent against mycelial fungi but poorly penetrates surface tissue. In addition, there may be some basis for using immunogenic products adjunctively.

The operative approaches currently used for guttural pouch mycosis are ligation of affected arteries on the cardiac (proximal) side of the lesion, or a combination of proximal ligation and arterial catheterization with a balloon-tipped catheter inserted on the distal side of the lesion. Basic to each approach is an accurate assessment of which arteries have lesions. That assessment may be very difficult, owing to poor visibility and anatomical distortion by the lesion and inflamed tissue. Of concern in the development of surgical procedures has been collateral blood flow through intracranial arterial channels into the circle of Willis, to which the internal and external carotid arteries connect. There is a risk that blood pressure in the circle of Willis may be sufficient to rupture an aneurysm if proximal ligation of the artery is the only surgical treatment. The clinical results of two published studies indicate that proximal ligation alone was satisfactory in 36 of 40 cases so treated. The second approach, utilizing the balloon-tipped catheter, is technically more demanding but probably a better method of treatment. Comparative studies of these two basic approaches have not been published. The reader is directed to the supplemental readings list for more specific information on the surgical treatment of guttural pouch mycosis and its historical development.

PROGNOSIS

If the diagnosis of guttural pouch mycosis is confirmed when there is only a unilateral mucoid discharge, the prognosis for a successful outcome is guarded with medical treatment or rest alone. Surgical treatment would help ensure a better prognosis. The presence of an aneurysmal lesion and epistaxis greatly increases the probability of fatal hemorrhage if the condition is not treated surgically soon after diagnosis. Accompanying neurological signs or pulmonary disease alter the overall prognosis, even with successful resolution of the guttural pouch mycosis lesion. Horner's syndrome or laryngeal hemiplegia do not necessarily affect the prognosis for life, but do affect the prospects for performance. The presence of dysphagia indicates a poor prognosis. Mycotic injury to the cranial nerves is rarely reversible, and affected animals frequently develop aspiration pneumonia. The recovery rate following even mild cases of dysphagia is no better than 25 to 35 per cent.

Supplemental Readings

Cook, W. R.: The clinical features of guttural pouch mycosis in the horse. Vet. Rec., 83:336, 1968.

Freeman, D. E.: Diagnosis and treatment of diseases of the guttural pouch: Part I. Compend. Cont. Ed. Pract. Vet., 2:S3, 1980.

Freeman, D. E.: Diagnosis and treatment of diseases of the guttural pouch: Part II. Compend. Cont. Ed. Pract. Vet., 2:S25, 1980.

Lane, J. G.: The management of guttural pouch mycosis. Equine Vet. J., 21:321, 1989.

McCue, P. M., Freeman, D. E., and Donawick, W. J.: Guttural pouch tympany: 15 cases (1977–1986). J. Am. Vet. Med. Assoc., 194:1761, 1989.

Epiglottic Entrapment and Cysts

R. Stuart Shoemaker, BATON ROUGE, LOUISIANA
Peter F. Haynes, BATON ROUGE, LOUISIANA

EPIGLOTTIC ENTRAPMENT

Epiglottic entrapment is characterized by envelopment of the rostral epiglottis and its margins by subepiglottic tissue and arytenoepiglottic folds. The etiology of epiglottic entrapment is not well understood. Although a congenitally hypoplastic epiglottis may predispose to epiglottic entrapment, entrapment may also occur as an acquired event in adult horses with a normal-sized epiglottis.

CLINICAL SIGNS

The clinical signs of epiglottic entrapment are variable and may include exercise intolerance, abnormal respiratory noise, and coughing during eating or exercise. Affected patients are usually asymptomatic at rest and occasionally asymptomatic during exercise. Entrapment may be associated with dorsal displacement of the soft palate, particularly when the epiglottis is short.

Endoscopic examination of the nasopharynx is usually diagnostic. The serrated margins and fine vascular pattern of the epiglottis are hidden by the entrapping tissue, which may be ulcerated and must be distinguished from palate displacement and epiglottic ulceration. Chronic entrapment may predispose to secondary malformation or shortening of the epiglottis. Although epiglottic entrapment is usually persistent, the diagnosis of intermittent entrapment may require sequential endoscopy at rest and following exercise.

Lateral radiographics of the nasopharynx should be considered to further characterize the epiglottis and epiglottic entrapment. An epiglottis that is less than 75 per cent of normal length is likely to also be associated with palate displacement, thus reducing the prognosis for full recovery following surgical treatment of entrapment.

THERAPY

Epiglottic entrapment is managed by surgical release of the entrapping tissue from the epiglottis. The operation entails conventional ventral laryngotomy, identification and stabilization of the entrapping tissue, and axial transection of the entrapping tissue to the epiglottic apex. The incisions are generally left to heal by secondary intention. Exercise may be resumed in 4 to 5 weeks, when the ventral laryngotomy incision has healed.

Other recently described surgical methods for management of entrapment include transnasal electrosurgical division, transnasal or transoral division with a hooked bistoury, and transnasal division with the neodymium:yttrium-aluminum-garnet laser (see p. 294). Potential complications of the hooked bistoury technique in the standing horse, such as iatrogenic soft palate division, can be reduced by providing short-term general anesthesia.

Perioperative therapy may include tetanus toxoid, nonsteroidal anti-inflammatory agents, and antimicrobials.

The prognosis for return to function following surgery for epiglottic entrapment is related to epiglottic length and is good when the epiglottis is of adequate length. Epiglottic malformation or hypoplasia or secondary palate displacement suggest a guarded to poor prognosis.

SUBEPIGLOTTIC CYSTS

Subepiglottic cysts are relatively uncomon in the horse. It is speculated that they are the congenital remnants of the thyroglossal duct. Alternatively, they may be of inflammatory or traumatic origin.

Clinical signs of upper respiratory obstruction often are not recognized until the horse is placed into training. However, abnormal respiratory noise, coughing, choking, dysphagia, pneumonia, and respiratory distress have been observed in foals.

The diagnosis is established by nasopharyngeal endoscopic visualization of a space-occupying mass ventral to the epiglottis. Occasionally the cyst may be hidden under the soft palate; however, repeated stimulation of the swallow reflex and nasopharyngeal radiography should permit an accurate diagnosis to be made.

Management of subepiglottic cysts entails surgical extirpation via a ventral laryngotomy. The epiglottis is retroflexed into the larynx to allow access to the cyst, and the cyst is carefully dissected from the subepiglottic mucosa. The mucosa is usually allowed to heal by secondary intention.

Postoperative care consists of tetanus toxoid, nonsteroidal anti-inflammatory drugs, and antimicrobials.

The prognosis following surgical removal of subepiglottic cysts is good. Complications following extensive subepiglottic mucosal resection may include cicatrix formation and abnormal epiglottic function.

Supplemental Readings

Boles, C. L., Raker, C. W., and Wheat, J. D.: Epiglottic entrapment by arytenoepiglottic folds in the horse. J. Am. Vet. Med. Assoc., 172:338, 1978.

Haynes, P. F.: Dorsal displacement of the soft palate and epiglottic entrapment: Diagnosis, management, and interrelationship. Compend. Cont. Ed. Pract. Vet., 5:S379, 1983.

Honnas, C. M., and Wheat, J. D.: Epiglottic entrapment: A transnasal surgical approach to divide the aryepiglottic fold axially in the standing horse. Vet. Surg., 17:246, 1989.

Koch, D. B., and Tate, L. P.: Pharyngeal cysts in horses. J. Am. Vet. Med. Assoc., 173:860, 1978.

Linford, R. L., O'Brien, T. R., et al.: Radiographic assessment of epiglottic length and pharyngeal and laryngeal diameters in the Thoroughbred. Am. J. Vet. Res., 44:1660, 1983.

Pharyngeal Lymphoid Hyperplasia and Pharyngeal Stricture

R. Stuart Shoemaker, BATON ROUGE, LOUISIANA

Peter F. Haynes, BATON ROUGE, LOUISIANA

PHARYNGEAL LYMPHOID HYPERPLASIA

Pharyngeal lymphoid hyperplasia, often referred to as pharyngitis or follicular hyperplasia, is a nasopharyngeal condition characterized by an increased size and occasionally coalition of the normal lymphoid follicle distribution. The condition is most frequently observed in horses 2 to 3 years old. Its contribution to clinical signs, including exercise intolerance and abnormal respiratory noise, remains unanswered. Nasopharyngeal lymphoid follicles are normal in young horses and regress with age, usually disappearing by 4 to 5 years of age. It is suggested that pharyngeal lymphoid hyperplasia may be enhanced by exposure to one or more of the respiratory viruses.

Recognition of pharyngeal lymphoid hyperplasia is established by endoscopic examination of the nasopharynx. A grading scale from 1 (mild) to 4 (severe) has been described. It has been suggested that pharyngeal lymphoid hyperplasia may contribute to pharyngeal pain and dorsal displacement of the soft palate.

Pharyngeal lymphoid hyperplasia remains very controversial, since its contribution to clinical disease is unclear. Treatment may be initiated in advanced cases and may include topical nasopharyngeal therapy, such as corticosteroids, dimethyl sulfoxide, glycerine, and antimicrobials (see *Current Therapy in Equine Medicine 2*, p. 610), frequent and repeated vaccination against equine influenza and rhinopneumonitis, (e.g., at 60- to 90-day intervals), systemic immunotherapy, topical cryogen application, and electrocautery.

Clinical impressions suggest that the extent of pharyngeal lymphoid hyperplasia may be reduced by early recognition and frequent use of respiratory vaccines. Associated disorders, including dorsal displacement of the soft palate, frequently resolve without therapy following resolution of the pharyngitis.

NASOPHARYNGEAL CICATRIX

Nasopharyngeal cicatrix has been reported in horses of all ages, sex, and breed. It is characterized by a stricturing web of tissue in the wall of the nasopharynx. Cicatrices may be transverse, circumferential, or hemicircumferential and may involve the dorsal nasopharynx and soft palate. Transverse cicatrices are most commonly located on a plane through the guttural pouch openings and the epiglottis. Longitudinal cicatrices have also been reported on the dorsal pharyngeal wall. Additional nasopharyngeal and laryngeal abnormalities, including arytenoid chondritis, laryngeal hemiplegia, epiglottic entrapment, and guttural pouch empyema, have been associated with nasopharyngeal cicatrices.

Although severe generalized ulcerating nasopharyngeal inflammation has been suggested as a potential cause, the precise etiology is unknown. Clinical signs of nasopharyngeal cicatrix are similar to those of other upper respiratory abnormalities and include exercise intolerance, abnormal respiratory noise, and abnormal vocalization.

Nasopharyngeal cicatrix is diagnosed by endoscopic examination. A detailed examination of the nasopharynx to identify other abnormalities is essential.

Specific therapy for cicatrices has not been reported, though ablation with the neodymium:yttrium-aluminum-garnet laser or electrosurgical excision of the constricting tissue may be considered.

Supplemental Readings

Cook, W. R.: Some observations on form and function of the equine upper airway in health and disease I. The pharynx. *In*: Proceedings of the 27th Annual Convention of the American Association of Equine Practitioners, 1981, pp. 335–392.

Raker, C. W., and Boles, C. L.: Pharyngeal lymphoid hyperplasia in the horse. J. Equine Med. Surg. 2:202, 1978.

Schumacher, J., and Hanselka, D. V.: Nasopharyngeal cicatrices in horses: 47 cases (1972–1985). J. Am. Vet. Med. Assoc., *191*:239, 1987.

Dynamic Pharyngeal Collapse

Normand G. Ducharme, ITHACA, NEW YORK

Abnormal respiratory noise (stridor) is a common problem in horses. Noise may be the only abnormality or it may be accompanied by exercise intolerance, a problem that may seriously interfere with the usefulness of horses for strenuous competitions such as racing and jumping. There are numerous causes of abnormal respiratory noise in horses. Endoscopy provides a ready diagnosis of most diseases that cause abnormal noise by inducing changes in upper respiratory tract morphology. Diseases such as laryngeal hemiplegia, subepiglottic cyst, epiglottic entrapment, and arytenoid chondritis are examples of such disorders. In other cases, the soft palate is seen dorsad to the epiglottic cartilage, leading to a diagnosis of soft palate displacement. In many horses with stridor, however, endoscopic examination in the resting animal reveals no overt abnormalities. In such cases, diagnosis of the cause of noise is speculative at best and endoscopic examination while the horse is exercising is indicated. With the advent of the high-speed treadmill and video endoscopy, treadmill endoscopy has become an acceptable diagnostic modality. During such examinations we have observed three abnormalities that we term dynamic pharyngeal collapse: dorsal displacement of the soft palate, unilateral or bilateral ventral displacement of the roof of the nasopharynx, and dorsal displacement of the epiglottis (Fig. 1).

DORSAL DISPLACEMENT OF THE SOFT PALATE

Unlike the majority of the upper respiratory tract, which is supported by a bony or cartilaginous framework, the nasopharynx is most susceptible to functional airway obstruction during exercise. Dorsal displacement of the soft palate has long been recognized as a source of functional pharyngeal obstruction in exercising horses (*see* Fig. 1A). The extent of this problem is uncertain, but it has been estimated that 1 per cent of horses have "soft palate paresis" (a term often used interchangeably with dorsal displacement of the soft palate). Others consider that the soft palate contributes to the clinical signs in a large percentage of horses with respiratory obstruction during exercise. The recent development of techniques allowing endoscopic examination of horses as they exercise on a high-speed treadmill has allowed diagnosis of intermittent dorsal displacement of the soft palate during exercise. Therefore the diagnosis of "choking down" can now be made more precisely. In exercising horses, we have observed dorsal displacement of the soft palate in four different circumstances: during expiration, during inspiration, induced by swallowing, and induced by coughing. We have also observed that the larynx moves craniocaudally during exercise, with the

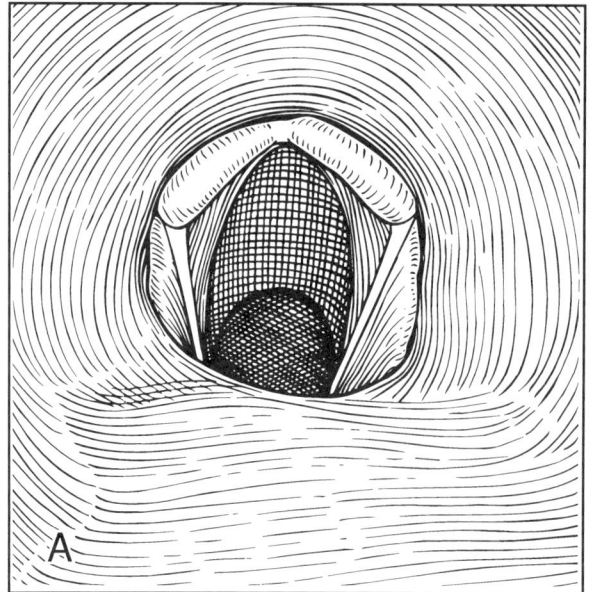
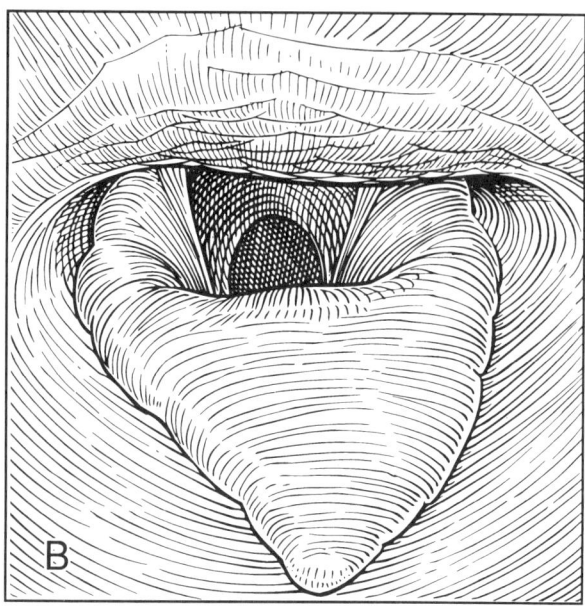
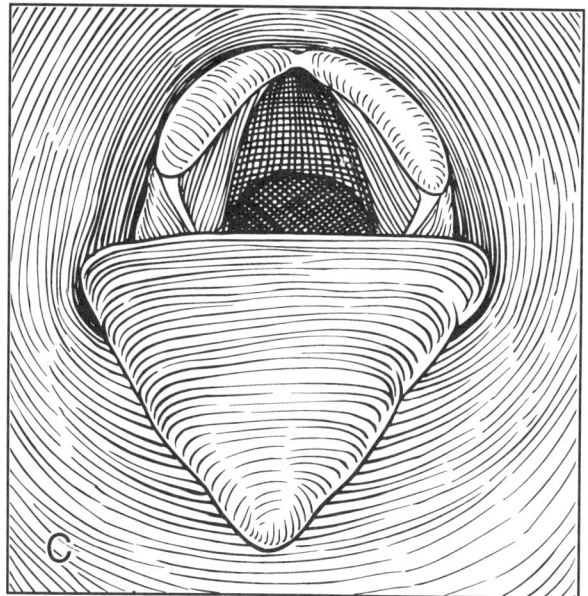

Figure 1. (*A*) Dorsal displacement of the soft palate during inspiration in an exercising horse. The epiglottis is hidden by the soft palate. (*B*) Ventral displacement of the roof of the nasopharynx late in the phase of expiration in an exercising horse. The arytenoid cartilages are hidden by the roof of the pharynx. (*C*) Dorsal displacement of the epiglottis in midinspiration in an exercising horse.

larynx displacing caudally in relation to the nasopharynx during expiration rather than during inspiration as in humans. We believe that this movement reflects the extension of the head as the front limbs make contact with the ground and the horse expires. Whether caudal traction is exerted on the larynx, associated with contraction of the strap muscles during inspiration, is unknown at this time.

This leads to the hypothesis that dorsal displacement of the soft palate may result from various abnormalities, and therefore no uniform treatment will be successful. Intermittent dorsal displacement of the soft palate may be divided into five types. Type I is due to an inappropriate laryngopalatal seal, allowing air to reach the ventral surface of the soft palate and displace it dorsally during expiration. Staphylectomy may be appropriate in these cases. Type II is observed during inspiration, perhaps as a result of caudal traction by the strap muscles, or perhaps because of increased negative pressure or increased pharyngeal compliance. Strap muscle resection may be appropriate in these horses. Type III is associated with the action of the root of the tongue. Limiting poll flexion or tongue tie is indicated in these horses. Type IV is a result of increased pressure or velocity of air flow in the pharynx associated with coughing. Treatment of the lower airway or tracheal irritation is appropriate. Type V is associated with malformation of the epiglottis (short, flaccid, narrow) requiring Teflon augmentation procedures.

VENTRAL DISPLACEMENT OF THE ROOF OF THE NASOPHARYNX

Unilateral or bilateral pharyngeal collapse has been observed in several horses exercising on a high-speed treadmill. These horses were seen for evaluation of upper respiratory noise. In most horses the roof of the nasopharynx obstructs the view of the dorsal aspect of the arytenoid cartilage without apparent obstruction of the rima glottidis. At this time we feel that this is a normal finding in exercising horses. However, in some horses, one to two thirds of the rima glottidis is obstructed by the roof of the nasopharynx, suggesting a functional obstruction (see Fig. 1B). The nasopharynx descends at the end of expiration and early in inspiration. The ventral displacement is bilateral in most horses. We know of no specific treatment for this condition.

DORSAL DISPLACEMENT OF THE EPIGLOTTIS

We have observed this abnormality in a few horses referred for upper respiratory noise during exercise. The displacement of the epiglottis results in obstruction of approximately half of the rima glottidis (see Fig. 1C). This obstruction occurs in the mid-phase of inspiration. We hypothesize that it is a result of either increased negative pressure in the nasopharynx or rostral displacement of the epiglottis (and larynx).

Supplemental Readings

Anderson, L. J.: Problems of the equine larynx and pharynx. NZ Vet. J., 25:387–388, 1977.

Cook, W. R.: The diagnosis of respiratory unsoundness in the horse. Vet. Rec., 77:516–528, 1976.

Cook, W. R.: Diseases of the auditive tube diverticulum (guttural pouch). In Robinson, N. E. (ed.): Current Therapy in Equine Medicine 2. Philadelphia, W. B. Saunders, 1987, pp. 612–618.

Cook, W. R.: Some observations on form and function of the equine upper airway in health and disease: I. The pharynx. In: Proceedings of the 27th Annual Convention of the American Association of Equine Practitioners, 1981, pp. 355–391.

Freeman, D. E.: Diagnosis and treatment of diseases of the guttural pouch: Part I. Compend. Cont. Ed. Pract. Vet., 2:S3–S11, 1980.

Goulden, B. E., Anderson, L. J., Davies, A. S., and Barnes, G. R. G.: Rostral displacement of the palatopharyngeal arch: A case report. Equine Vet. J., 8:85–98, 1976.

Haynes, P. F.: Dorsal displacement of the soft palate and epiglottic entrapment: Diagnosis, management, and interrelationship. Compend. Cont. Ed. Pract. Vet., 5(7):S379–S389, 1983.

Haynes, P. F.: Obstructive disease of the upper respiratory tract: Current thoughts on diagnosis and surgical management. In: Proceedings of the 32nd Annual Convention of the American Association of Equine Practitioners, 1986, pp. 283–290.

Koch, C.: Diseases of the larynx and pharynx of the horse. Compend. Cont. Ed. Pract. Vet., 5(2):S73–S79, 1980.

The Significance of Arytenoid Cartilage Movement

Richard P. Hackett, ITHACA, NEW YORK

Laryngeal hemiplegia is a common upper respiratory tract obstructive disorder affecting performance horses. It has been recognized for over a century that complete paralysis of the cricoarytenoideus dorsalis muscle results in functional upper respiratory tract stenosis and impaired racing performance. The disorder also typically causes an inspiratory noise, which may render horses used for less strenuous competition unsound of wind. In recent years, as endoscopic examination of horses has become more commonplace, it has become obvious that laryngeal hemiplegia is not an "all-or-none" disease. Endoscopic examination of many horses reveals arytenoid cartilage movement that is neither "normal," that is, synchronous and symmetrical, nor characteristic of laryngeal hemiplegia, that is, a dropped immobile left cartilage. These horses show various degrees of arytenoid cartilage asynchrony or asymmetry during endoscopic examination at rest. Significant controversy exists regarding the clinical significance of arytenoid cartilage asynchrony or asymmetry. This particularly applies to decisions regarding the disposition of sales yearlings determined to have such a condition and to determination of the clinical relevance and the need for corrective surgery of such findings in horses in training.

INCIDENCE OF LARYNGEAL HEMIPLEGIA

Laryngeal hemiplegia is diagnosed most commonly in Thoroughbred horses but is also a common problem in Standardbred horses, draft horses, warm bloods, and other large-statured horses. The disease is unquestionably related to physical size. One study determined that 95 per cent of affected horses were taller than 16 hands (160 cm). This was corroborated by another study, which determined that 83 per cent of affected horses were 160 cm or more in height and lent statistical support to the clinical impression that tall, young, male horses are most susceptible to idiopathic laryngeal hemiplegia. The disease rarely occurs in horses less than 15 hands (150 cm) tall and is almost never encountered in ponies. Estimates of the incidence of laryngeal hemiplegia have tended to focus on the Thoroughbred breed. Four recent surveys, which included large numbers of horses, predominantly or exclusively Thoroughbreds, recorded incidences of 2.6, 3.3, 4.7, and 8.3 per cent.

ETIOLOGY OF LARYNGEAL HEMIPLEGIA

Typically, the cause of dysfunction in cases of laryngeal hemiplegia is unknown. In a study of 127 horses with laryngeal hemiplegia, an inciting cause such as irritant perineural injection, guttural pouch mycosis, or toxicity was recognized in only 11 per cent of cases. For many years idiopathic laryngeal hemiplegia (ILH) was thought to be an isolated neuropathy that was somehow due to mechanical damage sustained by the left recurrent laryngeal nerve during its unique intrathoracic course around the root of the aorta. More recently, the identification of similar but less extensive abnormalities in the right recurrent laryngeal nerve of "roarers" and in long hind limb nerves has challenged the validity of this theory. Lesions observed in the peripheral nerves of roarers by light and electron microscopy support classification of the disease as a polyneuropathy, specifically a distal axonopathy. In similar motor neuron diseases in other species, the "dying back" process in the distal axon is the sequel to atrophy or abiotrophy of the nerve cell body. The disease process is manifested distally in the axon, because the cell body, upon which the axon depends for its health, fails to provide adequate sustaining or trophic influences. The longest and the largest axons are most severely affected. Many conditions—including metabolic diseases, intoxications, and genetic diseases—are capable of producing a distal axonopathy. Specific suggested etiologies for ILH in the horse include lead or plant intoxication, thiamine deficiency, and energy or antioxidant-dependent disorders. A pathogenic mechanism that links these disparate possibilities is one in which the primary defect occurs in the nerve cell body, the trophic center of the nerve.

It has long been suggested that ILH has a genetic basis. Analysis of breeding records and limited numbers of test matings lends support to the belief that hereditary factors are involved. Laryngeal hemiplegia has been observed in a foal, and neurogenic atrophy of the cricoarytenoideus dorsalis muscles has been observed in a fetal foal. While this evidence suggests that ILH may be a congenital disease, it does not account for the many horses that are diagnosed with the disease at 2 or 3 years of age or older. The exact role of inherited factors is unclear and it is possible that heredity exerts its influence through conformational characteristics such as neck length and body size or interacts with other, as yet unidentified factors.

ARYTENOID CARTILAGE ASYMMETRY AND ASYNCHRONY

Many horses have asynchronous or asymmetrical laryngeal function, suggesting paresis rather than paralysis of the cricoarytenoideus dorsalis. An endoscopic survey of Clydesdale horses found some degree of abnormal arytenoid movement in 50 per cent of animals over 1 year of age. Another endoscopic survey suggested that over 90 per cent of Thoroughbred horses have some degree of recurrent laryngeal neuropathy, as indicated by asynchronous laryngeal movements. The significance of a paretic type of laryngeal activity is controversial, because it is presently unknown whether horses with asymmetrical or asynchronous laryngeal movement are clinically impaired or will progress over time to become hemiplegic. Distal recurrent laryngeal nerve lesions in these horses are similar to those observed in hemiplegic horses, although less severe. Because the pathological lesions observed in the recurrent laryngeal nerves of hemiplegic horses and horses with paretic types of laryngeal movement are consistent with a progressive disease, a hemiplegic horse would be expected to pass through a paretic stage. Baker, however, concluded that horses with arytenoid asynchrony do not progress to hemiplegia in a 5-year study of Thoroughbred horses. Studies that corroborate this finding and address the question of progression in horses with arytenoid asymmetry are lacking. Until such studies are performed, the issue of progression must remain unresolved.

The performance consequences of altered movement of the arytenoid cartilages other than complete paralysis is likewise unclear. At least 40 per cent of large breed horses have some degree of laryngeal asynchrony or asymmetry, but the effect of such abnormality on an individual's athletic ability is often a matter of speculation. Many animals retain a substantial degree of activity in the left arytenoid cartilage but exhibit some degree of laryngeal asymmetry at rest or show some degree of asynchronous activity of the left arytenoid cartilage compared to the right (commonly referred to as "weak," "paretic," or "partially paralyzed"). There is limited basic knowledge of the effect of asynchronous or incomplete movements of the arytenoid cartilages on immediate and future performance. Some authors feel that asynchrony or partial paralysis precedes total paralysis. Others suggest that some horses with partial paralysis will undergo abductor muscle fatigue and suffer progressive compromise of the airway during exercise. A form of laryngeal cartilage movement termed asynchronous laryngeal abduction has been distinguished from partial laryngeal paralysis by some authors and has been considered to be a normal variation. Others, however, have stated that asynchronous abduction of the left arytenoid is conclusive proof of some degree of paralysis of the left cricoarytenoideus dorsalis muscle.

The above authors presumably viewed similar events but differ widely in their interpretation. We felt that studies of such problems were hampered by lack of well-defined descriptions of arytenoid cartilage activity during respiration and hence developed and validated the following grading system for assessment of laryngeal activity in resting horses:

I. Synchronous full abduction and adduction of the left and right arytenoid cartilages.

II. Asynchronous movement (hesitation, flutter, adductor weakness, etc.) of the left arytenoid cartilage during any phase of respiration. Full abduction of the left arytenoid cartilage (as compared to the right) inducible by nasal occlusion or swallowing.

III. Asynchronous movement (hesitation, flutter, adductor weakness, etc.) of the left arytenoid cartilage during any phase of respiration. Full abduction of the left arytenoid cartilage is *not* inducible and maintained by nasal occlusion or swallowing.

IV. Marked asymmetry of the larynx at rest and no substantial movement of the left arytenoid cartilage during any phase of respiration.

This scoring system was devised to give the examiners a frame of reference to grade laryngeal cartilage movement by a system more descriptive than "normal" or "abnormal." The grading system and the reliability of endoscopic examination as a diagnostic tool were tested using video recordings of the laryngeal activity of 108 unsedated resting horses. The recordings were obtained with the aid of a flexible video endoscope passed into the nasopharynx through the right ventral meatus. All video taped images were reviewed once and 72 were reviewed twice by three veterinarians. The mean intraobserver agreement was 83.3 per cent (range, 75.0 to 90.2 per cent) and the mean interobserver agreement was 79.0 per cent (range, 70.4 to 80.6 per cent). We concluded that the grading system was sufficiently reliable to aid clinicians and researchers in studies of laryngeal cartilage movements in horses.

An earlier version of this grading system included categories based on the assessment of resting laryngeal symmetry. This system had a very poor mean interobserver agreement (37 per cent). Observers could reliably determine asymmetry only in horses with complete paralysis. This required us to modify the system so that observers were no longer asked to assess resting laryngeal symmetry. This was the only difference between the two systems but led to substantially improved interobserver agreement (79 per cent). The improvement in agreement noted between the original and revised systems strongly suggests that the appearance of laryngeal symmetry in resting horses is highly variable and hence may be of limited clinical usefulness unless complete paralysis is present.

A computer program was developed to measure the left-to-right ratio of the rima glottidis. The mean left-to-right ratio for horses assigned a median laryngeal activity grade of I was 0.84 (range, 0.55 to 1.03). For grade II it was 0.82 (0.50 to 1.12), for grade III 0.59 (0.39 to 0.91), and for grade IV 0.24 (0.07 to 0.35). This measurement technique holds promise as a useful adjunct to subjective evaluation of laryngeal cartilage movement.

FACTORS AFFECTING RESTING ENDOSCOPIC EXAMINATION

In a companion study, our group looked at the effects of xylazine sedation, day of examination, and side of endoscope passage on the endoscopic appearance of the larynx in 20 horses. This study concluded that endoscopic evaluation of laryngeal cartilage movement is subjective and is influenced by sedation with xylazine, evaluation through the alternate nostril, and different day of examination. The most consistent evaluation was achieved by repeated examination through the left nostril. Sedation at either of two dosages of xylazine tended to make movements of the arytenoid cartilages more synchronous. Of particular clinical interest were two horses not capable of reaching full abduction of the left arytenoid cartilage during reexamination under xylazine sedation but had been originally capable of doing so. This led us to speculate that, had these been clinical patients, a laryngeal prosthesis might have been deemed indicated solely as a result of the effects of sedation. Conversely, however, one may wish to believe that two cases of laryngeal hemiplegia would have been missed had the horses not been sedated. Whether the findings in these horses were false positive or false negative could not be established by this study. In this study, computer measurement of the rima glottidis was less affected by the day of examination or the presence or absence of sedation than were subjective assessments.

ARYTENOID CARTILAGE MOVEMENT IN EXERCISING HORSES

In a third study, our group compared arytenoid cartilage movement in horses at rest with movement while horses were exercising on a high-speed treadmill. The goal was to assess the predictive value of our subjective grading system and computerized measurements with respect to arytenoid cartilage movement in the exercising animal, based on resting observation. Endoscopic examinations of the larynx were recorded on 49 horses both at rest and while exercising on a 5 per cent inclined high-speed treadmill for 8 minutes at a maximum speed of 8.5 m per second. Subjective laryngeal function scores for the resting animal were assigned using the grading system described above. Objective assessment of arytenoid abduction was obtained by measuring the rima glottis and expressing the results as a left-to-right ratio. Horses examined at rest and noted to have arytenoid cartilage asynchrony (grade II) could not be distinguished from normal horses (grade I) when exercising, because full abduction consistently occurred and was maintained throughout the exercise period. Five of six horses with incomplete left arytenoid abduction at rest (grade III) maintained full abduction during exercise, but one horse with grade III arytenoid cartilage movement showed dynamic collapse of the left hemilarynx. All horses with laryngeal hemiplegia (grade IV) at rest experienced dynamic collapse of the left hemilarynx during exercise. Horses with a resting left-to-right ratio of 0.71 or higher consistently showed complete arytenoid abduction at exercise. Horses with a left-to-right ratio less than 0.71 consistently showed dynamic collapse of the left hemilarynx at exercise. No difference in the exercising left-to-right ratio was noted between normal horses (grade I) and grade II horses or between grade I and grade III horses. These results suggested that horses with arytenoid asynchrony at rest do not suffer progressive compromise of the rima glottidis at exercise and that incomplete arytenoid abduction at rest is an unreliable predictor of such compromise.

CONCLUSIONS AND RECOMMENDATIONS

In summary, the following considerations and recommendations may be made for horses with various types of arytenoid cartilage movement:

GRADE I

Horses with grade I arytenoid cartilage movement are those classically considered "normal." In the treadmill study, all grade I horses exhibited full arytenoid abduction at exercise. Anecdotal reports indicate that a rare horse with normal movement at rest will exhibit dynamic collapse of the left arytenoid cartilage when exercised to exhaustion, but, based on accumulated evidence, such cases must be considered exceptional, if not unique. However, treadmill endoscopy is indicated in any horse with a history compatible with obstructive upper airway disorder in which no abnormalities can be identified on resting examination.

GRADE II

Horses with grade II arytenoid cartilage movement exhibit arytenoid asynchrony. It has been suggested that asynchronous movement is due to weakness of the laryngeal adductors and consequent imbalance between these muscles and the abductors. The "slap test" (see *Current Therapy in Equine Medicine 1*, p. 497) may reinforce this impression. Histological study of such horses has revealed degeneration of the recurrent laryngeal nerve, neurogenic atrophy in the abductors, and more advanced atrophy in the adductors. These findings suggest that asynchronous movement represents an early stage of hemiplegia. However, in a 5-year study of Thoroughbred horses Baker concluded that horses with arytenoid asynchrony did not progress to hemiplegia. This finding, coupled with our finding that all horses with grade II movement in the treadmill study exhibited full arytenoid abduction at exercise, supports the contention that horses exhibiting only asynchrony should be considered variations of normal. Surgical intervention for horses with grade II arytenoid cartilage movement based solely on resting endoscopic examination is inappropriate. In the exceedingly rare case, a horse may experience dynamic laryngeal collapse when exercised to exhaustion. This finding would be the only circumstance in which surgical treatment of a grade II horse would be indicated.

GRADE III

Horses exhibiting asymmetry as evidenced by inability to achieve and maintain full dilation of the rima glottidis with or without asynchronous arytenoid movement must be presumed to have somewhat more advanced degeneration of the left recurrent laryngeal nerve and consequent neurogenic atrophy of the laryngeal abductors and adductors. The reader is reminded that determinations of asymmetry are not reliable during resting respiration except in horses that are completely paralyzed. Incomplete abduction is an assessment made when movements of the arytenoid cartilages are exaggerated by nasal occlusion, swallowing, or recent exercise. Intuitively, it would seem likely that horses with grade III arytenoid cartilage movement would progress over time to complete hemiparalysis (grade IV). Such progression, however, remains to be documented. The clinical significance of grade III impairment can be determined only by endoscopy during exercise on a high-speed treadmill or immediately after exercise. The latter option is less satisfactory, because dynamic collapse of the rima glottidis terminates rapidly on cessation of exercise. In our treadmill study, 5 of 6 horses with grade III impairment exhibited full, symmetrical arytenoid abduction during strenuous but submaximal exercise on the treadmill. These horses were not considered candidates for corrective laryngoplasty. The sixth horse experienced dynamic collapse at work and was treated surgically.

GRADE IV

Horses with grade IV arytenoid cartilage movement are classical "roarers" and consistently demonstrate dynamic collapse of the left hemilarynx at exercise. Corrective laryngoplasty is indicated (see *Current Therapy in Equine Medicine*, p. 498).

Supplemental Readings

Baker, G. J.: Laryngeal asynchrony in the horse: Definition and significance. In Snow, D. H., Persson, S. G. B., and Rose, R. F. (eds.): Equine Exercise Physiology. Cambridge, England, Granta Editions, 1982, pp. 46–50.

Cook, W. R.: Recent observations on recurrent laryngeal neuropathy in the horse: Applications to practice. In: Proceedings of the 34th Annual Meeting of the American Association of Equine Practitioners, 1988, pp. 427–478.

Ducharme, N. G., Hackett, R. P., Fubini, S. L., and Erb, H. E.: Evaluation of the reliability of endoscopic examination in assessment of laryngeal function in horses: Part II. Influence of reexamination, side of examination, and sedation. Vet. Surg. (in press).

Hackett, R. P., Ducharme, N. G., Fubini, S. L., and Erb, H. N.: Evaluation of the reliability of endoscopic examination in assessment of arytenoid cartilage movement in horses: I. Subjective and objective laryngeal evaluation. Vet. Surg. (in press).

Rakestraw, P. C., Hackett, R. P., Ducharme, N. G., Nielan, G. J., and Erb, H. N.: A comparison of arytenoid cartilage movement in resting and exercising horses. Vet. Surg. 20:122, 1991.

Stick, J. A., and Derksen, F. J.: Use of videoendoscopy during exercise for determination of appropriate surgical treatment of laryngeal hemiplegia in a colt. J. Am. Vet. Med. Assoc., 195:619, 1989.

Arytenoid Chondritis

Frank A. Nickels, EAST LANSING, MICHIGAN

Arytenoid chondritis is a chronic, progressive condition of the larynx resulting in distortion of the arytenoid cartilage(s) and obstruction of the upper airway. The condition primarily involves the arytenoid cartilage, but the corniculate process may be involved secondarily. This abnormality is characterized by an enlargement of the cartilage, which restricts its normal motion and decreases airway diameter, resulting in exercise intolerance and a respiratory noise during strenuous exercise. The condition is most frequently unilateral and may be confused initially with laryngeal hemiplegia. The disease usually affects young racehorses, particularly Thoroughbreds, but has also been described in nonracing breeds.

The cause of arytenoid chondritis is unknown, but it is thought that laryngeal trauma may have a predisposing role. Although there are very few reports in the literature on the histological appearance of the affected cartilages, the pathological findings are generally consistent with a chronic recurrent inflammation. The presence of sinus tracts through the arytenoid cartilage suggests an underlying septic process. Increased mineralization of the laryngeal cartilages does occur and may extend into adjacent soft tissues.

CLINICAL SIGNS

Horses with arytenoid chondritis usually exhibit exercise intolerance at high speed and a respiratory noise during exercise. As in laryngeal hemiplegia, the noise is most pronounced on inspiration. Exercise intolerance has been reported to be more severe with arytenoid chondritis than with laryngeal hemiplegia. The history usually indicates a slowly progressive problem that develops over a period of weeks to months. In advanced cases, some horses may be incapable of exercise and may even be dyspneic at rest.

DIAGNOSIS

The diagnosis usually can be established from the history, clinical signs, and endoscopic examination findings. External palpation and laryngeal radiography may help define the nature and extent of the problem.

The endoscopic appearance of the arytenoid cartilage is usually conclusive for the diagnosis of the condition, even though the initial impression may be that of laryngeal hemiplegia. A limited range of motion of the corniculate process may be visualized concurrent with medial displacement of the affected cartilage. The main distinguishing feature of arytenoid chondritis is the presence of intraluminal projections covered with mucosa, which usually originate from the medial aspect of the arytenoid cartilage. These projections may cause contact erosions and granulating lesions on the contralateral cartilage (Fig. 1). Initially, the corniculate process of the affected cartilage may appear slightly thicker or wrinkled as a result of enlargement of the arytenoid cartilage caudally. Later, partial to full-thickness mucosal lesions may occur on the medial aspect of the corniculate process, which may become raised and reddened. These lesions may contact the opposite side, causing mucosal defects there also.

As the diseased cartilage becomes larger, it is forced into a more vertical position and projects into the airway; this causes the palatopharyngeal arch on the involved side to become more apparent. In advanced unilateral or bilateral involvement, the rima glottis is virtually obliterated, making visualization of laryngeal lumen difficult. Arytenoid chondritis should be high on the differential diagnosis list when right-sided laryngeal hemiplegia is diagnosed or bilateral "paralysis" is suspected.

External palpation of the affected larynx often reveals firm, large, less resilient laryngeal cartilages. Manual compression of the larynx often causes dyspnea and an audible noise at rest. Lateral laryngeal radiographs can be useful by demonstrating increased mineralization of the arytenoid cartilage. However, this mineralization must be distinguished from mineralization of the thyroid and cricoid cartilages and the muscular process of the arytenoid cartilage, which can be a normal radiographic finding. Radiographic evidence of extensive laryngeal cartilage mineralization reportedly is associated with a poor prognosis following surgical treatment of arytenoid chondritis.

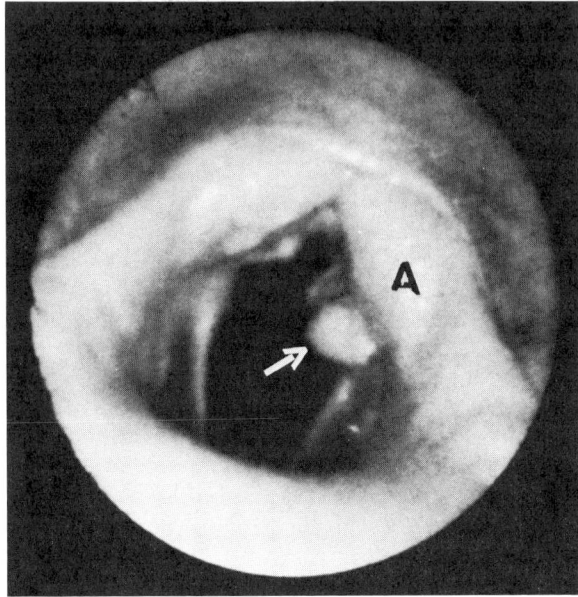

Figure 1. Arytenoid chondritis. The endoscopic view demonstrates a thickened left corniculate cartilage (*A*). Note the intraluminal projection *(arrow)* on the axial surface of the affected arytenoid cartilage and a granulating, contact lesion on the contralateral cartilage.

THERAPY

There are no published reports of successful medical management of arytenoid chondritis. Some anecdotal reports suggest that palliative treatments such as nonsteroidal anti-inflammatory drugs, steroids, antibiotics, and topical throat sprays may provide some short-term benefit when the cartilages are inflamed but lack obvious draining tracts.

Surgical therapy is not necessary in all cases of arytenoid chondritis, especially in mild cases where strenuous exercise is not required and progression of cartilaginous changes is slow. Surgical intervention is indicated when the rima glottidis is severely compromised by unilateral or bilateral involvement, or when athletic activity is desired. Arytenoidectomy is the surgical procedure of choice for the provision of a sufficient airway for maximal exercise. Methods of total, partial, and subtotal arytenoidectomy have been described. Because severe complications have been described following total arytenoidectomy, the partial and subtotal techniques are most commonly used. Partial arytenoidectomy entails removal of the entire arytenoid and corniculate cartilage except for the muscular process, whereas both the corniculate cartilage and the muscular processes are preserved in the subtotal procedure. Both techniques are adequately described in surgical texts. Reported modifications of the partial technique have included the use of Nd:YAG laser ablation, and performance of the technique without mucosal closure.

PROGNOSIS

Total arytenoidectomy as originally described in the late 19th century resulted in dysphagia and fatal aspiration pneumonia. In more recent experience that technique has proved unacceptable for similar reasons, although the complications were less severe. Other complications that have been reported are nasal discharge of food and water, coughing associated with either eating or exercise, and respiratory noise associated with exercise. A high incidence of postoperative complications has been reported following partial arytenoidectomy, especially when transection of the transverse arytenoid ligament was performed.

Although arytenoidectomy was considered only a salvage procedure in the past, many horses are able to return to competition and race successfully. It has been reported that both the partial and the subtotal procedures provide an adequate airway for maximal exercise, but objective evaluation of the subtotal method found that it failed to improve upper airway flow mechanics in exercising Standardbred horses with induced laryngeal hemiplegia.

Horses that present with excessive mineralization of the laryngeal cartilages or bilateral involvement of the arytenoid cartilages are not likely to return to competitive racing following surgical treatment.

Supplemental Readings

Belknap, J. K., Derksen, F. D., Nickels, F. A., Stick, J. A., and Robinson, N. E.: Failure of subtotal arytenoidectomy to improve upper airway flow mechanics in exercising standardbred horses with induced laryngeal hemiplegia. Am. J. Vet. Res. 51:1481, 1990.
Haynes, P. F.: Arytenoid chondritis in the horse. In: Proceedings of the 27th Annual Meeting of the American Association of Equine Practioners, 1981, pp. 63–69.
Haynes, P. F.: Subtotal arytenoidectomy in the horse: An update. In: Proceedings of the 30th Annual Meeting of the American Association of Equine Practitioners, 1984, pp. 21–33.
Haynes, P. F.: Surgery of the equine respiratory tract. In Jennings, P. B. (ed): The Practice of Large Animal Surgery. Philadelphia, W. B. Saunders, 1984, pp. 388–487.
Haynes, P. F., Snider, T. G., McClure, J. R., and McClure, J. J.: Chronic chondritis of the arytenoid cartilage. J. Am. Vet. Med. Assoc., 177:1135, 1980.
Orsini, P. G., Raker, C. W., Reid, C. F., and Mann, P.: Xeroradiographic evaluation of the larynx. J. Am. Vet. Res., 50:845, 1989.
Speirs, V. C.: Partial arytenoidectomy in the horse. Vet. Surg., 15:316, 1986.
Tate, L. P., Sweeney, C. L., Cullen, J. M., and Newman, H. C.: Nd:YAG laser partial arytenoidectomy and ventriculectomy in the horse. Vet. Surg., 16:104, 1987.
Tulleners, E. P., Harrison, I. W., and Raker, C. W.: Management of arytenoid chondropathy and failed laryngoplasty in the horse: 75 cases (1979–1985). J. Am. Vet. Med. Assoc., 192:670, 1988.
Tulleners, E. P., Harrison, I. W., and Raker, C. W.: Partial arytenoidectomy in the horse without mucosal closure. Vet. Surg., 17:252, 1988.
White, N. A., and Blackwell, R. B.: Partial arytenoidectomy in the horse. Vet. Surg., 9:5, 1980.

Upper Airway Flow Dynamics

John R. Pascoe, DAVIS, CALIFORNIA

Air flow is dependent on a number of factors, including the resistance to air flow and the strength of the pump moving the air (the respiratory muscular effort). The interrelationship between these parameters is illustrated in Figure 1. For a given resistance to air flow, a certain driving pressure is needed to generate the required flow (Fig. 1A). With exercise, air flow increases, so there must be a corresponding increase in driving pressure to accommodate this increased flow (Fig. 1B). In the normal horse, this increase in driving pressure is attenuated in part by a de-

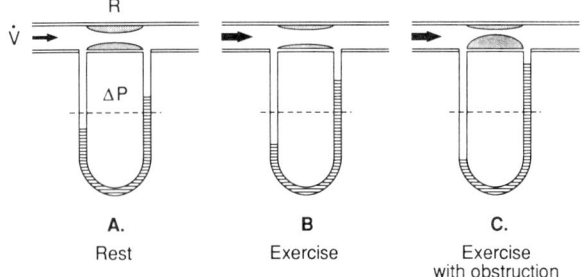

Figure 1. Schematic representation of changes in upper airway pressure and air flow at rest (*A*), during exercise (*B*), and during exercise with upper airway obstruction (*C*). The width of the arrow indicates the instantaneous air flow (V), the shaded area represents the airway obstruction (R), and the pressure manometer indicates the change in driving pressure (ΔP) needed to compensate for both the increased resistance to air flow offered by the obstruction and the increased air flow needed for exercise.

crease in flow resistance. This reduction in flow resistance is believed to be due to changes in airway shape (increased cross-sectional area) and compliance (increased tautness of the airway walls as a result of muscular activation and positional alignment of the head and neck). Consequently, the driving pressure needed to generate the required flow is lower than might otherwise be anticipated.

However, if the cross-sectional area of the airway is reduced by an obstruction, the resistance or impedance to air flow during exercise is increased (Fig. 1C). Thus the driving pressure, the respiratory muscular effort, must also increase if a comparable air flow is to be attained. Measurement of changes in airway pressure and flow can provide useful information about the severity of functional airway obstruction experienced during exercise.

PATHOPHYSIOLOGY OF UPPER AIRWAY OBSTRUCTION

Obstructions to air flow can be classed as fixed or nonfixed (variable). In general, fixed airway obstructions result in static increases in airway resistance during both inspiration and expiration. By contrast, nonfixed upper airway obstructions contribute to dynamic changes in airway resistance that generally have a more pronounced effect during inspiration, when airway pressures are negative (subatmospheric).

Structurally, some segments of the upper airway, such as the nasal cavity, are relatively rigid, and other segments, such as the pharynx, are elastic. Some of the elastic segments also have valvelike actions that are capable of markedly modifying the cross-sectional area of the airway. The principal valvelike structures in the upper airway are the nostrils, soft palate, and larynx. Although each segment of the airway is capable of undergoing some degree of change, the valvelike components have the most profound influence on resistance to air flow.

For an elastic segment of the airway, the tendency to collapse depends on the transmural pressure (the pressure across the airway wall), which in turn depends on the balance between the lateral airway pressure (the pressure perpendicular to the airway wall) and the tissue pressure (the pressure that the surrounding tissues can exert to counteract the tendency to collapse). The tissue pressure depends on the compliance of the tissues anchoring the airway walls and also on the degree of muscular activation tensing the airway walls. The lateral airway pressure is a function of the convective acceleration of the air, which is related to the square of the air flow velocity.

As an airway narrows, the bulk flow of air through the narrow region must be maintained and therefore the flow velocity increases. Consequently the lateral airway pressure decreases, becoming more negative, and if it becomes less than the surrounding tissue pressure, that segment of the airway wall begins to collapse inward until counteracted by the tension that develops in the surrounding tissue, the tissue pressure. However, as the airway wall begins to collapse, the cross-sectional area continues to decrease, further increasing the convective acceleration of the air at this site. Thus the lateral airway pressure becomes even more negative, thus accentuating the inward movement of the airway wall. If the airway wall is sufficiently compliant, this situation continues until there is complete collapse of the airway. Total obstruction to air flow ensues.

Video endoscopic studies of treadmill-exercised horses with left laryngeal hemiplegia have confirmed these concepts. A neuromuscular disease like recurrent laryngeal neuropathy impairs the ability of the dorsal cricoarytenoid muscle to stabilize the arytenoid cartilage and prevent collapse in the face of increasingly negative airway pressures. Consequently, with increased demand for air flow during exercise, there is progressive inward movement of the left arytenoid cartilage and vocal fold until toward the end of inspiration the left arytenoid is pulled across the midline and contacts the abducted right arytenoid cartilage and vocal fold. Thus, for an instant toward the end of inspiration, there is nearly complete obstruction of the airway at a time when it should be at its maximal cross-sectional area.

Compared with normal horses, horses with air flow obstruction have measurable increases in airway resistance and in upper airway pressure at the same air flow. Indeed, this has been demonstrated in treadmill-exercised horses and horses racing on a track. When the left recurrent laryngeal nerve is sectioned to induce left laryngeal hemiplegia, the inspiratory upper airway pressure needed to maintain flow is about 2.5 times that measured in horses with normal laryngeal function. Horses with naturally occurring left laryngeal hemiplegia have similar increases in inspiratory airway pressure when galloping at speeds greater than 15 m per second. There is essentially no change in expiratory upper airway pressure.

Other upper airway disorders produce lesser increases in airway pressure than occur with left laryngeal hemiplegia. For instance, left arytenoid chondropathy, which is primarily a fixed airway obstruction, results in about a twofold increase in inspiratory airway pressure at speeds greater than 15 m per second, as well as an increase in expiratory airway pressure. Epiglottic entrapment and subepiglottic cysts result in even smaller increases in airway pressure, and pharyngeal lymphoid hyperplasia appears to have no real effect on airway pressure. The influence of dorsal displacement of the soft palate (laryngopalatal dislocation) has not been studied.

It should be evident that the homeostatic response during periods of increasing air flow is to stabilize the collapsible segments of the airway to maintain adequate air flow. Since disease conditions either result in static or dynamic airway obstruction, treatment strategies must either restore the cross-sectional area of the airway, in the case of fixed obstructions, or stabilize the airway wall, in the case of dynamic obstructions. Recent studies have evaluated the efficacy of current surgical procedures in terms of their ability to meet these objectives.

It might be anticipated that surgical procedures that stabilize the left arytenoid cartilage and vocal fold should return airway pressures to near normal values. In fact, both treadmill and track studies have shown that laryngoplasty does improve airway mechanics to near normal levels. After surgery, there is still a slight increase in resistance and pressure above normal, probably reflecting the fact that the degree of abduction achieved at surgery is less than that achieved by the functionally normal larynx. Results with subtotal arytenoidectomy, both in induced "roarers" and in horses with arytenoid chondropathy, have been less dramatic. The observed results certainly support clinical experience and suggest that while arytenoidectomy may be useful for improving airway patency, it is of limited value for returning horses to athletic potential, since during exercise airway pressures and impedance are still elevated.

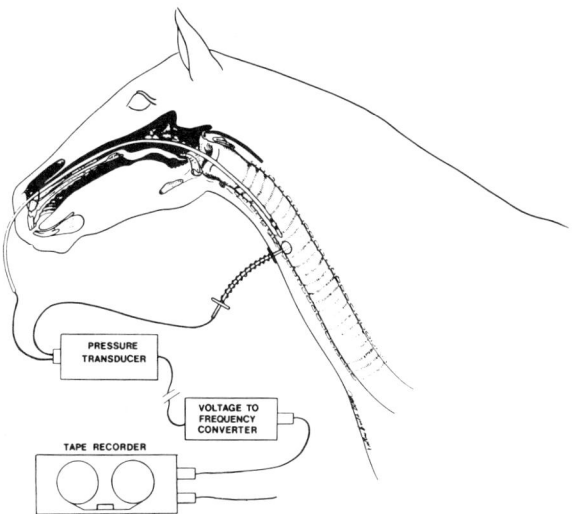

Figure 2. Schematic representation of recording systems for measurement of upper airway pressure in horses. The nasotracheal catheter system is less invasive than the transtracheal catheter system and is easier to maintain during exercise. (From Williams, J. W., et al.: Vet. Surg., 19:136–141, 1990. Reproduced by permission of J. B. Lippincott Co.)

TECHNIQUE FOR MEASUREMENT OF UPPER AIRWAY PRESSURE

Ideally, the measurement of interest when describing the mechanics of the upper airway is the resistance or impedance to air flow. To derive resistance it is necessary to know the instantaneous air flow and the driving pressure needed to achieve that flow. In a laboratory, both flow and pressure can be measured relatively easily, even in horses exercising on a treadmill. Unfortunately, flow meters suitable for use in horses galloping on a track are not available, so measurements have been restricted to changes in upper airway pressure. This requires a cannula, a differential pressure transducer, a recorder, and a pressure calibrating device (Fig. 2). Unfortunately, a portable system for recording upper airway pressure is not commercially available, but the interested reader can find details for construction of a custom system in a 1990 publication by Williams, Pascoe, et al. (see supplemental readings list).

Supplemental Readings

Belknap, J. K., Derksen, F. J., Nickels, F. A., Stick, J. A., and Robinson, N. E.: Failure of subtotal arytenoidectomy to improve upper airway flow mechanics in exercising Standardbreds with induced laryngeal hemiplegia. Am. J. Vet. Res., 51:1481, 1990.

Derksen, F. J., Stick, J. A., Scott, E. A., and Robinson, N. E.: Effect of laryngeal hemiplegia and laryngoplasty on airway flow mechanics in exercising horses. Am. J. Vet. Res., 47:16, 1986.

Morris, E. A., and Seeherman, H. J.: Evaluation of upper respiratory tract function during strenuous exercise in racehorses. J. Am. Vet. Med. Assoc., 196:431, 1990.

Pascoe, J. R.: Pathophysiology of upper airway obstruction. In White, N. A., and Moore, J. N. (eds.): Current Practice of Equine Surgery. Philadelphia, J. B. Lippincott, 1990.

Shappell, K. K., Derksen, F. J., Stick, J. A., and Robinson, N. E.: Effects of ventriculectomy, prosthetic laryngoplasty, and exercise on upper airway function in horses with induced left laryngeal hemiplegia. Am. J. Vet. Res., 49:1760, 1988.

Williams, J. W., Pascoe, J. R., Meagher, D. M., and Hornof, W. J.: Effects of left recurrent laryngeal neurectomy, prosthetic laryngoplasty, and subtotal arytenoidectomy on upper airway pressure during maximal exertion. Vet. Surg., 19:136, 1990.

Williams, J. W., Meagher, D. M., Pascoe, J. R., and Hornof, W. J.: Upper airway function during maximal exercise in horses with obstructive upper airway lesions: Effect of surgical treatment. Vet. Surg., 19:142, 1990.

Laser Surgery for Upper Respiratory Disorders

Eric Tulleners, KENNETT SQUARE, PENNSYLVANIA

In the past 20 years lasers have gradually gained widespread acceptance in surgery on humans. As more surgeons become properly trained and experienced in performing laser surgery, useful and clearly superior indications for the application of laser energy have become apparent. Surgical lasers also have unique applicability to upper respiratory tract procedures in the horse, often performed transendoscopically in the standing conscious patient. An increasing number of useful techniques have been described and put into practice by equine surgeons.

A laser is an electro-optical device capable of efficiently transmitting energy in the form of an intense beam of light. Depending on the wavelength, a very small diameter and highly focused laser beam can be delivered through a hand-held scalpel, a rigid or flexible fiber-optic endoscope, or guided by a micromanipulator through an operating microscope. Depending on the particular wavelength of light emitted, the energy density delivered, and the absorption characteristics of the tissue being irradiated, surgical lasers can cut, vaporize, coagulate, weld, or interstitially irradiate (i.e., deliver a homogeneous low level of radiation over a broad area). Selective destruction of targeted tissue is possible while healthy tissue in the light beam's pathway is spared. Photodynamic therapy is a technique that allows selective destruction of tumor tissue after it has absorbed a specific sensitizing agent and then is exposed to a specific laser light. Laser tissue welding has also been successfully performed to create totally sutureless patent anastomoses between any tubular hollow viscus such as blood vessels, vas deferens, fallopian tubes, ureters, and bowel. Some of the advantages to using lasers in surgery include a sterile incision; sealing of small vessels and lymphatics; reduced bleeding and operating time (particularly when incising highly vascular tissue); less postoperative edema, inflammation, and pain; and rapid healing with less scarring.

Factors that continue to restrain the use of lasers in surgery, particularly veterinary surgery, include equipment expense and special surgeon training. Surgical lasers purchased new may cost from $15,000 to more than $150,000, depending on the type and model. However, reliable good quality new equipment that is outdated for human surgery as well as used and reconditioned equipment is often available at substantial savings. Excellent didactic and hands-on training courses for physicians in human medicine are offered throughout the country at regular intervals and are readily available to veterinarians interested in learning about laser surgery.

GENERAL PRINCIPLES

Laser light interacts with tissue in four ways: reflection, transmission, scattering, and absorption. Only light that is absorbed by or scattered through tissue will create an effect. The wavelength of light in use (which is determined by the type of laser), the spectral absorption characteristics of the tissue being irradiated, and the laser's output power and beam spot size determine the three-dimensional thermal responses that will be induced.

Power density (watts per cm^2) is the power seen by the tissue and is a function of the number of watts delivered by the laser and the spot size of tissue irradiated. The total amount of laser energy delivered to tissue equals energy density (or fluence), which is defined as watts·seconds per cm^2 or joules per cm^2 and can be determined by knowing the power density and the amount of time that the tissue was irradiated. Power density can be altered by changing either the watts delivered by the laser or the spot size, but it is manipulated most dramatically by changing the spot size. For example, at a constant power, halving the spot size will quadruple the power density. The two surgical lasers widely used in human surgery are the carbon dioxide (CO_2) laser and the neodymium:yttrium-aluminum-garnet (Nd:YAG) laser, each named after the medium it uses.

CO_2 LASER

The CO_2 laser is an excellent and precise soft tissue cutter because its far infrared wavelength of 10.6 microns is strongly absorbed by water with minimal scattering. Virtually all CO_2 laser energy is absorbed within 200 microns of the tissue surface, since most tissue is more than 80 per cent water. The CO_2 laser creates a localized, intense thermal effect. It has fair coagulating capability but is not useful if active bleeding is present. Flexible optical fibers for the transmission of CO_2 laser light have recently become commercially available, but this laser typically is delivered to tissue via a rigid articulated arm with an arrangement of mirrors at each joint. The CO_2 laser with its line-of-site fire delivery has many applications in human general, otolaryngologic, neurologic, obstetric, and gynecologic surgery, but to date its usefulness in equine upper respiratory tract surgery has been extremely limited because of the horse's anatomy. Scientists and manufacturers have been working on light guides and flexible fibers for the CO_2 laser for at least 10 years. Some of the problems encountered include the cost and durability of the fibers, the amount of flexibility achievable, and the substantial dropoff in power that occurs as the laser energy traverses the articulated arm to the delivery in the tissue. The first commercially available flexible fiber for the CO_2 laser was introduced in 1990 and may have applications in transendoscopic surgery, but its usefulness in the equine upper respiratory tract has not been documented to date.

Nd:YAG LASER

Nd:YAG lasers emit laser energy in the near infrared spectrum of light at a wavelength of 1.06 micron. Nd:YAG laser energy is transmitted through water rather than absorbed, so it is useful even in fluid-filled cavities such as the urinary bladder. Nd:YAG light is strongly absorbed by protein molecules. It is an excellent coagulator even in the presence of active bleeding and on larger vessels. This wavelength is delivered to tissue through a long flexible optical fiber, so that its potential usefulness includes any endoscopically accessible body cavity. Nd:YAG light is delivered to tissue with the fiber tip 3 to 5 mm away from but not in contact with tissue (noncontact technique) or with the fiber tip directly in contact with tissue (contact technique). The principal drawback to noncontact Nd:YAG laser surgery is related to light scatter. With the noncontact, approximately 30 to 40 per cent of the energy is lost to backscatter. Forward and lateral scatter produces a broad, nonspecific thermal effect that may injure tissue to a depth of 3 to 5 mm from the beam's focal point. Used in this manner, Nd:YAG energy is an imprecise tissue cutter and results in a significant delayed thermal effect that may injure healthy tissue. Bulk heating of tissue is desirable, however, for photovaporizing large tumors, and this modality has been used extensively for the palliation of esophageal, tracheobronchial, colorectal, and urinary bladder cancer in humans. In equine upper respiratory tract surgery, transendoscopic Nd:YAG energy delivered in noncontact fashion has been effectively used on large ethmoidal hematomas, certain pharyngeal polyps and cysts, and pharyngeal and laryngeal granulation tissue, and for laryngeal sacculectomy.

In the contact technique, a synthetic sapphire probe is screwed onto a threaded metal connector attached to the tip of the fiber. These probes are available in different sizes and shapes and the tissue effect achieved is determined by the geometry of the probe in use. The probes have a melting point of 2,030° to 2,050° C, but coaxial cooling is still required with either sterile gas or fluid delivered through the fiber. In 1990 sculpted quartz fibers that have small diameters (0.6, 0.8, or 1.0 micron), specially shaped conical or hemispherical ends, and that do not require a synthetic sapphire probe were introduced and are reported to be useful in human nasal surgery, laparotomy, endometrial ablation, gastroenterology, urology, and general surgery.

Contact surgery reduces the amount of output power required by the laser by approximately 75 to 90 per cent when compared to the noncontact technique. Undesirable scatter is cut to less than 5 per cent, greatly improving precision and reducing thermal damage to healthy adjacent tissue. This means that smaller, more compact and portable machines with power outputs of less than 30 watts can be used to coagulate, vaporize, and incise tissue. Contact surgery restores the surgeon's tactile sense and permits delivery of a constant, focused spot size and a predictable power density.

CONTACT Nd:YAG LASER TECHNIQUE

Laser surgery to remove benign obstructive lesions in the horse's upper respiratory tract is an attractive alternative to conventional techniques, because it can often be performed transendoscopically on standing, conscious horses or as a relatively short general anesthetic procedure, usually on an outpatient basis. Aftercare is minimal, and depending on the condition being treated, the horse usually can return to unrestricted exercise in 7 to 14 days. For example, Standardbred and Thoroughbred racehorses have raced within 2 weeks after outpatient transendoscopic laser correction of epiglottic entrapment. At the University of Pennsylvania approximately 215 upper respiratory tract procedures were performed with the contact Nd:YAG laser between November 1986 and May 1990. The laser was dependable, and maintenance, consisting of approximately two preventive maintenance visits per year, has been minimal.

Most horses are treated as outpatients or day patients if general anesthesia is necessary. After initial endoscopic, physical, and, if necessary, radiographic examination the horse is given xylazine, 0.44 mg per kg intravenously (IV), and is positioned and cross-tied in a stocks. The windows are covered and warning signs designating that a class IV surgical laser is in use are posted at the entrance to each locked doorway. Before the horse is positioned in the stocks the surgical room nurse, who has been instructed in the safe use of the laser, has already moved the laser from the storage closet, warmed it up and checked that the fiber is properly calibrated.

All transendoscopic procedures are performed with either a fiber-optic or video endoscope with the image viewed on a television monitor. One assistant stands to the left of the horse to provide restraint if needed and one assistant stands to the right of the horse to maintain positioning of the endoscope. Topical anesthetic is sprayed on the lesion through polyethylene (PE) 240 tubing, which is passed through the endoscope biopsy channel. Protective goggles that filter out the Nd:YAG laser light and prevent possible retinal damage are worn by everyone in the room. Technically this precaution is not necessary since the endoscopic image is being viewed indirectly on the television monitor. An appropriate-sized (2.2 mm or 1.8 mm outer diameter) flexible fiber is passed through the biopsy channel until it can be seen protruding 5 to 8 cm from the end of the endoscope. If contact technique is being used, the contact probe must be screwed onto the metal coupler at the end of the fiber before the fiber is introduced into the biopsy channel. In most instances, a chisel, conical, or rounded probe is used. The surgeon uses one hand to control the vertical and horizontal endoscope positioning knobs and the other hand to turn the fiber on its longitudinal axis and to advance or retract the fiber within the biopsy channel. Wrapping several turns of 2.54-cm-wide adhesive tape to the fiber approximately 5 to 8 cm from its entrance into the biopsy channel (with 5 to 8 cm of fiber protruding from the distal end of the biopsy channel) makes it much easier for the operator to turn and to maintain accurate positioning of the fiber and attached probe.

Laser surgery relies on laser energy, not mechanical pressure, to create the desired tissue effect. The laser is activated by depressing the foot pedal and the fiber and probe are gently advanced as the desired effect is achieved. In most instances hemorrhage is negligible, so that surgery proceeds fairly rapidly. If additional sedation is needed, it is achieved with xylazine, 0.22 mg per kg IV. The lesion can be resprayed with topical anesthetic if the procedure lasts longer than approximately 30 minutes. Restraint with a twitch is rarely necessary except when large tissue fragments are retrieved with grasping forceps introduced into the pharynx, larynx, or proximal trachea through a custom-designed guide tube.

Most horses have been treated with the contact technique using a laser that delivers up to 60 watts,* a chisel probe,† and 15 watts of power delivered at 3-second intervals. Pharyngeal lymphoid polyps, epiglottic entrapment, dorsal epiglottic abscesses, intralaryngeal granulation tissue, tracheal ulcers, and chondromas have all been treated transendoscopically, for the most part on an outpatient basis. Subepiglottic cysts are excised transendoscopically and submucosally through an oral approach, usually on an outpatient basis, with the horse anesthetized and nasotracheally intubated. Guttural pouch tym-

---

*Surgical Laser Technologies, model CL-60, Malvern, PA
†Chisel probe contact tip, Md 2.5, Surgical Laser Technologies, Malvern, PA

panites has been treated transendoscopically in anesthetized foals. Ethmoid hematomas less than 5 cm in diameter have been treated transendoscopically with noncontact technique or with a chisel probe and forceps removal. Large ethmoidal hematomas have been excised through a frontal nasal bone flap using a 0.6-mm handheld laser scalpel with the horse under general anesthesia.

After surgery the horse is usually given phenylbutazone, 6 mg per kg IV. If indicated, the owner, trainer, or van driver is shown how to spray the pharynx with an anti-inflammatory, antibacterial pharyngeal mixture.° All horses are discharged with typed instructions and medication. In most instances the horse is given 1 week of confinement, with exercise restricted to hand-walking or paddock turnout. During this time phenylbutazone, 2 mg per kg, is given orally at 12-hour intervals for 6 days and 10 ml of the pharyngeal medication is sprayed into the pharynx via a No. 10 French catheter at 12-hour intervals for 7 days. Depending on the lesion being treated, if on endoscopic reexamination by the referring veterinarian approximately 7 days after surgery the surgical site is judged to be healing routinely and there is only an expected amount of residual inflammation, the horse can be returned to exercise if desired. If significant inflammation is present at 7 days, the horse is confined for an additional week and reexamined after this time. Nasal exudate is usually minimal, and rarely will a horse cough for more than a few days. To date no hemorrhage, respiratory distress, or deaths have been reported in horses operated on for obstruction of the upper respiratory tract.

CONCLUSIONS

A distinct advantage of Nd:YAG laser surgery is that the beam is transmitted through a flexible fiber, thereby affording transendoscopic access to the horse's upper respiratory tract. Custom-designed instruments are essential for obtaining nonsurgical access to the pharynx, larynx, and proximal trachea. Contact probes have greatly improved the cutting capability and precision of Nd:YAG energy, particularly when used on fairly vascular soft tissue; however, they are not as effective in cutting pale, dense, relatively avascular tissue such as the arytenoid cartilages. The Nd:YAG laser is capable of photovaporizing cartilage when used transendoscopically at higher powers in noncontact fashion, but it produces excessive thermal damage in normal tissue. Transendoscopic arytenoidectomy in the horse may require the use of other emerging lasers such as the holium:YAG or erbium:YAG laser, both of which have excellent hard tissue cutting capability. Because of its excellent cutting capabilities, the CO_2 laser will probably establish its niche in equine upper respiratory surgery as more equine surgeons begin using lasers and as the flexible fiber technology continues to improve.

The use of lasers in equine surgery has increased steadily in the past 6 years and laser surgery is just beginning to fulfill the promises it holds. The lay public is fascinated by lasers but often has unrealistic and unfounded expectations about what surgical lasers can achieve. We must not betray their confidence by using surgical lasers indiscriminately and ill-advisedly. The future of laser surgery for equine surgeons appears bright, but we must strive to maintain high standards for safety and surgeon training and discourage the inappropriate use of this new modality. The long-term results and complications of our surgical endeavors must be diligently monitored and scientifically reported so that clear-cut indications for the use of this unique tool are established and flagrant misuse is discouraged. Much as arthroscopic surgery has revolutionized the management of joint injuries in the horse during the past 15 years, laser surgery has the opportunity to revolutionize equine upper respiratory tract surgery and general surgery if appropriately utilized.

Supplemental Readings

Sharplan Lasers, Inc.: Focus on lasers and accessories. Surg. Prod., 9(5):15–16, 1990.

Surgical Laser Technology: Contact Laser Surgery in Endoscopy: An Introduction. Surgical Laser Technology, Inc., One Great Valley Parkway, Malvern, PA, 1984, pp. 1–16.

Tulleners, E. P.: Transendoscopic contact YAG laser correction of upper airway obstructions in the horse. In: Proceedings of the 35th Annual Convention of the American Association of Equine Practitioners, 1989, p. 341.

Tulleners, E. P.: Transendoscopic laser surgery of the respiratory tract. In: Traub-Dargatz, J. L., and Brown, C. M. (eds): Equine Endoscopy, St. Louis, C. V. Mosby Co., 1990, pp. 85–110.

Tulleners, E. P.: Transendoscopic contact Ybtrium Aluminum Garnet laser correction of epiglottic entrapment in standing horses. J. Am. Vet. Med. Assoc. 196:1971, 1990.

°Pharyngeal spray: 750 ml furacin, 250 ml DMSO, 1000 ml glycerin, 2000 mg prednisolone, prepared by the University of Pennsylvania Veterinary School Pharmacy, Kennet Square, PA

Section 7

LOWER RESPIRATORY TRACT DISEASES

Edited by Andrew F. Clarke

Diagnostic Techniques for Lower Respiratory Tract Diseases

Tim Mair, KENT, ENGLAND

The proper management of pulmonary, pleural, or mediastinal disease depends on accurate diagnosis. "Proper management" means not only the initiation of appropriate therapy but also informing the horse's owner or trainer of the nature of the disease and the prognosis. Because the clinical findings may be sufficiently characteristic to indicate the diagnosis, there is no substitute for routine physical examination and careful auscultation of the chest; however, in other cases further diagnostic procedures may be required. This chapter reviews some of the most useful and most commonly employed diagnostic tests for lower respiratory tract disease. This is not an exhaustive review, and some procedures such as lung function tests and radionuclide scintigraphy will not be considered here. Table 1 lists the more common lower airway diseases in the adult horse and their diagnostic features.

ENDOSCOPIC EXAMINATION

The principal indication for bronchoscopy in humans is to confirm or exclude a diagnosis of lung cancer. Although primary lung neoplasms are extremely rare in horses, endoscopic evaluation of the trachea and bronchial tree can also provide essential information for the diagnosis of lower airway and pulmonary diseases in the equine patient. The procedure is readily performed in the standing horse (sedated if necessary) but requires the use of an instrument of sufficient length to reach the area under investigation. A one-meter-long endoscope will permit examination of the proximal trachea, but an instrument 120 cm long is generally needed to allow visualization as far as the tracheal bifurcation. Longer instruments are necessary for examination of the bronchial tree. The endoscope

TABLE 1. DIFFERENTIAL DIAGNOSIS AND DIAGNOSTIC FEATURES OF THE MAJOR LOWER RESPIRATORY TRACT DISEASES IN THE ADULT HORSE

Disease	Diagnostic Features
Chronic obstructive pulmonary disease	Endoscopy: lower airway exudate and bronchial collapse Tracheobronchial aspiration: neutrophilia Bronchoalveolar lavage: neutrophilia
Exercise-induced pulmonary hemorrhage	Endoscopy: hemorrhage Tracheobronchial aspiration: free red blood cells, hemosiderophages
Lungworm	Endoscopy: larvae in bronchial tree Tracheobronchial aspiration: larvae, eosinophilia
Neoplasia	Radiography: thoracic mass, pleural fluid Ultrasonography: thoracic mass, pleural fluid
Pleuritis	Radiography: pleural fluid Ultrasonography: pleural fluid, pleural thickening Thoracocentesis: cytology, culture
Pneumonia/lung abscess	Endoscopy: lower airway exudate Tracheobronchial aspiration: neutrophilia Bronchoalveolar lavage: neutrophilia Transtracheal aspiration: Gram stain, culture Radiography: pulmonary consolidation, pleural fluid Ultrasonography: pulmonary consolidation, pleural fluid
Tracheal deformity	Endoscopy: airway narrowing Radiography: airway narrowing
Tracheobronchial foreign body	Endoscopy: foreign body, tracheitis/bronchitis
Tuberculosis/interstitial lung infiltrates	Tracheobronchial aspiration: neutrophilia, lymphocytosis Bronchoalveolar lavage: neutrophilia or lymphocytosis Radiography: miliary infiltrate Lung biopsy: histology

can be introduced through the larynx of most normal horses without eliciting a cough, but in animals with chronic lower airway disease the physical presence of the endoscope in the larynx frequently stimulates paroxysmal coughing, which impedes the examination and causes distress to the patient. Coughing can be reduced with the topical application of a local anesthetic solution (such as 2 per cent lidocaine). Similar applications at each bronchial division will aid the examination of the bronchi.

The main uses of endoscopy are listed in Table 2. Endoscopy is helpful in excluding upper airway lesions as causes of chronic coughing and in the diagnosis of certain lower airway diseases such as tracheal deformities and tracheobronchial foreign bodies, and sometimes *Dictyocaulus arnfieldi* infestation. The presence of exercise-induced pulmonary hemorrhage (EIPH) may be confirmed with the endoscopic identification of free blood in the airways, provided that the amount of hemorrhage is large enough to be grossly visible and the examination is carried out at an appropriate time after the hemorrhage.

Exudates are commonly present in many pulmonary diseases including chronic obstructive pulmonary disease (COPD), pulmonary abscesses, pneumonia, and lungworm infestation. Such discharges may be visible through the endoscope if they are sufficiently voluminous, and it may be possible to determine whether they are originating from all of the major bronchi (suggesting diffuse lung disease) or from an isolated lung segment (i.e., focal lung disease). The nature of the discharge may be assessed and small quantities of exudate identified by tracheobronchial aspiration. Exudates present in large amounts may be sampled directly by suction through a catheter passed down the biopsy channel of the endoscope. For small amounts of exu-

TABLE 2. PRINCIPAL USES OF ENDOSCOPY OF THE LOWER RESPIRATORY TRACT IN THE HORSE

Diagnosis of airway deformities (tracheal constriction/collapse, bronchial collapse)
Diagnosis of tracheobronchial foreign bodies
Diagnosis of lungworm infestation
Identification of airway discharges (hemorrhage, exudate, excessive mucus)
Tracheobronchial aspiration
Bronchoalveolar lavage
Bronchial and pulmonary biopsy
Removal of foreign bodies

date or a discharge too tenacious to be aspirated directly, lavage with 20 to 30 ml of sterile saline will aid the retrieval of a sample. If the saline is delivered to the level of the tracheal bifurcation it will tend to accumulate in the trachea at the level of the thoracic inlet, from where it may be aspirated. The principal use of such aspirates is for cytological examination. Diseases such as COPD, pneumonia, and lung abscesses are characterized by large numbers of neutrophils, whereas lungworm infestation stimulates an intense eosinophilic reaction; *D. arnfieldi* larvae may also be observed in some cases of lungworm infestation. The microbiological culture of tracheobronchial secretions is essential in cases of pneumonia or lung abscesses, but aspirates obtained endoscopically are unsuitable for this use since they invariably become contaminated by upper airway flora as the instrument passes through the nasopharynx. Samples suitable for culture may, however, be obtained if a guarded tracheal swab or catheter (where the distal end of the sampling device is protected by a cellulose plug) is utilized. Alternatively, the transtracheal aspiration technique may be used.

Tracheobronchial aspirates are derived from the larger airways, and the cytology of such fluids may not be entirely representative of secretions present in the small airways, which are the principal site of many diffuse lung diseases, including COPD. In addition, some apparently healthy horses may show a neutrophilic reaction in the tracheobronchial aspirates, which probably represents a nonspecific response to airborne pollutants. For these reasons, the analysis of such samples may give confusing results; this problem is largely overcome if secretions in the more distal airways are sampled (e.g., by bronchoalveolar lavage).

TRANSTRACHEAL ASPIRATION

A variety of needle–catheter combinations may be used to perform transtracheal aspiration. A convenient combination includes a 12-gauge, 3-inch over-the-needle cannula and a No. 5 French canine urinary catheter, or a 10-gauge, 3-inch cannula with a No. 8 French urinary catheter. An area over the middle third of the ventral cervical trachea is prepared for aseptic surgery and a bleb of local anesthetic agent is injected subcutaneously over the midline. A stab incision is made through the skin, the cannula is introduced into the tracheal lumen between two cartilage rings, the stylet is removed, and the urinary catheter is passed down into the tracheal lumen to the level of the thoracic inlet where the aspiration is performed with 20 to 30 ml of sterile saline. A very fine intravenous (IV) catheter can usually be introduced through the skin without using local anesthetic.

Samples obtained by transtracheal aspiration are suitable for routine cytology, Gram stain, and culture. Both aerobic and anaerobic cultures should be performed in cases of pneumonia or lung abscesses. Potential complications of transtracheal aspiration include subcutaneous abscess formation at the site of tracheal puncture, and pneumomediastinum.

BRONCHOALVEOLAR LAVAGE

Bronchoalveolar lavage (BAL) is safe and effective for sampling the small peripheral airways and alveolar spaces and has become popular for diagnostic and research purposes. The procedure may be performed through an endoscope (at least 2 meters long) or "blindly" using a commercially available or home-made catheter. The tube is wedged into a small bronchus (usually a fourth- or fifth-generation segmental bronchus), and approximately 300 to 500 ml of saline is introduced and retrieved in a single or multiple aliquots. The predominant cell types in BAL fluid from normal horses are macrophages and lymphocytes, but if smaller quantities of lavage fluid are used a higher proportion of neutrophils may be found (indicating more of a bronchial/bronchiolar lavage than a true bronchoalveolar lavage). Coughing may be a problem in horses with lower airway disease but can be minimized with heavy sedation or the sequential application of dilute lidocaine solutions as the catheter is advanced down the bronchial tree.

BAL samples secretions from a very small lung segment. If the procedure is performed blindly, the specific segment being sampled will be unknown. Although this may be unimportant in diffuse lung disorders such as COPD, in focal lung diseases such as pneumonia, lung abscesses, or EIPH a normal BAL sample may be obtained that is of no diagnostic value.

THORACIC RADIOGRAPHY

The large size of the thorax in a horse is associated with technical complications that limit the application of thoracic radiography in the assessment of disease. However, with the use of rare earth intensifying screens, high-speed radiographic film, and an air gap between the patient and cassette, it is possible to obtain radiographs of diagnostic quality covering much of the adult horse's chest with relatively low-powered x-ray equipment. Four overlapping films are generally necessary to demonstrate all of the thoracic structures in the adult horse (Fig. 1). An air gap between the patient and the cassette allows some of the low-energy scattered radiation to disperse and eliminates the need for a grid, greatly reducing the exposure factors. A focus-film distance of 2 meters is convenient, but if low-powered x-ray units are being used, this may have to be reduced to 1.5 or 1.0 meters so that the exposure time can be kept short enough (0.1 second or less) to avoid motion artifacts.

Lesions that are readily detectable with radiography include pulmonary consolidation/pneumonia; lung abscesses; EIPH lesions; lung infiltrates such as neoplasia, granulomas and fibrosis; and pleural effusions. It should be remembered that a large amount of lung tissue is hidden from view by the diaphragm and cardiac shadows, so that significant lung pathology may be present despite a normal radiographic appearance. Small airway diseases such as COPD often produce minimal radiographic changes.

DIAGNOSTIC ULTRASONOGRAPHY

Diagnostic ultrasonography is noninvasive and does not use ionizing radiation. The disadvantage is that both air and bone interfaces reflect practically all the incident beam so that it cannot usefully penetrate beyond the surface of the aerated lung. Ultrasonography is, however, well suited to examining the pleura. The volume and character of pleural effusions can be evaluated, although pleural fluid cytology should always be used to confirm its nature. Fluid loculations, fibrin tags, adhesions, and pleural thickening can also be identified. Consolidated areas of lung and other soft tissue lesions in the lung may be evaluated by this technique only if they extend to the pleural surface. Needle biopsy of such lesions may be performed under ultrasonographic guidance.

THORACOCENTESIS

Thoracocentesis is readily performed in the standing horse and is generally safe. Potential complications include pneumothorax, hemothorax, and cardiac puncture. The main indication is in the diagnosis or treatment of pleural effusions. The procedure may be performed on the right side at the seventh intercostal space, or on the left side at the seventh or eighth intercostal space. The precise level at which the chest is entered may vary with the level of the effusion. The area should be clipped and prepared aseptically, and the skin and intercostal muscles infiltrated with local anesthetic. A stab incision is made through the skin, and some form of cannula such as an IV cannula, teat cannula, or metal bitch urinary catheter is introduced into the pleural cavity along the cranial border of the rib. A three-way tap should be used to prevent aspiration of air into the cavity if no fluid is present. Samples of pleural fluid should be examined for cell count, cytology, protein and glucose levels, and aerobic and anaerobic culture.

LUNG AND PLEURAL BIOPSY

Lung or pleural biopsies are undertaken with the primary objective of establishing a histological or microbiological diagnosis in cases in which the diagnosis cannot be established with certainty by less invasive techniques. Percutaneous pleural or lung biopsy specimens are generally obtained using a cutting needle such as the

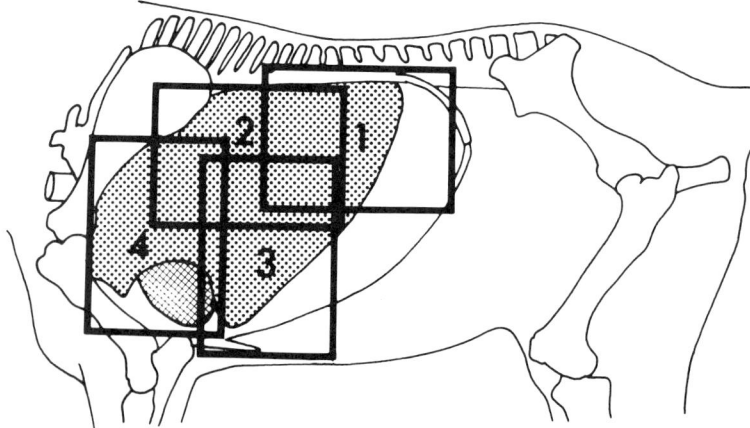

Figure 1. The four overlapping radiographic fields necessary to cover the entire thorax in the adult horse.

modified Vim disposable needle. The use of such wide-gauge needles (2 mm) carries the risk of potentially fatal complications, such as pneumothorax and hemorrhage, but in practice such complications appear to be rare.

Transbronchial lung biopsy is performed through the endoscope and is a viable alternative to percutaneous biopsy in cases of diffuse lung disease. The endoscope is wedged into a bronchus and the biopsy forceps advanced down a smaller bronchus until resistance is met. The forceps are advanced as far as possible during inspiration, then opened; the biopsy sample is taken as the airway narrows during exhalation. It is hoped that the forceps will have invaginated and torn away lung tissue as well as bronchial mucosa; a white fluffy-looking specimen that floats is likely to be a good one. Multiple biopsy specimens may be obtained in this manner.

PLEUROSCOPY

Pleuroscopy is the technique of examining the pleural cavity by endoscopy. It is a highly invasive technique and is usually limited to the confirmation of neoplasia in cases where this cannot be achieved by other procedures. An area over the selected intercostal space (which is assessed by radiography and diagnostic ultrasound) is clipped and prepared for surgery. The skin and tissues down to the parietal pleura are infiltrated with local anesthetic agents and an incision is made through the skin. The intercostal muscles are bluntly dissected and a teat cannula is pushed into the pleural space to create a pneumothorax. The ipsilateral lung will then collapse and an endoscope, preferably rigid, is introduced into the cavity. After the examination is completed the endoscope is removed and the intercostal muscles are sutured. A teat cannula is used to suck the air out of the cavity prior to closure of the skin.

Supplemental Readings

Beech, J.: Technique of tracheobronchial aspiration in the horse. Equine Vet. J., 13:136–137, 1981.
Bennett, D. G.: Evaluation of pleural fluid in the diagnosis of thoracic disease in the horse. J. Am. Vet. Med. Assoc., 188:814–815, 1986.
Mackey, V. S., and Wheat, J. D.: Endoscopic examination of the equine thorax. Equine Vet. J., 17:140–142, 1985.
Mair, T. S., and Gibbs, C.: Thoracic radiography in the horse. Vet. Rec. Suppl., 12:8–10, 1990.
Rantanen, N. W., Gage, L., and Paradis, M. R.: Ultrasonography as a diagnostic aid in pleural effusion of horses. Vet. Radiol., 22:211–216, 1981.
Raphel, C. F., and Gunson, D. E.: Percutaneous lung biopsy in the horse. Cornell Vet., 71:439–448, 1981.
Sweeney, C. R., Sweeney, R. W., and Benson, C. E.: Comparison of bacteria isolated from specimens obtained by use of endoscopic guarded tracheal swabbing and percutaneous tracheal aspiration in horses. J. Am. Vet. Med. Assoc., 195:1225–1229, 1989.
Whitwell, K. E., and Greet, T. R. C.: Collection and evaluation of tracheobronchial washes in the horse. Equine Vet. J., 16:499–508, 1984.

Therapeutics of the Respiratory Tract

Patrick M. Dixon, EDINBURGH, SCOTLAND

REST

The stresses of hard training, transport, and competition can exacerbate equine respiratory diseases. Rest, therefore, is an important aspect of the treatment for many equine pulmonary diseases. Unfortunately, there is little profit to be made from simply advising rest, and too few veterinarians promote and emphasize its enormous therapeutic benefit in respiratory disease. Viral respiratory infections in most cases cause more serious damage to the lungs than to the more obvious but less significant upper respiratory tract. Although the exact mechanisms are unclear, viral infections can cause continuing pulmonary disease in some animals for many months after the obvious signs of the infection have resolved and long after other infected animals have fully recovered. Rest is essential during the febrile period of viral disease but also for some weeks afterward until signs of pulmonary disease such as coughing and excessive tracheal secretions have greatly decreased.

Frequently, horses with lower respiratory

viral infection are dosed with antibiotics and anti-inflammatory drugs and kept in athletic training. As a consequence, and despite the antibiotic treatment, some horses get bacterial pleuropneumonias, or have delayed recovery or recrudescences of the viral diseases or possibly chronic bronchiolitis, which may predispose the animal to permanent exercise-induced pulmonary hemorrhage (EIPH) or chronic obstructive pulmonary disease (COPD). The higher incidence of pleuropneumonia in North America compared to Europe may in part reflect differences in the management of viral respiratory infections.

Hard exercise can exacerbate pulmonary inflammation by many mechanisms. In the galloping horse the increased respiratory rate and tidal volume cause large movements and stretching of the lung. Such physical stresses may be counterproductive to pulmonary healing. Hard exercise and the stress of travel also nonspecifically reduce the immune response by elevating plasma cortisol, epinephrine, and endorphin levels and specifically decrease equine pulmonary macrophage and lymphocyte activity. Recent work in humans has shown a reduction in the efficacy of the immune system of up to 70 per cent for 24 hours after hard exercise.

ANTIBIOTIC THERAPY

The aim of antibiotic therapy for bacterial respiratory infections is to safely achieve therapeutic levels of an effective antibiotic at the site of the infection, for an adequate period, and at reasonable cost. The practitioner should always consider whether antibiotic therapy is really indicated. Surveys of human medical practices have shown that up to two thirds of prescribed antibiotics are not indicated. Although increased numbers of bacteria can be isolated from the lower respiratory tract of many horses with viral respiratory diseases, these bacteria are rarely significant. With time and rest in a well-ventilated, dust-free box stall or outdoors in suitable climates, the pulmonary inflammation and bacterial numbers will regress. In primary viral infections, antibiotics have no effect on the course of the disease and may have adverse effects by potentially allowing the development of antimicrobial-resistant respiratory tract bacterial flora. High numbers of mainly gram-negative bacteria in association with a primarily neutrophilic cytology can be isolated from the lower respiratory secretions of many horses with COPD. These bacteria are not significant, and antibiotics have no clinical effect on the course of the disease.

These presumably opportunistic bacteria will regress spontaneously within weeks after the inhaled allergens are removed from the environment. A unilateral purulent nasal discharge usually indicates an upper respiratory lesion, and despite high levels of pathogenic bacteria such as *Streptococcus zooepidemicus* in these discharges, these infections are either secondary to poor natural drainage, for example, in primary sinusitis or guttural pouch empyema, or secondary to a tooth root abscess, maxillary cyst, upper respiratory tract tumor, or mycotic lesion. The temporary and usually incomplete decrease in the purulent nasal discharge following antimicrobial therapy is not in the patient's best interest as it just delays the establishment of a specific diagnosis and the institution of appropriate treatment of the primary cause, which is often surgical.

A pulmonary abscess, for example with *Rhodococcus equi* infection, forms an obvious physical barrier to antibiotic penetration, but chronic pulmonary infections can also prevent the diffusion of antibiotics from the blood to the site of lung infection. In acute respiratory infections, the bronchoalveolar barrier does not appear to prevent the diffusion of antibiotics. Antibiotics differ in their capacity to cross this barrier and their clinical efficacy is related more to their concentration in respiratory secretions rather than to serum levels. The aminoglycosides achieve poor levels in the lung in all species. Parenterally administered trimethoprim and sulfonamides have been found to achieve better levels in respiratory secretions in horses with chronic pulmonary disease than the penicillins, although further work is required in this field. The penicillins require increased dosage or frequency of administration in chronic lung disease to achieve adequate respiratory secretion levels. Some suggested antibiotic regimens for respiratory disease are shown in Table 1. Ideally, samples should be taken for culture and sensitivity testing (see p. 3) prior to implementing judicious antibiotic therapy while awaiting laboratory results. Although most bilateral nasal discharges are of pulmonary origin, they have variable and often high levels of upper respiratory tract contamination, as do most tracheal secretions collected by endoscopy or even bronchoalveolar lavage. Samples collected by transtracheal punctures or by protected endoscopic catheter techniques are most accurate. With unilateral nasal discharges, cultures and sensitivity testing are usually futile as the bacteria are commonly opportunistic and are quickly replaced by more resistant bacteria following antibiotic treatments.

TABLE 1. SUGGESTED ANTIMICROBIAL DOSAGE REGIMENS FOR EQUINE BACTERIAL RESPIRATORY INFECTIONS

Drug	Route	Dose	Interval (Hours)
Penicillin G sodium	IV, IM	20,000 units/kg	6–8
Procaine penicillin	IM	25,000 units/kg	12–24
Amikacin sulfate	IV, IM	4–7 mg/kg	8
Amoxicillin trihydrate	IM	6–10 mg/kg	8–12
Ampicillin sodium	IV, IM	10–20 mg/kg	6–8
Ampicillin trihydrate	IM	10–20 mg/kg	12
Chloramphenicol succinate	IV, IM	25 mg/kg	6–8
Chloramphenicol palmitate	PO	50 mg/kg	6
Cloxacillin sodium	IM	25–30 mg/kg	6
Erythromycin lactobionate	IV	5 mg/kg	8
Erythromycin estolate	PO	20–25 mg/kg	6
Gentamicin sulfate	IM, IV	3 mg/kg	12
Metronidazole solution, 0.5%	IV	20 mg/kg	12
Metronidazole	PO	20 mg/kg	12
Rifampin	PO	5 mg/kg	12
Streptomycin sulfate	IM	8–12 mg/kg	8–12
Trimethoprim-sulfonamide	IV, IM	15–25 mg/kg	8–12

ROUTE OF ADMINISTRATION

In the treatment of chronic pulmonary infections, a poor response to antibiotic treatment can sometimes be attributed to poor penetration of the antibiotic to the site of infection. Although increased dosage rates and frequency of administration can overcome this problem, care must be taken with some antibiotics (e.g., the aminoglycosides) to avoid overdosing and toxicity, particularly when used in foals with reduced renal function. Other attempts to increase pulmonary antibiotic levels include direct intratracheal antibiotic administration, which simply increases antibiotic concentrations in the larger airways. Aerosolized (nebulized) antibiotics, which are usually irritant to the airways and induce bronchoconstriction, can be given following bronchodilator treatment. Although the antibiotic-containing aerosol penetrates deeply into the lung, in normal horses only 10 to 15 per cent is deposited in the bronchioles. However, much less is deposited in diseased parts, owing to reduced air flow in such areas. The stability of the antibiotic aerosol ensures that most is exhaled, causing subsequent environmental contamination and human health risks.

DURATION OF TREATMENT

Many veterinarians use antibiotics for 1 to 3 days, which can result in unnecessary relapses and development of bacterial resistance. As a general rule, antibiotics should be given for at least 7 days for pulmonary infections. With these longer courses, there is a temptation to resort to oral administration, but many antibacterials are either poorly absorbed from the gastrointestinal (GI) tract (e.g., aminoglycosides) or are broken down by adult gut flora (e.g., trimethoprim in adult horses). Parenteral antibiotic administration is indicated where possible until further studies on the GI tract absorption of antibiotics in the adult horse show otherwise.

Prophylactic antibiotic administration may be justified during outbreaks of neonatal septicemia or in weak or dysmature foals, but in general this practice is undesirable. In addition to the risk of inducing antibiotic resistance, it can lead to a false sense of security and lax stable hygiene and management.

Intracellular bacterial infections such as *Rhodococcus equi* respond poorly to the usual range of antibiotics and a combination of erythromycin and rifampin that appears to be synergistic can be effective. With inhalation pneumonias, such as those associated with esophageal choke, pharyngeal dysphagias, or water inhalation, and in many cases of pleuropneumonia, anaerobic bacteria cause much of the pulmonary disease. These patients should be treated, preferably prophylactically, with drugs also active against anaerobic bacteria. Metronidazole is very effective against anaerobes only, but the intravenous form, unlike the oral form, is prohibitively expensive. The penicillins, chloramphenicol, and trimethoprim-sulfa combinations also have good activity against anaerobes, unlike the aminoglycosides or tetracyclines. Chloramphenicol, despite its short half-life, unpredictable oral uptake, and public health risks, is effective against most equine respiratory bacterial pathogens but should be kept as a reserve.

There is no consensus of opinion on the advisability of antibiotic treatment for strangles, but penicillin is the drug of choice, preferably given early in the course of the disease (see p. 324).

CORTICOSTEROIDS

In peracute bacterial or viral pneumonias there may be an indication for the use of these immunosuppressive drugs because of their anti-inflammatory effects, to reduce life-threatening pulmonary inflammation and exudation. Antibiotics used in combination with corticosteroids must be *bactericidal*. Rare cases of equine alveolitis with massive exudation may also respond well to corticosteroids. However, these drugs as well as nonsteroidal anti-inflammatory drugs (NSAIDs) are misused in equine respiratory disease, particularly in viral diseases, where they are used in combination with antibiotics to mask the signs in an attempt to get the animal back to work more quickly. The immunosuppressive effects of corticosteroids and the stress of a premature return to work can cause long-term pulmonary disorders.

In horses with COPD or summer pasture–associated obstructive pulmonary disease (SPAOPD), short-acting corticosteroids such as prednisolone can be given in severe cases to reduce lung inflammation, primarily affecting the delayed response and bronchial hyperreactivity. They are not bronchodilators or bronchomucotropic agents and have little effect on the acute phase inflammation of COPD. In combination with environmental changes they may speed clinical remission. Long-term corticosteroid therapy without environmental control will result in incomplete remission of signs, the usual potential side effects of chronic corticosteroid therapy, and, particularly in SPAOPD, the risk of development of laminitis in susceptible animals.

NONSTEROIDAL ANTI-INFLAMMATORY DRUGS

NSAIDs, particularly flunixin° but also phenylbutazone† and meclofenamic acid,‡ can also be used initially along with antibacterial therapy in peracute pneumonias as they can reduce life-threatening inflammation and are not immunosuppressive. They are not effective short- or long-term treatments for COPD.

°Banamine, Schering-Plough Animal Health, Kenilworth, NJ
†Butazolidin, Coopers Animal Health, Mundelein, IL
‡Arquel, Ford Dodge Labs, Fort Dodge, IA

BRONCHODILATORS

Three groups of drugs with bronchodilator effects have been used in horses.

MUSCARINIC RECEPTOR ANTAGONISTS—PARASYMPATHOLYTICS

Airway smooth muscle has rich parasympathetic innervation that causes bronchoconstriction when stimulated. Atropine blocks muscarinic receptors that are activated by acetylcholine release during parasympathetic nerve stimulation and thus causes bronchodilation. Although it is a most effective bronchodilator in the horse, its parasympatholytic effects are widespread and include tachycardia, mydriasis, decreased gut motility, and reduced output and increased viscosity of respiratory secretions. These side effects and its short duration of action precludes the widespread clinical use of atropine as a bronchodilator. The newer parasympatholytic drugs, ipratropium bromide° and oxytropium bromide,† are poorly absorbed from the respiratory system when given by nebulization and so have fewer systemic effects and no adverse mucokinetic effects. Because of their side effects, it is unlikely that these drugs will be of major clinical use in horses when used parenterally or orally.

β_2-ADRENOCEPTOR AGONISTS—SYMPATHOMIMETICS

Although only the tracheal smooth muscle is innervated by the sympathetic nervous system, all the airways are richly supplied with β_2 sympathetic receptors, which cause bronchodilation when stimulated by circulating catecholamines. Drugs such as isoprenaline, once widely used in humans, stimulate both β_1 (primarily cardiac) receptors as well as β_2 (primarily smooth muscle) receptors and have been largely replaced by a range of more specific agents, for example salbutamol‡ or terbutaline,§ that stimualte only β_2 receptors and thus have fewer side effects. Some of the newer β_2 sympathomimetics, for example clenbuterol∥ or mabuterol, have stronger and even more selective β_2 receptor binding, which will produce bronchodilation at low doses, result in fewer side effects, and provide longer duration of action. Given IV or by nebulization they

---

°Atrovent, Boehringer Ingelheim, Ridgefield, CT
†Oxivent, Boehringer Ingelheim, Bracknell, UK
‡Ventolin, Glaxo, Research Triangle Park, NC
§Bricanyl, Merrell Dow Pharmaceuticals, Cincinnati, OH
∥Ventipulmin, Boehringer Ingelheim, Mississauga, ONT

achieve maximal effects within minutes; most are absorbed well from the gut. These drugs also markedly increase mucociliary clearance in the horse and are potent pulmonary mast cell stabilizers. Clenbuterol is the only β_2 sympathomimetic approved for use in the horse; its effects are well documented in this species. The oral dose is 0.8 μg/kg b.i.d. If there is no improvement after three days of therapy, the dose can be increased to 0.16 μg/kg. The dose can be further increased to 0.24 and 0.32 μg/kg at three day intervals until a response is obtained. Horses failing to respond to 0.32 μg/kg can be considered to have irreversible bronchospasm. Do not begin with the high dose as it will cause excitement.

Methylxanthine Derivates

This group includes theophylline, theobromine, and caffeine. Theophylline is the most effective bronchodilator of this group, but because of poor solubility it is administered as various salts, for example, aminophylline or etamphylline. Although a more specific bronchodilator than theobromine or caffeine, theophylline also has widespread effects, including central nervous system, cardiac, and skeletal muscle stimulation and diuresis. The exact intracellular mode of action of these drugs is not fully understood; although once believed to act by increasing cyclic adenosine monophosphate levels in airway muscle cells through phosphodiesterase inhibition, more potent phosphodiesterase inhibitors have been found to have no bronchodilator effects. It has recently been suggested that they inhibit endogenously produced adenosine. Most theophylline salts are well absorbed from the equine gut, and newer slow-release GI preparations are now available. More rapid bronchodilation can be obtained by IV preparations. Studies in the horse suggest that although they are very effective bronchodilators, there is even a narrower therapeutic margin than in man, and toxic effects, especially hyperesthesia and excitement, can readily occur with overdosing, particularly with IV usage. Theophylline is also a very potent mucokinetic agent and a pulmonary mast cell stabilizer.

Clinical Use of Bronchodilators

These drugs, primarily the sympathomimetics such as clenbuterol and to a lesser extent theophylline, are widely and increasingly used in equine medicine, particularly in acute cases of COPD or SPAOPD, where bronchospasm of the larger airways plays a significant role in the respiratory dysfunction. However, the inflammatory changes in the smaller airways, i.e., cellular infiltration and mucus blockage, are not greatly affected by such drugs. Given IV or by nebulization in the case of sympathomimetics, they significantly reduce the increased airway resistance in most acute COPD or SPAOPD cases. With all bronchodilators the effects can be variable and individual variation in response is very marked. More prolonged courses of 1 to 2 weeks in conjunction with the environmental changes discussed on p. 310 will promote a more rapid resolution of clinical signs. Although the β_2 sympathomimetics and theophylline can inhibit the release of mast cell inflammatory mediators and increase mucociliary transport, these anti-inflammatory effects are not marked, and in the face of continuing antigenic challenge, as with prolonged bronchodilator administration without environmental control, these drugs will have only a partial therapeutic effect.

There may be a role for bronchodilators, particularly the sympathomimetics, as supportive therapy during viral respiratory infections. In addition to their ciliary mediated enhancement of mucokinesis, they relieve any bronchoconstriction resulting from virus-induced nonspecific airway hyperreactivity and thus further enhance mucociliary clearance, as well as relieving dyspnea. In severe pneumonias there is a risk that by inducing bronchodilation they may divert blood flow from well-ventilated to diseased parts of the lung and thus cause or exacerbate an acute ventilation-perfusion mismatching, which could worsen the animal's hypoxemia. Unless oxygen therapy is available these drugs should not be given IV to such patients. Recent work has shown that administration of sympathomimetics by an oxygen driven nebulizer can overcome this problem.

SODIUM CROMOGLYCATE

This unique drug acts by inhibiting both the immediate and late phase inflammatory response to antigen challenge in the susceptible lung. It is poorly absorbed from the gut and must be administered as a nebulized aerosol* or as a microfine powder. Some 85 to 90 per cent is deposited in the upper respiratory tract. Its exact mechanism of action is unknown, and an earlier belief that it simply acted as a mast cell stabilizer appears ungrounded, because some β_2 sympathomimetics are more potent mast cell stabilizers yet do not display the properties of sodium

---

*Intal, Fisons Consumer Health, Rochester, NY

cromoglycate. It is now thought likely to act as an inhibitor of platelet-activating factor (PAF), which is involved in both the early and late phases of pulmonary inflammatory response. In humans, cromolyn has little beneficial effect once exposure to antigens and clinical signs have occurred. In the horse, it is most beneficial if given to asymptomatic patients with COPD, but it can also be of some benefit during symptomatic periods. In the horse its clinical effects can last for many days, compared to hours in man. It is of value in some animals for long-term use where environmental control is genuinely impossible, such as a horse sharing a large open stable, or where environmental control is normally practiced but the patient must temporarily risk exposure to hay or straw, for example at competitions. The drug must be given by inhalation, which can be tedious and requires special equipment.

DRUGS ACTING ON MUCOCILIARY CLEARANCE (Mucokinesis)

Mucokinetic drugs, which by differing mechanisms increase the transport of the complex and incompletely understood airway secretions, are widely used in the treatment of equine pulmonary diseases. There is still limited scientific evidence on the clinical value of many of these agents both in humans and the horse, even though many have been shown to significantly increase mucociliary clearance. They can be divided into five groups according to mechanism of action, although many drugs have more than one mechanism of action. *Mucolytic drugs* increase mucokinesis by decreasing the viscosity of mucus, providing that ciliary action is effective. *Surface-acting drugs* are claimed to hydrate and emulsify airway secretions and promote their separation from airway walls. *Bronchomucotropic agents* (expectorants) increase the volume and reputedly decrease the viscosity of airway secretions by various vagally mediated reflexes or by direct mucous gland stimulation. *Cilia augmentors* increase the beat frequency of the respiratory cilia. *Bronchodilators* improve mucokinesis and also allow more productive coughing by dilating the airways.

Most of the effective mucolytic and surface-acting agents and some bronchomucotropic drugs must be given by aerosol. This is most effectively achieved by means of a nebulizer that produces an aerosol of droplet size less than 5 microns that reaches the distal airways. This involves costly equipment and prolonged administration times, usually many times daily, which are major disadvantages. Many of these agents will induce bronchoconstriction, and there is also the possibility that bacteria may be introduced, along with the aerosol, deep into a possibly immunocompromised lung. Some examples of these drugs are listed in Table 2. More than 30 other drugs are claimed to have mucokinetic effects, and hundreds of proprietary compounds containing various combinations of these are other drugs, including antihistamines, are widely and controversially used and misused in treating human and equine respiratory diseases.

Dehydration causes a reduction in the normal 95 per cent water content of airway mucus and the resultant increased viscosity reduces mucokinesis. For this and other obvious reasons, the maintenance of normal hydration whether by oral or IV route in horses with severe pulmonary disease is essential. Some published work has shown the clinical benefits of the bronchomucotropic drug bromhexine° in horses, which also increases antibiotic levels in airway secretions in other species. Clinical trials have shown the mucolytic dembrexine† to be of benefit in equine pulmonary disease. The β_2 sympathomimetics or theophylline promote mucokinesis by cilia enhancement, bronchodilation, and possibly bronchomucotropic effects. They also eliminate bronchoconstriction, which can occur nonspecifically with any airway inflammation, and stabilize pulmonary mast cells. These agents may prove to be the mucokinetic agents of choice in the horse. Clenbuterol has recently been shown to be an effective mucokinetic agent in equine COPD.

ANTIHISTAMINES

Although histamine levels in bronchoalveolar lavage fluid are sometimes increased in COPD, treatment with antihistamines has proved ineffective in the horse, which suggests that histamine is not a major inflammatory mediator in this disease.

RESPIRATORY STIMULANTS (Analeptics)

No drugs are available that will specifically stimulate the respiratory center, but some, such as nikethamide or doxapram, that stimulate all levels of the cerebrospinal axis also stimulate respiratory drive. They were once widely used in the treatment of respiratory failure in neonates or during anesthesia but are now believed to be

---

°Bisolvon, Boehringer Ingelheim, Bracknell, UK
†Sputolysin, Boehringer Ingelheim, Bracknell, UK

TABLE 2. MUCOKINETIC AGENTS WHICH HAVE BEEN USED IN THE HORSE

Agent	Dose	Administration	Mechanism	Side Effects/Disadvantages
MUCOLYTICS				
Sterile water	2–5 ml/50 kg q.i.d.	Aerosol	Rehydrates respiratory secretions	Requires nebulizer (bronchoconstriction)
Sterile saline	2–5 ml/50 kg q.i.d.	Aerosol	Rehydrates respiratory secretions	Requires nebulizer (bronchoconstriction)
Sterile saline	10 ml/kg	IV	Rehydrates respiratory secretions, bronchomucotropic at higher levels	Expense, possibility cardiac overload
Acetylcysteine, 10%	2–5 ml/50 kg q.i.d.	Aerosol	Disrupts sulfide bonds of mucus	Requires nebulizer, induces bronchoconstriction
Acetylcysteine, 10% with isoproterenol, 0.05%	5–10 ml/50 kg q.i.d.	Aerosol	Disrupts sulfide bonds of mucus	Requires nebulizer, induces bronchoconstriction
Sodium bicarbonate soln., 2%	3 ml/50 kg	Aerosol	Alkalinity disrupts mucous structure	Requires nebulizer, induces bronchoconstriction
Propylene glycol, 5%	3 ml/50 kg	Aerosol	Disrupts mucous structure + surface acting effect	Requires nebulizer, induces bronchoconstriction
Dembrexine	0.3 mg/kg	PO	Modifies mucus side chains, reducing viscosity	Not yet tested on pregnant mares
SURFACE-ACTING AGENTS				
Glycerol, 5%	2–5 ml/50 kg	Aerosol	Rehydrates and emulsifies mucus/frothy secretion	Requires nebulizer (irritation + bronchoconstriction)
Ethyl alcohol, 50%	5–10 ml/50 kg	Aerosol	Rehydrates and emulsifies mucus/frothy secretion	Requires nebulizer (irritation + bronchoconstriction)
BRONCHOMUCOTROPIC AGENTS				
Bromhexine HCl	0.1–0.25 mg/kg	PO	Unknown; also a mucolytic action	Low bioavailability and short half-life in horse
Potassium iodide	1 g/50 kg q.i.d.	PO	Gastropulmonary reflex	Iodism with long-term usage
Glycerol guaicolate	0.1–0.2 g/50 kg q.i.d.	PO	Vagally mediated and direct gland stimulation	Gastric irritation, dullness
Ammonium chloride	0.3 g/50 kg q.i.d.	PO	Gastropulmonary reflex	Gastric irritation, dullness
CILIA AUGMENTORS				
β sympathomimetics	See Bronchodilator section	PO, IV, aerosol	Possibly by altering periciliary fluid and mucus rheology	See Bronchodilator section
Xanthines	See Bronchodilator section	PO, IV, aerosol	Ciliary activity (also increases mucus production)	See Bronchodilator section
AIRWAY DILATORS				
β sympathomimetics	See Bronchodilator section	PO, IV, aerosol	Enlarges airways, more effective coupling	See Bronchodilator section
Xanthines		PO, IV, aerosol	Enlarges airways, more effective coupling	See Bronchodilator section

of little clinical value. The theophyllines increase medullary blood flow and are also effective analeptics.

ANTITUSSIVES

There is very little indication for these drugs in equine practice. Coughing is a protective reflex and indicates the presence of pulmonary disease, which should be diagnosed and specifically treated.

IMMUNOSTIMULANTS

Levamisole has been used in horses as an immunostimulant, often at lower doses and for much shorter periods than used in man. Recently a *Propionibacterium acnes* extract has also been promoted as an equine immunostimulant. There is little published evidence of the efficacy of either drug as an immunostimulant in the horse.

Supplemental Readings

Boushey, H. A.: Bronchodilators. *In:* Katzung, B. G. (ed.): Basic and Clinical Pharmacology, 4th ed. Norwalk, CT., Appleton & Lange, Inc., 1989, pp. 242–254.
Lehnert, B. E., and Schachter, E. N.: The Pharmacology of Respiratory Care. St. Louis, C. V. Mosby Co., 1980.
Rang, H. P., and Dale, M. M.: The respiratory system. *In:* Pharmacology. Edinburgh, Churchill Livingstone, 1987, pp. 297–308.

Environmental Monitoring in Relation to Equine Respiratory Disease

Andrew F. Clarke, GUELPH, ONTARIO, CANADA

The stabled horse is exposed to a wide range of respiratory pathogens. These include bacteria, viruses, mold spores, noxious gases, plant material, dust mites, and parasites. Their pathogenicity arises from their ability to initiate infection, induce allergy, behave as toxins or irritants, destroy tissue (e.g., migrating parasites), or simply overwhelm the lung's defense mechanisms, increasing the susceptibility to other pathogens. Furthermore, apart from initiating or increasing the likelihood of respiratory disease, the stable environment can affect the duration and severity of episodes of disease.

The likelihood of a pathogen inducing disease is dependent on its own pathogenicity, the level of challenge to which the host is exposed, and the susceptibility of the host. The stable environment, affected primarily by stable design and husbandry practices, can affect all of these factors.

In this chapter techniques and equipment that are appropriate for use by field veterinarians to objectively assess the stable environment are described. Guidelines for environmental criteria of stables are presented, along with methods of meeting these needs.

THE HORSES

A history of horses that have been housed, along with clinical details of horses currently in residence, should be the starting point. In relation to respiratory disease it may be necessary to carry out endoscopic examinations and lung washes (see p. 301). The involvement of viral and bacterial infections should also be assessed. This usually involves the collection of swabs from the horses for culturing or the analysis of sequential blood samples for changes in antibody titer levels (see p. 316). With the exception of *Rhodococcus equi*, which proliferates away from the horse, infectious agents are best sought directly from the horse rather than from air samples. This can be achieved using nasal or pharyngeal swabs or lung washes.

STABLE DIMENSIONS, WINDOWS, VENTS, AND DOORS

A tape measure provides some of the most useful information on stables. Guidelines for dimensions of stables and doors are given in Table 1.

TABLE 1. RECOMMENDED DIMENSIONS FOR STABLES (METERS)

Box stall	
Ponies	3.0 × 3.0
Horses	3.6 × 3.6
Foaling or isolation box	5.0 × 5.0
Tie stall	
Width minimum	1.7
Length	3.3
Rear passageway (minimum)	2.0
Door	
Height	2.4
Width	1.2

Measurements should be made (or taken from plans) of the dimensions of the buildings, the size and positioning of vents and windows, and the size of the skylight. Note should also be taken of the type of materials used and what provisions have been made for insulation. The dimensions of the building, the number of horses housed, and the level of insulation affect the ventilation requirements of a stable (Table 2). Skylights and windows allow sunlight, a potent killer of bacteria, viruses, and other microbes, including worm larvae, into stables. Ultraviolet translucent glass or plastic is preferable to normal glass. As a general guideline, the skylight should make up 10 per cent of the roof area.

Ethological studies have shown that horses prefer light stables. Increasing daylight is the primary factor that initiates the loss of winter coats and stimulates the mare to commence cycling (see *Current Therapy in Equine Medicine 2*, p. 491). Windows and open-top doors of box stalls allow horses to put their heads out into fresh air and also help to allay some of the boredom associated with being stabled for long hours.

VENTILATION

Closing a stable to keep it warm will increase the feed conversion efficiency of animals even though there is almost invariably an associated increase in respiratory disease. The short-term athletic ability and long-term welfare of horses are largely dependent on their respiratory well-being, so that fresh air takes precedence over feed conversion efficiency.

In a stable with clean forage and bedding, there is little advantage in having a ventilation rate of greater than 8 air changes per hour. In the vast majority of stables this can be achieved by natural forces of ventilation without mechanical intervention. There are three natural forces of ventilation: (1) the stack effect, i.e., air warmed by the horse rises and leaves the stable, drawing fresh air in; (2) aspiration: wind blowing across the top of a stable helps to draw stale air out of the building; and (3) perflation: wind blowing from side to side or end to end of a building aids ventilation.

Properly placed and adequately sized wall and roof vents are essential to make full use of these forces. Examples of the requirements for natural ventilation are given in Table 2. In designing new stables or improving existing buildings, calculations should be made for the individual structures. A meteorological survey will be of use in identifying particularly exposed walls and extremes of weather likely to be encountered.

For most box stalls an open-top door provides adequate inlet area for natural ventilation. However, allowances must be made for the situation when doors and windows are closed. A permanent vent can be placed above the front door. Most boxes should have a back wall vent as well to ensure proper air mixing and movement. For a monopitched roof this vent should be high in the back wall. Boxes with a peaked roof should have a capped chimney or covered ridge to act as an outlet for warm, stale air. Drafts can be cut down by baffling vents or covering them with plastic mesh such as Netlon. This will also prevent the entry of rain or snow into boxes. Vents should be well distributed to ensure thorough ventilation. This is especially critical in large barns.

One of the benefits of insulating stables is highlighted in Table 2. Insulation, by maintaining a slightly greater temperature difference between the inside and outside of the stable, allows smaller openings to be used to provide adequate natural ventilation in still air conditions. The benefits of insulation in terms of warmth within an average stable are not great.

Horses tolerate a wide range of temperatures. Those especially prone to cold include young foals and severely ill or malnourished animals. In such circumstances, additional sources of heating may be required. In large, airy stables and

TABLE 2. GUIDELINES FOR MINIMUM INLET AND OUTLET AREAS PER HORSE FOR BOX STALLS AND BARNS (METERS)

	Outlet Area	Inlet Area
Uninsulated box stall*	0.34	0.17
Insulated box stall*	0.27	0.14
Uninsulated barn†	0.46	0.23
Insulated barn†	0.38	0.19

Calculations should be made for individual structures (see Clarke, 1987).
*50 cu m of air space per horse, 1.0 m between inlet and outlet.
†85 cu m of air space per horse, 2.0 m between inlet and outlet.

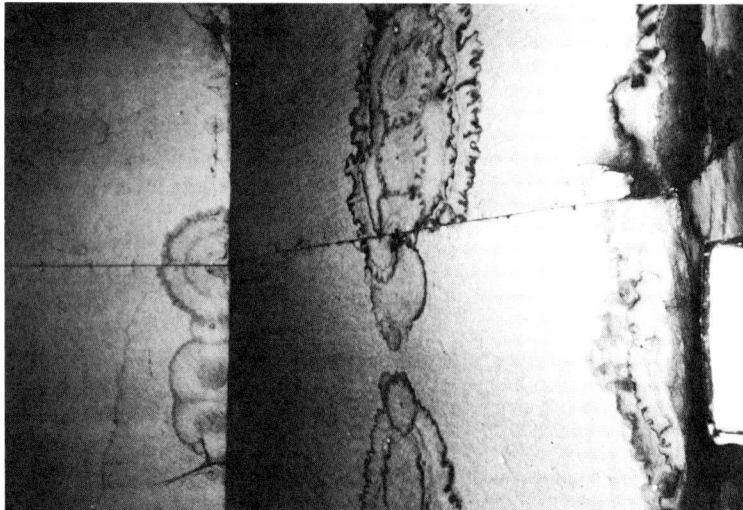

Figure 1. Pattern staining on the roof of a stable is a typical sign of poor ventilation. It usually occurs because of condensation but occasionally is seen with a leaking roof.

barns this can be most effectively achieved with the use of quartz-halogen heaters. The use of rugs, especially with the emergence of new, highly efficient materials that inhibit radiant heat loss,* cannot be overemphasized. A rug and a deep bedding will help to prevent conductive loss of heat when a horse or foal is lying down, with concrete-based floors being a particular cause for concern. Drafts increase convective heat losses, especially if the horse or foal has a wet coat. A draft is described as a windspeed of greater than 0.4 meters per second. An anemometer provides a ready method for quantifying air speed. Baffling vents or covering them with plastic mesh decreases the likelihood of drafts.

Condensation is a tell-tale sign of poor ventilation. Pattern staining seen in the roofs of stables (Fig. 1) is a sign of condensation, which can be avoided with improved ventilation and the use of a damp-proof membrane. In still, humid weather conditions where there are sudden changes in air temperature, some unavoidable condensation may occur on the walls of stables.

Graphic demonstrations of air flow patterns in stables and the adequacy of ventilation can be made with the use of smoke tubes or smoke pellets. The smoke tubes provide pinpoint sources of smoke that can be observed. Smoke pellets can be burned and fill a stable or barn with smoke. (Do not forget to turn off fire alarms.) Actual ventilation rates can be assessed by monitoring the clearance of the smoke with an airborne particle counter.†

---

*Flectarug, Chepstow, Gwent, UK
†Rion, Hawksley, Lancing, England

AIRBORNE PARTICULATE MATTER

In assessing the respiratory risks associated with dust there are four important points to consider: (1) The challenge should be quantified in absolute terms, depending on the types of samplers available; this is achieved by describing the mass of dust per unit volume of air (typically mg per cu m) or the number of particles per unit volume of (typically nos. per cu m). (2) Absolute challenge should be considered in relation to respirable and nonrespirable fractions, i.e., an indication of the amounts of dust capable of getting down deep into the lung; a rather arbitrarily chosen and widely accepted cutoff point being 5 μm. Owners often ask about the significance of the dust particles that are seen in the air of stables when fresh shavings or shredded paper are bedded down. By and large this dust consists of relatively large particles not capable of getting down deep into the lung. (3) The primary constituents of the dust should be identified; this can involve microscopic examinations, culturing samples, or even chemical analyses. (4) It is critical that the sampling technique identifies the challenges, especially high-level challenges to which horses are actually exposed. The highest levels of airborne contaminants in stables coincide with mucking out. Samples should be taken at quiet periods of the day and following mucking out. A mechanical sampler sitting on a table in the middle of a well-ventilated stable may record relatively low levels of dust while the horse eating its hay or sniffing at its bedding may be inhaling millions of respirable particles with each breath.

The simplest and least expensive types of samplers for assessing absolute challenge of airborne dust are units that collect dust from set volumes of air onto filter papers that are then weighed. More sophisticated (and expensive) units count and size particles using light dispersion techniques or piezoelectric balances to present data on masses of airborne dust.

The most common approach to collecting dust samples for microscopic examination involves the direct collection of particles onto gel-coated microscope slides. Exposing a slide to air and relying on particles to settle onto the slide will lead to disproportionate collection of large, nonrespirable dust particles such as plant fragments, because they fall from the air at a much greater rate than aerodynamically smaller, respirable mold spores. Similar limitations apply to "rotorod" collectors that rotate slides on a metal arm. Impactor samples draw air samples in through narrow slits and fire dust particles toward microscope slides; the efficiency of collection depends on the inertia of the particles. These samplers range from simple one-stage units to multistage units that deposit particles onto microscope slides according to their aerodynamic characteristics. The latter is costly in terms of capital outlay and laboratory time to count the large number of samples collected. The simple single-stage impactor discussed later is the most practical for field veterinarians.

Air samples can be examined for the presence of viable microorganisms by collecting samples into liquid and then plating out the samples onto culture media or using tissue culture techniques. Alternatively, the samples can be collected directly onto culture media. Exposing an open Petri dish to stable air will lead to disproportionate collection of large particles; this is especially relevant in relation to fungi and actinomycetes. Again, there is a wide variety of equipment such as impingers, cyclones, or impactor samplers that are aerodynamically more efficient than exposing an open Petri dish. Many of the infectious agents that cause respiratory disease in horses are short-lived when aerosolized, the collection procedures can cause damage to microorganisms, and the majority of pathogens require specific culture media and specific incubation temperatures to flourish. The best approach to identifying infectious agents causing respiratory disease is to take appropriate samples from the horses themselves. Airborne mold spores pose special problems for identification. The spores of many of the fungi and actinomycetes encountered in stables cannot be differentiated by microscopic examination. Culture techniques using Sabouraud's media with incubation temperature of 28° and/or 38° C will only allow a small proportion of potentially relevant species to develop. Appropriate media and incubation temperatures for these purposes are given in Table 3.

Horses are exposed to airborne particles ranging from mold spores to aerosols of bacteria and viruses. The primary sources of airborne particles in stables are the horse's feed (specifically forage) and its bedding. The highest exposures of respirable dust to which horses are exposed are associated with the mold-contaminated forage or bedding. In such circumstances dust levels at mucking out or in close proximity to the hay net may approach 10 to 15 mg per cu m, with between 20 per cent and 60 per cent of this fraction being respirable. There may be up to 3000 respirable particles of dust per milliliter of air (assuming a tidal volume of 4 litres, this challenge represents 12,000,000 particles per breath). Results of culture analyses reveal the presence of thermophilic and thermotolerant fungal and *Actinomyces* spp. Management practices that minimize the horse's exposure to these species of molds will decrease the total dust challenges described by up to 99 per cent.

A simple technique that allows on-the-spot assessments of mold of forage and bedding can help the clinician identify contaminated source materials and explain the problem to the client. The technique involves the use of a hand-held sampler that impacts dust onto a microscope

TABLE 3. MEDIA NECESSARY FOR THE GROWTH OF THE WIDE RANGE OF FUNGI AND ACTINOMYCETES TO WHICH THE STABLED HORSE IS EXPOSED (INCUBATION TEMPERATURES 28°, 38°, AND 58° C)

Fungal medium
  Malt extract, 20 gm
  Agar, 20 gm
  Distilled H_2O, 1 liter
  Penicillin,* 20 units ml^{-1}
  Streptomycin,* 40 units ml^{-1}
  Triton N101,† 0.05%
Actinomycete medium‡
  Oxoid nutrient agar, 14 gm
  Casein hydrolysate, 2 gm
  Agar, 10 gm
  Distilled H_2O, 1 liter
  Actidione,§ 50 µg ml^{-1}

*Suppresses bacteria.
†Alkylphenolpolyetheleneglycol (Fleuka Ag, Fluorochem Ltd., Peakdale Road, Glossop, Derbyshire, England) prevents overgrowth of the plate by rapidly spreading species of fungi.
‡Rifampicin at 5 µg ml^{-1} at 38° C is selective for *Saccharomonospora viridis*. Novobicin at 25 µg ml^{-1} at 55° C inhibits bacteria and favors growth of *Thermoactinomycetes vulgaris*.
§Actidione (cycloheximide), 50 µg ml^{-1}, inhibits fungi.

slide pre-coated with a gelatin-based mountant.°
A leaf from a bale of hay or straw is then agitated
and the sampler held in the dust cloud for 3 seconds. Loose materials such as wood shavings can
be shaken in a large paper bag prior to sampling
the dust directly from the bag. The microscope
slide is examined by light microscopy for the
presence of plant debris, pollen grains, fungal
spores, dust mites, and their excreta. Dust collected from forages and bedding that has not undergone significant molding is primarily of plant
origin (Fig. 2). In hay and straw samples these
consist primarily of irregularly shaped pieces of
leaf and stem, pollen grain, and plant hairs. Small
numbers of *Cladosporium* and *Alternaria* spores
are likely to be present, especially in "clean"
straw. When hay or straw is baled with a high
moisture content, prolific spore-producing species of thermotolerant and thermophilic fungi
and actinomycetes develop. Dust collected from
these source materials consists primarily of small
round mold spores in the 1 mm to 5 μm size
range (Fig. 3). A blood smear can be useful for
size comparisons, as an equine erythrocyte has a
diameter of approximately 5 μm. A similar picture is seen with plant-based bedding materials
that have molded in situ. There may also be evidence of dust mite contamination. The mites forage on mold spores, leaving characteristic feces.
Hay that has large numbers of mites or their fecal
pellets should be considered a potential health
hazard. Methods of providing horses with forage

°Equigiene, Wrington, Avon, England

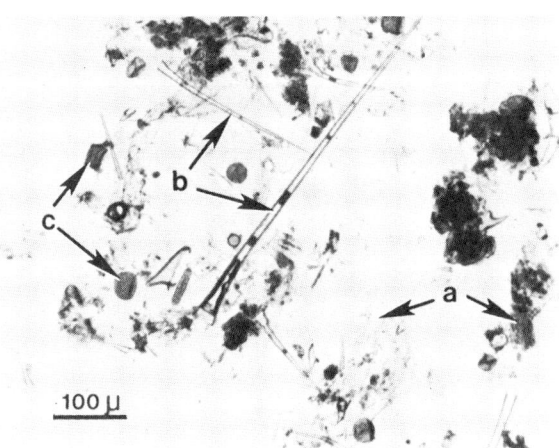

Figure 2. Photomicrograph of a typical dust sample collected from a "nonheated" hay sample. The primary dust constituents are of plant origin. (a = fragments of leaf material, b = plant hairs, c = pollen grains) (From Clarke, A. F.: Air hygiene of stables and chronic pulmonary disease in the horse. Ph.D Thesis, University of Bristol, 1986. Reproduced with permission.)

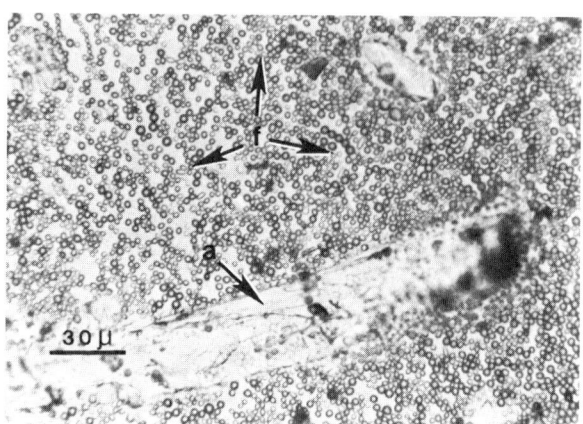

Figure 3. Photomicrograph of a typical dust sample collected from "heated" forage or bedding material. The primary dust constituents (f) are respirable mold spores; (a) is a piece of plant material. (From Clarke, A. F.: Air hygiene of stables and chronic pulmonary disease in the horse. Ph.D Thesis, University of Bristol, 1986. Reproduced with permission.)

and bedding material that avoid the risks of mold
spores are discussed in the chapter on chronic
obstructive pulmonary disease (see p. 330).

INFECTIOUS AGENTS

Levels of airborne bacteria, viruses, and fungal
spores that lead to an infection in previously unchallenged horses depend on the pathogenicity
of the agent and the resistance of the horse. The
highly contagious nature of infectious agents
such as the equine herpesviruses, the fact that
they are endemic in the horse population, and
their ability to be transmitted by means other
than aerosol dispersion make their control difficult. Furthermore, asymptomatic "carriers" can
act as ongoing or intermittent sources of disease.
Horses that pick up infections when away from
stables may shed bacteria and viruses for some
time before their own clinical signs develop.

Stable design and management are unlikely to
affect the incidence of episodes of highly contagious infectious disease. However, sound air hygiene practices will decrease the likelihood of
low-grade, less contagious infections. Furthermore, the air hygiene of stables can affect the degree and duration of respiratory tract infections;
this relates especially to ventilation, airborne
dust, and other pollutants including noxious
gases. The "open air factor" is a potent killer of
airborne microbes, as is the ultraviolet fraction
of sunlight.

Regular disinfection of stables, especially
when they are empty, will help to prevent the
persistence of a wide range of infectious agents.

There are three modes of disinfection: mechanical, physical, and chemical. Mechanical cleaning is necessary to remove organic material such as bedding, feces, or discharges that harbor or maintain pathogens and interfere with chemical and physical disinfection. Hosing or scrubbing surfaces with a detergent further decreases levels of contaminants.

Heat, dessication, and radiation form the basis for physical disinfection, with sunlight being particularly beneficial. The efficacy of steam cleaners can be enhanced with the addition of a detergent or chemical disinfectant to the steaming solution. Halogen compounds containing iodine and chlorine are effective against a wide range of microbes. The selection and use of specific disinfectants for specific types of pathogens is described more fully by Curtis (1983).

NOXIOUS GASES

Ammonia is the most commonly encountered noxious gas in stables; hydrogen sulfide is rarely seen. The absence of slurry pits and the low stocking density in stables, coupled with large air spaces and even moderate levels of ventilation, preclude problems with methane and carbon dioxide. Draegar tubes* offer a simple technique to assess levels of noxious gas in stables. Safe limits for horses are not known, although they should be below accepted levels for human exposure, which for ammonia and hydrogen sulfide are 5 and 20 ppm, respectively. High levels of ammonia are usually found in stables that are poorly drained or where deep litter bedding is used.

MECHANICAL GADGETRY

Mechanical gadgetry including air filters, ionizers, and spray systems for disinfectants are being increasingly advocated for use in stables. However, care should be taken to asses the real (if any) benefit such systems offer. Much of the work showing benefits of such gadgetry has been done on intensively housed livestock where feed conversion efficiency can be improved by closing up buildings and keeping the animals warmer, even though there are concomitant risks of increased respiratory disease. Fresh air takes priority over meat production efficiency with most stabled horses. Furthermore, most stables can be adequately ventilated without mechanical assistance, although fans may be beneficial in buildings that are excessively wide or long.

AIR FILTER SYSTEMS

Air filter systems can decrease the levels of airborne contaminants in closed buildings. The volumetric throughput of air, the filtering efficiency of the system (particles down to 1 μm must be filtered out of the air), and the often overlooked requirement for regular maintenance are their main practical limitations. Filter systems can be of benefit in ensuring that the dust generated in one area of the stables, such as with feed preparation, is prevented from spreading to the stable blocks. Filter systems that filter air before it enters stables may be appropriate when stables are in close proximity to unavoidable dust hazards.

IONIZERS

Benefits ranging from increased mucociliary clearance to reduced levels of airborne dust and killing airborne bacteria have been attributed to negative ions. There appears to be no real role for ionizers in well-ventilated stables.

SPRAY SYSTEMS

Fitted spray systems, similar to those used in greenhouses, and mist generators ("foggers"), have been advocated for use in stables to disperse disinfectants in the battle against infectious respiratory disease. The frequency of spraying varies from twice a week to twice a day. In a well-ventilated stable the disinfectant mist will be cleared quickly, well within an hour. The source of the majority of infectious agents in stables is the horses themselves, and brief encounters with disinfectant mists are unlikely to overcome this problem. The thin layers of disinfectant that would be deposited on walls and structures are not likely to penetrate globules of pus or other discharges sufficiently to be effective. Because of the airway hyperreactivity experienced by horses with damaged airway epithelium, care should be taken in exposing horses to potentially irritating aerosols.

Supplemental Readings

Bruce, J. M.: Heat loss from animals to floors. Farm Build. Prog., 55:1, 1979.
Clarke, A. F.: Management and housing practices in relation to *Rhodococcus equi* infection of foals. Equine Vet. Educ., 1:30–32, 1989.
Clarke, A. F.: Stable environment in relation to the control of respiratory disease. In: Hickman's Horse Management, 2nd ed. Orlando, Fla., Academic Press, 1987, p. 125.
Curtis, S. E.: Environmental Management in Animal Agriculture. Iowa City, Iowa State University Press, 1983.

---

*Draeger, Chesham, England

Druett, H. A.: The open air factor. In Hers, J. F., and Winkler, K. C. (eds.): Airborne Transmission and Airborne Infection. New York, John Wiley and Sons, 1973, p. 141.

Edwards, J. H., Trotman, D. M., and Mason, O. F.: Methods of reducing particle concentrations of *Aspergillus fumigatus* conidia and mouldy hay dust. Sabouraudia, 23:237–243, 1985.

Lioy, P. J., and Lioy, M. J.: Air sampling instruments for evaluation of atmospheric contaminants. Presented at the American Conference of Government Industrial Hygienists, 1983.

Respiratory Viral Disease
Jenny A. Mumford, NEWMARKET, ENGLAND

Specific antiviral therapeutic agents are not available for the treatment of equine viral diseases. The clinician's most powerful control measures remain sensitive diagnosis and the application of management procedures based on an understanding of the pathogenesis and epidemiology of these diseases. Of particular importance are vaccination programs, and quarantining procedures when horses are moved and mixed with new groups of animals. In the last two decades, respiratory disease in horses has received considerable attention from microbiologists, epidemiologists, and clinicians. Epidemiological surveys and the endoscopic investigation of respiratory disease have led to a better understanding of disease processes so that the long-term "loss of performance" episodes, once a major problem in racing animals, are now rarely reported. It is clear that many acute viral infections pass unnoticed by owner and trainer. Either the infection itself causes insufficient tissue damage to elicit overt clinical signs or vaccination restricts viral replication such that the infection is subclinical. It is now clear that lower respiratory tract inflammation, caused initially by respiratory viral infections, may go unnoticed for several weeks. The horse has a poor cough reflex, and clinical signs may not become apparent until the condition has become quite severe following secondary bacterial infection and inflammation of the airways. Endoscopy has increased the clinician's power to detect such lower respiratory tract disease. Examination of tracheal washes can reveal whether the horse is suffering from an acute viral infection, secondary bacterial infection, or chronic low-grade inflammation. Early detection of respiratory disease and cessation of heavy work programs until inflammation has resolved are central to the successful management of this problem. Antibiotic therapy based on the sensitivities of specific organisms isolated from tracheal washes will also speed the recovery process.

Vaccination and quarantine procedures remain the most effective measures of control. In the last decade there has been a major research effort in the development and evaluation of improved equine viral vaccines, with the result that realistic vaccination programs can be devised for some respiratory pathogens such as influenza virus. The development of an effective vaccine against equine herpesviruses 1 and 4 is proving more difficult but is the subject of intensive research effort. To date, vaccination has not been widely used for control of respiratory disease caused by equine viral arteritis or equine picornaviruses.

EQUINE INFLUENZA

Equine influenza, an acute respiratory disease of horses, is caused by infection with orthomyxoviruses of the influenza A type. Two antigenic subtypes have been recognized in the horse. A/equine 1 virus was first isolated in 1956 from a horse in Czechoslovakia and the prototype strain is denoted A/equine/Prague/56. A/equine 2 virus was isolated 7 years later from a horse in Miami, Florida, and thus the prototype strain is designated A/equine/Miami/63.

The two subtypes of equine influenza are differentiated on the basis of antigenic differences in the surface glycoproteins, the hemagglutinin, and the neuraminidase. The A/equine 1 virus carries an H7 hemagglutinin and an N7 neuraminidase. The A/equine 2 virus arose as a result of antigenic shift in which both surface glycoproteins were substituted for different antigenic types, i.e., an H3 hemagglutinin and an N8 neuraminidase.

Since the appearance of these viruses, both subtypes have exhibited antigenic drift as a result of minor changes in the amino acid composition of the surface glycoproteins. In the A/

equine 2 subtype, these changes have been sufficiently great that antigenic variants of H3N8 viruses are recognized, represented by the prototypes A/equine/Fontainebleau/79 and A/equine/Kentucky/81. A/equine 2 viruses have been the prevalent subtype affecting horses within the past two decades, with the last recorded outbreak of A/equine 1 infection occurring in 1979; nevertheless antibodies to A/equine 1 virus persist in unvaccinated Equidae, suggesting that the virus is still active in the population.

Pathogenesis

The clinical features of equine influenza in susceptible animals are often sufficiently characteristic to permit a tentative clinical diagnosis. In general the disease caused by A/equine 2 virus is more severe than that caused by A/equine 1 virus. Clinical signs include a dry harsh cough, pyrexia, nasal discharge, anorexia, and muscle soreness. Coughing is the most common sign and usually persists for 1 to 3 weeks in uncomplicated cases. The fever pattern may be biphasic during the purely viral phase of disease, with the height and duration of response reflecting both the subtype involved and the challenge dose received. Continuous fever beyond 4 or 5 days accompanied by increasing mucopurulent nasal discharge is indicative of secondary bacterial infection.

The A/equine 2 virus possesses more pneumotropic properties, with diffuse bronchiolitis, bronchitis, and pulmonary edema being possible features of infection. Within the respiratory tract, influenza virus replicates in epithelial cells, particularly of the trachea and bronchial tree, resulting in cellular necrosis and loss of cilia from large areas of the mucosal surfaces. This results in impairment of the mucociliary clearance mechanism and facilitates bacterial invasion and multiplication.

Mortality rates are usually very low in uncomplicated influenza infections, with the exception of infections in very young foals possessing no maternal immunity. In these animals, fatal pneumonias have been reported in which necrosis of the bronchioles, congestion of blood vessels, inflammation, neutrophil infiltration, edema, and alveolar collapse are features. In these foals and occasionally in adult animals, myocardial degeneration has also been reported, but mortality in adult horses is rare. Secondary complications following equine influenza are a common feature in stressed or ill-cared-for animals. Inadequate rest during the acute phase of disease, poor environmental conditions, or ineffective bacterial therapy may lead to chronic pulmonary disease or myocarditis.

Diagnosis

Although influenza infections in naive animals may be diagnosed with some certainty on the basis of clinical signs, in partially immune animals it is difficult to differentiate influenza from other viruses or bacteria involved in the respiratory disease complex. In these cases, laboratory tests are essential.

Virus Isolation and Detection

Influenza virus can be detected in nasal secretions by culture of infectious virus or by direct recognition of antigen using antibody-binding assays such as enzyme-linked immunoabsorbent assays (ELISA) or immunofluorescent staining (IF) techniques.

While culture of virus in embryonated hens eggs or Madin-Darby canine kidney (MDCK) cells remains the most sensitive approach, the success of this technique is dependent on the presence of viable virus. Thus nasopharyngeal swabs should be collected in the acute phase of the disease (preferably within 48 hours of pyrexia), placed in virus transport medium and maintained on ice during transport to a laboratory to ensure virus viability. This is not always practical, and therefore immunostaining methods that do not require the virus to be infectious are a useful diagnostic aid. Successful ELISA assays have been developed that use labeled monoclonal antibodies to detect virus nucleoprotein secreted into nasal fluids during an infection. Alternatively, infected epithelial cells recovered from tracheal washes or nasal scrapings may be detected by fluorescent antibody staining employing specific polyclonal antisera.

Serology

Infection may also be confirmed retrospectively using serological tests such as hemagglutination inhibition (EI) or single radial hemolysis (SRH). Serological diagnosis is dependent on the provision of acute and convalescent samples taken 14 to 21 days apart, but even then it may be difficult to diagnose infection in recently vaccinated horses where antibody levels are already high.

Epizootiology

During the past two decades, A/equine 2 has been the prevalent subtype worldwide. Major epidemics occurred in Europe in 1979 and 1989, in South Africa in 1986, and in India in 1987. In some parts of the world such as North America and France, the infection appears to be endemic, with localized outbreaks occurring in most years. To date equine influenza has not been recorded in Australia or New Zealand.

The use of air travel for horses provides a means by which equine influenza can spread long distances in a very short period of time. Vaccinated horses play an important role in the spread of this disease. Vaccination with inactivated vaccines reduces clinical signs of influenza in exposed animals without necessarily eliminating virus shedding. Thus, apparently healthy animals may be transported to foreign countries and mixed with susceptible animals while shedding virus. If quarantine procedures are inadequate the infection can be introduced into a naive population. The short incubation period and effective aerosolization of the virus by the frequent harsh cough result in the rapid spread of virus. The infection is believed to be carried almost exclusively from horse to horse, although recent evidence from South Africa and India indicates that virus can be transmitted by contact with contaminated water, transport vehicles, and personnel.

In naive animals, virus is shed for 7 to 10 days, but in animals immunized by previous infection, virus shedding is usually reduced to 2 to 3 days. It is not clear how the virus persists in the population between epidemics, and although long-term carriers have been postulated, they have not been proven. Immunity provided by previous infection is relatively short-lived, with clinical immunity lasting little more than a year.

Prevention and Treatment

As with all viral diseases, prevention is the best approach and vaccination is a key part of any preventive measures. Current influenza vaccines contain A/equine 1 and A/equine 2 viruses in an inactivated form, either as purified whole virus or subunit preparations. Both aqueous vaccines and adjuvant vaccines are available.

Most vaccines contain A/equine/Prague/56 or a more recent isolate of the H7N7 subtype. Additionally, they contain one or more isolates of the H3N8 subtype relating to the prototype virus Miami/63 and the recent variants Fontainebleau/79 and Kentucky/81. Traditionally, influenza vaccines have been prepared in embryonated eggs. More recently, products have become available that are prepared in tissue culture in an attempt to minimize contaminating material that may be poorly tolerated by the horse. Additionally, subunit vaccines have been developed, with the objective of minimizing reactogenicity.

The antibody response to inactivated influenza vaccine is strikingly short-lived, and a number of adjuvants (aluminum hydroxide, aluminum phosphate, oil, and saponin) have been incorporated into vaccines in an attempt to prolong immunity.

Recommended vaccination schedules vary but usually include two primary doses 4 to 6 weeks apart, followed by a 6-month booster injection, and then routinely 6 to 12 months thereafter. In some high-risk situations, vaccines are used much more frequently.

In the last decade the efficacy of influenza vaccines has been extensively tested in experimental challenge systems. By exposing horses to a nebulized aerosol of equine influenza, it is possible to reproduce clinical signs of disease, including pyrexia and the harsh dry cough. It has been clearly shown that the immunity provided by inactivated vaccines correlates closely with the level of circulating antibody to hemagglutinin as measured by the SRH test. Postvaccination antibody levels are determined by the antigenic content (potency) of the vaccine, the effectiveness of the adjuvant, the vaccination schedule, and the suitability of the vaccine strain. The precise level of antibody required for protection is influenced by the dose of challenge virus, but it is now possible to predict with some certainty the immune status of an individual based on measurement of circulating antibody to hemagglutinin.

It is particularly important to begin immunization programs at an early age, as repeated doses of vaccine eventually lead to an extended antibody response. The optimal timing of the first dose of vaccine in young foals depends on the immune status of the dam. On breeding farms where annual vaccination of mares occurs in the month prior to parturition, high levels of maternal antibody are transferred to foals and may persist for 4 to 6 months. In this group, primary vaccination is best begun at 6 months of age, as residual maternal antibody can interfere with an effective response to vaccination. In foals delivered to poorly immunized mares, vaccination should begin earlier, as recommended by vaccine manufacturers. During the epidemic of A/equine 2 in South Africa, foals were vaccinated at less than 1 month of age and were capable of developing an antibody response.

Many vaccine manufacturers recommend a period of rest following vaccination to minimize any possible adverse effects, such as transient pyrexia, depression, or localized swelling at the site of injection. It is possible that adverse reactions are related to the reactogenicity of the adjuvant or sensitization to egg proteins. It has also been noted that influenza vaccines containing tetanus toxoid are also more reactogenic.

Immunity provided by inactivated vaccines relies heavily on the presence of antibody to hemagglutinin. In contrast, immunity stimulated by infection with virulent or attenuated viruses is effective in the absence of circulating antibody and may be mediated by local respiratory tract antibody and cytotoxic T cell responses, which suppress viral excretion. Experimental vaccines using temperature-sensitive mutants or avian equine influenza reassortants may prove to be more effective products in the future.

The contribution of good management procedures to minimizing the effect of influenza should not be ignored. In an outbreak of influenza, early recognition of individuals incubating the disease and removal of such individuals can reduce the infection pressure on a group. The severity of disease is dose related, and reduction in the levels of challenge virus will reduce the clinical effects of infection. Immediate cessation of work programs will also allow recovery with minimal clinical involvement. Maintaining good stable hygiene and a dust-free, well-ventilated environment will also help to reduce the risk of secondary bacterial infections and subsequent bronchial hyperreactivity.

In cases of influenza not complicated by secondary bacterial infection, rest, hygiene, and nursing are sufficient to allow uneventful recovery without prolonged illness. Treatment with antipyretics such as nonsteroidal anti-inflammatory drugs is beneficial if the fever is severe or persists longer than 3 to 4 days. If pyrexia is prolonged and respiratory signs of coughing and nasal discharge worsen or fail to diminish, antibiotic therapy may be necessary to treat bacterial agents causing secondary infection.

EQUID HERPESVIRUS 1 AND 4

Until recently, equid herpesviruses 1 and 4 were known as equid herpesvirus 1, subtypes 1 and 2. Equid herpesvirus 1 (EHV-1) is the most virulent equine herpesvirus, capable of causing respiratory disease, abortion, foal death, and paralysis. Equid herpesvirus 4 (EHV-4) is usually associated with respiratory disease but occasionally has been recovered from individual cases of abortion. These two viruses can be distinguished genetically and antigenically, but nevertheless share many common features in relation to virus characteristics and disease processes.

Pathogenesis

Infections with EHV-1 and EHV-4 are transmitted via the respiratory route by inhalation of infectious aerosols or by direct contact with infectious secretions, utensils, or drinking water. These viruses replicate in the epithelial cells of the respiratory tract and rapidly localize in respiratory tract lymph nodes within 2 to 3 days of infection. EHV-1 also has a predilection for circulating leukocytes and endothelial cells.

First infections in young horses usually produce acute febrile respiratory disease characterized by rhinopharyngitis and tracheobronchitis. Typically there is a biphasic temperature response, anorexia and depression, enlarged submandibular lymph nodes, and a profuse serous nasal discharge becoming mucopurulent. In young foals with high levels of maternal antibody, clinical signs may be absent although viral replication and shedding still occurs. Occasionally, young foals may suffer a fatal bronchopneumonia. In partially immune, older animals, infections are often subclinical.

Respiratory infection with EHV-1 can have a number of important consequences. If pregnant mares become infected, abortion of an infected fetus may result. Following initial replication in the respiratory tract, virus circulates in the bloodstream within leukocytes and succeeds in infecting endothelial cells of blood vessels within the uterine wall, as well as other organs. This process occurs in the presence of high levels of circulating neutralizing antibody. Eventually the virus crosses the fetomaternal junction and infects the fetus, resulting in abortion.

The period between infection and abortion ranges from 9 to 120 days, with the majority of abortions occurring 10 to 20 days after infection. Most abortions occur in the last trimester of pregnancy. Infected fetuses are usually delivered precipitously with placental membranes intact. The fetus appears fresh and has probably died as a result of suffocation following separation of placental membranes. Occasionally, infected fetuses are delivered as early as 4 months of gestation and may be severely autolyzed.

Typical fetal lesions include bronchiolitis, pneumonitis, hepatic necrosis and inflammation, adrenal necrosis, and thymic and splenic white pulp necrosis. The thoracic and abdominal cavities may contain excessive amounts of clear, straw-colored transudate. Viral inclusion bodies are distributed widely in affected organs. Near-term foals infected in utero but born alive have extensive pulmonary, hepatic, lymphoreticular, and adrenal damage and normally succumb to bacterial infections in the first week of life.

Endometrial pathology is rarely reported in mares that have aborted as rapid recovery ensues and reproductive efficiency is not compromised.

An unusual consequence of respiratory disease with EHV-1 is neurological disease. It has not been established whether particular virus strains have paralytic potential or whether host factors play a role in the pathogenesis of this disease. The severity of the disease can vary widely from slight hind limb incoordination of a transient nature to quadriplegia and recumbency resulting in death. Neurological signs usually occur within 8 to 10 days of initial infection, when the primary temperature response and virus shedding has waned. The clinical signs are associated with the widespread dissemination of the virus throughout the body, localizing particularly in the endothelial cells of the blood vessels of the spinal cord and brain. This tropism results in vasculitis of the small blood vessels in the central nervous system (CNS), with secondary hypoxic degeneration and hemorrhage in adjacent neural tissue giving rise to areas of malacia associated with affected arterioles. Recovery of affected animals depends on the severity and extent of the CNS lesions and the speed with which these lesions resolve. Some animals recover completely, other individuals may suffer permanent impairment of locomotor function.

LABORATORY DIAGNOSIS

Virus Isolation and Detection

In first infections, equine herpesvirus is shed in large quantities in nasal secretions. In second or later infections the amount and duration of virus excretion are reduced. It is therefore important to collect nasopharyngeal swabs as quickly as possible after pyrexia is noticed, and to sample contact animals that may not as yet be showing clinical signs of infection.

Although nasal excretion may be short-lived in primed animals, subsequent cell-associated viremias of EHV-1 (and very occasionally, EHV-4) persist for days or even weeks following initial infection. It is therefore advisable to collect both nasopharyngeal swabs and heparinized blood samples.

EHV-1 can be cultured in a wide range of cells, including pig kidney, rabbit kidney, and equine fetal cells. EHV-4 has a much more restricted host range, and for successful primary isolation equine tissue culture is preferred.

Alternative methods for detection of EHV-1 and EHV-4 are becoming available. Detection of antigen in nasal secretions has been accomplished using monoclonal antibodies in antigen capture ELISA tests. Viral genome in tissues and body fluids can also be detected using the polymerase chain reaction method. This technique can detect latent viral genome as well as active infections.

Differentiation between EHV-1 and EHV-4 isolates is based on type-specific monoclonal antibodies or nucleotide differences in the viral genomes.

Identification of EHV-1 in an aborted fetus is routinely achieved by histology (detection of intranuclear inclusion bodies), immunostaining, or virus isolation. Fetal lung, liver, thymus, and adrenal are the preferred tissues for virus detection.

Cases of EHV-1 neurological disease can be difficult to diagnose if they occur in isolation. At the time ataxia or paralysis is first noticed, the animal has already responded immunologically to the infection. It is therefore difficult to isolate virus from nasal secretions, although cell-associated viremia may still be present. At postmortem examination it is sometimes possible to isolate virus from the CNS or other organs such as lung and spleen. Alternatively, virus may be detected in the endothelial cells of blood vessels by immunostaining.

Serology

Serological diagnosis of EHV-1 and EHV-4 can be difficult. First infections in foals often fail to stimulate a strong antibody response, with the result that fourfold increases in antibody titers between acute and convalescent serum samples cannot be demonstrated. This is particularly true for EHV-4 infections. The problem is compounded by the difficulty in recognizing the acute phase of infection in mild or subclinical cases and in truly acute phase sera. Furthermore, antibody responses in some individuals are slow to develop, with peak titers not reached until 6 weeks after infection.

In spite of the development of ELISA assays for the measurement of antibody to EHV-1 and EHV-4, the complement fixation (CF) test remains a useful tool. CF antibody is stimulated rapidly after infection, but also declines rapidly, so that high levels of CF antibody in convalescent samples may be regarded as indicative of recent exposure. At present it is difficult to identify the infecting virus (EHV-1 or EHV-4) from the specificity of serological responses. These two viruses share many common antigens, and in primed animals the antibody response is highly cross-reactive. The development of an antibody test that clearly differentiates between EHV-1 and EHV-4 would be extremely useful in assessing the potential dangers arising from cases of respiratory disease.

Serological tests should not be used to diagnose cases of individual EHV-1 abortions. Mares may deliver an EHV-1–infected fetus but show no sign of recent antibody activity. Alternatively, a mare producing a noninfectious fetus may have serological evidence of recent exposure to EHV-1 infection. A diagnosis can only be based on examination of the fetus.

In cases of paralysis, the extensive viral replication usually stimulates exceptionally high levels of antibody, which are present by the time signs of CNS involvement are noticed. Antibody titers can therefore be used as an indicator in cases of EHV-1 paralysis. While not all ataxic horses with high levels of antibody to EHV-1 are EHV-1 neurological cases, it is very rare to identify an EHV-1 neurological case with low or even moderate levels of antibody.

Epizootiology

The epizootiology of EHV-1 and EHV-4 is dominated by two factors, the ability of these viruses to infect without causing clinical signs and their ability to establish latent infections that may recrudesce and become productive under situations of stress. These features are common to both EHV-1 and EHV-4. It is now clear that a high proportion of the adult equine population carries both viruses in the latent form in respiratory tract lymph nodes. Circumstantial field evidence for latency has also been supported by experimental studies in which previous infections were stimulated to recrudesce by the application of corticosteroids.

Situations of stress, such as transportation, weaning, and castration, may cause recrudescence of latent infections. If EHV-4 is shed as a result of recrudescence, contact animals may suffer respiratory disease. If EHV-1 is shed from the respiratory tract, the clinical outcome may be more serious than new cases of respiratory disease, because abortions and paralysis may follow.

Despite the common features of subclinical infection and latency, the epizootiology of EHV-1 and EHV-4 differs in many respects. Differences in biological properties of EHV-1 and EHV-4 isolates have long been recognized, but with the advent of genetic analysis based on DNA restriction enzyme profiles it has become clear that these two viruses are associated with different disease syndromes.

EHV-4 is primarily a respiratory pathogen and is often recovered from the respiratory tract of foals and yearlings with "the snots." Only very rarely is this virus isolated from circulating leukocytes or aborted fetuses. It has not been associated with multiple abortions or cases of paralysis. Genetic fingerprinting has shown that within the EHV-4 virus type there are a number of genetic variants, but the significance of these differences in relation to pathogenicity or immunity has not been investigated. Infection with EHV-4 stimulates short-lived immunity, and young animals exposed to the virus are unlikely to enjoy any significant protection against subsequent reinfection with EHV-4 or EHV-1. Immunity stimulated by EHV-1 is probably more durable than immunity stimulated by EHV-4. It is very rare to record EHV-1 abortions in consecutive seasons in the same mare.

Although the relative incidence of EHV-1 and EHV-4 respiratory infections varies from year to year, it is unusual to isolate EHV-1 from foals with respiratory disease unless they have been in contact with cases of EHV-1 abortion or paralysis.

Within the EHV-1 virus type, two major DNA electrophoresis types have been identified. Between 1960 and 1980 the majority of EHV-1 abortions in Kentucky were caused by infection with the 1P genotype; more recently the 1B genotype has emerged. Both of these types have been recovered from abortions and cases of neurological disease. At present there is no way of recognizing an EHV-1 isolate with paralytic potential.

Rapid spread of EHV-1 and EHV-4 can occur, particularly among young animals sharing a common air space, and under stressful and crowded conditions such as at sales yards. More often the spread of these viruses from horse to horse is a slow process requiring close contact or common feeding and drinking facilities. When animals are pastured, the infection is rarely transmitted between animals in separate but adjacent paddocks if direct contact is prevented. Thus if EHV-1 is active on a breeding farm it may take several months before the infection has spread to all susceptible animals. This characteristic provides the opportunity for management intervention to limit the spread of the disease.

Treatment and Control

Rest and antibiotic therapy are the only treatment for EHV-1 respiratory infections at the present time. In the training animal it is important to identify the acute phase of infection with equine herpesviruses. Failure to identify this period and the continuation of stressful work programs during the course of the infection has been blamed as a cause of the long-term loss of performance. Certainly horses infected with EHV-1 may suffer long-term cell-associated viremias after the initial respiratory tract infection.

The clinician's most important role in control of EHV-1 infections is the limitation of EHV-1 abortions on a breeding establishment. This is achieved through sound management practices and the implementation of vaccination programs. Both approaches require an understanding of the epidemiology and the pathogenesis of the disease.

Two rather different epidemiological situations arise on breeding farms, both of which can result in abortion storms, although in one situation multiple abortions can be prevented by efficient management. EHV-1 infection may occur in a group of breeding animals as a result of the introduction of a new animal to the breeding farm without proper quarantine procedures. Such an animal may be shedding virus as a result of recrudescent infection, caused perhaps by the stress of transport or as a result of exposure to exogenous virus. Isolation of incoming animals for a period of 14 days with regular health monitoring should prevent such an occurrence. Alternatively, a resident mare on a farm may shed virus from the respiratory tract as a result of a recrudescent infection. The stress that precipitates such an event may not be apparent. Either situation can result in an infection of a large number of pregnant mares. The spread of infection may be completely without clinical signs until the first abortion occurs. Multiple abortions follow over a short period of time, and serological screening of contact animals will demonstrate that the infection has already spread within the group. In this situation the clinician can do little except ensure that the infection is not transmitted to other premises by the movement of horses.

The second course of events that may lead to an abortion storm is preventable with efficient diagnostic and management procedures. The recrudescence of a latent EHV-1 infection does not always result in viral shedding from the respiratory tract but may result in a cell-associated viremia. Although the mechanism of virus transfer from mare to fetus is not clear, it is believed that the cell-associated viremia is an essential component of the pathogenesis process.

During the viremic phase, such an animal is not necessarily a source of infection to her cohorts. It is only when the highly infectious fetus is delivered that contact animals are at risk. If there is a failure to recognize the fetus as an EHV-1 abortion, or a sickly foal is produced at term, the infection may be transmitted unwittingly by handlers or common stable equipment.

All fetuses or sickly newborn foals should be removed from contact with pregnant mares and the environment thoroughly disinfected and bedding removed and burned. Fetuses, placentas, and dead foals should be submitted to a laboratory for postmortem examination and virological diagnosis of EHV-1. If possible, in-contact and potentially exposed mares should be split into small groups and assigned separate handlers for a period of 2 to 3 weeks while laboratory tests are undertaken to confirm whether individual mares may have contracted the infection. If these management procedures are not adhered to rigorously, large numbers of contact animals may become infected by exposure to the fetus or foal. The pattern of subsequent abortions is different from the first situation referred to. There is usually a period of 10 to 20 days before the second abortion occurs, and then multiple abortions occur in a short time. The same principles of management intervention based on recognition of potentially infectious animals and separation of infected and noninfected animals can be applied to the containment of the neurological form of disease.

While vaccination programs are no substitute for good management practices such as hygiene, avoidance of stress, isolation, and rapid diagnosis of aborted fetuses, they nevertheless will help reduce the numbers of EHV-1 abortions. Two types of vaccine are available: inactivated whole virus combined with adjuvant and live attenuated virus. Both types of vaccine provide only short-lived immunity and at present do not incorporate EHV-4 antigens.

The inactivated vaccine, licensed for use against abortion, is administered to pregnant mares during the fifth, seventh, and ninth months of gestation. In young animals, two doses are recommended at an interval of 4 to 6 weeks, followed by boosters at 6-month intervals. Since this vaccine has been used regularly in breeding stock, particularly in the state of Kentucky, there is good evidence that the level of EHV-1 abortions has decreased.

The modified live vaccine is licensed for use in the control of respiratory disease, and requires a course of two primary injections at an interval of 4 to 8 weeks followed by booster vaccination at 6-month intervals.

Neither vaccine provides effective protection against respiratory disease, but repeated vaccination may reduce the severity of clinical episodes and the amount of virus shed into the environment. If vaccination programs are implemented, they should incorporate the majority of animals on a premises and are of little use if vaccinated individuals are surrounded by an unvaccinated population.

EQUINE VIRAL ARTERITIS

Equine viral arteritis (EVA) was first recognized as a separate viral disease within the equine influenza complex in 1953, following an outbreak of severe respiratory disease and abortion on a farm in Bucyrus, Ohio. The causative agent has been classified as a non-arthropod-borne togavirus with its own genus, arterivirus, although this classification is currently under review. With the possible exceptions of the British

Isles and Japan, the virus has a worldwide distribution, although disease outbreaks are rare.

PATHOGENESIS

EVA is an acute systemic disease involving a panvasculitis with virus replication occurring in most components of the cardiovascular system. Infection may result in high rates of abortion at any gestational age and severe respiratory disease, and in stallions can result in persistent viral shedding in the semen. Clinical signs can be very variable between individuals in an outbreak and between outbreaks, and it has been suggested that strains of high and low virulence may circulate in the equine population. Clinical signs include pyrexia, anorexia and depression, lacrimation and conjunctivitis, edema of the limbs, head, trunk and external genitalia in the stallion, skin rash, diarrhea, and congestion of the mucus membranes. Sometimes clinical signs are indistinguishable from those associated with other respiratory pathogens such as EHV-1.

The incubation period of the respiratory infection ranges from 3 to 14 days. Inhaled virus initially replicates in lung macrophages and spreads rapidly to local lymph nodes. The virus is then disseminated throughout the body via the circulatory system, replicating in endothelial cells and particularly medial cells of the small arteries. Resulting necrosis of the muscle cells leads to increased permeability of small arteries, generalized edema, and hemorrhage. Infectious EVA persists in the kidney and has been isolated from urine 2 to 3 weeks after infection. Virus can cross the placenta and infect the fetus, resulting in death. Abortion occurs as a result of lesions in the endometrium and detachment of the placenta. Fetuses are often autolyzed and do not generally show the typical arteritis seen in mature animals.

DIAGNOSIS

Because clinical signs of infection can be so variable, a clinical diagnosis is not possible. It is particularly important to differentiate between EVA, EHV-1 and EHV-4, and influenza virus, if breeding stock are involved.

A laboratory diagnosis may be achieved by isolation of virus from nasopharyngeal swabs or heparinized blood samples. Additionally, virus may be cultured from aborted fetuses, urine, and the semen of some affected stallions. The virus grows well in rabbit kidney cells and equine tissue culture. It may be identified by virus neutralization tests or immunofluorescent staining of infected tissue culture.

Serological diagnosis may be achieved using virus neutralization tests. Strong antibody responses develop 1 to 2 weeks after infection and persist for years.

EPIZOOTIOLOGY

Serological surveys have demonstrated the presence of EVA in North America, Europe, Africa, Australia, New Zealand, and the Middle East. Clinical outbreaks of disease are relatively infrequent but have been reported in Canada, the United States, Poland, and other European countries. The infection is endemic in Standardbred and Saddlebred horses, and outbreaks of respiratory disease attributed to EVA have been reported among horses on trotting tracks in the United States and Scandinavia. Nevertheless, many infections in young animals are subclinical. The prevalence of EVA among Thoroughbred horses is very low, less than 2 per cent in the United States, and it has not been detected in Thoroughbred horses in Britain or Japan. In 1984, however, EVA did affect Thoroughbred breeding stock in Kentucky.

Transmission of EVA can occur as a result of inhalation of infected aerosols or by contamination with infected fomites. Virus can be shed from the respiratory tract for up to 14 days after infection. On breeding establishments the stallion plays an important epidemiological role in the dissemination and perpetuation of EVA from year to year. A high proportion (30 to 50 per cent) of stallions infected with EVA become carriers. The duration of shedding is variable. Shedding may be a permanent feature in some horses, enabling them to infect mares at covering for several seasons. The existence of the carrier mare under natural conditions is less certain. However, EVA has been recovered from the urine of an experimentally infected mare over a period of 5 months; thus, urine should be considered as a potential source of infection.

TREATMENT AND PREVENTION

As with other respiratory viral infections, rest and the use of antibiotics to treat secondary bacterial infections are the only forms of treatment available. Control of infection must rely on hygiene, good management procedures, and vaccination in countries where a product is licensed.

EVA is an enveloped virus and is susceptible to standard disinfectants and detergents. Antibody screening will provide an initial indication of whether a stallion may be capable of shedding virus in semen. Approximately 30 to 50 per cent of seropositive stallions are carriers. Virus isolation tests on semen or test mating procedures are required to confirm whether an individual is capable of infecting mares at covering.

If breeding is to be attempted with a shedding

stallion, it is important that mares are first vaccinated. A live attenuated vaccine is available in the United States and has been in use since 1985, particularly among horses involved in the outbreak of EVA in Kentucky. Field evidence suggests that this vaccine is safe and provides protection in breeding stock.

EQUINE PICORNAVIRUSES

Equine picornaviruses include equine rhinovirus 1, 2, and 3 and an acid-stable picornavirus. The pathogenic potential of this group of viruses is unclear. While equine rhinovirus 1 has been associated with acute respiratory disease, it is also capable of infecting horses subclinically. Equine rhinovirus 2 and 3 and the acid-stable picornavirus have rarely been associated with acute disease. Foals may experience their first infection under the cover of maternal antibody; more frequently, young animals experience their first infection when they are weaned or mixed with other animals in breaking and training yards. Equine picornaviruses establish persistent infection and can be recovered from the oral cavity for long periods. They are less frequently isolated from the nasopharynx and only rarely from the blood. These viruses can be cultured on monkey or rabbit kidney cells as well as equine cells and are differentiated from each other by cross-neutralization tests using monospecific antisera. Antibody responses following infection can be measured using complement fixation and virus neutralization tests. Serological surveys have indicated that picornavirus activity often coincides with other virus infections such as equine herpesvirus. At present, there are no vaccines available for the control of these infections.

Supplemental Readings

Allen, G. P., and Bryans, J. T.: Molecular epizootiology, pathogenesis, and prophylaxis of equine herpesvirus-1 infection. In Pandey, R. (ed.): Progress in Veterinary Microbiology and Immunology. Basel, S. Karger, 1985.
Campbell, T. M., and Studdert, M. J.: Equine herpesvirus type 1 (EHV-1). Vet. Bull., 53:135, 1983.
Gerber, H.: Clinical features, sequelae and epidemiology of equine influenza. Proceedings of the 2nd International Conference on Equine Infectious Diseases, 1969, pp. 63–80.
Holmes, D. F., Kemen, M. J., and Coggins, L.: Equine rhinovirus infection: Serologic evidence of infection in selected United States horse populations. Proceedings of the 4th International Conference on Equine Infectious Diseases, 1978, pp. 315–319.
Kawaoka, Y., Bean, W. J., and Webster, R. G.: Evolution of the hemaglutinin of equine H3 influenza viruses. Virology, 169:283–292, 1989.
Mumford, J. A.: Preparing for equine arteritis. Equine Vet. J., 17:6, 1985.

Strangles
Frank G. R. Taylor, BRISTOL, ENGLAND

Strangles is an acute, highly contagious disease of the upper respiratory tract of horses. It is caused by *Streptococcus equi*, a gram-positive β-haemolytic streptococcus that is an obligate parasite of Equidae. The disease is characterized by inflammation of the nasopharyngeal and oral mucosa, a mucopurulent nasal discharge, and abscessation of regional lymph nodes. In most cases rupture and unimpeded drainage of abscesses leads to uneventful recovery. However, the contagion is of considerable economic importance due to extended recovery periods and occasional serious complications.

Strangles has a worldwide distribution and can occur in horses of any age, although youngsters (1 to 5 years old) are particularly susceptible. *S. equi* is transmitted in the discharges of infected horses by direct contact or via environmental contamination. Protected by moisture, it may remain viable for a month or more on bedding, pasture, feed, or utensils. The spread of infection is rapid and morbidity is high, often 100 per cent, in susceptible populations. However, mortality is low and is usually associated with the dissemination of infection to other organs. The protective immunity that follows an attack is short-lived and an individual can suffer repeated attacks at intervals of approximately 6 months if the challenge is virulent. In addition, horses that appear to have recovered from strangles may shed the organism intermittently in nasal secretions for a few weeks to several months. Consequently, there is an increased risk of strangles on premises where the horse population is high and movement is frequent.

Infection occurs by ingestion or droplet inhalation. The organism invades nasopharyngeal and oral mucosa, causing an acute pharyngitis and rhinitis. Spread occurs rapidly from tonsillar tissue to regional lymph nodes, typically the retropharyngeal and submandibular nodes. These develop abscesses that rupture and drain externally or, less commonly, internally into the pharynx or guttural pouches. Providing drainage is thorough, healing is usually uneventful.

A milder form of the disease, known as atypical or catarrhal strangles, is recognized in Great Britain, Australia, Canada, and Ireland and has been associated with a variant of *S. equi*. The atypical strain appears to lack capsular material rendering the organism more susceptible to phagocytosis, thus reducing its virulence. However, bacterial phenotype is not the sole criterion of atypical disease. Older horses or those suffering reinfection with *S. equi* may display atypical signs despite capsular forms being isolated from swabs, suggesting that the immune status of the host also influences the expression of disease. Young, immunologically naive animals are the most susceptible to severe strangles.

Complications are usually associated with the lymphatic or hematogenous spread of infection to other lymph nodes or organs ("bastard strangles"). Disseminated infection and abscessation have been recorded in most organs, including the lungs, mesentery, liver, spleen, kidneys, and brain. Regional spread may cause purulent lymphangitis or cellulitis of the head and neck. A rarer complication is purpura hemorrhagica, an immune-mediated vasculitis, which can develop in mature patients having very high antibody titers to antigens of *S. equi*.

CLINICAL SIGNS

Within 2 to 6 days of infection, depression, inappetence, and marked fever (103° to 105° F; 39.5° to 40.5° C) occur. Catarrhal inflammation of the upper respiratory tract results in painful swallowing, a soft, moist cough, and a nasal discharge that rapidly becomes mucopurulent. The head and neck are often held outstretched and the larynx is painful on palpation. Within 2 to 3 days the submandibular nodes swell and become hot and painful as abscessation develops. Swelling of the retropharyngeal nodes may be sufficient to cause respiratory obstruction and dyspnea, a feature that gave the disease its name. Rupture and drainage occurs some 10 to 14 days after the onset of clinical signs and resolution takes 3 to 6 weeks. However, in severe infections the convalescence is protracted, owing to chronic anemia and weight loss.

Atypical strangles is a milder form of the disease that is characterized by transient fever, a relatively modest nasal discharge, and occasional enlargement of submandibular lymph nodes.

Complications are infrequent and are usually associated with spread of infection to other parts of the body. Clinical signs therefore vary greatly, depending on the location and extent of purulent foci. Often the respiratory system is affected. Pneumonia may result from hematogenous spread of infection or from aspiration of pus following internal rupture of retropharyngeal nodes. Dysphagia associated with acute pharyngitis may also lead to aspiration pneumonia.

A rarer, aseptic complication is purpura hemorrhagica, in which there is an increased permeability of capillaries (see p. 510). The disease follows acute *S. equi* infection by several weeks, or may occur shortly after reinfection or after vaccination of previously infected animals. The reaction varies from mild and transient to severe and fatal, but consistent features are some form of subcutaneous swelling with petechiation or ecchymosis of mucous membranes. In mild cases there are widespread urticarial plaques, while in severe cases there is marked edema of the face, limbs, and abdomen.

DIAGNOSIS

A presumptive diagnosis is based on the history and development of clinical signs. Confirmation requires culture of *S. equi* from purulent material. Nasal or pharyngeal swabs may be submitted, but material from discharging lymph nodes is most likely to provide positive cultures.

THERAPY AND CONTROL

On suspicion of infection the horse should be isolated, kept warm and dry, and offered soft, palatable feedstuffs. The antibiotic of choice is penicillin, but its use in strangles is controversial. It is most effective during the earliest signs of infection before abscessation of lymph nodes is apparent. Procaine penicillin G (15,000 IU per kg) should be given intramuscularly (IM) twice daily until clinical signs have been absent for 5 days. During an outbreak the rectal temperatures of all contact animals should be monitored daily so that treatment can begin as soon as it is indicated.

If signs of abscess formation are apparent, antibiotics should be avoided since they tend to slow down abscess development. At this stage it is preferable to enhance maturation by applying hot fomentations or poultices to the intermandibular region. Once the center is sufficiently soft, it should rupture spontaneously, but it may be lanced if necessary. Afterward the cavity should be flushed regularly with 3 to 5 per cent povidone–iodine solution until it heals. Convalescence should occupy 4 to 6 weeks before a gradual return to work.

Throughout this period there should be strict attention to hygiene so that infection is not transmitted between horses. All utensils and tack should be thoroughly disinfected and the bedding burned. Contaminated stables should be scrubbed and disinfected or steam sterilized. After recovery some animals will continue to shed S. equi in nasal secretions for several weeks.

In a minority of cases complications may arise that threaten a successful outcome. If fever is prolonged or dyspnea develops as a result of extensive retropharyngeal node swelling, parenteral administration of penicillin is justified. In this instance an initial intravenous (IV) injection of aqueous penicillin G (40,000 IU per kg) may be combined with procaine penicillin (15,000 IU/kg IM) which should then be given twice daily. In upper respiratory obstruction, tracheostomy is indicated, and in cases of persistent anorexia or dysphagia, feeding by nasogastric intubation is necessary (see p. 724). Careful attention to fluid balance is also essential in dysphagic patients.

In cases of "bastard strangles" treatment is directed toward specific problems. Attempts to treat disseminated infection may be unrewarding and require high levels of antibiotic to be administered for protracted periods, at least several weeks. This often precludes parenteral treatment and the oral (PO) route should be considered. Potassium penicillin G (100,000 IU per kg PO) may be given three times daily. Where this drug is not available, trimethoprim–sulfadoxine may be injected twice (15 mg per kg IV, b.i.d.), followed by twice daily oral paste or in-feed powder (each 30 mg per kg). In apparently successful cases the withdrawal of treatment should be governed by the return of blood leukocytes and plasma fibrinogen concentrations to normal ranges, rather than relying on clinical criteria and demeanor alone.

Patients that develop purpura hemorrhagica are treated with corticosteroids in an attempt to resolve the vasculitis. Dosage is somewhat empirical and recommendations vary, but the length of treatment should be tailored to the response and withdrawal must be gradual. Soluble dexamethasone (5 mg per 100 kg IM) may be injected twice daily until the condition begins to improve, after which a single injection is given daily for up to a week, followed by a half dose (2.5 mg per 100 kg IM) on 2 or more alternate days. During this time parenteral penicillin is advisable to prevent secondary infection in compromised tissues. Supportive treatments include hematinics, but anemia is rarely severe enough to warrant transfusion.

PREVENTION

Strict quarantine is advised for all new arrivals on the premises and should occupy a period of at least 2 weeks and preferably a month. Vaccination may reduce the incidence and severity of disease, but it is not fully protective and immunity is short-lived. The failure of vaccines to protect probably reflects the absence of mucosal immunity that is known to follow natural infection. Proprietary vaccines are available in Australia and North America but not the United Kingdom. Two types of preparations are marketed: a killed S. equi culture, or bacterin,* and cell wall protein extracts.†,‡ Each is given by deep IM injection on two or three occasions during a primary course, with a booster added once each year or in anticipation of exposure. Occasional adverse reactions include inflammatory swellings at injection sites and, rarely, induction of purpura hemorrhagica in hyperimmunized individuals. In the United Kingdom bacterins have been prepared from young heat-killed cultures of current isolates during outbreaks. In all instances vaccination should only be undertaken as prophylaxis, either routinely or in the face of an outbreak. Horses that may be infected already should not be immunized.

Supplemental Readings

Sweeney, C. R., Benson, C. E., Whitlock, R. H., Meirs, D., and Whitehead, S.: Streptococcus equi infection in horses: Part I. Compend. Cont. Educ. Pract. Vet., 9:689–693, 1987.

Sweeney, C. R., Benson, C. E., Whitlock, R. H., Meirs, D., and Whitehead, S.: Streptococcus equi infection in horses: Part II. Compend. Cont. Educ. Pract. Vet., 9:845–851, 1987.

Timoney, J. F.: Shedding and maintenance of streptococcus equi in typical and atypical strangles. In: Equine Infectious Diseases. Proceedings of the 5th International Conference, 1987, pp. 28–33.

Yelle, M. T.: Clinical aspects of Streptococcus equi infection. Equine Vet. J., 19:158–162, 1987.

---

*Equibac II, Fort Dodge Labs., Fort Dodge, IA
†Strepvax, Coopers Animal Health, Kansas City, KS
‡Strepguard, Haver, Mobay Corporation, Animal Health Division, Shawnee, KS

Pleuropneumonia

Corinne Raphel Sweeney, KENNETT SQUARE, PENNSYLVANIA

Bacterial pleuropneumonia is defined as an infectious parenchymal pneumonia that extends and involves the visceral pleura and frequently results in a parapneumonic effusion. The first stage of the effusion is an exudative stage characterized by rapid outpouring of sterile pleural fluid into the pleural space in response to inflammation of the pleura. The associated pneumonic process is usually contiguous with the visceral pleura and results in increased permeability of the capillaries in the visceral pleura. If appropriate antimicrobial therapy is initiated at this stage, the pleural effusion may progress no further.

With progression the bacteria invade the pleural fluid from the contiguous pneumonic process and the second, fibrinopurulent stage evolves. This stage is characterized by the accumulation of large amounts of pleural fluid with many neutrophils, bacteria, and cellular debris. Fibrin is deposited in a continuous sheet covering both the visceral and parietal pleural in the involved area. As this stage progresses, the tendency is to loculation and the formation of limiting membranes. These loculations prevent extension of the empyema but make drainage of the pleural space with chest tubes increasingly difficult.

The last stage is the organization stage, in which fibroblasts grow into the exudate from both the visceral and parietal pleural surfaces and produce a nonelastic membrane called the pleural peel. This nonelastic pleural peel encases the lung and renders it virtually functionless. At this stage the exudate is thick.

For complete information on the pathogenesis, clinical signs, and diagnostic procedures in horses with pleuropneumonia, readers should refer to *Current Therapy in Equine Medicine 2*, pp. 592–593.

In horses with pleuropneumonia that show signs of tachycardia, jugular distention, forelimb pointing, and caudad displacement of the heart, the presence of a cranial thoracic mass as a sequela of infectious pleuropneumonia should be considered. Although the majority of such horses respond to conservative medical treatment with systemic antimicrobial therapy, invasive drainage of the thoracic mass may be needed for resolution of the problem. Though drainage can be attempted in a standing position, general anesthesia in a recumbent horse affords more effective and complete drainage.

Putrid discharges are the hallmark of anaerobic infection. Odor is considered a diagnostic indicator because aerobic bacteria do not typically produce such characteristic odor of putrefaction. However, the absence of a putrid discharge does not exclude anaerobic infections. Only two thirds of horses with anaerobic isolates have putrid odor.

The ultrasonographic findings in horses with pleuropneumonia include the presence of and character of pleural fluid (including fibrin, loculations, and gas echoes), pleural adhesions, changes in the pulmonary parenchyma (including compression atelectasis, consolidation, necrosis, and abscessation) and loculations. Survival of the horse with pleuropneumonia is significantly associated with the absence of pleural fluid, fibrin, loculations, parenchymal necrosis, and gas echoes. The absence of pulmonary parenchymal necrosis, gas echoes, and pleural fluid is associated with the best prognosis for return to previous performance.

THERAPY

ANTIMICROBIAL THERAPY

The most important treatment of bacterial pleuropneumonia is the use of systemic antimicrobial agents. Without bacterial culture results, broad-spectrum antibiotics should be used, because many horses have mixed infections of both gram-positive and gram-negative organisms. Commonly used therapy is penicillin (procaine penicillin G,* 22,000 IU per kg intramuscularly [IM] twice a day, or sodium penicillin G,† 20,000 to 40,000 IU per kg four times a day) combined with an aminoglycoside such as gentamicin‡ (2.2 mg per kg intravenously [IV] or IM four times a day), trimethoprim–sulfamethoxazole§ (30 mg per kg orally [PO] twice a day), ceftiofur,‖ or chloramphenicol¶ (20 to 50 mg per kg PO four times a day). Because of the need for long-term therapy, initial IV or IM therapy may need to be followed by oral antimicrobials. Antimicrobials are usually not administered orally until the

---

*Pfizer Inc., New York, NY
†Squibb, Princeton, NJ
‡Gentocin, Schering Corp., Kenilworth, NJ
§Tribrissen, Burroughs Wellcome Co., Research Triangle Park, NC
‖Naxcel, Upjohn, Kalamazoo, MI
¶Anacetin, Bio-Ceutic Laboratories, St. Joseph, MO

horse's condition is stable and improving, because blood levels obtained by this route are not as high as those achieved following IM or IV administration.

Treatment of anaerobic pleuropneumonia is usually empirical since antimicrobial susceptibility testing of anaerobes is difficult. While the majority of anaerobic isolates are sensitive to relatively low concentrations of penicillin, some members of the *Bacteroides* genus are known to produce beta-lactamases and are potentially penicillin resistant.

Metronidazole° has in vitro activity against a variety of obligate anaerobes including *Bacteroides fragilis*. Pharmacokinetic studies indicate that a dose of 15.0 mg per kg IV or PO four times a day is necessary to maintain adequate serum levels. Metronidazole is not effective against aerobes and therefore should always be used in combination therapy. Chloramphenicol is effective against most aerobes and anaerobes causing equine pleuropneumonia. Aminoglycosides should not be considered for the treatment of pleuropneumonia caused by an anaerobe unless they are used in combination therapy with penicillin.

DRAINAGE OF THE PLEURAL CAVITY

Following selection of an appropriate antimicrobial agent, the next decision to be made is whether to drain the pleural space. Ideally the decision is based on the ultrasonographic appearance of the pleural cavity.

Drainage of a pleural effusion can be accomplished by thoracocentesis, by using a cannula, by indwelling chest tubes, or by thoracostomy. The latter is reserved for severe abscessation of the pleural space. Thoracocentesis (see p. 302) is easily accomplished in the field and may not need to be repeated unless considerable pleural effusion reaccumulates. I have not encountered any problem from thoracocentesis performed every 48 hours. Indwelling chest tubes† are indicated when continued pleural fluid accumulation makes intermittent thoracocentesis impractical. If properly placed and managed they provide a method for frequent fluid removal and do not exacerbate the underlying pleuropneumonia or increase the production of pleural effusion. Description of the placement of the chest tube can be found in *Current Therapy in Equine Medicine 2*, p. 595.

OTHER THERAPY

Anti-inflammatory agents help reduce pain and may decrease the production of pleural fluid. This in turn may encourage the horse to eat and maintain body weight. Phenylbutazone (1 to 2 gm twice a day) or flunixin meglumine‡ (500 mg once daily) are commonly used for this purpose. Corticosteroids are *contraindicated* in bacterial pleuropneumonia. Intrapleural instillation of 250,000 IU streptokinase diluted in 100 ml of normal saline is sometimes used to treat humans with pleuritis, but the value of intrapleural enzymes in the treatment of equine pleuropneumonia has not been documented. Rest and an adequate diet are important components of the treatment of pleuropneumonia. Because the disease course and period of treatment are usually prolonged, attempts should be made to encourage eating.

PROGNOSIS

A guarded prognosis must always be given in cases of equine pleuropneumonia. With the improved ability to treat the disease, survival rates exceed 75 per cent. Most survivors do return to racing. One recent study showed that 50 per cent of pleuropneumonia survivors raced in the same or higher class while 50 per cent raced in a lower class than prior to their disease.

Supplemental Readings

Byars, T. D., Dainis, C. M., Seltzer, K. L., et al: Cranial thoracic masses in the horse: A sequela to pleuropneumonia. Equine Vet J. 23:3–4, 1991.

Reef, V.: Outcome and return to performance in horses with pleuropneumonia evaluated ultrasonographically. *In:* Proceedings of the 8th Annual Meeting of the American Veterinary Medical Association, 1990, pp. 573–575.

°Flagyl, Searle Pharmaceuticals, Chicago, IL
†Heimlick, Bard-Parker, Rutherford, NJ

‡Banamine, Schering Corp., Kenilworth, NJ

Chronic Obstructive Pulmonary Disease

Andrew F. Clarke, GUELPH, ONTARIO, CANADA

The classical picture of chronic obstructive pulmonary disease (COPD) is that of a severely dyspneic horse with flaring nostrils and marked abdominal effort on expiration. Such a horse is in distress while at rest and is incapable of any form of athletic exertion. These overt manifestations of disease are associated with bronchospasm, mucosal inflammation, and mucous plugging.

The above picture is the end stage or the most severe form of a disease complex capable of manifesting in many degrees. At the other end of the scale is a covert or minor degree of airway disease described as lower respiratory tract inflammation (LRTI), which only becomes apparent when the horse is put under extreme exertion. At the canter and the gallop, respiratory and locomotor cycles are locked in a 1:1 cycle. The galloping horse has less than half a second to inhale and exhale between 12 and 15 liters of air. Trotting horses by comparison have a 1:1 synchronization of respiration and stride frequency at submaximal exercise but at maximal exercise change over to a 1:3, 1:2, or 1:1.5 relationship that allows deeper tidal volumes. The galloper uses quicker, shallower breaths than the trotter. However, both need to move large volumes of air efficiently to perform to their fullest potentials. Minor degrees of bronchospasm or small increases in the amounts of mucus in the airways quickly take their toll at this level of performance, and although they are unlikely to be of immediate consequence to a pony used for pleasure riding, the disease is likely to become more severe with time so that even light exercise becomes distressing.

ETIOLOGY

COPD is associated with exposure to moldy hay and straw; it is more common in horses housed in badly ventilated stables and is often a sequela of bacterial and viral infections. A horse eating moldy hay or sniffing at contaminated bedding will inhale millions of mold spores with each breath. These spores are capable of reaching the deepest areas of the lung and it is believed that they trigger an allergic reaction that is responsible for the signs associated with COPD. Well-ventilated stables help to decrease the levels of airborne pollutants to which horses are exposed. The likelihood of bedding material molding in situ increases with poorly ventilated stables.

Lower respiratory tract inflammation associated with poor performance is usually seen in two situations. The first is where heavily contaminated forage or bedding such as "heated" hay or straw is introduced into a stable. The second is as a sequela to a bout of infectious respiratory disease. This may be a primary effect of the infection or it may be the result of the former lowering the horse's tolerance to previously insignificant levels of airborne pollutants such as dust and noxious gases.

PATHOLOGY AND PATHOPHYSIOLOGY

Pathological findings associated with COPD include diffuse bronchiolitis with epithelial hyperplasia, mucus cell metaplasia, inflammatory cell infiltration of the lamina propria of the bronchiole, and peribronchiolar fibrosis. Extensive emphysema, an irreversible destruction of alveolar septa, is rarely seen. With proper management, the vast majority of horses with COPD recover and remain asymptomatic. Pathophysiologically, bronchospasm, mucous plugging, and mucosal thickening lead to increased work of breathing and decreased levels of arterial oxygen. Airway hyperresponsiveness is of considerable importance in the treatment and management of horses with COPD and LRTI. Airway inflammation and damage to epithelial lining of the airways lead to a nonspecific hyperresponsiveness to all forms of inhaled pollutants, including dust, noxious gases, and even nebulized water. Fresh air is therefore of particular importance to horses with diseased airways, as their tolerance to inhaled pollutants will be much lower than normal.

CLINICAL SIGNS

Overt signs of COPD include a chronic cough, dyspnea, doubled expiratory effort with marked abdominal lifting, and exercise intolerance. The onset of disease may be sudden or gradual and may follow from an episode of infectious respiratory disease. The disease usually coincides with the horse being brought in from pasture to the stable, and owners often report that the horse is better while at pasture. Paradoxically, some horses exhibit signs of COPD while they are at pasture. This problem is known as summer pasture–associated obstructive pulmonary disease (SPAOPD) and is believed to be associated with exposure to pollens (see *Current Therapy in Equine Medicine*, p. 512). COPD is seen in horses of all ages, both sexes, and all breeds. There is an increasing incidence of disease with increasing age.

LRTI should be suspected in any cases of poor performance, especially when several horses in one stable are affected. Coughing need not be a clinical feature as the horse has a poor cough reflex. This point should be emphasized to owners, who often believe that there can be no lung disease without coughing. Observation of the horse's breathing while it is standing quietly in its box may reveal an increased lift of the abdomen with expiration. Auscultation of the chest at rest is often unrewarding, though light exercise or the use of a rebreathing bag may lead to audible moist rales and crepitous lung sounds. A diagnosis of LRTI is usually dependent on an endoscopic examination and a tracheal or bronchoalveolar lavage (see p. 301).

DIAGNOSIS

A provisional diagnosis of COPD can be made from a carefully taken history and clinical examination. Differential diagnoses and diagnostic techniques for horses with chronic respiratory disease are discussed on p. 300.

Intradermal antigen testing and serum precipitating antibody assessments are of little value. Endoscopy and lung washes are particularly applicable to the diagnosis of LRTI. Probably the simplest technique in aiding the diagnosis of COPD involves a response to therapy. The administration of a bronchodilator such as clenbuterol° intravenously (0.8 µg per kg) or via nebulization (10 ml containing 0.03 mg clenbuterol hydrochloride per ml) with an ultrasonic nebulizer† should provide relief of signs within 30 minutes. The easiest method of assessing lung function in the field involves the measurement of intraesophageal pressure changes, ΔPpl max.‡ The ΔPpl max of healthy horses at rest is between 2 and 4 cm H_2O. Blood gas analysis may also be carried out. An arterial Pa_{O_2} of less than 80 mm Hg is characteristic of COPD but can occur in the presence of many other lung diseases.

THERAPY, CONTROL, AND PREVENTION

Pharmaceuticals can be used to relieve the signs associated with LRTI and COPD and to speed the recovery of the affected horses. However, the treatment, control, and prevention of these airway diseases all entail reducing the horse's exposure to etiological agents.

PHARMACEUTICALS

Bronchodilators, mucolytics, and anti-inflammatory agents help to alleviate the signs of airway disease. Some cases of LRTI may be complicated by bacterial infections. Ideally, antibiotic therapy should be based on microbiological examinations of tracheal washes. The use of pharmaceuticals in the treatment of airway disease is described more fully on p. 303. Vaccines also play an important role in the control of some infectious respiratory disease. These are described in the sections on viral respiratory disease (see p. 316).

ENVIRONMENTAL CONTROL

The environmental control of any respiratory disease involves the maintenance of challenges below the threshold limiting value that will induce disease in the individual being challenged. The threshold limiting value for airborne dust, noxious gases, and infectious agents that will induce airway disease in horses is unknown. However, since the horse's response to these challenges is likely to be graded and since the mildest degrees of respiratory disease are likely to be associated with loss of performance, the horse's exposure to all airborne pollutants should be minimized at all times.

Ventilation

The level of airborne contaminants, including dust, noxious gases, and microorganisms, will depend on their rate of release into the air and their rate of clearance, primarily by ventilation (see p. 310). However, horses can still be ex-

---

°Ventipulmin, Boehringer Ingelheim, Animal Health, St. Joseph, MO
†Equigiene, Wrington, Avon, England

‡Ventigraph, Boehringer Ingelheim, Animal Health, St. Joseph, MO

posed to dangerous levels of airborne contaminants in the best ventilated stables.

The highest levels of respirable dust occur in stables at mucking-out time and horses should be kept out of the stables at this time. Horses can be exposed to high levels of respirable particles as they sniff at a contaminated bedding or eat a moldy hay. Clean source materials are therefore essential elements in minimizing the horse's exposure to the etiological agents of COPD and LRTI.

Bedding Materials

Straw is a particularly potent source of mold spores capable of causing COPD and LRTI. "Clean" alternatives to straw include wood shavings, peat, sawdust, shredded paper, and synthetic beddings (Table 1). Clean straw, under conditions of deep litter management or in hot, humid, poorly ventilated stables, may become a potent source of respirable mold spores. The other risks of deep litter management systems include build-up of the larval stages of gastrointestinal parasites and noxious gases along with accumulations of bacteria capable of causing primary and secondary infections.

Forage

Hay that has been baled with a high moisture content spontaneously heats and provides the conditions in which prolific spore-producing thermophilic and thermotolerant mold species develop. A horse eating this hay inhales millions of spores with each breath. Surveys have shown that up to 70 per cent of hay fed to horses in Great Britain and Scandinavia contain significant levels of mold contamination. The horseman's eye and nose is not a good guide to the quality of hay and objective assessments should be carried out. A simple technique involves the use of a hand-held sampler§ that collects dust particles onto a microscope slide (see p. 313).

Artificial drying of hay is one method that can decrease the risk of significant mold growth. The traditional approach to barn drying of hay has been to bale the hay and stack it with gaps between bales, which allows air to be blown around the bales. This approach is not particularly successful. Significant molding can still occur if the hay is baled with a high moisture content. Drying the hay before baling has proved to be very successful. Two approaches are taken. The first involves stacking the hay loosely into drying kilns and blowing air through it for 3 to 5 days until a suitably low moisture content is reached,

§Equigiene, Wrington, Avon, England

TABLE 1. AVERAGE ($\pm$SD) PARTICLE RELEASE RATES FROM VARIOUS FRESH BEDDING MATERIALS (PARTICLES/mg)°

Equibed†	Shredded Paper§	Shavings	Straw	Tissue Paper‡
19 (8)	46 (17)	144 (247)	10,619 (14,704)	53 (16)

°The counts are of respirable particles with aerodynamic diameter ≤5 µm.
†Equibed: Melcourt Industries, Tetbury, Glos., England (absorbent synthetic bedding).
§Diced newspaper: Shredabed, Exeter, England.
‡Tissue bedding: F. H. Lee, Bolton, Greater Manchester, England.

approximately 10 per cent. The second approach involves rapid, high-temperature drying of hay that has been cut and wilted in the field. Complete cubed diets or molasses and straw diets offer alternative ways of meeting the horse's forage needs. Alfalfa cubes, which act as a good nutritional balancer with oats, help to avoid the necessity of feeding hay. If horses on these diets develop stable vices or start to eat their droppings, other approaches will have to be taken.

Traditional silage or commercially available hayage products are minimal dust hay alternatives. Care should be taken if big bale silage is used. Broken or damaged bags, or silage containing dirt or having an ammonical smell should be discarded because of the risk of botulism. Bags should be used within 5 days of opening, especially in warm weather when it will mold quickly. Table 2 gives examples of particle release rates from various types of forage.

Soaking hay decreases the respirable challenge of spores. Spores can become airborne if the hay is allowed to dry out before it is fed. The hay should be thoroughly wet through, the simplest approach being to put the evening's hay in to soak when the horse's morning hay is fed and then in the evening put the morning's hay in to soak. Hay soakers are commercially available.° These units are plumbed in, hay is placed in situ, and the hay washed and drained. A further option is the use of hay cleaners. These machines agitate the hay and vacuum the dust away.† The former rather than the latter equipment is more applicable for use with relatively brittle alfalfa hay.

Storage and Shared Air Spaces

Hay and straw stored in close proximity to horses can be a potential source of inhaled re-

°Hay-Tek, Sohan, England
†Watts Hay, Wrington, Avon, England

TABLE 2. RELEASE RATES OF RESPIRABLE PARTICLES (AERODYNAMIC DIAMETER ≤ 5 μm) FROM VARIOUS TYPES OF FORAGES

	Ryegrass (clean)	Ryegrass (molded)	Alfalfa (clean)	Alfalfa (molded)	Hay-Tek*	Horsehage†	Silage
Particles per mg:	980	65,190	840	39,270	250	44	19

*Hay-Tek (air cured hay), Greens of Sohan, England.
†Horsehage, Westaway & Son, Paignton, England.

spirable mold spores, storage in lofts above stables being one of the main offenders. Apparently good air hygiene practices can break down because of dust generated in adjoining boxes or storage areas floating into the horse's air space. Manure piles of used bedding are another common offender. These are often positioned just behind stables in close proximity to back-wall vents. Used bedding is best placed in trailers and removed from close proximity to the stables every 2 or 3 days.

Supplemental Readings

Beadle, R. E.: Summer pasture associated obstructive pulmonary disease. *In* N. E. Robinson (ed.): Current Therapy in Equine Medicine 1. Philadelphia, W. B. Saunders, 1983, p. 512.

Burrell, M. H.: Endoscopic and virological observations on respiratory disease in a group of young thoroughbred horses in training. Equine Vet. J., 17:99–103, 1985.

Clarke, A. F.: Preserved forage: nutritional and respiratory aspects. Equine Vet. Educ., 1:65, 1989.

Clarke, A. F.: Stable environment in relation to the control of respiratory disease. *In:* Hickman's Horse Management, 2nd ed. Orlando, Fla., Academic Press, 1987, p. 125.

Clarke, A. F., Madelin, T. M., and Allpress, R. G.: The relationship of air hygiene in stables to lower airway disease and pharyngeal lymphoid hyperplasia in two groups of thoroughbred horses. Equine Vet. J., 19:524, 1987.

Derksen, F. J., Robinson, N. E., Armstrong, P.J., et al.: Airway reactivity in ponies with recurrent airway obstruction (heaves). J. Appl. Physiol., 58:598, 1985.

Kaup, F. J., Drommer, W., Damich, S., et al.: Ultrastructural findings in horses with chronic obstructive pulmonary disease (COPD): II. Pathomorphological changes of the terminal airways and the alveolar region. Equine Vet. J., 22:349, 1990.

McPherson, E. A., and Thomson, J. R.: Chronic obstructive pulmonary disease in the horse: I. Nature of the disease. Equine Vet. J., 15:203, 1983.

Robinson, N. E.: Airway obstruction in the horse. Equine Vet. Sci., 9:155, 1989.

Lung Parasites
M. Bailey, BRISTOL, ENGLAND

Parasites are a far more important consideration in the management of intestinal than respiratory disorders in the horse. However, a low level of exposure to parasitic infection can be regarded as part of the natural environment of the animal. Under ideal management conditions the level of parasite infection should not be sufficient to be associated with disease. When clinical signs do occur, they are likely to be due to a breakdown in husbandry procedures, which will be readily apparent during the preparation of a thorough clinical history.

Parasitic disease should be considered in a relatively susceptible animal or one that has been exposed to other animals that may be heavily infected. Thus, while horses of all ages may harbor parasites, young animals are more susceptible to associated clinical disease and the risk can be further increased in immunocompromised foals.

The degree of exposure can be assessed from the type of housing, the number of other horses sharing the accommodation, and the worming history of all the animals in the group. The presence of specific reservoirs should be identified. Donkeys are reservoirs for *Dictyocaulus arnfieldi*.

ETIOLOGICAL AGENTS

DICTYOCAULUS ARNFIELDI

The life cycle of *D. arnfieldi* is direct, implying the potential for direct horse-to-horse spread through infective larvae passed in feces. Such direct spread from horses may occur, since small numbers of adult worms have been found at necropsy in the lungs of horse grazed with no access to donkeys. However, the relatively low prevalence of patent infections in horses compared with donkeys means that the majority of lungworm infections in horses are acquired from grazing pasture shared with donkeys. Although no survival rate data are available for *D. arnfieldi* infection, small numbers of the infective larvae of *D. viviparus* may survive for several years in soil, which raises the possibility that pastures grazed by donkeys may remain contaminated for some time. Infection in donkeys appears relatively innocuous. In horses, however, *D. arnfieldi* in the lungs is associated with bronchitis, bronchiolitis, and accumulation of pus in the airways.

Parascaris Equorum

The life cycle of *P. equorum* is also direct, and horse-to-horse spread of eggs passed in feces is important in transmission. Following ingestion, larvae undergo tissue migration, passing through the liver, lung, and trachea before returning to the intestine. During the lung migratory phase, tissue eosinophila occurs and some eosinophils may accumulate in the lumen of the airways. Ascarid infections in horses and in other species results in good immunity, and respiratory disease is therefore a transient phenomenon seen in young animals. However, infection has been suggested as a predisposing factor in more severe, apical lobe pneumonias in young foals.

Strongylus Spp.

Larvae of the large strongyles are not normally considered respiratory pathogens. However, single migrating larvae have been reported from the lungs of infected foals and, in an extensive study of experimental infections with *S. vulgaris* diffuse, eosinophilic pneumonia was observed similar to that seen in *Parascaris*-infected foals.

Habronema

Larvae of the stomach worms *Habronema* spp. have been found in nodules in the lung tissue. No association with disease has been described.

Echinococcus Granulosus

Infection of horses with eggs of *E. granulosus* passed in feces of infected dogs can result in the development of large, space-occupying lesions that may occur in the lungs.

Pneumocystis Carinii

The protozoon *Pneumocystis carinii* has been recovered from the pneumonic lungs of young foals. An association exists with immunodeficiency, specifically with the combined immunodeficiency reported occasionally in Arab foals and rarely in other breeds. Infection with *P. carinii* is thus most likely to be secondary to an underlying problem.

DIAGNOSIS

The basis of all parasitological diagnosis is the examination of fecal samples for eggs or larvae. Such samples should be taken freshly and preferably directly from the rectum with a disposable glove to eliminate environmental contamination. Where parasites are considered as a cause of respiratory signs, samples should also be taken from suspected reservoirs, since *D. arnfieldi* infections are frequently not patent and respiratory signs are caused by migrating, not adult *P. equorum*. Examination of blood samples may not be of value: eosinophilia has been linked with "parasitic infection," but associations with particular species may be tenuous. Cytology on tracheal aspirates or bronchial lavage may be useful. Eosinophils are a feature of the pathology of all the nematodes parasitic within the lungs. However, parasitic pneumonias are also associated with neutrophil accumulation. Bronchoscopy has been used for direct demonstration of *D. arnfieldi* in the lungs. This may be of value where such infections are not patent.

THERAPY

The treatment of pneumonia associated with parasite infections is similar to that for other causes and is reviewed elsewhere. Direct control of parasite infections falls under two headings: anthelmintics and management.

Anthelmintics

Several of the benzimidazole derivatives have been used for treatment (Table 1). Mebendazole, given at 20 mg per kg for 5 days (twice the normal dose rate), is 75 to 100 per cent effective in reducing adult *D. arnfieldi* burdens in donkeys. Mebendazole has not been evaluated for treatment of migrating larvae of *P. equorum* but is effective against intestinal adults and can be used to minimize the risk to susceptible animals. Fenbendazole, 10 mg per kg per day for 5 days, is effective against migrating and adult *P. equorum* and *S. vulgaris* but not against adult *D. arnfieldi*. Albendazole, 50 mg per kg twice daily for 2 days, is effective against migrating *S. vulgaris* and at 25 mg per kg twice daily for 5 days has caused clinical improvement in ponies infected with *D. arnfieldi*. However, toxicity may be apparent at these doses. Albendazole is used for treatment of hydatid cysts in humans (9 to 15 mg

TABLE 1. DAILY DOSAGE AND DURATION OF THERAPY FOR ANTHELMINTICS EFFECTIVE AGAINST LUNG PARASITES

	Benzimidazoles			Ivermectin
	Mebendazole	Fenbendazole	Albendazole	
D. arnfieldi	20 mg/kg, 5 days (postmortem)°		25 mg/kg b.i.d., 5 days (clinical assessment)	200 μg/kg (postmortem)
P. equorum				
Adults	10 mg/kg	7.5 mg/kg		200 μg/kg
Larvae		10 mg/kg, 5 days (postmortem)		
S. vulgaris				
Adults	10 mg/kg	7.5 mg/kg		200 μg/kg
Larvae		10 mg/kg, 5 days (postmortem)	50 mg/kg b.i.d., 2 days (arteriography and postmortem)	200 μg/kg (postmortem)
Echinococcus			4–8 mg/kg b.i.d., 1 month (regression of lesions)	

°Techniques used for determining efficacy are indicated in parentheses.

per kg for 1 month followed by a 2-week break), but liver enzyme levels are monitored during treatment. The benzimidazole of choice is therefore mebendazole for *D. arnfieldi* and fenbendazole for larvae migrans. Resistance of intestinal small strongyles to benzimidazole derivatives has been reported, but the large strongyles are apparently not affected. No data are available for *D. arnfieldi*, but the more widespread cattle parasite *D. viviparus* has not as yet shown signs of resistance.

Recently ivermectin° has become popular for treatment of refractory infections. Ivermectin orally or by injection (200 μg per kg) appears to be effective against migrating *S. vulgaris* and against adult *D. arnfieldi*.

Management

Management for control of parasites capable of causing pulmonary signs is similar to that for intestinal parasites. Control hinges on elimination of reservoirs, that is, of animals shedding high levels of infective organisms. Conventional anthelmintic programs should be applied: (1) treatment with adulticidal drugs to reduce egg output at 6- to 8-week intervals during the periods favorable for transmission (warm, wet weather; spring to autumn in temperate climates); (2) a single treatment with a larvicidal drug once transmission has ceased, to eliminate developing or hypobiotic larvae and prevent carryover to the next year; (3) inclusion in the program of all animals grazed on the same pasture; and (4) control programs should be strongly enforced in the presence of young, susceptible animals. In addition, the control of *D. arnfieldi* requires the specific identification and treatment of (usually) infected donkeys.

Supplemental Readings

Lyons, E. T., Drudge, J. H., and Tolliver, S. C.: Ivermectin: treating for naturally occurring infections of lungworms and stomach worms in equids. Vet. Med., 80:58–64, 1985.

Lyons, E. T., Tolliver, S. C., Drudge, J. H., Swerczek, T. W., and Crowe, M. W.: Lungworms (*Dictyocaulus arnfieldi*): Prevalence in live equids in Kentucky. Am. J. Vet. Res., 46:921–923, 1985.

Turk, M. A. M., and Klei, T. R.: Effect of ivermectin treatment on eosinophilic pneumonia and other extravascular lesions of late *Strongylus vulgaris* larval migration in foals. Vet. Pathol., 21:87–92, 1984.

Vandermyde, C. R., DiPietro, J. A., Todd, K. S., and Lock, T. F.: Evaluation of fenbendazole for larvicidal effect in experimentally induced *Parascaris equorum* infections in pony foals. J. Am. Vet. Med. Assoc., 12:1548–1549, 1987.

°Eqvalan, MSD Agvet, Rahway, NJ

Exercise-Induced Pulmonary Hemorrhage

Andrew F. Clarke, GUELPH, ONTARIO, CANADA

Exercise-induced pulmonary hemorrhage (EIPH) is defined as the presence of blood in the tracheobronchial tree following athletic exertion. On some occasions a trace of blood may persist for several days. Endoscopic surveys of the respiratory tract of horses after competitive events have shown that a large number of horses suffer EIPH, while only a relatively low percentage (1 to 2 per cent) show blood at the nostrils (i.e., epistaxis). The reported incidences of EIPH range from approximately 30 per cent of Standardbreds to 60 per cent of Quarter Horses, with up to 75 per cent of Thoroughbred competitors being affected. Repeated examinations of populations of horses have shown a higher incidence of EIPH than is indicated by a single examination, with 95 per cent of horses examined two or more times showing evidence of EIPH on one occasion. It appears that EIPH is an unavoidable consequence of athletic exertion in the horse.

The presence of hemosiderophages (macrophages containing hemosiderin) in tracheal washes coincides with the beginning of fast work in 2-year-old Thoroughbreds and almost always occurs in racehorses once they have commenced fast work. There also appears to be an increasing trend for blood to be observed in the tracheobronchial tree of horses after exercise as they grow older. A grading system based on the amount of blood in the trachea has been developed in an attempt to characterize the degree of hemorrhage observed. However, this system has not been found to correlate the occurrence or degree of future hemorrhage to the occurrence of epistaxis or the horse's performance. In clinical terms it must be emphasized that there appears to be no clear relationship between EIPH and performance when large populations of horses have been examined. Unfortunately, endoscopic pictures that show blood in a horse's trachea are dramatic, especially when seen by an owner or trainer trying to explain the poor performance of a horse. The horse is labeled a "bleeder." It is my strong belief that extreme care should be taken before EIPH is accepted as the cause of loss of performance, except in the case of the horse that continually bleeds heavily.

Hemorrhage occurs from the dorsocaudal region of the horse's lung. There is considerable debate over the etiology of the hemorrhage. Some believe that there must be an underlying disease process, e.g., airway disease, while others argue that the dorsocaudal area of the lung is under such mechanical stress that hemorrhage can occur without disease. Postmortem examinations of old, retired racehorses have shown evidence of increased mucus and airway disease in the region of old lesions. Endoscopic surveys examining the presence of mucopus and EIPH have not established a clear relationship between the two, assuming of course, that mucopus is a true indicator of airway disease. What does remain clear is that in the dorsocaudal regions of the lungs of athletic horses there is a neovascularization associated with the body's attempts at healing. There is also the possibility of adhesions developing between the parietal and visceral pleura.

CLINICAL INVESTIGATION

When dealing with cases of EIPH the first step must be to take a full history and perform a thorough clinical examination. If the horse has suffered epistaxis the possibility of hemorrhage from the upper respiratory tract, for example from the guttural pouch, should be considered. If the horse has an elevated temperature there may be pneumonia, pulmonary abscesses or pleuropneumonia. Ultrasound scanning may facilitate a clearer diagnosis. Care should be taken in giving horses anti-inflammatory drugs if they have suffered EIPH. Damaged tissue makes an ideal locus for bacterial infections. If there is a bacterial infection, radiopaque shadows may be observed in the dorsocaudal corner of the lung of horses known to have had EIPH. In the majority of cases this shadow clears within a few days. However, in others it persists. My experience has been that these latter cases, though relatively rare, tend to remain problematical.

THERAPY

A wide range of therapeutic regimens have been advocated for the prevention or treatment of EIPH. To date these have all been based on anecdotal evidence and none has withstood scientific scrutiny.

Many of the early approaches were based on the assumption that there must be underlying coagulation defects or that normal coagulation could be enhanced by using estrogens, vitamin K, hesperidin, or citrus bioflannoids. However, no coagulation defects have been demonstrated to date, and controlled studies have proved this to be a fruitless approach.

BRONCHODILATORS

Limited studies carried out using bronchodilators have shown no efficacy in preventing EIPH. Indeed, the finding that EIPH does not affect performance would question that bronchoconstriction is a prerequisite of EIPH. Bronchodilators and mucolytics would clearly be indicated if airway disease was identified during the clinical examination, as would antibiotics if infection was identified.

FUROSEMIDE

Furosemide is the most widely used pharmaceutical for the treatment and prevention of EIPH. The origins of its use for EIPH remain unclear. The pharmacological basis for its use is tenuous but could could have evolved from the treatment of pulmonary edema. Furosemide apparently has a relatively short bronchodilatory effect when given to ponies with bronchoconstriction. However, bronchoconstriction has not been demonstrated or implicated in EIPH. Furosemide does have hemodynamic effects, at doses higher than those usually used for EIPH.

The use of furosemide as a prerace medication for bleeders has received considerable attention in recent years with several large studies being undertaken. By way of summary, these studies have shown no clear improvement in racing times following prerace administration of furosemide to horses with EIPH. Further, when furosemide was administered to 235 previously EIPH-negative horses, 62 (23.5 per cent) were found to be EIPH positive after racing. A recent study did show that geldings without EIPH had significantly faster racing times when given furosemide before racing than when furosemide was not given before racing.

MANAGEMENT

The debate regarding the significance of small airway disease in relation to EIPH will undoubtedly continue for some time. However, practices that decrease the horse's exposure to airborne contaminants should be maintained since small airway disease is a recognized cause of poor performance, and high levels of airborne contaminants could increase the risk of secondary infection developing at the site of hemorrhage. Air hygiene is dealt with in more depth in another section (see p. 310).

The use of gadgetry such as the equine transpirator, which exposes the horse to water vapor-saturated air, has failed scientific scrutiny.

Supplemental Readings

Clarke, A. F.: A review of exercise-induced pulmonary hemorrhage and its possible relationship with mechanical stress. Equine Vet. J., 17:166, 1985.

Clarke, A. F.: Comments on furosemide and exercise-induced pulmonary hemorrhage. Am. J. Vet. Res., 50:2183, 1989.

O'Callaghan, M. W., Pascoe, J. R., Tyler, W. S., et al.: Exercise induced pulmonary haemorrhage in the horse: Results of a detailed clinical, post-mortem and imaging study. VIII. Conclusions and implications. Equine Vet. J., 19:428, 1987.

Pascoe, J. R., and Raphel, C. F.: Pulmonary haemorrhage in exercising horses. Compend. Cont. Educ. Pract. Vet., 4:5411, 1982.

Sweeney, C. R., Soma, L. R., Maxson, A. D., et al.: Effects of furosemide on the racing times of thoroughbreds. Am. J. Vet. Res., 51:772, 1990.

Sweeney, C. R., and Soma, L. R.: Exercise-induced pulmonary hemorrhage in thoroughbred horses: Response to furosemide or hesperidin-citrus bioflavinoids. J. Am. Vet. Med. Assoc., 185:195, 1984.

Section 8

TOXICOLOGY

Edited by Francis D. Galey

Diagnostic Toxicology

Francis D. Galey, DAVIS, CALIFORNIA

Rapid, accurate diagnosis is critical to the treatment and prevention of diseases caused by toxic agents. Treatment of most toxicoses is supportive, and therefore prevention of further cases is usually the primary goal. The practitioner must determine if the horse's clinical signs are due to a toxic agent, the nature of the agent or its source, and the best way to minimize exposure.

The chapters in this section discuss therapy with an emphasis on understanding, identification, and exclusion of potential etiologies. Dose–response concepts (the amount of a poison needed to cause toxicosis) are included where appropriate. This section discusses correct, timely diagnosis as a means of preventing illness in additional animals. The discussion is not intended to be all-inclusive. Rather, it builds on information presented in earlier editions of *Current Therapy in Equine Medicine.* The topics were selected because of their relevance to the horse, the availability of new information, or their absence from earlier editions of this book.

Poisoning may affect many animals and may stimulate considerable emotion and publicity. Unfortunately, there is no magic test for all possible toxicants. Therefore, this chapter suggests a systematic approach to suspected poisonings. Examples are used where possible.

The approach to a toxicology case involves fitting together several pieces of a puzzle. Often parts of the story are not present. Negative findings may be as important as pathognomonic findings. Frequently no single pathognomonic finding will be present and a composite of several criteria must be evaluated in order to arrive at a diagnosis. The approach begins with a comprehensive history, followed by clinical examination, diagnostic pathology, analytical chemistry, and bioassay.

HISTORY

The history must include a description of the clinical syndrome; herd dynamics, including animal movement, location, and new introductions; management practices; the source and type of feed; the source of water; and environmental conditions. Questioning should be systematic, with findings carefully noted and maps drawn of the premises. Recent movements of animals and shipments of feed should be noted and all sources of feed, water, and bedding identified. Dates of most recent shipments should be recorded as appropriate. If the feed is mixed elsewhere, the practitioner should determine whether the mill also mixes feeds for other animal species. Incorporation of cow feed into a horse ration can result in potentially toxic exposure of horses to feed additives such as monensin or other antibiotics. The relationship between the time of initial exposure to a material and the onset of clinical signs can also provide clues to the diagnosis. More than 30 horses developed laminitis 12 hours after being bedded on a new shipment of shavings. The horses were rapidly removed from the shavings, which were later found to consist of 80 per cent black walnut *(Juglans nigra)*.

The regional environment, especially if industries or dumps are in the vicinity, must be investigated. Determine if animals are downstream or downwind from contaminated areas, such as piles of lead-laced mine tailings. The immediate environment should also be examined. Note where farm chemicals are stored, because feeding accidents have occurred when insecticides are stored near vitamin–mineral mixes. Observe feed preparation on site and at the mill, because mixing errors are a common source of toxicosis. Look for recently trimmed hedges or hedge clippings that are accessible to the horse. Clippings from some hedges such as yews *(Taxus* spp.) or oleander *(Nerium oleander)* can cause sudden death if eaten by horses. Examine fields for overgrazing or evidence of consumption of toxic plants.

Feeds should be sampled systematically. Samples of concentrates to be screened for toxicants must be obtained from the mixing bin and feed troughs. Feed ingredients should also be sampled. If screening of as-fed materials yields a positive result, then the various ingredients can be tested to determine the source of the toxicant.

Hay, forage, and pasture samples should be obtained and examined for potentially poisonous plants and evidence of consumption. Plants for identification should be sampled in their entirety, wrapped in a moist paper, and taken to a herbarium or cooperative greenhouse. Once the plant is identified, the practitioner can judge the potential hazard or consult with a veterinary toxicologist. If local identification is not possible, plants can be pressed, dried, and mailed to a diagnostic laboratory. Alternatively, the plant can be pressed onto a high-quality office copier. The resulting copy can then be faxed to the diagnostic laboratory for quick identification.

All samples of feed and forage should be representative of their original lot. Each bin should have several areas cored, or sampled and pooled. Several parts of several bales from each stack of hay should be sampled and pooled. Pooling is appropriate only for samples from the same bin or stack of hay; otherwise the samples should be kept separate. This is critical because toxicants are not always present uniformly in a bin. For example, some local concentrations of mycotoxins may be present in certain areas within a bin. Once the management, environmental, and feed records are complete, the clinician can concentrate on the clinical syndrome at hand.

CLINICAL EXAMINATION

Evaluation of clinical signs is the next step in piecing together the toxicology puzzle. The incidence of poisoning, the signalment of affected animals, and the nature, rapidity of onset, severity, and progression of clinical signs should all be observed. Some problems, such as ingestion of some plants and feeds, or improper or inappropriate injection of drugs or other chemicals, may result in sudden death with little evidence of specific intoxication. Other cases with nonspecific signs may be more insidious in onset, such as gradual weight loss from ingestion of locoweed or pyrrolizidine alkaloids. Conversely, clinical signs might be very specific, such as laminitis from exposure to black walnut shavings or paralysis due to botulism. Regardless of the type of clinical signs, it is important to rule out nontoxic causes of clinical signs and avoid focusing too rapidly on toxicology.

Clinical laboratory data may also be useful. Complete blood cell counts may suggest a type of anemia or infection, and serum biochemistry assays can help identify affected organ systems. A clinical biochemistry test that is especially useful in toxicology is the assay of acetylcholinesterase activity of whole blood. Depression of the activity of this enzyme suggests exposure to a carbamate or organophosphorus insecticide. Whole blood, serum, gastrointestinal (GI) contents, and urine are all useful for toxicology testing (Table 1).

PATHOLOGY

If animals have died, complete necropsies should be performed, because the toxicologic or forensic necropsy is usually critical to diagnosis of a toxicology case. In some instances, such as pyrrolizidine alkaloid toxicosis, histological examination may provide the only concrete diagnostic information. The necropsy (see p. 344) should be systematic and samples should be properly obtained for bacteriologic, virologic, histologic, and toxicologic examinations. Specimens that should be obtained for toxicology testing are listed in Table 1. It is often helpful to hold samples frozen until other testing is complete to ensure that the most useful and pertinent battery of chemical analyses is assigned. Not all samples will be needed, but it is easier to save samples and discard them later than to somehow "regenerate" them after the fact.

The samples should be examined before they are shipped. Parts of poisonous plants and frag-

TABLE 1. SAMPLES NEEDED FOR TOXICOLOGIC ANALYSIS

Sample	Amount	Condition	Examples
Antemortem Samples			
Whole blood	5 to 10 ml	EDTA anticoagulant	Lead, arsenic, selenium, acetylcholinesterase
Urine	100 ml	Plastic screw-capped vial	Drugs, some metals
Serum	10 ml	Remove from clot; use special trace element tubes	Trace elements, drugs, nitrates
Cerebrospinal fluid	1 ml	Clot tube	Sodium
GI contents	500 gm	Obtain representative sample	Pesticides, plants, metals, feed-associated toxicants
Hair		Rarely useful, call laboratory; wash prior to sampling	Occasionally chronic selenosis
Postmortem Samples			
Urine	100 ml	Plastic screw-capped vial	Drugs, some metals
Serum	20 ml	Remove from heart clot	Drugs, nitrates, electrolytes
Liver	250 gm	Plastic (foil if organics)	Pesticides, metals, botulinum
Kidney	250 gm	Plastic (foil if organics)	Metals
Brain	50%	Split sagittally, send half in formalin to pathologist, half frozen in plastic to analyst	Organochlorides, sodium, acetylcholinesterase
Fat	250 gm	Foil inside plastic	Accumulated organochlorines
GI contents	500 gm	Obtain representative sample	Pesticides, plants, metals, feed-associated toxicants
Ocular fluid	0.5 ml	Entire eye	Nitrates, magnesium
Bone	100 gm	One long bone	Fluoride
Miscellaneous		Injection sites, spleen	Some drugs
Environmental Samples			
Baits, etc.	200 ml or 200 gm	Clean mason jar (liquid, plastic)	Unidentified chemicals, feed additives
Concentrates	1 kg or more	Plastic sack, box; representative sample is imperative	Mycotoxins, feed additives, plants, pesticides, botulinum
Forage	1 kg or more	Plastic sack, box; representative sample is imperative	Plants, pesticides, botulinum
Plants	Plant	Fresh, or pressed and dried; send all plant parts	
Water	1 L	Clean mason jar, foil under lid for metals, plastic if organics	Metals, nitrates, pesticides, algae, sulfate

NOTE.—With the exception of whole blood and very dry samples (e.g., some feeds), all samples should be submitted frozen. When available, appropriate tissue samples, fixed in formalin, should also be submitted for histological analysis. Do not submit material in syringes.

ments of lead have been found in the GI contents of animals that have died suddenly. Specimens should be properly labeled, sealed, and frozen. Inclusion of a complete written history of the case with the samples will help the toxicologist order the appropriate tests and adequately interpret the results.

ANALYTICAL TOXICOLOGY

Analyses are readily available for several classes of toxicants, including heavy metals, pesticides, feed additives, drugs, and some natural toxins (see Table 1). Analytical chemistry involves much more than putting a minute amount of material into a machine. Analyses often require a great deal of preparatory chemistry and significant quantities of material. Thus, analyses for the most likely agents should be selected based on historical, clinical, and pathological data. A diagnostic laboratory should be consulted regarding the specimen sizes and times that are required for testing.

The best sample for analysis is often the feed source or GI contents. This is because the animal's body, especially the liver, has not had a chance to metabolize and dilute the parent compound. Following metabolism, many compounds (especially drugs) are concentrated in the urine during the excretory phase. This is why sampling from the source, GI tract, and urine is most valuable in obtaining a diagnosis.

BIOASSAY

There are two types of bioassay. In some situations, the response of affected animals to specific therapy is a legitimate diagnostic bioassay. This approach should be used with caution and only when the diagnosis is reasonably certain. Some therapeutic agents, such as atropine, which is used to treat organophosphorus or carbamate insecticide poisoning, are themselves potentially very hazardous to the horse.

The other category of bioassay involves feeding a suspected toxin or source of toxin to laboratory animals. This is done only when other diagnostic avenues have been exhausted.

PREVENTION AND TREATMENT

At the end of the initial toxicology case workup, the veterinarian will probably have formed some opinion of the source and nature of the intoxication. Exposure of horses to suspected material should be eliminated immediately. This may involve removal of animals from a pasture if plant toxicosis is suspected. If removal from the pasture is impractical, horses might be provided with adequate feed to prevent continued consumption of a noxious weed. If hay or grain are suspected sources, the feed remaining in troughs or racks should be completely replaced. Similar measures should be taken if bedding or water are suspected.

Once further exposure to a suspected agent has been prevented, horses must be clinically evaluated for possible treatment. Because many toxicants lack specific antidotes, treatment frequently consists of nonspecific support and alleviation of clinical signs. If appropriate, horses recently exposed to a suspected toxicant should be treated with an oral adsorbent such as activated charcoal (2 gm per kg body weight as a slurry in water, administered via nasogastric tube). Horses with impaired intestinal motility should receive mineral oil, but mineral oil and activated charcoal inactivate each other and should not be mixed. If a horse showing signs of colic has been treated with mineral oil and a toxicant is still suspected, activated charcoal can be administered 3 or 4 hours later if GI motility is normal.

Specific clinical problems are addressed next. When treating clinical problems, the practitioner must avoid administering drugs that are metabolized by, excreted by, or have an impact on the organs affected by the toxin. Once test results are complete and the toxicant has been identified, treatment can be modified accordingly.

Supplemental Readings

Blodgett, D.: The investigation of outbreaks of toxicologic disease. Vet. Clin. North Am. (Food Anim. Pract.), 4:145, 1988.
Hancock, D. D., Blodgett, D. J., and Gay, C. C.: The collection and submission of samples for laboratory testing. Vet. Clin. North Am. (Food Anim. Pract.), 4:33, 1988.
Osweiler, G. D., Carson, T. L., Buck, W. B., and Van Gelder, G. A.: Diagnostic toxicology. In: Clinical and Diagnostic Veterinary Toxicology, 3rd ed. Dubuque, Kendall/Hunt Publishing Co., 1985, pp. 44–51.

Toxicologic Implications of Sudden, Unexplained Death

John C. Haliburton, AMARILLO, TEXAS
William C. Edwards, STILLWATER, OKLAHOMA

The postmortem investigation is a valuable service provided to horse owners by the equine practitioner. If no imminent legal issues are associated with the death, many postmortem investigations require only a thorough necropsy and gross examination. Equine practitioners are frequently asked, however, to conduct or assist in a postmortem investigation where legal issues are associated with the death. These cases often require intensive laboratory examinations, including a comprehensive toxicologic workup.

Legal issues that most often arise in such cases

are generally related to the cause of death, the manner of death, and the question of insurance fraud. The cause of death is critical for equine insurance mortality claims because exclusions are commonly written into many policies. The manner of death defines how the death arose: by accident, from natural causes, or from intentional or malicious actions of an individual.

Equine insurance mortality claim investigations are in some respects the veterinary equivalent to human medicolegal investigations (i.e., forensic medicine). In both, the facts and findings of a scientific and medical investigation are used to resolve legal issues associated with the death.

Any sudden or unexpected death should be investigated, with the possibility of poisoning high on the list of probable cause. Table 1 lists some common causes of sudden death in horses that should be considered in the investigation of such cases. With few exceptions, all equine insurance mortality claims involving highly insured horses that have died suddenly, unexpectedly, or under suspicious circumstances are forensic cases requiring a comprehensive toxicologic evaluation. This chapter focuses on the logistics of conducting a forensic postmortem investigation on an equine insurance mortality claim in a manner that will ensure the highest degree of efficiency and cooperation with the toxicology laboratory. The discussion also addresses the role of the practitioner in forensic litigation.

POSTMORTEM EXAMINATION

Whenever an insurance mortality claim is filed, especially in the case of a highly insured horse, the insurance company will usually require a postmortem examination (i.e., necropsy) and a comprehensive pathology and toxicology laboratory examination before it will pay the claim (see p. 344). As a rule, the veterinarian selected to conduct the necropsy will be owner-appointed. The insurance company may also designate a veterinarian to witness the necropsy and to take custody of postmortem specimens. It is strongly recommended that the veterinarian retained to perform the necropsy, regardless of which party (owner or insurance company) has retained his or her services, request the presence of another veterinarian to witness or assist with the necropsy.

When contacted, the practitioner should immediately establish for whom his or her services have been retained—the owner or insurance company—and in what capacity he or she will be expected to function (as witness or as assistant in

TABLE 1. SOME CAUSES OF SUDDEN DEATH IN HORSES

Physical causes
  Trauma
  Electrocution
  Exsanguination
  Strangulation
  Gunshot
  Suffocation
  Heat stroke
  Exercise- or stress-induced cardiovascular failure
Natural causes
  Ruptured aortic aneurysm
  Cerebral vascular accident
  Hyperkalemic periodic paralysis
  Cardiac conductive disorders
Feed-related causes
  Colic–shock syndrome
  Blister beetle (cantharidin toxicosis)
  Ionophores
  Urea
  Cyanide
  Leukoencephalomalacia
Infectious causes
  Salmonellosis
  Anthrax
  Clostridial diseases
  Equine protozoal encephalomyelitis
Accidental drug-related causes
  Anaphylaxis
  Succinylcholine
  Anesthetic accidents
  Intra-arterial drug injections
  Iron injections
Malicious poisoning
  Strychnine
  Nicotine
  Arsenic
  Insulin
  Iron
  Barbiturates
  Potassium
  Magnesium
  Pesticides
  Exogenous insulin
Accidental poisoning
  Plant ingestion
  Oleander (*Neriin oleander*)
  Japanese yew (*Taxus*)
  Water hemlock (*Cicuta* spp.)
  Poison hemlock (*Conium* spp.)
  Blue-green algae (*Microcystis* spp.)
  Pesticides

the necropsy). The owner-appointed veterinarian may only be required to conduct the necropsy, whereas the veterinarian retained by the insurance company, in addition to witnessing the necropsy, is often asked to investigate the owners' management practices, health maintenance program, and physical facilities.

A brief case history should be obtained when the practitioner is first contacted about the case. Important information includes the name and age of the horse, name and address of the owner, and all available information on the circumstances associated with the death of the horse. This information is useful both for making the decision to accept or reject a case and for assessing possible conflicts of interest. If for any reason the practitioner feels that he or she cannot conduct an unbiased and objective postmortem investigation, the request should be declined. The practitioner should at this stage of the investigation evaluate and discuss with the client the feasibility of transporting the horse to an animal disease diagnostic laboratory that is staffed and equipped to conduct a comprehensive and thorough postmortem examination. Frequently the insurance company, and occasionally an owner, will designate a laboratory that the practitioner should contact prior to starting the necropsy. This is not done to question the competency of the practitioner but to ensure that all specimens required by the laboratory are collected, packaged, and transported to the laboratory in an acceptable and expedient manner. Laboratory tests are essential in forensic cases to confirm the diagnosis of the cause of death. The practitioner should be willing, therefore, to communicate with the designated laboratory in a timely and professional manner.

Often the toxicologist is presented with a collection of postmortem specimens and is asked to analyze them for "toxic substances," without any additional information provided such as the clinical and medical history, the circumstances surrounding the death, or the postmortem findings. That practice does not yield optimum results. Therefore, samples that are submitted should be accompanied by a complete, written account of the case, including the findings of the practitioner in the field.

Before the examiner starts the necropsy, a complete medical history should be obtained. Relevant data include vaccination history; medication received within the last 10 days; any previous injury, illness, or surgery; the approximate time the horse was last seen alive; parasite control program; and management practices. Information regarding rations or other feeds or supplements, approximate time the horse was fed prior to dying, and water source and availability should also be recorded. Photographs of the premises and several views of the animal should be taken. All photographs taken during a postmortem examination should be subsequently signed and dated. It should be established if the horse was moved after it died, and if so, the record should indicate who moved it, from where it was moved, how it was moved, and when and why it was moved. If the location of death is not the location where the horse is to be necropsied, the site of death should be inspected and any signs of terminal struggle noted. If evidence of foul play is apparent or suspected, local law enforcement authorities should be contacted for assistance before any physical evidence is disturbed.

A complete physical description of the horse including color, markings, tattoo numbers, and any physical defects is essential in all medicolegal cases. A portable cassette recorder and a 35mm camera with a flash are highly recommended for examiners who routinely conduct postmortem investigations.

SPECIMEN COLLECTION

Appropriate specimen selection, collection, and storage for toxicologic analyses is the responsibility of the veterinarian performing the postmortem examination. Practitioners are not expected to know what each individual toxicology laboratory prefers regarding the specimens to be submitted and how they should be submitted; therefore, it is best if the practitioner contacts the toxicologist for guidance and special instructions prior to conducting the postmortem examination. It is seldom possible to determine at the time of the necropsy exactly what specimens will be required for analysis. However, if the specimens and the quantities indicated in Table 2 are collected, a comprehensive toxicologic evaluation can be performed by most toxicology laboratories. The collection and subsequent analysis of stomach contents can be important in many cases of poisoning. The total amount of stomach content present should be

TABLE 2. RECOMMENDED SAMPLES AND AMOUNTS TO BE COLLECTED IN FORENSIC EXAMINATIONS

Specimen	Amount
Kidney	0.5–1.0 kg
Liver	0.5–1.0 kg
Lung	0.5 kg
Spleen	0.5 kg
Brain	½ of brain
Stomach content	1.0 kg
Intestinal content	1.0 kg
Urine	All
Blood°	100 ml
Vitreous humor	All
Fat	0.5 kg
Bone	Portion of long bone
Feces	0.5 kg
Muscle	Around suspected injection sites

°Blood from peripheral vessels and from the heart should be collected separately. A 10- to 20-ml aliquot of each should be preserved with sodium fluoride. Additional aliquots can be placed in EDTA tubes and clot tubes.

determined by weight or volume, mixed thoroughly, and divided into appropriately sized aliquots for submission to the laboratory. Duplicate samples for toxicologic evaluation should be placed in clean containers (Whirl-Pak bags are ideal) suitable for shipment and resistant to freezing, properly labeled, initialed, dated, and either refrigerated or frozen, depending on the length of time for transport and delivery to the laboratory.

In addition to the specimens listed in Table 2, it may be necessary to collect samples of feeds, water, drugs, plants, insects, chemicals, or bedding material. Analysis of these specimens may help solve a difficult case.

Forensic investigations of equine deaths not only require proper sample collection but also strict documentation of sample custody *(chain of custody)*. A chain of custody is a record of every aspect of the possession and transference of evidence from the time of collection to its ultimate introduction as evidence in court. The chain of custody specifically identifies each article of evidence, the time and date of receipt or transfer, and the names of all persons taking and transferring custody of the evidence. In addition, the law requires that evidence must be maintained in a secure location free from potential adulteration. Failure to maintain a chain of custody on all items of evidence could jeopardize a favorable judgment on an otherwise strong case.

Because of the large case load and limited storage facilities, most veterinary toxicology laboratories can keep forensic samples only for a relatively short period of time (e.g., 1 to 3 months). This situation, combined with the fact that most medicolegal cases may take 1 to 4 years to reach the courtroom, creates some major problems in litigation of many cases. There are two basic approaches to alleviating these potential problems. Most laboratories can store a limited number of forensic samples for an extended period of time. The practitioner should discuss this issue with the laboratory prior to sending or delivering any samples and should determine what samples can be stored and for how long. Alternatively, the practitioner can divide all of the specimens collected, giving one set of samples to the other party, one set to the laboratory, and keeping the third set in his or her possession in secure storage.

TRIAL PREPARATIONS

After the practitioner in a medicolegal case has completed the postmortem examination, submitted specimens to the laboratory, and filed an investigation report, the courtroom (including depositions) is the next stop. Court actions fall into one of two categories: civil and criminal. Civil cases, which are the predominant type of medicolegal cases encountered in veterinary medicine, are actions between two or more people, businesses, or governmental agencies. Civil cases are usually brought on breach of contract or a tort action. Criminal actions are cases in which criminal charges, state or federal, are brought against an individual by the government.

The practitioner may be called on to testify as a witness of fact (i.e., lay witness) or as an expert witness (see p. 343). As a lay witness the practitioner may only testify to what he or she did, said, smelled, touched, or heard (hearsay is not admissible evidence). The lay witness cannot give opinions or conclusions about any aspect of the case. The expert witness, on the other hand, can express opinions and conclusions on any issue within the scope of his or her expertise. The expert witness is an individual skilled in a specific art, trade, or profession, or is someone with special information or expertise in a particular subject area. The expert witness is presumed to be an impartial participant in a trial who, based on his or her qualifications as an expert, can explain the technical aspects of the case to the judge and jury. The practitioner who conducts the postmortem examination in an equine forensic case in which the cause of death is ultimately confirmed to be related to poisoning is most often called to testify as a witness of fact. However, depending on the circumstances, the practitioner may be called as an expert witness. Therefore, with the wide range of latitude existing in the two types of witnesses, it is very important for the practitioner clearly to understand his or her role in the testimony phase of a medicolegal case.

Regardless of the practitioner's role as a witness, a key to competent and professional demeanor in the courtroom is to maintain complete and accurate records of all activities and findings, including telephone conversations associated with the case. Do not attempt to rely on unaided memory. Not only is memory not documentable, it can become clouded and unreliable with the passage of time, and rarely will a medicolegal case make it to the courtroom without a delay of several months to years.

CONCLUSION

The procedures discussed in this chapter are fundamental to equine forensic investigations.

Proper sample collection, identification, and submission to the toxicology laboratory require some foresight and planning on the part of the practitioner and direct communication with the toxicologist. The quality of the specimens submitted will often be reflected in the usefulness of the toxicologic findings in medicolegal cases.

The diagnosis of poisoning or even an indication of a possible poisoning as the cause of death should not be issued or stated by the practitioner at the time of the necropsy. Rarely can the cause of death be accurately identified in a poisoning case solely from the necropsy findings. In clinical medicine, the practitioner, after obtaining a medical history, assessing clinical signs, and performing a physical examination, is accustomed to giving the client a diagnosis as to the cause of illness. The practitioner will often encounter this same inquisitive "want-to-know-now" owner or trainer during the necropsy of an insured horse. The practitioner should refrain from issuing a diagnosis or any conclusion at the time of the necropsy that implies poisoning as the cause of death, but should wait for the toxicology laboratory to issue its findings and conclusions. The comprehensive toxicologic testing that is often required in medicolegal cases can take several weeks to complete. Therefore, the practitioner must be patient and not be influenced or pressured into issuing a premature diagnosis as to the probable cause of death. This will prevent the practitioner from being personally and professionally humiliated by an opposing attorney in the courtroom for issuing an erroneous diagnosis or conclusion.

Supplemental Readings

Edwards, W. C., and Johnson, B. J.: A veterinarian's guide: Equine insurance examinations. Equine Pract., 8:19–22, 1986.
Meads, R.: Ready or not? Don't be afraid of litigation—Be prepared. Pet Vet., 2:12–14, 1990.
Osweiler, G. D., Carson, T. L., Buck, W. B., and VanGelder, G. A.: Clinical and Diagnostic Veterinary Toxicology, 3rd ed. Dubuque, Kendall/Hunt Publishing, Inc., 1985.
Poynter, D. F.: The Expert Witness Handbook: Tips and Techniques for the Litigation Consultant. Santa Barbara, Para Publishing, 1987.

Forensic Necropsy

Bill J. Johnson, DAVIS, CALIFORNIA

The practitioner is occasionally called on to perform a postmortem examination on a horse because it is insured for large sums of money or because the circumstances of the horse's death are likely to be the subject of a lawsuit. Typical veterinary necropsy training is oriented toward finding disease conditions or traumatic injuries. The trainee receives little information on how to handle malicious or potentially litigable cases in such a way as to protect the rights of all parties involved. The practitioner must be a neutral observer who is capable of making trained, intelligent observations and reporting findings without prejudice. Good planning and accurate record keeping are essential because these cases may end up in litigation 5 or 10 years after the original examination.

Forensic cases can be very time-consuming. If the practitioner does not have time to handle such a case, the client should be so informed and a referral suggested. Once the necropsy is performed the responsibility for the case has been accepted. Failure to follow accepted procedure in handling such a case may result in professional embarrassment in court or possibly a later lawsuit. If transportation is possible and postmortem decomposition during shipment is not a factor, it is best to send these cases to a qualified animal disease diagnostic laboratory. If this is not possible, the following guidelines should help protect the interests of all parties.

Obtain a thorough history and identify the legal owner of the horse. If the animal is insured, get the name and address of the insurance company and permission to communicate with them directly. The insurer should then be called to identify specific requirements in the policy that must be met before the company will settle a death claim. Inquire of the owner or attendant about previous health problems, present ration, changes in ration, previous medications, environmental changes, changes in the daily routine of the horse, and any clinical abnormalities present before death. Accept all of this information as opinion, not fact. Let the necropsy observations confirm or raise questions about the history.

Identify the horse as well as possible. Ask the

owner or the attendant if there are any identifying marks. If possible, photograph the animal, with pictures of the limbs, head, body, and any tatoos or lack of tatoos. Record, on the report, a description of markings and tatoos. Write only what can clearly be seen. If a tatoo is illegible, draw what remains. Clip the neck of Arabian horses and draw the figures just as they appear. Report only what you can testify to, not what is on the registration papers.

Start the necropsy without prejudices. It is fine to have a most likely diagnosis, but do not focus on that possibility to the point of ignoring other possibilities. Concentrate strictly on the matter at hand. From the clinical history, determine what organs or organ systems need particularly close scrutiny. A good systematic necropsy technique will ensure that all organs are examined and that any previously unforeseen problems will be recognized.

The obvious is not always as it seems. Ruptured stomachs and bloody intestines can be postmortem artifacts. When faced with a possible lesion, remember the process of inflammation. Any antemortem rupture should have areas of hemorrhage or fibrin release at the margins of the tear. Omentum or other organs should be lightly adherent to the edges of the ruptured organ. The serosa next to the tear may be dull and granular due to fibrin release, rather than its normal smooth and shiny appearance. What is often termed hemorrhagic enteritis is only blood-engorged capillaries and venules in the intestinal villi with postmortem imbibition of hemoglobin. Cases of enteritis should show some combination of necrosis, mural edema, adherent fibrin, or blood. On the other hand, do not be misled by normal-appearing intestines or organs. Inflammatory changes may be so subtle that they may only be seen microscopically in formalin-fixed sections.

Record the nutritional condition of the animal and its state of postmortem decomposition. Constantly ask questions based on what is being seen. Is there marked subcutaneous bruising? The presence of considerable bruising suggests a prolonged, agonal death, while the lack of any bruising suggests that the animal died suddenly, possibly due to malicious poisoning. Do necropsy findings match the owners' antemortem observations? Was the animal "just found dead"? In such cases, special attention should be paid to the jugular furrows and the intimal surfaces of the jugular veins for any evidence of an injection. Record all the organs that are examined, even though they appear normal. Five years hence on the witness stand, it may be difficult to remember if the adrenal glands were examined.

Carefully examine the organ system that makes the animal particularly valuable. If the horse is a valuable breeding stallion, examine the testicles and genital tract carefully. The limbs of valuable racing horses should be examined, especially the front limbs. The carpal and pastern joints are particularly susceptible to articular damage.

SPECIMEN COLLECTION

Collect 1-cm-thick sections in 10 per cent formalin for histopathological examination of any abnormal organs, plus sections of organs that could physiologically account for the clinical signs. If the animal was found dead, collect a wide assortment of tissues. In all cases, sections of kidney, spleen, liver, heart, lung, brain, stomach, small intestine, colon, and cecum should be collected. When the history or findings dictate, proper specimens should be collected for microbiological examination.

If there is even a hint that the horse's death is intentional or malicious, samples should be collected for toxicology. If possible, check with a toxicologist before performing the necropsy for any special samples or handling instructions. If this is not possible, use the guidelines on page 339 for collection, handling, and shipping of samples.

Finally, immediately record all findings. As an old proverb has it, "The historical accounts from the dullest pencil are clearer than those from the brightest mind."

Supplemental Readings

Edwards, W. C., and Johnson, B. J.: Equine insurance examinations. Equine Pract., 8:19, 1986.

King, J. M., Dodd, D. C., and Newson, M. E.: Necropsy of the horse: Parts 1, 2, 3. Mod. Vet. Pract., 59:897, 1978: 60:29, 60:109, 1979.

Taylor, R. F., and Sexton, J. W.: Medical-legal aspects of veterinary medicine. In: Proceedings of the 25th Annual Convention of the American Association of Veterinary Laboratory Diagnosticians, 1982, pp. 499–509.

Management of Toxicoses

E. Murl Bailey, Jr., COLLEGE STATION, TEXAS
Tam Garland, COLLEGE STATION, TEXAS

The prevention and treatment of equine toxicoses are common duties in veterinary practice. The constant threat of poisoning, accidental or intentional, makes client education imperative. Because of the multitude of intoxicants present in the environment or that may be introduced artificially, the practitioner should have a solid grasp of treatment and management procedures for dealing with toxicosis.

BASIC CONCEPTS OF TOXICOLOGIC THERAPY

The primary efforts in cases of intoxication are directed toward emergency intervention and preventing further exposure, establishing a tentative diagnosis upon which to base rational therapeutic measures, delaying further absorption, applying specific antidotes and remedial measures, hastening elimination of the absorbed intoxicant, administering supportive therapy, determining the source of the intoxicant, and educating the client.

When initiating therapy for animal toxicoses, veterinary clinicians should focus on treating the signs exhibited by the affected animals, unless the correct diagnosis is obvious. Preexisting conditions and the diagnosis should be determined after the patient's condition has stabilized.

It is important that neither the client nor the clinician wastes time. The animal should be examined by the veterinarian as soon as possible. The owners should be instructed to bring suspected toxic materials or their containers with them to aid in the diagnosis.

The most important aspect of treatment is to ensure adequate physiological function. This may include establishment of a patent airway and provision of ventilatory and cardiac support. Following stabilization of the animal's vital signs, the clinician may proceed with therapeutic measures.

Preventing the animal from absorbing additional toxicant is a major factor in treating cases of toxicosis. Removal of the animal from the affected environment is the first step to preventing further absorption; bringing the animal to the veterinary clinic or hospital may solve this problem. It may also be necessary to wash the animal's skin with a mild liquid detergent to remove the noxious agent. However, caution must be exercised to avoid the contamination of all persons handling the animal. Protective clothing, such as rubber aprons and gloves, is a necessity. In addition, the judicious use of adsorbents and cathartics will aid in preventing further absorption of ingested toxic materials. Absorption may be retarded by precipitation, inactivation, neutralization, oxidation, and chelation. Several of these mechanisms may be activated with carefully chosen locally acting chemical antidotes, as listed in Table 1.

Activated charcoal is probably the best adsorbing agent available for oral administration. Although it does not detoxify toxicants, it will effectively prevent absorption of a toxicant if properly utilized. Toxicants for which it is highly adsorptive include insecticides, herbicides, mercuric chloride, and strychnine. Many other toxicants, including morphine, atropine, barbiturates, and ethylene glycol, are also adsorbed.

Activated charcoal is available in several base formulations. The best type to use for treatment of toxicosis is of petroleum or vegetable origin.° Do not use mineral or animal formulated charcoal therapeutically for toxicosis. The appropriate technique for employing activated charcoal is as follows: (1) Make a slurry of the charcoal at a concentration of 1 gm per 3 to 5 ml of water (the dose is 1 to 3 gm per kg). (2) Administer the charcoal by stomach tube. (3) Immediately following the charcoal administration, a cathartic should be given. The dose should be repeated within 8 to 12 hours in many instances.

Either sodium sulfate or magnesium sulfate may be used as a cathartic in an emergency. Sodium sulfate is more efficient than magnesium sulfate and the preferred agent for evacuation of the bowel, especially with activated charcoal. With magnesium sulfate, there is some danger of central nervous system (CNS) depression due to the magnesium ion. The dose of sodium or magnesium sulfate is 1 gm of cathartic per kg body weight, dissolved in up to 4 liters of warm water.

°Toxiban, Vet-A-Mix, Shenandoah, IA

TABLE 1. LOCALLY ACTING ANTIDOTES AGAINST UNABSORBED POISONS

Toxicant	Antidote and Dose or Concentration
Acids, corrosives	Weak alkali–magnesium oxide solution (1:25 warm water) internally. *Never give sodium bicarbonate.* Milk of magnesia: 1–15 ml. Flush externally with water. Apply paste of sodium bicarbonate.
Alkali, caustic	Weak acid, e.g., vinegar (diluted 1:4), 1% acetic acid or lemon juice PO. Dilute albumin (4 to 6 egg whites to 1 qt. water) or give whole milk followed by activated charcoal and then a cathartic, because some compounds are soluble in excess albumin. Local: Flush with copious amounts of water and apply vinegar.
Alkaloids	Potassium permanganate (1:5000–1:10,000) for lavage or PO administration. Tannic acid or strong tea (200–500 mg in 30–60 ml of water) except in cases of poisoning by cocaine, nicotine, physostigmine, atropine, and morphine. Purgative should be used for prompt removal of tannates. Activated charcoal may be useful for some alkaloids, although its effectiveness remains to be proved (1 gm/kg body weight via stomach tube as a slurry in water).
Arsenic	Sodium thiosulfate, 10% solution PO (60–100 gm), followed by lavage. Protein: e.g., evaporated milk, egg whites.
Barium and bismuth salts	Sodium sulfate and magnesium sulfate (20% solution given PO). Dosage: 2–25 gm.
Carbon tetrachloride	Acacia or gum arabic as mucilage. Empty stomach, give high-protein and high-carbohydrate diet; maintain fluid and electrolyte balance. Hemodialysis is indicated in anuria. Epinephrine is contraindicated (ventricular fibrillation!).
Copper	Albumin: Use as for alkali intoxication. Magnesium oxide: Use as for acid intoxication.
Detergents, anionic (Na^+, K^+, NH_4^+ salts)	Milk or water followed by demulcent (oils, kaolin, acacia, gelatin, starch, egg white).
Detergents, cationic (chlorides, iodides)	Soap (Castile) dissolved in 4 times its bulk of hot water. Albumin: Use as for alkali intoxication.
Fluoride	Calcium (milk, limewater, or powdered chalk mixed with water) PO.
Formaldehyde	Ammonia water (0.2% PO) or ammonium acetate (1% for lavage). Starch: 1 part to 15 parts hot water added gradually. Gelatin soaked in water for ½ hour. Albumin: Use as for alkali intoxication. Sodium thiosulfate: Use as for arsenic intoxication.
Iron	Sodium bicarbonate: 1% for lavage.
Lead	Sodium or magnesium sulfate PO. See specific antidote. Albumin: Use as for alkali intoxication.
Mercury	Protein: Milk, egg whites (use as for alkali intoxication). Magnesium oxide: Use as for acid intoxication. Sodium formaldehyde sulfoxylate: 5% solution for lavage. Starch: Use as for formaldehyde intoxication. Activated charcoal: Use as for alkaloid intoxication.
Oxalic acid	Calcium: Calcium hydroxide as 0.15% solution. Other alkalis are contraindicated because their salts are more soluble. Chalk or other calcium salts. Magnesium sulfate as cathartic. Maintain diuresis to prevent calcium oxalate deposition in kidney.
Petroleum distillates (aliphatic hydrocarbons)	Olive oil, other vegetable oils, or mineral oil PO. After ½ hour, sodium sulfate as cathartic. Lavage is contraindicated for ingested volatile solvents, but petroleum distillates are used as carrier agents for more toxic agents.
Phenol and cresols	Soap-and-water or alcohol lavage of skin. Sodium bicarbonate (0.5%) dressings. Activated charcoal and/or mineral oil PO.
Phosphorus	Copper sulfate (0.2%–0.4% solution) or potassium permanganate (1:5000 solution) for lavage. Activated charcoal. Do not give vegetable oil cathartic. Remove fat from diet.
Silver nitrate	Normal saline for lavage. Albumin: Use as for alkali intoxication.
Unknown (e.g., toxic plants or other materials)	Activated charcoal: Replaces universal antidote; use as for alkaloid intoxication. Follow with a cathartic, and repeat procedure.

ELIMINATION OF ABSORBED TOXICANTS

Toxicants may be excreted by various routes, commonly the GI tract and lungs. Many absorbed toxicants are excreted via the kidneys and excretion is enhanced by the use of diuretics or by altering the pH of the urine.

The use of diuretics to enhance urinary excretion of toxicants requires adequate renal function and hydration of the affected animal. Once these conditions are established, diuretics are indicated. Monitoring of urinary output is essential, and a minimum urinary flow of 0.1 ml per kg per minute is necessary. The diuretics of choice are mannitol and furosemide. The dosage of mannitol is 2 gm per kg per hour; for furosemide it is 1.5 to 3.0 mg per kg, as needed.

Alteration of urinary pH to expedite the excretion of toxicants and foreign chemicals is a pharmacological technique that relies on the physicochemical phenomenon that ionized compounds do not readily traverse cell membranes and hence are not reabsorbed by the renal tubules. Consequently, acid compounds such as acetylsalicylic acid (aspirin) and some barbiturates remain ionized in acidic urine. As a result, urinary excretion of many toxic compounds may be enhanced by modifying the urinary pH. Sodium bicarbonate may be used as the alkalinizing agent.

Peritoneal dialysis is indicated in small animals with oliguria or anuria but is difficult to undertake in large animals. It is a time-consuming but effective technique for many conditions. The procedure requires the use of solutions that are exchanged every 30 to 60 minutes. Two dialyzing solutions are available: (1) 5 per cent dextrose in 0.45 per cent NaCl with 15 mEq per liter of potassium as potassium chloride, and (2) 5 per cent dextrose in water with 44.6 mEq of bicarbonate and 15 mEq of potassium. Ten to 20 ml per kg of dialyzing solution is infused into the peritoneal cavity, withdrawn after 30 to 60 minutes, and more fresh solution is infused. The infusion and withdrawal cycles should be maintained for 12 to 14 hours, or until normal renal function is restored. The pH of the dialyzing solutions may be altered to maintain the ionized state of the offending compound.

SUPPORTIVE MEASURES

The following supportive measures are critical in the treatment of intoxications: control of body temperature, maintenance of respiratory and cardiovascular functions, control of CNS signs, and control of pain.

BODY TEMPERATURE CONTROL

Hypothermia is controlled using blankets and keeping the animals in warm, draft-free stalls. Infrared lamps should be used with caution and constant observation to avoid burns. Hyperthermia is treated with ice bags, cold water baths, cold water enemas, or cold peritoneal dialysis solutions. Regardless of the type of temperature control required, the animal's body temperature must be constantly monitored to ensure that overcorrection does not occur.

RESPIRATORY SUPPORT

Appropriate respiratory support requires the presence of an adequate, patent airway. A patent airway may be achieved with a cuffed endotracheal tube for an unconscious animal or with a tracheostomy using a local anesthetic for a conscious animal. An emergency tracheostomy tube may be made from a cuffed endotracheal tube that has been shortened to reduce dead space.

The use of analeptic drugs in cases of severe respiratory depression or apnea is questionable because of the short duration of their effects and other undesirable side effects. Positive-pressure ventilatory support is of greater value than analeptic drugs. However, a large animal ventilator or large animal anesthetic equipment may not be available to all equine practitioners. The uses and dosages of several analeptic drugs are described later in the section on CNS depression.

CARDIOVASCULAR SUPPORT

Cardiovascular support requires the presence of adequate circulating volume, cardiac function, tissue perfusion, and acid–base balance. Circulating blood volume and cardiac activity are of immediate concern. Tissue perfusion and acid–base balance are not immediate concerns.

In the presence of hypovolemia due to loss of both red cells and plasma volume, whole blood is needed. A good rule is to give a sufficient quantity of whole blood to increase the packed cell volume to 75 per cent of the animal's estimated normal value. Cases of hypovolemia due to fluid loss alone can be treated by administering lactated Ringer's solution or plasma expanders. Central venous pressure may be monitored to prevent overloading the heart with too much volume, too rapidly. Tissue perfusion should also be monitored periodically to determine the adequacy of the replacement therapy. In some cases, it may be necessary to administer massive doses of intravenous (IV) corticosteroids (dexamethasone, 2 to 10 mg per kg). Vigorous fluid therapy should be maintained concomitant with large doses of IV corticosteroids.

The administration of inotropic and chronotropic drugs is necessary in most instances. One of these agents is calcium gluconate, which is infused IV (see p. 568) very slowly to effect. This agent is reported to be a good nonspecific agent to use in many toxicoses. Digoxin (0.002 to 0.006 mg/kg IV) can also be administered. Care must be taken not to give overdoses of cardioactive agents, as they are highly toxic to the myocardium.

ACID–BASE BALANCE

Control of acid–base balance problems consists primarily of physiologically maintaining an animal in a homeostatic condition. The most common acid–base disturbance in animals is metabolic acidosis. However, acidosis or alkalosis may occur in cases of intoxication.

In correcting metabolic acidosis, sodium bicarbonate administered IV at a rate of 2 to 4 mEq per kg every 15 minutes is the treatment of choice. Other alkalinizing solutions are one-sixth molar sodium lactate, 16 to 32 ml per kg; lactated Ringer's solution, 120 ml per kg; and Tromethamine buffer, 300 mg per kg. Bicarbonate is generally the easiest to administer because it requires the least volume and no metabolic conversion. Caution must be used in administering any alkalinizing agent to avoid inducing alkalosis.

Alkalosis, unless drug-induced, rarely occurs in animals. However, if alkalosis is present, the IV administration of 0.9 per cent NaCl (physiologic saline), 10 ml per kg, is usually sufficient for initial therapy. This should be followed by the oral administration of ammonium chloride, 200 mg per kg per day in divided doses. As with acidosis, the clinician should be cautious about overtreatment of alkalosis.

CENTRAL NERVOUS SYSTEM SUPPORT

Management of CNS disorders in cases of intoxication is simple in theory but complex in practice. The type of therapy depends on whether there is depression or hyperactivity. Depression can easily be changed into hyperactivity or vice versa by overzealous therapeutic measures.

CNS depression can be considered in the same way as respiratory depression because the management of the two conditions is very similar. Analeptic agents such as doxapram* (5 to 10 mg per kg), methetharimide (10 to 20 mg per kg), or pentylenetetrazol (6 to 10 mg per kg) are reported to be efficacious when administered IV. Their actions are short-lived, and CNS depression may return if the animals are not continuously monitored. Another disadvantage is that analeptics may induce convulsions. Artificial respiration or respiratory support is of greater value in animals exhibiting CNS depression and is often the treatment of choice.

CNS hyperactivity and convulsions can be managed by the administration of CNS depressants or tranquilizers. Pentobarbital sodium is generally the agent of choice for cases of CNS hyperactivity and convulsions. Care must be used in administration since a respiratory-depressing dose may be necessary to alleviate the CNS signs. In such cases, respiratory support is mandatory.

Inhalant anesthetics have been reported to be excellent for the long-term management of CNS hyperactivity, but their administration entails the use of the inhalant equipment for extended periods and thus they may not be practical in large animals. Centrally acting skeletal relaxants and minor tranquilizers have been reported for use in cases of convulsant intoxicants. Some of these drugs include methocarbamol,° 110 mg per kg IV; glycerol guaiacolate,† 110 mg per kg IV; and diazepam,‡ 0.5 to 1.5 mg per kg IV or IM. In cases of CNS stimulation due to extrapyramidal effects of phenothiazine tranquilizers, amphetamines have produced adequate control. Regardless of the regimen of therapy for CNS hyperactivity, the animals should be placed in a quiet, dark stall to prevent additional auditory or visual stimulation.

SYSTEMIC AND SPECIFIC ANTIDOTES

When a poison has been absorbed, use of a systemic antidote, if available, is indicated. In most situations it is advisable to treat immediately with a systemic antidote, to promote elimination (excretion), and to implement supportive therapy. However, specific antidotes are available for only a few poisons.

Systemic and specific antidotes and the dosages for each are listed in Table 2. The dosages and durations of treatments given in the table are only guidelines and must be adjusted according to the severity of the poisoning and the condition of the animal.

---

*Dopram, A. H. Robins, Richmond, VA

°Robaxin, A. H. Robins, Richmond, VA
†Guilaxin, A. H. Robins, Richmond, VA
‡Valium, Roche Labs, Nutley, NJ

TABLE 2. SPECIFIC SYSTEMIC ANTIDOTES AND DOSAGES

Toxicant	Systemic Antidote	Dosage and Method for Treatment
Amphetamines	Chlorpromazine	1 mg/kg IM, IP, IV; administer only half dose if barbiturates have been given: blocks excitation.
Arsenic, mercury and other heavy metals except cadmium, lead, silver, selenium, and thallium	Dimercaprol (BAL, Hynson; Wescott & Dunning)	10% solution in oil; give 2.5–5.0 mg/kg IM q. 4 h. for 2 days, b.i.d. for the next 10 days or until recovery. NOTE: In severe acute poisoning, 5 mg/kg dosage should be given only for the first day.
	D-Penicillamine (Cuprimine; Merck & Co.)	Developed for chronic mercury poisoning, now seems promising. No reports on dosage in horses. Dosage for humans is 250 mg PO q. 6 h. for 10 days (3–4 mg/kg).
Atropine, belladonna alkaloids	Physostigmine salicylate	0.1–0.6 mg/kg IM (do not overtreat; do not use neostigmine).
Barbiturates	Doxapram	2% solution: 3–5 mg/kg (0.14–0.25 ml/kg) IV only; repeat as necessary. NOTE.—The above is reliable only when depression is mild. In deeper levels of depression, artificial respiration (and oxygen) is preferable.
Bromides	Chlorides (sodium or ammonium salts)	0.5–1.0 gm/day for several days; hasten excretion.
Carbon monoxide	Oxygen	Provide pure oxygen at normal or high pressure, artificial respiration, blood transfusion.
Cholinergic agents	Atropine sulfate	0.02–0.04 mg/kg PRN. NOTE.—Atropine should be used in horses with extreme care to avoid potentially fatal ileus. A very slow drip is suggested, with constant monitoring of gastrointestinal status. *Avoid atropine toxicosis.*
Cholinesterase inhibitors	Atropine sulfate	0.02 mg/kg, repeated as needed for atropinization. Treat cyanosis (if present) first. Blocks only muscarinic effects. See note, above. *Avoid atropine toxicosis.*
Cholinergic agents and cholinesterase inhibitors (organophosphorus insecticides)	Pralidoxime chloride (2-PAM)	5% solution; five 20–50 mg/kg IM, IV injections (maximum dose is 500 mg/min), repeat as needed. 2-PAM alleviates nicotinic effect and regenerates acetylcholinesterase. Morphine, succinylcholine, and phenothiazines are contraindicated.
Copper	D-Penicillamine (Cuprimine)	See arsenic
Coumarin-derivative anticoagulants	Vitamin K_1 (Aqua-Mephyton, 5-mg capsules, Merck & Co.) (Vitamin K_1, Escahr, 25-mg capsules)	Give 3–5 mg/kg/day with food. Treat for 7 days for warfarin-type, treat for 21 to 30 days for second-generation anticoagulant rodenticides. Oral therapy is more efficacious than IV.
	Whole blood or plasma	Blood transfusion, 25 ml/kg
Curare	Neostigmine methylsulfate	Solution: 1:5000 or 1:2000. Dose is 0.001 mg/kg SC. Follow with IV injection of atropine (0.04 mg/kg).
	Edrophonium chloride (Tensilon; Roche)	1% solution: give 0.05–1.0 mg/kg IV.
	Artificial respiration	
Cyanide	Methemoglobin (sodium nitrite is used to form methemoglobin)	1% solution of sodium nitrite, dosage is 16 mg/kg IV (1.6 ml/kg). Follow with:

TABLE 2. SPECIFIC SYSTEMIC ANTIDOTES AND DOSAGES *Continued*

Toxicant	Systemic Antidote	Dosage and Method for Treatment
	Sodium thiosulfate	20% solution at dosage of 30–40 mg/kg (0.15–0.2 ml/kg) IV. If treatment is repeated, use only sodium thiosulfate.
	NOTE.—Both of the above may be given simultaneously as follows: 0.5 ml/kg of combination consisting of 10 gm sodium nitrite, 15 gm sodium thiosulfate in distilled water q. s. 250 ml. Dosage may be repeated once. If further treatment is required, give only 20% solution of sodium thiosulfate at 0.2 ml/kg.	
Digitalis glycosides, oleander	Potassium chloride	5–20 gm PO in divided doses, or in serious cases as diluted solution given IV by slow drip (ECG monitoring is essential).
	Diphenylhydantoin	25 mg/min IV until control is established.
	Propranolol (beta-blocker)	0.5–1.0 mg/kg IV or IM as needed to control cardiac arrhythmias (ECG monitoring is essential).
	Atropine sulfate	0.02–0.04 mg/kg as needed for cholinergic control. See note above. *Avoid atropine toxicosis.*
Fluoride	Calcium borogluconate	3–10 ml of 5%–10% solution.
Fluoracetate (Compound 1080; Sigma)	Glyceryl monoacetin	0.1–0.5 mg/kg IM hourly for several hours (total, 2–4 mg/kg), or diluted (0.5%–1.0% IV) (danger of hemolysis). Monoacetin is available only from chemical supply houses.
	Acetamide, pentobarbital	Experimental
	NOTE.—All treatments are generally unrewarding.	
Hallucinogens (LSD, phencyclidine [PCP])	Diazepam (Valium; Roche)	PRN. Avoid respiratory depression (2–5 mg/kg).
Heparin	Protamine sulfate	1% solution; give 1.0–1.5 mg by slow IV injection to antagonize each 1 mg of heparin. Reduce dose as time increases between heparin injection and start of treatment (after 30 min, give only 0.5 mg).
Iron salts	Deferoxamine (Desferal; Ciba)	Dose for animals not yet established. Dose for humans is 5 gm of 5% solution PO, then 20 mg/kg IM every 4–6 hours. In case of shock, dose is 40 mg/kg by IV drip over 4-hour period; may be repeated in 6 hours, then 15 mg/kg by drip every 8 hours.
Lead	Calcium disodium edetate, BAL, thiamide	See chapter on heavy metals.
Metaldehyde	Diazepam (Valium; Roche)	2–5 mg/kg IV to control tremors.
	Triflupromazine	0.2–2.0 mg/kg IV.
	Pentobarbital	To effect.
Methanol and ethylene glycol	Ethanol	Give IV, 1.1 gm/kg (4.4 ml/kg of 25% solution). Give 0.5 gm/kg (2.0 ml/kg) q. 4 h. for 4 days. To prevent or correct acidosis, use sodium bicarbonate, 0.4 gm/kg IV. Activated charcoal: 5 gm/kg PO if given within 4 hours of ingestion may help (although ability of activated charcoal to bind ethylene glycol is questionable).

Table continued on following page

TABLE 2. SPECIFIC SYSTEMIC ANTIDOTES AND DOSAGES *Continued*

Toxicant	Systemic Antidote	Dosage and Method for Treatment
Methemoglobinemia-producing agents (nitrites, chlorates)	Methylene blue	1% solution (maximum concentration), give by *slow* IV injection, 8.8 mg/kg (0.9 ml/kg); repeat if necessary. To prevent fall in blood pressure in case of nitrate poisoning, use a sympathomimetic drug (ephedrine or epinephrine).
Morphine and related compounds	Naloxone chloride (Narcan; Dupont)	0.1 mg/kg IV. Do not repeat if respiration is not satisfactory.
	Levallorphan tartrate (Lorfan; Roche)	Give IV, 0.1–0.5 ml of solution containing 1 mg/ml.
	NOTE.—Use either of the above antidotes only in acute poisoning. Artificial respiration may be indicated. Activated charcoal is also indicated.	
Oxalates	Calcium	23% solution of calcium gluconate IV. Give 3–20 ml (to control hypocalcemia).
Phenothiazine	Methylamphetamine (Desoxyn; Abbott)	0.1–0.2 mg/kg IV; also transfusion. Only available in tablet form.
	Diphenhydramine HCl	For CNS depression, 2–5 mg/kg IV for extrapyramidal signs.
Phytotoxic lectins (ricin, abrin, robin, crotin) and botulinum neurotoxin	Antitoxins often not available	Specific antitoxins such as botulinum antitoxin.
Red squill	As for digitalis and oleander	
Snake bite (rattlesnake, copperhead, water moccasin)	Antivenin (Wyeth) Trivalent Crotalidae (Fort Dodge)	Caution: equine origin. Administer 1–2 vials IV slowly, diluted in 250–500 ml saline or lactated Ringer's only if absolutely necessary to treat systemic effects; otherwise, avoid in horses. Also administer antihistamines. *Corticosteroids are contraindicated.*
Coral snake	(Wyeth antivenin, as above)	*Caution:* equine origin, use only if necessary. May be used as with pit viper antivenin.
Spider bite (black widow)	Antivenin (Merck & Co.)	*Caution:* equine origin. Administer IV undiluted.
	Dantrolene sodium (Dantrium; Norwich-Eaton)	1 mg/kg IV, followed by 1 mg/kg PO q. 4 h.
Spider bite (brown recluse)	Dapsone	1 mg/kg b.i.d. for 10 days. Also local treatment of site.
Strontium	Calcium salts	Usual dose of calcium borogluconate.
	Ammonium chloride	0.2–0.5 gm PO 3 to 4 times daily.
Strychnine and brucine	Pentobarbital	Give IV to effect. Higher dose is usually required than that required for anesthesia. Place animal in warm, quiet stall.
	Amobarbital	Give by slow IV injection to effect. Duration of sedation usually 4–6 hours.
	Methocarbamol (Robaxin; Robins)	10% solution; average first dose is 149 mg/kg IV (range: 40–300 mg). Repeat half dose as needed.
	Glyceryl guaiacolate (Guaiafenesin; Summit Hill Labs)	110 mg/kg IV as 5% solution. Repeat as necessary.
	Diazepam (Valium; Roche)	2–5 mg/kg to control convulsions. Evacuate stomach, then use other agents.

Systemic antidotes possessing specific actions are classified by the following mechanisms:

1. Complexing with a poison, rendering it inert (e.g., dimercaprol for arsenic poisoning)
2. Accelerating the metabolic conversion of a toxic product to a nontoxic product (e.g., thiosulfate for cyanide poisoning)
3. Blocking the metabolic formation of a poison from a nontoxic precursor
4. Specifically accelerating the excretion of a poison (e.g., chloride for bromide poisoning)
5. Competing with a poison for essential receptors (e.g., vitamin K_1 for coumarin derivative poisoning)
6. Blocking receptors responsible for toxic effects (e.g., atropine sulfate for cholinesterase inhibition)
7. Restoring normal function by repairing or bypassing the effects of a poison (e.g., methylene blue for methemoglobinemia)

Toxicity of Pharmacological Agents

Gordon W. Brumbaugh, COLLEGE STATION, TEXAS

Paracelsus (1493–1541) said, "All substances are poisons: there is none which is not a poison. The right dose differentiates a poison and a remedy." Paracelsus recognized the dose–response or dose–effect relationship of a drug in animals. Because no drug is totally safe, the clinical concern is of risk associated with use of the drug. The drug's benefits clearly influence the acceptability of its risks. It is therefore important to avoid an alarmist attitude regarding the toxicity of drugs. The risks of treatment may be acceptable for critically ill patients but not acceptable for patients in less desperate condition. Ill-informed criticism of drugs could restrict the use of potentially beneficial medication. Abstinence from the use of drugs avoids their toxic effects but is not in keeping with ethical treatment. Ignorance about drugs—using them when not needed, or in inappropriate dosages—can result in toxic effects.

Many adverse drug effects mimic signs of disease. Some understanding of the principles of toxicology is necessary for the recognition and management of a drug-induced toxicosis. Although specific situations surrounding each incident differ, there is usually evidence of exposure to a drug that can lead the veterinarian to suspect toxicity of that drug as a cause of the patient's signs.

Toxic effects of drugs, insofar as is possible, must be reversible, or the drugs would be prohibitively toxic. If the drug injures a tissue, the capacity of that tissue to recover largely determines the reversibility of the toxicity.

Unabridged, conclusive, accurate estimates of the incidence of toxic drug effects in animals, the nature and severity of those effects, and pertinent associated factors would be helpful but are not available. Drugs undergo rigorous testing before they are marketed; the incidence of adverse reactions, however, may be so low that thousands of patients must receive the drug before these data are available. It is therefore necessary that veterinarians be informed about the drugs they use, be able to recognize drug-induced complications, know how to evaluate the patient for evidence of drug-induced toxicity, report adverse effects of drugs to the respective manufacturer, and be prepared to provide medical support and antidotal treatment for a patient if toxicosis occurs.

GENERAL PRINCIPLES IN THERAPY OF DRUG-INDUCED TOXICOSES

There is no specific antidotal treatment for many drug-induced toxicoses. Supportive therapy is the most important aspect of treatment. The adage, "Treat the patient, not the poison," is the most basic and important principle. Supportive treatment should be directed toward maintaining function of vital organs, circulation, respiration, and fluid and electrolyte balance because the most efficient mechanisms for eliminating most drugs are the patient's own. Given enough time, those mechanisms will remove the offending drug, and if the drug is eliminated in timely fashion, healing will occur. Treatment must be adequately implemented so that vital organs and bodily systems are maintained before a specific antidote is administered. General principles for treatment of drug-induced toxicosis are the same as for treatment of other toxicoses and are summarized below.

IDENTIFY THE OFFENDING DRUG

If the history does not make the identity of the drug apparent, analysis of plasma, urine, and occasionally gastric contents or samples of tissues may be necessary to identify and quantify the drug before a definitive diagnosis of drug-induced toxicosis can be made. Appropriate analyses are frequently available at veterinary diagnostic laboratories, toxicologic laboratories, or clinical pharmacologic laboratories. Personnel at those facilities should be contacted regarding proper collection and submission of samples. Generally, samples should be obtained when toxicity is initially suspected.

PREVENT FURTHER EXPOSURE TO THE DRUG

Administration of the suspected drug should be discontinued immediately. Therapeutic monitoring of some drugs allows subsequent adjustments of the dosage regimen and reinstitution of the medication. If the drug was administered topically, the animal should be bathed; if it was administered orally, gastric lavage or orally administered adsorbents, such as activated charcoal (0.5 kg per 450 kg), may be helpful (see p. 340).

REDUCE CONCENTRATIONS OF THE OFFENDING DRUG IN CRUCIAL TISSUES

The concentration of an offending drug can be reduced by dilution; by interaction with other chemicals, which displaces it from the tissue formation of complexes; by chemical inactivation; or by enhanced biotransformation and elimination from critical tissues. When available, antidotes can also help.

USE SPECIFIC ANTIDOTES WHEN AVAILABLE AND INDICATED

Because antidotes are also drugs, their use must be justified. It is best, therefore, to reserve them for instances when toxicity to specific drugs has been confirmed. Otherwise they may compromise the patient further.

ENHANCE ELIMINATION OF THE DRUG

If possible, elimination of the offending drug should be accelerated. Biotransformation of the drug may be necessary before it is eliminated. Occasionally, biotransformation of a drug creates a metabolite that is responsible for the toxic reaction. In these instances, suppression of biotransformation helps to reduce toxicity. Laxatives, adsorbents, and maintenance of normal routes of elimination are usually sufficient for most drug-induced toxicoses in horses. Ion trapping, by alteration of urinary pH to keep excreted drugs in the ionized form and prevent reabsorption, can be used to enhance renal elimination of some drugs.

SPECIFIC AGENTS

ANTICOAGULANTS

The mechanism of the pharmacologic and toxicologic activity of coumarin congeners (e.g., warfarin) is similar; effects among the various drugs differ only quantitatively. These agents act only in vivo by interfering with hepatic synthesis of biologically active vitamin K–dependent clotting factors II, VII, IX, and X. The onset of clinical effects is delayed several hours because overt signs develop as a result of imbalanced rates of synthesis of biologically inactive coagulative factors and degradation of biologically active factors formed before introduction of the drug. Large initial doses of the drug can hasten the onset of hypoprothrombinemia only to a limited extent. The only significant difference in the ability of various coumarin congeners to produce and maintain hypoprothrombinemia is their respective half-life of elimination.

The fetus is quite susceptible to the effects of warfarin, because the drug crosses the placenta freely and the fetus has little capacity to synthesize clotting factors. Factors that enhance the hypoprothrombinemic response to these drugs include dietary and enteric microbial synthetic deficiencies, hepatic diseases, and hypermetabolic states. Drugs that can enhance the hypoprothrombinemic effect of warfarin by altering its pharmacokinetics include phenylbutazone, metronidazole, and trimethoprim-sulfamethoxazole. These drugs selectively prolong the elimination of levo-warfarin—the more potent isomer. Phenylbutazone and oxyphenbutazone can reversibly impair aggregation of platelets, displace warfarin from albumin, and cause gastrointestinal (GI) ulceration. These effects enhance the clinical activity of coumarin congeners.

Acetylsalicylic acid irreversibly inhibits aggregation of platelets and displaces warfarin from albumin. Heparin's antierythrocytic activity and its combined effect with coumarin congeners on one-stage prothrombin time could lead to hemorrhagic crises. Antimicrobial drugs can reduce enteric bacterial synthesis of vitamin K, but hypoprothrombinemia usually does not occur unless the diet is simultaneously deficient in vitamin K. Anabolic steroids and D-thyroxine can also increase the toxicity of these anticoagulants.

Multiple factors increase the risk of hemorrhagic crisis caused by coumarin congeners. These factors should be understood by clients and veterinarians, the patient should be monitored for toxic effects of the drug, and corrective therapeutic modalities should be available when these drugs are used.

Administration of the drug should be immediatley discontinued when hemorrhagic complications are suspected. Patients with mild adverse effects may respond to this approach alone or may require less aggressive management than more severely affected patients. Concomitant administration of drugs that could exacerbate hemorrhage should also be discontinued. Vitamin K_1 (phytonadione, 0.3 to 0.75 mg per kg) should be administered intravenously (IV) every 4 hours until hemorrhage is controlled. Vitamin K_3 (menadione) is much less effective as an antidote for coumarin congeners and, if administered parenterally, is toxic to the renal tubules. If hemorrhage is not reduced significantly within a few hours, fresh whole blood or frozen plasma should be administered in addition to vitamin K_1 (see page 517).

ANTI-INFLAMMATORY DRUGS

Toxicity caused by nonsteroidal anti-inflammatory drugs (NSAIDs) is believed to be related to inhibition of synthesis of prostaglandins. Lesions include necrosis of the medullary crest and renal tubules, and edema and ulceration of the GI tract. All NSAIDs can potentially cause toxicity, although relative risks or incidence may differ among drugs in this category. Toxicity appears to be dose-related, and differences of potency among these drugs obviously affect toxic doses of each.

Most is known about the toxicity of phenylbutazone and its major active metabolite, oxyphenbutazone; these drugs may be viewed as representatives of this class of drugs as a whole, keeping in mind the relative differences of potency. Phenylbutazone in dosages of 8 to 10 mg per kg body weight per day, administered orally (PO) or parenterally for several days, can produce toxic effects. Phenylbutazone and oxyphenbutazone are highly bound to proteins in plasma, have pKa values about 4.5, and have similar contraindications, toxicities, and interactions. Important interactions include displacement of other NSAIDs, oral anticoagulants, sulfonamides, and other drugs from proteins in plasma. The net result is an increased risk of toxicity for each drug. Phenylbutazone reversibly decreases activation of platelets, which can contribute to bleeding associated with a phenylbutazone–warfarin interaction, as described above. Hypovolemia, dehydration, preexisting renal disease, or other nephrotoxic compounds increase the risk of nephrotoxic effects induced by phenylbutazone. All relevant data should be considered before other nephrotoxic drugs are administered concurrently with phenylbutazone. Because other NSAIDs can cause similar toxicoses, concurrent administration of multiple NSAIDs is unwarranted and usually contraindicated. They compete for the same site of action, displace each other from transport proteins, and enhance the risk of toxicosis.

No antidote is available for toxicosis caused by phenylbutazone or other NSAIDs. Supportive therapy includes alkalinization of the patient's urine to enhance renal elimination of the drug by administering sodium bicarbonate–containing mixtures IV or PO.

ANTIMICROBIAL DRUGS

Several antimicrobial drugs can cause toxicosis. Sulfonamides and their acetylated metabolites can cause renal tubular nephrosis by precipitating from solution and forming crystals in renal tubules. Pyrimidine sulfonamides, such as sulfamerazine, sulfamethazine, and sulfadiazine, and their acetylated metabolites are more soluble and less prone to cause toxicosis. Concentrations of sulfonamides and acetylated metabolites in the tubular fluid and the pH of the tubular fluid influence precipitation. Supportive treatment for sulfonamide toxicosis is directed toward reducing precipitation. Alkalinization of the tubular fluid by administration of sodium bicarbonate and volume-induced diuresis enhance elimination of dissolved sulfonamides and reduce their precipitation.

Amphotericin B is an amphoteric molecule that causes nephrotoxicosis as a direct result of its pharmacologic action. It combines with sterols in the plasma membrane of renal tubular epithelial cells, which disrupts the continuity of the cell's membrane. Cytosolic contents leak, causing the damaged cell to die. Hypokalemia and metabolic acidosis may develop. Toxicity is related to the total dose of amphotericin B and can occur even with appropriate therapeutic doses. Prevention or treatment of toxicosis includes use of an appropriate dosage regimen, discontinuing treatment if signs of toxicosis develop, ensuring adequate hydration, and correcting abnormalities in acid–base balance and electrolyte levels.

The degree of nephrotoxicity caused by aminoglycoside is related to the specific aminoglycoside (neomycin is most toxic, streptomycin least toxic) and is dose-related. The total amount of drug administered and the trough concentration of the drug during a dosing interval are more relevant to toxicity than is the peak concentration.

Aminoglycosides are excreted by glomerular filtration, bind to the brush border of tubular epithelium, and translocate into cytoplasm and lysosomes of the cell. With toxicosis, disruption of lysosomes and brush border precedes tubular necrosis. Increased concentrations of enzymes in urine from tubular epithelial lysosomes and brush border usually herald the onset of tubular necrosis. Tubular casts in urine and elevated serum concentrations of urea nitrogen and creatinine are indications of overt renal damage. The risk of nephrotoxicosis consequent on aminoglycoside administration can be greatly reduced by adjusting dosage regimens according to the results of therapeutic drug monitoring.

While therapeutic efficacy has been attributed to high peak concentrations, the risk of toxicity can be reduced by low trough concentrations. Trough concentrations for gentamicin should decline to ≤ 1 μg per ml of plasma and for amikacin should be ≤ 2.5 μg per ml of plasma. Without therapeutic drug monitoring, prediction of those concentrations is inaccurate. With therapeutic drug monitoring, the dosage regimen can be adjusted specifically for each patient to *avoid* nephrotoxicity. Extremes of age, acidemia, hypotension, and concurrent administration of other nephrotoxic compounds are some factors that contribute to aminoglycoside nephrotoxicity. Alkalinization of the urine may reduce the risks of and aid in treatment of nephrotoxicosis caused by aminoglycosides.

Miscellaneous antimicrobial drugs can produce adverse effects by allowing suprainfection to develop, or by altering GI microflora. Of particular concern in horses are the lincosamides. Macrolides are perhaps of slightly less risk but should be used with caution. Accidental ingestion of lincomycin (50 ppm) in feed has resulted in necrotic, pseudomembranous colitis and death in horses; horses that survived were prone to develop laminitis. The pathogenesis of pseudomembranous colitis has not been precisely elucidated but is believed to be associated with overgrowth of *Clostridium difficile*, which produces toxins that cause the lesions.

Other antimicrobial drugs that can induce lethal enterocolitis include ampicillin, clindamycin, erythromycin, vancomycin, gentamicin, and cephalosporins. Tetracyclines and potentiated sulfonamides have been associated with diarrhea and death believed to be caused by drug-induced microfloral changes. Some antimicrobial drugs cause altered architecture of small intestinal mucosa, which can lead to malabsorption. Although architectural changes may be reversible, malabsorption may complicate enteric disorders already present. Renal tubular necrosis and hepatic fatty degeneration can occur following use of the tetracyclines and appear to be related to dose, duration of therapy, and status of the patient. Tetracycline's nephrotoxicity is enhanced by endotoxemia and its hepatotoxicity is enhanced by pregnancy. Cardiovascular collapse, associated with IV administered tetracylines, can result from the tetracycline in the formulation or its carrier, usually propylene glycol. Cardiovascular effects can be reduced experimentally by administering calcium-containing products or antihistamines (H_1-receptor blockers) prior to administration of the tetracycline. Clinically, these cardiovascular effects can be minimized by diluting the tetracycline-containing product in a calcium-free, isotonic fluid solution and administering it slowly.

Cardiovascular Drugs

Quinidine and digoxin are the most commonly used cardiovascular drugs in horses and can produce lethal toxicoses. Quinidine produces antiarrhythmic effects by interfering with transsarcolemmal flux of sodium. The net physiological effects of quinidine are a composite of direct actions on the heart and vasculature and indirect actions caused by its vagolytic activity and subsequent increased sympathetic tone. These net effects depend on autonomic tone and the dose of quinidine. Quinidine depresses spontaneous automaticity of the sinus node, slows conduction throughout the heart, and prolongs refractoriness. It also reduces peripheral vascular resistance by causing α-adrenoceptor blockade.

Orally administered doses of 10 gm to 450-kg horses every 2 hours for a total of four doses produce concentrations of 0.7 to 1.5 μg per ml of plasma. Therapeutic concentrations of quinidine (0.5 to 3.0 μg per ml of plasma) prolong the QRS and QT intervals, usually increase sinus rate, and resolve atrial fibrillation or other arrhythmias for which quinidine is indicated. Toxic doses produce marked slowing of conduction and prolongation of the PR, QRS, and QT intervals; in addition, atrioventricular and intraventricular blockade, ventricular extrasystoles, and wide QRS ventricular tachyarrhythmias may occur. Frequent side effects include poor capillary perfusion, hypotension, depression, nervousness, soft feces, diarrhea, and anorexia. Laminitis is also a complication that can appear after a single dose or at any time during a course of therapy. If any of these signs develop, administration of the drug should be discontinued. Because prolongation of the QRS interval is a sign of either therapeutic efficacy or toxicity, administration of quinidine should be discontinued when the QRS interval is prolonged by 25 per cent.

Sodium bicarbonate (0.5 to 1.0 mEq per kg IV) can temporarily reverse signs of toxicity because increased alkalinity of plasma lowers the concentration of potassium and increases the fractional binding of quinidine to protein, thereby decreasing the amount of active drug in plasma. Other treatments should be supportive and include IV administration of polyionic fluids to minimize the potential effects of negative inotropy and hypotension. Therapeutic monitoring of concentrations of quinidine is available at many human hospitals, veterinary diagnostic laboratories, and veterinary clinical pharmacology laboratories at teaching hospitals.

Digoxin is the digitalis glycoside most commonly used in horses. Its therapeutic effects depend on prevailing autonomic tone, direct myocardial effects, and indirect reflex cardiovascular effects. Digitalis glycosides sensitize pressure receptors, decrease sympathetic tone, and augment parasympathetic tone. They directly inhibit the $Na^+/K^+/ATPase$-dependent pump in the sarcoplasmic reticulum of cardiac cells. These effects result in decreased heart rate, prolongation of atrioventricular conduction, supraventricular antiarrhythmic activity, peripheral vasodilation, and increased cardiac contractility and output with improved peripheral blood flow.

The positive inotropic effects of digitalis glycosides are dose-related, and relatively small increases in concentrations of these drugs in plasma can lead to signs of toxicity. Signs include depression, anorexia, marked sinus bradycardia, disturbances in atrioventricular conduction, supraventricular and ventricular arrhythmias, widened QRS intervals, bundle-branch block, and increased atrial and ventricular excitability. Cardiac contractility increases during early stages of toxicity and leads to increased consumption of oxygen. Additionally, increased peripheral vascular resistance develops because of centrally mediated increased sympathetic tone. The net result of the latter changes is predisposition to cardiac ischemia and reduced cardiac output. Hypokalemia, hypoproteinemia, renal failure, dehydration, and interactions with other drugs increase digitalis glycoside toxicity. For example, quinidine and verapamil reduce renal clearance of digoxin and increase the plasma digoxin concentration.

Therapeutic concentrations of digoxin range from 0.5 to 2.0 ng per ml of plasma, and dosage recommendations should be used as guidelines to maintain concentrations in that range. The horse should be closely monitored for clinical signs of response or toxicosis. Therapeutic monitoring should be used to *avoid* the toxic effects of digoxin. Acute toxicosis can be treated by discontinuing the drug, enacting supportive measures, providing oral supplementation with potassium salts, and, if necessary, administering antiarrhythmic drugs.

Theophylline is a methylxanthine used primarily as a bronchodilator. It has several actions in common with other methylxanthines, such as caffeine. These actions include diuresis, stimulation of the central nervous system, tachycardia, variable vascular effects, and relaxation of smooth muscles in several tissues. Three basic cellular actions of methylxanthines are (1) enhanced translocation of Ca^{++} from the terminal cisternae of sarcoplasmic reticulum, (2) inhibition of cyclic AMP–phosphodiesterase, and (3) antagonism or blockade of adenosine receptors. Signs of toxicity of the methylxanthines are mainly referable to the central nervous and circulatory systems. Manifestations of toxicity in horses include restlessness, excitement, tremulous muscles, tachycardia (sometimes with extrasystoles), and tachypnea. These signs can occur with circulating concentrations of theophylline that are therapeutic in people; therefore, suggested therapeutic concentrations for horses (8 to 15 μg per ml of plasma) are lower than those for people.

Because individual variation occurs regarding "susceptibility" to toxic effects of theophylline, close clinical monitoring of the horse and of drug concentrations in plasma are very important when theophylline is used. Interaction with other drugs can enhance the toxicity of theophylline; of particular note are drugs that are highly bound to protein, displacing theophylline; and erythromycin, which decreases elimination of theophylline, causing it to accumulate to toxic concentrations.

Treatment of theophylline toxicosis is supportive. Neurological signs may be controlled with diazepam (0.10 to 0.15 mg per kg IV). Guaifenesin (5 per cent in 5 per cent dextrose) containing a thiobarbiturate (thiamylal, 2 mg per ml) administered IV, 1 ml per kg to effect, may also be effective. Elimination of theophylline can be enhanced by orally administered activated charcoal (0.5 kg per 450 kg body weight). Because the drug is highly lipid soluble and is distributed widely in the body, adsorption of the drug in the intestine may serve as a "trap" to aid its elimination.

Supplemental Readings

Beech, J.: Drug therapy of respiratory disorders. Vet. Clin. North Am. (Equine Pract.), 3(1):59, 1987.
Brumbaugh, G. W.: Rational selection of antimicrobial drugs for treatment of infections of horses. Vet. Clin. North Am. (Equine Pract.), 3(1):191, 1987.
Davis, L. E.: Adverse drug reactions in the horse. Vet. Clin. North Am. (Equine Pract.), 3(1):153, 1987.
Muir, W. W., and McGuirk, S.: Cardiovascular drugs. Their pharmacology and use in horses. Vet. Clin. North Am. (Equine Pract.), 3(1):37, 1987.
Osweiler, G. D., Carson, T. L., Buck, W. B., and Van Gelder, G. A.: Antibacterials. In: Clinical and Diagnostic Veterinary Toxicology, 3rd ed. Dubuque, Kendall/Hunt Publishing Co., 1985, pp. 205–224.
Osweiler, G. D., Carson, T. L., Buck, W. B., and Van Gelder, G. A.: Metals and metalloids.: In: Clinical and Diagnostic Veterinary Toxicology, 3rd. ed. Dubuque, Kendall/Hunt Publishing Co., 1985, pp. 67–142.
Rall, T. W.: Central nervous system stimulants. The xanthines. In Gilman, A. G., Goodman, L. S., and Gilman, A. (eds.): The Pharmacologic Basis of Therapeutics, 6th ed. New York, Macmillan Publishing Co., 1980, pp. 592–607.
Schentag, J. J., Simons, G. W., Schultz, R. W., Vance, J. W., and Williams, J. S.: Complexation versus hemodialysis to reduce elevated aminoglycoside serum concentrations. Pharmacotherapy, 4:374, 1984.
Schmitz, D. G.: Toxic nephropathy in horses. Compend. Cont. Ed. Pract. Vet., 10(1):104, 1988.

Industrial Toxicants
E. Murl Bailey, Jr. COLLEGE STATION, TEXAS
Tam Garland, COLLEGE STATION, TEXAS

Poisoned horses continually confront veterinary practitioners with therapeutic and prophylactic problems. The widespread use (and misuse) of pesticides and industrial chemicals in the United States causes accidental toxicoses in animals. The likelihood of toxicosis in horses makes it imperative that veterinarians attempt to educate their clients about the inherent dangers of chemicals and pesticides. Proper handling and storage techniques and appropriate usage of these compounds will lessen the number of intoxications. This chapter briefly identifies some common industrial toxicants and describes the therapeutic and management procedures that should be instituted to treat the resulting diseases.

INORGANIC CHEMICALS

Most inorganic chemicals, if ingested in sufficient quantities, will induce gastrointestinal (GI) signs. Acute intoxication with these agents is characterized by colic, tenesmus, profuse diarrhea, shock, dehydration, coma, and death. Until a proper diagnosis is obtained, fluids, analgesics, and antispasmodics should be used to maintain the life of the affected horse. Initial maintenance of life is more important than the subsequent application of appropriate antidotal therapy. Inorganic chemicals must be differentiated from other causes of acute abdominal pain such as blister beetle toxicity, various plants, including castor bean *(Ricinus communis)* and sesbania *(Sesbania vesicaria* and *S. drummondii)*, acute salmonellosis, colitis, intestinal torsion, and anterior mesenteric artery thrombosis. Unusual instances of chemical spills, drainage through dump sites, or leeching from mining operation may cause hazardous levels of certain heavy metals to appear in water offered to horses. Aluminum, beryllium, boron, chromium, cobalt, copper, iodide, iron, manganese, molybdenum, and zinc are examples of such potential metal contaminants.

FLUORIDES

Fluorine (F_2) rarely occurs in nature except in the form of fluorides. Fluorides are ubiquitous, occurring in varying amounts in soil, water, the atmosphere, vegetation, and animal tissues. Inorganic fluorides are the most important causes of fluoride toxicosis in animals. Organic fluorides occur in nature and in some commercial products but have not been implicated as inducing problems in horses.

Fluoride concentrations greater than 3 ppm in water will cause mottling of developing teeth.

Water containing more than 4 ppm of fluoride is only marginally safe for horses, and water containing more than 8 ppm should be avoided. Phosphorus feed supplements should be defluorinated and should not contain more than 0.3 per cent (3000 ppm) fluoride. A total daily dietary concentration of 40 ppm (calculated as dry matter) consumed for a prolonged period is considered the maximum tolerable level for horses.

Fluoride intoxication may be acute or chronic. The acute syndrome follows accidental ingestion of high levels of fluorides; the clinical signs are described later in this chapter. The sources of such poisonings in livestock usually are sodium fluorosilicate used as an insecticide, and contaminated water, vegetation, and feeds. The clinical signs associated with the predator toxin sodium fluoroacetate (Compound 1080) have no relationship to the clinical signs of either acute or chronic fluoride intoxication.

In horses chronic fluorosis is more common than the acute form. The variable and extended interval between ingestion and clinical signs complicates the diagnosis. An insidious onset and the nonspecific lameness and general debilitation cause fluorosis to be confused with other chronic diseases. Horses with moderate to marked fluorosis appear unthrifty even when ample amounts of quality feed are available. The hair coat becomes rough and dry, and winter coats are shed slowly in the spring. Horses with severe fluorosis often are lame.

The earliest and most sensitive indicator of fluorosis in young horses is dental lesions. Ingested fluoride affects enamel and dentine formation so that affected teeth have a characteristic mottling, staining, hypoplasia, and hypocalcification, and are subject to excesssive abrasion. There may be evidence of soreness and sensitivity to heat and cold in the teeth, resulting in quidding of the feed. The central portion of affected cheek teeth may be lost, allowing food particles to be forced into the pulp cavity. Mandibular abscesses may subsequently form. Infected areas are often 4 to 6 cm in diameter and can include a fistulous tract that drains from the ventral aspect of the mandible.

Fluoride is stored in bone without demonstrable changes in its structure and function. However, if excess fluoride is ingested for a prolonged period, structural and functional bone changes appear at sites of greatest metabolic activity and in bones under the greatest stress from weight-bearing and locomotion. The first palpable lesions are usually bilateral hyperostotic lesions on the metatarsal and metacarpal bones, mandibles, and ribs. The first and second phalanges may have abnormal periosteal hyperostosis, particularly at tendon insertions. Often the third phalanx is enlarged, with a layer of very rough-textured bone. This increases pressure within the hoof, leading to a laminitis-like syndrome. Although lameness problems may improve following removal of the fluoride, affected bones may not improve. Since fluorosis does not primrarily affect the intra-articular structures, it must be differentiated from the bony change in equine osteoarthritis, which is initially intra-articular, with marginal lipping in advanced cases.

When fluorosis is suspected and clinical signs are absent, urinalysis can aid diagnosis. Fluoride concentrations in urine appear to vary with specific gravity and should be standardized. Typically, urine values have been corrected to a specific gravity of 1.040, although other bases have been used. Normal urine fluoride levels are less than 6 ppm. Concentrations greater than 15 to 20 ppm are considered to be diagnostically significant.

Bone samples can be obtained by biopsy or at necropsy for analysis of fluoride content and gross and microscopic evaluations. Normal bone fluoride concentrations are 400 to 1200 ppm. Levels above 3000 ppm are diagnostically significant. Hair, skin, hooves, and soft tissues have no characteristic changes, and only small (less than 2.5 ppm) amounts of fluoride are retained in soft tissues. Correlating clinical findings, biopsy results, and necropsy observations with the fluoride content of the water and forage often helps substantiate or disprove suspected toxicosis.

There are no therapeutic or prophylactic measures that will completely prevent the toxic effects of excess fluoride ingestion, but aluminum salts such as aluminum sulfate, aluminum chloride, calcium aluminate, and calcium carbonate partially reduce fluoride effects. Although these measures will not eliminate a fluoride problem, they often ameliorate its severity.

Mercury

Mercury poisoning is rare in horses but has occurred sporadically, usually as a result of feeding seed grains treated with organomercurial fungicides. Mercury was banned as a seed dressing in 1970, but other sources of mercury poisoning have included mercurial ointments, batteries, and pharmaceuticals. Mercury persists in the environment, and some forms tend to accumulate in the food chain. The source and frequency of exposure to mercury determine the morbidity, which is generally high, with a guarded prognosis among affected animals.

Organic mercury is more readily absorbed

than the metallic or inorganic forms. Digestive tract irritation and subsequent kidney and central nervous system (CNS) effects may be seen, depending on the form of mercury and its concentration in the feed or water. Inorganic and phenylmercury compounds generally cause hyperemic to hemorrhagic and necrotic gastroenteritis and colitis, along with pale, swollen kidneys. Histologically, there is epithelial necrosis of alimentary mucosa and renal tubules. The severity and course of the toxicosis is reflected in the clinical pathology changes indicating renal damage. Alkyl (organic) mercury toxicosis produces mainly neurological lesions. Microscopically, focal malacia of the cerebral cortex, demyelination, astrogliosis, microgliosis, loss of granular cells in the cerebellum, and fibrinoid degeneration of CNS arterioles are evident.

Demonstration of a source of mercury is important in the diagnosis since the availability of this toxicant is limited. The maximum tolerable level of organic or inorganic mercury in the diet of horses is considered to be 2 ppm. Inorganic mercury has the highest tissue residues in the kidney, while both brain and kidney accumulate high concentrations of alkyl mercury. These tissues may be used for analysis. In acute disease, the kidney cortex and liver would be expected to contain in excess of 10 ppm mercury on a wet weight basis. Brain tissue should be collected for chemical and microscopic analyses if alkyl mercury poisoning is suspected. Mercury poisoning has been confused with viral encephalitides, salmonellosis, inorganic or organic arsenic poisoning, and lead poisoning.

Treatment of either inorganic or organic mercury toxicosis in livestock is often unsuccessful. No therapeutic regimens have been established for horses, but extrapolation from cattle dosages is recommended. Administration of a saline cathartic (sodium sulfate) at a rate of 3 gm per kg PO following removal from the source should be helpful. Sodium thiosulfate has been advocated, since mercurials may be complexed with the sulfhydryl radical. The recommended dosage for adult cattle is 30 gm PO in a 10 per cent solution. Dimercaprol,° a 10 per cent oil suspension, is given intramuscularly at 2.5 to 5.0 mg per kg every 4 hours for 2 days, three times a day on the third day, and then twice daily for 10 days or until recovery. An alternative therapy suggested for mercury toxicosis has been D-penicillamine† given PO, 3 to 4 mg per kg every 6 hours for 10 days.

°British Anti Lewisite (BAL),
†Cuprimine, Merck & Co., West Point, PA.

ORGANIC COMPOUNDS

Polyhalogenated Biphenyls

Polyhalogenated biphenyls (PHBs; polybrominated biphenyls [PBBs] and polychlorinated biphenyls [PCBs]) are extremely stable industrial chemicals sold under the trade names of FireMaster and Arochlor. The resistance of PHBs to degradation or metabolic transformation increases with the level of halogenation. Like other halogenated hydrocarbons, PHBs are highly lipophilic and are selectively deposited in body fat.

The toxic syndromes associated with PHBs in horses have not been defined. Disease syndromes and lesions in horses would be similar to those in cattle. In cattle, PBBs have produced various disease syndromes encompassing anorexia, decreased milk production, increased frequency of urination and lacrimation, and some lameness. Subsequent clinical signs included hematomas progressing to abscesses, weight loss (even though the ration had been changed and appetites were normal), abnormal hoof growth, matting and loss of hair, and thickened, wrinkled skin on the neck, shoulder, and thorax. Prolonged gestation, lack of udder development, dystocia (with large calves delivered dead or that died soon after birth), and postparturient metritis were common. Pathological lesions were consistent with the various disease syndromes.

There is no specific treatment available for PHB toxicosis. Sources of PBB should be eliminated, and animals exhibiting clinical signs of illness should be treated symptomatically.

Phenolics

Phenolic chemicals are very useful antimicrobials that are stable in the environment, soluble, and can mix with numerous other organic chemicals. Pure phenol is an excellent disinfectant but proved too toxic for routine environmental and animal applications. Phenol derivatives have less toxicity while retaining the germicidal properties. Chlorine and other radicals have been added to the benzene ring of phenol to develop a myriad of useful commercial materials such as disinfectants, fungicides, and components of multimixture materials that are likely to be disposed of and made available inadvertently to grazing animals.

Exposure to phenolic chemicals occurs by accidental application or direct exposure through the carelessness of an uninformed owner. Dietary contamination can occur through sprays applied in feeding areas or through mistaken chemical identity.

Phenolics are rapidly absorbed from the intact skin or from the digestive tract, and these tissues may show evidence of the corrosiveness of phenol. Early signs include incoordination, mild muscular fasciculation, depression leading to coma, and deepening coma with terminal respiratory failure. Increased red blood cell fragility and intravascular hemolysis may occur. Icterus is progressive until death. In mild cases clinical signs may occur and regress within 24 hours; more severe poisoning may result in death within 24 to 36 hours.

At necropsy, lesions consistent with the protein-coagulating properties of phenolic chemicals are seen. Congestion of internal organs and generalized icterus are apparent. The skin or digestive tract contents may have a characteristic phenol odor. Coagulation necrosis of epithelial cells, moderate hepatocyte degeneration, and nonspecific nephrotoxic changes are noted microscopically.

A history and evidence of contact with phenolic-containing materials are invaluable for the diagnosis of phenolic poisoning since clinical signs are not sufficiently specific. The presence of one or more animals with clinical signs should suggest the possibility of phenol toxicity. Urine from suspect animals may be used in a rapid test.

A specific treatment for phenolic intoxication is not available; however, further exposure should be prevented and supportive therapy initiated. Washing the exposed skin with soap and water and applying sodium bicarbonate bandages will reduce the topical effect, while administration of activated charcoal is effective in binding unabsorbed phenolic chemicals in the digestive tract. Glucose may have some benefit in reducing liver damage and maintaining renal function. Recovery from phenolic poisoning is still largely determined by the total dose absorbed and the animal's ability to detoxify and excrete the offending chemical.

Coal Tars

Coal tar poisoning, most often occurring in swine, is an acute, highly fatal disease. Death from this toxicosis may occur several decades after the last known pasture contamination with clay pigeons, since the toxic compounds are environmentally stable. Phenol, cresols, and a variety of aromatic hydrocarbons (naphthalene, naphthalene derivatives, anthracene, and anthracene oils) are the toxic agents found in plumbers' pitch and tarpaper materials. Young animals are most susceptible to poisoning.

The most common syndrome has a rapid clinical course culminating in sudden death, with no diagnostic signs. This is due to progressive destruction of the liver by the coal tar–pitch compounds. Thoracic and abdominal fluid increases, and sudden death is often associated with exertion. Occasionally a more chronic illness is observed, accompanied by anorexia, depression, weakness, a rough hair coat, anemia, and icterus. The characteristic lesion is a markedly swollen liver with a mottled appearance. Changes usually involve the entire liver, but in animals that survive for several days or in those with subclinical effects, the lesions may be confined to local or peripheral areas of the liver. There is no therapeutic regimen for coal tar intoxications other than symptomatic treatment with liver-sparing amino acids.

Herbicides and Fungicides

Treatment of most poisonings caused by herbicides and fungicides is symptomatic and supportive because of the lack of specific antidotes. Activated charcoal (1 to 3 gm per kg) and a saline cathartic (1 to 2 gm per kg) mixture should be given following oral exposure.

Animals intoxicated with sodium chlorate, which forms methemoglobin, should be given a 1 per cent intravenous solution of methylene blue at a rate of 8.8 mg per kg. This must be given slowly and the animal must be closely observed, because an overdose of methylene blue also causes methemoglobin formation.

Because sodium chlorate is not rapidly biotransformed, a poisoned animal may have to be treated for several days to ensure proper recovery. Other supportive measures should be instituted.

Hexachlorobenzine (HCB). This fungicidal agent for treatment of seeds occurs as a byproduct of a number of industrial processes and a variety of agricultural chemicals. Thus, HCB environmental contamination is extensive. HCB is a stable, persistent chlorinated hydrocarbon that is highly lipophilic and is selectively deposited in the body fat. The liver is the only tissue in which the metabolites, including pentachlorophenol and pentachlorothiophenol, tend to accumulate.

Signs of HCB intoxication during and after prolonged exposure are tremors, ataxia, weakness, paralysis, porphyria, possible photosensitization, and weight loss. Reported pathological changes are blood cell disorders, neurological abnormalities, and hepatomegaly. No specific treatment is available. Animals with clinical signs of HCB intoxication should be treated symptomatically.

Biomagnification of HCB occurs in animals so that tissue concentrations may reach 6 to 50 times the dietary level during long-term exposure. Therefore, concentrations in finished feeds should not exceed 0.02 to 0.05 ppm (depending on the duration of exposure). The Environmental Protection Agency has set an interim tolerance for HCB in cattle, sheep, goats, and horses of 0.5 ppm.

Pentachlorophenol Poisoning. Lumber that has been treated with wood preservatives, such as pentachlorophenol (PCP), creosote, and related phenolic compounds, is often used in the construction of animal facilities. Exposure occurs through skin contact with treated lumber, erroneous topical application of chlorinated compounds, licking or chewing on treated portions of stabling, or consumption of contaminated feeds. In unusual circumstances, respiratory exposure may occur if animals are housed in poorly ventilated barns that have been heavily treated with PCP. Pentachlorophenol uncouples oxidative phosphorylation and will induce the development of unusually high body temperatures. Clinical signs associated with PCP intoxication include hyperpnea and dyspnea, weakness, intense sweating, and tachycardia, leading to coma and death. Treatment for PCP intoxication is nonspecific but should include fluid therapy, cold water enemas, and generalized treatment for overheating. Once severe clinical signs develop, the prognosis is poor.

Tetrachlorodibenzodioxin (TCDD). Dioxins, highly toxic to rodents and birds, are less toxic to horses and humans. Dioxins are an example of how a chemical can unexpectedly occur in a horse's environment.

Many horses, birds, rodents, cats, and dogs died after being exposed to a horse arena in eastern Missouri. The clinical signs in horses included polydipsia, anorexia, severe weight loss, colic, alopecia, skin and oral ulcers, dependent edema, conjunctivitis, joint stiffness, and laminitis. Of 85 horses ridden in the arena, 58 became ill and 43 died.

The problem started 4 days after the arena had been sprayed with waste oil for dust control. It was subsequently discovered that the waste oil was a distillate residue from chlorophenol manufacture. This byproduct contained, among other substances, 300 to 356 ppm of 2,4,7,8-tetrachlorodibenzo-p-dioxin (TCDD), one of the most toxic synthetic substances known.

There is no known treatment for TCDD intoxication.

PETROLEUM PRODUCTS

Horses generally avoid feed, forage, or water containing petroleum products, and petroleum product intoxication in horses is rare. Most ingestions are minimally toxic. However, horses exhibiting pica or those confined to areas containing petroleum products may ingest these materials. Various petroleum or petroleum-based products may be used by owners to control insects, or as home remedies to treat skin conditions. Petroleum products include kerosene, gasoline, and other fuel oils, waste crankcase oil, and crude oil, or partially refined petroleum materials. Petroleum distillates may be used as vehicles for pesticides. Waste oily materials are used to reduce dust in arenas. Used petroleum materials may contain contaminants such as lead, PCP, or TCDD.

The clinical signs of petroleum product toxicosis depend on the product, its contaminants, and the route of exposure. Ingested petroleum products may produce salivation, blistering of the muzzle and mouth, colic, diarrhea, and 1 to 3 days of reduced appetite. Petroleum products applied to the skin produce local irritation with some hair loss. The horse may rub the involved areas, producing additional inflammation and possibly bleeding. Inhalation of toxic products, which may occur when stables are sprayed with petroleum products, may result in mild respiratory tract irritation. Coughing, increased respiratory rate, and pulmonary congestion may develop following heavy exposure.

The treatment for petroleum product toxicity varies with the type and extent of exposure. Conservative and supportive therapy is often sufficient, while in conditions such as aspiration pneumonia from petroleum product droplet inhalation, vigorous antibiotic and supportive therapy is indicated but often ineffectual. The horse should be removed from contact with the petroleum product as soon as possible. Osmotic cathartics should be used to empty the digestive tract, and soap and water should be used on the skin to remove topically applied petroleum products. In the case of severe GI irritation, parenteral fluid therapy or nasogastric tube feeding may be necessary. Soothing ointments may be used topically to protect irritated skin, and antibiotics may be employed to reduce the potential for systemic infections.

Supplemental Readings

Fowler, M. E., and Van Gelder, G. A.: Toxicology: *In* Mansmann, R. A., and McAllister, E. S. (eds.): Equine Medicine and Surgery, 3rd ed. Santa Barbara, American Veterinary Publishing, 1982, pp. 187–218.

National Research Council: Mineral Tolerance of Domestic Animals. Washington, DC, National Research Council–National Academy of Sciences, 1980.

Osweiler, G. D., Carson, T. L., Buck, W. B., and Van Gelder, G. A.: Clinical and Diagnostic Veterinary Toxicology, 3rd ed. Dubuque, Kendall/Hunt Publishing Co., 1985.

Heavy Metal Toxicosis

Larry J. Thompson, ITHACA, NEW YORK

Potentially toxic heavy metals (metals with a high specific gravity) discussed in this chapter are lead, zinc, and cadmium. Of these, lead is of greatest concern in veterinary medicine and will be emphasized, with zinc and cadmium covered in less detail. Other elements potentially toxic to horses, including arsenic, selenium, and mercury, were discussed in earlier editions of this text (see *Current Therapy in Equine Medicine 2*, pp. 668 and 670).

LEAD

Lead has been mined and used by man for centuries and is one of the most common causes of poisoning in veterinary medicine. Although lead toxicosis is still fairly frequently reported in cattle and dogs, lead toxicosis in the horse is relatively rare.

SOURCES OF EXPOSURE AND TOXICITY

The main route of entry of lead into the body is the digestive tract. Although only 1 to 2 per cent of ingested lead is absorbed into the body, it is excreted very slowly. Therefore, chronic exposure to small amounts may result in accumulation and subsequent toxicosis. Horses have more selective eating habits than cattle, so sources of lead that commonly cause toxicosis in cattle, such as lead-based paints, used motor oil from leaded gasoline–burning engines, lead storage batteries, and certain greases and caulking compounds, are not common sources of lead for horses. Most lead toxicoses in horses occur from ingestion of pasture or forage material that has been contaminated with lead from industrial mining, smelting, or lead reclamation operations.

Horses seem to be more sensitive than cattle to chronic low-level lead exposure. Clinical lead toxicosis has reportedly occurred in horses when cattle grazing the same pastures were unaffected. An overgrazing situation can increase the lead intake of the animal by direct ingestion of soil from short grasses or soil clinging to the roots of plants. Increased lead intake has occurred in horses pastured near heavily traveled highways. Exposure from forage near highways should diminish with the removal of lead from gasoline.

Lead in concentrations of less than 30 ppm on a dry matter basis is considered acceptable for forages (background = 3 to 7 ppm). Soil contamination with lead may increase the plant content to 15 to 30 ppm if there is no airborne contamination. Levels of 260 to 900 ppm and higher have been reported in forages grown near smelting operations (a source of airborne lead). Ingestion of forage with lead concentrations of greater than 80 ppm has been associated with chronic lead toxicosis in horses. Retrospective studies have shown that a lead intake of 1.7 to 2.4 mg per kg per day can cause chronic lead toxicosis in horses. Experimentally, single doses of 500 to 750 gm of lead acetate caused acute toxicosis in horses.

Most lead that is absorbed is transported in association with erythrocytes. Lead is initially distributed to all soft tissues of the body, with the highest concentrations found in the liver and the kidney cortex. The metal is eventually redistributed to bone and behaves similar to calcium in its deposition and mobilization. Small amounts of lead are excreted in the bile, milk, and urine. Unabsorbed lead is excreted in the feces.

Increased dietary zinc appears to help prevent the development of clinical lead toxicosis in horses. Additionally, lead deposition in bone appears to be decreased and retention in soft tissue increased by high dietary levels of zinc. Less than optimum amounts of dietary calcium and phosphorus have resulted in increased liver lead concentrations in growing horses.

CLINICAL SIGNS AND LESIONS

Inspiratory dyspnea caused by paralysis of the recurrent laryngeal nerve ("roaring") is the most commonly reported clinical sign in cases of chronic lead toxicosis. Exercise will often elicit a severe episode of dyspnea in horses that appear normal at rest. Choking and regurgitation of food or water through the nostrils may also occur and may lead to aspiration pneumonia. Depression and anorexia are common in affected horses. Other, less common clinical signs include weakness, incoordination, poor hair coat, lower lip paralysis, and stiff or swollen joints. Young animals are more susceptible to lead toxicosis than adults and seem to manifest bone or joint abnormalities more often. Diarrhea and colic can occur, and in cases with higher exposures complete paralysis or seizurelike activity may occur terminally.

Anemia in lead-poisoned horses may result from both increased fragility of erythrocytes and depressed cell production in the bone marrow. Basophilic stippling and other abnormalities of erythrocytes may also be seen. The action of ferrochelatase, an enzyme involved in heme synthesis, is inhibited by lead, causing an increase in zinc protoporphyrin in the blood. In man, the increase in zinc protoporphyrin is a sensitive indicator of lead toxicosis. Initial work with zinc protoporphyrin in the horse has indicated it may have diagnostic value in that species as well.

DIAGNOSIS

An accurate history, evaluation of likelihood of exposure, the presence of appropriate clinical signs, lack of specific pathological lesions, and chemical analysis are all important components in diagnosing lead toxicosis. Postmortem findings in lead-poisoned animals are nonspecific. The most dramatic finding may be lung lesions associated with aspiration pneumonia. Histologically, the renal tubular epithelial cells may show irregular acid-fast intranuclear inclusion bodies. Proper collection and submission of appropriate samples for lead analysis are critical for a diagnosis of lead toxicosis (see p. 339). A whole blood lead concentration of 0.30 ppm or greater, in the setting of compatible clinical signs, is consistent with lead toxicosis (background blood lead is below 0.10 ppm). A blood lead concentration in excess of 1.0 ppm warrants a poor prognosis. The anticoagulant of choice for blood lead analysis is edetate (EDTA), unless the diagnostic laboratory specifically recommends the use of heparin because of the analytical methodology employed. Lead concentrations in liver and kidney cortex in excess of 5 to 10 ppm on a wet weight basis also support a diagnosis of lead toxicosis.

THERAPY

The first step in the treatment of lead-poisoned animals is removal of the source of lead exposure. In mild cases, placing the animals in noncontaminated pastures or switching forage sources may allow recovery. Edetate calcium disodium (CaEDTA, CaNa$_2$EDTA [Calcium Versenate]) is used to chelate and quickly remove the body's excess lead burden in more severely exposed animals. The proper dose for the horse is 75 mg per kg body weight per day of CaEDTA given by slow intravenous (IV) infusion, divided b.i.d. or t.i.d. A 6.6 per cent solution of CaEDTA dissolved in normal saline or 5 per cent dextrose, which has been commercially available in the past, is recommended. With the 6.6 per cent solution, the daily dosage is equal to 1 ml per 0.9 kg body weight. More dilute solutions of chelating agent can also be used (see below). Treatment is continued for 4 or 5 days, then stopped for 2 days. If additional treatments are needed, the sequence of 4 days of treatment and 2 days of rest should be repeated. Adequate fluid and electrolyte balances must be maintained during the treatment period to reduce the risk of renal injury that can occur from EDTA chelation. A urine sample taken 24 hours after the initiation of chelation therapy will show greatly elevated concentration (10 to 100 times prechelation concentrations) if an animal has an increased body lead burden.

If edetate calcium disodium is unavailable from commercial sources, the veterinary practitioner may want to formulate a stock solution for emergency use. One formula that has been suggested is to make a 10 per cent stock solution by dissolving 101.1 gm of edetate tetrasodium (Na$_4$EDTA) plus 30 gm of anhydrous calcium chloride (CaCl$_2$) in distilled water up to a total volume of 1000 ml. Both compounds can be obtained from chemical supply companies. From the 10 per cent stock solution a 2.22 per cent working solution of CaEDTA for treating lead toxicosis can be made by mixing 220 ml of 10 per cent stock solution with 780 ml of distilled water. With the 2.22 per cent working solution, the daily dosage is equal to approximately 3.5 ml per kg body weight and should be divided into two or three separate administrations. Edetate tetrasodium, which is used as an anticoagulant, should never be administered as treatment for lead toxicosis as it may cause hypocalcemia. Only edetate calcium disodium should be used.

Magnesium sulfate or sodium sulfate (500 to 1000 gm) can be given as a 10 per cent oral solution to provide cathartic action and to decrease the availability of lead remaining in the gut. Activated charcoal (250 to 500 gm) can also be given orally as a 20 per cent slurry. Thiamine hydrochloride has been shown to decrease tissue lead accumulation in cattle and laboratory rats. Thiamine also increases the efficacy of CaEDTA in removing excess lead from rats chronically fed lead acetate. In experimental lead poisoning, calves have been dosed with thiamine at 2 mg per kg per day and adult cattle at 250 to 2000 mg per day IM or SC. Although thiamine is recommended for therapeutic use in the horse (e.g., in bracken fern toxicosis) at a dosage of 0.5 to 5 mg per kg, its use in equine lead toxicosis has not been evaluated.

ZINC

Although zinc is an essential trace element and dietary zinc has a wide margin of safety, both clinical and experimental cases of zinc toxicosis in horses have been reported. Zinc interacts with several trace elements and has been shown to increase copper excretion in horses. Most clinical problems of excess zinc have occurred in situations of environmental contamination of pastures or forages, similar to that described for lead toxicosis. Environmental zinc contamination has been reported near lead and zinc mines, zinc smelting operations, brass foundries, and other industries such as galvanized iron manufacturing plants. Other sources of excess zinc have included zinc oxide top-dressing of pastures to correct a soil zinc deficiency, excess zinc in concentrates due to mixing errors, and excess zinc in the water supply. Zinc may be released into the water from galvanized surfaces subjected to electrolysis, such as occurs when galvanized and copper pipes are joined.

Clinical Signs and Lesions

The young animal is much more susceptible to zinc toxicosis than the adult, with most reported cases occurring in foals or yearlings. Initial clinical signs include enlargement of the epiphyseal regions of the long bones, often with no apparent pain. The animal will subsequently develop lameness with a stiff gait or reluctance to move. Severely affected foals will often stand with the head held low, have an arched back, and will resist curving the spine laterally when turned to the side. Decreased weight gain or ill thrift along with progressive anemia have also been reported.

Joint abnormalities have occurred, including sterile effusions of the hock and radiographic findings of osteochondrosis dissecans. Pain and swelling can occur in the fetlock, carpal joint, hock, elbow, or stifle. Postmortem findings in zinc toxicosis have included erosions and roughened joint surfaces in the facets of the cervical vertebrae or in the articular cartilage of any of the limb joints.

Diagnosis

Normal forage concentrations of zinc generally range from 25 to 70 ppm. Forage concentrations associated with clinical zinc toxicosis have ranged from 102 to 3500 ppm. Zinc toxicosis has been produced experimentally in 4- to 8-month-old foals with a zinc intake of 184 mg per kg per day. A marked decrease in the growth rate of foals was noted when dietary zinc concentrations exceeded 3600 ppm. Liver concentrations of zinc greater than 200 ppm are considered above normal, and in clinical cases of zinc toxicosis liver concentrations have usually been greater than 500 ppm. Liver zinc concentrations have exceeded 1300 ppm and kidney cortex concentrations have exceeded 295 ppm in cases of experimental zinc toxicosis in horses.

Serum or plasma zinc concentrations must be interpreted with caution. Normal serum zinc concentrations generally range from 0.6 to 1.7 ppm. Serum zinc in great excess of 1 ppm is indicative of excess zinc intake and, when combined with appropriate history and clinical signs, may be compatible with zinc toxicosis. However, supporting samples such as feed or pasture forages should also be analyzed. Possible contamination of samples submitted for zinc analysis should always be considered. Contamination with zinc stearate from the rubber parts of most disposable syringes and blood collection tubes has been documented. The amount of contamination will vary with the contact time of blood or serum with the rubber part and from tube to tube within a package or lot. Thus, the use of an unused tube to control for contamination is not possible. The use of all-plastic disposable syringes and plastic screw-top tubes will avoid this rubber-associated zinc contamination. Any reusable glass syringes or tubes should be rinsed in acid before use and the tube stopper covered with plastic wrap. The use of special trace element blood collection tubes is recommended[*][†] Hemolyzed samples should be interpreted with caution, because zinc concentrations may be inappropriately elevated in those specimens.

Therapy

The treatment of animals with zinc toxicosis entails removing the source of excess zinc and providing a clean, high-quality diet. Supportive medical care should be provided as needed. The judicious use of copper or calcium supplements has been of benefit in certain instances. The lesions of zinc toxicosis are very similar to those produced by copper deficiency in same-age animals, and increased copper in the diet will help protect against the effects of excess zinc.

CADMIUM

In addition to lead and zinc, a third heavy metal associated with environmental contamination is cadmium. Cadmium is not considered an essential trace element. It occurs in nature with lead and zinc. Thus, sources may include mining or smelting operations as well as sewage sludge and iron plating industries. Acute cadmium toxicosis is rare in domestic animals, although horses are reported to have suffered a probable

---

[*]Vacutainer, Trace Element Tube, No. 6526 Royal Blue, Beckton Dickinson & Co., Rutherford, NJ

[†]Venoject Trace Element Tube, T200 SM, Royal Blue, Terumo Medical Corp., Elkton, MD

cadmium toxicosis from a cadmium-containing paint. The cadmium content of commercial diets for domestic animals reportedly ranges from 0.18 ppm to 0.7 ppm. With an adequate diet, dietary cadmium above 5 ppm is the level at which gross adverse effects may occur. Some disruption in mineral balance, especially in marginal deficiencies, can occur at 1 ppm dietary cadmium.

Cadmium has an extremely long half-life in the animal body and thus will accumulate with age. The liver and kidney are preferential sites of deposition, and high concentrations of the metal may accumulate in the kidney cortex. The horse accumulates cadmium in the kidney cortex to a greater degree than other animals. For that reason, tissue cadmium levels must be interpreted with consideration for both cadmium exposure history and the age of the animal.

Background concentrations of cadmium in liver and whole kidney of horses raised in the midwestern United States have been reported as 3.5 ppm and 2.5 ppm, respectively. These concentrations were 10-fold greater than for other species reported in the survey. Higher background concentrations of cadmium were found when only kidney cortex was analyzed. Cortical concentrations ranged from 12 ppm to 186 ppm of cadmium, with an average of 61 ppm for horses averaging 14.5 years of age. Mild microscopic changes in the kidney cortex were associated with the higher concentrations of cadmium in the kidney cortex. In man, kidney cortex concentrations of cadmium above 200 ppm result in glomerular and tubular damage, but the critical level in the horse has not been confirmed. Nephrocalcinosis has been reported in horses chronically exposed to zinc and cadmium contamination from smelting operations. In that incident cadmium concentrations in the kidney cortex were 156 ppm and 115 ppm in two affected animals, with liver concentrations reported as 30 and 15 ppm. Additional studies reported average kidney cortex concentrations of 111 ppm cadmium in foals raised on contaminated pastures, but no renal damage was found. However, lesions compatible with zinc toxicosis were evident in the foals.

Cadmium interacts with several other dietary trace elements. Cadmium is a known antagonist to dietary zinc and copper and will exacerbate deficiencies of these elements. Additionally, increased dietary zinc will decrease cadmium absorption. Dietary cadmium is also antagonistic to iron, selenium, manganese, and cobalt. Increased dietary cadmium may increase the severity of clinical signs and decrease survival in chronic lead toxicosis. Blood or serum concentrations of cadmium are extremely low and currently are not useful indicators of cadmium exposure.

At present, no treatment protocol is known for cadmium toxicosis in domestic animals.

Supplemental Readings

Ammerman, C. B., Fick, K. R., Hansard, S. L., and Miller, S. M.: Toxicity of certain minerals to domestic animals: A review. Gainesville, FL, Florida Agricultural Experimental Station Research Bulletin, No. AL73-6, 1973.
Edwards, W. C.: Preparation of calcium disodium EDTA for treatment of lead poisoning. Stillwater, OK, Okla. Anim. Dis. Diagn. Lab. Newslett., Winter, 1989.
Holm, L. W., Wheat, J. D., Rhode, E. A., and Firch, G.: The treatment of chronic lead poisoning in horses with calcium disodium ethylenediaminetetraacetate. J. Am. Vet. Med. Assoc., *123*:383, 1953.
National Academy of Sciences: Mineral Tolerance of Domestic Animals. Washington, DC, National Academy Press, 1980.
Osweiler, G. D., Carson, T. L., Buck, W. B., and Van Gelder, G. A.: Clinical and Diagnostic Veterinary Toxicology, 3rd ed. Dubuque, Kendall/Hunt Publishing Co., 1985.
Puls, R.: Mineral Levels in Animal Health. Clearbrook, British Columbia, Sherpa International, 1988.

Feed-Associated Poisoning

Merl F. Raisbeck, LARAMIE, WYOMING

Poisoning in horses most frequently results from ingestion. Although there are a large number and wide variety of potential contaminants, certain toxicants are much more frequent causes of equine poisoning than others. This results from use in other domestic species (e.g., feed antibiotics), extreme potency in horses (e.g., ionophores), or both.

IONOPHORES

The carboxylic acid family of ionophores, such as monensin, lasalocid, salinomycin, and narasin, are added to the rations of poultry, swine, and cattle as coccidiostats and to improve feed utilization. Chemically, the class is characterized by the ability to form lipid-soluble complexes with cations such as sodium or potassium. This property facilitates cationic diffusion across biological membranes. Although the ionophores have a good margin of safety in their target species, they are extremely toxic in Equidae, apparently because of slower metabolism.

The toxicity of the ionophores results from their ability to destroy transmembrane cation concentration gradients. Since many cellular homeostatic mechanisms such as adenosine triphosphate (ATP) production depend on such gradients, this process results in cell death. In Equidae, principal targets are mitochondria of highly energetic tissues such as the myocardium, kidney, diaphragm, and musculature. Many authors tout the relative toxicity, and thus the potential safety, of some ionophores in horses. However, the relative hazard, or the likelihood that poisoning will occur under field conditions with products formulated for use in poultry or cattle, does not differ greatly with the different ionophores. Horses and other Equidae should not be exposed to products containing ionophore feed additives under any circumstances.

Occasional horses may be poisoned as the result of access to cattle supplements while on pasture. More commonly, however, poisoning results from improper incorporation of medicated premixes into horse rations or contamination of mixing equipment or trucks.

CLINICAL SIGNS

The clinical signs of acute ionophore intoxication in horses are progressive and vary somewhat with dose and with the individual animal. Signs usually include anorexia, abdominal pain, profuse intermittent sweating, and posterior ataxia characterized by a stiff gait and reluctance to move. Tachycardia and hypotension may occur within 8 to 12 hours after exposure, especially in peracute cases. Terminally, some horses may become hypertensive. Polyuria and tenesmus occur soon after intoxication. Later, poisoned animals may become oliguric. Hematuria is evident after 24 hours in some animals. Death may result from hypovolemic shock compounded by electrolyte losses within 24 to 48 hours of intoxication. Individuals that survive sublethal acute doses may succumb to complications of myocardial necrosis and scarring weeks or months later.

There is no practical method available to detect the ionophores in vital samples from acutely poisoned horses. For therapeutic purposes, the diagnosis must be based on clinical signs, clinicopathological findings, and feed analysis. As signs develop, water loss from renal tubular damage is reflected in increased packed cell volume (PCV) and serum protein levels, and increased urine output of low specific gravity. The blood urea nitrogen (BUN) and creatinine levels may also increase. Somewhat later, increased creatine phosphokinase (CPK) and lactic dehydrogenase (LDH) levels suggest skeletal and myocardial muscle necrosis. Serum calcium and potassium levels fall soon after the onset of clinical signs, and some individuals become hyperglycemic. Diagnostically useful lesions may be absent in horses that die acutely. Later, necrosis and degeneration of the myocardium, skeletal muscle, and renal cortex may be present.

THERAPY

There is no specific antidote for ionophore intoxication. Vitamin E and selenium provide some protection against monensin intoxication in swine, but the therapeutic significance in the horse is dubious. Calcium channel blockers, which have been suggested for treatment of ionophore toxicosis, actually potentiate monensin effects in rodents.

As with any oral intoxication, the first priority should be blocking absorption of any toxicant remaining in the gastrointestinal (GI) tract. Activated charcoal (0.5 kg per 450 kg) or mineral oil given per os (PO) prevent uptake of the compound from the gut. Saline cathartics may also be useful to speed elimination, but autonomic cathartics and cardiac glycosides should be avoided. Supportive therapy includes aggressive parenteral administration of fluids to correct hypovolemia and support cardiovascular and renal function. If clinical laboratory support is readily available, it is desirable to use supplemental potassium to correct hypokalemia. However, supplemental calcium is not indicated unless hypocalcemia becomes severe.

Therapeutic management of horses that survive acute intoxication is primarily supportive. Horses that have apparently recovered from acute monensin intoxication have died peracutely weeks or months later. In my experience, in each instance excercise or some other stressor appeared to induce arrhythmias, and the animal "dropped dead" in midstride. Thus, nursing care and stress reduction are indicated for several months in convalescing animals. Additionally, owners should be warned against riding such animals for several months after apparent recovery and not until the animals have been exercised hard with no signs of cardiac damage.

ANTIBIOTIC-ASSOCIATED COLITIS

The unique nature of the equine digestive system renders horses especially vulnerable to antibacterial agents. Fatal colitis in horses and ponies has resulted from feeding lincomycin, tylosin, tetracycline, and neomycin. Other antibacterial feed additives may also be capable of causing antibiotic-associated colitis, but this has not yet been documented. The pathogenesis of antibiotic-associated colitis is very poorly understood. While there is agreement that the primary insult is antibiotic-stimulated overgrowth of toxigenic bacteria, the identity of such bacteria is controversial. Actually, there is no reason to doubt that different genera may be involved in different cases. The variable nature of antibiotic-associated colitis is substantiated by the experimental observation that lincomycin, 5 mg per kg PO, killed four of four ponies in one experiment but had no observable effect on four additional ponies 3 months later. It is likely that antibiotic-associated colitis results from synergistic effects between diet, environment, and antibiotic.

The onset of antibiotic-associated colitis is usually delayed 24 to 48 hours after oral exposure to contaminated feedstuffs. Initial clinical signs include profuse, watery, nonhemorrhagic diarrhea, anorexia, and lethargy. As the condition progresses, animals usually develop colic, moderate to severe tachycardia, dark mucous membranes, and fever. Borborygmi may be decreased or absent. Severely affected animals become prostrate and die within 3 to 5 days. Clinicopathological findings are typical of shock and dehydration. An initial, transient neutropenia may be seen, but most horses will not be examined until the hemogram has progressed to severe leukocytosis and neutrophilia. The PCV and total protein content are markedly increased. The principal gross lesions are an edematous colon distended with serosanguinous fluid and a hemorrhagic adrenal medulla. There may be diffuse ecchymotic hemorrhages on many of the visceral organs, and blood may clot poorly.

Although antibiotic residues may occasionally be detected in GI contents, the suspected feedstuff is the optimum sample for analysis. Most horses that survive the acute onslaught will later develop laminitis.

Since the bacterial agents responsible for the condition have not been conclusively identified, there is no specific antidote. Oral exchange resins such as cholestyramine, which ameliorates antibiotic-associated colitis in hamsters by preventing adsorption of bacterial toxins, have not been evaluated in horses. Activated charcoal and mineral oil may be useful. Intravenous (IV) fluid therapy should be tailored to replace fluid and electrolyte losses. The fluids should be used aggressively from the onset of clinical signs. Parenteral administration of gentamicin and flunixin appears beneficial in resolving the acute crisis, as is phenylbutazone in ameliorating the subsequent laminitis. Rest and supportive care must be extended throughout convalescence to prevent a relapse.

BLISTER BEETLE (Cantharidin) INTOXICATION

Historically, blister beetle (*Epicauta* spp.) poisoning in horses fed alfalfa has been a serious problem in the southern Great Plains states. Recent changes in alfalfa hay production have resulted in cases occurring as far north as Illinois and Minnesota. The active toxin (cantharidin) is contained in the lymph of adult beetles, which feed on alfalfa in mid to late summer. If the insects are trapped and crushed by crimping-type mowers, the toxin is incorporated into the hay, which may remain toxic for years. Experimentally, as few as two to five beetles may produce colic in horses.

CLINICAL SIGNS

Clinical signs vary with the dose of toxin from mild depression and anorexia to severe shock and death. Initial signs include anorexia, colic, apathy, and behavior that suggests oral irritation. Later, straining to urinate and diaphragmatic flutter may be evident. Clinicopathological findings include decreased serum calcium and magnesium levels, hypoproteinemia, low urine specific gravity, hematuria, and azotemia. Chemical analysis of urine or ingesta is necessary to confirm a diagnosis of blister beetle intoxication. Because of the very small concentration usually present in urine, several hundred milliliters may be necessary for detection.

THERAPY

Treatment is symptomatic. Mineral oil and osmotic diuresis will speed elimination of the toxin. GI protectants such as aluminum hydroxide (60 mg per kg PO) or magnesium sulfate (500 mg per kg PO) should be given to minimize damage and the associated pain. IV fluid replacement therapy should be tailored to the individual case by frequent monitoring of the serum electrolyte levels. If this is not possible, supplemental calcium (e.g., calcium gluconate, 24 mg Ca^{++} per kg body weight) and magnesium (e.g., magnesium sulfate, 6 mg MG^{++} per kg body weight) may be useful. These should be diluted in the first day's replacement fluids and given slowly IV. In horses that survive more than 24 to 48 hours, CPK levels may be used as a prognostic indicator of myocardial damage.

Alfalfa growers should inspect their fields before cutting when there is a possibility of insect swarms. Affected areas either should not be cut for hay or should be treated with malathion before cutting. The appropriate withdrawal time for the malathion must be observed. Horse owners should be aware of the potential hazard associated with feeding alfalfa and only buy hay from known, reputable sources.

FESCUE

Tall fescue *(Festuca arundinacea)* is a popular forage in warm temperate climates such as the southeastern United States, because it is a good forage producer and because it persists almost indefinitely and tolerates very poor grazing management. However, mares on fescue pastures experience increased incidences of agalactia, retained and thickened placentas, prolonged gestation, and stillbirths. The original, 1980 study revealed agalactia in 15 per cent of mares grazed on fescue but in less than 2 per cent of mares grazed on other pastures.

Initially, selenium deficiency was suspected because early anecdotal reports indicated that toxic pastures were deficient in selenium and that supplemental selenium alleviated the problem. However, controlled experiments have discredited this hypothesis. Most current evidence implicates ergopeptide alkaloids produced by *Claviceps*-like, endophytic fungi. Apparently these alkaloids inhibit prolactin release. This situation is analogous to that in cattle that develop agalactia when pastured on fescue that is heavily parasitized by endophyte. Pastures produced from endophyte-free seed are free from the adverse effects of contaminated pastures. Unfortunately, endophyte-free fescue strains are not as hardy as other varieties of fescue.

At present, prevention is more rewarding than therapy. The simplest procedure is to avoid feeding fescue pasture or hay to mares during the last 30 to 60 days of gestation. An alternative to avoiding fescue for pregnant mares is to supplement with legume hay. Heavy fertilization exacerbates the effects of the endophyte in cattle. Although this factor has not been experimentally confirmed in horses, it seems reasonable to use only the bare minimum of fertilization required for forage production. If the use of fescue is unavoidable, the level of contamination should be evaluated. Several laboratory methods have been devised for measuring the level of endophyte contamination of fescue pastures. One factor common to all is the absolute necessity of obtaining a completely randomized collection of up to 100 subsamples.

Experimentally, the dopamine antagonist perphenazine (fed at 0.5 mg per kg per day) reverses the effects of ergot alkaloids on prolactin concentrations and milk production when given from day 295 of gestation. Slightly higher doses produce hyperesthesia, sweating, and colic, so extreme caution should be exercised when using this drug in mares that are due to foal but have no mammary development. Other, less toxic antagonists may be identified in the near future.

AFLATOXIN

The aflatoxins (B_1, B_2, G_1, and G_2) are a highly toxic group of mycotoxins produced in grains by *Aspergillus* spp. The high moisture content and warm environmental conditions required for aflatoxin production make aflatoxicosis mainly a problem of tropical and subtropical areas. Nonetheless, episodes in cattle and swine have occasionally occurred in the northern United States. Relatively little information has been published on the effects of aflatoxins in horses, but there is no question that horses and other Equidae are susceptible to aflatoxin and that natural aflatoxicosis occurs in these species.

CLINICAL SIGNS

Aflatoxin produces both an acute hepatotoxic syndrome and several chronic conditions, including carcinogenesis, immunosuppression, and ill thrift. There is no reason to doubt that the latter conditions occur in horses, but at present, only the acute, hepatotoxic syndrome is well documented. Anorexia is the earliest and most consistent sign of acute aflatoxicosis. In a few instances, horses have died within 24 to 48 hours of the onset of anorexia without showing further signs. More commonly they become febrile and lethargic and exhibit tachycardia, rapid respiration, and abdominal straining to produce bloody diarrhea. Icterus may or may not be evident. Prolonged clotting times, bleeding, and anemia may be seen in animals that survive the initial stages of acute intoxication. Central nervous signs, including ataxia and convulsions, have been reported in some cases.

The most dramatic clinicopathologic findings include elevated clotting times, γ-glutamyl-transpeptidase (GT), alanine transferase (ALT), and aspartate aminotransferase (AST), and decreased total protein and anemia. Grossly, the liver may be enlarged, hemorrhagic, and friable or fatty. Hemorrhagic enteritis, pale, swollen kidneys, and diffuse petechial and ecchymotic hemorrhages are also common findings. In experimental poisonings and one clinical report the brain was swollen, as evidenced by compressed sulci. None of these findings is pathognomonic, and definitive diagnosis hinges on identification of aflatoxin metabolites in urine or tissue. Because the toxin is present at very low concentrations in urine, several hundred milliliters should be submitted for analysis.

THERAPY

Treatment of aflatoxicosis is frustrating. By the time the herdsman realizes there is a problem, the prognosis is grave. The first priority should be identification of the source of the toxin and its removal from the diet. Glutathione precursors such as L-methionine (50 mg per kg PO) and sodium thiosulfate (20 per cent, 0.22 ml per kg IV, slowly) may be beneficial if used early and aggressively. Increased high-quality protein and supplemental fat-soluble vitamins should be given to compensate for decreased utilization. Although administration of vitamin E and selenium in excess of nutritional requirements has not been beneficial therapeutically, deficiencies in these substances will potentiate the effects of aflatoxin. If there is any question about the vitamin E and selenium status of the animal, parenteral supplementation is in order. Transfusion may be indicated to supplement endogenous clotting factors in animals with serious bleeding. Concurrent infectious diseases should be aggressively treated with the appropriate antibiotics as the animal is likely to be immunosuppressed.

BOTULISM

Botulism is a neuroparalytic disease caused by one of seven immunologically distinct toxins produced by *Clostridium botulinum*. Although there are marked differences in equine susceptibility to different immunotypes and subtle differences in clinical signs, all share a common mode of action and general clinical syndrome. Toxin is taken up by peripheral cholinergic neurons, binds irreversibly to a receptor in the presynaptic neuron, and blocks exocytotic release of acetylcholine. This irreversible binding implies that recovery of nerve function involves replacement of the nerve terminal.

In horses, botulism results from ingestion of preformed toxin or from toxin production by the organism in septic wounds or damaged areas in the gut. Growth and toxin production requirements vary considerably among strains of *C. botulinum*, but all are anaerobic, will not tolerate pH less than 4.5, and require a moist substrate for growth. Thus, thoroughly cured, dry hay is an unlikely source of toxin unless contaminated by other substances such as rodent carcasses. Most reports of equine botulism implicate silage or excessively moist hay. In at least one instance, horses and donkeys were poisoned by drinking from a pond contaminated with animal carcasses.

CLINICAL SIGNS

The hallmark of *C. Botulinum* intoxication is a rapidly progressive, flaccid neuromuscular paralysis. Signs occur within 1 to 14 days of exposure and include weakness and tremors of the limbs. These often start in the hindquarters and progress craniad to eventually include paralysis of the jaw and throat (as evidenced by inability to retract the tongue), dysphagia, and roaring. In some cases, initial signs may involve the large muscles of the front limb and palpebral muscles. Initially, affected animals are reluctant to rise and lie in sternal recumbency with the head resting on the ground. Later, as respiratory muscles become paralyzed the victim lies on its side with head and neck extended to facilitate abdominal breathing. If forced to get up and move about, animals exhibit incoordination, stumbling, knuckling, and ataxia. Sensation and consciousness are retained until death. There may also be signs referable to autonomic dysfunction as a consequence of disruption of parasympathetic effector sites and autonomic ganglia.

Diagnosis is based on toxin identification in serum, feed, liver, or feces. Traditional bioassays based on mouse inoculation may lack adequate sensitivity to detect toxin in serum. Nevertheless, no practical assay with better sensitivity is available at present. Samples should be frozen immediately and assayed as quickly as possible after collection as activity may decrease when samples are kept at ambient temperature. Clinicopathological findings are typical of stress and muscle necrosis.

THERAPY

Specific therapy consists of administering antitoxin. However, antitoxin will not neutralize toxin that has already been bound to neurons. Antitoxin (5000 units IM in divided doses) *is* indicated to neutralize circulating toxin if the horse is sufficiently valuable to justify the expense. Limited evidence in rodents and humans suggests that 4-aminopyridine or 3,4-diaminopyridine (0.3 to 1 mg per kg by IV drip) may be of use in overcoming skeletal paralysis in some instances.

Supportive care is very important in the treatment of equine botulism. Purgatives should be given to eliminate the potentially large reservoir of toxin in the alimentary tract. Horses that cannot swallow should be given food and water by stomach tube. Recumbent animals should be supported in slings if possible or else kept on thick bedding and rotated two to three times daily to minimize decubitus and muscle injury. Care should be taken to avoid positions that might further compromise respiration. Antibiotics such as the aminoglycosides, which may adversely affect nerve function, should be avoided. Exercise should be avoided even in animals that can move, as it may exhaust limited neuronal stores of acetylcholine and thus accelerate the onset of paralysis.

Because of the very poor prognosis of equine botulism, prevention is imperative. Feedstuffs should be kept dry and free from contamination by rodent carcasses. If feeding silage, make sure that the pH is less than 4.5. Dead animals should be disposed of by deep burial in a well-drained area. Botulinum toxoid may be used to protect unaffected animals in the rare situation where it is not possible to identify and remove the source of toxin from the environment.

DICOUMAROL AND ANTICOAGULANT RODENTICIDES

Dicoumarol is a fungal metabolite of coumarins found in spoiled sweet clover hay. Once produced, the toxin may persist in hay for years. Although poisoning is most commonly reported in cattle, horses are also susceptible. Horses have also been poisoned by accidental incorporation of anticoagulant rodenticide baits in feedstuffs.

CLINICAL SIGNS

Clinical examination of affected animals reveals pale mucous membranes, a weak, rapid pulse, and generalized weakness. Bleeding and bruising are common; however, the particular sites affected are more a function of the probability of local injury than the toxin itself. Hematomas are commonly noted in areas of the neck, trunk, or limbs where there has been pressure or bruising and in joints. There may be blood in feces and around other orifices. Epistaxis is frequently one of the first signs in horses. Hematomas in various body cavities may result in blindness, paresis, lameness, and dyspnea.

Citrated blood may be evaluated for prothrombin (PT) and activated partial thromboplastin times (APTT). The activated clotting time (ACT) assay, however, may be more useful for the clinician, because that test has the dual advantages of being inexpensive and simple to run in the field or veterinary clinic. Definitive diagnosis requires identification of dicoumarol in blood, liver, or feed, but a prolonged APTT, PT, or ACT in the setting of exposure to spoiled sweet clover is sufficient reason to initiate treatment. Lesions seen on postmortem examination include pale or bruised musculature and accumulations of blood in the thorax and peritoneum.

THERAPY

Vitamin K_1 is the specific antidote for dicoumarol poisoning and will usually return the PT to normal within 12 to 24 hours. Dosage regimens are the subject of some controversy. If a case involves simple dicoumarol (sweet clover) poisoning, 1 to 2 mg per kg of vitamin K_1 given in divided doses subcutaneously is usually sufficient. If the animal was poisoned by one of the newer anticoagulant rodenticides such as diphacinone or brodifacoum, treatment should be repeated as indicated by the ACT for 2 to 3 weeks.

Menadione (vitamin K_3) is of little benefit in anticoagulant poisoning and may cause acute renal failure in horses. It is therefore not recommended. Although IV vitamin K_1 preparations are available, IV administration has been associated with a high incidence of adverse reactions. Phenylbutazone, salicylates, aminoglycosides, and sulfonamides may potentiate the anticoagulant effects of the related anticoagulant, warfarin, and thus are contraindicated.

Severely anemic patients should be transfused with whole blood. If possible, blood from the donor and recipient should be cross-matched before transfusion (see *Current Therapy in Equine Medicine 2*, p. 317). Cross-matching is especially important if the recipient has received transfusions previously. Transfusions of whole blood or plasma will reverse bleeding, but the transfused clotting factors are soon exhausted and bleeding will resume. Additional fluids may be indicated for the severely hypovolemic patient. Thoracocentesis may be necessary if a case involves severe dyspnea due to hemothorax.

Supplemental Readings

Ionophores

Amend, J. F., Mallon, F. M., Wren, W. B., and Ramos, A. S.: Equine monensin toxicosis: Some experimental clinicopathologic observations. Compend. Cont. Ed. Pract. Vet., 2: S173–S183, 1980.

Amend, J. F., Nichelson, R. L., King, R. S., Mallon, F. M., and Freeland, L.: Equine monensin toxicosis: Useful ante-mortem and post-mortem clinicopathologic tests. *In:* Proceedings of the 31st Annual Convention of the American Association of Equine Practitioners, 1985, pp. 361–371.

Antibiotic-Associated Colitis

Kohn, C. W.: Colitis-X. *In* Robinson, N. E. (ed.): Current Therapy in Equine Medicine. Philadelphia, W. B. Saunders Co., 1983, pp. 200–207.

Prescott, J. F., Staempfli, H. R., Barker, K., Bettoni, R., and Delaney, K.: A method for reproducing fatal idiopathic colitis (colitis x) in ponies and isolation of a *Clostridium* as a possible agent. Equine Vet. J., 20:417–420, 1988.

Whitlock, R. H.: Colitis: Differential diagnosis and treatment. Equine Vet. J., *18*:278–283, 1986.

Blister Beetle (Cantharidin) Intoxication

Schmitz, D. G.: Cantharidin toxicosis in horses. J. Vet. Intern. Med., 3:208–215, 1989.
Schoeb, T. R., and Panciera, R. J.: Pathology of blister beetle *(Epicauta)* poisoning in horses. Vet. Pathol., *16*:18–31, 1979, pp. 125–134.

Fescue

Johnson, M. C., Siegel, M. R., and Bush, L. P.: The endophyte of tall fescue. *In* Lacey, J. (ed.): Trichothecenes and Other Mycotoxins. New York, John Wiley & Sons, 1985.
Loch, W., Worthy, K., and Ireland, F.: The effect of phenothiazine on plasma prolactin levels in non-pregnant mares. Equine Vet. J., *22*:30–32, 1990.
Schillo, K. K., Leshin L. S., Boling, J. A., and Gay, N.: Effects of endophyte infected fescue on concentrations of prolactin in blood sera and the anterior pituitary and concentrations of dopamine and dopamine metabolites in brains of steers. J. Anim. Sci., *66*:713–718, 1988.

Aflatoxin

Angsubhakorn, S., Poomvises, P., Romruen, K., and Newberne, P. M.: Aflatoxicosis in horses. J. Am. Vet. Med. Assoc., *178*:274–278, 1981.

Asquith, R. L.: Biological effects of aflatoxins: Horses. *In* Diener, U. L., Asquith, R. L., and Dickens, J. W. (eds.): Aflatoxin and *Aspergillus flavus* in Corn. Auburn, Ala., Alabama Agricultural Experiment Station, 1983.
Cysewski, S. J., Pier, A. C., Baetz, A., and Cheville, N. F.: Experimental equine aflatoxicosis. Toxicol. Appl. Pharmacol. 65:354–365, 1982.

Botulism

Sakaguchi, G., Ohishi, I., and Kozaki, S.: Botulism: Structure and chemistry of butulinum. In Hardegree, M. C., and Tu, A. T. (eds.): Bacterial Toxins. New York, Marcel Dekker, 1988, pp. 191–216.
Tacket, C. O., and Rogawski, M. A.: Botulism. *In* Simpson, L. L. (ed.): Botulinum Neurotoxin and Tetanus Toxin. San Diego, Academic Press, 1989, pp. 351–378.
Thesleff, S.: Pharmacologic antagonism of clostridial toxins. *In* Simpson, L. L. (ed.): Botulinum Neurotoxin and Tetanus Toxin. San Diego, Academic Press, 1989, pp. 281–298.

Dicoumarol and Anticoagulant Rodenticides

Caspar H., and Willard, J.: Moldy Sweet Clover Poisoning. Extension monograph. Fargo, ND, North Dakota State University, 1986.

Toxic Plants

Mike Murphy, ST. PAUL, MINNESOTA
John Reagor, COLLEGE STATION, TEXAS

The toxic plants that an equine practitioner is most likely to encounter or those not discussed in earlier editions of *Current Therapy in Equine Medicine* are discussed below. Photosensitization and the following plants are not included herein, because they are discussed in previous editions of this book (see *Current Therapy in Equine Medicine 2*, p. 672): castor bean *(Ricinus communis)*, oak (*Quercus* spp.), water hemlock *(Cicuta* spp.), yellow star thistle *(Centaurea solstitialis)*, Russian knapweed *(C. repens)*, bracken fern *(Pteridium aquilinum)*, horsetail *(Equisetum arvense)*, death camas *(Zigadenus* spp.), poison hemlock *(Conium maculatum)*, chokecherry *(Prunus virginiana)*, St. Johnswort *(Hypercum perforatum)*, wild jasmine *(Cestrum diurnum)*, and sleepy grass *(Stipa* spp.). The effects of tall fescue *(Festuca arundinacea)* on equine reproduction were discussed in the previous chapter (see p. 369).

Most inquiries about toxic plants involve three broad areas: (1) recognition of the plant and the clinical syndrome; (2) toxicity of the plant, diagnostic methods, and treatment; and (3) methods of preventing reexposure to the animal(s) or control of the plant in the field. These concerns are addressed for each plant discussed in this chapter.

The geographic distribution of a plant, which must be ingested as a green forage to cause toxicosis, defines the areas of a country where poisonings due to that plant are observed. However, plants that retain toxicity after drying may cause toxicosis anywhere in the country, owing to the shipment of hay outside the native habitat. In general, plant toxicoses are more common the year of and the year following a drought. Toxic plant problems may occur, however, in any region and in any year since individual forage management practices vary widely.

As with other equine diseases, the gamut of classical clinical signs is rarely demonstrated by an individual animal, so a compilation of common clinical signs and associated plants is included for quick reference (Table 1). Sources such as veterinary diagnostic laboratories, weed specialists, and local weed surveys should be

TABLE 1. CLINICAL SIGNS AND ASSOCIATED TOXIC PLANTS

Sign	Plant
Abnormal stance	Singletary pea
Anorexia	Milkweeds, nightshades, pyrrolizidine alkaloids
Ascites	Pyrrolizidine alkaloids
Ataxia	Locoweeds, snakeroot/goldenrod
Bradycardia	Japanese yew, Oleander (cardiac glycoside)
Colic	Lantana, milkweeds, nightshades
Collapse	Japanese yew, oleander (cardiac glycoside)
Constipation	Pyrrolizidine alkaloids
Convulsions	Nightshades
Cyanosis	Maple
Death (not sudden)	Nightshades, pyrrolizidine alkaloids
Depression	Kleingrass, locoweeds, nightshades, pyrrolizidine alkaloids
Diarrhea	Hoary alyssum, Japanese yew, lantana, milkweeds, nightshades, pyrrolizidine alkaloids
Discolored urine	Maple
Dyspnea	Nightshades
Emaciation	Locoweeds, pyrrolizidine alkaloids
Fever	Hoary alyssum
Gait stiffness	Snakeroot/goldenrod, sorghum
Gastroenteritis	Lantana
Head pressing	Pyrrolizidine alkaloids
Hepatoencephalopathy	Kleingrass
Hind legs forward	Singletary pea
Hind limb ataxia	Sorghum
Hind limb paresis	Sorghum
Hyperexcitability	Locoweeds
Icterus	Kleingrass, maple, pyrrolizidine alkaloids, lantana
Incoordination	Japanese yew
Laminitis	Black walnut
Mania	Pyrrolizidine alkaloids
Methemoglobineamia	Maple
Muscle trembling	Nightshades, milkweeds (cardiac glycoside)
Paralysis	Locoweeds, nightshades
Partial throat paralysis	Snakeroot/goldenrod
Polypnea	Maple
"Poor doer"	Kleingrass
Rough hair coat	Kleingrass, pyrrolizidine alkaloids
Scleral petechiation	Maple
Severe sweating	Snakeroot/goldenrod
Skin edema/slough	Lantana
Sluggishness	Snakeroot/goldenrod
Stand in shade	Lantana
Stocking-up	Hoary alyssum
Stringhalt gait	Singletary pea
Sudden death	Japanese yew, maple, milkweeds, snakeroot/goldenrod, oleander (cardiac glycoside)
Tachycardia	Maple
Trembling	Japanese yew, locoweeds
Urine dribbling, scalding	Sorghum
Weakness	Nightshades
Wide-based stance	Snakeroot/goldenrod

consulted for plant identification. The toxicity of plants is commonly reported in terms of per cent body weight that must be ingested to cause either clinical signs or death. To put these values in perspective, the average horse on pasture can be expected to consume 2 to 2.5 per cent of its body weight on a dry matter basis in 24 hours. The detection of plant toxins in biological tissues is rarely possible. Therefore, identification of the plant in hay or pasture, evidence of its ingestion, the presence of appropriate clinical signs, and the presence of supportive laboratory data or lesions are all commonly used for the diagnosis of plant toxicoses.

Treatment for most plant-related toxicoses is general (such as administration of activated charcoal or mineral oil) and symptomatic. Preventing access to the plant and controlling it in the field are the most successful prophylactic measures. Some weed control measures are included as specific examples for certain areas; however, the local weed control specialist should be consulted for appropriate forage management practices in your locale.

WHITE SNAKEROOT (Eupatorium rugosum) AND RAYLESS GOLDENROD (Isocoma wrightii)

White snakeroot, also known as snakeroot or richweed, is found in the eastern half of the United States in wooded pastures, and along lakes and streams. Rayless goldenrod, also called Jimmy weed or burrow weed, grows in the Southwest in open pastures. Horses ingesting either plant may exhibit signs of sluggishness, gait stiffness, ataxia, wide-based stance, partial throat paralysis, severe sweating, or sudden death without any previous signs. Poisoning generally occurs on wooded pastures in October or November when forage is covered with snow and horses graze stalks available above the snow as their only forage source, or at any time of year when the weed is baled in hay. The toxin, tremetone, remains active in hay. Occasionally, newly introduced animals will ingest snakeroot or rayless goldenrod when other forage is available. On a dry matter basis, ingestion of 0.5 to 2 per cent body weight by a horse can be lethal. Affected animals commonly have marked elevations in muscle enzyme levels (creatine phosphokinase [CPK], aspartamine aminotransferase [alanine transferase, ALT], and lactate dehydrogenase [LDH]). Skeletal and myocardial degeneration and necrosis are seen histologically.

White snakeroot toxicosis of horses on pasture may be prevented by effective weed control or reduced by providing adequate supplemental feed immediately after a snow. The plant can be controlled with 2,4-D-amine or ester at 1 to 2 quarts per acre in bloom or beyond. Animals should be kept out of the area until the plant is completely dead.

HOARY ALYSSUM (Berteroa incana)

Hoary alyssum has recently been associated with limb edema ("stocking-up"), transient fever, and diarrhea in horses. The plant is commonly found throughout the northern half of the United States in waste areas, disturbed soils, and as a contaminant in alfalfa (and other) hay fields. The plant may be ingested in the spring and early summer when other forage is not available, or at any time of year when baled in hay. The toxin in hoary alyssum and its toxicity are currently unknown, but animals are reported to develop signs within 2 to 3 days of ingesting contaminated hay. Animals with limb edema normally recover within 2 to 4 days following removal from the source. The best control is proper management of pastures and hay stands. Repeated 2,4-D or dicamba applications in grass pastures or hexazinone in established alfalfa may chemically suppress but not control the plant.

BLACK WALNUT (Juglans nigra)

Black walnut is used in the furniture industry and consequently is incorporated into wood shavings or sawdust. Horses in contact with fresh wood shavings comprised in whole or in part of black walnut have developed limb edema, lethargy, or laminitis. Not all samples of black walnut shavings are toxic, but the use of these shavings in bedding is not advised. Aeration of shavings or the use of old shavings has been suggested as a means of preventing the problem, but is not recommended since toxicity is unpredictable. The toxicity of shavings from butternut (Juglans cinerea) and English walnut (Juglans regia) has not been determined; they should be considered potentially toxic. Removal of animals from the bedding and prompt treatment of laminitis commonly result in recovery.

PLANTS CONTAINING CARDIAC GLYCOSIDES

Milkweeds (Asclepias spp.), azalea (Rhododendron spp.), foxglove (Digitalis spp.), and oleander (Nerium oleander) are grouped together because of a common mechanism of action. Numerous species of milkweeds are found throughout the United States. The common names for these plants are even more numerous than the number of species. Fortunately, all of the common names include the term "milkweed." Azaleas or laurels are ornamental plants in the southern United States and houseplants throughout the country. Foxglove is a European native grown as an ornamental in the United States. Oleander is an ornamental plant found along roadways and in flower beds throughout the southern half of the United States.

The milkweeds are commonly seen in pastures throughout the country, but since they are highly unpalatable, they are ingested only under circumstances of severe overgrazing. The other three plant species are ingested when animals are allowed to graze yards or roadways, when trimmings are thrown over a fence to the horses, or when a frost causes the leaves to fall and blow into the pasture or paddock. Ingestion of any of the plants by animals often leads to sudden death. Rarely, anorexia, colic, or diarrhea may be observed. The plants contain one or more cardiac glycosides that are believed to interfere with the sodium/potassium-ATPase system, causing an atrioventricular block that progresses to asystole.

Cardiac glycosides are quite toxic. For example, some milkweeds are toxic to horses when 0.05 to 2 per cent body weight is ingested. Because of this extreme toxicity and the rapid onset of death, plant parts may be found in the stomach contents on necropsy. Treatment is rarely possible, leaving prevention as the only method of controlling toxicosis due to these plants.

YEW (Taxus spp.)

Yew or ground hemlock is commonly planted as an ornamental around foundations in the northern half of the United States. Any animal ingesting the plant is normally found dead. Rarely, signs of trembling, incoordination, collapse, diarrhea, bradycardia, and acute cardiac failure may be observed up to 2 days after ingestion, since the toxin acts by depressing conduction and myocardial depolarization. *Taxus* is readily consumed by livestock, especially in winter months when other forage is not available, or any time of year when the prunings are tossed over the fence to them. Yew is quite toxic, 0.1 to 0.5 per cent body weight being lethal, so a diagnosis of poisoning is commonly made by identifying plant parts in the stomach contents. Treatment is rarely possible, so prevention of exposure is the sole means of control.

MAPLE (Acer spp.)

The red maple, *Acer rubrum*, is classically associated with toxicity; however, field suspicions of other maples exist, so any *Acer* species (all maples) should be considered potentially toxic. Maples are native in northeast, north central, and southeastern regions; however, they are commonly planted as ornamentals throughout the country. Horses that ingest the wilted leaves may exhibit polypnea, tachycardia, icterus, cyanosis, scleral petechiation, brownish discoloration of the urine, methemoglobinemia, Heinz body formation, or acute death. The toxin responsible for the methemoglobinemia and Heinz body formation is not yet identified.

Poisoning generally occurs in September or October when the leaves wilt, fall, and cover other available forage in the pasture or paddock. Occasionally when a tree or branch is felled (lightning, hail storm, clearing land, etc.), the wilted leaves become available for ingestion. Lack of other forage exacerbates the problem. Ingestion of 1.5 and 3 pounds of wilted leaves by a 1000-pound horse is reportedly toxic and lethal, respectively. In a live animal, anemia, hemoglobinemia, Heinz bodies, and increased aspartate aminotransferase (AST), sorbitol dehydrogenase (SDH), plasma protein, and bilirubin are supportive of a diagnosis of maple poisoning. Histologically, icterus, centrilobular hepatic degeneration, pigment-induced renal degeneration, and erythrophagocytosis in the spleen, adrenal, and liver, in conjunction with comparable gross lesions, are observed. Transfusion of blood or fluids, or both, may be indicated in severe cases.

To prevent poisoning, eliminate access to wilted maple leaves. To reduce the likelihood of poisoning, provide adequate supplemental feed when wilted maple leaves are available. For the long term, maple trees should not be planted in horse pastures or paddocks.

PLANTS CONTAINING PYRROLIZIDINE ALKALOIDS

Hound's tongue (*Cynoglossum officinale*), groundsel (*Senecio* spp.), rattlebox (*Crotalaria* spp.), heliotropum (*Heliotropium* spp.), and fiddleneck (*Amsinckia* spp.) are grouped together because they have a common mechanism of action. Numerous common names exist for the *Senecio* species, including stinking willie, wooly groundsel, thread-leaf groundsel, Riddell's groundsel, bitterweed, and broom groundsel. *Amsinckia* is also commonly called fiddleneck.

Clinically, animals with minimal exposure to these plants and those with an early syndrome come to attention because of poor condition ("poor doers"). Those receiving greater exposure develop rough hair coats, depression, and anorexia. Signs can progress to icterus, ascites, emaciation, diarrhea or constipation, head pressing, mania, and eventually death.

Early in the syndrome, hepatic damage is reflected by elevations in serum SDH, ALT, and γ-glutamyl transferase (GGT) levels. Later in the syndrome, elevated bilirubin levels, decreased albumin levels, altered albumin to globulin ratios, and perhaps a compensatory polyclonal gammopathy are present. Histologically, lesions vary from hepatic necrosis and hemorrhage to liver fibrosis with biliary hyperplasia. Megalocytosis is characteristic for pyrrolizidine alkaloid poisoning. A latent period of at least 3 weeks following ingestion precedes the appearance of megalocytes. The hepatocyte nucleus increases in size without mitosis.

KLEINGRASS (Panicum coloratum)

Kleingrass is a recently introduced perennial grass found in improved pastures in the southwestern United States. It is utilized for both grazing and hay. Toxicity in horses is usually seen when the animals consume kleingrass hay as their only roughage source. The highest concentrations of hepatotoxic saponins are found during times of rapid growth. Thus, higher quality hay is likely to be more toxic than that containing overmature plants. Clinical signs are those associated with loss of liver function and vary from depression and poor performance to icterus and hepatoencephalopathy. The photosensitization commonly seen in sheep and goats with kleingrass poisoning is not usually present in horses. Affected animals have elevated ALT, LDH, alkaline phosphatase (AP), and bilirubin levels. There is no specific treatment. Poisoning can be prevented by not feeding kleingrass hay or forcing horses to ingest a large amount of the grass on pasture.

SINGLETARY PEA (Lathyrus hirsutus)

Singletary pea, also known as wild winter pea or caly pea, was at one time planted over a wide area of the southern, extreme western, and northwestern United States. It has become naturalized in many areas where there is adequate rainfall. The plant produces desirable, nutritious forage, and poisoning is confined to consumption of the seeds. Horses ingesting hay containing singletary pea in the seed pod stage of maturity for weeks to months develop clinical signs. Affected horses usually stand with their hind legs and feet too far forward. The hind legs are partially paralyzed, and animals that are forced to move will do so in a stringhalt fashion. Most animals recover when the source of singletary pea seeds is removed. To prevent the problem, hay containing singletary pea should be harvested prior to the setting of seed pods.

NIGHTSHADES (Solanum Spp.)

Various nightshades are found in many areas of the United States. They range from the ornamental Jerusalem cherry to the thorny buffalo bur. All are considered to be potentially toxic; however, they are not usually consumed by horses, even when they make up most of the available forage. Poisoning usually follows ingestion of contaminated hay. Clinical signs may involve either the central nervous system (CNS) or the gastrointestinal tract, or both. Gastrointestinal signs include anorexia, colic, and diarrhea. CNS signs include depression, dyspnea, muscle trembling, weakness, paralysis, or convulsions prior to death. Treatment is symptomatic. Therapy with dimethyl sulfoxide has reportedly alleviated severe neurological signs in some animals.

SORGHUM (Sorghum Spp.)

A small percentage of horses consuming large amounts of sorghum forage or hay develop sorghum cystitis. Most cases are the result of the animals grazing fields planted with a sorghum-sudan hybrid. Hind limb ataxia of varying degrees occurs in affected animals. Signs may progress from urine dribbling and scalding to complete paresis of the rear limbs. Because the syndrome is the result of nerve degeneration, affected animals do not recover. Prevention of the syndrome centers on restriction of access to sorghum pasture or hay.

LOCOWEEDS (Astragalus and Oxytropis Spp.)

Locoweeds are found in the western half of the United States. There are many species of *Astragalus*, and they vary greatly in toxicity (some are nontoxic). Horses must consume large amounts of the plant (30 per cent body weight) over a period of weeks to months to become affected. Affected animals have neurological signs that may vary from hyperexcitability and trembling to ataxia, depression, emaciation, and paralysis. Histologically, locoism is characterized by widespread cytoplasmic vacuolation of cells in the brain and visceral organs. "Loco" horses are dangerous to ride despite apparent recovery following removal of the plant. Although locoweeds are thought to be addictive, this assumption has been questioned. These weeds are not highly palatable, but once animals begin consuming them they must be moved to a "loco-free" range to discontinue exposure. Animals introduced to ranges containing locoweed are much more likely to be poisoned than horses raised on ranges containing the plant.

LANTANA (Lantana camara)

Lantana may be found as a volunteer ornamental shrub across the southern part of the United States. The clusters of blooms vary from pink and white to orange and yellow to orange and red. The toxicity is highly variable; plants with the darker flowers appear to be more toxic. Lantana causes liver damage, secondary photosensitization, gastroenteritis, and some loss of renal function. Affected animals avoid the sun due to edema of the unpigmented areas. This edema can progress to necrosis and epithelial sloughing. A mild to severe diarrhea may be present along with colic early in the syndrome. Serum activities of ALT, LDH, AP, and GGT are markedly elevated. Poisoning is prevented by proper pasture management, since the plant is not consumed in significant amounts unless other forages are not available.

Supplemental Readings

Beier, R. C., and Norman, J. O.: The toxic factor in white snakeroot: Identity, analysis and prevention. In: Proceedings of a Symposium on the Public Health Significance of Natural Toxicants in Animal Feeds, 1990, pp. 1–23.

Cheeke, P. R., and Shull, L. R. (eds.): Natural Toxicants in Feeds and Poisonous Plants. Westport, CT, AVI Publishing Co., 1985.

Kingsbury, J. M. (ed.): Poisonous Plants of the United States and Canada. Englewood Cliffs, NJ, Prentice-Hall, Inc., 1964.

Kownacki, A. A., and Tobin, T.: Plant Toxicities. In Robinson, N. E. (ed.): Current Therapy in Equine Medicine. Philadelphia, W. B. Saunders Co., 1983, pp. 595–607.

Oehme, F.: Plant Toxicities. In Robinson, N. E. (ed.): Current Therapy in Equine Medicine. Philadelphia, W. B. Saunders Co., 1987, pp. 672–682.

Equine Leukoencephalomalacia/ Hepatosis and Stachybotryotoxicosis

Val Richard Beasley, URBANA-CHAMPAIGN, ILLINOIS

This chapter describes two distinct mycotoxicoses. The first, equine leukoencephalomalacia/hepatosis, is associated with contamination of corn by *Fusarium moniliforme* and is common in the United States. The second, stachybotryotoxicosis, is attributed to *Stachybotrys* spp., primarily in hay or straw, and is a potentially important but presently unrecognized mycotoxicosis in the United States.

EQUINE LEUKOENCEPHALOMALACIA/ HEPATOSIS

Equine leukoencephalomalacia/hepatosis is a liquefactive necrosis of the white matter of the brain of horses, donkeys, and mules. It was first described in the United States in 1891 and is now known to occur in many parts of the world. The disease may present as equine leukoencephalomalacia, liver failure, or both. In some years, equine leukoencephalomalacia has killed thousands of horses worldwide. The major risk factor in the occurrence of equine leukoencephalomalacia is feeding of mold-damaged corn. *Fusarium moniliforme* is believed to be present in 80 to 100 per cent of the corn produced annually. Corn screenings, which contain stunted or broken kernels and debris, tend to be heavily contaminated by fungi and are especially hazardous. Inoculating sterilized corn with toxic strains of *F. moniliforme* and feeding the culture material to horses or donkeys has resulted in equine leukoencephalomalacia and liver failure. Damage to corn from insects, drought, floods, and wet harvest conditions may predispose to equine leukoencephalomalacia. Feeding a contaminated diet for one to several weeks may cause the disease.

CLINICAL SIGNS AND LESIONS

The neurological form of equine leukoencephalomalacia is manifested by an afebrile syndrome involving reduced responsiveness to external stimuli, incoordination, aimless wandering, head pressing, circling, recumbency, hyperexcitability, paresis, and potentially other locomotor, psychic, or autonomic disturbances. Horses with neurological effects usually die, often within 24 hours of the onset of clinical signs. Survivors may have life-long neurological deficits. Liver failure may cause icterus, edema, hemorrhage, elevated serum hepatic enzyme activities and bilirubin levels, and possibly hepatoencephalopathy. The hepatic effects are believed to be more reversible than the neurological derangements.

Equine leukoencephalomalacia is most often characterized by liquefactive necrosis of the subcortical white matter in one or both cerebral hemispheres. The lesions vary from microscopic to involvement of the majority of a cerebral lobe, and liquefied contents of these areas range from light yellow and clear to flocculent or blood-stained. The border between foci of malacia and the normal neuropil may be characterized by vascular congestion and thrombosis, perivascular edema, hemorrhages, and cuffs of eosinophils and mononuclear cells. Malacic lesions may also occur in the thalamus, brain stem, cerebellum, or medulla oblongata.

Hepatic lesions may include grossly evident yellow discoloration of centrilobular zones on both the capsular and cut surfaces. Typical microscopic lesions include marked centrilobular hepatocellular necrosis with inflammatory cell infiltrates, severe vacuolation of periportal hepatocytes, and mild to moderate periportal fibrosis.

Etiology

Strains of *F. moniliforme* may produce the cardiotoxin moniliformin, the estrogen mimic zearalenone, the phytotoxin fusaric acid, the mutagen fusarin C, the cytotoxin (in neoplastic cell lines) fusariocin C, gibberellins (plant hormones), malonic acid, benzoanthentrione pigments, kaurane diterpenoids, and phenolics. None of the above toxins, however, have been shown to cause equine leukoencephalomalacia/hepatotoxicosis in horses.

Another *F. moniliforme* toxin, fumonisin B_1, purified from a South African strain (MRC 826), has been used to reproduce equine leukoencephalomalacia/liver failure in horses. The reproduction of various degrees of the disease occurred after either intragastric, intravenous, or repeated oral administrations of the toxin or culture material containing fumonisin B_1 to horses. The toxin was isolated and identified as fumonisin B_1, using the ability of the compound to cause abnormal foci in the liver of rats as a bioassay. Drought-striken corn in various areas of the United States has recently been shown to contain up to 250 ppm of fumonisin B_1. Ten ppm has been found in corn associated with outbreaks of equine leukoencephalomalacia. Additional fumonisins are produced by *F. moniliforme*, but even less is known of their occurrence or toxicity at this time. Also, it is possible that other, structurally unrelated toxins may play an important role in these diseases.

Corn causing equine leukoencephalomalacia/liver failure in horses may also be quite hazardous to other species of animals. For example, rats administered culture material of *F. moniliforme* developed hepatic cancer, cirrhosis, intraventricular cardiac thrombosis, and nephrosis; sheep developed acute nephrosis and hepatosis; and swine experienced feed refusal and pulmonary edema. Recent experience from field cases involving swine exposed to naturally contaminated corn containing high concentrations of fumonisin B_1 (i.e., 50 ppm and higher) suggests that pigs of all ages may experience pulmonary edema and pleural effusions, and sows may abort.

Diagnosis

Tentative diagnoses are strengthened if corn is being fed, particularly if it is mold-damaged or screenings. Clinical signs, clinical chemistry findings, and lesions suggestive of equine leukoencephalomalacia/liver failure should be present. The absence of evidence indicative of other hepatotoxicoses supports a diagnosis of *F. moniliforme*–induced hepatosis. Abnormal elevations in blood ammonia levels may be present in animals with hepatoencephalopathy.

Finding fumonisin B_1 at approximately 10 ppm or greater would seem to be supportive of a diagnosis. However, until dose–response studies are performed using purified toxin, it will remain difficult to interpret the toxicologic significance of various concentrations of fumonisin B_1 in rations of horses. Furthermore, until a margin of safety is established based on observations from dosing studies and exposures in the field, it will be impossible to state that a given ration bears a negligible hazard.

Therapy and Prevention

No proven therapies for equine leukoencephalomalacia or *F. moniliforme*–associated hepatoses exist. B-vitamin therapy may be tried, but there are no data to indicate benefit. Symptomatic care including control of seizures may be attempted; however, the outcome of most cases of equine leukoencephalomalacia is death. This author is aware of one instance in which 3 horses with apparent equine leukoencephalomalacia seemed to stabilize in response to IV administration of dimethyl sulfoxide, but one cannot conclude on this basis alone that dimethyl sulfoxide is an appropriate therapy. Animals with hepatosis should be supported as indicated for other forms of potentially reversible liver failure.

A reliable way to avoid equine leukoencephalomalacia and *F. moniliforme*–associated hepatosis is to avoid corn in the diets of horses. If corn is fed, pelleted diets made with corn should generally be avoided; only healthy-appearing corn should be given and it should be screened before using. Corn screenings should not be given to equids. Analysis of feed for fumonisins is recommended, but failure to detect the toxins cannot be regarded as proof of a lack of hazard of these syndromes.

STACHYBOTRYOTOXICOSIS

Historically, thousands of horses have reportedly died from stachybotryotoxicosis in the Soviet Union, Europe, and South Africa. In Hungary, *Stachybotrys atra* was isolated from straw incriminated in stachybotryotoxicosis of horses and sheep; *S. chartarum* was implicated in toxicosis of sheep in South Africa. The condition has been reproduced by feeding of initially "clean" forage that had been incubated at high moisture with strains of *S. atra* obtained from outbreaks of stachybotryotoxicosis. *S. atra* is a soil fungus that produces dense, sooty accumulations of black spores in contaminated straw or hay. That fungus has been shown to produce potent macrocyclic trichothecene mycotoxins including satratoxins G and H, verrucarin J, and roridin E. Stachybotryotoxicosis can poison many species, such as horses, cattle, sheep, swine, and humans (by contact). Therefore, forages contaminated with stachybotryotoxins should not be diverted to other species as a means of disposal.

CLINICAL SIGNS, CLINICAL PATHOLOGY, AND LESIONS

The naturally occurring syndrome is initially afebrile in horses fed low levels of toxic feed. Fissures develop at the corners of the mouth, followed by deeper necrosis at the oral-mucocutaneous junction. In some cases, edema of the lips, hypersalivation, rhinitis, conjunctivitis, and enlarged tender lymph nodes occur. This may be followed by a quiescent period of approximately 5 days in which thrombocytopenia, reductions in blood clotting and clot retraction, leukopenia, and agranulocytosis develop. Subsequently, body temperatures may increase and thrombocytopenia, leukopenia, and coagulopathy can become severe. The pulse during the second phase of the syndrome may be weak and arrhythmic. Generalized oral necrotic lesions and colic develop, blood glucose level declines, and inorganic phosphorus may be reduced. Affected animals typically die after 5 to 6 days.

Another form of stachybotryotoxicosis is termed the atypical, or "shocking" form. Although this form of the syndrome usually follows higher levels of exposure, it also has been observed sporadically in groups of horses exposed to lesser levels of toxic feed. The "shocking" form was reproduced after 10 days of feeding of *S. atra*-infected straw. Affected horses had no signs referable to the oral cavity. Loss of reflexes, hyperesthesia, hyperirritability, blindness, stupor, reluctance to move, a wide stance, leg crossing, leaning against objects, anorexia, dysphagia, and polydypsia were noted. Often the gut became atonic, and occasionally diarrhea occurred. Some horses developed shock, rectal temperatures above 41° C, "shortness of breath," cyanosis, and hemorrhages in the visible mucosae.

Lesions may include generalized hemorrhage (sometimes involving the meninges and brain), necrosis and inflammation of the alimentary tract apart from the esophagus, enlarged lymph nodes depleted of lymphocytes, focal necrosis and depletion of granulocytes in bone marrow, and circumscribed areas of degeneration in the liver, kidneys, and myocardium. The adrenal cortex may be hypoplastic in the typical form and hemorrhagic in the acute form of the disease. As with the fumonisins, information is presently inadequate on the role of specific macrocyclic trichothecene mycotoxins and the concentrations at which the toxins pose a negligible hazard.

THERAPY

In other trichothecene-associated diseases, activated charcoal administration, supportive care including corticosteroids and fluids for shock, antibiotics for bacterial infections, and an uncontaminated, well-balanced diet with elevated protein content are of value. A similar approach seems appropriate for horses with stachybotryotoxicosis.

Supplemental Readings

Equine Leukoencephalomalacia/Hepatosis

Bezuidenhout, S. C., Gelderblom, W. C. A., Gorst-Allman, C. P., Horak, R. M., Marasas, W. F. O., Spiteller, G., and Vleggaar, R.: Structural elucidation of fumonisins, mycotoxins from *Fusarium moniliforme*. Chem. Soc. Commun. 743–745, 1988.

Buck, W. B., Haliburton, J. C., Thilsted, J. P., Lock, T. F., and Vesonder, R. F.: Equine leucoencephalomalacia: Comparative pathology of naturally occurring and experimental cases. Proc. Am. Assoc. Vet. Lab. Diag., 22:239–258, 1979.

Graham, R.: Cornstalk disease investigations: Toxic encephalitis or non-virus encephalomyelitis of horses. Vet. Med., 31:46–50, 1936.

Marasas, W. F. O., Kellerman, T. S., Gelderblom, W. C. A., Coetzner, J. A. W., Thiel, P. G., and Van Der Lugt, J. J.: Leukoencephalomalacia in a horse induced by fumonisin B1 isolated from *Fusarium moniliforme*. Onderstepoort J. Vet. Res., 55: 197–203, 1988.

Wilson, B. J., Maronpot, R. R., and Hildebrandt, P. K.: Equine leukoencephalomalacia. J. Am. Vet. Med. Assoc., 163:1293–1295, 1973.

Stachybotryotoxicosis

Forgacs, J.: Stachybotryotoxicosis and moldy corn toxicosis. *In* Wogan, G. N. (ed): Mycotoxins in Foodstuffs. Cambridge, Mass., MIT Press, 1965, p. 87.

Harrach, B., Mirocha, C. J., Pathre, S. V., and Palysik, M.: Macrocyclic trichothecene toxins produced by a strain of *Stachybotrys atra* from Hungary. Appl. Environ. Microbiol., 41:1428–1432, 1981.

Harrach, B., Bata, A., Bajmócy, E., and Benko, M.: Isolation of satratoxins from the bedding straw of a sheep flock with fatal stachybotryotoxicosis. Appl. Environ. Microbiol., 45:1419–1422, 1983.

Section 9

CARDIOVASCULAR DISEASE

Edited by Virginia B. Reef

Cardiovascular Problems Associated with Poor Performance

Virginia B. Reef, KENNETT SQUARE, PENNSYLVANIA

Although musculoskeletal and respiratory problems are the most frequent causes of poor performance in horses, cardiovascular disease may be associated with poor performance more frequently than is recognized. Congenital heart disease, valvular insufficiency, myocardial dysfunction, pericardial disease, arrhythmias, aortoiliac thrombosis, and jugular vein thrombosis may all affect performance. Changes in performance may range from a few seconds prolongation of racing time to staggering, ataxia, and collapse. A thorough physical examination should be performed in any horse being evaluated for poor performance, including careful cardiac auscultation, palpation of the peripheral arterial pulses (including the metatarsal arterial pulses), palpation of the veins for patency and refill, and evaluation of the mucous membranes and capillary refill time.

CONGENITAL CARDIAC DISEASE

A ventricular septal defect is the most likely congenital cardiac disease to affect performance in horses. Horses with more complex congenital cardiac defects usually grow slowly and have exercise intolerance that is detected at a young age. Ventricular septal defects are also the most common equine congenital cardiac anomaly and may go undetected until the animal is put into work. The size of the ventricular septal defect and its location determine the effect this lesion will have on the horse's performance. Horses with membranous ventricular septal defects that measure 2.5 cm or less in diameter often are performing up to the owner's expectations but are unlikely to be top racehorses. Horses with ventricular septal defects that are larger than 2.5 cm in diameter or located in the muscular portion of the interventricular septum are likely to perform poorly.

Diagnosis is based on auscultation of the characteristic murmur and echocardiographic confirmation of the defect. The characteristic murmur is a loud, band-shaped, pansystolic murmur with the point of maximal intensity over the right fourth intercostal space. The murmur is usually grade III to VI/VI in intensity. A similar though usually slightly softer murmur is auscultated over the pulmonic valve area. This murmur is usually more crescendo–decrescendo in quality and holosystolic. This is a relative pulmonic stenosis murmur caused by increased blood flow across the normal pulmonic valve.

Two-dimensional real-time echocardiography is the optimal diagnostic study as ventricular septal defects can readily be imaged in the membranous portion of the septum underneath the septal leaflet of the tricuspid valve and the right coronary cusp of the aortic valve in the right parasternal left ventricular outflow tract view (long and short axis). The interventricular septum should be scanned in all imaging planes, looking for alternative locations of the ventricular septal defect. Pulsed wave and color flow Doppler echocardiography can be used to localize the shunt associated with the ventricular septal defect. The shunt is usually left to right and should be depicted as a red to orange mosaic jet on color flow Doppler. Continuous wave Doppler echocardiography can be used to obtain the peak velocity of the jet; combined with a systolic blood pressure, the peak velocity can be used to estimate right ventricular pressures. High peak velocities of the ventricular septal defect jet are associated with normal right ventricular pressures and a small ventricular septal defect (2.5 cm in diameter or less). Lower peak velocities are associated with larger ventricular septal defects and a higher right ventricular pressure.

VALVULAR INSUFFICIENCY

Significant mitral regurgitation is more likely to affect performance than is insufficiency of the other equine heart valves. Moderate to severe mitral regurgitation results in an increased left atrial pressure, pulmonary hypertension, and pulmonary edema. Common presenting complaints are slower racing times (often 20 to 30 seconds slower), stopping at the ¾ pole, coughing (at rest or during exercise), prolonged recovery time to resting respiratory rate, and a long cooling out time. Occasional horses may have profuse exercise-induced pulmonary hemorrhage. Tricuspid regurgitation, although fairly common, is rarely associated with performance problems unless the tricuspid regurgitation is severe. Similarly, most horses with aortic regurgitation and volume-loaded left ventricles cope well until left ventricular dilation progresses and stretching of the mitral annulus occurs, resulting in mitral regurgitation. M-mode and two-dimensional real-time echocardiography are necessary to characterize the cardiac chamber enlargement and valvular abnormalities present with valvular insufficiency, while pulsed wave and color flow Doppler echocardiography are used to flow map the regurgitant jet and semiquantify its severity. The likelihood of a particular valvular insufficiency being associated with performance problems depends on which valve is affected, the degree of chamber enlargement and volume overload, and the size and distribution of the regurgitant jet.

MYOCARDIAL DYSFUNCTION

Performance-related problems are common if myocardial dysfunction exists and pump function is decreased (see p. 393). Performance problems are usually severe, with marked changes in racing times and clinical signs of weakness, staggering, or collapse associated with exercise. Pulmonary edema, dyspnea, and tachycardia may also be seen in horses with acute myocardial dysfunction associated with recent exercise. A heart rate monitor, radiotelemetry, or electrocardiogram during exercise will reveal heart rates that are significantly increased over normal for each level of exercise. Normal horses have heart rates of 70 to 120 bpm while trotting, 120 to 150 bpm while cantering, 150 to 180 bpm at a hand gallop, and above 180 bpm while galloping. Performance testing of horses with suspected myocardial disease on a treadmill may be indicated in more mildly affected animals. Other diagnostic tests and therapeutic interventions depend on the suspected underlying etiology of the myocardial dysfunction.

PERICARDIAL DISEASE

Pericardial effusion and constrictive pericarditis impair left ventricular filling and result in a decreased stroke volume and lower cardiac output associated with exercise. In mild cases the clinical signs may be minimal. As the impairment to ventricular filling worsens, an increased resting heart rate will be noted and heart rate will increase markedly with exercise. Venous distention and peripheral edema will be noted as the effusion or constrictive pericarditis worsens. Echocardiography provides a definitive diagnosis by demonstrating an echo-free space between the pericardium and epicardium or by demonstrating a thickened echogenic epicardial echo with poor ventricular filling (see p. 404).

ARRHYTHMIAS

Cardiac arrhythmias are the most frequent cardiovascular cause of poor performance in horses (see below). Atrial fibrillation often causes dramatic changes in performance with prolongations of racing times by 20 or 30 seconds or more. Weakness, ataxia, or collapse may occur in approximately 10 per cent of horses with atrial fibrillation. Frequent atrial or ventricular extrasystoles may also impair performance but often result in a change in performance of 3 to 5 seconds. Ventricular or supraventricular tachycardia that is sustained and occurs during exercise may cause more dramatic changes in performance, including collapse. Bradyarrhythmias such as advanced second-degree heart block, complete heart block, and sick sinus syndrome may also cause dramatic changes in performance and collapse. A resting electrocardiogram will reveal the electrocardiographic diagnosis in most cases. An exercising electrocardiogram obtained via radiotelemetry with the horse on a longe, under saddle, or in a performance test on a treadmill may be necessary to induce the arrhythmia or to determine the significance of arrhythmia associated with exercise.

AORTOILIAC THROMBOSIS

Aortoiliac thrombosis occurs infrequently in horses but causes significant performance problems (see *Current Therapy in Equine Medicine 2*, p. 175). The most common complaints include exercise-associated weakness, lameness, ataxia, staggering, or collapse. Hyperpnea or dyspnea may also be noted with the exercise bout. Physical examination findings may include a decreased metatarsal arterial pulse or decreased saphenous refill time in the affected limb. Successful treatment or management of aortic iliac thrombosis has occasionally been reported with the use of larvicidal dewormer, nonsteroidal anti-inflammatory drugs, and a controlled exercise program with gradual increases in exercise. In general, the prognosis for these horses is poor, because the disease is advanced by the time the diagnosis is made.

JUGULAR VEIN THROMBOSIS

Jugular vein thrombosis can also result in performance-related problems (see p. 406). Unilateral swelling of the head associated with exercise may result in significant upper respiratory tract obstruction and decreased performance. Head shaking has also been reported with exercise in some affected individuals. Physical examination findings include a corded thrombosed jugular vein that does not fill, and distention of the facial veins. Endoscopic examination of an affected horse after exercise usually reveals venous congestion in the pharynx and pharyngeal swelling. Ultrasonographic examination of the affected vessel reveals complete occlusion of the affected vessel by a thrombus.

Supplemental Readings

Muylle, E., Vandenhende, C., Oyaert, W., et al: Delayed monensin sodium toxicity in horses. Equine Vet. J., 13:107, 1981.
Pipers, F. S., Reef, V. B., Wilson, J.: Echocardiographic detection of ventricular septal defects in large animals. J. Am. Vet. Med. Assoc., 187:810, 1985.
Reef, V. B.: Heart murmurs, irregularities, and other cardiac abnormalities. *In* Brown, C. M. (ed.): Problems in Equine Medicine. Philadelphia, Lea & Febriger, 1989, pp. 122–137.
Reef, V. B., Levitan, C. W., and Spencer, P.A.: Factors influencing prognosis and treatment in horses with atrial fibrillation. J. Vet. Intern. Med., 2:1, 1988.
Reef, V. B., Roby, K. A. W., Richardson, D. W., et al: Use of ultrasonography for the detection of aortic-iliac thrombosis in horses. J. Am. Vet. Med. Assoc., 190:286, 1987.

Cardiac Arrhythmias

Johanna M. Reimer, KENNETT SQUARE, PENNSYLVANIA

Physiological arrhythmias such as first- and second-degree atrioventricular (AV) block, sinoatrial (SA) block, wandering atrial pacemaker, sinus bradycardia, and sinus arrhythmia are common in horses. Such arrhythmias occur at slow to normal heart rates and are abolished by excitement, exercise, or the administration of atropine. Pathological arrhythmias include atrial fibrillation, supraventricular premature contractions, supraventricular tachycardia, ventricular premature contractions, ventricular tachycardia, third-degree AV block, and advanced second-degree AV block.

Most arrhythmias are detected with careful cardiac auscultation. The history and physical examination may identify any predisposing causes or hemodynamic effects of the arrhythmia. Electrocardiography (ECG) is used to accurately characterize the arrhythmia. The base-apex ECG provides the best tracing, owing to minimal movement artifacts and larger wave forms. The right forearm (negative) electrode may be placed dorsal to the right scapula or in the right jugular groove two thirds of the way down the neck. The left forearm (positive) electrode is placed over the apex of the heart in the sixth intercostal space on the left side just above the point of the elbow. The right hind leg electrode, or ground, is placed anywhere on the body, remote from the heart. More than one lead may be necessary for ECG diagnosis of some arrhythmias, especially those that are more complex. In such cases, any of the standard unipolar or bipolar limb leads will suffice. The duration of the PR (0.22 to 0.56 seconds, lead II), QRS (0.08 to 0.17 seconds, lead II), and QT (0.32 to 0.64 seconds, lead II) intervals should be measured and the ST segment evaluated. It should be recognized that T wave changes occur frequently in normal horses and that the ECG is not useful as an indicator of cardiac size in the horse.

To determine the significance of an arrhythmia in relationship to performance, ECGs should be obtained at rest; during exercise with radiotelemetry if possible; and during recovery from exercise. Additional diagnostic tests include echocardiography, serum electrolyte measurements, serum cardiac isoenzyme measurements, and a 24-hour ECG recording via a Holter monitor. A 24-hour ECG may aid in more accurately determining the frequency and significance of an arrhythmia and may also document arrhythmias in horses with syncope.

PHYSIOLOGICAL ARRHYTHMIAS

Arrhythmias associated with high vagal tone occur at resting heart rates of 40 bpm or less and are abolished by exercise, excitement, or vagolytic drugs such as atropine sulfate. These arrhythmias are not associated with cardiac disease.

FIRST- AND SECOND-DEGREE AV BLOCK

Second-degree AV block is the most common physiological arrhythmia in the horse. A normal or low resting heart rate and a predominantly regular rhythm with occasional dropped beats is detected. An isolated fourth heart sound may be audible, immediately followed by a pause. The ECG demonstrates normal P-QRS-T complexes and occasional P waves not followed by a QRS-T complex.

Mobitz type I second-degree AV block (Wenckebach) is most common in horses and is characterized by progressively lengthening PR intervals preceding the dropped beat (Fig. 1). Mobitz type II second-degree AV block (constant PR intervals) is also observed. Occasionally two consecutive dropped beats may be observed in normal horses. Advanced second-degree AV block should be considered pathological if the arrhythmia persists at higher heart rates (above 50 bpm) or if syncope occurs in association with prolonged periods of second-degree AV block (greater than 6 to 10 seconds). Second-degree AV block is also a normal physiological response to supraventricular (atrial) or ventricular tachycardia.

WANDERING ATRIAL PACEMAKER

Wandering atrial pacemaker is a physiological arrhythmia most frequently seen with sinus arrhythmia and sinus bradycardia. Auscultation may reveal a regular or slightly irregular rhythm. The change in the morphology of the P wave seen on the ECG may be associated with a change in the PR interval. Wandering atrial pacemaker may occur concurrently with other physiological arrhythmias, including first- or second-degree AV block, sinus arrhythmia, and sinus block. This arrhythmia is abolished at higher heart rates and should not be confused with atrial premature depolarizations (APD); the P wave of the wandering atrial pacemaker will

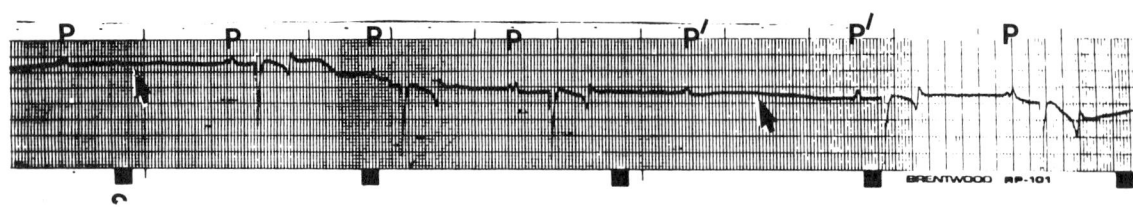

Figure 1. Base-apex ECG from a 3-year-old Standardbred filly with Mobitz type I (Wenckebach) second-degree AV block and a wandering atrial pacemaker. Note the slow heart rate (30 bpm), the two P wave morphologies (P = biphid sinus P waves, P′ = wandering atrial pacemaker), and second-degree AV block (arrows). Note the progressive lengthening of the PR intervals of the three complexes in the center of the strip before the dropped beat occurs. This arrhythmia was abolished when the horse was excited.

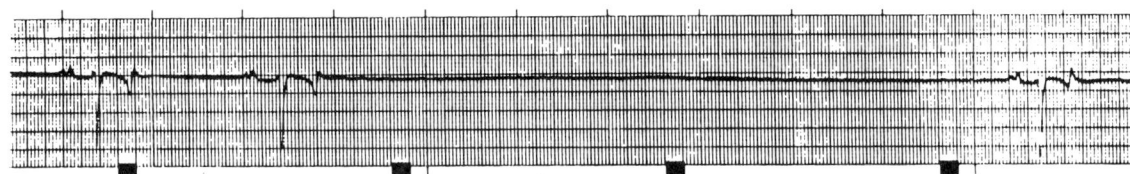

Figure 2. Base-apex ECG from a 2-year-old Thoroughbred filly with sinus arrest. Note the long period (6 seconds) in which there are no P waves on the ECG. The period in which there is no atrial activity is greater than two P-P intervals, and the arrhythmia is therefore termed sinus arest. This arrhythmia was abolished with excitement and atropine.

not occur earlier than the normal P-P interval, whereas the P wave of an APD will occur earlier than normal.

SINUS ARRHYTHMIA, SINOATRIAL BLOCK, SINOATRIAL ARREST

These arrhythmias are characterized by sinus bradycardia and are abolished at elevated heart rates. Sinus arrhythmia is characterized by a slightly irregular rhythm, which may be associated with the respiratory cycle. It is less common in the horse than in the dog. The ECG reveals variable P-P and R-R intervals. Sinus block and sinus arrest are characterized by long diastolic pauses, without P waves observed on the ECG. Sinus block is defined as a pause equal to or less than two P-P intervals, while sinus arrest (Fig. 2) is a pause longer than two P-P intervals. Occasionally, junctional or ventricular escape beats may be observed after a long pause.

PATHOLOGICAL ARRHYTHMIAS

Generally, pathological arrhythmias include premature depolarizations, erratic rhythms, tachycardia (excluding sinus tachycardia), or bradycardia (excluding physiological arrhythmias). Their clinical significance varies depending on the associated clinical signs or source of other cardiac disease. These arrhythmias may be classified as supraventricular (arising from the sinus node, atria, or AV junction) or ventricular in origin.

SUPRAVENTRICULAR ARRHYTHMIAS

Atrial Premature Depolarizations

APDs are characterized by a regular underlying rhythm interrupted by premature beats. The APDs may be followed by a compensatory pause. Atrial premature beats are difficult to distinguish from ventricular premature depolarizations on auscultation and are confirmed by ECG. APDs are characterized by premature P waves, which may differ in morphology from the sinus P wave (Fig. 3). The P wave may also be buried in the ST segment or T wave of the preceding complex, and may not be followed by a QRS-T (Fig. 4). The QRS-T is morphologically normal, although its amplitude may differ slightly or T wave changes may be seen.

APDs may be associated with atrial myocardial disease, noncardiac systemic disease, electrolyte and metabolic imbalances, hypoxia, or toxins. Fevers or viral respiratory infection (historical or concurrent) may be reported in association with viral myocarditis. Elevations in serum cardiac isoenzymes support active myocardial inflammation or injury. APDs may be detected at rest or during recovery from exercise but are unlikely to adversely affect performance unless they are observed during exercise. APDs may predispose horses to the development of atrial fibrillation.

THERAPY

Any suspected underlying cause of the arrhythmia (electrolyte or metabolic imbalance)

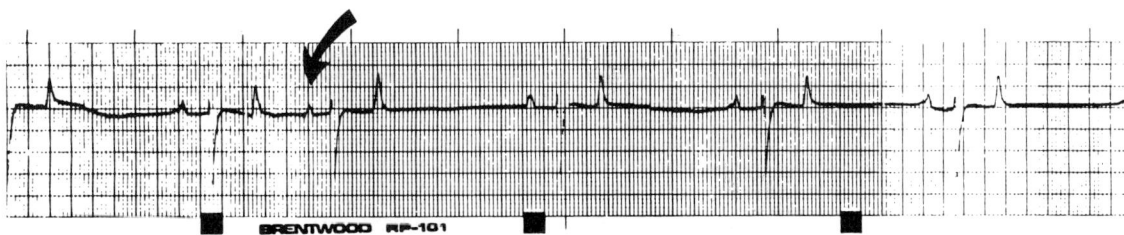

Figure 3. Base-apex ECG from a 5-year-old Standardbred stallion with atrial premature complexes. Note the premature P wave *(arrow)*, which is followed by a normal-appearing QRS-T complex. The premature P wave differs slightly in morphology from the sinus P wave.

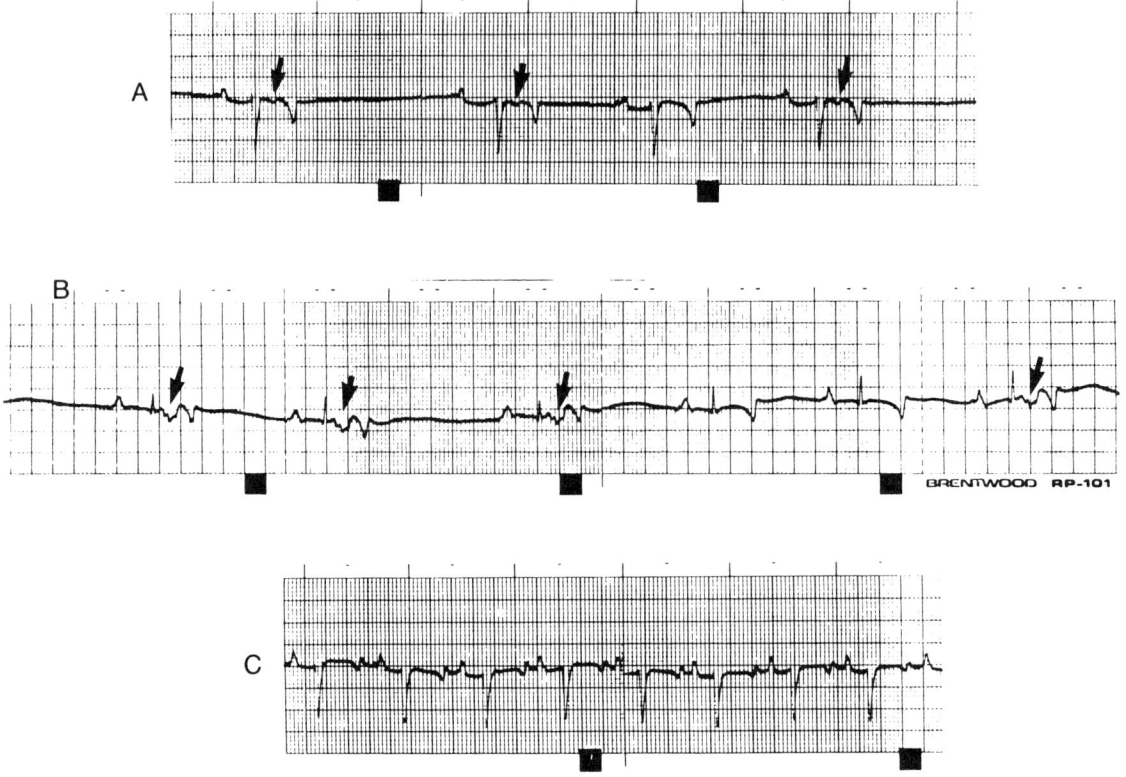

Figure 4. Base apex (A and C) and lead II (B) ECGs from a 10-year-old cross-bred gelding with atrial premature contractions (A and B) and paroxysms of atrial tachycardia (C). Note the inverted nonconducted P waves *(arrows)* within the ST segment of the QRS-T complex. Paroxysms of atrial tachycardia (80 bpm), not associated with any stimulation, were also noted (C).

should be corrected. If exercise intolerance or primary atrial myocardial disease is suspected, the horse should be rested for 1 to 2 months. If the APDs persist, additional rest is unlikely to be beneficial unless active inflammatory myocardial disease is present. Dexamethasone may be considered; however, its use in humans with myocarditis is controversial. Quinidine sulfate is usually effective in abolishing the arrhythmia; however, recurrence is common following discontinuation of the drug. Follow-up evaluation of horses with APDs should include ECG at rest and during and following exercise, and measurement of serum cardiac isoenzymes if initial results were abnormal.

Supraventricular (Atrial) Tachycardia

Supraventricular tachycardias may arise from an atrial ectopic focus or the AV junction (see Fig. 4C) and may be difficult to distinguish from sinus tachycardia. Sinus tachycardia is usually associated with excitement, exercise, pain, or other noncardiac disease or may be a compensatory response to myocardial failure. Horses with sinus tachycardia usually have a gradual change in heart rate (acceleration and deceleration) and it is not suppressed by vagal maneuvers.

Supraventricular tachycardia may be paroxysmal or sustained for more than 30 seconds. Supraventricular tachycardias are usually unifocal, rapid, regular rhythms that start and end abruptly. Variable second-degree AV block is frequently a feature of atrial tachycardia and is a normal mechanism suppressing conduction of APDs (Fig. 5). Auscultation of horses with atrial tachycardia and second-degree AV block reveals an irregularly irregular rhythm similar to atrial fibrillation. Isolated fourth heart sounds may be auscultated in these horses in quiet surroundings. Atrial tachycardia with variable second-degree AV block is common in horses undergoing treatment with quinidine sulfate for atrial fibrillation. This arrhythmia may be indicative of atrial myocardial disease and may be a poor prognostic indicator in horses that develop the arrhythmia while being treated for atrial fibrillation. These horses often have recurrences of atrial fibrillation, and conversion with quinidine sulfate may be unsuccessful.

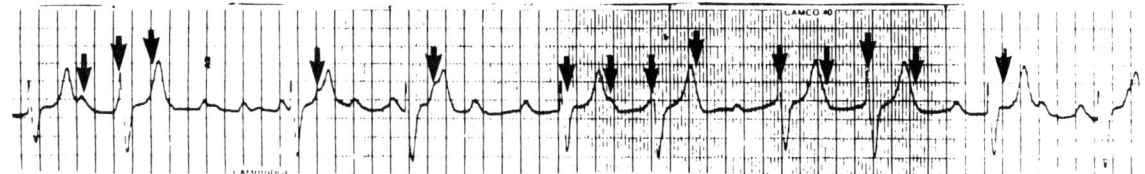

Figure 5. Base-apex ECG from a 6-year-old Thoroughbred gelding that developed atrial tachycardia with second-degree heart block while being treated with quinidine sulfate for atrial fibrillation. Note the rapid atrial rate (140/minute). Several P waves *(arrows)* are buried in the QRS-T complexes. There is variable second-degree AV block and varying PR intervals of the conducted beats, resulting in an irregularly irregular rhythm. Sinus rhythm was eventually restored; however, atrial fibrillation recurred 8 months later.

THERAPY

Quindine sulfate is the antiarrhythmic of choice for treatment of atrial tachycardia in the horse. A dosage of quinidine sulfate at 0.022 g per kg administered by stomach tube every 2 hours is given until the horse converts, gets toxic, or has received a total of five or six treatments in one day. Horses with atrial tachycardia may be more difficult to treat than those with atrial fibrillation and may require long-term (weeks to months) maintenance treatment to suppress the arrhythmia. In these horses quinidine sulfate can be given at a dosage of 0.022 g per kg every 6–12 hours (the longest treatment interval that is successful in suppressing the arrhythmia). If the resting heart rate is above 60 bpm or if myocardial dysfunction exists, digoxin should be administered to slow the ventricular response rate and for its positive inotropic effects. Quinidine is usually contraindicated in horses with congestive heart failure because of its hypotensive and positive chronotropic effects.

In horses that develop atrial tachycardia while undergoing treatment for atrial fibrillation (see Fig. 5), quinidine should be continued unless signs of quinidine toxicity are present. If the ventricular response rate is above 100 to 120 bpm, digoxin (0.002 mg per kg given intravenously [IV] or 0.01 mg per kg per os [PO]) should be given to slow the ventricular response rate.

Atrial Fibrillation

Atrial fibrillation is the most common clinically significant arrhythmia in horses and usually occurs without evidence of underlying cardiac disease. Atrial fibrillation is most frequently detected in racehorses, in which it significantly reduces performance, and may cause additional clinical signs, including pronounced exercise-induced pulmonary hemorrhage. The arrhythmia may also be detected as an incidental finding in horses used for less demanding sports. Horses with congestive heart failure frequently also have atrial fibrillation secondary to the atrial enlargement and underlying cardiac disease.

Auscultation reveals an irregularly irregular rhythm and heart sounds of variable intensity. The ECG reveals fibrillation (f waves) and irregularly spaced QRS-T complexes with normal configuration (Fig. 6). The resting heart rate is normal unless underlying cardiac disease and myocardial dysfunction exist. Grade III/V systolic murmurs suggestive of mitral or tricuspid insufficiency or a heart rate in excess of 60 bpm are negative prognostic indicators in horses with atrial fibrillation. The duration of atrial fibrillation may be difficult to determine, but it may be inferred from the horse's performance history. Horses with a short duration of atrial fibrillation are more likely to convert to sinus rhythm with quinidine sulfate, often require a smaller dose to effect conversion, and are less likely to have side effects from the quinidine sulfate or a recurrence of the arrhythmia.

THERAPY

Horses with congestive heart failure and atrial fibrillation should be treated with digoxin and furosemide. The goal of treatment is not to restore sinus rhythm but to provide medical management of the congestive heart failure. Quinidine may exacerbate congestive heart failure due to its hypotensive and positive chronotropic effects. The prognosis for these horses is grave due to the underlying cardiac disease and congestive heart failure.

Mitral regurgitation is the most common valvular insufficiency in horses with atrial fibrillation. Horses with tricuspid or mitral regurgitation with normal myocardial function and normal resting heart rates may, in general, be amenable to treatment with quinidine sulfate. Echocardiography should be performed to evaluate chamber sizes and myocardial function. Doppler echocardiography may also be used to confirm and map regurgitant jets. Horses with valvular regurgitation resulting in atrial dilation are at an increased risk for recurrence of atrial fibrillation.

The majority of horses with atrial fibrillation have no evidence of significant underlying cardiac disease and are candidates for treatment

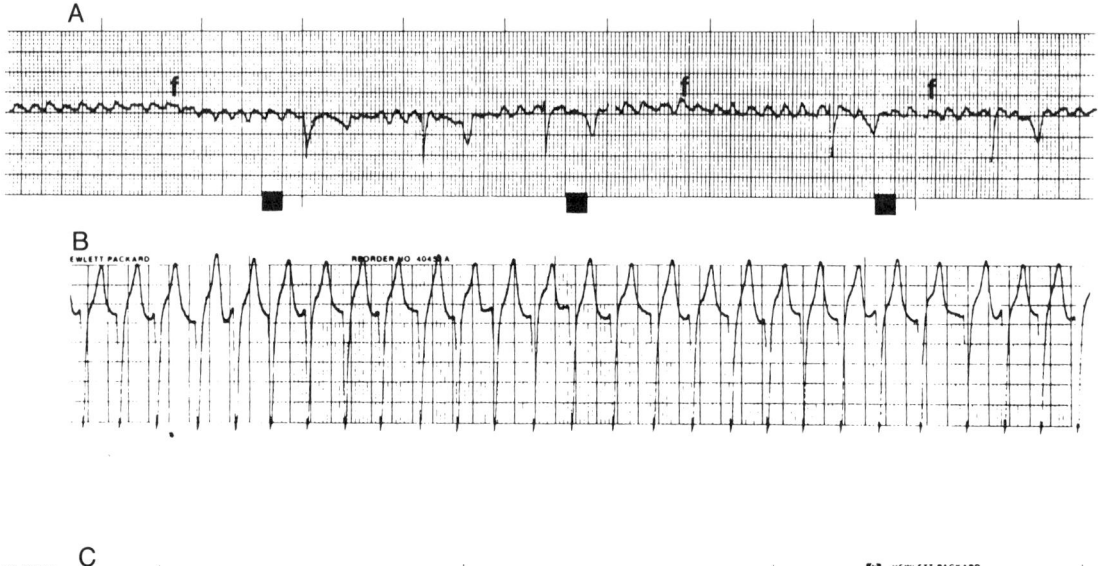

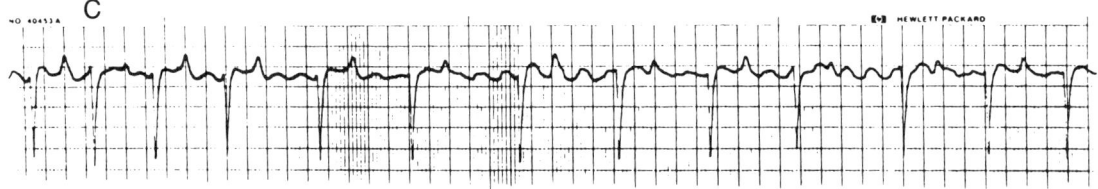

Figure 6. Base-apex ECG from a 5-year-old Standardbred stallion with atrial fibrillation (A). Note the fibrillation waves (f) and irregular ventricular response rate. After three doses of quinidine sulfate given 2 hours apart, supraventricular tachycardia (160 bpm) developed (B). Following treatment with digoxin (1 mg IV) and sodium bicarbonate (150 mEq IV), the heart rate slowed, was irregularly irregular, and fibrillation waves were evident (C). Digoxin therapy was continued and the horse successfully converted to sinus rhythm with quinidine sulfate (three doses given 2 hours apart) the following day.

with quinidine sulfate. Conversion to sinus rhythm usually results in a return to the previous level of performance. Occasionally, horses will spontaneously convert to sinus rhythm within 24 hours. In acute cases of atrial fibrillation (less than 1 week in duration), quinidine gluconate (2.2 mg per kg IV given as a bolus every 10 minutes, up to 8 to 10 mg per kg total dose) may be administered to restore sinus rhythm. If sinus rhythm is not restored, quinidine sulfate (0.022 mg per kg via stomach tube) should be given every 2 hours until sinus rhythm is restored (a total of five to six treatments has been given in one day) or evidence of toxicity such as diarrhea, urticaria, ataxia, nasal mucosal edema, or tachycardia is observed. The ECG should be monitored before each treatment for widening of the QRS. Quinidine treatment should be discontinued if the QRS duration increases by more than 25 per cent of the pretreatment value, as quinidine levels are likely to be in the toxic range. Inappetence and depression are commonly observed in horses given quinidine sulfate. Laminitis has not been observed at the currently recommended dosage. Horses should not be moved during treatment because of quinidine's hypotensive effects and the potential for rapid supraventricular tachycardias, both of which may result in collapse. There are occasional reports of sudden death associated with quinidine sulfate administration.

The heart rate should be monitored carefully during treatment. If the heart rate rises above 100 to 120 bpm (see Fig. 6B), digoxin (0.002 mg per kg) should be administered IV. Occasionally, horses may develop rapid supraventricular tachycardias (200 to 300 bpm). The rapid heart rate in combination with quinidine's hypotensive effects may cause collapse and death if not corrected immediately. Digoxin should be given IV in an attempt to slow the ventricular response rate. Sodium bicarbonate (1 mEq per kg) may also be given to increase protein binding of free quinidine and thereby lower active drug levels. Phenylephrine (10 mg in 500 ml of 0.9% saline administered as a fast drip) and large volumes of IV fluids should be administered to alleviate hypotension. Activated charcoal or oil could also be administered PO to limit further absorption of quinidine sulfate from the gastrointestinal (GI) tract.

Although quinidine and digoxin compete for

the same plasma protein binding sites and digoxin toxicity may develop, short-term use of both drugs simultaneously rarely produces adverse effects. Ideally, quinidine and digoxin concentrations should be monitored during treatment. The therapeutic range for digoxin is 0.5 to 2.0 ng per ml and for quinidine sulfate is 2.0 to 5.0 µg per ml.

If sinus rhythm is not restored after five or six treatments given at 2-hour intervals, the dosage interval may be increased to every 6 hours. Digoxin (0.01 mg per kg PO) may also be administered on day 2 if conversion has not occurred. Once sinus rhythm has been restored, quinidine and digoxin should be discontinued. An ECG should be obtained approximately 24 hours later to check for supraventricular premature depolarizations once the quinidine level has dropped below the therapeutic range. APDs indicate an increased risk for recurrence of atrial fibrillation. Continued antiarrhythmic therapy (quinidine or digoxin), anti-inflammatory therapy (corticosteroids), and rest may be considered in these horses. Horses may be returned to training after conversion unless active atrial myocardial disease is suspected. If an active myocarditis is present, if adverse effects developed during treatment, or if the horse had a history of pronounced exercise-induced pulmonary hemorrhage or myopathy associated with atrial fibrillation, an additional period of rest may be warranted before training is resumed.

Once converted, the heart rhythm should be monitored regularly before exercise to ensure that atrial fibrillation has not recurred. The heart should be ausculted carefully if the horse trains poorly or develops exercise-induced pulmonary hemorrhage or myopathy. If atrial fibrillation recurs and does not spontaneously resolve within 24 hours, treatment should be undertaken as soon as possible. Horses with atrial fibrillation that are used in less demanding sports such as dressage, show jumping, or pleasure riding or as breeding animals may perform without problems, providing significant underlying cardiac disease is not present. In such cases, there may be little benefit in treating these horses for atrial fibrillation.

Pre-excitation

Ventricular pre-excitation has been reported infrequently in horses. Auscultation is normal unless it is associated with bouts of supraventricular tachycardia (Wolff–Parkinson–White syndrome). Pre-excitation may be an incidental ECG finding and diagnosed on the basis of a shortened PR interval (<.22 seconds) at a normal resting heart rate (Fig. 7). The QRS complexes may or may not be abnormal in configuration. Supraventricular tachycardia associated with pre-excitation (Wolff–Parkinson–White syndrome) has not been recognized in the horse. Pre-excitation did not appear to affect performance in the horses in which it has been reported.

Advanced Second-Degree and Third-Degree AV Block

These arrhythmias are uncommon in the horse and are usually associated with inflammatory or

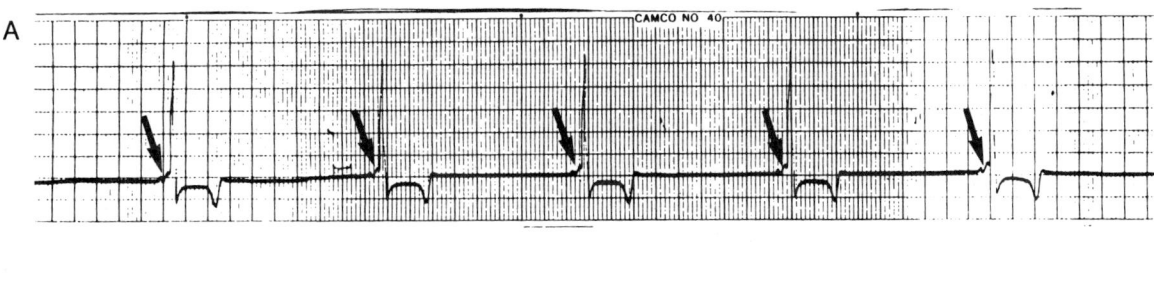
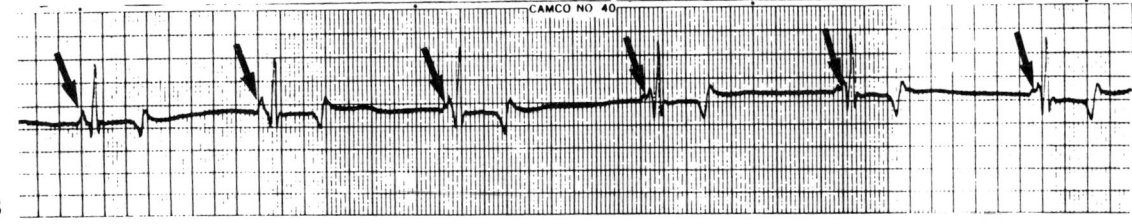

Figure 7. Base-apex (A) and lead II (B) ECGs from a 3-year-old Thoroughbred colt with ventricular pre-excitation. Notice the extremely short PR interval *(arrows)*. Aberrant ventricular conduction is particularly noticeable in the base-apex ECG, where the QRS is positive rather than negative. The pre-excitation was initially detected on an ECG obtained during an elective surgical procedure.

degenerative AV nodal disease. Horses may have syncopal episodes or may be severely exercise intolerant with advanced second-degree or complete heart block. Auscultation reveals a low-normal or very slow heart rate that does not increase in response to exercise, excitement, or atropine. In advanced second-degree AV block the ECG reveals frequent P waves not followed by QRS and T complexes with occasional conducted beats (Fig. 8). Occasionally, junctional or ventricular escape complexes may be seen. In complete or third-degree AV block, P waves are detected without associated QRS-T complexes (AV dissociation) with an independent and slower junctional or ventricular escape rhythm. Junctional depolarizations have a normal QRS morphology and an abnormally premature or absent P wave, occurring 20 to 30 times per minute. The P waves may occur before, during, or after the premature QRS. Ventricular depolarizations have an abnormal QRS configuration (widened and bizarre) with the T wave usually oriented in the opposite direction to the QRS. The idioventricular rhythm is approximately 10 to 20 bpm. The definitive treatment is a cardiac pacemaker, which has been implanted successfully in the horse. Corticosteroids may be of benefit if active inflammatory AV nodal disease is suspected. Dobutamine or vagolytic drugs may occasionally be of benefit in the short-term management of these arrhythmias, particularly in those that develop under anesthesia.

VENTRICULAR ARRHYTHMIAS

Ventricular Premature Depolarizations

Ventricular premature depolarizations (VPDs) occur less frequently than APDs in the horse. Auscultation reveals premature beats, usually followed by a compensatory pause. VPDs may be detected in horses with systemic disease, primary myocardial disease, toxemia, electrolyte or metabolic imbalances, or hypoxia. Horses may present with exercise intolerance or VPDs may be detected as an incidental finding. The ECG (Fig. 9) reveals premature QRS-T depolarizations which differ morphologically from the normal QRS-T, with the T wave usually oriented in the opposite direction to the QRS. The VPDs may be normal or wider in duration than the normal QRS-T. The VPDs may occur at fixed or varying intervals following the normal QRS.

THERAPY

If VPDs are associated with other systemic disease and do not cause significant hemodynamic alterations, specific antiarrhythmic therapy is unnecessary. If VPDs are suspected to be associated with poor performance in otherwise healthy horses, an ECG should be obtained during exercise. A 24-hour Holter monitor may also be considered to more accurately determine the frequency of the VPDs. Elevated serum cardiac isoenzyme levels may indicate active myocardial disease. VPDs are likely to be significant if they

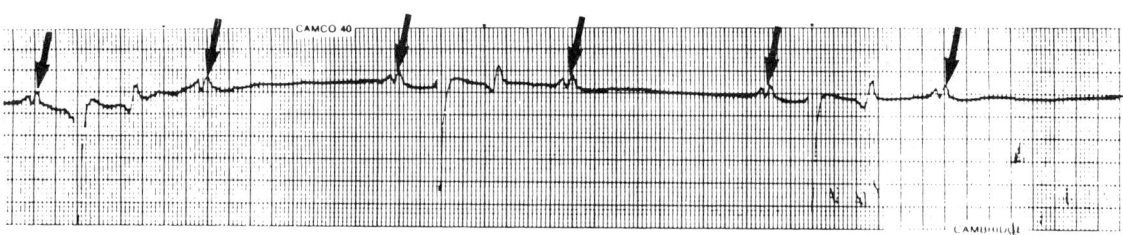

Figure 8. Base-apex ECG from a 7-year-old Quarter Horse gelding following treatment with dexamethasone for multiple episodes of syncope associated with complete heart block (ECG not shown). The rhythm was temporarily converted to 2:1 second-degree AV block. Note the slow heart rate (20 bpm) and the P waves *(arrows)*, which are conducted at every other beat.

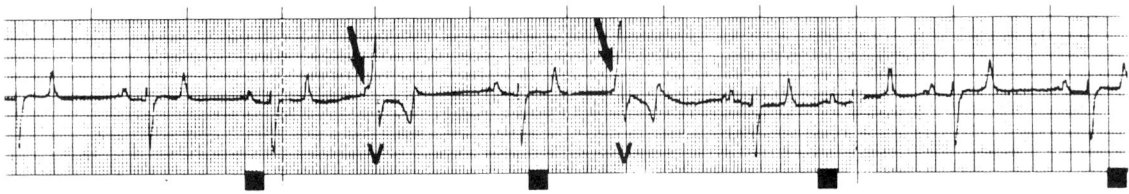

Figure 9. Base-apex ECG from a 20-year-old Thoroughbred gelding with ventricular premature depolarization (VPD) (v). The P waves are partially buried in the QRS of the VPDs *(arrows)*.

are frequent, multifocal, the R-on-T phenomenon exists, or if they increase in frequency with exercise or result in exercise intolerance. VPDs may be a reflection of primary myocardial disease and, if frequent, the horse should be stall rested, with monthly reevaluation. Corticosteroids may be indicated if myocarditis is suspected. Antiarrhythmic therapy is usually not indicated unless the arrhythmias are life-threatening (see Ventricular Tachycardia below). Most horses with VPDs without evidence of significant cardiac disease have a good prognosis and the VPDs resolve without specific antiarrhythmic therapy. If significant primary myocardial disease exists, digoxin and furosemide may be required for treatment of myocardial failure, although digoxin may exacerbate ventricular arrhythmias.

Ventricular Tachycardia and Accelerated Idioventricular Rhythm

Ventricular tachycardia is defined as four or more VPDs ocurring in succession. Ventricular tachycardia may be paroxysmal or sustained, uniform (one VPD waveform) or multiform. An accelerated idioventricular rhythm is defined as four or more successive VPDs occurring at a rate similar to the sinus rate (in the horse, 50 VPDs per minute or less). Ventricular tachycardia and accelerated idioventricular rhythms (Fig. 10) are most commonly associated with extracardiac systemic disease. Ventricular arrhythmias may also be associated with toxemia, metabolic imbalances, trauma, toxins (such as monensin), drugs (such as digoxin), and inhalation anesthetics. In horses with GI disease, the arrhythmia often is not noticed until 24 to 48 hours after the onset of clincal signs.

THERAPY

The majority of these arrhythmias will resolve as the underlying disease is corrected; however, antiarrhythmic therapy is warranted in horses with rapid ventricular tachycardia (greater than 100 bpm), multiform VPDs, or R-on-T phenomenon. Any electrolyte or metabolic imbalance should also be corrected, as it may have a role in the genesis of the arrhythmia or reduce the efficacy of antiarrhythmic drugs. The arrhythmia should be treated if it causes clinically significant hemodynamic effects. If the animal is hypovolemic, correcting the arrhythmia may improve the patient's hemodynamic status. Thus a systemically normal horse with ventricular tachycardia of 80 bpm may tolerate the arrhythmia with minimal hemodynamic effects, whereas a horse with severe diarrhea may be more hemodynamically compromised by the arrhythmia.

Antiarrhythmic therapy may include quinidine sulfate, quinidine gluconate, or lidocaine hydrochloride (Table 1). Quinidine gluconate may be given by IV bolus or drip. Administration of the drug as a drip may minimize quinidine's hypotensive effects. Lidocaine may also be administered as an IV bolus and continued as an IV drip if it appears to be effective. Lidocaine may cause central nervous system excitability in horses; however, it may be best for treating ventricular arrhythmias on an emergency basis, and in treating horses with severe myocardial dysfunction. Quinidine sulfate may be given PO to horses with minimal hemodynamic compromise, normal GI function, and ventricular arrhythmias that do not require immediate resolution. Phenytoin is reportedly most effective in restoring sinus rhythm in animals with digoxin-induced ventricular and supraventricular arrhythmias. Propranolol may also be effective in controlling supraventricular and ventricular tachyarrhythmias; however, there is little information regarding its efficacy in the horse. Because of its negative inotropic effects propranolol should not be used in horses with depressed myocardial function. Magnesium sulfate (up to 10 gm IV) has been used successfuly in the treatment of ventricular arrhythmias in human beings with normal and decreased serum magnesium levels. Magnesium sulfate appears to be beneficial for the treatment

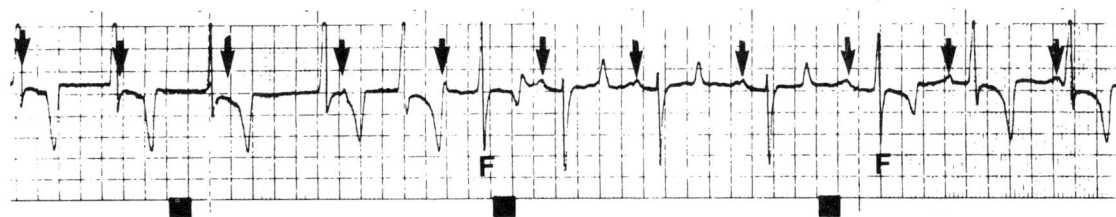

Figure 10. Base-apex ECG from a 12-year-old Thoroughbred mare with sinus tachycardia and paroxysmal uniform ventricular tachycardia that developed 24 hours after surgery for an ileal impaction. The ventricular premature depolarizations (VPDs) (positive QRS complexes) occurred at a rate of 60 to 75 per minute. There is a sinus tachycardia (negative QRSs) of approximately 60 bpm. Note the two fusion beats (F), and the P waves *(arrows)*, many of which are buried in the VPDs. The arrhythmia resolved within 12 hours without treatment.

TABLE 1. DRUGS USED IN THE MANAGEMENT OF CARDIAC ARRHYTHMIAS IN THE HORSE

Drug	Dose	Indications	Adverse Effects	Drugs to Counteract Adverse Effects
Digoxin	IV: 0.002 mg/kg (1 mg/450 kg) b.i.d. PO: 0.01 mg/kg (5 mg/450 kg) b.i.d.	Congestive heart failure, supraventricular tachycardia	Supraventricular ventricular tachycardia, depression, anorexia	Phenytoin (for arrhythmias)
Quinidine	PO: 0.022 mg/kg (10 gm/450 kg) q. 2–6 h. IV: 2.2 mg/kg bolus every 10 minutes to 8–10 mg/kg total IV drip: 0.064% solution,° 0.7–3 mg/kg/hr (½–2 L/hr/450 kg)	Supraventricular (atrial fibrillation) and ventricular arrhythmias	Supraventricular tachycardia, hypotension, depression, anorexia	Digoxin, sodium bicarbonate, phenylephrine (0.5–1 mEq/kg)
Lidocaine	IV: 0.5 mg/kg IV bolus every 5 minutes to 2.0–4.0 mg/kg total	Ventricular tachycardia	CNS excitability, seizures	Valium, phenobarbital
Propranolol	PO: 0.38–0.78 mg/kg (175–350 mg/450 kg) t.i.d. IV: 0.05–0.16 mg/kg (25–75 mg/450 kg) b.i.d.	Tachycardia	Bradycardia, AV block	Atropine
Phenytoin	PO: 10–22 mg/kg (4–10 gm/450 kg) b.i.d.	Digoxin-induced arrhythmias	Sedation, head twitching	
Atropine	IV: 0.01–0.015 mg/kg (5–7 mg/450 kg)	Bradycardia	Tachycardia, ileus	
Dexamethasone	IV or PO: 0.02–0.2 mg/kg (10–100 mg/450 kg) in decreasing doses	Suspected immune-mediated myocarditis (VCPs, APCs), advanced 2nd-degree or complete heart block	Laminitis, iatrogenic adrenal insufficiency, exacerbation of bacterial and viral myocarditis and other infections	

° A 0.064% solution of quinidine gluconate may be made by mixing 3.2 gm of quinidine gluconate (four 800-mg vials) in a 10-liter bag of isotonic intravenous fluids.

of ventricular arrhythmias in the horse; however, more clinical experience is needed before dosage recommendations and comments regarding efficacy can be made.

Supplemental Readings

Hilwig, R. W.: Cardiac arrhythmias in the horse. J. Am Vet. Med. Assoc., 170:153, 1977.

McGuirck, S. M., and Muir, W. W.: Diagnosis and treatment of cardiac arrhythmias. Vet. Clin. North. Am. (Equine Pract.), 1:353–370, 1985.
Muir, W. W., and McGuirck, S. M.: Ventricular preexcitation in two horses. J. Am. Vet. Med. Assoc., 183:573, 1983.
Reef, V. B., Levitan, C. W., and Spencer, P. A.: Factors affecting prognosis and conversion in equine atrial fibrillation. J. Vet. Intern Med., 2:1, 1988.

Myocardial Disease

Virginia B. Reef, KENNETT SQUARE, PENNSYLVANIA

Myocardial disease occurs infrequently in horses, although it may be more common than previously reported. Prior to the advent of equine echocardiography myocardial disease in horses was usually diagnosed at postmortem examination. Myocardial degeneration, necrosis, inflammation, and fibrosis were also reported in association with exposure of horses to the ionophore antibiotics, particularly monensin. Myocardial injury may result from toxic, viral, bacterial, traumatic, ischemic, hypoxic, or metabolic insults, from aberrant parasite migration, or by extension from a preexisting pericarditis or endocarditis. Abnormal myocardial function may be associated with poor performance and may complicate therapy for other disease processes.

CLINICAL SIGNS

A wide variety of clinical signs may be exhibited by horses with myocardial dysfunction, ranging from mild changes in performance to collapse and congestive heart failure. In many horses the change in performance is small, such as a few seconds longer race time, or the horse stops near the end of the race. After exercise, a prolonged time to return to resting respiratory rate and a long time to cool out are common complaints. Exercise-induced weakness or ataxia are frequent, owing to poor cardiac output. Cardiac arrhythmias, either supraventricular or ventricular, occur frequently in horses with myocardial disease. Pulmonary edema, venous distention, and peripheral edema are signs of advanced myocardial disease.

Auscultation may be normal or murmurs of valvular insufficiency, particularly atrioventricular valvular insufficiency, may be detected in horses with congestive heart failure. Peripheral arterial pulses are often weaker than normal, and systolic blood pressure is usually normal or low. Harsh lung sounds may be detected on auscultation of the thorax. The resting heart rate is usually normal unless congestive heart failure is present. Venous distention, jugular pulsations, peripheral edema, and pulmonary edema are present in horses with congestive heart failure. Premature supraventricular or ventricular depolarizations or atrial fibrillation may be detected.

DIAGNOSIS

Echocardiography is the method of choice for diagnosing myocardial disease in the horse. Both M-mode and two-dimensional real-time echocardiography are useful in assessing the degree of impairment of left ventricular (LV) function (see *Current Therapy in Equine Medicine 2*, p. 139). The heart should be examined carefully for any evidence of coexisting valvular or pericardial disease. Reduced ejection fraction, shortened ejection time, and reduced fractional shortening are characteristically found in horses with myocardial disease (Fig. 1). LV enlargement with increased end-diastolic and end-systolic dimensions and volumes is also frequently detected. Right ventricular enlargement is uncommon unless congestive heart failure or advanced myocardial disease is present. Mitral valve motion may be abnormal in diastole due to diminished LV compliance and elevated end-diastolic pressure. Spontaneous contrast may be seen in the LV in the presence of very poor LV function (Fig. 2). Abnormalities of the myocardium itself are infrequently seen except in horses that have been exposed to the ionophore antibiotics. In some horses with cardiac arrhythmias, echogenic

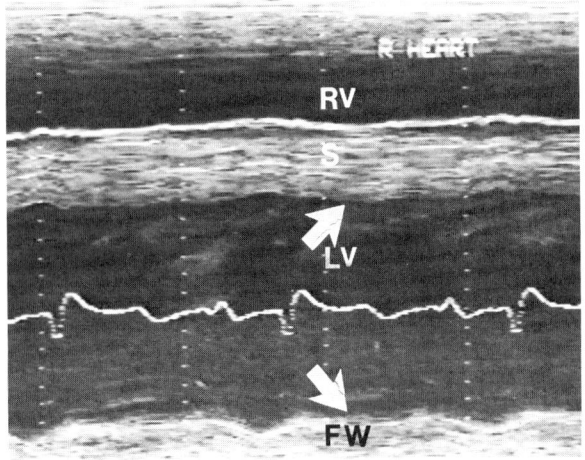
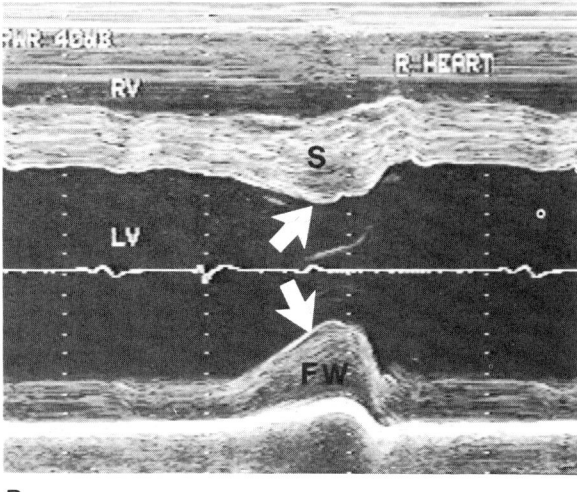

Figure 1. M-mode echocardiograms obtained at the right parasternal left ventricular position. (A) M-mode echocardiogram of a 4-year-old Thoroughbred gelding with acute monensin toxicosis. Note minimal thickening (arrows) of the left ventricular free wall (FW) and the interventricular septum (S) in systole (compare Fig. 1B). The shortening fraction was 8%. The electrocardiogram (base apex lead) is superimposed for timing. (RV = right ventricle, LV = left ventricle.) (B) M-mode echocardiogram of a normal 3-year-old Thoroughbred filly. Note thickening of the interventricular septum (S) and left ventricular free wall (FW) in systole (arrows). The shortening fraction was normal at 40%. The electrocardiogram (base apex lead) is superimposed for timing. (RV = right ventricle, LV = left ventricle.)

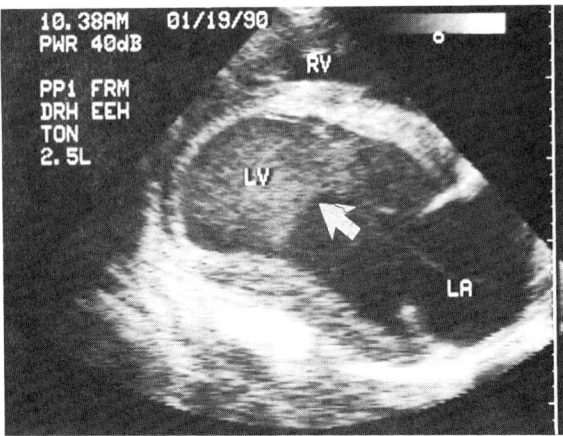

Figure 2. Real-time two-dimensional echocardiogram obtained at the right parasternal four-chamber position from a 4-year-old Thoroughbred gelding with acute monensin toxicosis. Note spontaneous appearance of contrast (arrows points to echogenic blood) at the apex of the left ventricle (LV). (LA = left atrium, RV = right ventricle.)

Figure 3. Real-time two-dimensional echocardiogram obtained at the right parasternal four-chamber position in a 10-year-old Thoroughbred gelding with acute onset of exercise intolerance at a combined training event. Auscultation of the heart revealed frequent ventricular premature contractions. An echogenic mass (black arrow) was imaged in the interventricular septum (IVS). (RV = right ventricle, LV = left ventricle.) White arrow points to the septal leaflet of the mitral valve (MV).

areas within the interventricular septum (Fig. 3) or LV free wall have been imaged but occasionally these may be an incidental finding in an otherwise normal animal.

Electrocardiography (ECG) should be performed in all horses with suspected myocardial disease. Abnormalities of the ST segment and T wave may be detected in horses with acute myocardial necrosis. Both supraventricular and ventricular arrhythmias may occur in the presence of acute and chronic myocardial injury. In some horses sinus tachycardia is present at rest with no other ECG abnormalities. If the resting cardiovascular examination is normal an exercise ECG may be indicated. Heart rates inappropriate for each level of exercise or sustained tachycardia following exercise are indications of myocardial dysfunction. Immediate postexercise echocardiography may also be useful in diagnosing mild functional abnormalities. Significant decreases in fractional shortening and ejection fraction may be detected and may be associated with the development of fatigue on exercise.

Cardiac isoenzyme determinations may also be useful in horses with acute myocardial injury. The isoenzymes of creatine phosphokinase (CKMB) and lactic dehydrogenase (LDH 1 and 2) may be elevated in horses with significant myocardial cell injury, usually myocardial necrosis. However, normal values for these isoenzymes does not rule out the possibility of myocardial disease.

The horse should be carefully evaluated for the presence of other disease processes or other metabolic abnormalities such as electrolyte imbalances, endocrine disorders, nutritional disorders, and other disease processes that may all result in abnormal myocardial function (Fig. 4). Paired serology for a rising titer to equine respiratory viruses may be indicated if a viral etiology is suspected. In many horses, however, the viral disease precedes the onset of clinical signs by weeks to months and a rising titer is no longer demonstrable. The horse's feed should be carefully evaluated to rule out possible exposure to ionophore-contaminated feed, either through accidental mixing at the feed mill or exposure of the horse to feed formulated for poultry or beef cattle.

THERAPY

Therapy for horses with myocardial disease should include stall rest and antiarrhythmic therapy when indicated. Correction of any underlying electrolyte abnormalities or treatment of any underlying disease processes should be performed and may result in the resolution of myocardial diseases associated with these etiological agents. Corticosteroid therapy may also be indicated if an immune-mediated myocarditis is suspected but should not be used if an active viremia is likely. The use of corticosteroids is controversial, as corticosteroids are known to be associated with the recrudescence of viral diseases. However, clinical responses to the use of corticosteroids in horses with myocardial dysfunction have been noted.

If exposure to a toxic substance is suspected the horse should be treated with mineral oil or charcoal administered through a stomach tube, if consumption of contaminated feed was recent. Vitamin E may have a protective effect in acute myocardial injury and should be considered if an acute toxic insult is suspected. Symptomatic therapy with positive ionotropic agents may be indicated in horses with severe myocardial injury. However, digoxin is contraindicated in horses with acute monensin toxicosis.

Horses must be given a guarded prognosis for recovery until response to therapy can be evaluated. Horses without significant cardiac enlargement have the best prognosis for recovery and return to normal function if the underlying disease can be successfully treated or the inciting insult is sublethal. If severe LV dilation has occurred, return to normal cardiac function is unlikely except in unusual cases such as severe hypocalcemia. However, horses with acute congestive heart failure and acute severe myocardial dysfunction have recovered completely and been able to return to racing with aggressive supportive and positive inotropic therapy. Often the etiological agent cannot be determined definitively but a variety of drug hypersensitivities or adverse drug reactions must be considered, particularly in the racing individual.

Supplemental Readings

Cranley, J. J., and McCullagh, K. G.: Ischaemic myocardial fibrosis and aortic strongylosis in the horse. Equine Vet. J., 13:35, 1981.

Doonan, G. R., Brown, C. M., Mullany, T. P. et al.: Monensin poisoning in horses: An international incident. Can. Vet. J., 30:165, 1989.

Else, R. W., and Holmes, J. R.: Cardiac pathology in the horse: 2. Microscopic pathology. Equine Vet. J., 4:57, 1972.

Mollenhauer, H. H., Rowe, L. D., Cysewski, S. J., and Witzel, D. A.: Ultrastructural observations in ponies after treatment with monensin. Am. J. Vet. Res., 42:35, 1981.

Van Amstel, S. R., and Guthrie, A. J.: Salinomycin poisoning in horses: Case report. Proceedings of the 31st Annual Convention of the American Association of Equine Practitioners, 1985, p. 373.

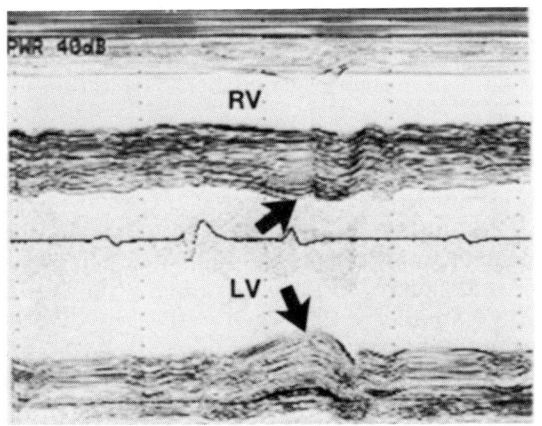

Figure 4. M-mode echocardiogram obtained at the left ventricular position in a 4-year-old Standardbred gelding with poor racing performance. The horse had exercise-induced weakness, ataxia, and a shortening fraction of 20%. Note poor thickening of the interventricular septum and left venticular free wall (arrows) during systole. The electrocardiogram (base apex lead) is superimposed for timing. The primary underlying disease in this horse was thoracic lymphosarcoma. (RV = right ventricle, LV = left ventricle.)

Acquired Valvular Heart Disease

Celia M. Marr, KENNETT SQUARE, PENNSYLVANIA

Degenerative lesions on equine heart valves are commonly found on postmortem examination, but the prevalence of clinical valvular heart disease is low. Inflammatory changes have been reported infrequently. In most instances the heart compensates for the valvular disease and performance is not affected. However, valvular disease can result in reduced performance and cardiac failure. The clinical impact of a valvular lesion depends on which valve is affected and on the severity of regurgitation.

Valvular disease can affect cardiac function in two ways: a lesion may affect the competence of the valve, rendering it insufficient; or it may produce an obstruction to forward flow (stenosis). Stenotic lesions are uncommon in horses and valvular heart disease is primarily manifested as acquired valvular insufficiency.

MURMURS

Cardiac murmurs are produced by disruption of laminar blood flow. They are common in horses and ponies of all types, with frequencies of up to 66 per cent reported in Thoroughbred racehorses. These murmurs are usually functional or physiological, the result of normal hemodynamic events. Careful auscultation and evaluation of the timing of the murmur, its intensity, point of maximum intensity, radiation, and the quality of the murmur will usually allow the clinician to separate individuals that have a functional murmur from those that require further investigation.

Physiological murmurs that are heard during systole are usually related to the ejection of blood from the ventricles into the great vessels and are often described as ejection murmurs. These murmurs are most commonly detected over the aortic and pulmonic valve areas and vary from grade I to grade III/VI in intensity. Exercise or excitement may increase or decrease the intensity of the murmur. Ejection murmurs are usually localized, early to midsystolic or holosystolic, and have a crescendo-decrescendo quality. In contrast, a regurgitant systolic murmur usually has its point of maximal intensity over one of the atrioventricular valves, radiates over a wider area (usually dorsad to the respective atria), is grade II to grade VI/VI, is holosystolic or pansystolic, and is band-shaped or crescendo in quality. Functional murmurs are also common in early diastole, grade I to grade III/VI, decrescendo or musical, and are loudest at the heart base. Holodiastolic murmurs are not physiological but are associated with semilunar valvular insufficiency, which is most commonly aortic.

ECHOCARDIOGRAPHY

Echocardiographic examination is recommended in any horse in which valvular heart disease is suspected. Two-dimensional images may demonstrate valvular abnormalities, volume overload, chamber enlargement, and abnormalities of cardiac function. M-mode echocardiography is useful for characterizing abnormalities of valve motion and for measurements of chamber and vessel size. Flow mapping is performed with pulsed wave or color flow Doppler echocardiography. However, the demonstration of valvular regurgitation does not imply that a lesion is clinically significant. Color flow Doppler studies in normal horses have confirmed that small regurgitant jets may occur commonly at the aortic and tricuspid valves and less frequently at the mitral and pulmonic valves. All echocardiographic findings must be interpreted in conjunction with the history, clinical examination, and other findings to characterize the hemodynamic and clinical impact of valvular regurgitation.

LEFT ATRIOVENTRICULAR VALVULAR INSUFFICIENCY

Postmortem studies have reported that the left atrioventricular (AV) (mitral) valve is the second most common site for degenerative valvular disease in the horse. However, mitral regurgitation is the most likely valvular insufficiency to cause impaired performance, exercise intolerance, congestive heart failure, and death.

CLINICAL SIGNS AND DIAGNOSIS

Presenting signs of left AV valvular insufficiency may vary from an incidental finding on a prepurchase or insurance examination to acute respiratory distress, coughing, and pulmonary edema. Elevated resting respiratory and heart rates, prolonged recovery time to resting respiratory and heart rates, and atrial fibrillation may be reported. Degenerative lesions usually progress slowly, while acute decompensation occurs with ruptured chordae tendineae. An insidious onset may not be appreciated by the owner until exercise intolerance is extreme or until congestive heart failure ensues.

The murmur of left AV valvular regurgitation is usually grade II/VI or louder, pansystolic or holosystolic, with its point of maximal intensity in the left fifth intercostal space. It radiates toward the heart base and is usually harsh and crescendo or band-shaped. A precordial thrill is palpable at the point of maximum intensity if the murmur is grade IV/VI or louder. If pulmonary edema is present, the respiratory rate and effort are often increased and harsh breath sounds are usually auscultated. Dependent edema, jugular distention, and pulsations may accompany respiratory signs in horses with degenerative mitral valve disease and slowly deteriorating cardiac function. Rupture of the pulmonary artery has been seen in horses with chronic mitral regurgitation secondary to dilation of the pulmonary artery by chronic pulmonary hypertension.

Echocardiographic findings include thickening of the valve cusps, a vegetative lesion, prolapse of a portion of the valve into the left atria, and/or ruptured mitral chordae tendineae. Left atrial and ventricular volume overload increases as the mitral regurgitation becomes more severe (Fig. 1). The extent of the regurgitant jet is mapped with pulsed wave or color flow Doppler echocardiography to semiquantify its severity. This study is most easily performed from the left cardiac window.

AORTIC VALVULAR INSUFFICIENCY

The aortic valve is the most common site for degenerative valve lesions reported at postmortem examination in the horse. Nodular or fibrous band lesions running parallel to the free edge of the valve cusps and generally involving the left coronary cusp are most frequently described. Diastolic murmurs of aortic insufficiency are common in adult horses, particularly older individuals, but the disease is usually well tolerated and clinical signs associated with it are infrequent.

CLINICAL SIGNS AND DIAGNOSIS

The aortic regurgitation murmur is holodiastolic, grade II/VI or louder, with its point of maximal intensity over the aortic valve area and radiating toward the left apex. It may be soft and decrescendo, harsh or musical. With left volume overload, the arterial pulses are bounding or hyperkinetic due to the falling diastolic pressure and the large difference between peak systolic and end-diastolic pressure. Usually performance is not affected. However, in horses with severe aortic insufficiency, poor performance may be noticed.

Echocardiographic examination may demonstrate nodular, parallel fibrous band, or endocarditis lesions, prolapse, or a flail cusp (Fig. 2). The

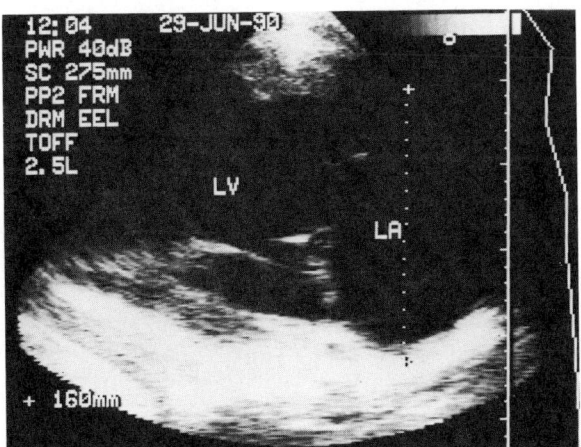

Figure 1. A long-axis echocardiogram illustrating left atrial (LA) and left ventricular (LV) dilation in a 5-year-old Thoroughbred with moderate mitral regurgitation. The size of the left atrium (160 mm) can be assessed most accurately from this image. The electronic callipers (+) indicate the measurement points.

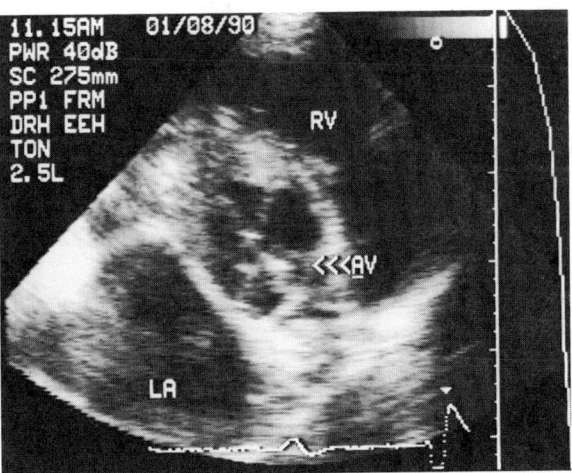

Figure 2. A right parasternal short-axis echocardiogram of the aortic valve in a 26-year-old Thoroughbred gelding. Note echogenic nodules (arrows) on the left coronary cusp of the aortic valve (AV). (RV = right ventricle, LA = left atrium.)

398 / ACQUIRED VALVULAR HEART DISEASE—continued

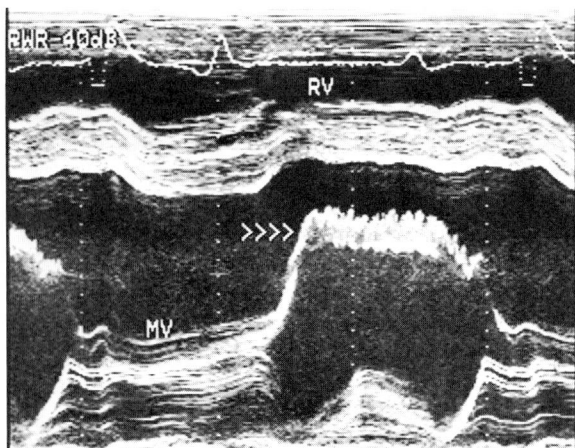

Figure 3. An M-mode echocardiogram of the mitral valve in a 26-year-old Thoroughbred gelding with aortic insufficiency. The septal leaflet of the mitral valve (MV) is fluttering in diastole (arrows). There is also early closure of the mitral valve. (RV = right ventricle.)

left ventricle (LV) may be volume overloaded with a large end-diastolic diameter, rounded apex, and exaggerated motion of the septal wall and free wall. Diastolic flutter of the mitral valve septal leaflet is detected in nearly all horses, whereas early systolic closure of the mitral valve is seen only in horses with more severe aortic regurgitation (Fig. 3). Doppler echocardiography (pulsed or color flow) is useful to determine the extent of the regurgitant jet and to semiquantify its severity. Flow mapping may be performed from the right or left cardiac window; the left cardiac window is usually better in the case of LV dilation.

RIGHT ATRIOVENTRICULAR VALVULAR INSUFFICIENCY

Although murmurs are frequently detected in systole in the tricuspid area, lesions are less commonly seen there on postmortem examination. Rupture of the chordae tendineae occurs occasionally and tricuspid insufficiency is a common sequel to mitral regurgitation and pulmonary hypertension.

CLINICAL SIGNS AND DIAGNOSIS

The murmur of tricuspid regurgitation has its point of maximal intensity in the right fourth intercostal space and radiates craniad and dorsad. It is holosystolic or pansystolic and is generally harsh, crescendo or band-shaped, and grade II/VI or louder. Jugular pulsations and venous distention are characteristic of severe tricuspid regurgitation and may be accompanied by dependent edema. With mild to moderate tricuspid regurgitation, many horses perform up to their owners' expectations.

Echocardiographic examination may demonstrate a valvular lesion and confirm the existence of a regurgitant jet (Fig. 4). Dilation of the right atria and ventricle accompanied by paradoxical septal motion indicate moderate to severe regurgitation.

PULMONIC VALVULAR INSUFFICIENCY

The pulmonic valve is the least common site for valvular pathology in the horse. The murmur of pulmonic regurgitation is heard best in the left

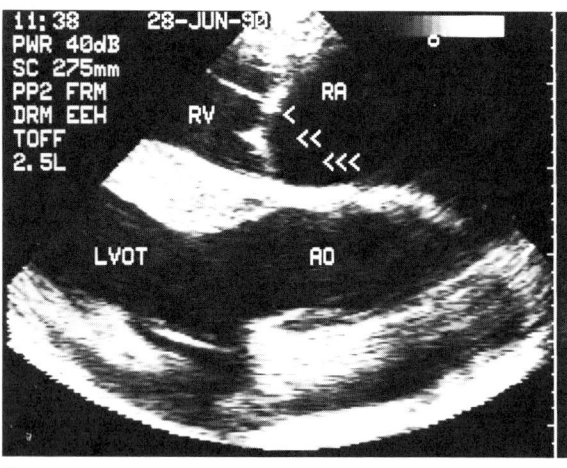
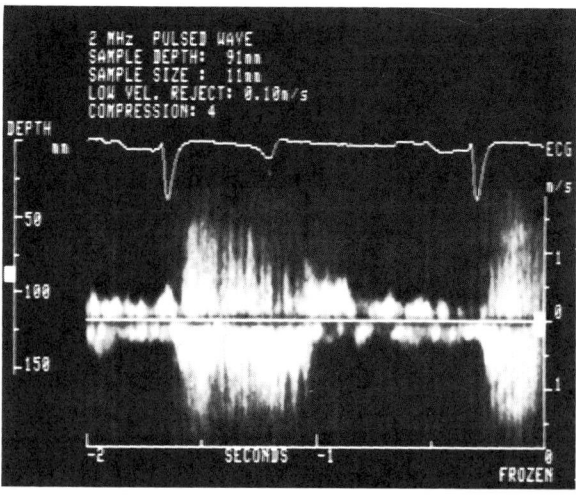

A B

Figure 4. (A) Left parasternal long-axis echocardiogram of the left ventricular outflow tract (LVOT), aorta (AO), right ventricle (RV), and right atrium (RA) in a 5-year-old Thoroughbred gelding with tricuspid regurgitation. Arrows indicate the location of the regurgitant jet detected by pulsed wave Doppler echocardiography. (B) Pulsed wave Doppler echocardiogram of the tricuspid regurgitant jet, obtained in the right atrium. Note high-velocity, aliased blood flow during systole.

third intercostal space and is usually grade II/VI or louder, holodiastolic, harsh, and decrescendo. Echocardiographic findings of right ventricular dilation occur with moderate to severe pulmonic regurgitation, and valvular pathology may be imaged.

MANAGEMENT AND PROGNOSIS

Repeated echocardiographic examination is the most objective method of assessing the rate of progression of valvular disease. Reevaluations should be performed at 6- to 12-month intervals, depending on the severity of the regurgitation and the type of valvular disease detected. In horses with slowly progressive, degenerative lesions, the useful life expectancy may be reduced by 2 to 3 years, if at all. More rapid progression usually occurs in horses with ruptured chordae tendineae or a flail cusp, resulting in poor performance and a markedly reduced life expectancy. The diameter of the pulmonary artery should be compared with that of the aorta, because dilation of the pulmonary artery indicates the presence of significant pulmonary hypertension and precedes pulmonary artery rupture. Horses with moderate to severe atrial enlargement are at risk for development of atrial fibrillation. In horses with severe aortic insufficiency, LV dilation may result in disruption of the mitral annulus, leading to mitral regurgitation and left-sided congestive heart failure.

Horses with acute, left-sided or biventricular congestive heart failure have a grave prognosis for life but may be supported medically for a time. Furosemide (0.5 to 2 mg per kg intravenously [IV], 1 to 2 mg per kg orally [PO], b.i.d. or t.i.d.) is indicated in congestive heart failure. Afterload reducers may be of benefit as they increase cardiac output. The arterial vasodilator hydralazine decreases total peripheral and pulmonary vascular resistance and increases cardiac output in normal horses at a dose of 0.5 mg per kg IV. Promazine may also be effective as an afterload reducer and can be given in the feed (1.5 mg per kg PO, b.i.d. or t.i.d.). Digoxin, a positive inotrope, is administered at 0.002 mg per kg IV or 0.01 to 0.011 mg per kg PO b.i.d. and appears to be clinically useful. It is indicated if myocardial function is reduced or in horses with concurrent atrial fibrillation (see p. xx). Salt supplements should also be avoided in horses with congestive heart failure. These horses should not be ridden and should receive stall rest or be turned out in a small paddock.

Supplemental Readings

Bonagura, J. D., Herring, D. S., and Welker, F.: Echocardiography. Vet. Clin. North Am. (Equine Pract.), 1:311–333, 1985.

Else, R. W., and Holmes, J. R.: Cardiac pathology in the horse 3: Gross Pathology. Equine Vet. J., 4:1–8, 1972.

Long, K. J.: Doppler echocardiography in the horse. Equine Vet. Educ., 2:15–17, 1990.

Reef, V. B., Lalezari, K., De Boo, J., et al: Pulsed-wave Doppler evaluation of intracardiac blood flow in 30 clinically normal Standardbred horses. Am. J. Vet. Res., 50:75–83, 1989.

Reef, V. B., and Spencer, P.: Echocardiographic evaluation of equine aortic insufficiency. Am. J. Vet. Res., 48:904–909, 1987.

Bacterial Endocarditis

Chrysann Collatos, ATHENS, GEORGIA

Bacterial endocarditis occurs uncommonly in horses. Vegetative lesions develop most often on the aortic or mitral valves, although masses involving the right atrioventricular valve, the pulmonic valve, and the left atrial wall have been reported. Multiple sites can be affected in a single animal. Affected animals range in age from 2 months to 15 years. No breed or sex predilection is known. The disease carries a poor prognosis.

HISTORY AND CLINICAL SIGNS

Horses with bacterial endocarditis typically have a history of depression, poor appetite, and intermittent pyrexia. Exercise intolerance, shifting leg lameness, and weight loss may be reported. Although a site of previous bacterial infection is rarely documented, organisms must circulate in the blood to initiate bacterial endocarditis. Animals with septic processes such as thrombophlebitis secondary to indwelling jugular catheters are at increased risk. Bacterial endocarditis should be considered in any animal with recurrent fevers of unknown origin, once more common causes have been ruled out.

Clinical signs observed consistently in affected animals include fever, tachycardia, and cardiac murmurs. Harsh, holosystolic or holodiastolic murmurs loudest over the left heart base are heard most often. The index of suspicion increases if other signs of cardiac disease are present. These include peripheral edema, arrhythmias, venous distention, jugular pulsation, and tachypnea.

DIAGNOSIS

The diagnostic plan must include a thorough physical examination, complete blood cell count, total serum protein concentration, serum albumin concentration, plasma fibrinogen concentration, blood cultures, electrocardiography, and echocardiography. The inflammatory process may be reflected in laboratory data indicating anemia, hypergammaglobulinemia, hyperfibrinogenemia, or, less commonly, leukocytosis and neutrophilia.

Blood for microbiological culture is obtained to document bacteremia and as an aid to antimicrobial therapy. Skin over the jugular vein should be clipped and cleaned as for sterile surgery. Blood is collected by venipuncture using careful aseptic technique and inoculated into blood culture media. Media should be kept at room temperature until processed. At least three samples obtained 2 hours apart should be submitted for culture. Bacteremia is often intermittent and precedes the onset of temperature elevation. Therefore, if the patient has a history of cyclic pyrexia, samples should be obtained over the 6-hour period prior to the next expected fever. Whenever possible, blood for bacterial culture should be collected before antimicrobial therapy is initiated.

Electrocardiography should be performed to characterize arrhythmias that may occur secondary to myocardial pathology. Vegetative lesions may involve the myocardium directly, or embolism from a vegetation to the coronary circulation may cause focal myocardial ischemia or myocarditis. Such abnormalities in the myocardium may alter electrical conduction; arrhythmias exhibited most commonly by animals with bacterial endocarditis are ventricular premature contractions and atrial fibrillation.

Two-dimensional real-time echocardiography

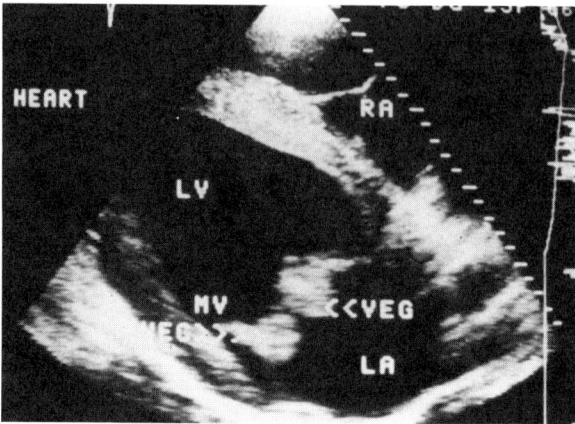

Figure 1. Two-dimensional echocardiogram of a large vegetative lesion (arrows) on the septal and free wall leaflets of the mitral valve. (LA = left atrium, LV = left ventricle, RA = right atrium, MV = mitral valve, IVS = interventricular septum.) (From Dedrick, P.: Treatment of bacterial endocarditis in a horse. J. Am. Vet. Med. Assoc., 193:339–342, 1988. Reproduced by permission.)

is the most sensitive diagnostic tool for identifying vegetative cardiac lesions. The affected valve leaflet is thickened, with a globular, irregular, usually hyperechoic mass seen most frequently at the free edge (Fig. 1). Mural lesions are visualized as echogenic masses protruding from the endocardial surface of the atria or ventricle. Abnormal blood flow through the affected valve can be demonstrated with Doppler echocardiography. Chamber size and myocardial contractility should be assessed to identify secondary cardiac disease. Chamber enlargement occurs with chronic valvular insufficiency.

THERAPY

Bacteriological cure is the goal of therapy for bacterial endocarditis. The vegetative mass is composed of fibrin, platelets, bacteria, and cellular debris. Poor penetration of antimicrobials into vegetations, high numbers of bacteria at the site of infection, and slow growth of deep-seated bacterial colonies all hinder the effectiveness of antimicrobial therapy. Intravenous (IV) administration of broad-spectrum bactericidal antimicrobials with excellent tissue penetration at high dosages is indicated.

Bacteria isolated from vegetative lesions at postmortem examination or from the blood of horses with bacterial endocarditis include streptococcal spp., *Actinobacillus equilli*, *Escherichia coli*, *Pseudomonas aeruginosa*, and *Erysipelothrix rhusiopathiae*. Fungal infection by *Candida parapsilosis* also has occurred. Insufficient cases have been reported to allow generalized predictions regarding the causative pathogens in equine bacterial endocarditis. In addition, blood culture may be unsuccessful, necessitating institution of empirical therapy.

In animals with suspected bacterial endocarditis and negative blood cultures, or pending receipt of blood culture results, initial therapy with potassium penicillin (44,000 IU per kg IV every 6 hours) and gentamicin (2.2 mg per kg IV every 6 hours) is recommended. Although gentamicin does not have excellent tissue penetration, its synergism with penicillin, broad spectrum of action, and reasonable cost warrant its use in empirical therapy. Adequate duration of antimicrobial therapy is not known, but treatment should be continued for a minimum of 4 weeks.

If a pathogen is identified, specifically directed therapy should be instituted. The use of rifampin against sensitive organisms is recommended in human patients with bacterial endocarditis. Rifampin penetrates tissues very well and can be administered orally (PO). It should always be used in combination with another agent (e.g., rifampin and penicillin, rifampin and a cephalosporin), as microbial resistance to rifampin develops rapidly. Pharmocokinetic studies in horses indicate that most gram-positive isolates are sensitive to rifampin administered at 10 mg per kg PO every 12 hours. When gram-negative isolates are identified, the combination of an aminoglycoside with a cephalosporin should be considered. Because the risk of nephrotoxicity can be increased in this situation, careful monitoring of serum creatinine concentrations and serum drug levels is indicated, and maintenance of adequate hydration is particularly important.

The ability of penicillins, certain cephalosporins, and rifampin to penetrate endocardial vegetations has been demonstrated in infected human valves removed at surgery. Bacteriological cure was documented in one horse with valvular bacterial endocarditis and *Streptococcus* spp. bacteremia using 50,000 IU potassium penicillin per kg IV every 4 hours and in a foal with mural endocarditis and *Escherichia coli* bacteremia using cefotaxime, a third-generation cephalosporin, at 40 mg per kg IV every 6 hours. In the second case, the organism isolated demonstrated in vitro sensitivity to gentamicin and cefotaxime; however, pyrexia persisted during gentamicin therapy, but resolved 36 hours after administration of cefotaxime. This may have been due to the superior penetrating ability of the cephalosporin over gentamicin. Both animals concurrently received additional antimicrobials to ensure broad-spectrum coverage.

If a bacterial pathogen is isolated from a patient with bacterial endocarditis, effective antimicrobial dosages may be determined using the serum inhibitory concentration. Serum inhibitory concentration is determined by testing the ability of patient serum dilutions collected just before the next antimicrobial dose to inhibit growth of a standard inoculum of bacteria isolated from the patient. Serum inhibitory concentrations of 1:16 or greater have been associated with high cure rates in people with bacterial endocarditis. Because of the cost of pharmaceuticals in large animal patients and the low incidence of positive blood cultures, such an ideal therapeutic regimen is rarely feasible.

In addition to antimicrobials, nonsteroidal anti-inflammatory agents are useful in therapy for bacterial endocarditis. Either phenylbutazone (up to 4.4 mg per kg per day) or flunixin meglumine (up to 1.1 mg per kg every 12 hours) will improve the patient's attitude through their antipyretic and anti-inflammatory effects. Minimum clinically effective dosages should be utilized as these agents can be toxic to the renal and gastrointestinal systems. The elimination rate of phenylbutazone is increased by rifampin's stimulation of hepatic microsomal enzymes. In gram-negative infections, flunixin meglumine is recommended for it antiendotoxin effects. Although controlled studies have not been conducted, the use of aspirin (17 mg per kg PO every other day) to decrease platelet aggregation may be considered.

COMPLICATIONS

Horses exhibiting certain arrhythmias or heart failure due to chamber dilation require additional pharmacological therapy. Intermittent premature ventricular contraction without significant compromise of cardiac output, indicated by frequent pulse deficits and poor peripheral perfusion, does not require treatment. Atrial fibrillation may occur due to focal myocardial disease or secondary to chamber enlargement. Atrial fibrillation alone is not life-threatening in the resting horse; therefore, the underlying cardiac disease must be addressed prior to attempting conversion to normal sinus rhythm (see p. 387).

Digoxin should be administered to horses with valvular insufficiency or myocardial dysfunction secondary to vegetative lesions if cardiac output is compromised significantly (see p. 392). These animals are identified by the presence of clinical signs of heart failure or evidence of decreased cardiac contractility with chamber enlargement on echocardiography (see p. 393). Drug interactions with digoxin are common. Drugs that induce hepatic microsomal enzyme activity, such as rifampin, may shorten the duration of effective digoxin serum levels. Administration of quinidine to digitalized patients may cause a 40 to 60 per cent increase in digoxin serum concentration, causing signs of digoxin toxicity.

Embolic disease may occur in any body system of animals with vegetative bacterial endocarditis. Left-sided lesions are associated most commonly with renal infarcts or pyelonephritis, while right-sided vegetations may cause pulmonary complications. Ventricular arrhythmias are most frequently associated with embolism from left-sided lesions, particularly those involving the aortic valve. Other potentially affected structures include synovial membranes, retina, and the brain. Repeated clinical and laboratory evaluation of all body systems should be performed to ensure early detection of such problems. Embolic disease should be considered likely in animals with persistent pyrexia despite improvement in cardiac-related signs.

ASSESSMENT AND PROGNOSIS

Progress is assessed on the basis of serial echocardiographic examinations, the incidence of pyrexia, repetition of microbiological culture of peripheral blood, changes in the CBC, and alterations in clinical signs. Cardiac auscultation alone cannot be used to evaluate changes in a vegetative mass. Murmur quality may change as the mass contracts or enlarges; resolution of a previously auscultable murmur is a good prognosticator, but the persistence of a murmur does not necessarily indicate therapeutic failure. Signs of successful therapy include resolution of pyrexia, a decrease in the size of the vegetation on ultrasound examination, and a return to normal heart rate and rhythm.

The long-term prognosis for bacterial endocarditis is poor. Therapy should not be undertaken without a serious commitment to prolonged, extremely expensive treatment. Unfortunately, even when bacteriological cure is achieved, progressive contraction of the affected valve leaflets during the healing process or secondary to rupture of the chordae tendineae may result in permanent valvular insufficiency. The volume-overloaded heart compensates initially, but eventually fatal myocardial failure ensues.

Animals with mural vegetations have a better prognosis for long-term survival if valvular involvement is absent, because chronic valvular insufficiency may not occur. One foal with an atrial mural lesion, *E. coli* bacteremia, gross cardiomegaly, myocardial dysfunction, and atrial fibrillation responded to therapy and entered race training at 2 years of age.

Supplemental Readings

Collatos, C., Clark, E. S., and Reef, V. B.: Atrial fibrillation, cardiomegaly, left atrial mass and R. equi septic osteoarthritis in a foal. J. Am. Vet. Med. Assoc. *197*:1039, 1990.

Dedrick, P., Reef, V. B., Sweeney, R. W., and Morris, D. D.: Treatment of bacterial endocarditis in a horse. J. Am. Vet. Med Assoc., *193*:339, 1988.

Kasari, T. R. and Roussel, A. J.: Bacterial endocarditis: Parts I and II. Compend. Cont. Educ. Pract. Vet., *11*:655, 1989.

Robbins, M. J., Eisenberg, E. S., and Frishman, W. H.: Infective endocarditis: A pathophysiologic approach to therapy. Cardiol. Clin., *5*:545, 1987.

Pericardial Disease

Bill Bernard, LEXINGTON, KENTUCKY

Jean Lamb, LEXINGTON, KENTUCKY

Pericarditis, inflammation of the visceral and parietal pericardium, is an uncommon cardiovascular disease in the horse which can, however, lead to life-threatening cardiovascular abnormalities. An understanding of the pathophysiology and associated clinical manifestations can result in rapid recognition and appropriate therapeutics.

The pericardium is a thin, highly vascular membrane that doubly envelops the heart and the proximal portion of the great vessels. Comprised of visceral and parietal components, the pericardium encloses a potential space that contains a small amount of lubricating fluid. The pericardium functions to allow smooth, frictionless motion of the heart in relation to other mediastinal structures and also serves as a barrier to infection or inflammation of other thoracic organs. It provides a ligamentous function in maintaining optimal functional position of the heart while preventing excessive cardiac displacement.

Unlike many other types of cardiac disease that affect the contractility or systolic pumping ability of the heart, the primary effect of pericarditis is on ventricular filling. The normal pericardium plays an important role in maintaining diastolic ventricular compliance. The nondistensibility of the diseased pericardium decreases diastolic ventricular compliance and impairs ventricular filling, thereby reducing diastolic ventricular volume and cardiac output.

As pericardial effusion progresses sufficiently to raise pericardial pressure above pleural pressure, cardiac tamponade occurs. There is pressure on the heart, and stroke volume is reduced from decreased ventricular filling. Initially, cardiac output is maintained by increased rate. If venous pressure becomes substantially elevated, clinical signs of right-sided heart failure develop. Decreased left ventricular output may result in diminished arterial pulses, fatigue, and weakness.

Constrictive pericarditis and fibrosis may occur secondary to purulent or fibrinous pericarditis. Pericardial fibrosis results in pericardial constriction. If sufficient fibrosis occurs, limitation to ventricular filling results in the same progression of events as cardiac tamponade, eventually resulting in right-sided heart failure.

ETIOLOGY

In horses, causes of pericarditis include bacterial and viral infections, often secondary to pneumonia or pleuritis; and traumatic injuries, either blunt or penetrating. Other causes may include abscessation, such as may occur subsequent to septic endocarditis; neoplasia, or idiopathic etiologies. Sepsis appears to be the most frequent cause of pericarditis; however, isolation of the causative agent is rare and results of both antemortem and postmortem bacterial cultures are often negative. Pericardial mesothelioma with pericardial effusion has also been reported in the horse.

CLINICAL SIGNS AND DIAGNOSIS

Clinical signs of pericarditis are variable and depend on the amount of pericardial effusion and the rate of pericardial fluid accumulation. Clinical signs also vary according to the etiology of the disease. Presenting features may include upper respiratory infection, pneumonia, pleuritis, colic, fever, lethargy, depression, anorexia, tachypnea, ventral edema, and weight loss.

The clinical examination of a horse with suspected pericarditis should include careful auscultation and thorough evaluation of the cardiovascular system. Small pericardial effusions may be very difficult to detect during routine examination. Larger effusions result in diminished or muffled heart sounds on auscultation. The palpable apex beat may also be diminished; however, this may also occur with obesity, pleural effusions, or masses. Other signs of cardiovascular compromise including tachycardia, peripheral venous (usually jugular) distention, and arterial hypotension or palpably diminished pulse pressures are most significant when cardiac compression exists. Other indications of cardiac tamponade include signs of right-sided heart failure, such as pleural effusion and ventral edema.

Other than diminished heart sounds and pericardial friction rubs, auscultable cardiac abnormalities, such as murmurs and arrhythmias, are usually absent. Pericardial friction rubs are a result of the rubbing of the visceral and parietal pericardium. Friction rubs are most commonly identified when small amounts of effusion are in contact with a roughened, fibrinous pericardial surface. Friction rubs may be absent if the pericardial effusion is large. Pericardial friction rubs must be differentiated from murmurs and pleural rubs. Pleural friction rubs are associated with respiration while pericardial friction rubs are usually triphasic, associated with the cardiac cycle, and may be differentiated from murmurs by their coarse, grating quality.

The definitive diagnosis of pericardial effusion is made with B-mode or M-mode echocardiography (Figs. 1 and 2). The epicardium is separated from the pericardium only in systole if the effusion is small. With severe effusions, epicardial echoes are separated from the corresponding pericardial echoes in all phases of the cardiac cycle (see Figs. 1 and 2). A thickened pericardium or fibrin tags may be identified (see Fig. 1).

Hematology may reveal an inflammatory leukogram, elevated white blood cell count, and fibrinogenemia, suggesting an inflammatory process. Prerenal azotemia may be present. Serology may be useful if viral infection is suspected.

Thoracic radiography may be useful in demonstrating pericardial effusion with the appearance of an enlarged, pumpkin-shaped cardiac silhouette. However, the frequent concomitant pleural effusion often obliterates the cardiac silhouette. Therefore, radiography is not a reliable technique with which to confirm the presence of pericardial effusion.

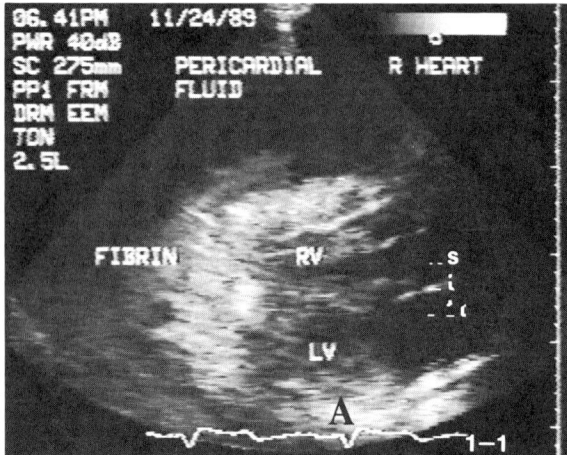 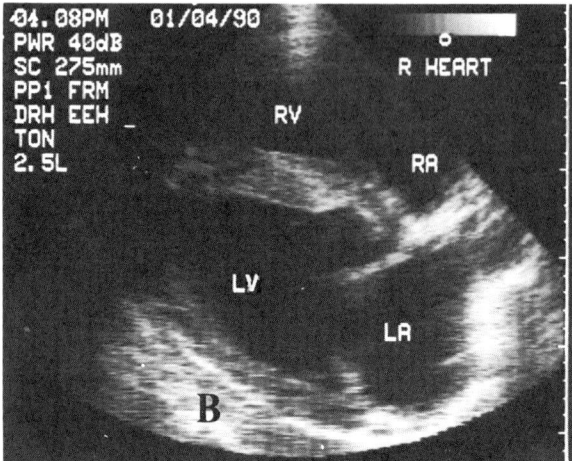

Figure 1. Ultrasonograms of the heart at the right third intercostal space in a horse with pleural effusion at presentation (A) and 40 days after initiation of treatment (B). (LV = left ventricle. RV = right ventricle. RA = right atrium, LA = left atrium.) Pericardial fluid and fibrin are labeled in A. B reveals resolution of pleural effusion.

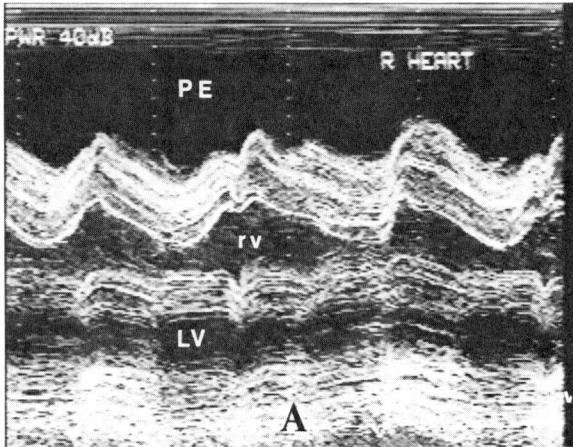 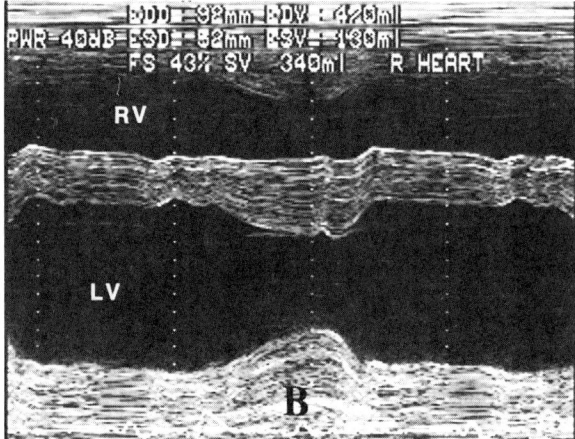

Figure 2. M-mode ultrasonograms of the heart at the right third intercostal space in a horse with pleural effusion (A) and 40 days after initiation of treatment and resolution of effusion (B). (PE = pericardial effusion, RV = right ventricle, LV = left ventricle.)

Electrocardiography (ECG) may support the diagnosis of pericardial effusion. Diminished QRS voltage is a consistent finding in horses with pericardial effusion and is attributed to the short-circuiting effect of the pericardial effusion. Electrical alternans, a variation in QRS amplitude related to the swinging action of the heart in a pool of pericardial fluid, is another common ECG finding and is more specific for pericardial effusion. Nonspecific ST segment changes may be identified.

Pericardiocentesis is useful in determining the etiology of the pericardial effusion. Normal pericardial fluid is present in small amounts and consists of a fluid low in protein (less than 2.5 gm per dl) and with a low total nucleated cell count (less than 1500 nucleated cells per μl). Alterations in the protein content and cell count of the fluid can lead to classification as a modified transudate or exudate. Pericardial fluid can be further classified as to cell type: neutrophilic, lymphocytic, monocytic, eosinophilic, or neoplastic. Neutrophils can be further classified as degenerative (karyolytic) or well preserved. Karyolytic neutrophils indicate the presence of a septic process, while well-preserved neutrophils represent an aseptic inflammatory process. Nonseptic effusions may be compatible with idiopathic pericarditis (eosinophilic, histiocytic), viral pericarditis (well-preserved neutrophils, lymphocytes), or neoplasia (histiocytic, lymphocytic, mesothelial cell increase.) Further evaluation of pericardial fluid should include culture and cytological evaluation for microorganisms. Examination for cellular inclusions and special staining may prove useful in the future for identifying viral diseases.

Pericardiocentesis is best performed over the left fourth, fifth, or sixth intercostal space 6 cm below the point of the shoulder. Ultrasound examination can be used to determine the most appropriate site for centesis. The site should be clipped and aseptically prepared and local anesthetics used. Depending on the patient, sedation may be required. Spinal needles, over-the-needle intravenous catheters, teat cannulas, or argyle chest drains can be used for the centesis. ECG monitoring during the procedure is important as premature ventricular contractions may indicate contact with ventricular myocardium. Prolonged ventricular irritation may induce life-threatening arrhythmias, and appropriate doses of lidocaine or quinidine (see p. 392) should be at hand.

THERAPY

The prognosis for recovery from pericarditis has improved in the past few years. Appropriate, early aggressive therapy, including pericardial drainage, has improved the outcome even in horses with severe pericarditis. Reports of successful treatment of both idiopathic, nonseptic pericarditis and septic pericarditis have been recently published. Initial treatment of pericarditis will vary with the severity of the condition and the degree of cardiac tamponade. If cardiac compression is severe and right-sided heart failure exists, immediate removal of pericardial fluid is required. Concurrent pleural effusion often exists in the majority of pericarditis cases and drainage of excessive pleural fluid may be required to improve cardiac and respiratory function.

Diuretics such as furosemide are rarely indicated, as pulmonary edema is infrequent and diuretics rarely help remove excess pericardial fluid. Cardiac inotropes will not improve cardiac output as they do not influence the inappropriate ventricular filling resulting from cardiac compression. Additional treatment should include supportive care, fluid therapy, correction of existing acid–base or electrolyte abnormalities, anti-inflammatories, and analgesics, if needed.

Results of pericardiocentesis, in an attempt to determine the etiology of the disease, are required to guide subsequent treatment. Idiopathic pericarditis with aseptic effusion has responded well to parenteral corticosteroids or pericardial drainage. Suspected septic pericarditis can be treated systemically with broad spectrum antimicrobials. Penicillin–aminoglycoside combinations provide a broad spectrum of activity against many gram-positive and gram-negative organisms. Indwelling pericardial drains (16 to 20 French) may be used if pericardial effusion persists subsequent to initial drainage. Echocardiography is used to select the optimal site for drain placement from the left cardiac silhouette, usually the fifth intercostal space 6 cm below the point of the shoulder. ECG should be performed during placement of the drain to check for arrhythmias. Placing an indwelling drain is not without complications. Laceration of an intercostal artery, coronary artery, or lung; arrhythmias; or puncturing the heart are possible. However, with ultrasound guidance and care, this is a fairly safe procedure.

Indwelling drains allow repeated drainage, lavage, and instillation of antibiotics. Lavage and instillation of antibiotics can be repeated twice daily and drains may be removed when minimal effusion is obtained over a 48-hour period. The removal of fibrin, bacteria, and inflammatory cells and their by-products appears to be beneficial in resolution of the persistent effusion. Although concentrations of antimicrobial agents in the pericardial fluid are equal to or in excess of serum concentrations 2 hours after intravenous administration, direct instillation of antimicrobial agents into the pericardial sac increases the drug concentration in pericardial fluid above that in serum.

Therapeutic pericardiectomy has not been reported in horses, although surgical treatment of constrictive pericarditis in the cow has been described.

Supplemental Readings

Bernard, W. B., Reef, V. B., Clark, S. et al.: Pericarditis in horses: Six cases (1982–1986). J. Am. Vet. Med. Assoc., 196:468, 1990.

Dill, S. G., Simoncini, B. S., Bolton, G. R., et al.: Fibrinous pericarditis in the horse. J. Am. Vet. Med. Assoc., 180:266, 1982.

Freestone, J. F., Thomas, W. P., and Carlson, G. P. et al: Idiopathic effusive pericarditis with tamponade in the horse. Equine Vet. J. 19:38, 1987.

Reef, V. B., Gentile, D. G., and Freeman, D. M.: Successful treatment of pericarditis in a horse. J. Am. Vet. Med. Assoc., 185:94, 1984.

Wagner, P. C., Miller, R. A., Merrit, F., et al.: Constrictive pericarditis in the horse. J. Equine Med. Surg., 1:242, 1977.

Jugular Vein Thrombophlebitis

Sarah Y. Gardner, RALEIGH, NORTH CAROLINA
William J. Donawick, KENNETT SQUARE, PENNSYLVANIA

Jugular vein thrombophlebitis is a well-recognized clinical problem in the horse. It is frequently associated with intravenous (IV) injections and inflammation due to chemical irritation, IV catheterization, and mechanical trauma to the vascular wall intima, or a coagulopathy. Septic jugular vein thrombophlebitis may develop from needle or catheter contamination during insertion, migration of bacteria along the catheter from the skin, contaminated IV solutions, or hematogenous spread from another focus of infection. Complications of jugular vein thrombophlebitis include extensive edema, endocarditis, pulmonary thromboembolism, and septicemia.

CLINICAL SIGNS

On palpation of the affected vein, a firm, intraluminal, cylindrical mass is usually felt or the vein may feel corded. When the horse's nares are occluded and it exhales forcefully (Valsalva maneuver), the vein fails to distend if the lumen is completely occluded with thrombus, or distends slowly if the lumen is partially occluded. Venous occlusion may result in distention of superficial veins on the affected side and may lead to edema in the pharyngeal, laryngeal, and facial areas and congestion of the oral and nasal mucous membranes. If both jugular veins are affected, edema may be extensive, possibly resulting in dyspnea and dysphagia. Septic jugular vein thrombophlebitis should be suspected in horses that have perivascular swelling, heat, or pain on palpation of the affected vein. Pyrexia, anorexia, or depression may also indicate sepsis. With sepsis of the perivascular tissues, purulent exudate may drain from the affected site.

DIAGNOSIS

If a catheter is in place at the time of onset of jugular vein thrombophlebitis, it should be removed immediately. The skin should be cleaned at the skin–catheter junction with alcohol and allowed to dry before removal of the catheter. A smear can be made from the catheter and gram-stained, and the catheter can be submitted for bacteriological culture by the semiquantitative method. Isolates recovered should be tested for antimicrobial sensitivity.

Hematology may reveal an inflammatory leukogram and hyperfibrinogenemia, especially in horses with septic thrombophlebitis. If septicemia is suspected, blood cultures should be performed and antimicrobial sensitivity determined.

ULTRASONOGRAPHIC EXAMINATION OF THE JUGULAR VEIN

Ultrasonography is a useful aid in the diagnosis of jugular vein thrombophlebitis. The normal jugular vein is an anechoic tubular structure. The vein distends during the Valsalva maneuver and collapses when pressure is exerted with the transducer probe; these dynamic events are decreased or absent when the vein lumen is filled with thrombus. Ultrasonographically, thrombosis appears as an echogenic mass within the vein. Ultrasonography may be used to specifically characterize the nature of the thrombus. An aseptic thrombus appears relatively uniform with low or medium amplitude echoes, whereas a septic thrombus appears heterogeneous with anechoic to hypoechoic areas representing fluid or necrosis within the thrombus, or hyperechoic areas representing gas. Ultrasonography can be used to sequentially follow venous thrombi to document resolution or progression. If sepsis is suspected, an aspirate should be obtained aseptically from a fluid-filled (anechoic or hypoechoic) area within the thrombus under ultrasonographic guidance. The aspirate should be gram-stained and cultured for aerobic and anaerobic bacteria with antimicrobial sensitivity testing.

THERAPY

Treatment of jugular vein thrombophlebitis should include local hydrotherapy of the affected area. Topical application of dimethyl sulfoxide or ichthammol° may be helpful.

Nonsteroidal anti-inflammatory drugs (phenylbutazone, 2 mg per kg orally [PO] twice a day, or flunixin meglumine, 1 mg per kg PO twice a day) may be useful in severe cases and should be administered for a few days.

If sepsis is suspected, appropriate antimicro-

°Ichthammol 20% ointment, J. A. Webster, Billerica, MA

bial therapy should be selected based on bacteriological culture results and antimicrobial sensitivity testing. Aerobic or anaerobic bacteria, or both, may be involved. The most commonly isolated gram-positive organisms include β-haemolytic *Streptococcus* spp., α-haemolytic *Streptococcus* spp. (not group D), and *Staphylococcus aureus*. The most commonly isolated gram-negative organisms include *Pasteurella–Actinobacillus* spp., *Escherichia coli*, and *Klebsiella pneumoniae*. If bacteriological culture is not possible or if culture results are negative but other clinical parameters indicate sepsis, broad-spectrum antimicrobial therapy should be initiated. Recommended antimicrobial therapy is penicillin (sodium or potassium penicillin G, 20,000 to 40,000 IU per kg IV or intramuscularly (IM) four times a day, or procaine penicillin G, 22,000 IU per kg IM twice a day), combined with an aminoglycoside. Amikacin sulfate (7 mg per kg IV or IM three times a day) is preferable to gentamicin sulfate (2.2 mg per kg IV or IM four times a day). Trimethoprim–sulfamethoxasole (30 mg per kg PO twice a day) has the advantage of oral administration but is effective against only 50 per cent of isolates. Metronidazole (15 mg per kg PO four times a day) should be added to the treatment regimen if hyperechoic areas representing gas are imaged within the thrombus.

The affected vein should not be used for drug administration or blood sampling. Ideally the opposite jugular vein should be preserved and not utilized either. Other veins that may be used for catheterization, drug administration, and blood sampling include the lateral thoracic, cephalic, median, and saphenous.

Antimicrobial therapy should be continued until all signs of inflammation (pain, heat, swelling, pyrexia) and fluid pockets within the thrombus on ultrasound examination have resolved and the leukogram and fibrinogen values are normal. Surgical excision of the vein should be considered in cases that are nonresponsive to medical therapy or are complicated by septicemia and toxemia.

PREVENTION

Precautions can be taken to decrease the risk of development of jugular vein thrombophlebitis. Before any drugs are injected into the jugular vein, the skin overlying the vein should be wiped with alcohol. This will not sterilize the skin but will remove any gross debris that may be present. The injection should be as atraumatic to the vessel wall as possible. The injection of irritating drugs should be avoided or the drugs should be diluted.

For catheterization of the jugular vein, the practitioner should be familiar with the catheterization technique and observe strict asepsis. Select the least thrombogenic catheter material available (silicone rubber < polyurethane < polytetrafluoroethylene < polyethylene < polypropylene) with as small a bore as feasible. Clip the hair at the catheter site and scrub the skin with an antiseptic (preferably an iodine-containing solution.) Wash hands with an antiseptic soap and wear sterile gloves. Insert the catheter as atraumatically as possible, tunneling it subcutaneously before penetrating the vein. Secure the catheter with suture or cyanoacrylate* glue to reduce movement. A topical polyantimicrobial ointment at the skin–catheter junction and a sterile vapor-permeable dressing may be applied to the site. Record the date and time of catheterization.

For maintenance of jugular catheters, disinfect ports before entry. If a continuous infusion is not being used, flush the catheter with sterile heparinized (10 IU per ml) saline and inspect the site every 6 to 8 hours. Visual inspection is not necessary if the site is palpated gently through the intact dressing, no pain or tenderness is present, and the horse is afebrile. Remove the catheter in 72 hours or when it is no longer needed. Change IV tubing used for drug or fluid administration every 48 to 72 hours. Change IV tubing used for hyperalimentation every 24 to 48 hours. IV tubing should be changed immediately after the administration of blood products or lipids, and once started all parenterals and lipids should be administered within 12 hours. Change the entire IV system immediately if contamination occurs or septic thrombophlebitis is noted or strongly suspected. In the case of phlebitis without signs of infection, change the catheter.

PROGNOSIS

Nonseptic thrombophlebitis usually resolves and recanalization of the affected vein occurs over time. Septic thrombophlebitis may resolve after appropriate antimicrobial therapy, and in some horses resolution will result in the return of a fully functional vein. In other horses the resulting fibrosis will lead to partial to complete occlusion and decreased blood flow. Stricture of the vein may also occur. Over time, collateral circulation will develop. In some horses antimicrobial therapy is unsuccessful and surgical excision of the affected vein is necessary. The surgery requires an experienced surgeon.

---

*Duro Super Glue, Loctite Corp., Cleveland, OH

Supplemental readings

Bayly, W. M., and Vale, B. H.: Intravenous catheterization and associated problems in the horse. Compend. Cont. Educ. Pract. Vet., 4:S227, 1982.

Deem, D. A.: Complications associated with the use of intravenous catheters in large animals. Calif. Vet., 6:19, 1981.

Gardner, S. Y., Reef, V. B., and Spencer, P. A.: Ultrasonographic evaluation of 46 horses with jugular vein thrombophlebitis: 1985–1988. A retrospective study. J. Am. Vet. Med. Assoc. (in press).

Morris, D. D.: Thrombophlebitis in horses: the contribution of hemostatic dysfunction to pathogenesis. Compend. Cont. Educ. Pract. Vet., 11:1386, 1989.

Congenital Cardiovascular Disorders

Frank S. Pipers, NORTH GRAFTON, MASSACHUSETTS

Although the prevalence of congenital cardiovascular disorders in horses has never been precisely established, it is generally considered to be less than 5 per cent. This may be due to the fact that little is done to perpetuate life in affected horses, thereby permitting natural selection to prevail. Nevertheless, the detection of fetal and congenital abnormalities is economically crucial with respect to potential obstetrical problems and culling from a pool of potential athletes. Recent developments in diagnostic ultrasonic technology and its use in clinical practice greatly facilitate the detection of problems in the perinatal and postpartum periods.

DIAGNOSIS

Clinicians routinely evaluate the cardiovascular system of neonates and young horses as part of their physical examination or in response to problems suspected or detected. Signs of respiratory difficulty, exercise intolerance, weakness, stunting of growth, and poor condition are common complaints and causes for concern. The physical examination usually begins with inspection of the patient followed by the evaluation of the mucous membranes for color and capillary refill time, observation of the jugular furrow for venous distention or pulsation, and palpation of the arterial pulses for rate, rhythm, and character abnormalities.

Auscultation of the left and right hemithoraces for murmurs and rhythm abnormalities is important for the detection of cardiovascular problems. Left basilar systolic ejection murmurs (grade III/VI or less) are common findings in foals less than a week or so of age. These murmurs are often attributed to physiological causes such as ejection turbulence or a patent ductus arteriosus that did not close completely for 2 to 3 days post partum. Unlike in other species these ductal murmurs are not usually continuous but simply systolic. The patent ductus and the murmur rarely persist or create a clinical problem. Very loud murmurs, murmurs that radiate diffusely over the hemithoraces, and murmurs that persist past 1 week of age should be of concern and provoke further, more extensive examinations.

In addition to abnormal murmurs and transients, irregular heart rates and rhythms are also subjects for concern. Neonatal foals typically have heart rates of approximately 80 to 100 bpm (the rate decreases over the next few months) entrained in a regular rhythm. Excitement due to handling often transiently elevates the rate but once the foal relaxes the rate typically returns to normal. Persistent tachycardia or rhythm irregularity warrants further investigation.

At this juncture the clinician can proceed in a number of directions to acquire additional information pertaining to the competency of the cardiovascular system. Classical approaches include blood work, electrocardiography (ECG), phonocardiography, radiography, cardiac catheterization, and echocardiography. However, the best option for determining the location, severity, and consequences of the problem is echocardiography (Fig. 1). The ultrasound examination begins with identification of the specific chambers affected and quantifying the degree of cardiac chamber enlargement. Each chamber and great vessel should be identified for its anatomical characteristics and their interrelationships determined. Subsequently the muscular walls should be evaluated for integrity, thickness, and functional capacity (per cent Δ d). Next the cardiac valves are evaluated for competency and structural integrity. Finally, the pericardium

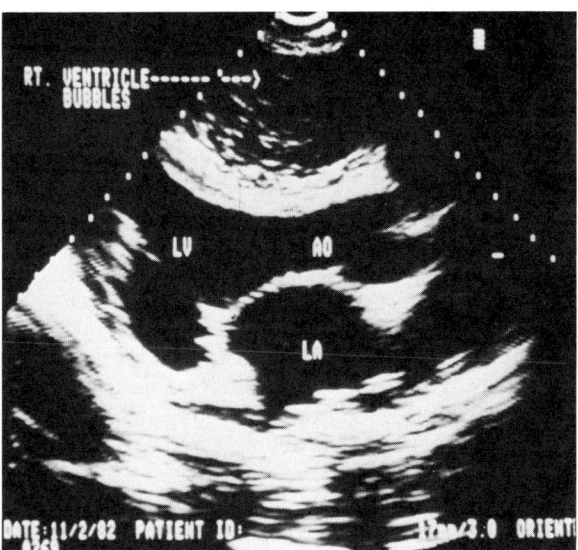

Figure 1. Right parasternal long-axis echocardiographic view of the heart of a normal horse. (LA = left atrium, LV = left ventricle, AO = aortic outflow tract.)

should be evaluated for thickness and fluid accumulation. Normal values for cardiac dimensions of adult horses and foals are available. If the heart is of normal size and functioning normally, one can assume either there is no cardiac disease or the lesion is hemodynamically insignificant. In the presence of cardiac arrhythmias (auscultated or detected echocardiographically), ECG may be useful to ascertain whether the rhythm disturbance is originating from the ventricles or above the ventricles. This determination generally dictates medical therapy.

Many authors discuss the use of multiple leads for the acquisition of electrical information even though the usefulness of these data has never been substantiated. By contrast, simply attaching both arm leads 1 inch apart over the skin on the left jugular furrow and both leg leads 1 inch apart over the left apex of the heart will produce an easy to interpret "monitor lead" for ECG interpretation.

After evaluating the physical, auscultatory, electrophysiological, and echocardiographic information, the practitioner is in a position to diagnose many of the congenital disorders and their consequences. Doppler echocardiography and contrast echocardiography are some relatively new, noninvasive methods of extracting additional information. Although these procedures can theoretically be performed in the field, they require the help of a trained specialist and some unique equipment. For disorders that defy detection by the methods described above, cardiac catheterization at university referral centers remains as an option. This is primarily of academic interest, as few surgical procedures are available as a form of therapy.

VENTRICULAR SEPTAL DEFECTS

By far the single largest category of congenital defects are the ventricular septal defects (VSDs). These defects occur as single entities or as part of more complex congenital anomalies such as tetralogy of Fallot and the tricuspid atresia complex. In rare instances there may be more than one VSD in the same heart; these often appear in the muscular septum.

Most frequently VSDs present as single lesions high in the membranous septum. The severity of the lesion is a function of the size of the defect and of resistance to flow through the defect. Pathophysiologically, VSDs lead to pulmonary overcirculation, resulting in a left heart volume overload which, if severe enough, induces left heart failure. In severely protracted cases of pulmonary overcirculation, pulmonary vascular remodeling (media hypertrophy and intimal thickening) occurs and results in pulmonary hypertension. This ultimately leads to an increase in right ventricular pressure and a diminution or reversal of the shunting. This progressive pulmonary hypertension usually results in right heart failure, compounding the left heart failure, and the subsequent demise of the patient.

Clinical presentations of VSD are diverse and apparently dependent on the size and location of the lesion and the work load imposed on the horse. Although many VSDs are detected on routine physical examinations of patients with no signs of disease, in a large subgroup of neonates respiratory distress related to heart failure is part of the presentation. It is also common to see athletic horses at the training stage in which VSDs have eluded detection. Clinical signs develop when the work load exceeds the cardiac reserve.

Clinical signs include exercise intolerance, poor growth, respiratory distress, weakness, ataxia, syncope and nonspecific signs of malaise. Severely affected patients in heart failure may have dyspnea, subcutaneous edema, pale mucus membranes, prolonged capillary refill times (>2 seconds), jugular distention and pulsation, rapid pulses, and precordial thrill over the right sternal, apical and left basilar regions. Auscultation of the thorax reveals systolic murmurs at the right sternal border, tricuspid region, and left base (pulmonic valve area). The intensity and characteristics of the murmur vary with the severity of the disease but are usually loud (grade III/VI or louder) and band shaped. As the degree

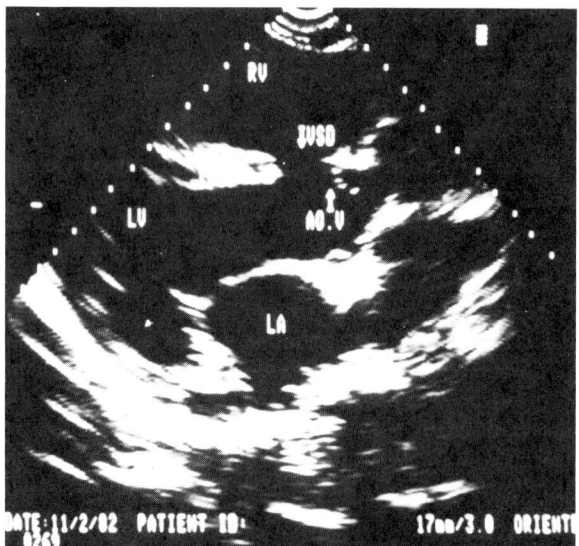

Figure 2. Right parasternal long-axis echocardiographic view of a foal with a ventricular septal defect (VSD). (RV = right ventricle, LV = left ventricle, AOV = aortic valve, LA = left atrium.)

of turbulence increases the murmur intensifies and is accompanied by a palpable precordial thrill on the hemithorax.

Echocardiographic examinations of the heart from the right parasternal window (Fig. 2) usually reveal the defect in the membranous septum. The defect is usually located ventral to the aortic valve and the septal leaflet of the tricuspid valve. Occasionally the tricuspid valve flutters in response to the shunting of blood across the defect. If the defect is very small (a few millimeters in diameter), it may not be visible with routine two-dimensional echocardiography. Sophisticated noninvasive techniques such as spectral and color flow Doppler echography are needed for definite diagnosis. When the lesions are small the consequences of the defect are usually insignificant; the horse has no clinical signs and may race successfully, although usually in lower classes of races.

Patients with large VSDs and large shunts are rarely successful in racing or other strenuous performance. The author has seen a few successful show horses with large (4 cm), previously undetected defects. The disease is diagnosed later in life during a prepurchase or insurance examination.

A few other congenital lesions have been reported, including patent ductus arteriosus, tetralogy of Fallot, tricuspid atresia, truncus and pseudotruncus arteriosus, persistent fetal circulation, transposition of the great vessels with or without inversion of the ventricles, and endocardial cushion defects. Of prime importance to the client is whether the heart is defective and the implications of the congenital defect for the future of the horse.

Regarding most complex congenital diseases, there is often stunting of growth and lethargy in addition to the classical signs of heart failure previously mentioned. Loud left hemithoracic murmurs, possible systolic and diastolic murmurs, cynosis with exercise, polycythemia, and low arterial Po_2 are compatible with complex anomalies and may distinguish them from a VSD.

Supplemental Readings

Lombard, C. W., Evans, M., Martin, L., and Tehrani, J.: Blood pressure, electrocardiogram and echocardiogram measurements in the growing pony foal. Equine Vet. J., 16:342–347, 1984.

Machida, N., Yasuda, J., Too, K., and Kudo, N.: A morphological study on the obliteration processes of the ductus arteriosus in the horse. Equine Vet. J. 20(4):249–254, 1988.

Pipers, F. S., and Adams-Brendemuehl, C. S.: Techniques and applications of transabdominal ultrasonography in the pregnant mare. J. Am. Vet. Med. Assoc. 185(7):776–771, 1984.

Pipers, F. S., Reef, V. B., and Wilson, J.: Echocardiographic detection of ventricular septal defects in large animals. J. Am. Vet. Med. Assoc., 187:810, 1985.

Stewart, J. H., Rose, R. J., and Barko, A. M.: Echocardiography in foals from birth to three months old. Equine Vet. J., 16:332–331, 1984.

Section 10

FOAL DISEASES

Edited by Benjamin J. Darien

Identification and Early Management of the High-Risk Neonatal Foal

Barbara D. Brewer, GAINESVILLE, FLORIDA

The past decade has witnessed growing interest and considerable advances in equine neonatal critical care, so that it is now possible to save the lives of foals that formerly would not have survived. Sick foals treated early and aggressively, before they require intensive support, have a far better prognosis for survival with future athletic soundness than those treated heroically. Treatment costs are also less if sick foals are identified early. A cooperative effort involving farm owners, managers, night watchmen, and the veterinarian will optimize prenatal and perinatal care of the mare and her foal.

Newborns of all species need different and more fastidious care than their adult counterparts. Their immune systems are immature and easily overwhelmed. They do not exhibit the early signs of shock or sepsis seen in adult horses, and thus their condition may suddenly deteriorate and death may ensue without warning. Newborns lack many of the compensatory mechanisms available to adults experiencing metabolic and thermal derangements, and their nutritional requirements are high, owing to their rapid growth and high metabolic rates. They rarely exhibit a single problem at a time, and even straightforward illnesses may be complicated by secondary problems. For these reasons, increased emphasis on the equine perinatal period is recommended. Problems can be anticipated before they occur, thus avoiding disappointment and disasters.

IDENTIFYING THE HIGH-RISK FOAL

By anticipating that a mare might have a difficult delivery or that the foal might not be normal, the practitioner can prepare for close observation and rapid intervention. The peripartum period can be divided into three time segments, each requiring the oversight of all members of the team, including owners, managers, and the veterinarian.

BEFORE BIRTH

Mares that have lost previous foals or given birth to sick or premature foals may do so again. This may be due to inadequate colostrum production, inability to carry a foal to term, uterine infection, poor mothering instinct, or other reasons. Maiden mares foal 5 days earlier on average than experienced mares, and their udders do not fill in advance. Old mares, frequently possessing poor conformation, may be more prone to uterine infection or insufficient placentation and thus may produce infected or small for gestational age foals.

If colostrum is observed leaking from the mare's teats, the foal may need colostral supplementation. Premature lactation may also be a sign that placentitis or placental insufficiency is present and that the foal might be infected or dysmature. The following are also considered risk factors if they occur in the last months of pregnancy: maternal fever, purulent vaginal discharge, endotoxemia, surgery, hydrops allantois, or long-term use of any medication, even at an appropriate dosage. Malnourished mares or mares in suboptimal environments can be expected to produce abnormal foals.

DURING BIRTH

The following factors concerning labor and delivery have been associated with adverse outcomes. Dystocia is a well-recognized cause of a weak or asphyxiated foal at risk of rapidly decompensating or developing an infection. Prolonged gestation, longer than 365 days, may rarely produce a large foal causing a difficult birth, or more likely will result in a small for gestational age foal that poorly tolerates the stress of labor, delivery, and the neonatal period. Foals born prematurely are frequently infected in utero or have been poorly nourished by an inadequate placenta. Many are at increased risk for the development of a host of respiratory, metabolic, thermoregulatory, hormonal, and infectious problems after birth. Prolonged or difficult labor can lead to fetal asphyxia and its potentially fatal consequences. Untimely induction of labor and cesarean sections have also been associated with considerable morbidity and mortality in newborns. Extremely rapid delivery, particularly when the mare is standing, may result in early cord rupture with potential depletion of blood volume and consequent anemic hypoxia. Similarly, immediate clamping of the cord or blood loss at birth may decrease the foal's blood volume. Premature placental separation, indicated by a red, basketball-like structure at the vulva, can cause fetal death or severe hypoxic consequences unless the foal is delivered rapidly. Foals born stained or covered with meconium-contaminated amnionic fluid are likely candidates for meconium aspiration pneumonia.

Observation of the placenta may lead the clinician to suspect infection or fetal hypoxia. Discrete pale areas in the freshly delivered placenta are suggestive of premature placental separation and possible fetal hypoxia. Placentas that look grossly thickened or otherwise abnormal and weigh more than 11 per cent of the foal's body weight may be indicative of an infected foal.

AFTER BIRTH

Twin foals, particularly the smaller of the two, or orphan foals must be considered high risk, as must the foal that appears to be premature. Regardless of their gestational age, premature or dysmature foals are recognized by their curly ears, small size, lax tendons, silky hair coat, and domed head. Foals that have any abnormality on initial physical examination, including those that are apparently healthy but cannot rise because of contracted tendons, should be worked up as will be described. Foals with delayed colostral intake or any other abnormality in their behavioral profile (Table 1) should also be examined and monitored closely. Exposure to infectious diseases and trauma resulting in open wounds to the neonate are obvious risk factors. The mare should be checked after foaling for signs of trauma suggestive of a difficult delivery during an unwitnessed birth. Udders should be carefully scrutinized. The presence of good-quality colostrum followed by adequate milk production should be noted. Although a thick yellow secretion from the udder does not guarantee that good colostrum is available, thin, watery or milky secretions almost always indicate the absence of colostrum. The udder should be monitored for infection. An udder that is too full suggests that the foal is not sucking, an early sign of illness.

DIAGNOSTIC PROCEDURES RECOMMENDED FOR HIGH-RISK FOALS

While it has been suggested that all newborn foals should be tested for failure of passive transfer, it is most crucial that this test be performed on high-risk foals and that low immunoglobulin status in these foals be corrected (see page 422). A sepsis score, backed up with blood cultures, has been a useful tool in our hands, predicting the presence of infection or septicemia correctly 93 per cent of the time and the absence of either 88 per cent of the time (Fig. 1). Laboratory data

TABLE 1. NORMAL BEHAVIORAL PROFILE OF THE NEONATAL FOAL

Behavior	Time (Range)
Suck reflex present	20 min
Stands	57 min (15–165)
Suckles	111 min (35–420)
Is alert, can see, responds to its environment, and follows its dam	

Sepsis Score

Foal's Name _____
Case Number _____
Age _____

Date _____

Total Score† _____
Check One:
____ At admission?
____ Day subsequent to admission?
Indicate day
#: ____

Number of points to assign:

Information collected:		4	3	2	1	0	This case
I. CBC 1. Neutrophil count (NOT TOTAL WBC!)	Record exact #		<200/mm³	2000-4000 or >12,000	8000-12,000	Normal	
2. Band neutrophil count			>200/mm³	50-200		<50	
3. Doehle bodies, toxic, granulation, or vacuolization in neutrophils			Marked	Moderate	Slight	None	
4. Fibrinogen mg/dl				>600	401-600	≤400	
II. Other Laboratory Data 1. Blood glucose mg/gl				<50	50-80	>80	
2. IgG quick test mg/dl*		<200	200-400	401-800		>800	
III. Clinical Examination 1. Petechiation or scleral injection not secondary to eye disease or trauma			Marked	Moderate	Mild	None	
2. Fever				>102°F	<100°F	Normal	
3. Hypotonia, coma, depression, convulsions				Marked	Mild	Normal	
4. Anterior uveitis, diarrhea, respiratory distress, swollen joints, open wounds				Yes		No	
IV. Historical Data 1. Placentitis, vulvar discharge prior to delivery, dystocia, long transport of mare, mare sick, foal induced, gestation > 365 d				Yes		No	
2. Prematurity			<300 days	300-310	311-330	>330	

Figure 1. The sepsis score. A score of 11 or higher correctly predicts sepsis 93% of the time. 1. If a foal is more than 12 hours old, compute the score using the zinc sulphate turbidity (ZST) value obtained. 2. If the foal is less than 12 hours old, use a +2 for the ZST if there is a history of nursing what appeared to be good colostrum. Give the foal a +4 if it has not nursed or if in doubt.

utilized include the total neutrophil count, band neutrophil count, presence of toxic changes within neutrophils, fibrinogen, blood glucose levels, and IgG status. Physical examination parameters to be noted include temperature, appearance of the sclerae, mentation, the presence of diarrhea, open wounds, anterior uveitis, respiratory distress, and swollen joints. Historical data, including gestational age, is utilized as well.

Any abnormal foal should undergo chest radiography. Newborns with moderate to severe lung disease typically do not have abnormal lung sounds on auscultation. Ultrasonography has proved useful for the evaluation of the foal's umbilicus, and this structure should always be assessed in cases of fever of unknown origin. Arterial blood gas values are valuable in assessing lung function. Samples are usually readily obtained from the great metatarsal artery.

MANAGEMENT

Management of the high-risk foal involves a keen eye for detail and close monitoring. These foals are best approached with the expectation that they presently are ill or will likely become ill. Close observation of behavior, particularly the amount of time spent down and spent sucking, as well as detailed records of the foal's vital signs are invaluable in thwarting a catastrophe. Foals found to be sick should have their problems treated rapidly and aggressively.

Secondary problems such as entropion, corneal ulcers, hypothermia, and hypoglycemia should be anticipated and immediately treated. Since high-risk foals are typically immunocompromised, the diligent application of sterile technique and exceptional hygiene are crucial. The importance of providing adequate nutrition, either parenterally or enterally, cannot be overstated. Malnutrition works steadfastly against the recovery process.

Supplemental Readings

Brewer, B. D., and Koterba, A. M.: Development of a scoring system for the early diagnosis of equine neonatal sepsis. Equine Vet. J., 20:18–22, 1988.

Koterba, A. M.: Identification and early management of the high risk neonatal foal: Averting disasters. Equine Vet. Educ., 1:9–14, 1989.

Koterba, A. M.: Diagnosis and management of the normal and abnormal neonatal foal: General considerations. In: Koterba, A. M., Drummond, W. C., and Kosch, P. C. (eds); Equine Clinical Neonatology. Philadelphia, Lea & Febiger, 1990, pp. 3–15.

Koterba, A. M., Drummond, W. H., and Kosch, P. C.: Intensive care of the neonatal foal. Vet. Clin. North Am. (Equine Pract.), 1:3–34, 1985.

Sonea, I.: The sick neonatal foal. In Brown, C. M. (ed.): Problems in Equine Medicine. Philadelphia, Lea & Febiger, 1989, pp. 256–285.

Varner, D. D., and Vaala, W. E.: Equine perinatal care: Part II. Routine management of the neonatal foal. Compend. Cont. Educ. Pract. Vet., 8:S81–S94, 1986.

Neurological Examination of the Neonatal Foal

Susan Shaftoe, MADISON, WISCONSIN
Susan D. Semrad, MADISON, WISCONSIN

Neurological examination of the newborn foal is an integral part of the total physical examination. Findings on neonatal neurological examination differ from those in the adult. Additionally, subjective evaluation of individual foals between veterinarians may differ, and findings will change as the foal grows older. The examination should be systematic and repeated in the same manner each time so that some areas of the nervous system are not inadvertently omitted. Evaluation begins with the examiner observing the foal from a distance, followed by a close-up scan proceeding from the head to the tail. Gait analysis can then be pursued. By proceeding in this way, the examiner can determine whether any lesions exist above the foramen magnum. Additional lesions may be found on evaluation of the spinal cord, peripheral nerves, or musculoskeletal system; if so, integration of brain deficits with more peripheral ones should be considered. Attempts should be made to localize a lesion to one area of the nervous system, with the knowledge that a multifocal and diffuse neurological disease may also be present. After deciding on the anatomic sites of the neurological deficits, the examiner formulates a list of differential diagnoses and establishes the most likely etiology of the disease.

HISTORY

It is important to elicit from the owner as much historical information as possible about the dam and the foal. Although the foal may have signs of neurological disease while the dam appears normal, the mare's history is relevant. Length of gestation is important, as the premature foal may have a less mature nervous system than a full-term foal. Previous abnormal foalings should be noted. Premature lactation is of concern if partial or complete failure of passive transfer of immunoglobulins occurs with concurrent septicemia and secondary meningitis or encephalitis. Neurological deficits may occur in combination with diseases of other organ systems in these cases. Information about maternal problems during gestation or during the periparturient period, such as vaginal discharge, excessive abdominal enlargement, gastrointestinal upsets, colic, or respiratory disease, is relevant, as is the history of tetanus, influenza, and rhinopneumonitis vaccinations.

Historical data on the foal should include the onset, duration, and progression of neurological signs and how long it took the foal to stand, move around the stall or pasture, and nurse after birth. Affinity between the mare and foal should be ascertained. Ability to stand and find the udder appropriately varies with each foal and gestational age. From the behavioral information and later clinical evaluation, the examiner may determine that the neurological derangement is due to traumatic episodes, vascular accidents, metabolic disturbances, congenital abnormalities, multisystemic septicemia, or idiopathic causes.

PHYSICAL EXAMINATION

In the last 10 years, much has been learned about the equine neonate, but there is still a lot to learn about the premature and dysmature foal. Even though studies on neuronal myelination have shown that the full-term foal is "neurologically" mature at birth and that the normal foal can stand, ambulate, and nurse soon after birth, this does not mean that the neurological system is entirely developed.

A neurological deficit may first manifest with behavioral or gait abnormalities. It is important to recognize, however, normal differences between the foal and dam. Foals sleep or lie in lateral or sternal recumbency more than the dam. Nonetheless, they are easily aroused. Lack of arousal following stimuli may indicate abnormal mentation. The foal holds its head in a more flexed position than the dam, and during both standing and moving, the normal foal has an exaggerated head movement, especially after being stimulated by touch or vision. The motion is not unlike the "intention tremors" seen in adult cerebellar disease or in cerebellar abiotrophy of the foal.

Hypermetria, an exaggerated flexion of the limbs, that may be noted when the dam and the foal are observed walking side by side, may also be normal in the neonate. A premature or weak foal may exhibit flexor tendon laxity in the limbs, most particularly in the pastern or fetlock region, resulting in walking on the palmar or plantar region of the limbs. It is important to differentiate between a weak, sick foal and one that has true laxity associated with immaturity, dysmaturity, or congenital abnormalities.

Restraint is usually required to perform a thorough neurological examination of the standing foal. Placing one hand around the cervical region and the other around the perineal region may initiate struggling and then intermittent "flopping" into the restrainer's arms. This should be distinguished from "floppiness," in which the foal sinks down because of generalized weakness or tendon laxity associated with generalized musculoskeletal abnormalities.

CRANIAL NERVES

Cranial nerve evaluation elicits some responses that are unlike those in the adult horse. Although the response to a menace is usually absent until 1 to 2 weeks of age, visual sense is normal at birth. Withdrawal from a bright light is accompanied by an exaggerated jerking of the head. Funduscopic examination of the eyes and leading the animal through an obstacle course will identify true blindness secondary to a lesion of cranial nerve II (optic), cranial nerve III (oculomotor), or the tracts leading to and from the cerebrum. The pupillary light response is present at birth, although an anxious, excited foal may not exhibit this reflex. Ventromedial positioning of the pupil in the neonatal foal often occurs, in contrast to the slight ventrolateral rotation of the pupil in the adult horse. This strabismus may be noted for up to 2 weeks or longer. In order to evaluate the pupillary position, it is necessary to hold the head in a horizontal position. Tactile stimuli around the face provoke exaggerated movement away from the stimuli.

A foal with neurological disease may not be able to suckle and swallow appropriately. Causes of dysphagia include white muscle disease, trauma, weakness associated with septicemia, or the presence of a foreign body. A normal foal or a weak foal often holds its tongue outside the mouth. To distinguish this normal finding from abnormal cranial nerve XII (hypoglossal) function or cerebral dysfunction, tongue strength is tested by grasping the tongue. The normal foal retracts the tongue, but abnormal foals are unable or slow to retract. Many other cranial nerve responses resemble those in an adult horse. Foals that are recumbent due to illness may exhibit abnormal function of the seventh (facial) cranial nerve if continual pressure is placed on one of its branches.

CERVICAL LESIONS

Manipulation of the head and neck should be undertaken with caution in animals with suspected neurological disease as an unexpected rearing up, painful response, or collapse may be elicited, or the neurological signs may worsen if there is neck injury. A click heard when the neck is moved may indicate an occipito-atlantoaxial malformation. Pain or swelling over the head or spinal cord or blood emission from the ears may suggest trauma. Pain may be indicative of osteomyelitis of the vertebrae or joints in a previously septic foal. Malalignment of the vertebral column, suggesting a congenital problem, should be assessed by palpation. Endoscopic examination is necessary to observe the abduction of the arytenoid cartilage occurring when the withers is slapped on the contralateral side. This reflex, tested with the slap test, is usually observed by the time the foal is 2 weeks old.

LIMB REFLEXES

Passive manipulation of the limbs in the very young recumbent normal foal will reveal the exaggerated flexibility of the forelegs and hind legs. The tip of the toe of the forelimbs will flex to touch the scapula and the hind limb cannon bone will approximate with the tibial tuberosity. This flexibility normally disappears a day or so after birth, particularly if the foal can exercise. Premature or dysmature foals and foals with musculoskeletal abnormalities will exhibit this flexibility for a longer time.

Spinal reflexes should be assessed when the foal is in lateral recumbency, a procedure that may entail catching the alert, ambulatory foal. Spinal reflexes in the foal are more readily elicited and appear hyperactive when compared to the adult horse. In general, the foal has exaggerated tone.

The extensor thrust reflex is manifested by extension of limb joints and toe in response to pressure on the sole of the hoof. Although others have observed this reflex to be most prominent in the pelvic limbs, we have also observed the response in the thoracic limbs. This reflex usually disappears 18 to 24 hours after birth. The withdrawal reflex (flexor reflex), elicited by applying pressure to the distal limb, is present, as is a crossed extensor reflex. The latter gradually diminishes and disappears by 2 to 4 weeks of age. The crossed extensor reflex is characterized by extension of the lower thoracic or pelvic limb when pressure is placed on the contralateral upper limb. Such a reflex in the adult would suggest a significant upper motor neuron lesion.

In the forelimbs, the biceps and triceps reflexes are often noted, though the ability to elicit them decreases over time. In the hind limb, the patellar and flexor reflexes are usually hyperactive when compared with the adult. Clonus may be observed after eliciting the patellar reflex. Additionally, the gastrocnemius and cranial tibial reflexes are commonly present in the neonate, but are not normally noted in the adult horse. It is common to see these exaggerated limb reflexes up to 2 to 4 weeks of age, although it has been suggested that the limb responses may vary with the amount of exercise the foal receives. The more exercise, the less pronounced will be the limb reflexes.

GAIT

Gait analysis is difficult in the neonatal foal because it cannot be handled easily. With maturity and handling, the foal is easier to manage and gait analysis is simpler. It is important to eliminate maneuvers that can compromise the foal, whether it be fear that results in falling or rearing, or movements of the body that exacerbate a spinal cord lesion. In many cases the foal's gait is appraised by watching it follow the dam. Ataxia should be noted, although it should be remembered that the neonate has a short-strided, awkward, or "gawky" gait in comparison to the dam. As the foal grows older and more accustomed to moving around, the gait more closely resembles that of the dam. Pastern or fetlock laxity decreases if there are no underlying congenital abnormalities and if the foal is not premature with immature cuboidal bones and cartilaginous damage.

Weakness is difficult to evaluate unless it is extreme. Due to their size, foals are easily pushed and pulled from side to side, and the response to pressure applied to the withers or gluteal region may be exaggerated. Depending on the cooperation of the patient, hemiwalking, hopping on the hind limbs, and wheelbarrowing procedures can be performed on a soft surface to test proprioception.

ADDITIONAL TESTING

Ancillary evaluation of the equine neonate with suspected neurological disease includes cerebrospinal fluid analysis and electromyography. Blood tests must rule out metabolic disease (hypoglycemia or acidosis), hypoxemia, musculoskeletal disease (white muscle disease), and trauma. Radiography is indicated if there is evidence of a fracture or osteomyelitis. Radiographs of the neonate must be interpreted carefully, as the physeal plates are open and may mimic a fracture line. Even with portable x-ray equipment, congenital abnormalities or trauma can be diagnosed. Results of cerebrospinal fluid analysis (Table 1) resemble those of the adult horse, except for a higher total protein content, the high-

TABLE 1. NORMAL RANGE OF CEREBROSPINAL FLUID VALUES IN NEONATAL FOALS*

Parameter	Value
Color	Clear
Total protein	100 mg/dl ±50 (biuret method) trace to +2 (quantitative reagent stick), 1.3347 to 1.3350 (refractive index)
Glucose	80% of blood glucose value
pH	7.34 to 7.40
WBC count	< 5 cells/μl
RBC count	0 to 500/μl
Creatine kinase, IU/L	15.2 ± 9.2
Sodium, mmol/L	142.6 ± 2.8
Potassium, mmol/L	3.6 ± 2.1
Chloride, mmol/L	109 ± 3.4

From Koterba, A. M., Drummond, W. C., and Kosch, P. C. (eds.): Equine Clinical Neonatology. Philadelphia, Lea & Febiger, 1990, p. 501. Reproduced by permission.
*Values may vary depending on technique of analysis.

est reported being an average of 138 mg per dl. This discrepancy between foals and adults has been attributed to a less mature blood–brain barrier in the young animal. Electromyography should be performed whenever muscle atrophy is ascertained on clinical examination.

A complete blood cell count, including a white blood cell differential and an assay for partial or complete failure of absorption of immunoglobulins, should be routine in a young neonate when sepsis and secondary meningoencephalitis are suspected. Biochemical analysis may help rule out other systemic diseases, especially those with concurrent metabolic disturbances. An elevated creatine phosphokinase level will aid in diagnosing white muscle disease as a cause of weakness. This enzyme may also be elevated secondary to trauma, though not usually to the extent that it is in white muscle disease.

Supplemental Readings

Adams, R.: Neurologic examination of the newborn foal. *In* Robinson, N. E. (ed.): Current Therapy in Equine Medicine 2. Philadelphia, W. B. Saunders, 1987, pp. 199–202.

Green, S. L., and Mayhew, I. G.: Neurologic disorders. *In* Koterba, A. M., Drummond, W. H., and Kosch, P. C. (eds.): Equine Clinical Neonatology. Philadelphia, Lea & Febiger, 1990, pp. 496–530.

Mayhew, I. G.: Large Animal Neurology: A Handbook for Veterinary Clinicians. Philadelphia, Lea & Febiger, 1989, pp. 15–47.

Reed, S. M.: Neurologic examination of neonatal foals and diagnostic testing useful to evaluate normal foals with neurological problems. *In:* Proceedings of the American College of Veterinary Internal Medicine, 8th Annual Forum, 1990, pp. 601–606.

Ultrasonographic Evaluation and Diagnosis of Foal Diseases

Virginia B. Reef, KENNETT SQUARE, PENNSYLVANIA

There are innumerable applications of diagnostic ultrasonography (US) in the equine neonatal and pediatric patient. Evaluation of neonatal umbilical remnant structures, bladder, and much of the gastrointestinal (GI) viscera is possible in addition to more standard imaging of the abdominal organs (liver, kidney, and spleen) and the thoracic viscera (heart and lungs). US is well tolerated by the equine neonatal or pediatric patient as the examination is noninvasive and can usually be performed in the unsedated animal. The only patient preparation required is clipping of hair from the skin over the structures that are to be examined to obtain optimal image quality. The skin is cleaned and a coupling gel is applied for the subsequent examination.

UMBILICAL INFECTION

Infection of the internal umbilical remnant structures occurs frequently in the absence of palpable abnormalities of the external umbilical remnant. Most affected foals are referred for US evaluation because of septicemia, infection at a site other than the umbilicus (particularly septic arthritis), an unexplained persistent leukocytosis, neutrophilia, or hyperfibrinogenemia, or palpable abnormalities of the external umbilical remnant. The majority of foals with internal umbilical remnant infection are 1 to 4 weeks old when referred for US evaluation. However, numerous younger foals and a few older than 4 weeks have been identified with internal umbilical remnant infection. The oldest reported horse with internal umbilical remnant infection was 16 months old when the condition was detected. Most foals have more than one internal umbilical structure involved, and bacteriological culture of fluid or exudate from the affected structures usually yields multiple organisms. Blood cultures or bacteriological cultures obtained from joint aspirates or other infected sites usually yield at least one organism cultured from the infected umbilicus.

Imaging of the umbilicus is best performed with a 7.5-MHz transducer containing a built-in fluid bath or using a hand-held standoff. All four internal umbilical structures can be imaged with US in the normal foal up to 4 to 8 weeks of age. The umbilical vein can be found on the midline from the external umbilical remnant to the liver and normally measures 6.0 ± 2.0 mm in diameter. The urachus and both umbilical arteries can be scanned from the external umbilical remnant to the bladder and measure 17.5 ± 4.0 mm at the bladder apex. Each umbilical artery can then be imaged along the bladder, measuring 8.5 ± 2.0 mm at this location. Enlargement of the structures indicates infection. The lumen of the umbilical vein, umbilical arteries, or urachus may be filled with sonolucent, hypoechoic, or echogenic fluid (Fig. 1) and may contain hyperechoic gas echoes if gas-forming organisms (usually anaerobes) are involved.

Both medical and surgical treatment has been successful in affected foals. Medical treatment is usually recommended for foals with no signs of disease other than laboratory abnormalities (leukocytosis, neutrophilia, or hyperfibrinogenemia), mild enlargement of the internal umbilical remnant structures, or foals in which only one internal umbilical remnant structure is affected. Foals with septicemia, septic joints, internal umbilical remnant structures greater than twice normal size, or multiple infected internal umbilical remnant structures are surgical candidates. If medical therapy is selected, the internal umbilical remnant structure should be followed with serial US studies performed every 2 to 3 days, as changes in these structures may occur rapidly. If the internal umbilical remnant structures enlarge, changing antimicrobials or surgical resection is indicated. In most foals, broad-spectrum antimicrobial therapy should be considered with agents effective against both gram-positive and gram-negative organisms. If gas echoes are seen within the internal umbilical remnant structures, antimicrobial drugs should be selected that have efficacy against anaerobic organisms as well.

The prognosis for foals with internal umbilical remnant infections is usually good and successful outcomes have been reported with both medical and surgical therapies. If the umbilical vein is enlarged and purulent material can be detected at its entrance to the liver, a more guarded prognosis should be given. Surgical resection in these foals may lead to abdominal contamination and possible subsequent peritonitis or adhesions.

HERNIAS

US evaluation of umbilical and scrotal hernias is a useful addition to the physical examination and case management. The herniation of GI viscera can be diagnosed (Fig. 2) and the motility and wall thickness of the herniated portion of intestine evaluated. The compromised herniated intestine has a thickened edematous wall and decreased to absent peristaltic movement. If the swelling is hot and painful, an abscess may be associated with the hernia, particularly umbilical hernias. The extent and involvement of any internal umbilical remnant structures or intra-abdominal structures can be determined. Measurement of the hernial diameter may also aid the surgeon in the decision about hernial closure.

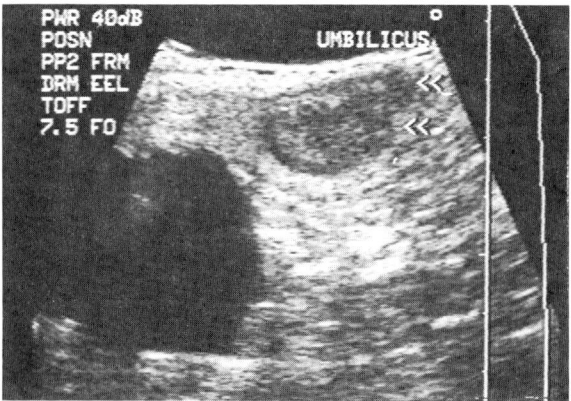

Figure 1. Long-axis sonogram of the urachus of a 4-day-old Standardbred colt obtained with a 7.5-MHz sector scanner transducer (Microimager 2000 Ausonics, Universal Medical Systems, Yonkers, NY) containing a built-in fluid bath. The external umbilical remnant is to the right of the image (not shown) and the bladder is the anechoic structure on the left of the image. The infected urachus *(arrows)* is filled with hypoechoic (purulent) material.

URINARY TRACT DISORDERS

US examination of the bladder and urachus can speed up the diagnosis of a ruptured bladder. Affected foals are usually 1 week old or less and

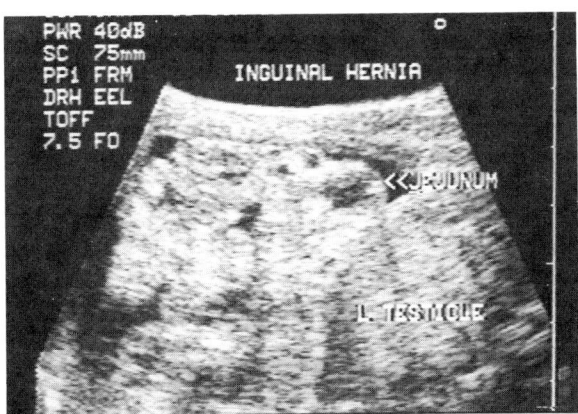

Figure 2. Long-axis sonogram of the scrotum of a 14-day-old Thoroughbred colt with a scrotal hernia. The sonogram was obtained with a 7.5-MHz sector scanner transducer containing a built-in fluid bath. Note loops of small intestine (jejunum) and the left testicle within the scrotum.

exhibit signs of depression, lethargy, and increasing abdominal distention. US evaluation reveals a large fluid-filled abdomen and a collapsed bladder (Fig. 3). In many instances, the actual tear in the bladder wall is visible and fluid can be seen going from the bladder into the abdominal cavity. The fluid within the abdominal cavity is usually anechoic, consistent with a uroperitoneum. The small and large intestinal viscera can be seen floating within the clear sonolucent fluid.

Although uroperitoneum is most frequently caused by a ruptured bladder, tears in the urachus or ureters may also result in uroperitoneum. If the urachus is the source of the uroperitoneum, the bladder will be filled with anechoic fluid (urine), and anechoic fluid may be imaged leaking from the urachus or dissecting into the retroperitoneal space along the falciform ligament and along the urachus. Ureteral ruptures result in a uroperitoneum with a small intact bladder. The ureters are not routinely visible on US in foals. Therefore, this diagnosis must be suspected in foals with a large fluid-filled abdomen, an intact bladder, and normal urachus.

Persistent patent urachus and urachal diverticulum are also easily detected with US. With a persistent patent urachus, fluid extends from the bladder apex into the urachus to the external umbilical remnant. As the patent urachus closes, a urachal diverticulum often forms. This is most easily visualized with a full bladder as an outpouching of the bladder apex between the two umbilical arteries that does not communicate with the external umbilical remnant. Some authors have suggested that a persistent patent urachus may predispose to the development of urachitis, and thus repeated US evaluation is probably indicated in these foals.

In foals with a history of hematuria or excessive hemorrhage of the umbilicus at parturition, US examination of the urachus, umbilical vessels, and bladder may be indicated. Several septicemic foals with histories of hematuria have had a large blood clot in the bladder detected with US. The same organisms were obtained on bacteriological culture of urine and blood. Surgical intervention in these foals for removal of the blood clot as well as prophylactic removal of the internal umbilical remnant structures has been performed successfully.

US evaluation of the foal's kidney is also useful in characterizing renal dysfunction. Large, swollen sonolucent kidneys are imaged in foals with acute renal failure. Echogenic kidneys are seen with infiltrative disease and usually indicate chronicity. Congenital renal abnormalities may also be detected but occur rarely in foals.

US evaluation of the right kidney is most successfully performed from the right 14th to 16th intercostal space, centering on the 15th intercostal space. The kidney is usually located between two lines level with the dorsalmost and ventralmost aspects of the tuber coxae. The left kidney is optimally scanned in the 17th intercostal space or in the cranial portion of the paralumbar fossa. This kidney is normally slightly more ventral in location, medial to the spleen, and usually is imaged between a line level with the dorsal border of the tuber coxae to a line level with the tuber ischii. If a renal biopsy is desirable, it can be performed under US guidance. A 5-MHz transducer is usually optimal for scanning foal kidneys.

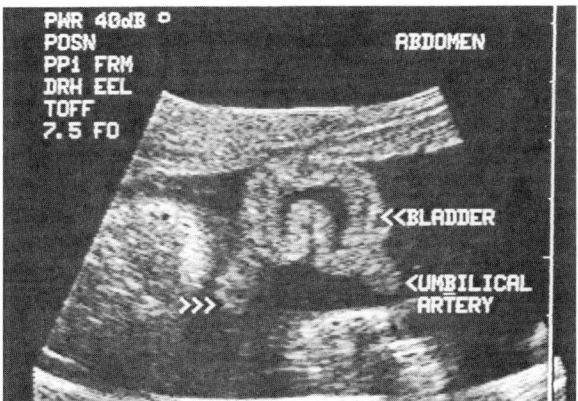

Figure 3. Short-axis sonogram obtained in a 6-day-old Thoroughbred colt with uroperitoneum and a ruptured bladder. The sonogram was obtained with a 7.5-MHz sector scanner transducer containing a built-in standoff. Note large amount of anechoic fluid in the abdomen, collapsed bladder, and right and left umbilical arteries.

US EVALUATION OF THE FOAL WITH COLIC

Because of the preponderance of small intestinal lesions in foals presenting with colic, US evaluation of the foal abdomen is a very helpful part of the diagnostic workup. Differentiation between a medical and surgical lesion can often be made based on the US appearance of the GI tract.

Small intestinal intussusceptions in foals have a characteristic target or bull's-eye appearance when imaged. The targetlike appearance is caused by scanning through the apex of the intussusception. The thick outer hypoechoic rim is caused by severe edema of the entering and exiting walls of the intussusceptum. When the entering and exiting walls of the intussusceptum are scanned on cross-section where edema is less severe, the intussusception may appear as two concentric rings with an inner circular area or as double concentric rings with a central echogenic core. The central echogenic core represents the inner lumen of the intussusceptum. The small intestinal segments proximal to the area of the intussusception appear distended with fluid; the wall thickness is more normal.

With a small intestinal volvulus, the entire small intestine is distended with fluid and the wall is thickened, edematous, and hypoechoic. Peristalsis is not visualized in the small intestine with a complete volvulus. Other partial strangulations may be imaged, with affected portions of small intestine having thickened edematous hypoechoic walls and distended, fluid-filled lumina (Fig. 4). Little or no motility is seen in the affected segments, whereas a normal small intestinal wall with GI motility is usually seen in the unaffected segments.

Meconium and ascarid impactions can also be successfully imaged in many foals. A small colon filled with echogenic material and accompanied by distention of the more proximal portions of intestine is consistent with a meconium impaction. Numerous ascarid worms are usually imaged in foals with ascarid impaction. The ascarid worms can be imaged individually within the small intestine or as a ball or mass. Fluid distention of the more proximal portion of the intestine makes visualization of the ascarids easier.

Nonsurgical lesions such as peritonitis and enteritis have characteristic appearances on US. With enteritis, fluid distention of the intestinal tract is visualized. Both the small and large intestine may be involved. The walls of the small and large intestine may be normal or thickened, edematous, and more hypoechoic than normal, particularly in foals with severe inflammatory bowel diseases such as clostridial enteritis or salmonellosis. Active motility of these affected portions of the small intestine is usually noticed, making a surgical lesion unlikely. Peritonitis is usually associated with excessive hypoechoic to echogenic abdominal fluid accumulation. Fibrin tags or adhesions between the serosal surface of the bowel and peritoneum or between abdominal organs is often imaged. Free gas visualized within the peritoneal cavity suggests an anaerobic component to the bacterial peritonitis or the possibility of a ruptured viscus.

Abdominal US of a colicky foal often reveals a fluid- and gas-distended large intestine. The amount of distention in the large bowel may preclude further US evaluation. Many of these foals have spasmodic or gas colic without large intestinal displacement, and surgery often is not indicated. Gastric distention is also readily visualized as an enlarged fluid-filled stomach immediately caudad to the liver in the proximal portion of the abdomen.

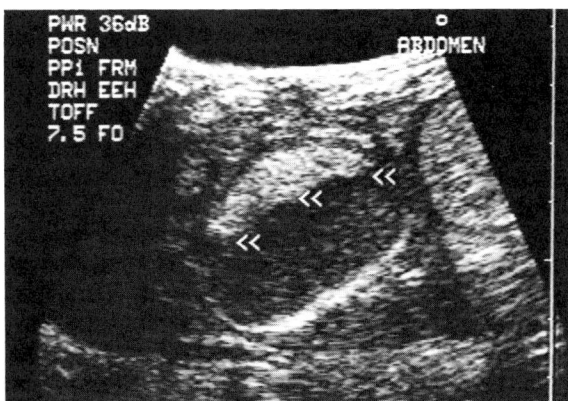

Figure 4. Sonogram of the ventral abdomen of a 1-month-old Arab foal with colic and abdominal distention. The sonogram was obtained with a 7.5-MHz sector scanner transducer containing a built-in fluid bath. *Arrows* point to mural thickening in a small segment of the jejunum. The remaining small intestinal wall appears normal. This foal had multifocal mural abscesses in this portion of jejunum, which was surgically removed.

HEPATIC DISORDERS

The hepatic parenchyma is easily evaluated in foals, and this imaging study should be done in any foal with suspected hepatic disease. The liver is detected ventral to the lung margins on the entire right side from the 6th to the 15th intercostal spaces, on the left side from the 7th to the 9th intercostal spaces, and may be imaged caudad to the xiphoid. A 5-MHz transducer is usually used for optimal image quality. Foals with proximal duodenal or gastric ulcers or strictures often have elevated biliary enzyme levels. In these foals, biliary distention, thickening of the bile ducts, and increased echogenicity of the hepatic parenchyma have been visualized, associated with obstruction of the biliary tree, cholangitis or cholangiohepatitis. Multiple pinpoint echogenic foci have also been seen in several foals with widespread miliary microabscesses. These foals were referred for US because of the presence of icterus and elevated liver enzyme levels. Congenital hepatic anomalies, portacaval shunts, or diaphragmatic hernias in which the hepatic parenchyma may have herniated into the thoracic cavity or pericardial sac may also be successfully imaged.

THORACIC US

Thoracic US is particularly useful in foals with suspected pleural effusion, pleuritis, consolidating pneumonia, or abscessation. Pleural fluid is readily visualized by scanning in the intercostal spaces with the 5-MHz transducer. Anechoic or hypoechoic fluid surrounding the floating pulmonary parenchyma is imaged. Foals with a history of thoracic trauma should be scanned, as hemothorax is common in this group. Pleuritis and pleural effusion is less common in foals than in the adult horse but should be evaluated in foals with marked cranial ventral dullness on auscultation and percussion, pleurodynia, or pleural friction rubs.

US infrequently shows pulmonary parenchymal abnormalities in many of the acute interstitial pneumonias in foals because of the interstitial nature of this disease. However, older foals with consolidating bacterial pneumonia often have large sonolucent portions of lung. Fluid-filled cavitated areas of the lung may also be seen in foals with *Rhodococcus equi* pneumonia. However, these abscesses may not always be imaged with US owing to their multifocal distribution. Thus, thoracic radiography should be included as part of the diagnostic workup in any foal in which lower respiratory tract disease is suspected.

CARDIAC DISEASES

Echocardiography is particularly useful in the evaluation of suspected cardiac disease and is the method of choice for the diagnosis of congenital cardiac disease in foals. Bacterial endocarditis, pericardial effusions, and fibrinous pericarditis are also readily imaged with echocardiography in affected foals (see p. 408).

MASSES

US is extremely useful in assessing swellings or masses and in selecting a site for aspiration or biopsy. Abscesses, hematomas, cysts, and soft tissue masses can be distinguished by their US appearance. Abscesses are cavitated areas containing sonolucent, hypoechoic, or echogenic debris with no recognizable internal echoes other than those associated with the fluid. The echogenicity of the fluid varies from sonolucent to echogenic. Echogenic masses may be seen within the abscess if necrotic muscle or foreign material is present within the abscess. Foreign bodies appear as echogenic to hyperechoic masses, usually casting acoustic shadows, and are surrounded by fluid. A tract may often be found extending down from the skin to the abscess containing the foreign body.

Sonolucent loculated fluid is most consistent with a hematoma. On occasion, echogenic material may be seen within, consistent with internal clot formation. A large cavity of sonolucent fluid with or without distinct septation and acoustic enhancement of the far wall suggests a cystic structure. Cysts are unusual in foals and are a less likely diagnosis than abscess or hematoma. Soft tissue masses may have a homogeneous appearance or a complex pattern of echogenicity, depending on the tissue making up the mass. US guidance may be used to perform aspiration or biopsy.

Diagnostic US is useful in the evaluation of a wide variety of foal diseases and should be included in a comprehensive workup of any foal with peripheral swelling of unknown origin, clinical pathological evidence of diseases affecting one of the internal organs, colic, or auscultable abnormalities of the respiratory or cardiovascular system. A thorough knowledge of normal anatomy is necessary to perform US successfully. The major limitations to successful US scanning include normally aerated structures, such as normal lung or gas-filled colon, and bony structures such as ribs. The noninvasive nature of US makes it an important part of the diagnostic armamentarium in the evaluation of foals with a wide variety of problems.

Supplemental Readings

Bernard, W. V., Reef, V. B., Reimer, J. M., et al.: Ultrasonographic diagnosis of small intestinal intussusception in three foals. J. Am. Vet. Med. Assoc., 194:395–397, 1989.

Byars, T. D., and Halley, J.: Uses of ultrasound in equine internal medicine. Vet. Clin. North Am. (Equine Pract.), 2:253–258, 1983.

Rantanen, N. W.: Diseases of the abdomen. Vet. Clin. North Am. (Equine Pract.), 2:67–88, 1986.

Reef V. B., and Collatos, C.: Ultrasonography of umbilical structures in clinically normal foals. Am. J. Vet. Res., 49:2143–2146, 1988.

Reef V. B., Collatos, C., Spencer, P. A., et al. Clinical, ultrasonographic, and surgical findings in foals with umbilical remnant infections. J. Am. Vet. Med. Assoc., 195:69–72, 1989.

Passive Transfer of Immunity to Foals

Susan L. White, ATHENS, GEORGIA

Transfer of circulating maternal antibodies to the foal during gestation is prevented by the diffuse epitheliochorial placentation of the mare. Although the foal is immunologically competent at birth and capable of mounting an immune response, it is immunologically naive due to the lack of antigenic challenge in utero. Consequently, except for small amounts of IgM, the foal is agammaglobulinemic at birth. Maternal transfer of immunoglobulins occurs postnatally via ingestion and absorption of immunoglobulin-rich colostrum by the foal. Lack of adequate transfer of immunoglobulins predisposes the foal to infection by pathogenic or opportunistic organisms in the environment and is the most common factor associated with sepsis in the foal.

PASSIVE TRANSFER OF IMMUNITY

Colostrum is produced by selective secretion of circulating immunoglobulins into the mammary gland during the last month of gestation, with the majority of immunoglobulin concentration occurring in the last 2 weeks. Stimulation for the production of colostrum is believed to be triggered by changing levels of estrogen and progesterone during the last 4 weeks of gestation. Colostrum is produced only once during each pregnancy; premature lactation by the mare may result in partial or complete loss of colostrum. Over 80 per cent of the immunoglobulins concentrated in presuckle colostrum are of the IgG and Ig(T) classes, with the remainder of the IgM and IgA classes. Colostrum also contains low molecular weight proteins that enhance the efficacy of absorption of macromolecules and may also provide complement and lactoferrin, which aid in the defense against microorganisms.

With the exception of IgA, which is manufactured by the mammary gland and is present in milk, a rapid decline in immunoglobulins occurs when mares are suckled. IgG and IgG(T) concentrations are negligible by 12 hours in mares suckled by vigorous foals and absent in all mares by 24 hours after parturition. The volume of colostrum ingested by active lightbreed foals is 3 to 5 L during the first 12 hours of life.

Immunoglobulins are absorbed by specialized villous epithelial cells present throughout the small intestine at birth. Uptake occurs by pinocytosis, with each cell accumulating a maximum amount of protein in large macroglobules prior to discharging it into the intracellular space at the base of the cell. The proteins pass into the local lacteals and into the systemic circulation via the thoracic duct. The process of protein absorption is nonselective. The large amount of immunoglobulins absorbed by the foal is controlled by the selective concentration of immunoglobulins in colostrum. Immunoglobulins are present in the foal's serum by 6 hours of age and reach adult levels by 24 to 48 hours.

The maximum capacity for protein absorption is present immediately after birth and is greatest before 6 to 12 hours of age. The capacity for protein absorption declines linearly and the intestine is "closed" by 18 to 24 hours. Closure occurs because of sloughing of the specialized enterocytes and replacement by more mature epithelial cells incapable of protein absorption. Loss of the specialized enterocytes begins immediately after birth and occurs regardless of the ingestion of colostrum or other sources of nutrition by the foal.

The concentration of serum immunoglobulins obtained by passive transfer in the foal is dependent on the concentration of immunoglobulins in the colostrum and the volume of colostrum ingested. Maximal levels are present at 24 to 48 hours after birth and subsequently decline, owing to dilution by the increasing plasma volume of the foal and by a steady-state catabolism. The half-life of maternally derived IgG and IgG(T) is 23 days and 20 days, respectively. The concentration of passively acquired immunoglobulins is usually below levels for adequate protection against infection by 1 to 2 months and has disappeared by 5 or 6 months. Autogenous or actively formed immunoglobulins, first detectable in the foal's serum at 1 to 2 weeks of age, gradually increase, reaching adult levels by 6 months. Total immunoglobulin concentration is lowest in the foal at 8 to 12 weeks of age as maternal levels rapidly decline and autogenous levels slowly rise. During this period the foal is most vulnerable to infections; however, in a fully functioning immune system the total immunoglobulin concentration remains above the minimal protective level. In foals that receive some but less than adequate passive transfer of immunity, the decline in total immunoglobulin concentration to below adequate levels occurs earlier and the foal is in particular danger of acquiring infections at 3 to 6 weeks of age.

FAILURE OF PASSIVE TRANSFER

Failure of passive transfer is the most common immune disorder of the foal and the leading cause of sepsis. Failure of passive transfer can occur because of maternal factors or foal factors. Maternal factors include nonformation of colostrum, low immunoglobulin concentration in colostrum, or loss of colostrum in premature lactation. Foal factors include failure to ingest colostrum or failure of intestinal absorption of immunoglobulins (Table 1).

Mares with a gestational length less than 320 days may not form colostrum because of the lack of time for concentration of immunoglobulins in the mammary gland or because of disruption of the normal sequence of hormone levels in the final stages of gestation. Premature foals born prior to 320 days of gestation should be able to absorb colostrum because the specialized enterocytes necessary for absorption appear early in fetal development. In the southeastern region of the United States, mares ingesting endophyte-infected fescue grass or hay during the last trimester of gestation may be agalactic or may have a significantly delayed onset of lactation. Serious illnesses in the mare in the periparturient period may also cause failure of colostral production. Delayed milk letdown occasionally occurs in maiden or nervous mares, depriving the foal of colostrum during the time of maximal immunoglobulin absorption. Mares may produce colostrum with inadequate levels of immunoglobulin for adequate passive transfer. Factors affecting the concentration of immunoglobulins in colostrum are unknown but are believed to be genetically controlled. Although wide variations in immunoglobulin concentrations in colostrum have been reported both between breeds and within breeds, presuckle colostrum immunoglobulin concentration should be at least 3000 mg per dl. Colostral immunoglobulins may be measured by single radial immunodiffusion (SRID) assay of the whey fraction or estimated by a commercial colostrometer.*

Premature lactation is the most common cause of poor-quality colostrum. It is relatively common in multiparous, older mares and has been associated with placentitis, premature placental separation, and twinning. The onset of premature lactation has been attributed to abnormal hormone changes in placental disorders, but in the majority of cases no known mare factors can be identified. Since colostrum is produced only once, significant loss of immunoglobulins can occur during steady dripping of colostrum over several hours to days.

Foals may fail to ingest colostrum because of weakness due to prematurity or illness, congenital abnormalities that prevent standing or suckling, rejection by the mare, or accidental factors such as inadvertent separation of the mare and foal after birth. Malabsorption of colostrum has been incriminated as a cause of failure of passive transfer in foals known to ingest colostrum containing sufficient immunoglobulins. Since glucocorticosteroids cause changes in the permeability of the small intestine and interfere with the uptake of macromolecules in other species, it has been hypothesized that stresses on the foal af-

TABLE 1. MAJOR CAUSES OF FAILURE OF PASSIVE TRANSFER IN FOALS

Maternal factors
  Gestational length < 320 days
  Premature lactation
  Agalactia
    Fescue toxicosis
    Severe parturient illness or death
  Inadequate concentration of immunoglobulins in colostrum
  Behavior aberrations
    Rejection of foal
    Inadequate milk letdown
  Known isosensitization of the mare
Foal factors
  Weak or sick foals
  Congenital abnormalities delay or prevent suckling
  Intestinal malabsorption of immunoglobulins

---
*Lane Manufacturing Co., Denver CO

fecting glucocorticosteroid levels may account for early closure or marked malabsorption. To date no studies have verified this hypothesis, and causes remain unknown.

The minimum level of serum IgG required for passive protection of the foal ranges from 400 to 800 mg per dl. Less than 200 mg per dl of IgG reflects complete failure of passive transfer. Partial failure of passive transfer is considered to be 200 to 400 or 800 mg per dl IgG. The concentration of IgG that constitutes protection from infection depends on several factors. An IgG concentration of 400 mg per dl has been shown to be adequate for healthy foals raised in a clean environment under good management conditions with no stresses. Foals with one or more risk factors for infection (see p. 411) or already showing signs of infection often are not protected by serum IgG concentrations of 400 to 800 mg per dl. Crucial to the foal but not considered in total IgG concentrations are the presence and titer of specific antibodies to pathogens encountered by the foal.

The incidence of failure of passive transfer in a variety of farm studies varied from 2.9 to 24 per cent. Farm management practices are the most important determinant in the occurrence of failure of passive transfer. However, prompt recognition of failure of passive transfer and appropriate management of the foal figure importantly in the reduction of severity of illness or death and a decrease in economic loss.

EVALUATION OF PASSIVE TRANSFER

Observation of foaling and the immediate postparturient period by a trained attendant ensures early detection of failure of passive transfer due to failure of the foal to ingest colostrum or agalactia in the mare. Observation of the mare and foal may also identify foals at risk for failure of passive transfer and allow for early therapeutic management. The healthy foal should stand and nurse by 2 hours after parturition. Early colostrum may be evaluated for IgG content by a colostrometer, a hydrometer that measures specific gravity. The correlation between the specific gravity and IgG concentration of colostrum is excellent. Colostrum should have a minimum of 3000 mg per dl IgG or a specific gravity of 1.060 or greater.

A variety of methods are available for evaluation of the foal's IgG concentration (Table 2). The foal is tested at 18 to 24 hours of age to allow for completion of the absorptive process and passage of the immunoglobulins into the foal's circulation. Evaluation may be performed

TABLE 2. METHODS OF TESTING FOR FAILURE OF PASSIVE TRANSFER IN FOALS

Method of Assessment	Comments
Farm management	Identifies agalactia or failure to nurse
Colostral specific gravity	Simple, quick, effective; will not identify foals with intestinal malabsorption
Protein fractionation by electrophoresis	Separates gamma-globulins from other proteins but requires specialized laboratory equipment, extensive time, expensive
Single radial immunodiffusion	Monospecific quantitative assay of IgG, requires 24 hours, expensive
Zinc sulfate turbidity	Simple, "foal side"; hemolysis interferes with test; requires 1 hour; may overestimate IgG concentrations <400 mg/dl
Latex agglutination	Simple, "foal side"; uses whole blood or serum; completed in 10 minutes; does not differentiate values of IgG >400 mg/dl
Enzyme immunoassay	Simple, "foal side"; uses whole blood or serum; completed in 10 minutes; semiquantitative to 800 mg/dl IgG

throughout the first month of life; however, early diagnosis of failure of passive transfer is desirable because of the severe consequences, particularly in foals with one or more risk factors for infection. Plasma proteins read on a refractometer or total serum protein content are not reliable indicators of failure of passive transfer because of the wide range of values found in foals with adequate IgG concentrations.

Protein fractionation by serum electrophoresis separates the globulin fractions (alpha, beta, and gamma) and albumin. When the total serum protein is known (determined by biuret method), values for each fraction can be obtained. Although useful, this method is generally performed in a commercial clinical pathology laboratory as it requires specialized equipment and technical expertise. It is expensive and time-consuming.

The SRID assay* is a specific quantitative assay for IgG. Foal serum is placed in a well on an agarose gel plate containing monospecific antibody to equine IgG. With migration and precipitation, antigen–antibody complexes form a ring; the diameter of the ring correlates with IgG concentration. SRID is the most accurate method for de-

---

*Veterinary Medical Research and Development, Inc., Pullman, WA; Miles Scientific, Elkhart, IN

termining IgG concentration and is the standard against which all other methods are compared. Disadvantages of SRID include the 18 to 24 hours required to complete the test and inaccuracy of results if strict adherence to technical procedures is not followed. Commercial kits have multiwell plates and are expensive if only one or a small number of foals are tested at one time. If plates are reused for multiple tests at different times, interference from migration lines of previous tests may yield inaccurate results.

The zinc sulfate turbidity test is a semiquantitative test that measures total immunoglobulin (IgG and other classes) in serum by the formation of a visible precipitate when the immunoglobulins combine with zinc ions in solution. The opacity of the resulting solution is read on a spectrophotometer or visually estimated by the operator. A commercial test kit‡ is available, or the reagent may be made by the practitioner. Reagents are easily altered by exposure to air, rendering the test inaccurate, and therefore must be handled carefully. The test requires one hour at room temperature for completion. Precipitates are fragile and samples must be carefully handled. Hemolysis interferes with the test, and overestimation of the immunoglobulin concentration has been reported to occur commonly in foals with less than 400 mg per dl IgG, resulting in inability to recognize foals with partial failure of passive transfer.

The latex agglutination test° estimates the IgG concentration by the degree of agglutination between latex beads coated with monospecific antibodies to equine IgG and IgG in foal's blood or serum. The agglutination occurs in 10 minutes and is unaffected by hemolysis. The test accurately identifies IgG concentrations less than 400 mg per dl; however, the maximum end point of 400 mg per dl IgG does not allow for determination of IgG values between 400 and 800 mg per dl, which is desirable for the sick foal or the foal at risk for infection.

The enzyme immunoassay test is a semiquantitative assay which utilizes development of a color spot with calibration standards corresponding to concentrations of 200, 400, and 800 mg per dl IgG built into the test. The commercial kit† utilizes whole blood or serum and requires 3 minutes of incubation. Approximately 10 minutes is required to perform the entire test. Excellent correlation exists between results from the enzyme immunoassay and SRID and no errors of overestimation of IgG occur.

THERAPEUTIC MANAGEMENT

Farm Management

Mares that foal away from home should arrive at the foaling farm 2 to 4 weeks prior to parturition to allow development of specific antibodies to environmental organisms. Vaccination of the mare 2 to 4 weeks prior to foaling increases the titer of specific immunoglobulins in colostrum. Observation of foaling by a trained attendant allows for evaluation of presuckle colostrum for IgG concentration and ensures that the foal nurses within 3 hours of birth. For foals identified with failure or partial failure of passive transfer, efforts should be directed toward minimizing the foal's exposure to pathogens, decreasing stresses on the foal, and optimizing the environment, as well as instituting careful monitoring of the foal for early signs of infection.

Foals Less Than 12 Hours Old

When inadequate ingestion of colostrum can be anticipated due to premature lactation, agalactia, low specific gravity of colostrum, or a weak or orphaned foal, the foal may be given colostrum orally. Two hundred to 250 ml of colostrum may be collected from mares after their own foals have suckled 2 to 3 times and frozen ($-4°$ F or $-20°$ C) for future needs. Colostrum should not be collected from mares that have prelactated and should contain a minimum of 3000 mg per dl IgG, or ideally at least 6000 mg per dl IgG, as estimated by a colostrometer or measured by SRID of the whey fraction. Frozen colostrum may be stored for 1 year without loss of quality. Although the immunoglobulins are stable for longer than 1 year, other components in the colostrum deteriorate with prolonged storage.

The amount of colostrum needed depends on the size of the foal, the degree of failure of passive transfer, time of administration and quality of the colostrum. As a general rule, a foal should receive 2 to 3 liters of colostrum within the first 12 hours of life. Ideally, the colostrum should be administered in aliquots of 500 ml with at least 1 hour between each administration.

If the foal is more than 6 hours old at the time of colostral supplementation, absorption of immunoglobulins is significantly decreased and the resulting IgG concentration in the foal's serum may be inadequate. Local protection of the gastrointestinal tract by oral colostrum still warrants its administration.

---

‡Equiz Z, Veterinary Medical Research and Development, Inc., Pullman, WA
°Foalcheck, Haver-Lockhart, Shawnee, KS
†CITE-Foal IgG Test, Agritech Systems, Inc., Portland ME

Equine plasma or serum may be substituted for colostrum. Because of the low total immunoglobulin content of plasma (mean IgG = 500 mg per dl) compared to colostrum, much larger quantities must be used.

A concentrated equine serum containing high antibody titers to *E. coli* for oral prophylactic use within 12 hours of birth has recently become available.° Although the product is not meant as a substitute for colostrum, it may be beneficial in foals with known failure of passive transfer.

Foals deprived of colostrum from their dam for prevention of neonatal isoerythrolysis should only be given colostrum or plasma from mares known to be free of anti-erythrocyte antibodies. All foals given oral colostrum or plasma should be tested at 24 hours of age to ensure absorption of adequate immunoglobulins.

FOALS GREATER THAN 12 HOURS OLD

It is unlikely that foals 12 to 24 hours old will absorb enough immunoglobulins from oral colostrum to correct significantly low IgG levels. If the foal's IgG concentration is below the acceptable level at 24 hours of age, IgG supplementation should be given intravenously. Sources of exogenous IgG are plasma harvested from a local donor, commercial fresh frozen plasma, or commercial concentrated serum. Plasma harvested from a local donor has the advantage of containing antibodies to local environmental organisms and pathogens. Several criteria should be met when choosing a donor horse. The horse should test negative on an agar gel immunodiffusion test for equine infectious anemia and should be free of antibodies to equine RBCs. The prospective donor's plasma can be screened for lysins and agglutins to all known equine blood types by a blood typing laboratory (see p. 431). Since it is common for RBCs to contaminate plasma separated from blood by sedimentation, the donor horse should also be blood group Aa and Qa negative, as these blood types are most commonly associated with cases of neonatal isoerythrolysis. If harvested by the practitioner, the use of commercial blood collection bags with a transfer pack for plasma† minimizes the handling of the blood and plasma and helps ensure sterility. Care should be taken to completely fill the blood collection bags, or excess citrate from the anticoagulant may induce hypocalcemia in the foal. The major disadvantage of plasma harvested under general practice conditions, particularly if plasma is obtained at the time of need, is that the concentration of IgG is unknown. Most commercial sources of plasma and serum currently available are labeled with the minimal mg per dl of IgG present in each unit. Commercial sources of fresh frozen plasma†,‡ are convenient, save time, are free of diseases, are negative for red cell antibodies, may originate from horses immunized against specific pathogens of the horse (e.g., *Rhodococcus equi*) to which commercial vaccines are unavailable and originate from animals with known immunoglobulin levels. The major disadvantage of commercial plasma is that it may not have high titers to specific organisms in the foal's environment. Commercial equine serum§,‖ has the advantage of not having to be kept frozen. Studies have shown serum to be equivalent to fresh frozen plasma in providing adequate levels of immunoglobulins in foals with failure of passive transfer.

Appropriate dosage levels of exogenous IgG are still unclear and are dependent on whether or not treatment is for an established systemic infection or for prophylaxis. Marked decreases in serum IgG concentrations have been observed in foals within 24 hours of administration of exogenous IgG in which the amount administered was calculated on the basis of the plasma volume of the foal and the concentration of IgG in the foal's serum and donor plasma. Possible reasons for this decrease are clearance of denatured IgG, clearance of IgG complexes formed by infused IgG and existing antigens, change in the catabolic rate or destruction of IgG, or redistribution of IgG to extravascular sites. The most important reason for early reduction in circulating IgG levels in healthy foals treated prophylactically for infection is probably redistribution. The importance of this loss of IgG from the circulation is unknown. In septicemic foals, accelerated loss of IgG occurs at an unpredictable rate due to increased catabolism secondary to infection and an increased use of IgG.

Healthy foals with no signs of current infection given exogenous IgG should receive 200 to 400 mg of IgG per kg of body weight, dependent on the severity of the failure of passive transfer and the minimal acceptable concentration of IgG for the particular foal. Foals already suffering from infection should receive 400 to 500 mg of IgG per kg body weight. In all cases of exogenous IgG administration, the IgG concentration of the foal's serum should be remeasured in 1 to

---

°Coli Endotox, Grand Laboratories, Larchwood, IA
†Fenwall Labs., Deerfield, IL

†Polymune (1500 mg per dl IgG), Veterinary Dynamics, Inc., Chino, CA.
‡HiGamm-Equi (2500 mg per dl IgG), Lake Immunogenics, Ontario, NY
§Endoserum (3000 mg per dl IgG), Imvac, Columbia, MO
‖Proimmune-E (4000 mg per dl IgG), American Veterinary Reference Labs., Addison, IL

3 days and as deemed necessary thereafter, depending on the foal's condition. Foals with established infections may need several administrations of IgG over the course of their illness.

Serum IgG levels are not an indication of specific antibody titers. Foals with low serum IgG levels may remain healthy if specific antibody titers to organisms they encounter are adequate. Conversely, very high serum IgG concentrations in a foal do not preclude infection. In the future we may realize even greater success with exogenous immunoglobulin therapy if products with known titers to specific organisms become available in concentrated form.

Supplemental Readings

Baldwin, J. L., Vanderwall, D. K., Cooper, W. L., and Erb, H. N.: Immunoglobulin G and early survival of foals: A three-year field study. In: Proceedings of the 35th Annual Convention of the American Association of Equine Practitioners, 1989, pp. 179–186.

Bertone, J. J., Jones, R. L., and Curtis, C. R.: Evaluation of a test kit for determination of serum immunoglobulin G concentration in foals. J. Vet. Intern. Med., 2:181–183, 1988.

Koterba, A. M., Brewer, B., and Drummond, W. H.: Prevention and control of infection. In Beech, J. (ed.): Neonatal Equine Disease. Vet. Clin. North Am., 1:41–50, 1985.

LeBlanc, M. M.: Responses to plasma transfusion in clinically healthy and clinically ill foals. In: Proceedings of the 33rd Annual Convention of the American Association of Equine Practitioners, 1988, pp. 755–761.

LeBlanc, M. M., McLaurin, B. I., and Boswell, R.: Relationships among serum immunoglobulin concentration in foals, colostral specific gravity, and colostral immunoglobulin concentration. J. Am. Vet. Med. Assoc., 189:57–60, 1986.

White, S. L.: The use of plasma in foals with failure of passive transfer and/or sepsis. In: Proceedings of the 35th Annual Convention of the American Association of Equine Practitioners, 1989, pp. 215–218.

Hemostasis in the Newborn Foal

Benjamin J. Darien, CORVALLIS, OREGON
Bernard F. Feldman, BLACKSBURG, VIRGINIA

This chapter reviews the aspects of the hemostatic system that differ in newborns compared with foals 7 to 14 days old; discusses the most frequently encountered primary and secondary conditions that affect hemostasis; lists the practical laboratory tests used to evaluate acquired and congenital hemostatic disorders; and describes the relevant therapeutic regimens for certain hemostatic disorders.

NEONATAL MATURATION OF THE COAGULATION SYSTEM

Normal hemostasis is maintained by an interaction between the vascular endothelium, platelets, blood proteins, and fibrinolytic system. Alterations in hemostasis (hemorrhage and thrombosis) are not uncommon complications in the sick neonate. In such cases, accurate interpretation of clinicopathological data is predicated on an understanding of the physiology of hemostasis and is germane to formulating an appropriate therapeutic regimen. Hemostasis is briefly reviewed here for the reader's convenience.

The endothelial cells play an important role in maintaining hemostasis by balancing anticoagulant properties (maintaining blood flow and preventing thrombotic events) with procoagulant activities (generation of thrombin and platelet-activating factor). Platelet interaction with von Willebrand factor is necessary for the normal adhesion of platelets to the exposed subendothelial collagen of injured blood vessels. Thus, the interaction between injured vessel walls and blood platelets results in the formation of a primary hemostatic plug and constitutes primary hemostasis. Fibrin generated by the coagulation proteins is complexed within the aggregated platelets to form a fibrin–platelet plug and constitutes secondary hemostasis. Dissolution of the fibrin clot occurs by adsorption of tissue plasminogen activator (tPA) onto the fibrin clot, the generation of plasmin, and the subsequent degradation of fibrinogen and fibrin into fibrinogen degradation products (FDPs).

To regulate the hemostatic response, the activity of the procoagulant and fibrinolytic proteases are modulated by numerous inhibitors, antithrombin III (AT-III), protein C, α_2-antiplasmin (α_2-AP), and tPA inhibitor (tPA-I). AT-III appears to be the most important of the procoagulant inhibitors as it accounts for 75 per cent of the thrombin-inhibiting activity in plasma and has activity against factors in both the intrinsic and common pathways. Thus, hemostasis is maintained only when an intricate balance exists among insult, such as vascular injury, platelet aggregation, or coagulation cascade activation, response (fibrin platelet plug), regulation by inhibitors (AT-III and tPA-inhibitor), and endothelial repair.

Levels of specific liver-derived coagulation factors vary with postnatal development (Table 1). The immature liver of neonates results in decreased amounts of vitamin K–dependent procoagulant factors VII and IX. Factor VII is approximately 70 per cent of normal adult levels at birth, while factor IX is approximately 40 per cent. Factor VII approximates adult levels by 2 days of age, is elevated by 2 weeks of age, and remains elevated through 5 months of age. Factor IX approximates normal adult levels by 2 to 4 weeks of age. Von Willebrand's factor (vWf:Ag) and factor VIII procoagulant (VIII:C) are elevated in term foals and remain so through the first 5 months of life.

Fibronectin, a glycoprotein that promotes cellular adhesion, aggregation, and agglutination and is involved in the pathogenesis of infections from inception to the final stages of healing, is approximately 60 per cent of normal adult levels at birth and reaches adult levels by 7 days of age.

The natural circulating inhibitor AT-III is approximately 75 per cent of adult levels at birth, decreases another 10 per cent by 24 hours, and reaches adult levels by 7 days of age. Levels for protein C, α_2-AP, and tPA-I have not yet been determined.

The platelet count and fibrinogen levels in newborn foals are essentially the same as adult values. However, qualitative disorders in platelet function (diminished response to several agonists) are present at birth and may help explain the slightly prolonged bleeding time seen in newborn foals with normal platelet counts. The prothrombin time (PT), which is used to evaluate the extrinsic and common pathways, is within the adult normal range at birth. PT is prolonged by deficiencies of factors V, VII, X, II (thrombin), or I (fibrinogen), or by the presence of inhibitors against any one (or more) of these proteins. The activated partial thromboplastin time (APTT), which is used to evaluate the intrinsic and common pathways, is only slightly prolonged in the newborn and is well within the adult normal range by 2 days of age. However, APTT is not a sensitive monitor of factor deficiencies because abnormalities or inhibitors of any of the associated factors may offset the deficiencies, resulting in an APTT that may be supranormal (shortened) or prolonged.

DIAGNOSIS AND TREATMENT OF CONDITIONS THAT AFFECT HEMOSTASIS

Historical factors related to the mare, parturition, or the foal relevant to acquired or congenital disorders of hemostasis in the foal are listed in Table 2. The history and physical examination will usually provide more useful information regarding the diagnosis and need for specific therapy than will laboratory tests. Physical examination findings associated with hemostatic disorders include petechial and ecchymotic hemorrhages in the pinna of the ear and mucous membranes of the oral cavity and vulva. Such findings are consistent with septicemia, vascular fragility, platelet abnormalities or disseminated intravascular coagulation (DIC). Episcleral hemorrhage and jaundice are consistent with infection, neonatal isoerythrolysis, or liver disease,

TABLE 1. NORMAL RANGES FOR LABORATORY SCREENING TESTS FOR HEMOSTASIS PROBLEMS IN FOALS

Age	Platelets ($\times 10^9$/L)	PT (sec)	APTT (sec)	BT (min)	Fibrinogen (gm/L)	FDP (μg/ml)	AT-III (%)	VII (%)	VIII:C (%)	IX (%)	vWf:Ag (%)	pFN (μg/ml)
Birth	—	12.7	56.3	—	—	80	77/77	68.7	210	38	380	230
+3 hr	208 (91–325)	10.1/12.6 (8.5–11.7)	40.7/54.1 (33.9–47.5)	—	0.155/0.115 (0.091–0.219)	40	75.9/73 (58.7–96.8)	69.4	174	39	275	250
+24 hr	129–409	12.5	57.8	6.8–12.8	0.129	—	63.9	72.7	135	39	163	265
+48 hr	105–353	11.9	47.4	—	0.156	—	71.1	94.1	164	50	155	350
+7 days	111–387	12.3	47.6	1.7–8.1	0.149	—	94.1	129.9	196	66	135	390
+14 days	133–457	12.0	47.9	2.5–5.8	0.149	—	98.0	142.2	193	89	235	322
Adults	100–350	13.1 (7–19)	47.0 37–54	1.0–5.0	0.137 (0.1–0.4)	<10	100.0 (71–129)	100.0	100	100	100	397

NOTE.—Values in parentheses represent means ± 2 SD. Ranges of normal values may vary among laboratories, depending on the reagents and the equipment employed.

PT = prothrombin time, APTT = activated partial thromboplastin time, BT = bleeding time, FDP = fibrinogen degradation products, AT-III = antithrombin III (equine), VIII = factor VIII, VIII:C = functional factor VIII, IX = factor IX, vWf:Ag = von Willebrand factor: antigen, pFN = plasma fibronectin.

TABLE 2. CONDITIONS OCCURING IN THE MARE, DURING PARTURITION, OR IN THE FOAL THAT CAN HAVE A PRIMARY OR SECONDARY EFFECT ON HEMOSTASIS IN THE FOAL

Condition	Primary or Secondary Effect on Hemostasis
Mare	
1. Fever or infection	1. Septicemia/endotoxemia
2. Enterocolitis	2. Septicemia/endotoxemia
3. Hydrops allantois	3. Fetal anemia
4. Medications (NSAIDs, antibiotics, DMSO)	4. Hepatoxicity/hypoxia, drug-induced coagulopathy or hemolysis
5. Bleeding problems in previous offspring	5. Inherited abnormalities of clotting factors or platelet function
6. Vaccination status	6. EHV-1 infection, hepatic necrosis
Parturition	
1. Premature separation of placenta	1. Hypoxia, acidemia, anemia
2. Cesarian section, premature rupture or clamping of the umbilical cord	2. Blood loss anemia, hypoxia, acidosis
3. Dystocia	3. Neonatal stress, aspiration pneumonia, septicemia, intra-abdominal or intrathoracic hemorrhage
Foal	
1. Colostral intake	1. Neonatal isoerythrolysis, FPT
2. Medications (NSAIDs, antibiotics, DMSO)	2. Gastroduodenal ulceration, hepatotoxicity, intravascular hemolysis
3. Infection	3. Septicemia/endotoxemia, vascular fragility, hepatic dysfunction, altered platelet function, DIC

NSAIDs = nonsteroidal anti-inflammatory drugs, DIC = disseminated intravascular coagulation, DMSO = dimethyl sulfoxide, FPT = failure of passive transfer

while large bruises or hematomas are consistent with clotting factor deficiency, liver disease, platelet abnormality, or DIC. Characterizing the foal as "sick" or "well" tends to be very useful in prioritizing a list of differentials. Sick foals are often recumbent, anorexic, depressed, and febrile. Prematurity, dysmaturity, perinatal infection, respiratory distress, metabolic derangements, and birth asphyxia are common primary conditions affecting the foal and can result in secondary conditions that affect hemostasis, such as hypoxia, acidosis, endotoxemia, hepatocellular dysfunction, vascular injury, and coagulation cascade and platelet activation. The "well" foal is usually full term and without obvious clinical disease. Foals with neonatal isoerythrolysis appear well initially but rapidly progress to the "sick" group. In well foals, the underlying disorder is diagnosed on physical examination (hemarthrosis, hematomas, large bruises, petechiae or ecchymoses) or there is laboratory evidence of impaired hemostasis. Such foals are encountered far less frequently and generally have inherited abnormalities of clotting factors or platelet function.

PRIMARY CONDITIONS AFFECTING HEMOSTASIS

Factor VIII deficiency (classic hemophilia A) is a sex-linked recessive trait that has been described in Thoroughbred and Standardbred colts. On laboratory examination, an abnormal factor VIII concentration, prolonged APTT, and normal PT would be consistent with this condition. Additionally, deficiencies in factors XI, IX, VIII, VII and thrombin have been reported in Arabian foals. Treatment of these conditions is palliative at best. However, confirmation of carrier females of the affected line and genetic counseling should be performed to reduce the incidence of recurrence.

Platelet response to agonists is attenuated in the newborn foal but returns to normal by the first week of life. The change in bleeding time from 1 day of age to after 7 days of age is consistent with this change in platelet function. No therapy is usually required unless secondary factors exacerbate the condition.

SECONDARY CONDITIONS AFFECTING HEMOSTASIS

Neonatal isoerythrolysis is an important immunological condition of newborn foals that, if not diagnosed early and treated effectively, can result in a fatal hemolytic crisis. Neonatal isoerythrolysis results from absorbing colostral antibodies (alloantibodies) directed against the foal's red blood cells (RBCs). The antibodies are produced by the mare in response to foreign RBC antigens (foal's RBCs), which leak into the maternal circulation during parturition (alloimmunization). In subsequent pregnancies the alloantibodies are produced by the mare, concentrated in the colostrum, and absorbed with other immunoglobulins when the foal acquires passive immunity. Mares that do not have the Aa or Qa antigen are at risk of producing neonatal isoerythrolysis–causing antibodies (more than 90 per cent of cases of neonatal isoerythrolysis are the result of absorbing Aa and Qa alloantibodies). Mares that do not have the Ca or Aa antigen but have antibodies to Ca are less likely to initiate an immune response to the Aa blood group antigen (antibody-mediated immunosuppression) on the foal's RBCs.

Foals that develop neonatal isoerythrolysis appear normal for the first hours of life but develop clinical signs between 12 hours and 4 days of age with the severity of the clinical signs determined by the amount of anti-RBC antibody absorbed. Typical foals with neonatal isoerythrolysis become weak, lethargic, depressed, and icteric. The cardiovascular response (heart and respiratory rate) and hematological changes (RBC less than 6×10^6, packed cell volume [PCV] less than 25 per cent, and hemoglobinuria) usually parallel the severity of clinical signs.

A diagnosis of neonatal isoerythrolysis is supported by laboratory confirmation of an incompatible minor agglutination cross-match, positive hemolytic cross-match between the foal and dam, or a positive Coombs test on the foal's blood. The latter test is not specific for a diagnosis of neonatal isoerythrolysis as other immune-mediated conditions also result in IgG- or C3-mediated agglutination of erythrocytes. Because the alloantibodies responsible for neonatal isoerythrolysis act more strongly as hemolysins than they do as agglutinins, diagnostic tests which demonstrate hemolysis are preferred for laboratory confirmation of this condition. However, these tests require an exogenous source of rabbit complement, are complicated, and thus are best suited for blood typing diagnostic laboratories. Some laboratories that perform these tests are listed at the end of the chapter.

Testing mares for alloantibodies (neonatal isoerythrolysis–causing antibodies) during late gestation (within 30 days of foaling) is best done with a hemolytic assay. Mare's serum mixed with test horse RBCs possesing blood group antigens known to cause neonatal isoerythrolysis is considered positive for alloantibodies when complete hemolysis occurs at dilutions greater than 1:16. Testing stallions for compatibility to mares requires a cross-match with the stallion's RBCs, or the mare's antibodies can be compared with the stallion's blood group. Testing for neonatal isoerythrolysis at the time of foaling requires a minor cross-match (the foal's erythrocytes and the mare's serum), or a "jaundice foal agglutination" test, which is described in Table 3.

The best therapy for neonatal isoerythrolysis is prevention; however, this is not always possible. When the diagnosis is made prior to parturition, the condition can be prevented by milking-out the mare for the first 24 to 48 hours, muzzling the foal during this same period, and providing alternative colostrum to ensure adequate transfer of antibodies. In affected foals, supportive care should include enteral nutrition, intravenous polyionic fluids and plasma (in cases of failure of passive transfer). In severely affected foals—those with a PCV less than 12 per cent or an erythrocyte count less than 3×10^6 per μl—a whole blood transfusion (1 to 2 liters) should be performed. In these cases, a single treatment with a corticosteroid (dexamethasone, 0.1 to 0.2 mg per kg) appears to be beneficial. Antimicrobial therapy (e.g., ampicillin or trimethoprim–sulfa), as an aid in preventing secondary bacterial infections, is indicated and should be included in the therapeutic regimen.

SEPSIS

Several risk factors (gram-negative enteric organisms, opportunistic respiratory pathogens,

TABLE 3. JAUNDICED FOAL AGGLUTINATION TEST

Materials
1. Centrifuge capable of spinning blood tubes at 300 to 600 × gravity.
2. Test tube rack.
3. Test tubes: Either 13 × 100 mm disposable tubes or blood collection tubes.
4. Pasteur pipettes and rubber bulbs or another pipette system to deliver 1.0-ml volumes.
5. Saline at room temperature.
6. Serum or colostrum from mare and RBCs from mare and foal, preferably in EDTA anticoagulant.

Methods
1. Collect colostrum from the mare.
2. Collect a blood sample in anticoagulant from the foal.
3. Make serial dilutions of colostrum: 1:2, 1:4, 1:8, 1:16, 1:32. The total volume in each tube should be approximately 1 ml.
4. Add one drop of foal's whole blood to each tube and mix.
5. Centrifuge tubes for 2 to 3 minutes at medium speed (300 to 500 × gravity).
6. Invert each tube, pouring out liquid contents. Observe the status of the button of RBCs at the bottom of the tube:
   a. Complete agglutination causes the cells to remain tightly packed in the button.
   b. Strong agglutination causes the cells to remain in large clumps.
   c. Weaker agglutination causes the cells to remain in smaller clumps as they run down the side of the tube.
   d. No agglutination causes the cells to easily flow down the side of the tube.

Notes
1. Two controls should also be run. The cells should be tested with saline to be certain that the cells do not agglutinate by themselves.
2. The colostrum should be tested with the dam's own cells to be certain that it is not the conditions of the test or the viscosity of the colostrum that is causing the agglutination. These controls need only be run when there is a positive reaction in the JFA test for the foal's RBCs.

From Bailey, E., Conboy, H. S. and McCarthy, P. F.: Neonatal isoerythrolysis of foals: An update on testing. In: Proceedings of the 33rd Annual Convention of the American Association of Equine Practitioners, 1987, pp. 341–353. Reproduced by permission.

periparturient stress, failure of passive transfer) increase the foal's propensity to develop infection and result in neonatal septicemia. Failure to contain the infection to an organ system by host defense mechanisms or therapeutic intervention can result in systemic dissemination and altered hemostasis. Elevations in fibrinogen and FDP levels and consumption of coagulation inhibitors (AT-III, protein C) is evidence of a hypercoagulable state, the progression of which, if not attenuated, will be DIC. Appreciating the significance of systemic amplification of a disease condition (pneumonia to pleuritis and septicemia; necrotizing enterocolitis to peritonitis and septicemia; septicemia to hepatitis, endocarditis, or nephritis) is the first step in understanding the pathogenesis of hemostatic disorders, the laboratory findings, and the rationale for therapy.

Activation of the coagulation cascade (plasma protease) system is an early phenomenon in severe infection and septicemia. Disruption of the balance between activating and inhibitory coagulation proteases may lead to hypercoagulability, hemorrhagic tendency, or disturbances in vascular tone and permeability. Cellular damage as a consequence of these events and the generation of mediators of inflammation contribute to the development of septic shock and the multiple organ failure syndrome.

Laboratory findings in foals with hemostatic disorders secondary to septicemia are listed in Table 4. Increased accute phase reactants (fibrinogen, factor VIII:C, and vWf:Ag), consumption of protease inhibitors (AT-III, protein C), and generation of FDPs support a diagnosis of hypercoagulation even though the platelet count APTT, and PT may be within the reference range. The primary objective in treating the hypercoagulable condition is to treat the underlying disease process. This usually includes intravenous administration of polyionic fluids to improve organ perfusion, hydration, electrolyte imbalances, and minor acid–base derangements; nasal insufflation of oxygen or ventilation; and broad-spectrum antimicrobials. Anti-inflammatories, histamine H_2 antagonists, parenteral nutrition, and bicarbonate therapy may also be included in the therapeutic regimen on an as-needed basis. In conditions where systemic dissemination of the infectious and inflammatory process results in altered hemostasis, the key to correcting the consumptive coagulopathy is replacing the inhibitory proteases which maintain the hemostatic balance. In the foal, this requires the administration of fresh (or fresh frozen) platelet-rich plasma (PRP, 1 to 2 liters). Although the use of heparin in conjunction with PRP remains controversial, the administration of sodium heparin (40 IU per kg IV once, followed 2 hours later by 40 IU per kg SC, twice a day for 3 days) appears to be beneficial. In addition to evaluating the patient for clinical improvement, serial (daily, at least in the acute phase) coagulation profiles for assessing improvement or deterioration are recommended.

LABORATORIES THAT PROVIDE BLOOD TYPING SERVICES FOR NEONATAL ISOERYTHROLYSIS

Serology Laboratory
University of California
Davis, CA 95616
(916) 752-2211

Stormont Laboratory, Inc.
1237 East Beamer Street, Suite D
Woodland, CA 95695
(916) 661-3078

Dr. Melba Ketchum
Shelterwood Equine Laboratories
Box 215
Carthage, TX 75633
(214) 693-6424

Veterinary Laboratory, Inc.
1033 N. Limestone
Lexington, KY 40505
(606) 252-0415

Dr. Jill McClure
Veterinary Clinical Sciences
School of Veterinary Medicine
Louisiana State University
Baton Rouge, LA 70803
(504) 346-3297

Supplemental Readings

Bailey, E., Conboy, H. S., and McCarthy, P. F.: Neonatal isoerythrolysis of foals: An update on testing. *In:* Proceedings

TABLE 4. LABORATORY FINDINGS IN FOALS WITH DISEASE CONDITIONS RESULTING IN ALTERED HEMOSTASIS

Test	Hypercoagulable State
Platelet count	Normal to decreased
Activated partial thromboplastin time	Supranormal to normal to prolonged
Prothrombin time	Normal to prolonged
Fibrinogen degradation products	Increased
Antithrombin III	Decreased
Plasma fibronectin	Decreased
Fibrinogen	Increased (may be decreased in acute conditions)

of the 33rd Annual Convention of the American Association of Equine Practitioners, 1987, pp. 341–353.
Becht, J. L., and Semrad, S. D.: Hematology, blood typing, and immunology of the neonatal foal. Vet. Clin. North Am. (Equine Pract.), 1:91–116, 1985.
Green, R. A.: Clinical implications of antithrombin III deficiency in animal diseases. Compend. Cont. Educ. Pract. Vet., 6:537–545, 1984.
Morris, D. D.: Hemostatic function tests in horses: Current and future trends. In: Proceedings of the 33rd Annual Convention of the American Association of Equine Practioners, 1987, pp. 331–340.
Shappell, K. K., and Lock, T. F.: Hematologic parameters after neonatal isoerythrolysis in a foal. Compend. Cont. Educ. Pract. Vet., 8:867–872, 1986.

Neonatal Maladjustment Syndrome

Christopher M. Brown, EAST LANSING, MICHIGAN

The term *neonatal maladjustment syndrome* was originally coined to describe foals with a spectrum of gross behavioral abnormalities. These abnormalities had been recognized for many years, and the foals had been variously described as "barkers," "wanderers," or "convulsives." Foals with infections and premature foals were excluded from the description. However, as more observations were made, these narrow limits were found to be too restrictive. Many foals with infections and many premature foals may show signs identical to those of classical neonatal maladjustment. In this chapter, the term will be used broadly and will be applicable to most neonatal foals with severe behavioral abnormalities. The description focuses on the behavioral and neurological aspects of the diseases, but the presence of concurrent problems should not be overlooked, particularly as these additional problems markedly influence the prognosis.

CLINICAL SIGNS

The following is a description of a classical case of neonatal maladjustment syndrome. By no means all cases will have all of these signs, and foals with additional problems may have other signs that may alter or overshadow the neonatal maladjustment signs.

Foaling is usually normal, and the foal stands and nurses well for the first 24 hours. Depending on how closely the foal is observed, various behavioral abnormalities may be noticed. The foal may become disoriented, wandering around the stall and occasionally becoming stuck in a corner. It may stop nursing and appear not to recognize the mare. It may appear blind. Limb, neck, and body movements are often jerky. This period may last for several hours, but is usually short if convulsions are to follow.

The onset of convulsions is usually sudden. The signs are dramatic, with spasm of the limbs, neck, and tail, progressing to tonic–clonic convulsions. The foal usually falls, and may flip over backward. Opisthotonos with extensor rigidity may occur. Some foals lie and paddle, often violently banging the head on the floor. Some grind their teeth, and some make strange barking sounds. If untreated, seizures may continue for 30 minutes or more, and some foals may die at this point. Between convulsive periods the foals may be comatose or semicomatose, but often respond abnormally to stimuli. Seizures may be induced by mild tactile or auditory stimuli. Unfed comatose foals die. This post- or interconvulsive period may last hours to days. Some untreated foals, and many treated foals without complications, show a slow gradual recovery. Initially they may be able to stand with assistance. Walking is often aimless and the foal may be weak. The foal appears blind and will not suckle. They often will not lie down spontaneously, but when placed in lateral recumbency they sleep. Finally, the ability to see and nurse returns. This slow recovery may take 7 to 10 days, although foals not improving by 4 to 5 days usually die. Recovery is not always complete and some foals are left with residual deficits in sight, mentation, or nursing ability. Not all foals pass through all of the above stages, and, even when present, signs are not always pronounced and may only be noticed by astute close observation.

The above progression is for a classical case. Many foals may present with similar clinical signs but do not conform to this pattern. These foals have different or additional problems, which may be related to prematurity, infections, trauma, metabolic derangements, congenital problems, or combinations of these. Foaling may have been complicated or protracted, and clinical signs of central nervous system (CNS) dysfunction may be present from birth. They may be weak, unable to stand or suckle, be febrile, and have other signs consistent with multisystemic problems. In addition, varying components of the neonatal maladjustment syndrome may be present. These complicated atypical neonatal maladjustment cases have a poor prognosis.

CAUSES

The cause or causes of neonatal maladjustment syndrome are unknown. Many suggestions have been made, but all evidence is circumstantial. Possible causes include trauma to the CNS during parturition, CNS anoxia, and CNS hemorrhage. It is most likely that many factors are involved in the cause. CNS lesions are variable and correlate poorly with the clinical signs. Lesions observed include subarachnoid and parenchymal hemorrhages, neuronal necrosis, malacia, and edema of the brain and spinal cord. As some of these changes may develop in animals that have undergone severe and repeated seizures, it is impossible to say which lesions cause the seizures and which are the results of seizures.

In the nonclassical cases of neonatal maladjustment syndrome additional causative factors include hypoglycemia, electrolyte disorders, and acid–base abnormalities. Septicemia, particularly that leading to meningitis, may be involved in some cases.

DIAGNOSTIC AIDS

In classical cases the signs and history are the most helpful clues. Clinicopathological data are nonspecific and may reflect the resulting stress. In more complicated cases, laboratory data may reflect additional organ system involvement. If facilities and budget permit, routine hematology, serum biochemistries, arterial blood gas determinations, serum IgG measurement, cerebrospinal fluid (CSF) analysis, and blood culture should help define the extent of the additional problems.

DIFFERENTIAL DIAGNOSIS

As neonatal maladjustment syndrome is a vaguely defined condition it cannot always be clearly differentiated from many concomitant or similar problems. For the most part this is not too important, as management in many cases is empirical. Convulsions or coma, or both, may develop in foals with septic meningitis. These foals may be persistently febrile, with increased neutrophils, protein, and bacteria in the CSF. Hematological changes are usually consistent with an infectious process. Some severely hypoglycemic foals may be comatose and convulse. Causes of hypoglycemia include sepsis and fulminating liver disease such as Tyzzer's disease. Laboratory and clinical data help differentiate these conditions. In addition, premature and dysmature foals may be weak, depressed, and reluctant to suckle. A history of early birth and the physical examination findings may help differentiate these foals.

THERAPY

Management of neonatal maladjustment centers on four main areas: controlling seizures, maintaining nutritional intake, correcting metabolic abnormalities, and treating or preventing infections. Although this list of objectives is apparently straightforward, their fulfillment can be very frustrating and labor-intensive, and hence potentially very expensive. The foal may need continuous support and therapy for many days.

The foal should be kept with its dam, although it may be completely disinterested in her. This is important, as the mare–foal bond should not be broken. The objective is to have the foal return to nursing the mare. The mare should be milked out frequently and her milk fed to the foal. As these foals initially have no suckle reflex, they must be fed by stomach tube. Foals with neonatal maladjustment syndrome often violently resent handling of the head, so repeated passage of the stomach tube should be avoided. The stomach tube should be taped in place and stoppered when not in use. For adequate growth, a foal needs mare's milk equal to about 20 per cent of its body weight daily. Initially milk should be given hourly, but by the time the foal is 3 to 4 days old the frequency can be reduced to every 2 or 3 hours, with increased individual dosages.

If the foal is totally disoriented, it may be necessary to partition off a portion of the stall to contain and protect the foal. This can be done with straw bales or padded mats. This keeps the mare close to the foal. Convulsing foals suffer head trauma, particularly to the eyes, and a padded helmet may be useful to reduce the trauma. As the foals are often hyperreactive, extraneous stimuli should be kept to a minimum. The foal should be disturbed as little as possible. The area should be quiet and fairly dimly lit, and all movement or handling should be deliberate but quiet. Ideally, with medical therapy the foal should be able to be left mostly undisturbed except for feeding and nursing care. Control of convulsions is best achieved with medication. Attempts to control by physical restraint alone usually make matters worse and rapidly exhaust both foal and handler. As many of the agents used are given intravenously (IV), an indwelling jugular venous catheter is invaluable for the management of these foals. Venipuncture in convulsing foals is difficult.

Diazepam is the drug of choice for immediate short-term control of seizures. A slow IV infusion of 5 to 20 mg is given to effect (approx. 0.1 to 0.4 mg per kg). In many foals only a short period of control is achieved with diazepam, and if more than three or four doses are given, longer-acting agents should be selected.

Phenobarbital, 5 to 20 mg per kg in 30 ml of saline, is given over 20 to 30 minutes as the initial dosage. Dosage is based on effect. The maintenance dosage is about 9 mg per kg given every 8 hours. Foals may be sedated and ataxic. The dosage should be adjusted to achieve control of seizures with the fewest side effects.

Phenytoin, initially at 5 to 10 mg per kg IV and subsequently at 1 to 5 mg per kg IV, intramuscularly (IM), or per os (PO) every 2 to 4 hours, may also be used. Phenytoin is more expensive than phenobarbital and must be given more frequently. However, if the oral route is used the drug can be given at feeding time down the stomach tube.

Foals with uncontrollable seizures or those in which the cost of therapy is important may be treated with IV sodium pentobarbital given to effect, approximately 2 to 4 mg per kg. Marked sedation or even anesthesia may occur at higher or more frequent dosages. Assessing the clinical course of the problem in heavily sedated foals is difficult, and making decisions for changing therapy is not easy.

Phenothiazines should not be used in convulsing foals. They lower the seizure threshold and they are hypotensive and long-acting. Also, xylazine should not be used as it is hypertensive and thus may exacerbate cerebral hemorrhage.

The selection of an anticonvulsive agent and duration of therapy is somewhat empirical. Occasional foals only need one or two treatments with diazepam. In many, however, longer-acting agents must be given for 2 or more weeks, after which time medication is gradually withdrawn. If convulsions recur, the initial loading dosage should be given and the protocol repeated.

Medications to reduce cerebral edema may be helpful. Hyperosmotic solutions such as mannitol should be avoided, as they may exacerbate edema when cerebral hemorrhage has developed. In addition, these agents may exacerbate electrolyte abnormalities. Dimethyl sulfoxide may be of value in the acute stage of cerebral edema. The dosage is 0.5 to 1.0 gm per kg dissolved in 5 per cent dextrose to yield a 10 per cent solution that is given IV. High concentrations can cause intravascular hemorrhage.

If sepsis is likely or is proven based on blood or CSF culture results, appropriate antibiotics should be given. Fluid, electrolyte, and acid–base abnormalities should be corrected with appropriate fluids, and if failure of passive transfer has been confirmed, it should be treated with IV plasma.

PROGNOSIS

There are few data to guide the clinician and owner when assessing the possible outcome of these cases. In one study, 80 per cent of foals with classical neonatal maladjustment syndrome and no other problems survived. However, less than 30 per cent survived if the foal had one or more of the following problems: positive blood culture, serum IgG less than 400 mg per dl, diarrhea, radiographic thoracic abnormalities, abnormal behavior at birth, fecal blood, blood in gastric reflux fluid, or prematurity.

Foals that do not improve within 3 to 4 days rarely recover. Some foals that recover have residual neurological problems, but most recovered foals grow well and behave normally. Some owners feel that these recovered foals are more "people-oriented" than other foals. This is probably due to the close nursing attention they received in the first few days of life.

Supplemental Readings

Clabough, D. L., and Martens, R. J.: Equine neonatal maladjustment syndrome. Compend. Cont. Educ. Pract. Vet., 7:S497–S505, 1985.

Clement, S. F.: Convulsive and allied syndromes of the neonatal foal. Vet. Clin. North Am. (Equine Pract.), 3:333–344, 1987.

Collatos, C.: Seizures in foals: Pathophysiology, evaluation and treatment. Compend. Cont. Educ. Pract. Vet., 12:393–399, 1990.

Palmer, A. C., Leadon, D. P., Rossdale, P. D., and Jeffcott, L. B.: Intracranial haemorrhage in pre-viable, premature and full term foals. Equine Vet. J., 16:383, 1984.

Vaala, W. E.: Diagnosis and treatment of prematurity and neonatal maladjustment syndrome in newborn foals. Compend. Cont. Educ. Pract. Vet., 8:S211–S224, 1986.

Neonatal Septicemia

Lynn Rolland Hovda, FALCON HEIGHTS, MINNESOTA

Septicemia, a generalized systemic disease associated with the presence of microorganisms or their toxins in the blood, is one of the most common conditions affecting foals less than 7 days old. Despite medical advances, the mortality remains high, ranging from 50 to 75 per cent. Early recognition and treatment are essential for survival of the foal and prevention of complications that may impair future athletic or reproductive performance.

The pathogenesis of neonatal septicemia is multifactorial and involves the development of one or more predisposing factors. These may occur in utero, during parturition, or early in postnatal life. In utero factors affecting fetal development include abnormal fetal maturation, fetal stress and hypoxia, and placental insufficiency. Abnormal fetal maturation may occur secondary to inadequate nutrition during pregnancy or poor health of the mare. Uterine-placental derangement or, more rarely, maternal systemic disease are associated with fetal stress and hypoxia. Intrauterine infection is the most common cause of placental insufficiency. Microorganisms such as *Escherichia coli* and β-haemolytic *Streptococcus* spp. are present in the genital tract, environment, and on the skin of normal horses, and generally enter the uterus through the cervix.

Induction of parturition, prolonged parturition, or dystocia may result in the birth of weak foals or foals born prior to transfer of antibodies to the colostrum. Other factors at parturition associated with the development of septicemia include early rupture of the umbilical cord, premature placental separation and cesarean section.

A number of conditions may predispose to the development of septicemia early in postnatal life. Management and environmental factors such as overcrowding, poor ventilation or sanitation, inadequate umbilical care, or inappropriate use of antimicrobial agents result in increased exposure to high concentrations of bacteria or the development of resistant bacteria in the environment. The most significant factor in the development of neonatal septicemia is failure of passive transfer (FPT) of maternal antibodies (see p. 422). Foals are born agammaglobulinemic and require colostrum to obtain maternal antibodies for prevention and control of infection. Conditions causing FPT can be associated with either the mare or foal. Mares with premature lactation may drip colostrum for hours to days before parturition. If parturition is premature, there may have been insufficient time for the mare to concentrate antibodies in the colostrum. Low colostral antibodies sometimes occur without physical evidence of premature lactation or parturition or abnormally low antibody concentration in the mare's blood. The cause is unknown, but the condition is more common in maiden mares than in experienced mares. Colostrum may be deliberately withheld from foals to prevent neonatal isoerythrolysis. Premature foals or those that are orphaned, rejected, sick, or suffering from neonatal maladjustment syndrome or congenital abnormalities may consume insufficient amounts of colostrum during the first 24 hours of life. After this time, further colostrum intake is useless as antibody absorptive function in the small intestine has ceased. Foals observed to nurse well from a mare known to have good-quality colostrum may still develop FPT. Decreased antibody absorptive capacity of the intestinal mucosa early in postnatal life may be responsible for this condition.

Etiological agents vary from region to region. The variation may reflect true geographic differences in bacterial populations or differences caused by management practices, such as the indiscriminant use of prophylactic antibiotics. The placenta, umbilicus, respiratory tract, and gastrointestinal (GI) tract all serve as portals of entry. Although the umbilicus is most often incriminated, entry through the respiratory or GI tracts probably occurs more frequently.

The overwhelming majority of infections are caused by gram-negative microorganisms. One recent retrospective study reported gram-negative microorganisms in 100 per cent of the cases by antemortem blood culture or necropsy. Mixed infections occurred in 55 per cent of the cases; pure gram-positive infections did not occur. *Escherichia coli*, *Klebsiella pneumoniae*, *Salmonella* spp., and *Actinobacillus* spp. are the most commonly isolated microorganisms, with the prevalence varying according to geographic location. Less frequently occurring gram-negative microorganisms are *Pseudomonas* spp., *Enterobacter* spp., *Pasteurella* spp., *Listeria* spp., *Serratia* spp., and *Proteus* spp. Gram-positive agents include β-haemolytic (especially *Streptococcus zooepidemicus*) and α-haemolytic *Streptococcus* spp., *Staphylococcus* spp. (especially *Staphylococcus aureus*), *Bacillus* spp., *Coryne-*

bacterium spp., and *Clostridium* spp. (especially *Clostridium perfringens*).

CLINICAL SIGNS

The clinical picture reflects the pathogenicity of the etiological agent, the foal's immune status, and the duration of illness. Some foals exhibit signs at birth or shortly thereafter, but most foals appear normal until 2 to 4 days, when deterioration suddenly occurs. Early signs are usually vague, nonspecific, and frequently missed by inexperienced observers. Foals may be weak, lethargic, mildly depressed, reluctant to move, or inappetent. The mare's udder may be engorged or the foal's face stained with milk. Dehydration is usually mild, with slightly sunken eyeballs and little increase in skin turgor. Fever is not a good indicator of early septicemia since hypothermia or normothermia are just as likely to occur. Signs of advanced septicemia are more obvious, but by the time they are noted the prognosis for a full, uncomplicated recovery is poor. Increased respiratory effort often results in rapid, shallow breathing. Petechial and ecchymotic hemorrhages may develop on the vulva, pinna of the ear, or oral mucous membranes. Episcleral hemorrhages not associated with trauma may become prominent. Extremities may be cool and clammy. Hypotonia, behavioral changes, convulsions, or coma may occur. Localizing signs such as diarrhea, pneumonia, omphalophlebitis, anterior uveitis, swollen or painful joints, or meningitis may be present and obscure identification of generalized septicemia.

DIAGNOSIS

An early diagnosis of neonatal septicemia is difficult as no single laboratory test repeatedly identifies the disease. The diagnosis is best made using a combination of historical data, physical examination, and laboratory findings. A scoring system incorporating these factors has been developed by the University of Florida (see p. 413). It is helpful in establishing the diagnosis and monitoring the disease course.

HISTORY

A thorough and complete history should be obtained. An accurate gestational age is essential as a gestation shorter than 320 days or longer than 360 days places the foal at high risk for septicemia. The quantity and quality of colostrum, as well as the time ingested, should be noted. Colostrum should be ingested within 6 to 8 hours of birth. Other important historical data include an abnormal placenta, vulvar discharge prior to foaling, and any maternal illness 30 days before foaling.

PHYSICAL EXAMINATION

The importance of a careful and systematic physical examination cannot be overemphasized. If emergency care is required, the examination can be postponed but should not be neglected. The pinna of the ear and the mucous membranes of the oral cavity and vulva should be examined closely. Petechial and ecchymotic hemorrhages may be associated with defects in coagulation, and muddy, red, oral mucous membranes with a hyperemic rim around the teeth are associated with toxemia. A capillary refill time greater than 2 seconds and cold, clammy extremities indicate poor peripheral perfusion or septic shock. Eyes should be checked for jaundice, episcleral hemorrhages, and the presence of hyphema, hypopyon, or fibrin in ventral aspects of the anterior chamber. Blepharospasm, photophobia, lacrimation, miosis, and ciliary injection are hallmarks of anterior uveitis. The umbilical stump should be examined thoroughly for warmth, swelling, purulent material, abscessation, or a patent urachus. The absence of signs, however, does not exclude the presence of an infection, as bacteria can ascend the umbilical cord and cause an abscess in the urachus or umbilical vessels. The thorax should be auscultated and percussed even though significant lung pathology frequently occurs in the setting of relatively normal lung sounds and a slight increase in respiratory rate. Coughing, nasal discharge, dyspnea, and abnormal lung sounds such as crackles and wheezes signify the onset of more serious lung disease. Pleuritis may be associated with quiet or absent lung sounds. All joints, especially the shoulder and hip, should be palpated thoroughly for distention, pain, or periarticular edema, and ambulatory foals should be observed for lameness. Examination of the GI tract includes auscultation for borborygmus, estimation of the quantity and quality of fecal material, and passage of a nasogastric tube. Fecal material should be saved for further analysis. Urination should be noted, particularly if the foal has received large amounts of intravenous (IV) fluids, and a sample saved for routine urinalysis. Despite the time and difficulties involved, a complete neurological examination should be performed. Deficits such as behavioral changes, depression, convulsions, and coma may be associated with meningitis or other factors such as acidosis or hypoglycemia (see p. 414).

LABORATORY ANALYSIS

The definitive antemortem diagnosis of neonatal septicemia is made only with positive blood culture. The recovery rate of microorganisms is fairly good, reaching 81 per cent in one recent study. Based on necropsy findings, however, an appreciable number of microorganisms, especially gram-negative agents, are not recovered. Failure to isolate all etiological agents should be suspected when the culture yields only gram-positive microorganisms or when improvement does not occur with antibiotic therapy selected according to culture and sensitivity testing results. The procedure for obtaining blood for culture is simple. The jugular vein is clipped and surgically prepared. Blood (10 ml) is withdrawn using aseptic technique and sterile needles and syringes. The sample is transferred aseptically to two sealed culture bottles of trypticase soy or peptone broth and one bottle is vented with a needle. Both bottles are incubated at 37° C. Most positive samples show turbidity at 24 hours, but some samples require 48 to 72 hours for growth to appear. Positive samples are subcultured for microorganism identification and antibiotic sensitivity. Ideally, blood cultures should be done more than once on untreated foals, but therapy should not be delayed to obtain a second blood culture. Foals previously treated with antibiotics should be cultured because positive results are often obtained. The use of an absorbent resin suspension to remove antimicrobial agents is controversial and currently not recommended. Culture of feces, joint or cerebrospinal fluid, tracheal washes, body cavity exudates, or urine may be helpful in identifying a microorganism. Foals with diarrhea as the presenting sign should be further evaluated with five serial fecal cultures for *Salmonella* spp. Most successful cultures are obtained early in the disease or just as feces become firm. A cerebrospinal tap is justified if neurological signs remain prominent after hypoglycemia, metabolic acidosis, and electrolyte abnormalities are corrected. Cloudy fluid with elevated total protein and increased white blood cell (WBC) count is indicative of an infectious agent. Culture and sensitivity testing of a tracheal aspirate may identify a pathogenic microorganism. The procedure may be intolerable to an already compromised foal, so careful individual assessment must be done prior to use. If indicated by physical examination, thoracocentesis, abdominocentesis, or arthrocentesis with culture and sensitivity testing of the fluid can be performed.

Since most cases of neonatal septicemia are associated with partial or complete FPT, assessment of the foal's immune status is mandatory. A variety of diagnostic tests are available. Zinc sulfate turbidity and latex agglutination are rapid, easy screening tests but not as quantitative as the single radial immunodiffusion assay (see p. 424). The minimum acceptable immunoglobulin level in premature, hospitalized, or sick foals is 800 mg per dl. Despite what has been written, levels between 400 mg per dl and 800 mg per dl may not provide adequate protection for high-risk foals.

A complete blood count (CBC) determined once is not specific for septicemia. Serial CBC are useful for monitoring changes, identifying trends, and determining prognosis. The hemogram varies with the stage of illness, offending microorganism, and immune status. Absolute segmented neutrophil counts are more diagnostic for septicemia than the total WBC count. Hematological abnormalities that correlate with septicemia include neutropenia (less than 4000 segmented neutrophils per μl) or neutrophilia (greater than 8000 segmented neutrophils per μl), increased immature (band) neutrophils (greater than 200 per μl), toxic changes in neutrophils such as Dohle bodies, basophilic cytoplasm, toxic cytoplasmic granulation or foamy vacuolation, and elevated (greater than 0.05) ratios of band forms to total neutrophil count.

The serum fibrinogen level varies with the stage of illness and may be normal, increased, or decreased. It is often normal early in disease, because the fibrinogen response does not manifest for 48 to 72 hours. When infection is acquired in utero, the fibrinogen concentration is frequently elevated at birth. Persistently elevated fibrinogen levels are usually present in foals with localized sites of infection; persistently low levels may suggest disseminated intravascular coagulopathy.

Packed cell volume (PCV), hemoglobin concentration, and red blood cell (RBC) values vary according to the severity and duration of disease. They are often increased early in disease in proportion to shock and dehydration. Normal postpartum changes, decreased hematopoietic activity from bacterial toxins or hemolysins, chronic infection, or the development of neonatal isoerythrolysis cause these parameters to decrease and make interpretation difficult.

Total plasma protein concentration is an inaccurate measure of hydration unless monitored frequently and interpreted in conjunction with the PCV. Poor absorption of colostral antibodies causes artificially low values; shock is associated with artificially high values.

Serum chemistry values are more important in therapy than in the initial diagnosis of septicemia. Variation depends on the age of the foal (see p. 825), cardiovascular status, dehydration, and concurrent focal sites of infection. Elevations in creatinine and serum urea nitrogen levels may reflect inadequate renal perfusion, dehydration, or localization of bacteria (especially *Actinobacillus equuli*) in the kidneys. Normal foals often have a moderately elevated bilirubin level early in life. Severe elevations may occur secondary to septicemia and other diseases such as hepatitis or neonatal isoerythrolysis. The blood glucose concentration in septicemic foals is often low, and frequent monitoring is encouraged.

Arterial blood gas analysis usually shows nonspecific abnormalities. In general, metabolic acidosis and low arterial oxygen tension are present, but these may vary depending on the respiratory status.

Protein, WBCs, or RBCs may be found on routine urinalysis secondary to bacterial nephritis. Culture of the urine may identify the offending microorganism. Proteinuria in very young foals should be interpreted with caution, as it is normally present after colostrum ingestion.

ANCILLARY AIDS

Many special procedures are used in the diagnosis of septicemia and evaluation of sequelae. Due to lack of abnormal lung sounds and frequency of lung pathology, thoracic radiographs are recommended for most septicemic foals. Thoracic radiographs and ultrasonography are useful in the detection of pleuritis. Internal umbilical or urachal abscesses can usually be identified with abdominal ultrasonography. Esophageal and gastroduodenal endoscopy or contrast radiography may show inflammation, erosions, or ulcers. Osteomyelitis or fractures may be identified by radiographic examination of distended joints. Radiographs should be repeated in 3 to 4 days if osteomyelitis is suspected but is not evident on initial films.

THERAPY

The management of neonatal septicemia includes supportive care, treatment of generalized infections, and treatment or prevention of localized infections. This is best accomplished with good supportive care, nutritional support, plasma infusions, fluid and electrolyte therapy, and aggressive use of broad-spectrum antibiotics.

SUPPORTIVE CARE

Of all therapeutic goals, this is the most challenging and time-consuming, yet absolutely necessary for foal survival. Recumbent foals should be kept on a soft mattress, water bed, or air bag and maintained in sternal position. If this is not possible, turning every 2 hours minimizes hypostatic lung congestion, atelectasis, and the development of decubital ulcers over bony prominences. Heating pads, heated water beds, radiant heat lamps, or blankets are helpful for hypothermic foals or those with decreased peripheral perfusion, but warming should be done slowly. If the foal is ambulatory but spends a significant amount of time lying down, straw is the preferred bedding, as shavings can be aspirated and may be a source of *Klebsiella* spp. infection.

Recumbent foals may have to be removed from the mare. If the foal is expected to return to the mare, milking every 2 to 3 hours is necessary to maintain lactation. Strict attention to hygiene will prevent mastitis or introduction of microorganisms into the milk.

The perineal area of diarrheic foals should be cleaned several times each day with a mild soapy water solution. Irritated skin requires a protectant such as vitamin A & D ointment or zinc oxide. Black, tarry feces should be examined for occult blood.

Application of sterile eye lubricants every 2 to 3 hours prevents corneal drying, especially when intranasal oxygen is used. Daily ophthalmic examinations allow early detection and treatment of corneal ulcers, which may occur secondary to dryness, trauma, or entropion.

Foals that are mildly hypoxemic but breathing well may respond to intranasal oxygen at 5 to 10 L per minute. If response is poor, more specialized respiratory support is required (see p. 478).

Thrashing or convulsing foals are dangerous to themselves and others and require adequate physical or chemical restraint. Intravenous (IV) diazepam (0.05 to 0.4 mg per kg body weight) provides good tranquilization and may be repeated as needed. Other agents such as phenobarbital, pentobarbital, and phenytoin are also useful and discussed elsewhere (see p. 434).

The umbilicus, particularly in recumbent foals, should be kept clean and dry. Treatment once or twice daily with a dilute povidone–iodine solution is preferred. If a patent urachus develops, early detection and cauterization with silver nitrate sticks or Lugol's solution may result in closure. The urachus should be treated twice daily for 3 or 4 days. Prompt surgical resection is recommended if closure does not occur during this time.

Foals born to mares not vaccinated with tetanus toxoid in the last 30 days of gestation or foals with FPT should receive equine origin antitoxin and tetanus toxoid simultaneously at separate sites. Owners should be advised of the possibility of antitoxin-associated hepatopathy.

NUTRITION

The provision of adequate nutrition is often overlooked in septicemic foals. Foals able to stand and nurse should be encouraged and assisted. Those too sick to nurse are usually hand-fed mare's milk, milk replacer, or goat's milk with a nipple bottle. A variety of nipples, including some designed for human infants, may be tried before one is accepted by a foal. If the foal is too weak or otherwise unable to nurse, feeding is best accomplished through an indwelling nasogastric tube. The nasogastric tube is placed in the esophagus, advanced into the stomach for each feeding, and returned to the esophagus. Tubes left in the stomach between feedings cause gastric dilation and reflux of stomach contents around the tube. Esophagitis or pharyngitis may occur if tubes are left in place for longer than 72 hours. The volume provided depends on the foal's age and ability to tolerate oral feedings. Ideally, foals should receive 10 per cent of their body weight per day on day 1 and up to 25 per cent of body weight per day by day 10. This may not be feasible in septicemic foals and the volume should be adjusted according to individual response.

An alternate method of providing oral nutrition that is gaining acceptance in some teaching hospitals is the use of enteral products designed for human use (see p. 744). They are administered either by nipple bottle or by indwelling small-bore esophageal feeding tube. Depending on the product and the foal, tolerance may be good and the incidence of esophagitis, bloat, or ileus decreased.

Partial or total parenteral nutrition (see p. 747) provides a good alternative for foals unable to tolerate enteral feeding. The IV route provides adequate calories, fluid, electrolytes, vitamins, and trace minerals until oral feeding can be reinstituted. Parenteral nutrition is frequently used in septicemic foals with severe diarrhea or decreased GI motility resulting in bloat or gastric reflux. The immature or diseased GI tract is bypassed, allowing time for rest and repair.

PLASMA INFUSIONS

Foals with a history of poor colostrum intake, laboratory diagnosis of partial or complete failure of passive transfer, positive sepsis score, or hypercoagulable condition require a *prompt* plasma transfusion. Plasma may be purchased commercially or obtained from an adult horse. Most septicemic foals require a minimum of 40 ml per kg, or about 2 to 4 liters of plasma. If the concentration of immunoglobulins per liter of plasma is known, a calculated dose of 500 mg per kg body weight is recommended.

FLUID AND ELECTROLYTES

Dehydration, electrolyte abnormalities, hypoglycemia, and metabolic acidosis are common in septicemic foals. A balanced polyionic solution such as lactated or acetated Ringer's solution is a good fluid choice until laboratory results are known. The volume of fluid necessary to correct dehydration can be quickly calculated from the formula: body weight (kg) × dehydration (per cent) = liters of fluid. For example, a 50-kg foal that is 10 per cent dehydrated requires 5 liters of fluid to correct dehydration. This may be administered rapidly over 4 to 6 hours, if respiratory and renal function are good. Once dehydration is corrected, a maintenance rate of 75 to 90 ml per kg body weight per 24 hours (about 175 ml per hour) is adequate unless losses through diarrhea or reflux are excessive.

Foals have limited glycogen reserves and quickly become hypoglycemic, especially if oral therapy is stopped and parenteral nutrition is not instituted. Either 5 or 10 per cent dextrose can be used to maintain euglycemia, depending on personal preference and response to therapy. Dextroxe 5 per cent is isotonic and less irritating to veins. It can be alternated with lactated or acetated Ringer's solution or administered as a slightly hypertonic solution of 5 per cent dextrose with ½ strength lactated or acetated Ringer's solution or 0.45 per cent sodium chloride. If the foal continues to be hypoglycemic, 10 per cent dextrose can be infused at 4 to 8 mg per kg body weight per minute. This solution is moderately hypertonic, and jugular veins should be palpated several times a day for warmth and swelling. Parenteral nutrition is recommended if the response to 10 per cent dextrose is poor.

Metabolic acidosis persisting after volume expansion should be treated with isotonic (1.3 per cent) sodium bicarbonate. Hypertonic (5 per cent) sodium bicarbonate solutions are not necessary and may cause paradoxical central nervous system (CNS) acidosis or hypernatremia. The amount of bicarbonate required is calculated from the formula: 0.5 × body weight (kg) × base deficit. (An estimation of base deficit can be obtained from blood gas analysis; subtract mEq of bicarbonate from 24 mEq.) For example, a 50-kg foal with a bicarbonate of 17 mEq would have a base deficit of 7 and require 175 mEq of bicarbonate to correct the total deficit. Generally, only one-half of the total calculated deficit is administered at maintenance flow rates. Repeated blood gas analysis is used to monitor response to therapy and calculate further bicarbonate requirements.

ANTIBIOTIC THERAPY

Early and appropriate antibiotic therapy is necessary to control infection and prevent complications. Ideally, the antibiotic choice is based on the results of culture and sensitivity testing. This is not possible in septicemic foals, however, as therapy would be delayed by 48 to 72 hours. Broad-spectrum antimicrobial therapy at the correct dose is indicated for any foal suspected of having septicemia. Bactericidal drugs are used because neonatal foals are immunologically naive, reticuloendothelial systems are immature, phagocytic function is inefficient, complement levels are variable, and stress and sepsis may depress immunocompetency. Drug combinations should be additive or synergistic. Parenteral administration (IV or IM) is preferred. Absorption of orally administered drugs in neonatal foals is erratic and may result in abnormally high or low blood levels. In generalized septicemia, the duration of antibiotic therapy is normally 10 to 14 days. If localizing signs or complications develop, antibiotics are continued for 2 weeks after all signs have resolved.

The most frequently used antibiotic combination in neonatal septicemia is penicillin G or ampicillin and an aminoglycoside such as gentamicin or amikacin (see Table 1 for recommended doses). Penicillin G has a narrow spectrum of action but provides good coverage against most gram-positive cocci, anaerobes, and many gram-positive rods. Caution is advised in premature foals or those with hemostatic defects, since very high doses of penicillin impair platelet aggregation. The spectrum of action of ampicillin is broader and includes activity against some gram-negative microorganisms. Many of these organisms, however, have become resistant to ampicillin.

The limiting factor in the veterinary use of aminoglycosides is the development of nephrotoxicity. Aminoglycosides are excreted by glomerular filtration and concentrate in the proximal tubules of the renal cortex with secondary interstitial damage. Many foals receiving an aminoglycoside for longer than 4 to 5 days will develop mild renal impairment that reverses when the antibiotic is discontinued. Aminoglycosides should be discontinued at the first sign of nephrotoxicity. Recent research has shown enzymuria (particularly γ-glutamyltransferase) to be an early indicator of nephrotoxicity. In a clinical setting, the earliest indicator of renal tubular damage is the presence of protein, RBCs, and hyaline or granular casts in the urine. A decrease in glomerular filtration rate and rise in serum creatinine level (even as small as 0.3 mg per dl for gentamicin) are hallmarks of significant renal accumulation. It is not unusual for the serum creatinine level to continue to rise after drug therapy has ceased. The importance of frequent urinalyses with sediment examination in foals receiving aminoglycosides cannot be overemphasized.

Aminoglycoside peak and trough levels are used in humans to establish an appropriate dose and prevent nephrotoxicity. Nephrotoxicity has occurred with "normal" levels, so these values are best interpreted in conjunction with urinalysis findings and serum creatinine levels. Levels are normally measured every 3 to 4 days and are especially useful in identifying trends. Rising trough levels are better indicators of impending nephrotoxicity than high peaks. Suggested gentamicin peak and trough levels in foals are 10 μg per ml and 1–2 μg per ml, respectively. Amikacin peak and trough levels for foals have not been established in the literature, but human recommendations are peak concentrations of 15 to 30 μg per ml and trough concentrations of 5 to 8 μg per ml, depending on the microorganism. In general, most foals do well when the peak does not exceed 15 to 25 μg per ml and the trough remains below 5 μg per ml. Because the volume of distribution is larger and t½ is longer in foals, lengthened dosage intervals result in high peaks with prolonged low troughs.

As a general rule, this means that aminoglycosides (i.e., gentamicin) should be administered twice a day instead of three times a day in foals, while the total dosage administered per day (in milligrams) remains the same. If larger concen-

TABLE 1. ANTIBIOTIC DOSAGE RECOMMENDATIONS FOR SEPTICEMIC FOALS*

Antibiotic	Dose, Interval, and Frequency
Sodium penicillin G	25,000–50,000 IU/kg IV q. 6–8 h.
Potassium penicillin G	25,000–50,000 IU/kg IV q. 6–8 h.
Procaine penicillin G	25,000–50,000 IU/kg IM q. 12 h.
Sodium ampicillin	20 mg/kg IV q. 6–8 h.
Gentamicin sulfate	2.2 mg/kg IV or IM q. 8–12 h.
	3.3 mg/kg IV or IM q. 12 h.
Amikacin sulfate	7 mg/kg IV or IM q. 8-12 h.
	11.5 mg/kg IV or IM q. 12 h.
Trimethoprim–sulfa	15 mg/kg IV q. 12 h.
Sodium cephalothin	20–30 mg/kg IV q. 6 h.
Sodium cefazolin	20 mg/kg IV q. 8–12 h.
Sodium cefuroxime	20–30 mg/kg IV q. 8–12 h.
Sodium cefotaxime	20–30 mg/kg IV q. 6 h.
Sodium ceftazidime	20–30 mg/kg IV q. 8 h.
Sodium ceftizoxime	20–30 mg/kg IV q. 8 h.

*The smaller dose or longer dosing interval is often used for premature foals or foals less than 7 days old.

trations are necessary to achieve adequate peaks, the dose should be divided and given twice a day.

Septicemic foals are at high risk for developing aminoglycoside-induced nephrotoxicity. This is due to a combination of factors including prolonged duration of therapy, renal insufficiency, concurrent drug therapy (particularly with cephalothin), volume depletion, and hypokalemia. Aminoglycosides can be used successfully in septicemic foals if careful attention is paid to these factors and adequate fluid is provided for diuresis.

Trimethoprim–sulfonamide combinations are generally accepted as bactericidal agents. These combinations are effective against a broad spectrum of gram-positive and gram-negative microorganisms, although resistance, especially to *Enterobacter* spp., is rising. Sulfonamides are oxidizing agents and should be used cautiously in neonates. Foal RBCs are sensitive to oxidation, and hemolysis or methemoglobinemia can occur. Other reported side effects in adult horses that may be important in foals are acute toxic enteritis, transient neutropenia, transient ataxia, and sudden death.

Cephalosporins have been classed into three different generations based on their spectrum of action. Cefazolin and cephalothin are two frequently used first-generation agents active against most aerobic gram-positive cocci, many anaerobic cocci and bacilli, and some gram-negative bacteria. Cephalothin has the greatest reported incidence of nephrotoxicity. These drugs are normally used in combination with an aminoglycoside and are most effective against septicemia caused by *Staphylococcus* spp., *Streptococcus* spp., and *Escherichia coli*. As with other widely used antibiotics, resistance has limited the usefulness of this group.

Second-generation cephalosporins retain most gram-positive and anaerobic coverage and have expanded gram-negative coverage. In this group, cefuroxime has the most potential in neonatal septicemia, especially when resistance has developed to first-generation cephalosporins or an aminoglycoside cannot be used.

Moxalactam, cefotaxime, cefoperazone, ceftizoxime, ceftriaxone, and ceftazidime are all third-generation cephalosporins. Gram-negative coverage is greatly expanded with these agents, but anaerobic and gram-positive action is less. Ceftazidime, cefotaxime, and ceftizoxime have good CNS penetration and are recommended for treatment of bacterial meningitis. Hypoprothrombinemia and platelet dysfunction have been reported, particularly with moxalactam, so close monitoring is advised. The use of third-generation cephalosporins in neonatal septicemia is increasing, especially as resistance to other antibiotics continues to develop.

SEQUELAE

Localized infections may develop in various body systems if the foal survives the initial septicemic episode. The GI tract, respiratory tract, and umbilicus are most frequently affected. Diarrhea, although generally a sign of a specific disease, may develop secondary to systemic disease and may result in dehydration, electrolyte imbalances, and metabolic acidosis. Vigorous IV therapy and good supportive care are the cornerstones of therapy. Pneumonia is common in septicemic foals and if poorly treated progresses to a chronic state. Treatment consists of an appropriate systemic antibiotic, supportive care, and minimization of stress. Omphalitis or omphalophlebitis is characterized by pain, warmth, or discharge from the umbilicus. If an abscess is present externally or visible ultrasonographically, surgical resection may be necessary.

Meningitis is caused by hematogenous spread of bacteria from a primary site such as the umbilicus. Foals may appear dull, depressed, and disoriented or develop convulsions or coma or both. A third-generation cephalosporin is the antibiotic of choice. Aminoglycosides have poor CNS penetration even when the meninges are inflamed and are ineffective in the treatment of bacterial meningitis.

Anterior uveitis may develop as a sequela to systemic disease. Photophobia, blepharospasm, lacrimation, miosis, and ciliary injection are signs of anterior uveitis. In addition to systemic antibiotics, local treatment is necessary. Local therapy includes a mydriatic such as atropine, a topical steroid such as dexamethasone, and a broad-spectrum antibiotic such as gentamicin or bacitracin/polymyxin/neomycin.

Septic arthritis and osteomyelitis are common sequelae and may be a cause for euthanasia in advanced cases. Early recognition and treatment are necessary to prevent permanent damage. Treatment consists of the appropriate systemic antibiotic, articular rest, and irrigation and large-volume lavage of affected joints (see p. 455). Most antibiotics have good penetration to inflamed synovial membranes and closely adjacent bone. Penetration to deeper areas of osteomyelitis is poor.

Septicemic foals are highly stressed from disease and frequent handling and consequently are at risk for gastroduodenal ulcers. Diagnosis is generally based on the presence of bruxism, profuse salivation, abdominal pain, and occult blood in reflux or feces. Many therapeutic options have been described, but successful treatment usually includes sucralfate and an H_2-receptor antagonist such as cimetidine or ranitidine (see p. 184).

Septic shock is the most common sequela of septicemia in neonatal foals. Septic shock is characterized by decreased peripheral capillary perfusion and tissue hypoxia and may result in sequestration of fluid and decreased effective circulating blood volume. Vigorous IV fluid therapy at 30 to 40 ml per kg body weight (about 2 liters per hour in a 50-kg foal) is required. Dopamine is indicated if cardiac output and peripheral perfusion remain poor after adequate rehydration. Normally, a dopamine solution administered at 3 µg per kg per minute causes vasodilation of renal and mesenteric circulation. Use should be monitored closely and the infusion slowed or stopped if blood pressure increases excessively. Doses higher than 5 µg per kg per minute can cause vasoconstriction and are usually contraindicated. Corticosteroids are currently not routinely used in septic shock. Nonsteroidal anti-inflammatory drugs such as flunixin meglumine are beneficial but have been associated with gastroduodenal ulcers and nephrotoxicity in volume-depleted foals and need to be used with caution. Fresh, platelet-rich plasma (40 ml per kg body weight) is indicated if hemostatic abnormalities, such as venous thrombosis, petechial hemorrhage, altered coagulation profile, and a positive sepsis score exist.

PROGNOSIS

Without early recognition and vigorous medical intervention, the prognosis for recovery is poor. The development of disseminated infection, especially meningitis, results in a grave prognosis. Highly localized infections such as omphalitis, gastroenteritis, and pneumonia have a better prognosis because progression is slower, and localization indicates that some immune function may be present. Without early and aggressive treatment, septic arthritis and osteomyelitis carry a very poor prognosis. Generally the more joints affected, the worse the prognosis. The initial WBC and differential do not provide a prognosis. A poor prognosis is associated with persistence of laboratory abnormalities such as neutropenia with toxic changes, leukocytosis, or elevated fibrinogen levels.

Supplemental Readings

Adland-Davenport, P., Brown, M. P., Robinson, J. D., and Derendorf, H. C.: Pharmacokinetics of amikacin in critically ill neonatal foals treated for presumed or confirmed sepsis. Equine Vet. J., 22:18–22, 1990.
Baggot, J. D., Love, D. N., Stewart, J., and Raus, J.: Gentamicin dosage in foals aged one month and three months. Equine Vet. J., 18:113–116, 1986.
Brewer, B. D., and Koterba, A. M.: Bacterial isolates in foals in a neonatal intensive care unit. Comp. Cont. Ed. Pract. Vet., 12:1773–1781, 1990.
Caprile, K. A., and Short, C. R.: Pharmacologic considerations in drug therapy in foals. Vet. Clin. North Am. (Equine Pract.), 3:123–144, 1987.
Carter, G. K., and Martens, R. J.: Septicemia in the neonatal foal. Compend. Cont. Educ. Pract. Vet., 8:S256–S270, 1986.
Sojka, J. E., and Brown, S. A.: Pharmacokinetic adjustment of gentamicin dosing in horses with sepsis. J. Am. Vet. Med. Assoc., 189:784–789, 1986.
Wilson, W. D., and Madigan, J. E.: Comparison of bacteriologic culture of blood and necropsy specimens for determining the cause of foal septicemia: 47 cases (1978–1987). J. Am. Vet. Med. Assoc., 195:1759–1763, 1989.

Hepatic Disease in Foals

Erwin G. Pearson, CORVALLIS, OREGON

Hepatic disease in foals is not common, and clinical signs may not be apparent until some liver functions have failed. The liver has a large reserve, and up to 80 per cent of the hepatocytes may have to be damaged before failure occurs. However, some liver functions may not be as developed in the neonate as they are in the adult. Both infectious and toxic agents can cause hepatic disease either in utero or postnatally.

ETIOLOGY

Tyzzer's disease is an infectious, necrotizing hepatitis that occurs in foals from 7 to 42 days of age. Mares may be carriers. It is caused by *Bacillus piliformis*, and the experimental incubation period is 3 to 7 days. This is a very acute illness; some foals are just found dead, and the duration of clinical signs in many others is from 2 to 12 hours, but occasionally depression is noted for up to 48 hours. Rectal temperature may be subnormal terminally or may be elevated to 42° C in earlier stages. A few foals are icteric, but this condition has not had time to develop in most cases. Most cases are diagnosed on postmortem examination. The finding of multifocal necrotizing hepatitis and identification of gram-positive filamentous rods in hepatocytes at the margins of the necrotic areas are presumptive evidence of Tyzzer's disease. A Warthin–Storry silver stain of the tissue will help identify the long slender bacilli. Most foals die despite therapy.

Equine herpesvirus 1 can cause a multifocal necrotizing hepatitis in foals, but the more frequent signs are related to the interstitial pneumonia caused by the virus. The infection is thought to be acquired in utero and causes abortion in most cases. Fetuses that survive and are born weak may have respiratory signs such as rapid and labored respirations, or radiographic changes in the lungs. A few are depressed and icteric as a result of the hepatic damage. The diagnosis is made by finding intranuclear inclusion bodies in hepatocytes or by identifying the virus by fluorescent antibody techniques.

Cholangiohepatitis can occur along with some of the foal septicemias and with infections of the bowel such as salmonellosis. In most of these cases the other signs produced by the infection are more predominant. Liver failure may nevertheless occur and may be life-threatening. An extrahepatic cholestasis can occur as a result of duodenal ulcers with strictures.

The best-documented toxic cause of hepatic disease is ingestion of paste containing ferrous fumarate. If this iron-containing paste is given shortly after birth and before colostrum is consumed, the foal will usually show clinical signs in 2 to 5 days. The most pronounced signs are related to hepatic encephalopathy and include depression, ataxia, aimless wandering, head pressing, and other abnormal behavior. Icterus may be seen if the foal does not die peracutely. Liver function test results are abnormal, and histologically the liver will have massive areas of hepatocyte necrosis, some bile duct hyperplasia, and perhaps early portal fibrosis. Most affected foals die if hepatic failure is evident.

Other hepatotoxic agents could potentially damage the liver of young foals. Table 1 lists some hepatotoxic agents to which a foal may be exposed. There are however, few documented cases of poisoning by these agents in foals. Pyrrolizidine alkaloid from consumption of *Senecio* and other plants is toxic to horses, but *Senecio* usually is not consumed by foals. It is transferred to the milk if consumed by the dam, but experiments in feeding pyrrolizidine alkaloid–containing goat's milk to calves did not produce hepatic lesions.

A few anomalies of the hepatobiliary system have been described in foals. Portosystemic shunting has been reported in horses, but most animals are at least several months old. In these animals the serum bilirubin and γ-glutamyl-transpeptidase levels are elevated, but the concentrations of ammonia and bile acid in the serum are disproportionately high. Congenital biliary atresia has caused cholestasis and hepatic failure.

TABLE 1. SOME POTENTIAL HEPATOTOXINS FOR FOALS

Drugs
   Corticosteroids
   Tetracycline
   Erythromycin
   Rifampin
   Anesthetic gases
   Phenothiazine tranquilizers
Chemicals
   Iron
   Copper
   Carbon tetrachloride
   Chlorinated hydrocarbons
   Coal tar pitch

CLINICAL SIGNS AND DIAGNOSIS

The clinical signs of hepatic failure in foals are not consistent or specific. In addition, concurrent diseases may mask the signs, or the foal may not live long enough for them to develop. Liver failure may be suspected in foals that have severe depression, abnormal behavior, or are icteric. Since these signs are produced more frequently by other neonatal foal diseases, liver function tests are necessary to confirm hepatic damage. Most foals with hepatic failure are hypoglycemic. Blood ammonia levels are elevated and blood urea nitrogen levels may be low or normal. Prolongation of the prothrombin time and partial thromboplastin time occurs in many foals with hepatic failure even though there is some reserve for production of the clotting factors. However, none of the changes in these products is specific for liver disease or liver failure.

Serum bilirubin is usually increased, due mainly (80 to 90 per cent) to unconjugated bilirubin unless there is some bile duct obstruction. The elevation in serum bile acids is specific for liver disease or portal shunting, but normal

TABLE 2. DIFFERENTIAL DIAGNOSIS OF ABNORMAL LABORATORY FINDINGS IN FOALS WITH HEPATIC DISEASE

Observation	Nonhepatic Cause
Hypoglycemia	Malnutrition, septicemia, hypothermia
Prolonged prothrombin time or partial thromboplastin time	Disseminated intravascular coagulation, congenital coagulation defect
Blood ammonia elevated	Negative nitrogen balance, abnormal bowel
Bilirubin elevated	Hemolysis, neonatal isoerythrolysis
Bile acid increased	Portosystemic shunt
Alkaline phosphatase increased	Bone, gut, placenta
Aspartate aminotransferase increased	Muscle damage
Bromsulphthalein clearance increased	Competition with bilirubin from hemolysis

ranges for foals have not been well documented. Levels above 20 µmol per liter should be considered significant. The ratio of plasma aromatic to branched-chain amino acids will probably be increased, but the analysis is expensive and not performed by most laboratories. Table 2 lists some parameters likely to be abnormal in foals with liver disease and gives some other causes of these abnormalities.

Serum levels of liver-produced enzymes are often increased in foals with liver disease, but normal values for some of these enzymes are higher in foals (Table 3). The dehydrogenases such as sorbitol dehydrogenase and glutamate dehydrogenase are specific for the liver, but the half-life is short and serum concentrations may return to normal a few days after the insult. Serum γ-glutamyltransferase levels are often increased severalfold but are normally higher in young foals than in adults. Serum alkaline phosphatase is increased in most cases but the increase is not specific for liver disease.

Histopathological examination of liver biopsy tissue is the most diagnostic procedure. Liver biopsy is performed on foals fairly easily and without excessive risk. It can be accomplished in the standing or recumbent foal using a notch-cutting biopsy needle at least 4½ inches long. The preferred site is on the right side where a line drawn from the point of the shoulder to the tuber coxae crosses the 13th or 14th intercostal space. Ultrasonography may demonstrate enlarged bile ducts or a change in liver texture.

THERAPY

Treatment of liver failure in foals is not often rewarding, but treating liver disease before the liver has failed may be useful. Foals with massive hepatocyte necrosis or fibrosis that bridges between lobules are unlikely to have a lasting response to therapy. Before treatment is instituted it is important to stop exposure to the causative agent, whether it is infective or toxic.

Therapy directed against the specific disease should be initiated if possible. If Tyzzer's disease is diagnosed ante mortem, the foal should be given 0.1 ml per kg of a 50 per cent dextrose solution intravenously (IV), followed by a 10 per cent dextrose solution administered over a longer period of time. Antibiotics effective against *Bacillus piliformis* should be given IV. Possible effective antibiotics are penicillin, tetracycline and erythromycin. Antibiotics may also be needed to treat the cholangihepatitis that may occur with salmonellosis and other septicemias.

Foals born with equine herpesvirus 1 infections usually do not survive, but supportive therapy may help. Foals with massive hepatocyte necrosis from toxins will not survive in most cases, even though the liver has an excellent ability to regenerate. Support must be given to keep the foal alive long enough for some regeneration to take place. This may include ventilation and other respiratory supports, as described on page 478.

Supplying adequate metabolizable energy is perhaps the most important consideration in the general treatment of hepatic disease in foals.

TABLE 3. NORMAL RANGES FOR HEPATIC TESTS IN HORSES OF VARIOUS AGES[°]

Test	Age				
	<12 hr	1–3 days	2–3 wk	6 mo	Adult
γ-Glutamyl transferase, IU/L	16–52	13–67	20–104	32–42	8–30
Alkaline phosphatase, IU/L	<1200	861–1563	295–615	161–253	73–194
Aspartate aminotransferase, IU/L	36–156	147–341	160–520	181–253	150–270
Sorbitol dehydrogenase, IU/L	NA	1.1–2.9	0.5–3.7	0.8–2.2	1.9–5.8
Total bilirubin, mg/dl	1.6–3.8	1.5–3.3	0.6–2	0.5–2	0.4–2
Bromsulphthalein clearance, t ½	NA	<5 min	<3.5 min	<3.5 min	<3.5 min
Serum bile acid, µmol/L	NA	NA	NA	<15	<15

[°]Broadest range from several references. NA = not available

Since most affected foals are hypoglycemic and do not have hepatic glycogen stores, a continuous source of glucose or other energy is needed. It is often best to place the foal on total parenteral nutrition unless it is hyperlipidemic.

Since there is an increase in the ratio of aromatic to branched-chain amino acids in the blood, IV solutions should be high in branched-chain amino acids. Human preparations are available that contain predominantly branched-chain amino acids, but they are expensive.*† Oral pastes and solutions with high concentrations of branched-chain to aromatic amino acids can be formulated and force fed. High levels of aromatic amino acids relative to branched-chain amino acids are involved in the production of hepatic encephalopathy; they are thought to be precursors of false neurotransmitters, or abnormal amounts of certain neurotransmitors. These amino acid ratios are especially important if neurological signs are present.

If the foal can be kept in a positive energy balance and in an anabolic state, thiamine,‡ 0.002 to 0.003 ml per kg given intramuscularly (IM); vitamin K_1, 0.5 to 2.0 mg per kg IM§ daily; and folic acid, 75 mg total dose IM, repeated every 4 to 7 days, should be given. If there are coagulation problems, 1 to 2 liters of fresh plasma may be useful. It may also dilute the ammonia and aromatic amino acid concentrations in the blood. In other species use of laxatives and oral antibiotics such as neomycin has been recommended to reduce the amount of ammonia in the bowel, but the efficacy of this approach in the foal has not been proved. In humans, lactulose is given to reduce the ammonia absorbed from the gut, and might help in foals. In humans a 50 per cent syrup is given until diarrhea develops, but this seems inappropriate in foals.

If neurological signs are present becasue of hepatic encephalopathy, some sedation may be needed to control the foal before other treatment can be started. Diazepam may be given at a dose of 5 to 10 mg or to effect, and repeated when needed at a lower dose. Sometimes the dextrose administration alone will reduce neurological signs.

Supplemental Readings

Bauer, J. E., Asquith, R. L., and Kivipelto, J.: Serum biochemical indicators of liver function in neonatal foals. Am. J. Vet. Res., 50:2037–2041, 1989.

Brown, C. M., and Mullaney, T.P.: Tyzzer's disease in foals. *In* Smith, B. P. (ed): Large Animal Internal Medicine. St. Louis, C. V. Mosby, 1990, pp. 848–849.

Divers, T. J.: Neonatal hepatic failure. *In* Smith, B. P. (ed): Large Animal Internal Medicine. St. Louis, C. V. Mosby, 1990, pp. 848.

Humber, K. A., Sweeney, R. W., Saik, J. E., Hansen, T. O., and Morris, C. F.: Clinical and clinicopathologic findings in two foals infected with *Bacillus piliformis*. J. Am. Vet. Med. Assoc., 193:1425–1428, 1988.

Mullaney, T. P., and Brown, C. M.: Iron toxicity in neonatal foals. Equine Vet. J., 20:119–124, 1988.

---

*FreAmine III, Kendal McGraw Labs., Irvine, CA
†Travasol, Baxter Health Care Corp., Deerfield, IL
‡Thiamine HCl, Veterinary Labs., Lenexa, KS
§Phytonadione, Vedco, St. Joseph, MO

Gastrointestinal Diseases of the Neonatal Foal

Susan D. Semrad, MADISON, WISCONSIN
Susan Shaftoe, MADISON, WISCONSIN

Diseases of the gastrointestinal (GI) tract are common in neonates and foals less than 6 months of age. The majority of these conditions may be managed medically, as only a small percentage of foals (less than 1 per cent) develop life-threatening abdominal disorders requiring surgical intervention. Although GI dysfunction may be a primary problem, commonly it occurs secondary to septicemia in the neonate. Twenty-six per cent of deaths during the first 2 months of life are due to neonatal infections complicated by diarrhea. Detailed assessment is necessary, as several conditions can cause abdominal distention and pain, and multiple organ disease is common in young foals. Quick and accurate differentiation between surgical and nonsurgical conditions is imperative as young foals have few reserves with which to withstand the cardiovascular alterations and endotoxemia that often accompany severe GI dysfunction. Secondary life-threatening hypoglycemia, hyperkalemia, or hypokalemia and metabolic acidosis may develop quickly in the compromised young foal.

The majority of foals with GI problems present with either abdominal pain (colic) and distention or diarrhea. Often the foal has been depressed, lying down more frequently or nursing less aggressively before signs of abdominal disease are noted. Signs of abdominal discomfort may be subtle, such as tail switching, frequent attempts to defecate or urinate, standing with legs camped under or stretched out behind, treading, pawing, bruxism, difficulty lying down, or looking at flank; or the signs may be dramatic, such as biting at the flanks, rolling from side to side, lying on the back with the legs in an abnormal position, frequently getting up and down, or throwing itself down. Abdominal discomfort after eating is suggestive of a high obstruction or gastroduodenal ulcer with abnormal gastric emptying. Common causes of abdominal pain with or without abdominal distention in the young foal include meconium retention, congenital anomalies, uroperitoneum, viral enteritis, gastroduodenal ulcers, intestinal displacement, intussusception, scrotal, umbilical, or abdominal hernia, foreign body ingestion, impaction, and peritonitis.

MECONIUM RETENTION

Meconium is dark green mucilaginous material that accumulates in the lower intestinal tract during gestation. It consists of intestinal gland secretions, cellular debris, and digested amniotic fluid. Meconium may be passed as early as 4 hours after birth. In most foals the bowel is emptied of meconium within 24 to 48 hours of birth, although some foals continue to pass meconium until 96 hours of age. Meconium is considered to be retained if the foal makes frequent attempts but fails to produce meconium by 12 hours of age.

Meconium retention or impaction is the most common cause of abdominal discomfort in the newborn foal, with approximately 1.5 per cent of all foals suffering from the condition and requiring treatment. Meconium usually becomes impacted in the small colon or rectum. Colts are more commonly affected, possibly due to their narrow pelvic canal. Other factors predisposing to meconium retention include maternal malnutrition, delayed colostrum intake with loss of laxative effect, conditions that compromise the foal, such as asphyxiation, dystocia, prematurity, or low birth weight, intestinal disease or hypomotility of the colon, and dehydration. Mild clinical signs are initially apparent within 6 to 24 hours of birth. As abdominal distention and intestinal pain become more pronounced, the severity of clinical signs increases. Commonly observed signs include depression, decreased nursing, restlessness, frequent posturing to defecate, straining to defecate, tail switching, elevated tail, standing with the back arched while contracting the abdominal muscles, lying down, and rolling. Tachycardia and tachypnea are observed as the abdominal discomfort increases. Colonic meconium impaction is often accompanied by more severe abdominal pain than is rectal meconium obstruction. Auscultation and percussion of the abdomen may reveal colonic tympany even before abdominal distention is obvious. In some foals, the urachus may reopen as a result of straining to defecate.

Clinicopathological alterations are minimal in the early stages of meconium retention. As the foal decreases its oral intake and sweats due to abdominal discomfort, dehydration and prerenal azotemia result. A stress leukogram may become evident. Leukopenia, with a left shift and toxic changes in the white blood cells (WBCs) and an elevation in peritoneal fluid WBC count and protein may be seen with severe meconium obstruction if the surrounding bowel becomes compromised.

Diagnosis of meconium retention is made on the basis of failure to pass meconium, clinical signs, and digital examination. Digital examination may reveal firm meconium pellets within the rectum and helps to rule out atresia or agenesis of the rectum or colon. Abdominal radiographs may define the extent of the obstruction and degree of gas accumulation as well as assist in ruling out other causes of intestinal obstruction. Contrast radiography (barium enema) or proctoscopy may be performed if further confirmation is needed.

Therapy

Therapy is aimed at removal of the meconium obstruction without traumatizing the surrounding colon or rectum. The majority of foals will respond to medical intervention, including stool softeners or laxatives, intravenous (IV) fluids, and analgesics. Warm water or saline, soapy water enemas (with or without mineral oil or glycerin added), or 10 ml of a 5 per cent solution of dioctyl sodium sulfoccinate (DSS) diluted in warm water may be administered through soft flexible rubber tubing. The enema tube should not be advanced more than 10 to 12 inches into the rectum and the fluid should flow by gravity. Overdistention of the rectum, use of irritating chemicals, and excessive manipulation of the rectum during enema administration may lead to rectal trauma and atony or urethral irritation, especially in colts. Manual extraction of hard meconium pellets should be undertaken with caution so as not to damage or tear the surrounding intestine. If no response is noted after two to four enemas an alternative approach should be considered. Commercial Fleet enemas may be used but should not be repeated more than twice.

Mild oral laxatives including 4 to 6 ounces of mineral oil or olive oil may be given via nasogastric tube to help soften the stool. Oral laxatives are almost always 100 per cent effective in relieving the impaction when administered before GI motility has been attenuated by gas distention and persistent colic. Harsh laxatives such as DSS or hypertonic saline are irritating to the bowel and should be avoided. Stool may also be softened by IV administration of a balanced electrolyte solution to establish normal hydration status. Electrolyte imbalances, including hypokalemia and hypocalcemia, should be corrected to encourage intestinal motility. In anorectic foals, IV glucose may serve as a temporary energy source.

Analgesics may be indicated once the source of the abdominal discomfort has been established. Because they may cause gastric ulcers, nonsteroidal anti-inflammatory agents should be used judiciously in foals, especially if their hydration status is not optimal. Narcotic analgesics may decrease aboral movement of ingesta, prolong meconium retention, and contribute to fecal water loss.

Surgical intervention is warranted in refractory cases accompanied by abdominal pain, progressive abdominal distention, or bowel compromise or if the underlying cause of the continued abdominal discomfort cannot be clearly defined. The prognosis for simple meconium impaction without bowel compromise is good.

OBSTRUCTIVE GI DISEASE AND ILEUS

Obstructive GI disease may be mechanical or functional in origin. The incidence of intestinal accidents is relatively low in the foal except for intussusception and small intestinal volvulus. Frequently these conditions occur secondary to enteritis or diarrhea. Less commonly, cecal torsion, colonic torsion, or incarcerated hernias may cause acute abdominal discomfort and tympany. Often it is difficult to differentiate pain and abdominal distention due to an intestinal accident or mechanical obstruction from discomfort secondary to functional ileus induced by enteritis or septicemia.

Abrupt dietary changes, enteritis, or parasite infestation may result in alterations in intestinal motility and predispose to intestinal intussusception. Intussusception occurs in foals 1 week to 6 months of age, with foals 3 to 5 weeks of age most commonly affected. Two clinical syndromes have been described. Most frequently intussusception is an acute syndrome with abdominal pain, abdominal distention, decreased borborygmi, dehydration, anorexia, and cardiovascular compromise. Blood and peritoneal fluid alterations are consistent with bowel compromise and endotoxemia. Less commonly, intussusception may present as a subacute syndrome with anorexia, depression, intermittent abdominal pain, diarrhea, and weight loss.

Small intestinal volvulus has also been associated with parasite migration, dietary changes, and excessive roughage in the foal's diet. Affected foals, usually 2 to 4 months old, develop severe, persistent abdominal pain accompanied by abdominal distention and rapid cardiovascular compromise. When the intestine is compromised and necrotic, leukopenia, left shift, toxic WBCs, elevated hematocrit, elevated, decreased, or normal serum protein, metabolic acidosis, and electrolyte imbalances are consistent with endotoxemia. Peritoneal fluid protein concentration and WBC count increase and the neutrophils appear degenerate. Evidence of fulminant peritonitis may be present. Abdominal radiographs reveal multiple loops of dilated small intestine. Fluid lines apparent at different levels are suggestive of small intestinal volvulus.

Indications for surgical intervention include acute, persistent or uncontrollable pain, persistent tachycardia greater than 120 bpm, progressive abdominal distention, an increase in peritoneal fluid protein content or WBC number or change in WBC character, radiographic or ultrasonographic evidence of bowel obstruction, and continuous gastric reflux. Fluid therapy to correct electrolyte and metabolic derangements and circulating volume is necessary to stabilize the foal prior to surgical correction of an intestinal obstruction.

Although often difficult, it is imperative to differentiate intestinal accidents from functional ileus, the loss or absence of intestinal motility, or primary tympany of the GI tract due to fermentation of colostrum or milk. Ileus in foals has been associated with prematurity, GI dysfunction secondary to asphyxia, enteritis, septicemia, peritonitis, and impaired autonomic nerve function secondary to electrolyte imbalance, metabolic derangement, intestinal inflammation, or defective innervation.

Clinical signs of ileus, including abdominal discomfort and distention, will vary in severity depending on the degree of gas and fluid accumulation within the intestine. Intolerance to feeding, gastric reflux, and decreased borborygmi are usually evident. Severe abdominal distention providing pressure on the diaphragm may lead to secondary respiratory distress.

Electrolyte abnormalities can include hypokalemia and hypochloremia if gastric reflux is present; hypokalemia, hyponatremia, hypochloremia, and hypocalcemia if enteritis/diarrhea is present; and other metabolic derangements. However, normal electrolyte values are frequently seen. The gastric fluid pH is elevated if reflux of small intestinal contents occurs. Multiple gas-distended loops of bowel may be evident on abdominal radiography or ultrasonography (see p. 420). Peritoneal fluid may be normal or may reflect the degree of intestinal inflammation and compromise.

THERAPY

Treatment of functional ileus can be extremely difficult. Correction of the primary underlying cause is paramount. A medical approach is best unless either extreme bowel distention leads to persistent, uncontrollable pain and bowel compromise or a mechanical obstruction cannot be ruled out. In this case, surgical intervention to decompress the bowel may be of some benefit. Medical management for ileus includes removal of gastric reflux through a nasogastric tube and fluid therapy to correct hydration and electrolyte and metabolic imbalances and to provide energy. Enteral feedings are usually decreased in volume or discontinued to provide intestinal rest. In such cases parenteral nutrition is necessary to provide adequate caloric intake for the foal (see p. 747). Exercise may encourage intestinal motility. Analgesic agents are administered as needed to relieve abdominal discomfort. Care must be taken to avoid the use of analgesic agents that decrease intestinal motility or are ulcerogenic. Use of intestinal stimulants, such as metoclopramide* is controversial, not without risk, and of questionable benefit.

CONGENITAL DEFECTS OF THE GI TRACT

Stricture, atresia, or agenesis may occur anywhere along the intestinal tract. Developmental anomalies generally mimic intestinal obstruction from meconium retention and result in abdominal pain and distention. The onset of clinical signs may occur within the first 12 hours of life or later. Foals with high obstruction due to stenosis or stricture of the pylorus or upper duodenum often exhibit pain and may regurgitate milk after nursing. Antiperistaltic esophageal waves, gastric reflux, and reflux esophagitis may also be noted. Progressive tympany and distention of the abdomen accompany lesions involving the cecum and distal intestinal tract.

Anal atresia is relatively common in foals and may occur as a single defect or in association with anomalies of the urogenital system. The rectum may end blindly a significant distance from the anus or, less commonly, a thin membrane may separate the anus from the rectum. The anus may be well developed with sphincters or may be only a small depression. The diagnosis is made by careful examination of the anus and rectum, or by barium enema examination and contrast radiography.

In the foal with colonic atresia, any portion of the large colon may be atretic and represented only as a thin membranous wall with no teniae. The distal portion of the small intestine or the proximal portion of the small colon may be atretic. The diagnosis is usually confirmed at surgery. Attempts at surgical correction have met with variable success. There is some evidence that the condition is heritable in foals.

Ileocolonic aganglionosis or lethal white foal syndrome occurs in white, blue-eyed, pink-skinned foals born to matings of overo-Paint horses. The disease is characterized by absence of myenteric and submucosal neuronal ganglia in the terminal portion of the ileum, cecum, or entire colon. Affected foals are normal at birth but become colicky within 5 to 24 hours. The diagnosis is suspected from the color pattern of the dam, sire, and foal. Abdominal radiographs, surgical exploration, and necropsy findings confirm the diagnosis. Attempts at surgical correction have not been successful. The mode of inheritance is unknown but has been demonstrated not to result from a single recessive gene.

Congenital inguinal and diaphragmatic hernias may result in abdominal pain in young foals. Inguinal hernias in colts are characterized by enlargement of one or both sides of the scrotum. Herniation of small intestine into the scrotum often spontaneously corrects within the first few weeks of life. Intervention may not be required unless bowel becomes incarcerated within the hernia. Signs associated with congenital diaphragmatic hernias will depend on the amount and viability of the abdominal viscera in the thoracic cavity. Affected foals may exhibit dyspnea, pleurodynia, or labored breathing. Radiography

---

*Reglan, A. H. Robins, Richmond, VA

or ultrasonography of the cranial abdomen and thorax help to confirm the diagnosis. Attempts at surgical correction have been disappointing.

ENTERITIS/DIARRHEA

Diarrhea is the most common GI disturbance of young foals. Up to 80 per cent of foals have at least one episode of diarrhea during the first 6 months of life. The majority of diarrheal episodes in foals are mild, transient, and not life-threatening. Affected foals, however, must be closely monitored for depression, dehydration, discomfort, and other signs of compromise, as physical status may deteriorate rapidly and death losses may be significant unless foals are treated promptly.

Foal Heat Diarrhea

Foal heat diarrhea is a mild, self-limiting diarrhea with few systemic effects that occurs in suckled or artificially raised foals between 6 and 14 days old. Previously this diarrheal syndrome was thought to be associated with hormonal changes in the dam and changes in milk composition during first postpartum estrus, hence the name foal heat diarrhea (FHD). Infection with *Strongyloides westeri* acquired through nursing from infected mares was another debated cause. Changes in milk composition and strongyloidosis have been disproved as causes of FHD through studies on foals raised on artificial diets and in controlled environments. Attempts to identify viral agents and cryptosporidia in the feces of affected foals have produced inconsistent results. Currently, FHD is thought to reflect adaptive changes in the foal's intestinal tract as the foal begins to ingest more fiber (hay and grain) and indulge in coprophagy. These activities require adjustment in digestive processes and help to establish new bacterial flora and ciliates in the foal's intestinal tract.

The fecal consistency of affected foals is usually soft to watery and the stool may have a slightly fetid odor. Affected foals are active, alert, afebrile, continue to nurse, and show little discomfort or straining during passage of feces. The diarrhea usually resolves in less than a week. In most cases no therapy is indicated other than nursing care to prevent perineal scalding. If the diarrhea persists for longer than several days but the foal remains normal in other respects, intestinal protectorants may be beneficial. If the diarrhea persists or the foals becomes depressed, dehydrated, hypophagic, or febrile, other causes of diarrhea should be investigated. Blood work and fecal evaluation to rule out septicemia and infectious causes of diarrhea should be performed.

Nutritional Diarrhea

Nutritional diarrhea in foals may result from (1) milk engorgement, which can result when the foal nurses after a period of separation from the dam, or when an orphaned foal is overfed; (2) improperly prepared artificial diets that are too concentrated or too dilute; (3) transient lactase deficiency in a premature foal or in a sick foal off feed for a period of time or suffering from viral enteritis; or (4) ingestion of foreign substances such as roughage feeds, sand, or feces. The first three may result in improper digestion of milk lactose in the small intestine. Incompletely digested milk passes into the large intestine, ferments, and draws water into the intestine, resulting in osmotic diarrhea. Ingestion of sand, dirt, or feces may induce diarrhea by intestinal irritation. Early ingestion of hay has also been incriminated as a cause of diarrhea, attributed to inability of the large colon to adapt to fibrous material.

The diagnosis of nutritional diarrhea is based on the foal's history and age and presence of diarrhea without evidence of systemic illness. If transient lactase deficiency is suspected, an oral lactose tolerance test may be performed to support the diagnosis. Foals with diarrhea persisting after correction of suspected nutritional causes or with signs of systemic involvement should be evaluated for alternative causes of the diarrhea.

Diarrhea induced by the increased osmotic load that results from overly concentrated artificial milk products may lead to dehydration and electrolyte disturbances. Correction of the dietary formulation or changing to a different milk source such as goat's milk may resolve these problems. If this is not adequate or dehydration is severe, balanced polyionic fluids given IV may be necessary to establish normal hydration and electrolyte balance. When a transient lactase deficiency is suspected, milk may be treated with a commercial lactase preparation* prior to feeding. Alternatively, yogurt with active cultures may be fed.

Viral Diarrheas

Rotavirus is the most common cause of viral enteritis in young foals; 30 to 60 per cent of foals with diarrheal syndromes are infected with rotavirus. Much less is known about the incidence of other viral agents and their relationship to en-

---

*LactAid, LactAid Inc., Pleasantville, NJ

teritis/diarrheal syndromes in foals. Coronavirus, adenovirus, and parvovirus-like particles have been isolated from feces of foals with diarrheic stool. Some of these agents have been isolated in conjunction with rotavirus.

While clinical disease due to rotavirus is primarily noted in foals less than 6 months of age, serological surveys have shown that virtually 100 per cent of healthy adult horses tested have antibody titers to rotavirus. Thus, it is possible that adult horses serve as asymptomatic carriers of the virus and a potential source of infection for susceptible foals. Isolation of rotavirus from the feces of apparently healthy foals has also been reported. Other potential sources of infection include the environment, as rotavirus may remain viable for up to 9 months; foals shipped to the farm while in the incubation phase of the disease; and clinically affected foals or foals recovering from rotavirus infection. Rotavirus has been identified in the feces of affected foals from 2 days before onset of diarrhea to 6 days after recovery. Intermittent shedding of virus for up to 8 months post infection has also been reported.

Rotavirus diarrhea may be endemic on a farm, with a few foals being affected yearly; or outbreaks of epidemic proportion may occur. The extent of the infection is determined in part by the number of susceptible animals on the farm, the degree of contamination of the premises, predisposing factors such as poor management or overcrowding, level of antiviral colostral antibodies acquired by the foal, and methods taken to contain the infection.

Diarrhea associated with rotavirus enteritis results from a combination of mechanisms. Viral invasion of villous epithelial cells of the small intestine results in loss of absorptive cells and brush border enzymes, villous atrophy, and proliferation of crypt cells. These changes result in malabsorption/maldigestion, increased secretion, transient lactose intolerance, and increased movement of fluid into the colon, fostering an osmotic component to the diarrhea.

Foals with rotavirus diarrhea display varying degrees of depression, hypophagia, or anorexia, mild to profuse watery diarrhea, and commonly a fever (39° to 41° C). The onset of diarrhea usually occurs 12 to 24 hours after the foal first appears depressed and hypophagic. Severe abdominal discomfort and signs of colic may be observed before the onset of diarrhea in some foals. Generally, younger foals are most severely affected and usually have voluminous, nonodorous, profuse watery diarrhea. These foals have a higher mortality rate if not treated aggressively. Foals older than 30 days may have only fever and mild depression, with or without diarrhea. In the majority of foals, clinical signs resolve within 3 to 4 days, but may persist longer in the more severely compromised animals. Depending on the severity of infection and the presence of secondary bacterial infection, affected foals will show varying degrees of weight loss, dehydration, electrolyte imbalances such as hyponatremia, hypochloremia, and sometimes hypokalemia, and metabolic acidosis. Anorexic young foals may also be hypoglycemic. Foals may develop clinical signs of gastroduodenal ulcer syndrome (see p. 184), while recovering foals may appear unthrifty for a period of time.

Feces for diagnostic evaluation should be collected close to the onset of the disease as the virus is shed heavily during early infection. Both rotavirus serotypes (H1 and H2) associated with diarrhea in foals may be detected by commercially available tests or electron microscopy. The ELISA° and the latex agglutination tests† show good correlation with electron microscopy. A stool sample should be submitted for culture to identify any contributing bacterial agents. In foals with abdominal pain and signs of colic, diagnostic procedures including abdominocentesis, abdominal radiography, and blood tests should be undertaken to rule out intestinal accidents requiring surgical intervention.

Management of foals with rotavirus diarrhea is aimed at maintaining hydration and electrolyte and acid–base status, reducing abdominal discomfort or intestinal irritation, preventing secondary bacterial infections, and preventing spread of the infection to other foals. Mildly affected foals that continue to nurse effectively may require no intervention other than close observation and isolation. Mild dehydration and electrolyte imbalances may be corrected by administration of oral electrolyte solutions. As most young foals will not voluntarily consume adequate amounts of these solutions, they should be given via bottle or nasogastric tube. In foals with loss of intestinal absorptive capacity, IV fluid administration may be required. Balanced polyionic electrolyte solutions are usually adequate unless the foal is severely acidotic, hyponatremic, hypokalemic, or hypoglycemic. In acidotic and hyponatremic foals, administration of isotonic bicarbonate may be necessary. Potassium and glucose may be added to the fluids to correct the hypokalemia and hypoglycemia, respectively.

Foals that are anorectic or intolerant of oral

°Rotazyme II ELISA, Abbott Labs., North Chicago, IL
†Virogen Rotatest, Wampole Labs., Cranberry, NJ

feedings will require parenteral nutrition to supply energy and electrolytes. Foals with suspected transient lactose intolerance may be fed mare's milk that has been preincubated with a commercial lactase preparation allowing degradation of lactose into its component monosaccharides.

Intestinal protectorants*,† have been recommended as coating, anti-inflammatory, and antisecretory agents. The use of these agents is controversial, as they may cause ulcers due to their salicylate component and antiprostaglandin activity.

Nursing care involves keeping the perineal area clean and dry. Zinc oxide ointments applied to the perineal area after cleaning and drying may help to decrease scalding from the diarrhea.

Quarantine, strict isolation procedures, and reduction of overcrowding are necessary to prevent the spread of infection. Ideally, separate caretakers are assigned to care for the healthy foals and their dams and affected foals. If this is not possible, healthy foals and mares should be tended to before the ill foals. Affected foals and their dams should be housed away from healthy animals. Gloves, boots, and separate coveralls should be worn when handling affected animals and their manure and disinfected after each use. Rotavirus in feces is resistant to many commonly used disinfectants. Quaternary ammonium compounds and chlorine are inactivated by the presence of organic matter and thus not effective in killing the virus. Phenol compounds are effective. Commercially available cattle rotavirus vaccines give variable results when used in foals and are not reliably protective.

BACTERIAL CAUSES OF DIARRHEA

Bacterial agents, most commonly *Clostridium* spp. and *Salmonella* spp., may cause peracute or acute enteritis and septicemia in the foal; death often occurs before the onset of diarrhea. Affected foals present with severe toxemia and rapidly develop shock and cardiovascular collapse. Intestinal perforation and peritonitis may also occur. Therapeutic attempts are commonly unsuccessful.

Enteric infection with *Clostridium perfringens* A, B, and C causes depression, severe abdominal pain, abdominal distention, and fetid, bloody diarrhea, followed by death within 24 to 48 hours. Foals are affected during their first 2 days of life and death losses are high. *Clostridium welchii, C. sordelli*, and *C. difficile* may cause similar clinical signs. *C. difficile* has also been associated with severe watery diarrhea in non-antibiotic-treated foals 2 to 5 days old. Diarrhea associated with *C. difficile* varies from mild to severe and may be accompanied by hemorrhagic necrotizing enteritis. Depression, weakness, anorexia, and abdominal discomfort are also noted. Fecal shedding of *C. difficile* is only recognized in foals with diarrhea. Clostridial infections are usually sporadic but occasionally a farmwide outbreak may occur.

Clostridial organisms can be cultured on anaerobic agar plates. *C. difficile* may be grown on *C. difficile* agar plates (cycloserine–cefoxitin–fructose agar). As clostridia occur normally within the intestinal tract, demonstration of their presence alone is not sufficient to confirm the diagnosis. The presence of clostridial toxin is demonstrated through toxin neutralization tests in mice. Commercial tissue cytotoxicity neutralization kits are available for detection of *C. difficile* toxin. Postmortem lesions that are fairly specific for clostridial enteritis in foals include extensive mucosal necrosis of the small intestine with massive intraluminal hemorrhage.

Salmonella is probably the most common cause of bacterial enteritis in the foal. *S. typhimurium, S. saintpaul, S. newport*, and other serotypes have been isolated from affected foals. In foals less than 2 weeks old acute septicemic salmonellosis often results in death before diarrhea develops. Early stages of salmonellosis are characterized by depression, weakness, anorexia, neutropenia, and degenerative changes in the neutrophils. Pyrexia is not a consistent finding. Foals with septicemic salmonellosis may survive with intensive management only to develop secondary septic arthritis, pneumonia, nephritis, or meningitis.

Enteritis due to virulent Salmonella strains results in ileus with bowel distention, sequestration of fluid in the gut lumen, hypoproteinemia, and mucosal edema due to protein loss into the bowel wall. Depression, severe abdominal pain, abdominal distention, toxemia accompanied by a leukopenia, left shift, and toxic granulation of WBCs, dehydration, and serum electrolyte losses of sodium, chloride, potassium, and bicarbonate often precede the onset of diarrhea. Peritonitis may or may not be present. As diarrhea may not develop for 12 to 36 hours after the onset of other clinical signs, acute salmonellosis may be difficult to differentiate clinically from intestinal accidents in foals. Once present, the diarrhea is often profuse, watery, and may have a pungent offensive odor. Invasion of the bowel by less virulent strains of Salmonella may result in a milder clinical syndrome. Although the clin-

---

*Pepto-Bismol, Procter & Gamble, Cincinnati, OH
†Corrective Mixture, Smith Kline Beecham Animal Health, Philadelphia, PA

ical signs and clinicopathological alterations are similar, they are less severe. The diarrhea is mild and more responsive to therapy. Concurrent bacteremia may or may not be present. Chronic salmonellosis is uncommon in foals, but in a small percentage of infected foals, diarrhea may persist for several weeks to months.

Clinical diagnosis is made on the basis of presenting signs, physical findings, and clinicopathological alterations, although these are nonspecific. Isolation of a *Salmonella* spp. through culture of feces, blood, or intestinal tissue is required to confirm the diagnosis. Isolation of the organism from rectal mucosal biopsy is possible, but the sample may be difficult to obtain due to the size of the foal. As fecal shedding may be intermittent, at least five fecal cultures are required. Fecal samples taken before diarrhea develops or as stool returns to a formed consistency appear to have a higher yield of positive cultures. Approximately 5–10 gm of feces is superior to rectal swabs for culture of the organism. Isolation of the organism is facilitated by use of selective media for *Salmonella* spp., for example selenite F enrichment broth. The presence of fecal leukocytes correlates with disruption of the distal intestinal mucosa and supports a diagnosis of bacterial enteritis.

Sepsis scoring (see p. 413) in foals less than 10 days old and blood cultures should be performed as bacteremia frequently accompanies enteritis in neonates. In foals with abdominal distention, radiography and ultrasonography (see p. 420) may help differentiate between dynamic ileus secondary to enteritis and obstructive disease.

Although *Escherichia coli* is a common isolate from the blood of septicemic foals, enteritis and diarrhea due to enterotoxigenic *E. coli* is uncommon in the horse. Enterotoxins and pili associated with enteropathogenic strains of *E. coli* affecting calves and piglets have been isolated from the feces of foals with diarrhea. Although K88 receptor sites have been identified in foal epithelium, challenge with *E. coli* K88 does not produce diarrhea without concurrent viral infection. Thus, it is unlikely that enterotoxigenic *E. coli* is a major primary cause of enteritis in foals.

Enterotoxigenic *Bacteroides fragilis* has been isolated from young foals with naturally occurring diarrhea. Affected foals range from 2 to 60 days of age, but the majority are less than 7 days old. Clinical signs include depression, lethargy, colic, and diarrhea ranging from acute hemorrhagic or watery to chronic. Affected foals are often concurrently positive for rotavirus. Foals respond well to intense supportive care.

Rhodococcus equi infection occasionally causes diarrhea in foals 1 to 4 months of age. Diagnosis is based on elimination of other causes of diarrhea and is facilitated if the foal also has *Rhodococcus equi* pneumonia. Isolation of the organism from the feces is not diagnostic as it is a normal inhabitant of the equine intestinal tract. Characteristic lesions include ulceration of lymphoid aggregates in the wall of the large colon.

Campylobacter jejuni has been isolated from the feces of healthy and diarrheic foals. The overall significance of *Campylobacter* spp. as an enteric pathogen in the horse has not been determined. Other bacteria sporadically implicated in foal diarrhea include *Actinobacillus, Klebsiella, Streptococcus durans,* and *Yersinia.*

Parasite-Related Diarrheas

The true incidence of diarrhea in foals associated with *Strongyloides westeri* infestation is unknown. Foals commonly become infected by ingestion of milk containing larvae and less frequently by larvae penetrating the skin. The prepatent period is 8 to 14 days. Mild enteritis may develop in infected foals. The correlation between fecal egg count and the incidence of diarrhea is poor; thus, foals with high egg counts may be asymptomatic. Experimental infection of foals with large numbers of larvae has caused severe diarrhea, fever, and death. Patent infections can be diagnosed through fecal flotation with salt or sugar solutions. The typical embryonated eggs are approximately one-half the size of a *Strongylus* egg.

Anthelmintic treatment of the dam shortly after foaling helps to decrease the incidence of *Strongyloides westeri* infections in foals. Anthelmintics reportedly effective include ivermectin,[*] 200 μg per kg; thiabendazole,[†] 44 to 50 mg per kg; oxibendazole,[‡] 10 mg per kg; and cambendazole,[§] 20 mg per kg.

Young foals may develop diarrhea, fever, and abdominal discomfort in association with *Strongylus vulgaris* infestation when exposed to an overwhelming larval challenge. These signs may be observed after experimental challenge of foals or in foals housed in a heavily contaminated environment. Clinical signs may be observed during the prepatent period of infection as the larvae migrate through the arteries supplying the intestine 14 to 20 days after infection. Fecal examination does not reflect the degree of parasite infestation, owing to the long prepatent period (6 months). Strongyle eggs observed in the feces

---

[*]Ivomec, MSD AGVET, Rahwey, NJ
[†]Equizole, MSD AGVET, Rahwey, NJ
[‡]Anthelcide, Norden Labs, Lincoln, NE
[§]Camvet, MSD AGVET, Rahway, NJ

of foals less than 6 months of age most commonly are a result of coprophagy and do not represent a patent intestinal infection.

Cryptosporidium is an important cause of enterocolitis in many species and has been identified in the feces of immunodeficient and immunocompetent foals with diarrhea. Transmission is by the fecal–oral route. The incubation period appears to be 3 to 7 days with diarrhea usually evident for 5 to 16 days in most species. The organism completes its life cycle intracellularly but extracytoplasmically at the apical border of intestinal epithelial cells. Intestinal lesions associated with cryptosporidial infection in foals include villous blunting, fusion and atrophy with cryptitis and hypercellularity of the lamina propria. Due to loss of absorptive surface, weakness, malabsorption, and diarrhea are observed in affected foals. Severe dehydration and electrolyte and acid–base imbalances may develop in some foals, whereas in others the infection appears to be self-limiting.

Investigations of the association between diarrhea and shedding of oocytes in the feces of foals have given various results. Of 82 foals studied, 16 per cent shed *Cryptosporidium* oocytes but diarrhea did not appear to be associated with the period of oocyst shedding. In other studies, pony foals removed from their dams at 25 hours of age and raised in a helminth-free environment shed oocytes in their feces from 2 to 18 days. The appearance of oocytes in these foals corresponded with episodes of diarrhea. Thus, the true relationship between cryptosporidial infection and intestinal disease in the foal is not fully understood.

Detection of *Cryptosporidium* by fecal examination may not be easy. On direct fecal smear the oocytes stained with a dimethyl sulfoxide modified acid-fast stain appear bright pink. The use of auramine-O-fluorochrome dye on direct fecal smears has also proved effective, but fluorescent microscopy is needed to identify the organism. Fresh postmortem intestinal tissue samples may be routinely fixed and stained for identification of the organism.

Management of foals with cryptosporidiosis is supportive as there is no proven effective treatment. The primary goal is to prevent spread of the infection. Isolation techniques and good sanitation are paramount. *Cryptosporidium* is resistant to most disinfectants, but formalin (10 per cent), ammonia (5 per cent), and sodium hypochlorite have been shown to have some efficacy against the oocytes.

Although *Eimeria leuckarti* is found in the feces of foals 1 to 4 months of age, the significance of this agent in causing intestinal disease is unknown. To date this protozoon has not been linked to diarrheal disease.

Management of Foals with Enteritis/Diarrhea

Foals with acute enteritis and diarrhea usually present with dehydration, electrolyte imbalances, and metabolic acidosis. Hyponatremia and hypochloremia are common. Potassium status is variable, depending on the degree of metabolic acidosis and renal compromise. The majority of foals are hypokalemic and are often hypoglycemic. These abnormalities are relatively consistent regardless of the underlying cause and vary more in severity than character. Endotoxemia or septicemia, indicated by leukopenia, left shift, toxic neutrophils, and lymphopenia, is commonly seen in foals with acute bacterial enteritis or severe viral enteritis.

Initial therapy is aimed at restoring circulating volume and correcting electrolyte and metabolic imbalances. Unless the metabolic acidosis is severe, IV administration of a balanced polyionic electrolyte solution such as acetated Ringer's solution or lactated Ringer's solution is adequate. If the foal is moderately to severely acidotic and hyponatremic, isotonic sodium bicarbonate (1.3 per cent; 12.5 gm of sodium bicarbonate per liter of distilled water) may be required. Rapid administration of a hypertonic solution with a high sodium content to a foal with a significantly subnormal serum sodium level may induce acute neurological signs and cerebral hemorrhage. Potassium, not in excess of 3 to 5 mEq per kg per day or 0.5 mEq per kg per hour, may be added to the fluids if the foal is hypokalemic. Dextrose, 1 to 2.5 per cent, will help move potassium into the cell and will provide some energy source, though not meet the foal's caloric needs. For foals with a low glucose level and unknown electrolyte and acid-base status, a 2.5 per cent dextrose and 0.45 per cent saline solution has been recommended. In less severely affected foals, use of oral electrolyte solutions, as discussed under viral diarrheas, may be adequate.

Caloric intake must be maintained either through nursing, supplemental feeding with a bottle or nasogastric tube, or parenteral alimentation. Normally, nursing foals ingest 10 to 11 liters (20 to 25 per cent of body weight) of mare's milk each day. The foal's body weight should be monitored daily to assess the adequacy of daily feed intake.

If clostridial enteritis is suspected, milk feedings should be withheld. Hydration status, electrolyte concentrations, and plasma glucose levels may be maintained by administration of oral or parenteral fluid, or both. Glucose and electrolyte solutions provide 25 per cent or less of the foal's caloric needs, and therefore should not be used as a means of total support for more than 24 hours. Caloric needs may be met by parenteral alimentation with glucose, lipids, and amino acids. Parenteral alimentation requires placement of a jugular catheter extending into the central vein, strict adherence to feeding protocol, and careful monitoring of the foal's blood glucose levels, hydration status, and electrolyte and acid–base balance (see p. 747).

Intestinal protectants often exert a beneficial effect in foals with diarrhea, especially when the foal is otherwise clinically normal. Preparations containing bismuth subsalicylate seem superior to those containing kaolin, pectin, or activated charcoal. Bismuth subsalicylate° neutralizes bacterial toxins, has some antibacterial activity, and may exert an antisecretory effect by its antiprostaglandin action. It can be administered at a dosage of 4 to 6 ounces every 6 to 8 hours and results in darkened feces. If the intestinal protectant does not exert a beneficial effect within 48 hours, continued administration is not warranted. Caution must be used when administering antidiarrheal agents to foals with clinical or clinicopathological evidence of toxemia. Delay or cessation of fecal passage in toxemic animals may lead to increased time for absorption of endotoxin and other toxins from the gut. In some toxic animals, a rapid deterioration in clinical status may be noted after administration of intestinal protectorants and other antidiarrheal agents.

Hypoproteinemia is common in infections caused by invasive organisms such as *Salmonella*. This may be especially obvious in foals with inadequate or marginal passive transfer of colostral antibodies. When plasma protein content decreases to less than 4 or 4.5 gm per dl, administration of 1 to 3 liters of plasma may have a beneficial effect on the foal. Alternatively, administration of *Salmonella typhimurium* antiserum† to hypoproteinemic, endotoxemic foals will not only help to restore normal protein levels, but will also increase IgG levels and help to neutralize circulating endotoxin.

Broad-spectrum antimicrobial therapy with penicillin and an aminoglycoside or penicillin and trimethoprim–sulfa drugs is indicated in foals with suspected primary or secondary bacterial enteritis or bacteremia. Parenteral antimicrobials are preferred as oral agents may potentiate or induce diarrhea. Blood cultures should be obtained before initiation of antimicrobial therapy. If clostridial enteritis is suspected, IV administration of potassium penicillin at recommended (22,000 IU per kg IV four times a day) or higher doses is indicated. When enteritis due to *Bacteroides fragilis* is suspected, metronidazole (15 to 20 mg per kg PO or IV four times a day) should be added to the treatment regimen.

Nonsteriodal anti-inflammatory agents have been advocated for use in enteritis due to their anti-inflammatory, analgesic, and possibly antisecretory effects. These agents must be used cautiously in ill and especially dehydrated foals, because they can cause gastric ulcers and be nephrotoxic. Reduced doses of flunixin meglumine (0.25 mg per kg IV two or three times a day) may be of benefit in endotoxemic foals. Concurrent therapy with agents that prevent ulcers (see p. 184) may be advisable for foals receiving NSAIDs.

NECROTIZING ENTEROCOLITIS

Necrotizing enterocolitis is an acquired GI disorder characterized by abdominal distention and pain, gastric reflux, passage of bloody stool, ileus, and generalized sepsis. Although commonly seen in human premature infants, the condition has infrequently been reported in compromised equine neonates. Passage of bloody stool has not been a consistent feature of the disease in the foal.

The etiology of the disease is multifactoral. Three factors important to the development of necrotizing enterocolitis have been recognized: (1) ischemic/hypoxic insult to the bowel associated with placental insufficiency or premature separation, dystocia, cardiopulmonary disease, or shock and hypotension; (2) bacterial colonization of damaged bowel wall; and (3) availability of substrate for the bacteria to metabolize. Bacteria commonly isolated from infants with necrotizing enterocolitis include *E. coli* and *Klebsiella* spp. These bacteria colonize the intestinal wall and produce gas but not extensive mucosal damage. Clinical signs characteristically become evident after initiation of enteral feeding. Bowel perforation is common and usually occurs within 24 to 48 hours following onset of clinical signs.

Diagnosis in foals with a compatible clinical history and signs is made on the basis of radiographic findings. Demonstration of air within the bowel wall, pneumatosis intestinalis, is the pathognomonic sign. The intramural air may present as radiolucent localized cystic collections, diffuse linear strips, or ring-shaped areas. Gas-

---

°Pepto-Bismol, Procter & Gamble, Cincinnati, OH
†Endoserum, Immvac, Columbia, MO

eous bowel distention is also observed. Free air in the abdomen may be observed if bowel perforation has occurred.

Once necrotizing enterocolitis has been diagnosed, enteral feedings are withheld until radiographic signs resolve. Nutritional requirements must be met during this time by parenteral alimentation. Broad-spectrum antimicrobial therapy is initiated. Supportive care and close monitoring of the neonate for signs of intestinal perforation are essential. Surgical intervention is required if bowel perforation occurs.

PERITONITIS

Peritonitis in the neonate may develop secondary to uroperitoneum, systemic bacterial infection, invasive bacterial enteritis, ruptured gastric ulcer or bowel, rupture of or leakage from an umbilical abscess, bowel compromise with an acute intestinal accident, or parasite migration. Reported causes of hemoperitoneum in the foal include rupture of the umbilical vessels, splenic or liver laceration, mesenteric aneurysm or hematoma, and rupture of a juvenile granulosa cell tumor.

Depression, abdominal discomfort and distention, dehydration, signs of toxemia, and fever may be observed. Respiratory effort may be compromised if the peritoneal effusion is severe enough to cause pressure against the diaphragm, transmigration of fluid into the pleural cavity, or hypoproteinemia. The former two events may mechanically interfere with respiration, while the latter may predispose the foal to pulmonary edema. The presence of peritoneal effusion is confirmed by abdominocentesis, abdominal radiography, or ultrasound evaluation. Analysis of the fluid sample may help to determine the primary disease process. Evaluation of peripheral blood and peritoneal fluid electrolyte and creatinine concentrations will help confirm the presence of uroperitoneum (see *Current Therapy in Equine Medicine 2*, p. 722). Alteration in the peripheral blood cell count may reflect the presence of primary septicemia or toxemia secondary to the underlying cause. Ultrasound examination may be used to assess the size and integrity of the umbilical vessels and the presence of an urachal abscess (see p. 418). Abdominal radiography may reveal bowel distention or displacement consistent with an intestinal accident requiring surgical intervention.

Management of peritonitis includes stabilizing the foal, treatment of the underlying disease process, broad-spectrum antimicrobial therapy, relief of abdominal distention and interference with breathing, and supportive therapy (see discussion of peritonitis, p. 236).

Supplemental Readings

Austin, S. M., DiPietro, J. A., and Foreman, J. H.: *Cryptosporidium* spp.: A cause of diarrhea in immunocompetent foals. Equine Pract., *12*:10–14, 1990.
Geor, R. J., and Papich, M. G.: Medical therapy for gastrointestinal ulceration in foals. Compend. Cont. Educ. Pract. Vet. *12*:403–412, 1990.
Higgins, W. P., Gillespie, J. H., and Schiff, E. I.: Equine rotavirus: Three epizootics. Equine Pract., *12*:15–18, 1990.
White, S. L.: Diagnosis and management of foal colic. *In* Gordon, B.J., and Allen, D. (eds.): Colic Management in the Horse, 1st ed. Lenexa, KS, Veterinary Medicine Publishing Co., 1988, pp. 177–188.
Wilson, J. H., and Cudd, T. A.: Common gastrointestinal diseases. *In* Koterba, A. M., Drummond, W. H., Kosch, P.C. (eds.): Equine Clinical Neonatology, 1st ed. Philadelphia, Lea & Febiger, 1990, pp. 412–430.

Septic Arthritis and Osteomyelitis

Pamela C. Wagner, CORVALLIS, OREGON
Barbara J. Watrous, CORVALLIS, OREGON
Benjamin J. Darien, CORVALLIS, OREGON

Septic arthritis or osteomyelitis in a foal less than 2 months old is most often of hematogenous origin. Frequently the orthopedic manifestation is secondary to an infection of the respiratory or gastrointestinal (GI) tract or umbilicus. Blood-borne bacteria may colonize the synovium or developing ossification centers while the primary infection goes undetected. Early signs of septic arthritis may be nonspecific and often the owner suspects a traumatic incident because of the rapidity of onset. Delays in diagnosis and treatment may preclude obtaining the best results in this syndrome.

Trauma, with introduction of infection by direct penetration of the joint or physis, is also a frequent cause of septic arthritis or osteomyelitis. Early diagnosis is often easier in these cases because of the obvious wound. Although the pathogenesis of traumatic and septic arthritis differ, treatments are similar.

In 1983, Firth introduced the classification of septic arthritis and osteomyelitis of hematogenous origin that forms the basis of the current classification. Prior to that time, "joint ill" was used to refer to cases of infectious arthritis, with or without osteomyelitis, and to septic physitis or metaphysitis. Five types, based on location, clinical signs, prognosis and treatment, seem appropriate (Fig. 1).

S TYPE

This type, infectious synovitis, affects the neonatal foal by the first 10 days of age. Often the foal is systemically ill and multiple joints are affected. There are few, if any, radiographic changes; however, soft tissue swelling around the affected joint(s) is identified (Fig. 2). The effusion contains a high number of white blood cells, most of which are neutrophils. The most common organisms isolated are *E. coli*, *Klebsiella* spp., β-haemolytic streptococcus, *Salmonella* spp., and *Actinobacillus equuli*. Although the foal shows signs of synovitis without macroscopic evidence of osteomyelitis, at necropsy the cartilage is often affected.

E TYPE

Foals with this type of septic arthritis (joint and adjacent epiphysis) are somewhat older (usually several weeks of age) than foals with the S type. Multiple joints can be affected and lameness often develops following the appearance of

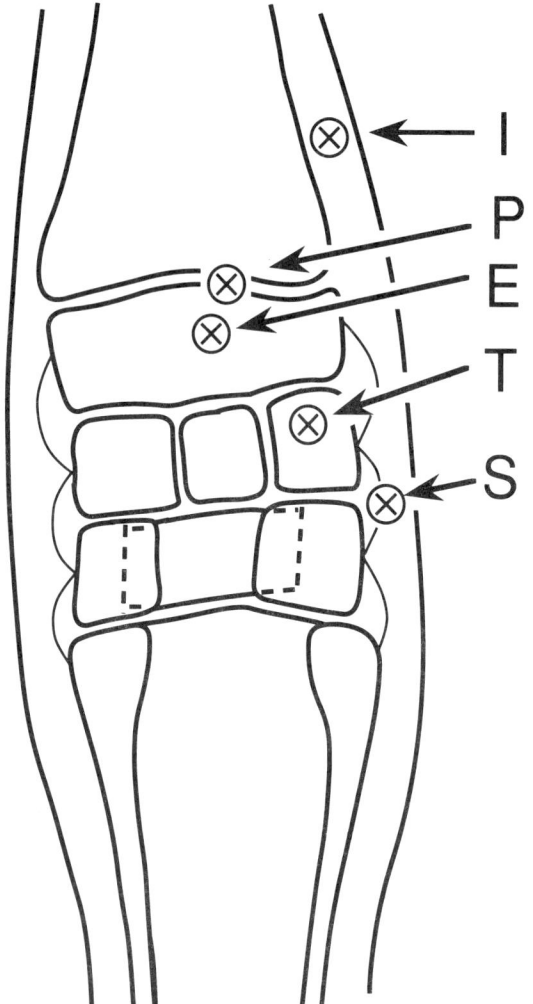

Figure 1. The five types of septic arthritis and osteomyelitis, based on location of lesion, clinical signs, prognosis, and treatments. I, invasive type; P, physeal type; E, epiphyseal type; T, tarsal type; S, synovial type.

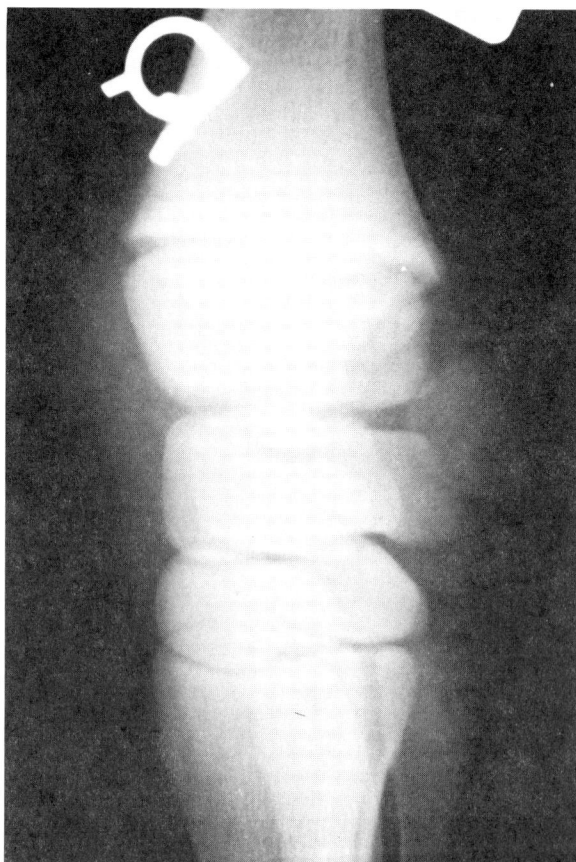

Figure 2. Soft tissue swelling localized to the radiocarpal joint without osseous involvement is characteristic of S type synovitis.

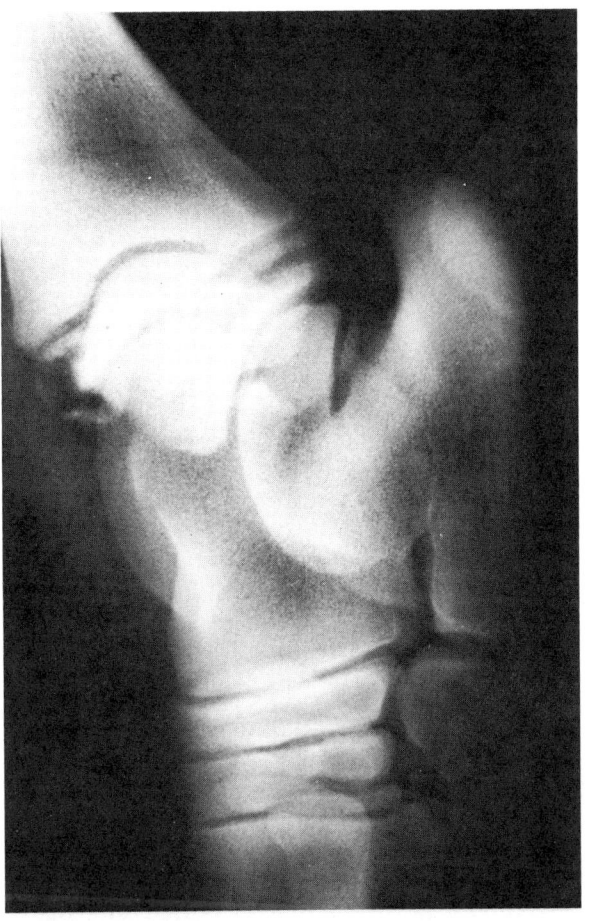

Figure 3. Joint distention is associated with focal bone lysis of the distal tibial epiphysis, in this case representing E type septic arthritis and synovitis.

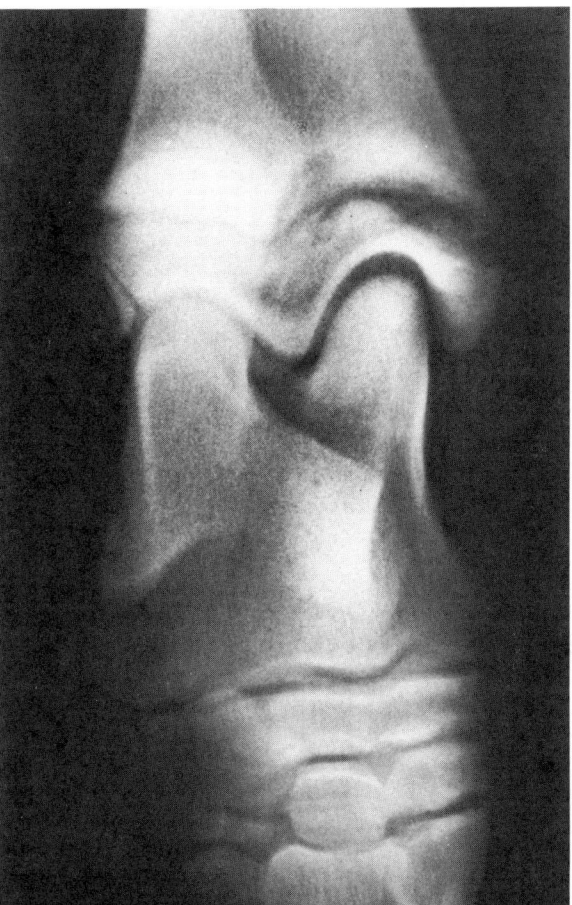

Figure 4. Hematogenous infection of the distal tibial physis with adjacent bone lysis of the metaphysis and epiphysis as the infection spreads proximally and distally from the growth plate.

other systemic diseases. Differentiation of E and S types is based on radiographic evidence of osteomyelitis of the epiphysis (Fig. 3). Purulent involvement of the synovial membrane may arise either as a primary hematogenous infection of the epiphysis with secondary synovitis or as an extension of joint sepsis to the adjacent epiphysis. The most common organisms identified are *E. coli*, β-haemolytic streptococcus, and *Salmonella*.

P TYPE

The age of foals with this physeal type of hematogenous infection has been reported to be 9 days to 4 months. An affected foal is often healthy, and characteristically only one limb is affected. The lesion is at first confined to the physis and metaphysis or the epiphysis and there is very little effusion. Persistence of the lesion in close proximity to a joint may result in a sterile synovitis or "sympathetic effusion" in that articulation. P type lesions are identified radiographically in the metaphysis, physis, or epiphysis (Fig. 4). They may result in pathological fracture or may extend into the joint, causing a secondary septic synovitis. The most common organisms identified are β-haemolytic streptococcus, *Salmonella* spp., and *Rhodococcus equi*.

T TYPE

Recently, osteomyelitis of the small tarsal or carpal bones has been called the T type (Fig. 5). Involvement of flat bones (ribs, pelvis, etc.) and nonarticular traction apophyses also occur. Infection in the small tarsal bones is most frequently encountered and may lead to collapse of the central or third tarsal bone. The common organisms encountered are *E. coli* and *Salmonella* spp. In most cases multiple joints are involved.

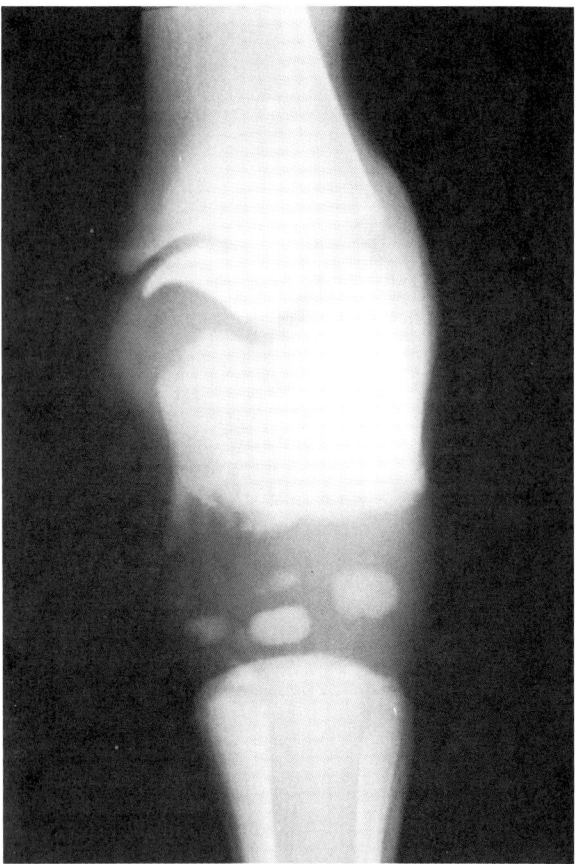

Figure 5. Osteomyelitis of the cuboidal bones (T type osteomyelitis) resulting in dissolution of numerous tarsal bones.

I TYPE

Invasion into a physis or joint from a periarticular soft tissue abscess is referred to as the I type. It is most commonly encountered adjacent to the hip and shoulder. Clinical signs of lameness occur prior to the joint invasion. Large soft tissue masses may be identified radiographically (Fig. 6A) or ultrasonographically. If the abscess is diagnosed and treated aggressively, septic arthritis (Fig. 6B) may be avoided.

PATHOGENESIS

Susceptibility of a foal to infections of the joints is dictated by host factors such as failure of passive transfer, stress in the perinatal period, and immaturity at birth. External factors that may increase susceptibility include the cleanliness of the perinatal environment, climatic conditions, attention to care of the umbilical stump, onset of standing and suckling, and the health of the dam.

Septicemia in foals is the primary predisposing factor to the development of septic arthritis/osteomyelitis (synovial membrane and/or periarticular bone) syndrome. Twenty-five per cent of cases of septic arthritis examined at necropsy have evidence of vasculitis of the umbilical arteries (arteritis) or vein (phlebitis).

The pathogenesis of S and E type arthritis is a septicemia that results in colonization of bacteria in the synovial membrane or epiphyseal bone, respectively. The vascular supplies to the synovium and the epiphysis are extensive yet arise from common vessels: the metaphyseal arteriole loops and epiphyseal arteries. The metaphyseal vascular loops juxtapose the epiphysis via transphyseal vessels while the periarticular arterioles give rise to a capillary network that supplies the joint capsule and synovial membrane. The slowing of blood through the transphyseal vessels and capillary network permits transmural migration of bacteria and colonization of the epiphysis and synovial membrane, respectively.

Growth of bacteria within the synovium causes periarticular synovitis and capillary thrombosis, which results in synovial cell ischemia and death. As the synoviocyte's ability to dialyze plasma and produce hyaluronic acid decreases, the resultant synovial fluid becomes copious, acidic, higher in leukocyte number and proteolytic enzymes, and lower in substrates necessary for cartilage nutrition. Cartilage degradation is a sequel to reduced nutrition and increased enzymatic destruction, while cartilage degradation products induce the release of mediators that augment the synovitis.

In some cases of E or T type arthritis, it is sometimes difficult to determine if the synovial effusion is infectious or inflammatory. If the bone infection has not entered the joint, the prognosis for recovery is better. A reactive synovitis may be present, i.e., there are no bacteria within the joint but the inflammatory reaction is present. Treatment aimed at reducing the inflammation and stopping cartilaginous damage is the same as if there were bacteria within the synovial membrane.

In P type lesions, the bone lesion occurs before the synovium becomes involved. At presentation, the infection may still be limited to the physis and thus therapy and prognosis would be different.

In I type lesions, the articular or bone lesion is a result of the direct extension and invasion from a regional abscess. Because animals with these lesions usually are clinically lame prior to any bone involvement, foals with persistent undiagnosed lameness warrant extensive diagnostic evaluations.

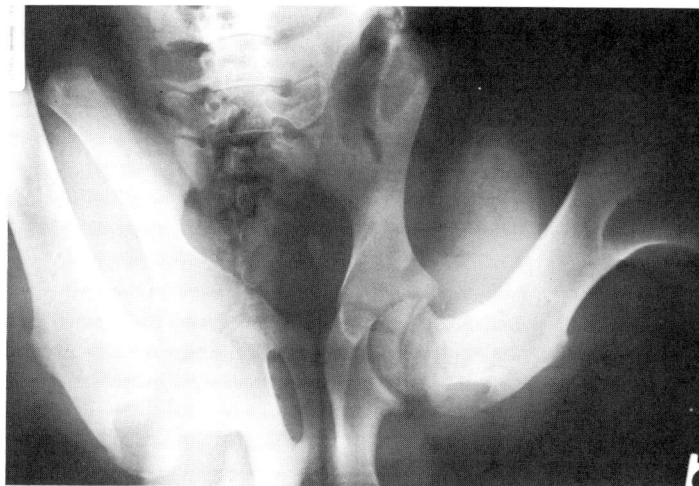
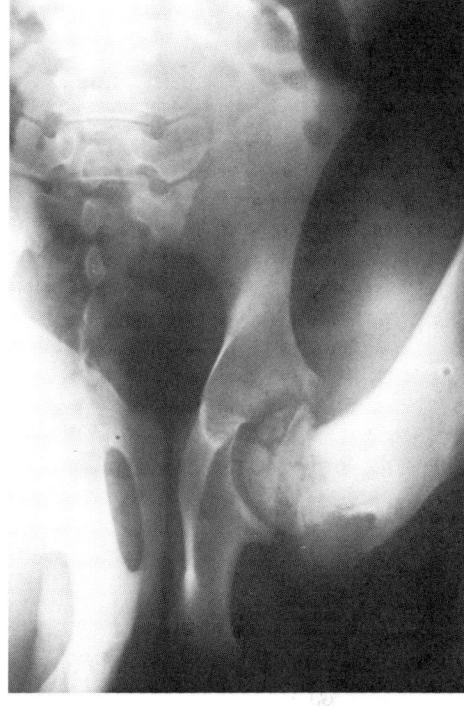

Figure 6. (A) An abscess located in the gluteal muscles can be identified radiographically by the numerous small gas bubbles associated with the focal infection. (B) Without proper treatment, diffuse invasion (I type septic arthritis and osteomyelitis) of the coxofemoral joint occurred.

RADIOGRAPHIC FINDINGS

Radiographic signs in the acute phase often lag behind the clinical signs of septic arthritis or osteomyelitis. With hematogenous septic arthritis (S type) the radiographic changes are limited to increased periarticular soft tissue swelling, but the study serves to rule out fracture as a source of acute lameness. Rarely, soft tissue gas may be identified, indicating the presence of a juxta-articular abscess. Serial radiography is often required to verify the development of bone involvement and monitor progress of treatment. The earliest anticipated changes include bone lysis (visible with optimum film quality at 3 to 5 days following initial seeding of bone by infection or infarction) and periosteal new bone formation. Sites for periosteal new bone formation include joint capsule attachments to bone (S and E types) and adjacent to cortical localization of septic emboli (P and E types). Bone lysis is initially subtle and usually unmarginated. Any location may be affected; however, careful evaluation should be directed to subchondral bone of the joint surfaces and metaphyseal and epiphyseal trabecular bone adjacent to metaphyseal growth plates. Progression occurs from patchy lysis to an enlarged, poorly or well-marginated focus. Islands of mineralized bone may be located with the lytic focus and may represent sequestra. Response to therapy with resolution of infection may leave a discrete lytic focus interpreted as a bone cyst. Large lesions may precipitate pathological fracture or collapse of joint surfaces.

Radiographic evaluation of suspect I type lesions is indicated to identify existing secondary bone invasion. Additionally, serial films help monitor bone response to therapy when involvement is recognized. Radiographic survey of multiple joints and physes may be indicated in cases of suspicion of widespread septicemia and bone localization. Alternatively, when available, bone scintigraphy may provide a sensitive diagnostic tool for early bone involvement when radiographic signs are negative.

Ultrasonography can be used to examine synovial effusions. The presence of septic debris, fibrin, and cartilage fragments may be identified as small echogenic foci suspended in the otherwise anechoic synovial fluid. Sonography may also reveal soft tissue abscesses and rule out a preexisting umbilical abscess as the nidus of infection.

Arthroscopy may be used to determine the degree of damage present prior to or at the onset of treatment. The use of the arthroscope to evaluate the damage to cartilage in S type lesions or the extension of E, T, P, or I type lesions into the joint is indicated whenever such a diagnosis may alter the decision to treat the animal.

THERAPY AND PROGNOSIS

Once diagnosed, septic arthritis and osteomyelitis must be treated immediately to ensure the best possible outcome. Although the regimen may vary with the type of septic arthritis diagnosed, the treatment goals are similar: to remove the infectious agent, to minimize cartilaginous damage due to the infectious process or the therapeutic regimen, and to minimize reactive new bone formation.

S Type

Systemic antibiotic therapy is required and is based on Gram stain results initially and culture results as they become available. Until such data are available, broad-spectrum antibiotics (Table 1) should be used promptly and continued for at least 3 weeks.

Drainage of the synovial space by aspiration may be adequate to treat early cases, but most S type infections benefit dramatically from joint distention and lavage with the foal tranquilized or anesthetized. Lavage should be copious (3 liters per joint every other day for at least three treatments). The most effective lavage solution is a pH-adjusted buffered electrolyte solution such as lactated Ringer's solution adjusted to a pH of 7.4. If possible, the fluids should be administered under pressure to allow joint distention. This enables lavage of the crevices of the joint as well as the more accessible surfaces. Large-bore ingress and egress cannuli facilitate removal of debris and adequate fluid application. Intra-articular administration of antibiotics at the end of lavage may be helpful initially in achieving high concentrations within the joint. The most commonly administered antibiotic is gentamicin (50 mg per ml), which should be buffered with sodium bicarbonate (1 mEq per ml). A near-normal pH can be achieved by adding 2 ml of sodium bicarbonate to 1 ml of gentamicin.

Intra-articular therapy with sodium hyaluronate increases the concentration of hyaluronic acid within the joint, increases synovial membrane lubrication, and decreases inflammation. Such therapy should commence after the infection has been successfully controlled. Three treatments of sodium hyaluronate at weekly intervals has been recommended.

If the condition has existed for more than a week, lavage may be inadequate to remove the debris. Surgical debridement of the joint via arthrotomy or arthroscopy may be indicated in such cases. As the incision is closed, a closed suction system may be installed to maintain constant joint decompression. Periodic lavage through the system may be considered if it can be assured that the unit remains sterile.

A combination of stall confinement during the therapy period and exercise restriction for sev-

TABLE 1. DOSAGE RECOMMENDATIONS FOR COMMON ANTIMICROBIAL DRUGS USED IN FOALS

Agent	Dose/kg	Frequency	Route
Amikacin sulfate	7.0 mg	b.i.d. or t.i.d.	IV,IM
	10.0 mg	b.i.d.	IV,IM
Ampicillin			
Sodium	11–22 mg	q.i.d.	IV,IM
Trihydrate	20 mg	t.i.d.	PO
Cephadroxil°	25 mg	q.i.d. (q. 4 h.)	IV
Cephalothin°	18 mg	q.i.d.	IV,IM
Cephapirin	20–30 mg	q.i.d.	IM
Cephoxitin°	20 mg	q.i.d. (q. 4 h.)	IV
Erythromycin			
Estolate	25 mg	t.i.d. or q.i.d.	PO
Ethylsuccinate	25 mg	t.i.d.	PO
Gentamicin sulfate	3.3 mg	b.i.d.	IV,IM
	2.2 mg	b.i.d. or t.i.d.	IV,IM
Kanamycin sulfate°	7.5 mg	b.i.d.	IV
Metronidazole°	10–15 mg	q.i.d.	PO
Penicillin G			
Procaine	22,000 U	b.i.d. or s.i.d.	IM
Sodium or potassium°	22,000—100,000 U	q.i.d.	IV,IM
Rifampin	5–10 mg	b.i.d. or s.i.d.	PO
Ticarcillin	44–50 mg	q.i.d.	IV,IM
Trimethoprim–sulfonamide	15 mg	b.i.d.	IV,PO

Modified from Koterba, A. M., Drummond, W. M., and Kosch, P. C. (eds.): Equine Clinical Neonatology. Philadelphia, Lea & Febiger, 1990.
°Dosage recommendation based on studies in adult horses.

eral weeks during the convalescent period is recommended. Physiotherapy (passive limb movement) during the confinement period may minimize fibrin adhesion formation and tendon contracture. The use of nonsteroidal anti-inflammatories should be judicious, recalling that gastric ulceration in such patients is the rule rather than the exception.

If it is suspected that failure of passive transfer is the cause of the spread of bacterial infection to joints, plasma transfer should be considered. If the umbilical stalk appears to be enlarged, infected, or inflamed on clinical examination or ultrasonography, the umbilicus should be surgically removed.

E Type or T Type

When the bone of the epiphysis or cuboidal bones of the tarsus or carpus is involved, the prognosis is more guarded. In some cases, the infection has started in the epiphysis but has not entered the joint via the articular cartilage. Visualization of the joint via arthroscopy or analysis of synovial fluid for sepsis, as in cases of tarsal or carpal osteomyelitis, is helpful in determining if the cartilage is still intact. In these cases, surgical curettage is of debatable value. In cases where there is improvement with lavage and antibiotics, the surgeon should resist the temptation to open the joint and curette the lesion. Long-term therapy with antibiotics has been successful in resolving the infection in the bone. The accompanying synovitis should be treated as described under S type lesions.

With tarsal or carpal infection (osteomyelitis and synovitis) joint lavage is less successful due to the complexity and size of the joint cavities. Cuboidal bone collapse may be a sequel to bone lysis.

P Type

This type of osteomyelitis has a somewhat better prognosis than the E type due to its location distant from the joint surface. Severe lesions in the physis, however, may cause premature closure with possible angular deformities even if the lesions resolve with antibiotic therapy and

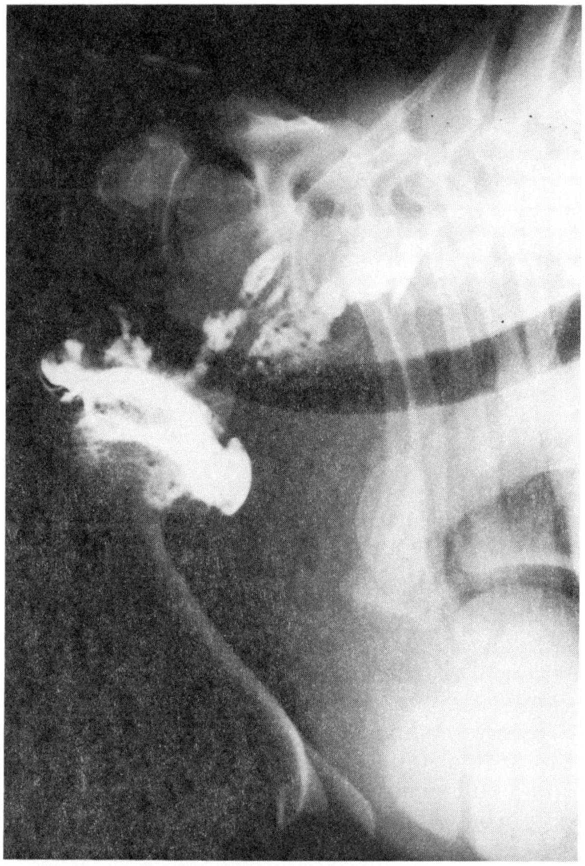

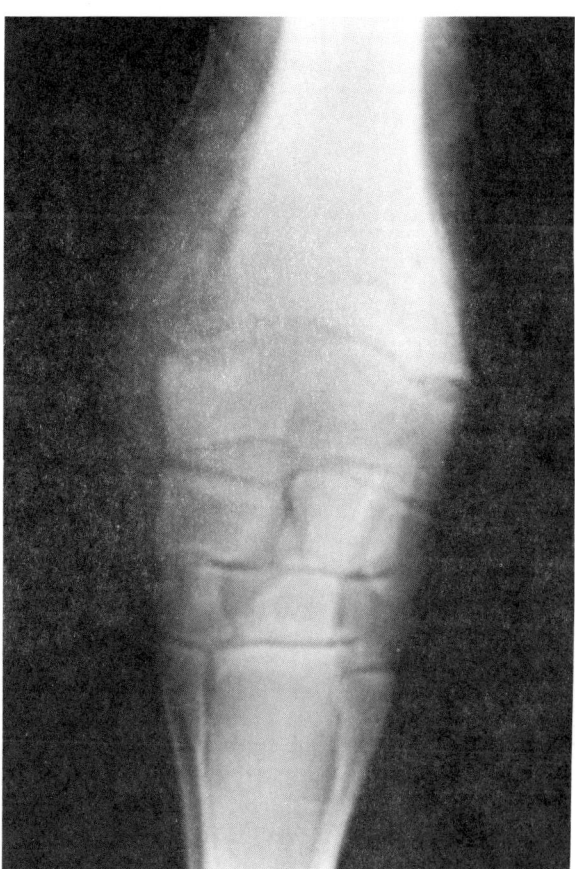

Figure 7. Contrast arthrography demonstrating communication between the septic periarticular soft tissue and shoulder joint, indicating loss of integrity of the joint capsule and septic arthritis.

Figure 8. A soft tissue wound resulted in underlying osteomyelitis and septic physitis in this foal. Early surgical debridement usually results in a good outcome.

curettage. Metaphyseal lesions can be drilled and curetted with favorable results in most cases. Usually the adjacent joint is not infected, although it may have an inflammatory, nonseptic synovitis that should be treated with lavage and intra-articular sodium hyaluronate as described for S type.

I TYPE

Large soft tissue masses located near joints in foals should be suspected of being abscesses. Diagnosis is confirmed via peripheral blood evaluation, physical examination, ultrasonography, and percutaneous aspiration. Contrast arthrography of the joint may be helpful in determining if invasion of the joint has already occurred, indicating a poorer prognosis (Fig. 7). If invasion has not occurred, drainage of the abscess, isolation of the organism, and appropriate antibiotic therapy are indicated.

In instances where an abscess or traumatically introduced infection has caused infection of the metaphysis or physis (Fig. 8), early debridement of soft tissue and curettage of the infected bone is indicated.

Supplemental Reading

Adams, R.: Polyarthritis and osteomyelitis. In Koterba, A. M., Drummond, W. H., and Kosch, P. C. (eds.): Equine Clinical Neonatology. Philadelphia, Lea & Febiger, 1990, pp. 317–330.

Baird, A. N., Taylor, J. R., and Watkins, J. P.: Debridement of septic physeal lesions in 3 foals. Cornell Vet., 80:85–95, 1990.

Carter, G. K., and Martens, R. J.: Septicemia in the neonatal foal. Compend. Cont. Educ. Pract. Vet., 8:S256–S270, 1986.

Hanie, E. A.: Antibiotic therapy for infections of skeletal and synovial structures: Part II. Equine Pract., 11:7–14, 1989.

Martens, R. I., Auer, J. A., and Carter, G. K. Equine pediatrics: Septic arthritis and osteomyelitis. J. Am. Vet. Med. Assoc., 188:582–585, 1986.

Risk Factors Associated with Developmental Orthopedic Disease

M. Amy Williams, AUBURN, ALABAMA

Diseases of bone and cartilage are of primary interest to those responsible for the management and feeding of brood mares and foals. New knowledge has accumulated over the past decade about a group of debilitating bone diseases that commonly occur in young, healthy, rapidly growing horses. These conditions, originally referred to as metabolic bone disease, have recently been renamed developmental orthopedic disease. Several investigators have reported an increasing incidence in developmental orthopedic disease, both in Europe and the United States, and have estimated as much as a tenfold increase in this disease in the past decade. Because of similarities in pathogenesis, developmental orthopedic disease presently includes osteochondrosis, subchondral bone cyst, osteochondritis dissecans, physitis, flexure deformities, angular limb deformities, and cervical vertebral malformation. None of these conditions has a single etiology; however, genetics, trauma, nutrition, and endocrine imbalances have all been suggested as contributing factors. A description of this disease complex and the proposed etiologies are presented.

OSTEOCHONDROSIS

During skeletal growth, the transition from cartilage to bone (endochondral ossification) is a highly organized process. Rapid, orderly proliferation of new cartilage cells is followed by hypertrophy, calcification, invasion of blood vessels, and new bone formation. The primary lesion of osteochondrosis occurs within this region of complex events.

In osteochondrosis, there is a disturbance of the normal differentiation of the cartilage cells and a failure of cartilage transition to bone. Calcification of the matrix does not take place, vessels from the bone marrow do not penetrate the cartilage, and endochondral ossification ceases.

Areas of thickened cartilage are often retained. Osteochondritic lesions may be small, incidental findings at necropsy or serious defects capable of producing lameness, arthritis, and pathological fractures.

Islands of retained cartilage in subchondral bone are subject to cyst formation. The medial condyle of the distal femur is the most commonly reported site. Other sites include the carpus, fetlock, pastern, and tibial condyles. Joint effusion and gait abnormalities are common with cystic lesions, though some are asymptomatic.

OSTEOCHONDRITIS DISSECANS

An alternative outcome to thickened retained cartilage is osteochondritis dissecans. Cracks and fissures form in the thickened articular cartilage and eventually extend to the joint surface. Joint pressure can lead to avulsion of a cartilage flap, which may or may not stay attached.

Osteochondritis dissecans may be manifested by lameness, which may occur before or after training begins. The femoropatellar and tibiotarsal joints are the principal sites of osteochondritis dissecans in the horse. Other sites include the scapulohumeral and humeroradial joints. Fluid distention of the joint capsule is generally marked. Lesions are commonly found bilaterally, even when lameness is unilateral. Radiographic changes may be incidental findings without clinical signs.

PHYSITIS

Osteochondrosis of the metaphyseal growth plate is generally referred to as physitis. In physitis, the transition of cartilage to bone loses its orderly longitudinal process. The addition of physical stress results in microfractures of new bone trabeculae and hemorrhage in the zone of calcification. This disturbance in growth results in bone being laid down transversely.

Radiographic evidence of physitis includes abnormal physeal widening and irregularity. Increased density and sclerosis in the metaphysis give the growth area a flared appearance. Additional enlargement may occur from periosteal proliferation on either side of the physis. Large islands of cartilage retained within the metaphysis may appear as radiolucent areas.

Clinically, physitis is manifested as physeal enlargement with or without lameness and occurs during a rapid growth phase of a physis. The most common sites include the distal radius, distal metacarpal and metatarsal bones, proximal first phalanx, and distal tibia. Clinical physitis may indicate a concurrent risk of osteochondrosis occurring at articular sites or secondary physeal complications (such as limb angulation or flexure deformities).

ACQUIRED ANGULAR LIMB DEFORMITY

Acquired limb angulation in foals may be due to delayed or defective endochondral ossification and generally occurs at the sites common to physitis.

Angular limb deformities are characterized radiographically by metaphyseal flaring and sclerosis, physeal widening and irregularity, and epiphyseal wedging and asymmetry. Hypoplasia of the cuboidal carpal and tarsal bones may also occur, especially in the immature foal.

ACQUIRED FLEXURE DEFORMITY

Acquired flexure deformities in foals are commonly associated with pain. Conditions such as painful physitis and osteochondrosis dissecans of the scapulohumeral and femoropatellar joints have been implicated. Because of this association, flexure deformities are considered a manifestation of developmental orthopedic disease. Pain in the limb may reduce weight-bearing and initiate reflex withdrawal. Shortening of the suspensory ligament and flexor tendons occurs as ground force decreases.

Acquired flexure deformities can be unilateral or bilateral and usually occur at the metacarpophalangeal, metatarsophalangeal, or distal interphalangeal joints.

CERVICAL VERTEBRAL MALFORMATION

Cervical vertebral malformation of horses is characterized by spinal cord compression and neurological dysfunction. Osteochondritic lesions have been seen in the articular surfaces as well as in the vertebral body growth plates of horses with cervical vertebral malformation. Clinical signs of cervical vertebral malformation in young horses generally appear between 6 months and 5 years of age; however, cervical vertebral lesions have been observed at necropsy in foals as early as 90 days after birth.

PROPOSED ETIOLOGIES

GENETICS

A genetic study of osteochondritis dissecans in Swedish horses reported that certain sires produced offspring with a significantly higher frequency of osteochondritis dissecans than the progeny of other stallions. The investigators concluded that developmental orthopedic disease probably has a multifactorial background, of which genetic factors constitute one part. The utilization of or requirement for nutrients may have a genetic association. Examples of genetic–nutrient interaction in various species have been presented in the literature for requirements of copper, selenium, and vitamin E. A relationship between rapid growth and occurrence of osteochondrosis has been described for various species and may be genetically linked. However, most equine studies suggest that factors other than those regulating size seemed to be involved in the pathogenesis of developmental orthopedic disease.

Trauma

Trauma may influence developmental orthopedic disease in horses. Compression of the growth plate by unbalanced weight distribution, as occurs in conformational abnormalities or unilateral lameness, is known to inhibit endochondral ossification. Results of a recent survey of Quarter Horse weanlings suggest that mechanical stress, such as working very young horses on treadmills, lunging, or ponying, might predispose to developmental orthopedic disease. On the other hand, stall confinement and lack of exercise have also been associated with increased severity of developmental orthopedic disease.

Endocrine

Many endocrine factors control the metabolism of growing cartilage. Growth hormone, insulin, and insulinlike growth factor I stimulate the production of new cartilage cells. Direct, indirect, and local actions of these hormones are important in maintaining synchrony of the growth of muscle, fat, and skeletal tissue.

The latter stages of chondrocyte maturation appear to be dependent on the thyroid hormones. Hypothyroidism in foals produces delayed appearance of ossification centers, delayed endochondral ossification, and lesions consistent with osteochondrosis.

Nutrition

Overfeeding (Energy and/or Protein)

The rate of growth in young horses is dependent on the level of energy and protein, as well as adequate amounts of minerals and vitamins. Daily levels of digestible energy (Mcal per day) and crude protein (gm per day) recommended by the National Research Council (NRC) are intended to be used as guidelines for growing horses. However, weanlings and yearlings given free access to high-quality rations generally consume quantities greater than those recommended. Such overfeeding of energy or protein is frequently suggested to cause developmental orthopedic disease.

Calcium and Phosphorus Imbalances

Calcium and phosphorus are essential macrominerals for proper bone growth and development in horses. In young, growing animals, a simple calcium deficiency results in rickets; in adults the disease is called osteomalacia. Lack of bone mineralization also occurs from deficiencies of phosphorus and vitamin D, or incorrect ratio of calcium to phosphorus. However, the lesion produced by such simple deficiencies is histologically different from the lesion of developmental orthopedic disease. Calcium and phosphorus are likely to be components of a multifactorial disease complex exerting influence on trace minerals and endocrine factors.

Copper and Zinc

The most commonly reported trace mineral deficiency to cause naturally occurring skeletal disease in young horses is copper. There are reports that erosion-like lesions involving the articular cartilage in the joints of foals were prevented by feeding supplemental copper in the ration. Similar bone disorders were reported in foals with environmental exposure through the diet to abnormally high levels of zinc and molybdenum, thereby inducing a copper deficiency. Recent field surveys and feeding trials support an association of high dietary copper concentrations with a decreased incidence of developmental orthopedic disease.

Vitamins

Bone development in growing animals in modulated by vitamin A. Green forages contain ample concentrations of vitamin A precursors; however, these concentrations decrease with maturity and storage. For this reason, the vitamin most likely found inadequate in horse rations is vitamin A. However, potential danger from inappropriate vitamin A supplementation has been suggested. Similar associations with excessive vitamin D supplementation have been observed. Although vitamin E is required in the equine diet, more research is needed to determine optimal levels for growth.

RECOMMENDATIONS

Based on the present extent of knowledge, the following recommendations are offered as a guide to reduce the risk of developmental orthopedic disease in foals.

Avoid extremely rapid growth rates. Adjustments in dietary energy and protein concentrations must be suited to each individual foal in order to account for genetic variations. Monthly measurements of height (from ground to withers) and weight (by scale or girth tape) should be recorded and compared to standard growth curves for the particular breed.

Avoid inconsistent growth rates. Growth "spurts" created by periods of undernutrition followed by periods of overnutrition are more likely to be associated with developmental orthopedic disease. Such periods may occur at weaning, following an illness, or after a transition from grass pasture to legume hay.

Assess foals weekly for proper bone formation, joint enlargement, or gait abnormality. Early identification and treatment of problems is extremely important to successful outcome.

Weigh amounts of grain and hay fed daily. Keep the ratio of grain to hay below 60:40 for weanlings and below 50:50 for yearlings. A high proportion of nonstructural dietary carbohydrate is more likely to alter insulin activity and to interfere with endocrine regulation of bone development. Divide the daily grain allotment into smaller, more frequent feedings. Separate foals from one another at feeding time in order to control the amount of grain consumed.

Determine the proper grain formulation to match the hay being fed. Obtain a reliable laboratory analysis of the hay for protein, energy, and mineral concentrations. Laboratory analysis of hay is necessary due to variations in soil and harvesting conditions. A consistent hay source must be maintained to prevent ration imbalances.

It is essential that adequate and balanced levels of macro- and microminerals be supplied in the concentrate fed. It should not be assumed that horses will consume their mineral requirements from mineralized salt blocks or loose minerals (Table 1). Avoid oversupplementation of vitamins A, D, and E.

Do not subject individuals less than 1 year old to artificial forms of exercise such as lunging, ponying, or treadmill work. These animals should be allowed to exercise freely at least 12 hours per day.

TABLE 1. ESTIMATE OF DAILY NUTRIENT REQUIREMENTS FOR WEANLING AND YEARLING HORSES WITH EXPECTED MATURE WEIGHT OF 500 KG

Nutrient	6 mo.	12 mo.
Daily dry matter intake	5.5–6.5 kg	7.5–8.5 kg
Digestible energy	16 Mcal	20 Mcal
Crude protein	800 gm	900 gm
Calcium	40 gm	40 gm
Phosphorus	30 gm	30 gm
Magnesium	5 gm	6 gm
Potassium	13 gm	18 gm
Sodium	5 gm	7 gm
Sulfur	8 gm	10 gm
Iron	350 mg	400 mg
Copper	150 mg	150 mg
Manganese	300 mg	300 mg
Zinc	300 mg	300 mg
Selenium	2.0 mg	2.0 mg
Iodine	.8 mg	.8 mg
Cobalt	.8 mg	.8 mg
Vitamin A	10,000–12,000 IU	16,000–18,000 IU
Vitamin D	5,000–6,000 IU	6,000–7,000 IU
Vitamin E	500 IU	700 IU

The daily nutrient requirements are given on an as-fed basis.

Avoid selection of bloodlines with a predisposition to developmental orthopedic disease. Give careful consideration to dietary mineral concentrations in brood mare rations, particularly during the last 3 months of gestation.

Supplemental Readings

Bridges, C. H., and Moffitt, P. G.: Influence of variable content of dietary zinc on copper metabolism of weanling foals. Am. J. Vet. Res., 51:275–280, 1990.

Glade, M. J.: The role of endocrine factors in equine developmental orthopedic disease. Proc. 33rd Ann. Conv. Am. Assoc. Equine Pract., 1987, pp. 177–189.

Hintz, H. F.: Factors which influence developmental orthopedic disease. Proc. 33rd Ann. Conv. Am. Assoc. Equine Pract., 1987, pp. 159–162.

Hintz, H. F.: Some myths about equine nutrition. Compend. Cont. Educ. Pract. Vet., 12:78–81, 1990.

Kronfeld, D. S., Meacham, T. N., and Donoghue, S.: Dietary aspects of developmental orthopedic disease in young horses. Vet. Clin. North Am. (Equine Pract.), 6:451–465, 1990.

National Academy of Sciences: Nutrient Requirements of Horses, 5th ed. Washington, D.C., National Academy of Sciences—National Research Council, 1989.

Foal Pneumonia

W. David Wilson, DAVIS, CALIFORNIA

Pneumonia in foals more than 1 month of age causes significant economic loss to the equine industry worldwide in terms of mortality, growth and performance retardation, diminished value, and the expense associated with treatment and prophylaxis. Mortality rates of 5 to 15 per cent are common, but up to 80 per cent of affected foals have died in some outbreaks, especially when *Rhodococcus equi* was the pathogen involved. Disease prevalence varies from year to year and between different geographic locations, emphasizing the importance of climatic and management factors.

ETIOLOGY

The etiology of foal pneumonia is complex and appears to involve the interaction of a number of predisposing factors with a variety of microorganisms. The overwhelming majority have bacterial pneumonia at the time of presentation, but viral agents such as equine herpesvirus 1 and 4 (EHV-1 and -4), influenza, rhinoviruses, adenoviruses, and possibly others are thought to be important predisposing factors in individual cases. These viral agents, frequently considered to cause disease restricted to the upper respiratory tract, also compromise pulmonary defenses by causing ulceration of the respiratory epithelium and impairment of pulmonary alveolar macrophage function and mucociliary clearance. Primary viral pneumonia due to influenza is recognized occasionally in young foals and can prove fatal in severe cases. Foals born with congenital EHV-1 infection frequently have severe pneumonic lesions with or without pleural effusion, a condition that has a high mortality rate. Outbreaks of EHV-1 and EHV-4 are common in suckling and weanling foals, with more severely affected foals showing pneumonic signs during the primary disease or after secondary bacterial infection. Parasite control is an important part of the overall management scheme since parasitism causes unthriftiness and increased susceptibility to infection. Ascarid larvae also cause pulmonary damage and a mild pneumonia during migration through the lung. The role of mycoplasma and chlamydia has not been fully established. Protozoa such as *Pneumocystis carinii* and various fungal agents have been isolated from pneumonia cases on rare occasions, but these are generally associated with immune deficiency states. Most fungi isolated from tracheobronchial aspirates of pneumonic foals are insignificant environmental contaminants.

Pneumonia in *neonatal* foals is usually associated with generalized sepsis and has a high mortality rate. Etiological agents are those associated with septicemia and include *Escherichia coli*, *Actinobacillus suis* spp., *Klebsiella pneumoniae*, *Actinobacillus equuli*, other gram-negative bacteria, and β-haemolytic streptococci. Clinical recognition of pneumonia in these patients is difficult, and treatment for the pneumonia is only part of the intensive care protocols necessary to save these septic foals (see p. 435).

The majority of bacterial pneumonias involve older foals and are caused by opportunistic pathogens that are normal inhabitants of the equine upper respiratory tract or the gastrointestinal (GI) tract, or are environmental contaminants. The frequency of isolation of each bacterial species varies between different geographic locations and polymicrobic infections are common. β-haemolytic streptococci, especially *S. zooepidemicus*, are the most frequent isolates in all geographic locations. *S. equi*, although a common cause of strangles in foals and young horses, is rarely isolated from the lungs of foals with pneumonia. Gram-negative nonenteric bacteria, including *Actinobacillus suis* spp., other *Actinobacillus* spp., *Pasteurella* spp., and *Bordetella bronchiseptica*, are also frequently isolated, either alone or in combination with *S. zooepidemicus* or other organisms. *Rhodococcus equi*, a gram-positive pleomorphic rod (coccobacillus), occurs sporadically but is enzootic on some breeding farms and is the most devastating cause of foal pneumonia under these circumstances. Gram-negative enteric bacteria, for example *Klebsiella pneumoniae*, *E. coli*, and *Salmonella* spp., and *Pseudomonas aeruginosa* are involved in some cases, particularly in younger foals that become infected as neonates. Other aerobic bacteria such as *Staphylococcus* spp. and anaerobic bacteria are the etiological agents in a small percentage of cases, but anaerobic species are isolated much less frequently than is the case with bacterial pneumonia in adult horses.

EPIDEMIOLOGY

The majority of pneumonia cases are seen in foals between the ages of 6 weeks and 4 months, although younger foals may be affected, particularly when predisposed by partial or complete failure of passive transfer of colostral antibodies. Pneumonia is common in foals with immune deficiency disorders, such as combined immune deficiency in Arabians, but most affected foals have no demonstrable immunological defect.

Of the interactive environmental and management factors that appear to predispose foals to the development of pneumonia, high ambient temperature, with or without high humidity, is important, especially when dry dusty conditions prevail. Dust irritates the respiratory tract and can compromise respiratory defenses as well as acting as a fomite for potential pathogens such as R. equi. Severe fluctuations in ambient temperature (hot days and cold nights) may exacerbate the problem. In colder climates, chilling and overprotection from the cold, for instance with blankets or by reducing ventilation in a barn, are also detrimental. Overcrowding stresses foals and increases the concentration and transmission of pathogens both indoors and at pasture.

Indoors, warmth and humidity promote survival of pathogens and stabilization and transmission of infective aerosols. Bedding, as well as being a potential source of dust and allergens, may act as a culture medium for certain bacteria and fungi. Poor stall drainage and sanitation, high temperatures, and poor ventilation contribute to the build-up of noxious gases such as ammonia that compromise pulmonary defense. The common practice of transporting mares and foals to other farms for breeding and the mixing of visiting mares and foals or show horses with the resident foal crop also increase the likelihood of acquiring infections.

The epidemiology of R. equi infections is not well understood, although recent work on the ecology of R. equi promises to shed considerable light on the subject. The organism is a coprophilic soil inhabitant that is resistant to many disinfectants and tolerates a wide range of soil pH and desiccation, especially in the presence of herbivore feces. The organism can survive in soil containing equine fecal material for at least 12 months. Replication increases with increasing temperature, the optimal temperature for growth being 30° C. R. equi has been isolated from the GI tract of most grazing herbivores and appears to multiply in the GI tract of foals. After passage of feces, the organism proliferates rapidly in the aerobic environment of the fecal pat.

The feces of dams and the soil environment appear to be important sources of R. equi for the colonization of the foal intestinal tract during the first few weeks of life. The coprophagic behavior of foals may be important in fecal shedding by foals, which, along with reduced moisture and increased environmental temperatures, promotes multiplication of R. equi in fecal pats. Dry, windy conditions during the summer months promote dispersion of an increased number of organisms in the air, resulting in an increased aerosol challenge dose at a time when a large number of susceptible foals are present. Preventive measures aimed at reducing or avoiding focal areas of fecal contamination are important in control to break the environmental cycle, which relies on amplification of R. equi in fecal pats. Despite the presence of a large number of horses that are shedding R. equi in their feces, many farms do not experience disease problems, suggesting that variations in virulence between different strains of the organism as well as management, environmental conditions, and other factors are important in determining disease incidence.

PATHOGENESIS

Most infections leading to foal pneumonia are acquired by inhalation of aerosolized or dustborne pathogens, but hematogenous seeding of the lung secondary to septicemia also occurs, especially in neonates. Infectious agents suspended in aerosols or on dust particles tend to be deposited on the mucosa of terminal and respiratory bronchioles. Colonization of the bronchiolar epithelium by bacteria occurs when pulmonary defense mechanisms are overwhelmed by massive challenge or are compromised by factors such as viral infection, dust, or noxious gases. The resulting inflammatory response is characterized by the influx of neutrophils and other inflammatory cells into the airways and pulmonary parenchyma. Interference with gas exchange occurs in the bronchopneumonic areas and, if severe enough, results in ventilation–perfusion mismatch, hypoxemia, and clinical manifestations of respiratory disease.

Unlike most other bacteria that cause pneumonia in foals, R. equi possesses specific characteristics that enhance its pathogenesis. The polysaccharide capsule of R. equi appears to inhibit phagocytosis and killing and further facilitates infection by helping the organism adhere to cells. R. equi is a facultative intracellular parasite that can survive and actively multiply in alveolar macrophages by inhibiting normal phagosome–lysosome fusion and perhaps by causing nonspecific degranulation of lysosomes. The organism appears to be more effectively phagocytosed and killed by neutrophils, but the presence of specific anti-R. equi opsonic antibody, and perhaps complement, appears to be important in this regard. Ingestion, phagosome–lysosome fusion, and killing in macrophages is also greatly enhanced by opsonic antibody and lymphocyte factors. Continued influx of macrophages and neutrophils leads to chronic pyogranulomatous inflammation, destruction of pulmonary parenchyma, and formation of pyogranulomatous mass lesions. This process appears to progress relatively slowly so that signs may not become apparent until several weeks after infection. Incubation periods of 2 to 3 weeks or longer have been noted in natural and experimental infections. Ingestion of large doses of the organism, either from the environment or from swallowed respiratory tract secretions, may lead to GI lesions, particularly ulcerative enterocolitis, in a small proportion of foals, but this is not thought to be a major portal of entry for respiratory tract infections. Significant pyogranulomatous lesions may develop in the hilar, mediastinal, or mesenteric lymph nodes, and secondary bacteremia occurs occasionally with serious sequelae, including septic osteomyelitis, arthritis, uveitis or panophthalmitis, or generalized infection.

Survey cultures of feces and tracheal wash samples in endemic herds indicate that the intestinal tract of the majority of foals becomes colonized with *R. equi*, and substantial numbers of foals acquire subclinical pulmonary *R. equi* infections. These exposures may serve to effectively immunize the majority of foals under these circumstances. It is thought that foals that develop pneumonia and become ill do so because they receive an overwhelming challenge at a time when passive humoral protection is waning and prior to the development of an adequate specific immune response by the foal. Serological studies using a sensitive enzyme-linked immunosorbent assay (ELISA) indicate that specific anti-*R. equi* antibodies are common in the horse population and are passively transferred to foals in the colostrum. The decline in levels of passively acquired antibody results in an "antibody trough" at 8 to 10 weeks of age, or earlier if passive transfer is suboptimal, after which levels rise to those seen in adult horses by 6 months of age.

CLINICAL SIGNS

The history and clinical presentation of foals with pneumonia vary considerably, depending on the chronicity and severity of the condition, the etiological agents involved, and environmental conditions. The spectrum ranges from an otherwise normal-appearing foal with intermittent coughing and mild mucopurulent nasal discharge to one with a high fever, profuse purulent nasal discharge, severe respiratory distress, and cyanosis. Tachypnea and altered respiratory character are typical features that are best assessed at rest during the cool part of the day, since ambient temperature, exercise, and restraint have a significant effect on respiratory rate and character. Increased intercostal effort, often characterized by asynchronous rib excursion, or rippling of the rib cage, is a subtle but frequent early sign. More severely affected foals also show nostril flaring, increased abdominal effort, or frank abdominal breathing with minimal costal excursion. These foals are exercise intolerant, have an anxious expression, and may develop signs of severe respiratory distress and cyanosis if stressed or forced to exercise.

Coughing, although not invariably present, is an important clinical sign. In early cases, coughing is generally most obvious in the morning when the foal is disturbed or restrained after lying down, or after brief exercise. The nature of the cough varies from intermittent, moist, and shallow to paroxysmal, deep, and hacking. Almost all pneumonic foals will cough when a rebreathing bag is applied, whereas normal foals rarely do so. A bilateral mucopurulent nasal discharge is a frequent finding, but some foals, especially those with *R. equi* pneumonia, have a nonproductive cough and no nasal discharge. Exudate from the lower airways may be swallowed and not appear at the nose as a nasal discharge. Fever is a common but not invariable finding. Rectal temperature in affected foals is generally in the range of 38.8° to 40.0° C (102° to 104° F), but can be in excess of 40.5° C (105° F). Demeanor and appetite are highly variable and do not necessarily reflect the severity of underlying pulmonary pathology. Some foals have a normal demeanor and appetite, others show severe depression and anorexia. Most affected foals are well grown and in good flesh, but weight loss and stunting may become apparent with chronicity.

The majority of clinical cases of *R. equi* pneumonia represent the chronic form of the disease with a smaller percentage representing a more fulminant subacute form. Even with the chronic form of the disease, respiratory signs are frequently of acute onset, reflecting the insidious progression of the disease process until sufficient lung is damaged to cause respiratory failure. In addition, the subtle early signs of disease are frequently missed or ignored by horsemen, allowing the condition to progress to a more advanced stage before veterinary help is sought.

Auscultation, both at rest and after application of a rebreathing bag, if not precluded by severe respiratory distress, is helpful in defining the presence and, to a lesser degree, the extent and nature of lung involvement when findings are interpreted in the context of other signs, such as respiratory rate and character. The lung sounds in pneumonic foals vary considerably. Mildly affected foals have increased tracheal sounds and increasing audibility and harshness of expiratory bronchovesicular sounds. Occasional inspiratory and expiratory wheezes and crackles are usually audible over involved areas, which are most often located cranioventrally. In many cases adventitious sounds are audible only when a rebreathing bag is used. In more severely affected foals, increased tracheal and bronchovesicular sounds are accompanied by fine and coarse crackles and widespread polyphonic wheezes. Lung sounds are diminished over areas of severe consolidation, extensive abscessation, or pleural effusion. Foals with a large amount of tenacious exudate in the trachea often have an audible and palpable tracheal rattle. In some cases, wheezes are audible at the nostrils, with the inciting turbulence also palpable on the chest wall. Pleuritis is a complicating condition in a small number of cases, but pleuritis secondary to pneumonia is much less common in foals than in adult horses. However, chest percussion remains a useful diagnostic procedure.

DIAGNOSIS

Important features in the history of affected foals include age; season; duration and progression of signs; response to treatment; previous cases in the herd including the agents isolated, antibiotic susceptibility, and response to treatment; other cases in the herd, herd history of viral respiratory disease and vaccination; movement of horses on and off the farm; parasite control; general herd management; and other clinical signs such as diarrhea and lymphadenopathy. In addition to examination of the respiratory system, a general physical examination should be performed, paying particular attention to hydration status, mucous membranes, umbilicus, joints, and the lymph nodes of the head and neck. *R. equi* infections may cause diarrhea, and up to 30 per cent of foals with *R. equi* pneumonia also show a chronic, active, nonseptic synovitis characterized by joint distension with minimal or absent lameness. In neonatal foals, pneumonia is frequently a manifestation of more generalized, usually gram-negative, sepsis.

Tracheobronchial aspiration with cytological examination and bacteriological culture of aspirated material is the most definitive diagnostic procedure available. In the field setting it is not always practical or desirable to obtain transtracheal aspirates from all pneumonic foals. On breeding farms where multiple cases are likely to occur, especially if *R. equi* has been a problem in previous years, a reasonable approach is to obtain tracheal aspirates in the first few cases of an outbreak to establish which organisms are involved and their antibiotic susceptibility patterns. Thereafter, aspirates should be obtained in any foal not responding to the chosen therapy, foals with atypical signs, and foals with other evidence (e.g., radiographic) of *R. equi* pneumonia. At least 3 to 5 days are necessary to assess response to initial treatment and the foal should be off antibiotics for at least 24 hours, if possible, before performing the tracheal aspiration on nonresponding foals. When an individual foal is involved, the severity of signs and the experience of the clinician will help determine the need for tracheal aspiration. The recent introduction of aspiration catheters that can be passed through the biopsy port of an endoscope has facilitated collection of appropriate diagnostic samples and provides an alternative to the transtracheal technique.

On cytological evaluation of smears of the cell pellet from tracheobronchial aspirates one should pay particular attention to cell types and numbers, their state of degeneration, and the presence, number, location (intra- or extracellular), morphology, and staining characteristics of bacteria. Accurate cytological evaluation will aid diagnosis and assist selection of initial antibacterial treatment before final culture results are available. In foals that have already been treated with antibiotics, bacteria are often seen on a direct smear but fail to grow in culture. In *R. equi* infections, false negative culture results have been noted, but in at least 50 per cent of cases, cytological examination of tracheobronchial aspirates demonstrates the characteristic pleomorphic gram-positive rods both intra- and extracellularly. Bacteriological cultures, both aerobic and anaerobic, and susceptibility testing of isolates are indicated. Because the number as well as species of bacteria may be important, quantitation of growth should be attempted.

Complete blood cell (CBC) count, including plasma protein and fibrinogen, will in most cases show evidence of a moderate to marked inflammatory response characterized by leukocytosis with neutrophilia, with or without a left shift, and an elevated fibrinogen level. However, with the possible exception of fibrinogen concentration, there does not seem to be a high degree of correlation between the severity of clinical signs and the magnitude of CBC changes. Sequential measurement of plasma fibrinogen concentration provides a useful means of monitoring response to therapy. The adequacy of colostral antibody transfer should also be determined in foals less than 1 month of age (see p. 422).

Radiography is a useful diagnostic technique, especially in more severe cases in which consolidation or abscessation is suspected or when *R. equi* is the suspected or confirmed pathogen. The procedure is also very helpful in evaluating the response to therapy. The use of rare earth screens and the air-gap technique makes it possible to take chest x-rays in smaller foals using some portable machines (Table 1). A high index of suspicion of *R. equi* pneumonia is warranted when there is a herd history of previous *R. equi* cases, when auscultation and percussion findings are compatible with anteroventral consolidation or consolidating lesions elsewhere in the lung, and when these findings are confirmed radiographically by the presence of air bronchograms in the cranioventral lung field, an increase in interstitial density, variously sized "cotton ball" or cavitary densities in the lung field, and hilar lymphadenopathy.

Other procedures that are useful in the diagnostic evaluation of pneumonic foals in selected situations include bronchovalveolar lavage, blood culture, virus isolation, serology for respiratory viruses, fecal flotation, immune function testing, thoracentesis, and ultrasonography. Culture of blood frequently yields bacterial growth in pneumonic neonatal foals, and *R. equi* may be isolated from the blood of affected foals with signs of systemic infection. A bronchodilator response test may be helpful in foals that continue to show signs of obstructive lung disease after the bacterial pneumonia has resolved.

A thorough necropsy examination, including culture and susceptibility testing of pneumonic lesions, abscesses, and exudates, should be performed on any foal that dies. In *R. Equi* pneumonia, the cranioventral portions of the lung, particularly the right lung, are affected by a consolidating bronchopneumonia. Variously sized pyogranulomas are found in these areas as well as in the caudodorsal portions of the lung. These lesions may contain inspissated material or they may drain pus when sectioned. Mediastinal lymph nodes are frequently enlarged and reactive and may show pyogranulomatous lesions. Similar lesions are present in the mesenteric lymph nodes and intestinal mucosa in a limited number of affected foals, the majority of which have intractable diarrhea for varying periods before death. Bacteremia with dissemination to joints, long bones, the eyes, and other organs, and accompanying inflammatory sequelae, are observed in a small number of cases.

THERAPY

An integrated approach to treatment is required so that, as well as destroying the causal organisms, the aim should be to improve respiratory function, minimize stress, and maximize patient comfort and environmental quality. Restricting exercise is important initially in more severe cases to reduce ventilatory demands. In milder cases and in those that are improving with treatment, limited exercise may be helpful in promoting expectoration. Confinement with the dam in a cool, clean, dust- and odor-free, well-ventilated enclosure is indicated to minimize activity and exposure to the elements. Screened doors and wall panels promote ventilation at foal level. Sprinklers can be used to control dust in paddocks and pastures, and feeders should be moved to a grassy area if possible. Barns with poorly insulated roofs can be cooled with water sprinklers on the roof on hot days. Confinement in an air-conditioned stall may be necessary for foals with marked respiratory distress.

Systemic antibacterial treatment should be based on the nature and severity of clinical signs, the results of culture and susceptibility testing of tracheobronchial aspirates, experience within the herd and locale, and the properties of the chosen drugs that determine their distribution to affected lung in therapeutic concentrations. In

TABLE 1. TECHNIQUE CHART FOR THORACIC RADIOGRAPHY OF THE FOAL WITH A MIDTHORACIC MEASUREMENT OF 24 CM

Machine Capacity	Focus–Film Distance (in.)	Air Gap	Film	Screen	mA	Time (sec)	mAs	kVp
30 mA, 100 kVp	32	Yes	Medium speed	Regular speed°	10	0.3	3.0	100
30 mA, 100 kVp	32	Yes	Medium speed	Rare earth	10	0.05	0.5	100
20 mA, 80 kVp	32	Yes	Medium speed	Rare earth	20	0.1	2.0	80
20 mA, 80 kVp	32	Yes	Medium speed	Rare earth	10	0.2	2.0	80

From Martens, R. J., et al.: Foal pneumonia: A practical approach to diagnosis and therapy. Compend. Cont. Educ. Pract. Vet., 9:S361–S373, 1982. Reproduced by permission.
°Note the prolonged exposure time when regular-speed screens are used.
Abbreviations: mA = milliampere, mAs = milliampere second, kVp = kilovolt peak.

addition, the required route and frequency of drug administration, toxicity, and relative cost of therapy are important considerations.

Because β-haemolytic *Streptococcus* spp. are the most common bacteria isolated from pneumonic foals more than 30 days of age, penicillin G is a logical choice for initial treatment in circumstances where *R. equi* has not previously been a problem. This drug also shows activity against many isolates of gram-negative nonenteric organisms such as *Actinobacillus* spp. and *Pasteurella* spp. When involvement of penicillin-resistant gram-negative organisms is suspected or confirmed, an effective antibiotic that is compatible with penicillin should be included in the regimen. Aminoglycosides such as gentamicin, amikacin, or kanamycin are logical choices, but these agents should not be used alone because of their poor activity against β-haemolytic streptococci. In addition, they are expensive and potentially nephrotoxic, especially in animals with reduced renal output secondary to dehydration. Trimethoprim–sulfonamide combinations have a broad spectrum of activity, which includes many of the causal agents of foal pneumonia, and can be administered by the oral route (15 to 30 mg of combination per kg every 12 hours). Table 2 provides further guidelines for antibiotic selection but should not be used as a substitute for susceptibility testing of individual isolates. Antibiotic treatment should be continued for 5 to 7 days after the foal is clinically normal. If the foal does not show clinical improvement within 3 to 5 days following initiation of treatment, the therapeutic regimen should be reevaluated, including a repeat tracheal wash. Chronic cases will generally respond more slowly than acute cases.

The treatment of *R. equi* pneumonia poses special problems in that the disease is frequently of insidious onset and by the time signs are noticed the condition is often chronic, with extensive bronchopneumonia and pyogranuloma (abscess) formation. *R. equi* is susceptible in vitro to a wide range of antibiotics; however, the dramatic increase in recovery rates since the introduction of oral treatment with erythromycin and rifampin makes this the therapeutic approach of choice. These lipid-soluble agents show synergistic ac-

TABLE 2. SELECTION OF INITITAL ANTIBIOTIC BASED ON ORGANISM INVOLVED AND PRACTICAL CONSIDERATIONS (COST, EASE OF ADMINISTRATION, TOXICITY)

Organism	Antibiotic of Choice	Alternate Antibiotic*
Streptococcus spp., β-haemolytic	Penicillins	TMP-sulfa or erythromycin (±rifampin)
Streptococcus spp., nonhaemolytic	Penicillin + kanamycin, penicillin + gentamicin	TMP-sulfa or erythromycin
Coagulase-positive *Staphylococcus* spp. (non-penicillinase-producing)	Penicillin	Ampicillin or TMP-sulfa or rifampin and/or erythromycin or cephalothin
Coagulase-positive *Staphylococcus* spp. (penicillinase-producing)	Cephalothin or gentamicin	Rifampin and/or erythromycin or oxacillin
Actinobacillus suis spp.	TMP-sulfa or gentamicin	Penicillin or ampicillin or tetracycline or cephalothin
Actinobacillus spp.		
Pasteurella spp.		
Bordetella bronchiseptica	Gentamicin	TMP-sulfa or kanamycin or tetracycline
Rhodococcus equi	Erythromycin and rifampin	Gentamicin and penicillin or erythromycin
Escherichia coli	Gentamicin	Amikacin† or ticarcillin or cephalothin or TMP-sulfa
Salmonella spp.	Gentamicin†	Amikacin or ticarcillin + clavulanic acid or 3rd-generation cephalosporin or TMP-sulfa
Klebsiella spp.	Gentamicin† or amikacin†	Cephalothin or 3rd-generation cephalosporin or ticarcillin + clavulanic acid
Enterobacter spp.	Gentamicin† or amikacin†	3rd-generation cephalosporin or ticarcillin + clavulanic acid
Proteus mirabilis	Penicillin	Cephalosporins
Proteus spp. (other than *P. mirabilis*)	Kanamycin or gentamicin	Ticarcillin or cephalosporin
Pseudomonas aeruginosa	Amikacin† or ticarcillin	Carbenicillin or gentamicin or ticarcillin + clavulanic acid or 3rd-generation cephalosporin
Anaerobic bacteria (other than *Bacteroides fragilis*)	Penicillin	Metronidazole or tetracycline or cephalothin
Bacteroides fragilis	Metronidazole	Penicillin or cephalothin

This table should be used only as a guideline for initial therapy and should not replace susceptibility testing.
*TMP-sulfa denotes trimethoprim–sulfonamide combination preparations. Third-generation cephalosporins include ceftizoxime, cefotaxime.
†May need to combine with a broad-spectrum penicillin (e.g., ampicillin), an antipseudomonal penicillin (e.g., tircarcillin), or cephalosporin.

tivity in vitro; both effectively penetrate cell membranes to achieve therapeutic concentrations in the lung, bronchial secretions, and within phagocytes; and both appear to be active in the environment of pyogranulomas, thus sterilizing them. Because resistance to rifampin can develop rapidly during therapy, it is not used alone to treat infections in any species. The severe consolidating pulmonary lesions that characterize *R. equi* infections necessitate early recognition and prolonged treatment for resolution. Relapses are common if treatment is prematurely discontinued. Improvement in clinical signs and WBC counts, normalization of plasma fibrinogen concentrations, and radiographic resolution of lesions are used to guide the duration of therapy, which generally ranges between 3 and 12 weeks, rarely longer. A positive clinical response within 7 days suggests a favorable prognosis. The superior efficacy of the erythromycin and rifampin combination over other regimens for treating *R. equi* contributes to a shorter duration of therapy, which to a large extent offsets the cost of this regimen. The acid-stable estolate or ethylsuccinate esters of erythromycin at a dose of 25 mg per kg PO every 6 to 8 hours, combined with rifampin at a dose rate of 3 to 5 mg per kg PO every 12 hours, are used to initiate therapy. Rifampin causes reddish discoloration of urine, and the erythromycin–rifampin combination frequently causes the fecal consistency to soften. The occurrence of the latter side effect does not necessitate discontinuing treatment, but these foals should be monitored carefully since a small but significant number will develop depression, severe diarrhea, dehydration, and electrolyte loss necessitating intensive therapy and cessation of treatment with rifampin–erythromycin. Similar side effects have been noted on occasion when rifampin is used in combination with penicillin G or trimethoprim–sulfonamide. These signs are most likely to occur between the second and fourth day of treatment but can develop at any time during treatment. In addition, idiosyncratic reactions characterized by hyperthermia, tachypnea, and increased liver enzyme levels have been seen in foals being treated with erythromycin. High doses of potentiated sulfonamide drugs (30 mg of combination per kg PO every 8 to 12 hours) have proved therapeutically effective in early, mild cases, as has the combination of gentamicin (2.2 mg per kg every 8 hours) with penicillin G administered parenterally.

Maintenance of adequate hydration is important to promote mucociliary clearance and expectoration by reducing the viscosity of tenacious bronchial secretions. This can usually be accomplished by the provision of clean water, but parenteral therapy with balanced electrolyte solutions may be indicated in some cases. Expectorants such as iodides, guaiacol, volatile oils, and sulfonamides are often beneficial by helping mobilize respiratory secretions. Mucolytics such as bromhexine hydrochloride or a newer derivative,° can also be beneficial in cases with large amounts of mucopus in the airways. The use of cough suppressants is generally contraindicated in the treatment of foal pneumonia.

Nebulization is helpful in foals with tenacious secretions or a nonproductive cough but is contraindicated in foals with voluminous moist secretions. The major functions of nebulization are to liquefy secretions, relieve bronchospasm, decrease mucosal edema, and kill bacteria. Ultrasonic nebulizers that disperse droplets less than 5 μm in diameter should be used since larger droplets are filtered out in the upper respiratory tract and do not reach the terminal airways. Nebulized agents include bland carrier solutions, bronchodilators, mucolytics, and antibiotics. The aerosol is delivered through a loose-fitting mask, such as a gallon or half-gallon plastic jug, with 30-minute exposures at 6- to 8-hour intervals. The following has been reported to be a useful nebulizing formula for foals with pneumonia caused by *R. equi* or gram-negative organisms: (1) bland solution: half-strength saline (180 ml); (2) mucolytic: acetylcysteine 20 per cent (5 to 10 ml); (3) bronchodilator: isoproterenol (2 ml) or isoetharine HCl (1 ml); and (4) antibiotic: gentamicin sulfate (150 mg) or kanamycin sulfate (400 mg). Polymyxin sulfate can also be used as the antibiotic when gram-negative organisms are involved.

Oxygen therapy is indicated in foals with severe respiratory distress. Nonsteroidal anti-inflammatory drugs (NSAIDs) such as phenylbutazone or flunixin meglumine have a euphoric effect and are useful in treating highly febrile, depressed, anorectic foals. However, they negate the value of temperature in monitoring the effectiveness of therapy. These cases should be monitored carefully and NSAIDs should be discontinued when the foal's attitude and appetite improve.

Foals judged to have widespread bronchoconstriction on the basis of clinical findings or the results of bronchodilator response tests may benefit considerably from bronchodilator therapy. Aminophylline (5 to 10 mg per kg PO every 12 hours) terbutaline (0.02 to 0.06 mg per kg PO every 12 hours) or clenbuterol (0.8 μg per kg PO

°Sputolysin, Boehringer Ingelheim, Bracknell, England.

or IV every 12 hours) have proved beneficial in selected patients, particularly those with an abnormal respiratory character (increased expiratory effort) and adventitial lung sounds after the bacterial component has been eliminated with antibiotic therapy. Culture-negative cases of this type appear to be suffering from hyperreactive small airways disease with excess mucus secretion similar to that seen in adult horses with chronic obstructive pulmonary disease. Aminophylline treatment should be short term and should be monitored carefully since clinical signs may deteriorate in some foals due to cardiotoxicity and increased ventilation–perfusion mismatch. In addition, the elimination of erythromycin, and perhaps other antibiotics, may be altered by aminophylline. If the response to environmental improvement, dust-free management, and bronchodilator treatment is poor, short-term low-dose steroid treatment, such as dexamethasone, 0.02 to 0.05 mg per kg given once daily for 4 to 7 days, may be necessary to break the inflammatory, mucus-secreting cycle and promote resolution.

PREVENTION

The cornerstone of prevention is good herd management. This involves good hygiene and sanitation, maximizing environmental quality, avoiding overcrowding, reducing dust, enforcing strict parasite control, vaccinating early to prevent viral respiratory infections, enforcing rest if viral respiratory infections do occur, maintaining fixed herd groups, separating resident horses from visiting horses, and isolating new arrivals and clinically ill horses. Foaling management is also very important, in particular the booster vaccination of mares against respiratory pathogens before foaling, ensuring adequate early colostral intake by foals, attention to the foal's umbilicus at foaling, and avoiding transportation and mixing of young foals from different sources. Adequate shade is important for horses pastured in hot sunny climates. Extreme care must also be taken when transporting foals, especially those with respiratory disease, during the summer months, since the interior of horse trailers can become extremely hot, particularly when the trailer is parked. Early diagnosis of pneumonia cases is important if treatment is to be cost-effective and successful.

Routine preventive measures outlined for the control of foal pneumonia, while helpful, have not prevented serious outbreaks of *R. equi* pneumonia on individual breeding farms. Bearing in mind the coprophilic nature of *R. equi*, the use of clean paddocks for foals, strict attention to removal of feces from the foaling and foal paddocks, and dust control are indicated to reduce the level of challenge experienced by susceptible foals. Despite the mixed results achieved by vaccinating foals or their dams (pre-foaling) with *R. equi* bacterins, recent evidence indicates that passive antibodies may be important in conferring resistance to infection. A program whereby hyperimmune plasma is administered to foals during the first month of life may reduce the incidence of *R. equi* pneumonia on problem farms. Such hyperimmune plasma is now commercially available.°

BRONCHOINTERSTITIAL PNEUMONIA IN FOALS

A rapidly progressive, high mortality syndrome characterized by the acute onset of severe respiratory distress, pyrexia, and cyanosis has been described in older foals and weanlings. Laboratory findings include neutrophilic leukocytosis, hyperfibrinogenemia, hypoxemia, hypercapnia, and respiratory acidosis. Radiographic findings are variable but include prominent interstitial patterns with mixed bronchial and alveolar patterns of varying severity throughout the lung fields. Pathological findings include severe diffuse suppurative bronchiolitis, severe interstitial pneumonia, type II cell hyperplasia, and hyaline membrane formation. The syndrome constitutes a respiratory emergency necessitating intensive therapy. Oxygen administration, corticosteroids, diuretics, anti-inflammatory agents, bronchodilators, and antibiotics have all been used with varying degrees of success. The mortality rate remains high.

Supplemental Readings

Beech, J.: Respiratory problems in foals. Compend. Cont. Educ. Pract. Vet., 8:S284–S290, 1986.

Darien, B. J., Brown, C. M., Walker, R. D., Williams, M. A., and Derksen, F. J.: A tracheoscopic technique for obtaining uncontaminated lower airway secretions for bacterial culture in the horse. Equine Vet. J., 22:170–173, 1990.

Martens, R. J., Martens, J. G., Fiske, R. A., and Hietala, S. K.: *Rhodococcus equi* foal pneumonia: Protective effects of immune plasma in experimentally infected foals. Equine Vet. J., 21:249–255, 1990.

Sweeney, C. R., Sweeney, R. W., and Divers, T. J.: *Rhodococcus equi* pneumonia in 48 foals: Response to antimicrobial therapy. Vet. Microbiol., 14:329–336, 1987.

Zertuche, J. M. L., and Hillidge, C. J.: Therapeutic considerations for *Rhodococcus equi* pneumonia in foals. Compend. Cont. Educ. Pract. Vet., 9:965–971, 1987.

°Polymune R., Veterinary Dynamics Inc., Chino, CA.

Sedation and General Anesthesia of the Foal

Sheilah A. Robertson, EAST LANSING, MICHIGAN

For purposes of anesthetic management, it is convenient to categorize foals as neonates (birth to 1 month old) or juveniles (1 to 3 months old). Anesthesia may be provided for healthy foals undergoing procedures such as correction of angular limb deformities and congenital hernias or for sick foals undergoing exploratory celiotomy or repair of a ruptured urinary bladder.

Neonatal foals are physiologically different from adult horses and from neonates of other species. Thus, scaled-down adult anesthetic techniques, or extrapolation across species boundaries, is no longer valid. In order to develop an anesthetic plan, the practitioner must have a basic knowledge of equine neonatal physiology and how this influences the action of anesthetic drugs.

PHYSIOLOGY AND PHARMACOLOGY

It is important to know normal values for the variables that are assessed prior to anesthesia, and those that are monitored intraoperatively.

A machinery murmur is normal on auscultation of foals up to the third day of life and is caused by blood flow through a still patent ductus arteriosus. Up to 40 per cent of foals have systolic murmurs until 3 months of age; these are considered innocent if they are restricted to the left heart base and do not exceed a grade II murmur, on a scale of I to V. Mean heart rate is 100 beats per minute (bpm) during the first month of life, decreasing to an average of 70 and 60 at 2 and 3 months of age, respectively.

Mean arterial blood pressure (MAP) values depend on the measurement technique employed. If indirect techniques such as ultrasonic Doppler recording or electronic sphygmomanometry are used, calculated MAP may be as low as 50 mm Hg in normal 1-day-old foals, rising to 60 to 70 mm Hg at 2 to 3 weeks of age. The MAP in 3-month-old foals is only 75 mm Hg by these techniques, and adult values are 100 to 120 mm Hg. Direct measurement of MAP via an arterial catheter reveals consistently higher values, but an increase in blood pressure with age is still apparent. Direct MAP should be between 70 and 90 mm Hg from 1 to 10 days of age, increasing to 105 mm Hg in 1-month-old foals. For consistency, blood pressure should always be measured by the same technique and with the foal in the same position. Regardless of the technique used, pony foals have a slightly lower arterial blood pressure than Thoroughbred foals. In adults, cardiac output can be improved by an increase in heart rate or stroke volume, or both. Despite echocardiographic evidence that left ventricular function is similar in foals and adults, it is believed that cardiac output is primarily rate dependent in neonates.

Normal respiratory rate is rapid at birth, 70 per min, and progressively slows with increasing age. Expected respiratory rate in a 1-week-old foal would be 40 to 50, declining toward adult values of 30 to 40 by 1 month of age.

The arterial oxygen tension (Pa_{O_2}) of foals is low by adult standards. Pa_{O_2} values range from an average of 65 mm Hg at 1 day of age to 85 mm Hg at 1 week, after which they gradually attain values of 95 to 100 mm Hg. Body position has a significant influence on Pa_{O_2} in foals, with values up to 14 mm Hg higher in standing or sternally recumbent animals than in laterally recumbent foals. Response to oxygen administration also changes with age. It is normal to see only a twofold to threefold increase in Pa_{O_2} in foals less than 3 days old breathing 100 per cent oxygen, whereas by 1 week of age, a fourfold to fivefold increase is expected. These responses are similar whether a face mask or intranasal catheter is used for oxygen administration. Oxygen consumption ($\dot{V}_{O_2}$) is 6 to 8 ml per kg per minute in the first week of life. This is two to three times greater than in adults and is likely due to the greater metabolic rate required for thermoregulation in foals. This fact is of practical importance if, as discussed later, a closed or low-flow inhalational anesthetic technique is used. Arterial partial pressure of carbon dioxide (Pa_{CO_2}) is similar in foals and adults (40 to 45 mm Hg).

The functional residual capacity (FRC), which buffers changes in inspired gases, is low in foals, and this, combined with a relatively greater blood flow to vessel-rich organs, including the brain, results in faster induction of anesthesia when inhalational agents are used.

A so-called physiological anemia of the newborn is a normal phenomenon observed in foals. Packed cell volume (PCV) at birth averages 43 per cent, falling to about 34 per cent over the first 2 weeks of life, most likely a result of intravascular hemolysis. Changes in the hematocrit over the next 12 months are minimal. Hemoglobin shows a parallel decline from a mean of 15.4 gm per dl at birth to 12.6 gm per dl at 2 weeks of age. From birth, foals have adult total plasma protein (TPP) values (60 ± 8 gm per L).

Recent studies have shown that while foal kidneys may be structurally immature, they are functionally mature, and the glomerular filtration rate (GFR) and effective renal plasma flow at 2 days of age are not significantly different from those of adults. Foals are able to handle an electrolyte load, with fractional excretion and clearance rates for sodium being similar to those of adults, and those for potassium and calcium being higher. Data from pharmacokinetic studies of renally excreted antibiotics, including amoxicillin and ampicillin, also indicate that renal function is mature at an early age in foals.

Blood urea nitrogen values of less than 2 mmol per L are normal up to 3 months of age (normal mean adult value is 3.5 mmol per L). Rapid incorporation of amino acids into proteins is thought to be the cause of the low value in foals. Because foals excrete a very dilute urine compared to other species, their fluid requirements are greater than for other neonates. Foals will drink up to 25 per cent of their body weight per day.

As a percentage of their body weight, foals have greater total body water, blood, plasma, and extracellular fluid (ECF) volumes than adults. In foals up to 2 months of age, the ECF accounts for 35 to 40 per cent of body weight, compared to 25 per cent in adult horses. Therefore, on a milliliter per kilogram basis, foals require considerable volumes of intravenous (IV) crystalloids to expand or maintain their vascular volume, and it must be remembered that only one third of administered crystalloids is retained within the vascular space.

Indirect evidence indicates that foal's livers also mature early, since the pharmacokinetics of chloramphenicol, an antibiotic that requires hepatic metabolism for its elimination, are similar in one- to nine-day-old foals and adults. The integrity of the blood–brain barrier, which limits diffusion of drugs into the central nervous system (CNS), has not been studied in foals. Clinically, foals show more rapid and profound responses to sedative agents such as diazepam° and xylazine†, and it is likely that similar to neonates of other species, their blood–brain barrier is immature.

Body fat accounts for only 2 per cent of body weight in foals compared to 5 per cent in adults. This, combined with their large surface area to body weight ratio, predisposes them to hypothermia. In addition, sedatives, tranquilizers and general anesthetics obtund hypothalamic control of thermoregulation. Shivering can increase the already high $\dot{V}o_2$ of foals by up to fourfold and could result in hypoxemia. For these reasons, it is important to maintain body temperature in foals by employing techniques that include circulating water blankets, elevated environmental temperatures, warm IV fluids, and radiant heaters. Of these, radiant heaters are best, as they both supply heat and inhibit shivering.

SEDATION OF THE FOAL

Foals may require sedation for several reasons, including radiography, bandage and cast changes, IV catheter placement, intensive care procedures, and general anesthetic premedication. Low doses of diazepam (0.05 to 0.1 mg per kg IV) will cause recumbency and sedation sufficient for radiography and minor procedures in most foals. This agent provides no analgesia, and if painful procedures are to be performed, local anesthetic techniques should also be employed. Recently, antagonists have become available for the benzodiazepine group of drugs, of which diazepam is a member. Flumazenil° is a safe antagonist, devoid of any agonist activity, and 0.5 to 2.0 mg (total) given slowly IV should antagonize the sedative effects of diazepam in foals.

There are no significant differences in the cardiopulmonary responses to high doses of IV xylazine (1.1 mg per kg) in healthy 10- and 28-day-old foals. Unlike adults given a similar dose, most foals become recumbent. Foals' heart rates fall by about 20 to 30 per cent, but the second-degree atrioventricular block so typically seen in adults does not occur in foals. A biphasic (initial increase followed by a decrease) change in blood pressure, similar to that in adult horses, occurs, but the MAP does not fall below 60 mm Hg, the value considered necessary for perfusion of vital organs. It would be prudent to avoid xylazine in hypovolemic foals, as marked hypotension may accompany the bradycardia. Respiratory rhythm is markedly disrupted after xylazine administration in foals. Frequent upper airway noise indicative of respiratory obstruction occurs for up to 20 minutes, after which time respiration becomes slow and regular. Despite this response,

---

°Valium, Roche Labs., Nutley, NJ
†Rompun, Mobay Corp., Shawnee, KS

°Anexate, Hoffman LaRoche, Basel, Switzerland

healthy foals show no changes in Pa_{O_2} or Pa_{CO_2}. Foals with respiratory disease, including those with upper airway obstructions, may not be able to compensate for these respiratory insults and should not be given xylazine.

Rectal temperature falls significantly after xylazine administration in foals but not adults. It is important to know that temperature may be depressed for more than 2 hours following administration, long after the sedative effects have abated. Rectal temperature should be monitored in all foals given xylazine, and they should not be exposed to extremes of environmental temperature.

The sedative effects of xylazine (1.1 mg per kg IV) last 60 to 90 minutes but, if this is longer than desired, lower doses or a reversal agent can be employed. Yohimbine° (0.1 mg per kg slowly IV) reverses the sedative and cardiopulmonary effects of xylazine in adult horses and should be equally effective in foals.

The actions of the potent α_2 agonist detomidine† are similar to those of xylazine in adult horses. This agent is less desirable than xylazine for sedation and analgesia of young foals, as even low doses (10 to 40 µg per kg IV) are associated with a 60 per cent incidence of arrhythmias.

If long-term sedation is required, phenobarbital‡ would be the drug of choice; 20 mg per kg diluted in saline and infused over 25 to 30 minutes is safe in healthy foals. Onset of sedation occurs within 20 minutes and lasts 8 hours, during which time foals are ataxic and sleepy but arousable.

GENERAL ANESTHESIA OF THE FOAL

Even although the focus of attention is on the foal, one must not forget about the mare. The presence of the dam at induction of anesthesia is extremely valuable and reduces the stress imposed on the foal. After the foal has lost consciousness, the mare can be housed nearby but must be sedated to prevent the agitation that is caused by separation from the foal. Xylazine (0.3 to 0.5 mg per kg IV) provides rapid onset and profound sedation. Acepromazine (0.04 mg per kg IM) given simultaneously provides several hours of sedation after the effects of xylazine wane.

Although most evidence suggests that foals can metabolize and excrete injectable anesthetic drugs from an early age, inhalational anesthesia is the technique of choice in neonatal foals. Inhalant agents provide safer, more controllable anesthetic conditions and a faster recovery.

Foals are permitted to suckle prior to anesthesia as this ensures adequate blood glucose levels, and regurgitation or vomiting is not a problem in foals. Sedation is seldom necessary, but uncooperative foals may be sedated with one of the previously described agents. Inhalational agents can be delivered via a face mask, but this practice is often complicated by gastric distention, exposure of personnel to anesthetic gases, and struggling by the foal due to the smell of the anesthetic agent. Also, mask induction does not provide a secure airway in the event of an emergency. For these reasons, nasotracheal intubation is the preferred technique. Long (55-cm), cuffed, soft, silicone rubber tubes° ranging from 7 to 11 mm internal diameter (30 to 71 French) will be suitable for the smallest to the largest of foals. Both the tube and the foal's nostril are liberally lubricated with lidocaine jelly.† The tube is then passed 1 to 2 inches along the ventral meatus, at which time the foal usually struggles a little. After a pause, an assistant should extend the foal's head and neck so that the tube can be advanced toward the nasopharynx and into the trachea. When the foal has been successfully intubated, breath sounds are clearly audible and condensation forms on the inside of the tube with each expiration (Fig. 1). If misplaced in the esophagus, the tube can often be palpated on the left side of the neck.

Once in the trachea, the tube is advanced until the nasotracheal tube connector is flush with the foal's nostril, and the cuff is inflated. After the tube has been secured with a gauze tie or tape it is connected to the anesthetic circuit. A circle system with high fresh gas inflow rates (3 to 4 liters per minute) is suitable for induction. Initially, oxygen alone is administered and then the vaporizer is turned on; it is best to start at the lowest setting and increase by 0.5 per cent increments with every three to four breaths. The foal is supported until it becomes weak, when it can be positioned appropriately. Anesthesia may be maintained via the nasotracheal tube, or the foal may be reintubated orally. Reintubation is necessary only if nasotracheal intubation was accomplished with a very small diameter tube.

Once the desired level of anesthesia has been achieved, a closed system is advisable. With this technique, only enough oxygen to meet meta-

---

°Yobine, Lloyd Labs., Shenandoah, IA
†Dormosedan, Norden Labs., Lincoln, NE
‡Phenobarbital Sodium Injection, Elkins-Sinn Inc., Cherry Hill, NJ

°Aire Cuf, Bivona Surgical Instruments, Gary, IN
†Xylocaine 2% Jelly, Astra, Westborough, MA

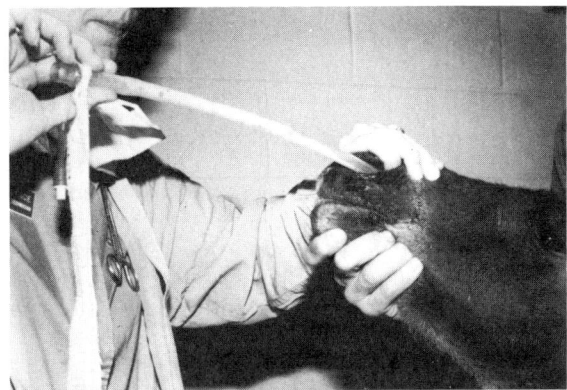

Figure 1. The foal's head and neck are extended to facilitate intubation. When successfully placed in the trachea, condensation forms within the tube during each expiration.

bolic requirements is supplied to the circle system. The pop-off valve is closed and the oxygen flow meter initially set to provide 6 to 8 ml per kg per minute (higher than in adults). If the rebreathing bag becomes distended, oxygen is being delivered in excessive quantities and the flow meter setting should be lowered. If the bag becomes empty, the flow meter setting must be increased to meet oxygen requirements. Closed-system inhalational techniques are economical and assisted ventilation is simplified, because the anesthetist does not have to continually manipulate the pop-off valve. Also, rebreathing of warmed and humidified gases minimizes heat loss and desiccation of the respiratory passages. An anesthetic breathing circle system designed for small animals or humans will suffice for foals up to 100 kg if a double CO_2 absorber canister is used. At weights above 100 kg, conventional equipment designed for adult horses is required.

The inhalational agent of choice is isoflurane[*] because of its rapid induction and recovery characteristics, lack of arrhythmogenicity, minimal metabolism, and higher therapeutic index. Compared to halothane,[†] it causes less cardiopulmonary depression. Recent studies indicate that the minimum alveolar concentration (MAC, the alveolar concentration required to prevent 50 per cent of patients responding to a painful stimulus) of isoflurane is constant in foals between 1 and 6 weeks of age and is less than adult isoflurane requirements.

The previously held belief that IV dextrose therapy is required in all foals during anesthesia is false. Normal foals have adult glucose levels (7 to 8 mmol per L) at less than 12 hours of age, and in the absence of feeding, these levels are maintained for at least 2 hours. Foals should only be given supplemental dextrose if blood glucose analyses indicate hypoglycemia. Unnecessary administration may cause a surge of insulin release and rebound hypoglycemia when dextrose is withdrawn. Lactated Ringer's solution should suffice for most routine procedures. The rate of administration depends on blood loss and clinical assessment but may be as high as 10 ml per kg per hour. The PCV should be monitored periodically to prevent excessive hemodilution.

Older and less easily restrained foals may be induced with injectable agents. Popular and safe techniques include premedication with xylazine or diazepam and induction with a mixture of guaifenesin (GGE) and ketamine (1 gm of ketamine added to 1 liter of 5 per cent GGE), or guaifenesin and thiamylal (2 gm of thiamylal added to 1 liter of 5 per cent GGE), infused IV to effect.

MONITORING

Foals should be monitored closely during anesthesia. Physical monitoring should include palpation of the peripheral pulse and auscultation of the heart with an esophageal stethoscope. Blood pressure can be measured directly or indirectly as previously described. Direct blood pressure monitoring has the disadvantages of being invasive, technically demanding, and expensive, but it is recommended in physiologically compromised foals and if prolonged surgery or substantial blood loss is anticipated. The actual value (mm Hg) at which hypotension is diagnosed will depend on the monitoring technique employed. Also, trends in blood pressure values are more informative than single, isolated recordings. Low blood pressure is first managed by decreasing the level of anesthesia and increasing the rate of fluid administration. IV glycopyrrolate (0.01 mg per kg) or atropine (0.02 mg per kg) should be given if bradycardia is the cause. Occasionally inotropic agents such as dopamine or dobutamine (1 to 5 μg per kg per minute) may be necessary. Electrocardiographic monitoring will reveal arrhythmias if they arise.

Oxygenation status is less easy to monitor. Mucous membrane color is very unreliable and techniques such as transcutaneous oxygen monitoring have been disappointing. At present, the only reliable method is analysis of arterial blood samples, but pulse oximetry shows some promise as a continuous, noninvasive method of monitoring hemoglobin saturation. Adequacy of alveolar ventilation can be monitored continuously and noninvasively by capnography (analysis of end-

---

[*]Aerrane, Anaquest, Madison, WI
[†]Halothane USP, Halocarbon Labs., Hackensack, NJ

tidal CO_2), since expired CO_2 values correlate closely with the arterial partial pressure of carbon dioxide (Pa_{CO_2}).

General supportive care should include careful positioning, use of protective eye lubricant, and heated water blankets. The immune status of many foals is compromised, so invasive techniques such as IV and intra-arterial catheterization must be done aseptically. If it is anticipated that an IV catheter will be required for several days postoperatively, the catheter of choice is a 16- or 18-gauge L-cath.° Cyanoacrylate† works effectively to secure catheters in place and obviates the need for invasive suturing techniques.

Anesthetic management of septic or metabolically deranged foals differs little from that already outlined, provided that stabilization is accomplished prior to surgery. This includes rehydration and, in the case of a ruptured urinary bladder, correction of hyperkalemia. Most sick foals will not resist nastotracheal intubation and inhalational techniques.

°Lumed, Luther Medical Products, Inc., Santa Ana, CA
†Super Glue, Super Glue Corp., Hollis, NY

RECOVERY

Foals should be allowed to recover in a warm environment and placed in sternal recumbency to optimize their Pa_{O_2}. If they shiver, supplemental oxygen must be provided to prevent hypoxemia. Foals often recover faster when stimulated by their dam, which can be brought to the recovery area. As soon as they can be assisted to stand, they should be allowed to suckle to maintain their fluid and caloric intake and preserve maternal bonding.

Supplemental Readings

Adams, J. G., and Trim, C. M.: Plasma glucose concentrations in anesthetized foals. Equine Pract., 12:25–29, 1990.
Caprile, K. A., and Short, C. R.: Pharmacologic considerations in drug therapy in foals. Vet. Clin. North Am. (Equine Pract.) 3:123–144, 1987.
Carter, S. W., Robertson, S. A., Steele, C., and Jourdenais, D. A.: Cardiopulmonary effects of xylazine sedation in the foal. Equine Vet. J. 22:384–388, 1990.
Robertson, S. A., Carter, S. W., Donovan, M. and Steel, C.: Effects of intravenous xylazine hydrochloride on blood glucose, plasma insulin and rectal temperature in neonatal foals. Equine Vet. J., 22:43–47, 1990.
Webb, A. I.: Nasal intubation in the foal. J. Am. Vet Med. Assoc., 185:48–51, 1984.

Respiratory Support of the Newborn Foal

Dennis R. Geiser, KNOXVILLE, TENNESSEE

Respiration is defined as the transport of oxygen from the atmosphere to the cells and the transport of carbon dioxide from the cells to the atmosphere. Adequate respiration depends not only on normal pulmonary function but also on normal cardiovascular and hematological function. Ventilation is a part of the respiratory process that involves the actual inflow and outflow of air between the atmosphere and alveoli. Alveolar ventilation is the rate of exchange of alveolar air with atmospheric air each minute. Ventilation is dependent on respiratory rate and tidal volume [rate × (tidal volume − dead space volume)]. Factors that directly influence pulmonary ventilation in the neonate include function of the respiratory muscles, compliance of the lung, surfactant production, airway resistance, central nervous system (CNS) regulation, residual lung volume, and dead space volume. Hypoventilation, an inadequate renewal of alveolar air by atmospheric air, can result from several causes (Table 1).

NEONATAL RESPIRATORY ADAPTATION

Several important events must occur for a fetus to adapt to the extrauterine environment and become a normal neonate. In the horse, the transition from the fluid uterine environment to an air-filled environment is explosive and quick. Since the lungs are fluid-filled in utero, successful transition to breathing air requires the expulsion and absorption of fluid from the lungs. The initiation of spontaneous ventilation is dependent on chest expansion after expulsion from the birth canal and adequate external stimulation to activate the CNS. Alveolar expansion distributes surfactant over the alveolar surfaces, reducing surface tension and facilitating further alveolar

TABLE 1. CAUSES OF RESPIRATORY DEPRESSION AND FAILURE IN THE NEONATAL FOAL.

Respiratory Depression (Respiratory causes)	Respiratory Depression (Nonrespiratory causes)	Respiratory Failure
Prematurity	Shock, hypovolemia	Idiopathic apnea of prematurity
Respiratory distress syndrome (surfactant deficiency)	Anemia	Dystocia, prolonged birth, asphyxia
Upper airway obstruction	Persistent fetal circulation	Cesarean section
Pneumothorax	Acidosis, hypoglycemia	Trauma
Meconium aspiration	CNS disease, cerebral edema, cerebral hypoxia	CNS disease, hypoxia, seizure, coma, meningitis
Pneumonia	Drugs	Shock, hypoxemia
Atelectasis	Muscle disease	Cardiovascular disease
Aspiration		Sepsis/endotoxemia
Pulmonary edema		Hypoglycemia
Pleuritis, pleural effusion		Hypocalcemia
Diaphragmatic hernia		Hypothermia
		Hypoxic pulmonary hypertension
		Persistent fetal circulation

expansion. In addition, fetal circulatory shunts must be eliminated to produce a normal circulatory pattern. In general, the vascular resistance of the fetal lungs must be reduced to allow increased blood flow, and the vascular shunts (ductus arteriosus and foramen ovale) should close. Body temperature and acid–base status should favor proper hemoglobin saturation in the lungs and desaturation at the tissue level. Abnormal alterations in these adaptive processes, such as persistent fetal circulation, hypoxic pulmonary hypertension, hypothermia, or surfactant deficiency, may result in respiratory compromise in the neonate.

NEONATAL RESPIRATORY DISTRESS

Respiratory compromise in the foal may be divided into critical and noncritical respiratory depression. Critical respiratory depression includes the syndromes that produce an acute or immediate life-threatening situation. Apnea is usually the primary presenting sign in these patients. Noncritical respiratory depression includes the problems that are not immediately life-threatening but require respiratory support. Noncritical respiratory depression may become acutely critical or may progress to a life-threatening state if proper therapy is not instituted.

Apnea is the complete cessation of respiratory efforts and can be divided into primary and secondary apnea. Primary apnea is diagnosed when the lack of ventilatory efforts is easily alleviated by the initiation of spontaneous breathing through external stimulation. In most cases, cardiovascular parameters are normal. Heart rate may be decreasing but remains within normal limits. Blood pressure usually remains normal. Secondary apnea usually occurs if the initial cessation of ventilation goes uncorrected and asphyxia continues. Secondary apnea may be characterized by periodic deep gasps ending in total anoxia. Sensory stimuli fail to initiate rhythmic ventilatory efforts. Intermittent positive-pressure ventilation is required.

Noncritical respiratory depression is usually characterized by hypoxemia and hypercapnia in the presence of spontaneous ventilatory efforts. Methods of therapy depend on the cause and degree of respiratory depression (see Table 1).

DIAGNOSIS

The diagnosis of equine neonatal respiratory disease in a field situation is based mainly on physical examination. When apnea is detected the cardiovascular system should also be evaluated, including the presence or absence of a heartbeat, quality of peripheral pulse, heart rate, mucous membrane color, and capillary refill time. Since there is an intimate relationship between the pulmonary and cardiovascular systems, ventilatory therapy may also require cardiovascular support. Initially during an apneic episode, tachycardia with good pulse quality and capillary refill time may be present. However, if apnea continues, bradycardia may occur, pulse quality will decline, capillary refill time will increase, and cyanosis will be evident. Cardiac arrest may then ensue.

Physical aspects of respiratory evaluation include respiratory rate and quality or pattern, pulmonary sounds, and mucous membrane color (Table 2). A low respiratory rate may not produce abnormal blood gas tensions if tidal volume is adequate. Tachypnea may be characterized by low tidal volumes, movement of only dead space air, and blood gas abnormalities. It may be di-

TABLE 2. NORMAL VALUES OF RESPIRATORY VARIABLES IN THE NEONATAL FOAL

Parameter Measured	Value	
Temperature	99.0–101.5° F	
Heart rate		
Postpartum	>60 bpm	
Days 1–5	80–120 bpm	
Resp. rate		
Postpartum	60–80 breaths/min	
12 hours	30–40 breaths/min	
Blood Gases	0–24 hours old	>24 hours old
Pa_{O_2} (mm Hg)	40–50	80
Pa_{CO_2} (mm Hg)	52–60	48
pHa	7.20–7.30	7.40
HCO_3^- (mEq/L)a	24.0–26.0	28.0
Pv_{O_2} (mm Hg)		40–45
Pv_{CO_2} (mm Hg)		45–52
pH_v		7.380
HCO_3^- (mEq/L)v		28.0–30.0

rectly related to the degree of respiratory disease or influenced by extrapulmonary disease. Low respiratory rates are the exception in the foal but may occur in association with some situations such as CNS disease and hypothermia. Auscultation of the chest will normally reveal increased vesicular sounds when compared to adult animals. However, auscultation is not a reliable method for determining the presence of respiratory disease in the equine neonate. Mucous membrane color also does not correlate well with the degree of hypoxemia or hypercapnia in the neonate. Cyanosis may occur only at oxygen tensions less than 40 mm Hg in the neonate or when severe cardiac shunts are present.

Because the presence or absence of pulmonary abnormalities in the neonate cannot be reliably determined by routine physical examination, special diagnostic methods, such as radiography, blood gas analysis, clinical pathology, and ultrasonography, are often employed. Thoracic radiology is a part of a routine neonatal data base and is important for the diagnosis and monitoring of foal respiratory disease.

Evaluation of blood gas tensions is important in diagnosing respiratory failure, determining the severity of the disease, developing a therapeutic strategy, and monitoring the effects of therapy. Arterial blood may be obtained from the carotid, lingual-facial, transverse facial, and great metatarsal arteries. Difficulty in obtaining samples may occur in fractious patients and in cases of severe hypotension. Arterial catheters may increase the ease of frequent sampling but must be properly maintained as they are potential sources of sepsis and hemorrhage. Blood gas samples should be held in an ice slush if the analysis is delayed for more than 30 minutes. Factors that should also be considered when evaluating blood gas results are summarized in Table 3.

Arterial blood gas is necessary for accurate evaluation of the pulmonary system. However, with respiratory arrest it is usually not practical or necessary to obtain blood gas samples as it can be assumed that oxygen and carbon dioxide values are abnormal and ventilatory support should be instituted. After the restoration of respiratory function, blood gas analysis is critical for determining adequacy of ventilation and for continued monitoring of therapy.

Venous blood may be used to evaluate metabolic acid–base status and may indicate severely low arterial gas tensions when an excessive venous hypercapnia (Pv_{CO_2} greater than 60 mm Hg) or hypoxemia (Pv_{O_2} less than 20 mm Hg) exists. The most frequent blood gas abnormalities noted in neonatal respiratory disease are hypercapnia and hypoxemia. Arterial CO_2 tension is used to determine adequacy of ventilation. Hypercapnia contributes to an acidemia and may be responsible for producing tachypnea in the neonate. Hypocapnia is unusual in the neonate but may occur during hyperventilation, which may be either spontaneous or the result of controlled ventilation. Hypoxemia may result from inadequate ventilation, cardiovascular shunting, diffusion abnormalities, and ventilation–perfusion ($\dot{V}/\dot{Q}$) mismatching. Three blood gas aberrations may occur in the neonate: (1) hypoxemia, normocapnia, (2) severe hypoxemia with normocapnia or hypocapnia, and (3) severe hypoxemia and hypercapnia. In the latter two categories both tachypnea and abnormal breathing patterns may be evident.

Clinical pathological examination includes a complete blood cell count and fibrinogen levels. The hematocrit, hemoglobin, and red blood cell count may be helpful in determining the oxygen-carrying capacity of the blood. The white blood cell profile and fibrinogen levels may indicate the presence or absence of sepsis. Ultrasonography may be helpful in diagnosing extrapulmonary causes of respiratory dysfunction in the neonate.

TABLE 3. FACTORS THAT SHOULD BE CONSIDERED WHEN EVALUATING BLOOD GAS RESULTS

1. Venous or arterial sample
2. Signalment and vital signs
3. Position of foal during sampling (sternal or lateral recumbency)
4. Amount of activity during sampling
5. Inspired oxygen concentration
6. Proper collection and handling of sample

THERAPY

Therapy may be divided into primary and secondary strategies. Primary therapy includes the establishment of a patent airway, support of ventilation, and oxygen enrichment of inspired air. Secondary treatments include all measures used for additional support of the respiratory system as well as general supportive care of the foal. These measures may include airway hygiene, drug therapy, inhalation therapy by nebulization, coupage, sternal positioning, temperature maintenance, cardiovascular support, fluid therapy, and nutritional support.

When apnea is diagnosed, rapid institution of therapy is required. External stimulation should be attempted initially. Vigorous rubbing, stimulation of the nasal mucosa or skin of the ear canal with a straw, and flexion and extension of the limbs may be used in an attempt to initiate ventilatory efforts. If these measures fail after 30 to 60 seconds, some form of ventilatory support should be instituted.

Airway patency should be determined. If a large amount of pharyngeal fluid is present, suctioning may be helpful. This can be accomplished in the field by using a small, soft, rubber or latex catheter and 60-cc syringe. Excessive negative pressure should be avoided and suctioning should be intermittent. More sophisticated suction devices are available for use with portable or central vacuum systems. Postural drainage is difficult in the foal and may aggravate ventilatory distress by increasing abdominal pressure on the diaphragm. Placing the foal on a slight incline during resuscitation may allow drainage of a portion of the airway fluid. Orotracheal or nasotracheal intubation* is ideal when pulmonary resuscitation is necessary.

Mouth to nose resuscitation is done by closing the foal's mouth and lips, occluding one nostril with the hands, and blowing into the other nostril. Observation of the extent of thoracic excursions will provide a rough evaluation of adequate tidal volume. This method only provides short-term ventilatory assistance without oxygen enrichment.

The human adult ambu bag† is adequate for ventilating equine neonates. It can be used with a snug-fitting canine mask or with an endotracheal tube. If an oxygen source is available most ambu bags have an adaptor for providing oxygen enrichment of the inspired air.

Another method for providing short-term ventilation of the foal is the use of a demand valve.‡ It assists the spontaneously breathing patient by providing oxygen when a certain amount of negative pressure is applied to it or allows the clinician to administer a positive-pressure breath at a chosen interval. A practical kit for short-term emergency field resuscitation of foals would include a small "E" oxygen tank, oxygen line, endotracheal tubes, and a demand valve or ambu bag.§

Chemical stimulation of ventilation may be attempted. However, because of the variability of response to drugs such as doxapram hydrochloride,‖ it is better to first initiate external resuscitation and then attempt chemical stimulation. Chemical stimulants are usually not effective in cases of secondary apnea. If emergency resuscitation is successful in initiating spontaneous breathing, enrichment of the inspired air with oxygen should be provided until the effectiveness of the patient's ventilation can be evaluated.

OXYGEN INSUFFLATION

Oxygen enrichment of inspired air may be accomplished by taping or suturing in place a small, soft, plastic tube in the nasopharynx. The oxygen flow should range between 5 and 10 liters per minute and, if continued for more than 15 to 30 minutes, the oxygen should be humidified to prevent airway drying. Other supportive measures such as removal of excessive airway secretions and maintenance of a sternal body position should be instituted in conjunction with insufflation. Oxygen insufflation is indicated in foals with low blood oxygen tensions, less than 60 mm Hg. Insufflation will often be effective in elevating arterial oxygen tensions in mild to moderate cases of $\dot{V}/\dot{Q}$ mismatching and diffusion abnormalities in the lung. In cases of severe cardiac shunts and pulmonary disease, insufflation may be of little benefit in elevating blood oxygen tensions. Pre- and posttreatment blood gas analysis is ideal in monitoring response to insufflation and may help in diagnosing the presence or absence of extrapulmonary abnormalities. Insufflation will not improve ventilation or decrease high blood CO_2 tensions.

Blood oxygen tension should be maintained between 70 and 100 mm Hg. Oxygen tensions greater than 100 mm Hg for prolonged periods of time may produce oxygen toxicity. As the clin-

---

*Aire Cuf Bivona Inc., Gary, IN
†PMR-2 manual resuscitator, Puritan Bennett, Kansas City, MO
‡Demand value, Hudson, Temecula, CA
§Portable emergency oxygen unit, Puritan Bennett, Kansas City, MO
‖Dopram V Inj., A. H. Robins, Richmond, VA

ical signs or laboratory data indicate improvement in respiratory function and blood oxygenation, the neonate should be gradually weaned from the insufflated oxygen.

MECHANICAL VENTILATION

Long-term mechanical ventilation of the foal is a time-consuming and technical endeavor that requires intensive labor and monitoring. Before long-term neonatal ventilation is attempted, adequate equipment should be on hand and personnel should be trained in proper respiratory therapy. A knowledge of neonatal respiratory physiology is crucial to effective mechanical ventilation.

Mechanical ventilators are generally divided into two classes: volume limited and pressure limited. This means that either a volume or pressure value is preset for inspiration, and inspiration is terminated when that value is reached.

Volume-limited Ventilator

This type of ventilator can be adjusted to deliver a predetermined tidal volume at a constant flow rate. The pressure developed in the airways is dependent on the volume delivered, the resistance of the airways, and respiratory compliance. For example, a tidal volume of 5 ml per lb (10 ml per kg) will produce a higher inspiratory pressure in a patient with a very stiff, noncompliant lung or chest than in a patient with a very compliant lung.

Pressure-limited Ventilator

This type of ventilator is generally more complex in design and consequently more difficult to operate. The function of this type of ventilator is not regulated by a preset volume but depends on the development of a preset pressure in the proximal airways. The volume of air delivered, then, depends on the driving pressure, inspiratory flow rate, inspiratory time, resistance of the airways, and pulmonary compliance. For example, if the proximal airway pressure is set at 22 mm Hg, air will continue to flow into the alveoli and develop a tidal volume until the airway pressure reaches 22 mm Hg. In a patient with a stiff lung or high airway resistance the preset proximal airway pressure may be reached very rapidly, before an adequate tidal volume is generated.

Other ventilator characteristics that are necessary for long-term neonatal respiratory support include the ability to humidify and warm the air, the ability to vary the inspired oxygen concentration (FI_{O_2}), or oxygen blending, and the ability to produce positive end-expiratory pressure (PEEP). Human hospitals and dealers in used and reconditioned equipment may serve as sources of less expensive ventilator units; some sources are listed at the end of the chapter.

Indications for the need to mechanically ventilate a foal include hypercapnia (Pa_{CO_2} above 60 mm Hg), hypoxemia (Pa_{O_2} less than 50 mm Hg), and apnea. Neonates with marginal blood gas values, hypoxemia plus normocapnia or hypocapnia, that do not respond to oxygen supplementation by insufflation are also candidates for ventilatory support. It is important to inform clients that mechanical ventilation of the neonate usually necessitates a long hospitalization period and requires a substantial financial commitment.

PATIENT PREPARATION AND MANAGEMENT

After the decision to ventilate has been made, an airway must be established. This can be accomplished by nasotracheal intubation or tracheostomy. Nasotracheal intubation is preferred (see p. 476). If the patient is severely depressed from the disease process it may be possible to initiate mechanical ventilation without chemical restraint. However, in many cases, chemical and physical restraint may be necessary for adequate ventilation. Sedation of the neonate can be accomplished by the use of several different drugs (Table 4). Phenobarbital° is an oxybarbiturate with anticonvulsant properties. Barbiturates may be administered in hypnotic or sedative doses and in anesthetic doses. Phenobarbital, when administered in hypnotic doses, produces minimal cardiopulmonary depression. A slight decrease in respiratory rate, heart rate, and systemic blood pressure may be experienced and may accentuate the hypotensive effect of shock. The administration of a dose of phenobarbital should be followed by a waiting period of 15 minutes before additional drug is administered, because repeated injections may produce excessive CNS depression and overdosage. It is prudent to use only the minimal amount required for the desired level of restraint.

Pentobarbital§ has the disadvantage of a short duration of action. At high doses, pentobarbital is anesthetic and may produce cardiovascular depression.

Diazepam† has been used for short-term or acute control of seizures in the foal. The disadvantage of diazepam to produce restraint for mechanical ventilation is its short duration of action and low level of sedation.

The use of the sedative hypnotics xylazine‡

°Phenobarbital sodium USP, Wyeth Ayerst Labs., Philadelphia, PA
§Pentobarbital sodium, Ft. Dodge Labs., Ft. Dodge, IA
†Valium Inj., Hoffman LaRoche, Nutley, NJ
‡Rompun, HaverLockhart, Mobay Corp., Shawnee, KS

TABLE 4. DOSAGES OF VARIOUS DRUGS FOR CHEMICAL RESTRAINT DURING MECHANICAL VENTILATION

Drug	Dose and Route	Comment
Phenobarbital°	1) 10 mg/kg IV (loading dose) 5 mg/kg IV (maintenance dose) 2) 2–9 mg/kg IV t.i.d.	Adjust as needed; give each dose to effect
Diazepam	0.02–0.04 mg/kg IV	Not for prolonged sedation
Pentobarbital	2.0–4.0 mg/kg IV	Short-acting, cardiovascular depression, slow to achieve effect
Chloral hydrate	3–10 gm/50 kg IV	Lag period, cardiovascular depression, slow to achieve effect
Xylazine	0.4–1.0 mg/kg IV	Cardiovascular depression, for use in refractory cases
Detomidine	0.005–0.02 mg/kg IV	Cardiovascular depression, for use only in very refractory cases
Pancuronium	0.04–0.066 mg/kg IV†	Short-acting, requires cardiovascular monitoring
Atracurium	0.04–0.07 mg/kg †	Short-acting, requires cardiovascular monitoring

NOTE—The exact doses of these drugs for restraint of the foal will vary. The dosages recommended here should be considered only guidelines.
°Drug of choice.
†Doses described in adult horses under general anesthesia.

and detomidine§ in the sick foal has not been recommended, due to the cardiopulmonary depression produced by these drugs. However, in patients that do not respond to routine sedatives, these drugs may be employed as a last resort. Because of their rapid onset of action they should be titrated to effect. Chloral hydrate‖ has also been used for the restraint of neonates. Although chloral hydrate is a reliable sedative, its margin of safety is very low. Severe dose-dependent cardiovascular depression may occur. This drug, if used, should be given to effect. Chloral hydrate is slow to cross the blood–brain barrier, and consequently a 10- to 15-minute lag period may occur before the full CNS effect is achieved. This drug may be employed only when other drugs have failed to produce adequate restraint.

A nasogastric tube¶ should be placed in each patient receiving mechanical ventilation to allow removal of gas that may accumulate in the stomach. Nasogastric tubes designed for adult humans work well for this purpose. These tubes are generally small, soft, nonirritating, and well tolerated for long periods. The nasogastric tube should be sutured to the nostril. Suction may be applied to the tube when gas distention occurs.

Foals receiving mechanical ventilation will usually require intravenous alimentation, because complete oral alimentation may contribute to gas distention and colic. However, it may be beneficial to administer small amounts of enteral nutrition to maintain the integrity and function of the gastrointestinal tract.

Ventilation Protocol

The ventilator settings will be dictated by each individual case and type of pulmonary disease present. The diseased lung may require more intense ventilation than the normal lung to maintain normal blood gas values. The different modes of ventilation that can be provided depend on the type of ventilator used (Table 5). Routine positive-pressure ventilation may be administered continuously in neonates that have no spontaneous respiratory efforts or that require continuous ventilation to maintain blood gas values within normal limits. In some cases only intermittent positive-pressure ventilation may be necessary to supplement the neonate's spontaneous respiratory efforts. Other modes provided by some ventilators that are beneficial in providing adequate respiratory support include posi-

TABLE 5. MODES OF MECHANICAL VENTILATION THAT CAN BE USED FOR NEONATAL RESPIRATORY SUPPORT

PPV Positive-pressure ventilation: The production of air flow into the lungs by creating a pressure difference between proximal airway and the alveoli.

IPPV Intermittent positive-pressure ventilation

IMV Intermittent mandatory ventilation: Patient is allowed to breath spontaneously but controlled breaths are delivered at a preset interval or rate.

SIMV Synchronous intermittent mandatory ventilation: Allows patient to breath spontaneously via a demand valve system but delivers a mandatory breath at a preset interval and volume. May also deliver a mandatory breath if patient becomes apneic when the next positive-pressure breath is due.

PEEP Positive end-expiratory pressure: The maintenance of positive pressure (1–5 cm H_2O) in the airways at the end of expiration. Prevents airway closure by maintaining alveolar volume between breaths.

CPAP Continuous positive airway pressure: Provision of positive end-expiratory pressure during spontaneous respiration. The patient exhales to a preset expiratory pressure. This modality maintains lung volume for improved gas exchange.

Sigh: Periodic breath or breaths having a volume 1.5 to 2 times greater than the normal tidal volume.

---

§Dormosedan, Norden Labs., Lincoln, NE
‖Chloral hydrate, Fisher Scientific, Atlanta, GA
¶Internal replacement feeding tubes, Corpak Co., Wheeling, IL

tive end-expiratory pressure (PEEP), continuous positive airway pressure, and intermittent sighing to prevent atelectasis and activate surfactant. Guidelines that may be used for initial ventilator setting include the following: (1) tidal volume of 10 to 12 ml per kg, (2) ventilatory rate of 20 to 25 breaths per minute, (3) peak proximal airway pressure of approximately 20 to 25 cm H_2O, (4) intermittent mandatory ventilation mode should be used initially in cases where spontaneous respiration is present, (5) PEEP of about 2 mm Hg, and (6) two to three sighs every 15 minutes. Adjustments are then made based on blood gas analysis. Positive airway pressure or PEEP may be necessary to decrease CO_2 or increase oxygenation. Initially, 100 per cent inspired oxygen (FI_{O_2}) may be required; however, the inspired concentration should eventually be reduced to the minimum concentration that will maintain arterial oxygen tensions between 80 and 100 mm Hg.

Hygiene during mechanical ventilation is very important in preventing secondary complications. Hygienic procedures should include: 1) aseptic suctioning of the endotracheal tube six to eight times per day, (2) maintenance of a closed breathing circuit, (3) changing the delivery hoses of the circuit daily, (4) personal hygiene, such as hand washing, (5) sterilization of endotracheal tubes and delivery apparatus and replacement of any ventilator filters between patients, and (6) use of sterile water in the humidifier of the ventilator.

As the neonate's condition improves, weaning from the ventilator should be done slowly and systematically. It is important to continue monitoring vital signs and blood gas values during the weaning process. The first step is to reduce or eliminate positive airway pressure or PEEP if it was employed. The next step is to reduce FI_{O_2} in small increments until a value of approximately 30 to 40 per cent is reached without producing abnormal arterial oxygen tension. The third step is to reduce the rate until the foal is breathing spontaneously. Once the ventilator is disconnected, oxygen insufflation should be provided until normal blood gas tensions can be ensured. As the foal is weaned from the ventilator it should be weaned concurrently from any sedatives or other chemical restraining agents.

RESPIRATORY SUPPORT AND TRANSPORTATION

An apneic neonate or one with severe respiratory difficulty may have to be transported to an intensive care facility. Support of ventilation during transport can be achieved in several ways. In cases of apnea, manual ventilation by means of demand valve and ambu bag will be required, and the owner or farm personnel should be instructed in the use of support equipment for the trip. Neonates that make spontaneous respiratory efforts may be supported by insufflation alone. A small "E" oxygen tank contains approximately 670 liters of oxygen. At 5 to 10 liters per minute, a tank lasts approximately 1 to 2 hours.

In addition to respiratory support, all other necessary supportive measures should be employed, including the provision of warmth, fluids, and glucose. Hypothermia may adversely affect the oxyhemoglobin dissociation curve by shifting it to the left.

SOME SOURCES OF NEW OR USED EQUIPMENT FOR RESPIRATORY SUPPORT OF THE NEONATE

Universal Hospital Services
Bloomington, MN 55437

DRE Inc.
Louisville, KY 40243

Bear Medical Systems
Riverside, CA 92507

Ohmeda
Louisville, CO 80027

PPG Rrisa Marketing
PPG Biomed Inc.
Lenexa, KS 66215

Hamilton Medical
Reno, Nevada 89250

Bird Corporation
Palm Springs, CA 92262

Puritan Bennett Corp.
Kansas City, MO 64106

Monaghan Med. Corp.
Plattsburgh, NY 12901

Siemens Life Support
Chicago, IL 60173

JH Emerson Co.
Cambridge, MA 02140

Erika-Gambro Engstrom
Lincolnshire, IL 60069

Supplemental readings

Collatos, C. O.: Seizures in foals: Pathophysiology, evaluation, and treatment. Compend. Cont. Educ. Pract. Vet., 12:393–399, 1990.

Koterba, A. M., Drummond, W. H., and Kosch, P. C.: Equine clinical neonatology, Philadelphia, Lea and Febiger, 1990.

Lough, M. D., Doershuk, C. F., and Stern, R. C.: Pediatric Respiratory Therapy, 3rd ed. Chicago, Year Book Medical Publishers, 1985.

Madigan, J. E.: Manual of Equine Neonatal Medicine. Woodland, Calif., Live Oak Publishers, 1987, pp. 64–71.

Martens, R. J.: Neonatal respiratory distress: a review with emphases on the horse. Compend. Cont. Educ. Pract. Vet., 4:S23–S33, 1982.

Sonea, I.: Respiratory distress syndrome in neonatal foals. Compend. Cont. Educ. Pract. Vet., 7:S462–S469, 1985.

Section 11

HEMATOPOIETIC DISEASES

Edited by Debra Deem Morris

Diagnostic Approach to Anemia

Michelle M. Henry, ATHENS, GEORGIA

Anemia, defined as an absolute reduction in the circulating red blood cell (RBC) mass, is a common clinical problem in horses. Because differences in the rate of onset, severity, and duration of anemia induce wide variation in clinical and hematological responses, the etiological diagnosis of anemia and the appropriateness of the physiological response can be difficult to assess. Furthermore, several features unique to the equine erythron complicate the accurate diagnostic assessment of anemia. This discussion reviews the clinical signs of anemia, features particular to the equine erythron, and the diagnostic approach to anemia.

CLINICAL SIGNS OF ANEMIA

The rapidity of development and extent of RBC loss determine the clinical signs of anemia. The response to anemia directly reflects the degree of impairment in the oxygen-carrying capacity of the blood caused by a reduction in the RBC mass. Thus, the major physiological response to acute anemia is an attempt to increase oxygen delivery to the tissue, manifested by peripheral vasoconstriction, tachycardia, and tachypnea. Mucous membrane pallor also results from the decrease in blood hemoglobin content. A grade I or II systolic murmur may be audible, presumably due to blood flow turbulence resulting from decreased blood viscosity. The compensatory increase in cardiac output may obscure obvious clinical signs of anemia until the horse is stressed or exercised, whereupon weakness, exercise intolerance, or sudden collapse occurs. The increased metabolic demand on the cardiovascular system and tissue hypoxia may cause a rise in core body temperature. Acute severe anemia may also cause blindness or dementia and oliguria as a result of cerebral and renal hypoxia, respectively.

Clinical signs of anemia can be useful in determining the etiological diagnosis. Hypovolemic shock frequently accompanies acute, severe blood loss. Clinical signs of external blood loss such as epistaxis, melena, hematochezia, hematuria, or trauma are usually obvious; however, internal hemorrhage (intrathoracic or intra-abdominal hematomas) may be difficult to detect. Intrathoracic hemorrhage may cause tachypnea or dyspnea (or both). Acute intra-abdominal hemorrhage may cause ileus or colic (or both). Coagulopathy may be manifested clinically as frank or occult bleeding, petechial or ecchymotic hemorrhages, or both.

Icterus is a clinical feature of increased RBC destruction when the total serum bilirubin concentration exceeds 3 mg per dl. Icterus must be carefully evaluated in horses as it also is a clinical feature of anorexia and hepatopathy. Furthermore, because the presence of icterus depends on the rate and extent of RBC destruction in relation to hepatic clearance of bilirubin, lack of icterus does not preclude hemolysis. Intravascular hemolysis is more likely to cause icterus than is extravascular hemolysis. Hemoglobinuria may attend intravascular hemolysis if the renal threshold is exceeded.

The clinical signs of chronic anemia are more obscure because of well-established compensatory responses. Pallor of the mucous membranes, lethargy, or exercise intolerance usually accompanies chronic anemia. Anemia secondary to chronic disease, the most common type of anemia in horses, may be accompanied by anorexia, weight loss, dullness of the hair coat, fever, and depression.

DIAGNOSIS OF ANEMIA AND EVALUATION OF THE ERYTHRON

The diagnosis of anemia is confirmed by laboratory demonstration of reductions in the packed cell volume (PCV), hemoglobin concentration, and RBC count. The accuracy of the PCV, hemoglobin concentration, and RBC count depends on proper blood collection and transportation and laboratory techniques. A reduction in these indices that is not associated with clinical signs warrants reassessment. As in any species, evaluation of the equine erythron depends on assessment of the hydration status.

Several features unique to the equine erythron may complicate accurate determination of anemia. The PCV and erythrocyte count vary with age (Table 1), breed (Table 2), and use of the horse. The PCV of equine neonates less than 2 days old is similar to that of mature adult horses. However, the PCV of foals decreases rapidly in the first week of life and remains below adult values until approximately 18 months of age. The speculative causes of the lower PCV in foals and yearlings are transformation of fetal to adult hemoglobin, a functional iron deficiency, and rapid growth rate at this stage of life. In general, well-conditioned or warm-blooded horses have a greater PCV than poorly conditioned or cold-blooded horses.

The PCV also is highly variable among individual horses, owing to the large reserve of erythrocytes in the spleen. The equine spleen is a highly muscular and well-innervated organ that may contain up to one third of the circulating RBC mass. Because splenic contraction can increase the PCV by as much as 50 per cent, the diagnosis of anemia may be obscured by release of erythrocytes from the spleen under the influence of stress, excitement, apprehension, pain, or exercise. Finally, the tendency for rouleaux formation causes rapid sedimentation of equine blood and necessitates its thorough mixing prior to determination of the RBC count.

Once anemia is confirmed by an absolute decrease in the erythrocyte count, an etiological diagnosis must be made so that appropriate therapy may be instituted. Although historical information and clinical signs alone may be sufficient for accurate etiological diagnosis of anemia, additional tests may be necessary (Table 3). The three major mechanisms of anemia are blood loss, hemolysis, and inadequate erythropoiesis. Further pathophysiological classification of anemia as regenerative or nonregenerative depends on the appropriateness of the bone marrow's response to the reduced RBC mass. Blood loss and hemolysis generally result in regenerative anemias. A regenerative anemia is one in which the bone marrow responds appropriately to the RBC reduction by increasing RBC production and releasing more RBCs into the circulation. Unlike those of other domestic species, equine erythrocytes remain in the bone marrow until fully mature, even in the setting of intense erythropoiesis. Therefore, peripheral evidence of erythrocyte regeneration such as reticulocytosis, macrocytosis, anisocytosis, polychromasia, basophilic stippling, and nucleated RBCs is rarely found in responsive anemias in horses.

TABLE 1. INFLUENCE OF AGE ON NORMAL ERYTHRON VALUES (MEANS ± 1 SD) OF HOT-BLOODED HORSES

Parameter Measured	Age				
	1 day	8–14 Days	8–18 Mo	3–4 Yr	≥5 Yr
RBC, $\times 10^{-6}/\mu l$	10.5 ± 1.4	9.0 ± 0.8	8.6 ± 0.58	9.1 ± 1.2	8.6 ± 1.0
Hgb, gm/dl	14.2 ± 1.3	11.8 ± 1.2	11.8 ± 1.6	14.3 ± 1.4	14.4 ± 1.6
PCV, %	41.7 ± 3.6	34.9 ± 3.7	34.5 ± 3.8	40.8 ± 4.3	40.8 ± 0.1
MCV, fl	40.1 ± 3.8	39.1 ± 2.2	40.1 ± 2.9	44.8 ± 3.4	47.8

Adapted with permission from Jain, N. C. (ed.): Schalm's Veterinary Hematology, 4th ed. Philadelphia, Lea & Febiger, 1986.
RBC = red blood cell count, Hgb = hemoglobin, PCV = packed cell volume, MCV = mean corpuscular volume.

TABLE 2. INFLUENCE OF BREED ON NORMAL ERYTHRON VALUES (MEANS ± S.D.) IN ADULT HORSES

Breed	RBC ($\times 10^{-6}/\mu l$)	Hgb (gm/dl)	PCV (%)	MCV (fl)	MCH (pg)	MCHC (%)
Thoroughbred	9.35 ± 1.05	14.8 ± 1.3	41.7 ± 3.8	44.7 ± 3.4	15.9 ± 1.4	35.8 ± 1.4
Standardbred	8.37 ± 1.02	13.6 ± 1.6	38.3 ± 3.5	46.1 ± 4.0	16.3 ± 1.4	35.5 ± 1.6
Quarter Horse	8.26 ± 1.02	13.3 ± 1.6	38.0 ± 4.0	46.2 ± 3.9	16.1 ± 1.7	34.9 ± 1.6
Appaloosa	8.60 ± 1.11	13.3 ± 1.6	38.4 ± 4.7	44.8 ± 4.4	15.5 ± 1.3	34.5 ± 0.8
Arabian	8.41 ± 1.21	13.8 ± 2.1	39.3 ± 5.0	46.9 ± 1.9	16.4 ± 0.9	34.9 ± 1.0
Clydesdale	7.30 ± 0.87	12.4 ± 1.1	33.0 ± 3.0	44.6	—	38.1
Percheron	7.39 ± 1.08	11.7 ± 1.4	—	—	—	—

Adapted with permission from Jain, N. C. (ed.): Schalm's Veterinary Hematology, 4th ed. Philadelphia, Lea & Febiger, 1986.
RBC = red blood cell count, Hgb = hemoglobin, PCV = packed cell volume, MCV = mean corpuscular volume, MCH = mean corpuscular hemoglobin, MCHC = mean corpuscular hemoglobin concentration.

Howell–Jolly bodies, sometimes seen in responsive anemias in other species, may account for up to 0.1 per cent of the total RBCs in normal horses and are not indicative of responsive anemia. Because there is lack of peripheral evidence of erythropoiesis, the erythrocyte indices are not highly useful in horses, although a moderate increase in mean corpuscular volume (MCV) and anisocytosis may occur in responsive anemia. In general, an increased MCV is more likely to occur after hemolytic anemia than after blood loss anemia and usually does not occur until at least 2 weeks after the onset of anemia. Increased mean corpuscular hemoglobin (MCH) indicates the presence of free hemoglobin subsequent to in vivo or in vitro hemolysis. Microcytic, hypochromic, and macrocytic states are seldomly observed in the horse, though moderate to severe iron deficiency may cause microcytic, hypochromic anemia.

The availability of advanced multichannel blood cell counters has provided additional RBC indices useful in the evaluation of erythropoiesis. The RBC volume distribution width (RDW), a coefficient of variation of erythrocyte volume, increases in responsive anemias in the horse. Asymmetry of RBC size on histograms also may help predict responsiveness of the bone marrow or classification of anemia.

Biochemical assays, developed in an attempt to predict erythropoiesis in horses, include quantitation of RBC creatine and glucose-6-phosphate dehydrogenase concentrations. Elevations in both of these products correlate well with increased MCV and the presence of young RBCs in the peripheral blood. Although these as-

TABLE 3. DIAGNOSTIC TESTS FOR ANEMIA

Cause	Tests
I. Blood loss anemia	I. Bone marrow regenerative, usually no icterus, hypoproteinemia
A. Acute	A. Clinical signs of hypovolemic shock
1. Extracorporeal	1. Frank bleeding, epistaxis, melena, hematochezia, no icterus, hypoproteinemia
2. Intracorporeal	2. Paracentesis, ± hyperbilirubinemia, normal to low plasma protein, coagulation profile
B. Chronic	B. Clinical signs obscure in sedentary horse
1. Extracorporeal	1. Fecal occult blood, fecal float for parasite ova, urinalysis; microcytic, hypochromic anemia (nonregenerative); heavy burden of external parasites
2. Intracorporeal	2. Paracentesis, coagulation profile, transtracheal wash
II. Hemolytic anemia	II. Bone marrow regenerative, icterus
A. Intravascular	A. History, clinical signs, hemoglobinemia, hemoglobinuria, hyperbilirubinemia, normal to increased plasma protein, Heinz bodies, coagulation profile, liver evaluation (SDH, GGT, BSP), creatinine, urinalysis, Coombs test
B. Extravascular	B. Generally hyperbilirubinemia without preceding hemoglobinemia, normal to increased plasma protein, Giemsa stain, Coombs test, Coggins test, *Babesia* titer
III. Inadequate erythropoiesis	III. Bone marrow nonresponsive, no icterus
A. Chronic secondary	A. History, clinical signs, rectal examination, CBC, fibrinogen, serum protein electrophoresis, creatinine, glucose, electrolytes, calcium, urinalysis, SDH, GGT, BSP, abdominocentesis, transtracheal wash, liver biopsy, fecal float
B. Other	B. Bone marrow and peripheral blood evaluation

CBC = complete blood count, BSP = bromosulfophthalein, GGT = γ-glutamyltransferase, SDH = sorbitol dehydrogenase.

says are promising, the responses may be erratic and not widely available.

The most reliable measure of the bone marrow's responsiveness to anemia in horses requires evaluation of the bone marrow (see below). Typically, the diagnosis of blood loss or hemolytic anemia can be determined without bone marrow evaluation.

BLOOD LOSS ANEMIA

Blood loss anemia may be either acute or chronic, intracorporeal or extracorporeal. Acute blood loss of more than 30 per cent of blood volume is manifested clinically as hypovolemic shock. Acute extracorporeal blood loss (epistaxis, trauma, melena, hematochezia) is generally obvious; however, the PCV and total plasma protein concentration will not accurately reflect the degree of RBC loss for 24 to 48 hours since both RBCs and plasma are lost. The release of erythrocytes into the circulation via splenic contraction may further obscure the extent of RBC loss. Subsequent mobilization of extracellular fluid and water intake in the next 24 to 48 hours restore the plasma volume and cause the PCV and plasma protein concentration to decrease. Depending on the degree of blood loss, complete restoration of the PCV may take 2 to 3 months. Because plasma replacement occurs more rapidly than erythrocyte regeneration, the PCV often remains disproportionately lower than the plasma protein concentration during this period. In the absence of an obvious cause of acute blood loss a complete clotting profile is indicated to rule out blood loss secondary to coagulopathy.

Acute intracorporeal blood loss into thoracic or abdominal cavities or muscle masses may require paracentesis and cytological demonstration of peripheral blood elements (platelets, eosinophils, erythrocytes) or evidence of erythrophagocytosis. Rapid absorption of protein from body cavities may obscure the diagnosis of acute intracorporeal blood loss. A moderate increase in the total serum bilirubin concentration often accompanies intracorporeal blood loss as the RBCs are phagocytized by mononuclear phagocytes. Because iron is available for reutilization in erythropoiesis, the bone marrow response to intracorporeal blood loss tends to be more rapid than that to acute extracorporeal blood loss.

Chronic blood loss generally results in slowly developing anemia, because the bone marrow has a chance to regenerate erythrocytes as they are lost. Furthermore, physiological adaptations to chronic anemia tend to mask obvious clinical signs until the PCV drops below 15 per cent. Loss of iron in chronic extracorporeal blood loss may rarely result in nonresponsive iron deficiency anemia. Chemical assays for occult blood in feces and urine, cytological examination for hemosiderin-laden macrophages in body cavity effusions or a transtracheal aspirate, a coagulation profile, and bone marrow examination may be helpful in evaluating chronic blood loss anemia.

HEMOLYTIC ANEMIA

Hemolytic anemia may be acute or chronic, intravascular or extravascular. Acute intravascular hemolysis causes hemoglobinemia and subsequent hemoglobinuria, if the renal threshold of hemoglobin is exceeded. Because hemoglobin is rapidly cleared from the plasma and converted to bilirubin, icterus may be the only detectable evidence of recent hemolysis. New methylene blue–stained blood smears should be examined for Heinz bodies to rule out oxidant-induced hemolysis. A coagulation profile and assessment of liver and renal function may be useful in the diagnosis of microangiopathic hemolysis. Because some bacterial species such as *Clostridium*, *Staphylococcus*, and *Leptospira* excrete potent hemolysins, the horse should be carefully examined for evidence of infection.

Although hemolysis may occur intravascularly, most diseases associated with hemolysis cause increased extravascular erythrocyte destruction and hyperbilirubinemia without preceding hemoglobinemia. Diagnostic evaluation of suspected extravascular hemolysis should include peripheral blood smear evaluation for morphology, agglutination, and blood parasites; a direct Coombs test; and a Coggins test. Spherocytes, small round cells that lack central pallor, are rarely present in immune-mediated anemia of horses. Macro- and microscopic autoagglutination may occur in immune-mediated anemia; however, extensive rouleaux formation of equine erythrocytes is easily confused with autoagglutination. Because rouleaux formation is dependent on the plasma protein concentration, dilution of the blood with saline (1:4) will disperse rouleaux formation, while true agglutination will persist. A direct Coombs test may be positive in cases of immune-mediated hemolysis. Because the end point of the Coombs test is agglutination, this assay is unnecessary if agglutination is already evident. Heparin therapy also may cause erythrocyte agglutination in horses; thus, reductions in PCV and increases in MCV must be carefully scrutinized in horses receiving this drug. Intense icterus and anemia in neonates warrant hemolytic cross-match testing with the dam to rule out neonatal isoerythrolysis.

Because *Babesia* spp. can easily be overlooked

on routinely stained peripheral blood smears, Giemsa or methylene blue staining should be used. Since parasitemia precedes hemolysis, absence of parasitized erythrocytes does not rule out babesiosis, the diagnosis of which is more accurately based on positive serology. An agar gel immunodiffusion (Coggins) test for equine infectious anemia should be performed whenever chronic anemia is accompanied by icterus, weight loss, or intermittent fever. Because the Coggins test can be negative during early infection and in approximately 5 per cent of chronic cases, a negative test does not necessarily rule out this diagnosis.

A rapid reduction in the RBC mass that can occur with either acute blood loss or hemolytic anemia is often accompanied by fever and mature neutrophilia. Renal hypoxia or pigment-induced nephropathy may cause acute renal failure. Serum creatinine and electrolyte evaluation and urinalysis may be useful to guide therapy and prognosis. Hepatic hypoxia secondary to acute anemia may cause modest elevations in serum concentrations of sorbitol dehydrogenase (SDH) and γ-glutamyltransferase.

ANEMIA DUE TO INADEQUATE ERYTHROPOIESIS

Anemia due to inadequate erythropoiesis occurs when the rate of erythrocyte maturation is inadequate to replace the normal loss of aged erythrocytes from the blood. Because the problem lies within the bone marrow, these anemias are classified as nonregenerative and generally develop slowly since the equine erythrocyte life span is approximately 5 months. The slow onset of anemia allows ample time for adaptation and may obscure obvious clinical signs in the sedentary horse. The diagnosis of inadequate erythropoiesis is confirmed by bone marrow evaluation.

The most common cause of hypoproliferative anemia in horses is chronic disease. The anemia is generally mild to moderate (PCV 20 to 30 per cent) and clinical signs may reflect the primary disease process. Thorough and systematic physical and laboratory evaluation is necessary. If obvious clinical signs are lacking, the initial laboratory evaluation should include a complete blood cell count; plasma fibrinogen determination; serum protein electrophoresis; serum creatinine, glucose, electrolyte, calcium, sorbitol dehydrogenase, and γ-glutamyltransferase determinations; and urinalysis. Additional tests such as a transtracheal wash, thoracic radiography, thoracocentesis, abdominocentesis, bromosulfophthalein clearance test (BSP), or liver biopsy may be useful. Other causes of inadequate erythropoiesis (aplastic or myelophthisic anemia) are rare in horses but may be determined from the history, clinical signs, and examination of the bone marrow and peripheral blood.

In adult horses, bone marrow may be obtained from the sternum, rib, or ileum. Aspirates for cytology are most conveniently collected from the sternum by the following method. Clip and aseptically prepare a small area of skin on the ventral midline centered around a transverse line drawn between the point of both olecranons. A 3½-inch, 18-gauge disposable spinal needle, with stylet in place, is briskly inserted through the skin perpendicular to the flat sternal plate, in the cleavage between the deep pectoral muscles. While grasping the hub firmly with one hand and stabilizing the needle with the other, advance the needle until its tip reaches bone. At this point, slowly rotate the tip into the bone. Once the tip of the needle is well embedded into bone, remove the stylet and attach a 20-ml syringe. While stabilizing the needle in the bone, pull the syringe plunger rapidly to the 10-ml mark and release it. Repeat this maneuver two or three times. If blood is seen in the hub of the syringe, immediately release suction. The object is to exert negative pressure and break apart the marrow stroma without allowing blood to enter the collection site, as that would dilute the marrow specimen and interfere with accurate evaluation. Once marrow is observed in the hub, immediately stop aspiration and remove the needle and syringe together. If marrow is not obtained, reinsert the stylet, advance the needle, and repeat the aspiration.

Once a sample is obtained, thin smears should be promptly prepared to preserve cellular morphology. Place a drop of marrow near the edge of the slide, then place another clean slide face down over the drop, allowing it to spread in a thin layer between the slides. Pull the slides apart to create a thin smear on both. The slides should be promptly air dried, fixed, and stained. Wright's stain may be used for morphological evaluation, new methylene blue for determination of reticulocytes, and Prussian blue stain for semiquantitation of iron storage.

The myeloid–erythroid ratio (M:E) of a bone marrow aspirate is determined by counting at least 500 cells. The normal M:E ratio in horses ranges from 0.5 to 1.5. Although the M:E ratio may not always indicate the true status of erythropoiesis in the presence of anemia in horses, ratios less than 0.5 are generally consistent with an appropriate response. Evaluation of erythropoiesis involves counting the number of reticulocytes per 1000 erythrocytes. Reticulocyte counts greater than 2 per cent are indicative of erythroid regeneration. The maturity of the erythroid compartment also may be assessed. In normal horses, 70 to 90 per cent of erythroid cells are rubricytes and metarubricytes. The presence or absence of megakaryocytes or "abnormal" cells should be noted.

Supplemental Readings

Harvey, J. W., Asquith, R. L., Sussman, W. A., and Kivipelto, J.: Serum ferritin, serum iron, and erythrocyte values in foals. Am. J. Vet. Res., 48:1348, 1987.

Jain, N. C. (ed.): Veterinary Hematology, 4th ed. Philadelphia, Lea & Febiger, 1986.

Radin, M. J., Eubank, M. C., and Weiser, M. G.: Electronic measurement of erythrocyte volume and volume heterogeneity in horses during erythrocyte regeneration associated with experimental anemias. Vet. Pathol. 23:656, 1986.

Zinkl, J. G.: Pathophysiology of Anemias. In: Proceedings of the American College of Veterinary Internal Medicine, 1989, pp. 3–6.

Blood Loss Anemia
Michelle M. Henry, ATHENS, GEORGIA

ACUTE BLOOD LOSS

If more than 30 per cent of the blood volume (10 to 12 liters in a 450-kg horse) is lost acutely or the packed cell volume (PCV) decreases suddenly below 15 per cent, hypovolemic shock occurs. Acute blood loss is usually due to rupture or laceration of a major blood vessel, usually an artery, in the wake of trauma, surgery (e.g., castration), necrosis, or inflammation. Acute extracorporeal blood loss is obvious clinically as hemorrhage, epistaxis, melena, hematochezia, or hematuria.

A horse with necrotizing vasculitis of the carotid artery associated with guttural pouch mycosis may present with acute unilateral epistaxis. Pulmonary arterial necrosis secondary to severe pneumonia or pulmonary abscessation, or rupture of an ethmoid hematoma can cause acute bilateral epistaxis. Blood loss from the gastrointestinal (GI) tract secondary to a bleeding ulcer or cranial mesenteric artery aneurysm may rarely cause acute massive bleeding. Occasionally hemostatic disorders such as dicoumarin toxicity, congenital coagulation defects such as hemophilia or prekallikrein deficiency, immune-mediated thrombocytopenia, liver failure, or disseminated intravascular coagulation may cause acute external hemorrhage; however, these conditions generally result in internal hemorrhage and subacute to chronic blood loss.

The clinical signs of acute intracorporeal hemorrhage may be limited to hypovolemic shock. Acute hemothorax may result subsequent to thoracic trauma or rupture of a pulmonary abscess without evidence of epistaxis. Acute intra-abdominal hemorrhage may occur subsequent to trauma (e.g., splenic rupture), rupture of the cranial mesenteric artery during *Strongylus* larval migration, neoplastic lesions, intra-abdominal abscesses, rupture of an ovarian follicle, or rupture of the uterine artery during parturition.

THERAPY

The initial treatment for acute blood loss should be arrest of the hemorrhage when possible. External bleeding may be controllable by direct application of pressure or ligatures. Internal hemorrhage is often impossible to control since patient risk and time make general anesthesia unreasonable. Hypovolemic shock must be promptly treated with intravenous balanced crystalloid solutions to increase vascular volume. The necessary volume of fluid replacement usually is several times greater than the actual volume of blood lost, owing to extravascular equilibration of fluids. Careful monitoring is necessary to prevent overzealous dilution of the blood and exacerbation of the anemia and hypoproteinemia. Reduction in the heart rate and respiratory rate and improvement in the capillary refill time, pulse strength, and jugular distensibility are indications of improved cardiovascular status.

Administration of small volumes (4 ml per kg) of hypertonic crystalloid solutions (7 per cent NaCl) may be beneficial in the acute treatment of hemorrhagic shock; however, this therapeutic modality has not been fully evaluated in horses. Colloidal solutions such as dextran, albumin, or plasma may be more beneficial than isotonic solutions, but the necessary volume is often prohibitively costly.

Regardless of the cause, if anemia becomes life-threatening, and the PCV drops below 10 per cent over 24 to 48 hours, a whole blood transfusion is necessary. Donor selection, blood collection, and administration are discussed elsewhere (see p. 517). Transfused erythrocytes survive only 2 to 4 days; thus, the benefits of whole blood transfusion are only temporary. Furthermore, the increased PCV caused by a transfusion will blunt the bone marrow's initial response to the anemia.

Once the hemorrhage or hypovolemic shock has been controlled, the horse must be carefully monitored for signs of anemic hypoxia. The reduced oxygen-carrying capacity of the blood may cause renal hypoxia and acute renal dysfunction, necessitating additional fluid therapy. Administration of dopamine (3 µg per kg per minute) promotes renal vasodilation and may improve renal blood flow and oxygenation without causing excessive blood dilution. Because the reduction in oxygen-carrying capacity is due to decreased content of hemoglobin, oxygen therapy will not be beneficial.

Acute intracorporeal blood loss does not necessitate iron supplementation since iron is reabsorbed and reutilized. Acute extracorporeal blood loss may benefit from iron supplementation, but it is rarely necessary.

CHRONIC BLOOD LOSS

Chronic blood loss results in slowly developing anemia and obscure clinical signs. Chronic intermittent epistaxis may result from guttural pouch or nasal mycosis; ethmoid hematoma; nasal polyps or neoplasia; exercise-induced pulmonary hemorrhage; pulmonary abscessation, necrosis, or neoplasia; or hemostatic dysfunction. GI blood loss is usually occult in horses and rarely causes melena. Chronic GI blood loss may result from strongyles, gastric ulceration, nonsteroidal anti-inflammatory drug (NSAID) toxicity, coagulopathies, and neoplasia, especially squamous cell carcinoma. Blood loss from the urogenital system is uncommon and typically chronic. Chronic intermittent hematuria is most commonly seen with cystic or renal calculi, but it may also result from renal papillary necrosis due to NSAID toxicity, neoplasia of the kidney or bladder, renal abscessation, pyelonephritis, or vascular anomalies in the kidney. Severe louse or tick infestations may also cause chronic extracorporeal blood loss.

Chronic intracorporeal blood loss is difficult to identify and is usually the result of internal neoplasia or abscessation. Coagulation factor deficiencies (which may be congenital or due to liver failure), dicoumarin toxicity, and disseminated intravascular coagulation typically cause chronic low-grade intracorporeal (muscle, synovial joint, body) or extracorporeal (ecchymoses, epistaxis, hematuria, melena) bleeding. However, blood loss also may be acute. Platelet disorders, including congenital platelet disorders, disseminated intravascular coagulation, and immune-mediated thrombocytopenia, are associated with petechial hemorrhages as well as with internal and external hemorrhage.

THERAPY

Because the anemia is usually secondary, management of chronic blood loss necessitates identification and treatment of the primary disease process. Chronic extracorporeal blood loss rarely results in iron deficiency anemia in horses. Because the quantity of iron in the diet usually exceeds actual requirements, iron supplementation is generally not necessary. Parenteral iron dextran preparations can result in fatal reactions in horses and should be avoided. Oral dietary supplementation with ferrous sulfate is much safer than parenteral administration. Yearlings and weanlings with extracorporeal blood loss may benefit from oral iron supplementation since horses at this age have relatively small iron stores. Because acute hepatic failure and death have been reported in equine neonates given iron supplements, iron preparations should be avoided in foals less than 7 days old.

Supplemental Readings

Harvey, J. W., Asquith, R. L., Sussman, W. A., and Kivipelto, J: Serum ferritin, serum iron, and erythrocyte values in foals. Am. J. Vet. Res., 48:1348, 1987.

Jain, N. C. (ed.): Schalm's Veterinary Hematology, 4th ed. Philadelphia, Lea & Febiger, 1986.

Morris, D. D.: Review of anemia in horses: Part II. Pathophysiologic mechanisms, specific diseases and treatment. Equine Pract., 11:34, 1989.

Schmall, L. M.: Hypertonic saline therapy in horses and foals. In: Proceedings of the American College of Veterinary Internal Medicine, 1989, pp. 480–483.

Anemia Due to Inadequate Erythropoiesis

Michelle M. Henry, ATHENS, GEORGIA

Definitive diagnosis of anemia due to inadequate erythropoiesis requires cytological or histological (or both) evaluation of the bone marrow (see p. 491). Because the normal equine red blood cell (RBC) life span is approximately 5 months, these anemias are generally of mild to moderate severity and develop slowly. Anemia due to inadequate erythropoiesis may be caused by chronic disease, nutritional deficiency, myelophthisic disease, or bone marrow aplasia.

ANEMIA OF CHRONIC DISEASE

Anemia of chronic disease, the most common cause of anemia, may occur with any chronic infectious, inflammatory, or neoplastic condition. Systemic diseases in horses often associated with secondary anemia include internal abscessation; pneumonia; pleuritis; chronic liver or kidney failure; chronic bacterial, viral, or parasitic diseases; chronic immune-mediated diseases; and granulomatous diseases and internal neoplasia. These anemias are usually clinically silent, with the only clinical signs ascribed to the primary disease process.

At least three factors contribute to the development of anemia of chronic disease: (1) shortened RBC survival time, (2) sequestration of iron in the mononuclear phagocyte system, and (3) impaired bone marrow response to anemia. Hyperplasia and increased activity of the mononuclear phagocyte system in chronic inflammatory disease may result in an increased rate of RBC sequestration and destruction. RBCs may also be damaged or lysed as they pass through inflamed or injured tissue. Sequestration of iron in mononuclear phagocytes as hemosiderin, a storage form of iron less available for mobilization, contributes to impaired bone marrow responsiveness and low serum iron concentration during chronic disease. The decrease in serum iron concentration is accompanied by normal to decreased total iron-binding capacity (TIBC) and reduced per cent saturation of transferrin. Because iron is a crucial constituent of hemoglobin as well as a cofactor for several enzymes involved in erythropoiesis, iron sequestration suppresses erythropoiesis. Inadequate erythropoietin synthesis may contribute to anemia during chronic renal disease; however, no definitive evidence substantiates this proposal.

Therapy for anemia of chronic disease must be directed at the primary disorder. Because total body stores of iron are adequate, supplemental iron therapy is valueless and may be toxic.

ANEMIA FROM NUTRITIONAL DEFICIENCY

Nutritional deficiencies in protein, vitamins, or trace minerals that result in anemia are relatively uncommon in horses but may occur during starvation. Folic acid deficiency could potentially occur after long-term therapy with drugs that inhibit folate metabolism, such as trimethoprim, the sulfonamides, or pyrimethamine.

A deficiency in trace minerals—iron, copper, cobalt—is also quite rare in horses since legumes or soil have adequate concentrations of these substances. Trace mineral deficiency results in maturation defect anemia. Iron deficiency anemia is most common and usually secondary to chronic extracorporeal blood loss. Young foals, weanlings, and yearlings may be more susceptible to iron deficiency anemia because milk is a poor iron source and young horses have fewer iron stores than mature horses.

Early iron deficiency is characterized by normocytic, normochromic anemia, whereas microcytic, hypochromic anemia occurs with moderate to severe iron deficiency. The serum iron concentration and per cent transferrin saturation are usually decreased, with normal to elevated TIBC. Bone marrow cytology reveals a predominance of late rubricytes and metarubricytes and depletion of iron storage.

Treatment of iron deficiency anemia should be directed toward correcting the underlying disorder, which is usually chronic blood loss. Oral ferrous sulfate may be safely used after the seventh day of life, but generally good-quality forage is adequate treatment for iron deficiency. Parenteral administration of iron dextran to horses should be avoided.

APLASTIC ANEMIA

Aplastic anemia is a stem cell disorder that rarely occurs in horses. Typically, hypoplasia of all hematopoietic precursors results in pancytopenia, although selective erythroid aplasia has been reported in other species. Bone marrow aplasia may be due to (1) congenital or acquired failure of bone marrow stem cells to differentiate because of intrinsic damage or interruption of interaction with their microenvironment, or (2) immunologically mediated damage of normal precursor cells. Often the cause of aplastic anemia remains unidentified; however, predisposing causes in humans include bacterial or viral infections, chronic renal or liver disease, pregnancy, neoplasia, immune-mediated diseases, irradiation, estrogens, and drugs such as analgesics, antimicrobials, and sedatives. Phenylbutazone has been implicated as a cause of aplastic anemia in horses.

The clinical features of aplastic anemia are generally attributable to absence of granulocytes and platelets, which have a shorter life span than erythrocytes. Neutropenia increases susceptibility to bacterial infections, and thrombocytopenia often results in hemorrhage. The diagnosis of aplastic anemia depends on hematological evidence of pancytopenia, such as anemia, thrombocytopenia, and leukopenia, and cytological evidence of hypoplastic bone marrow. Bone marrow aplasia should be confirmed by histological examination of a bone marrow biopsy specimen. A positive Coombs test suggests an immune-mediated pathogenesis.

Treatment of aplastic anemia requires identification of the underlying cause. Recently used pharmacological agents should be discontinued or replaced by chemically dissimilar substitutes. Corticosteroids may be useful if an immune-mediated etiology is suspected. Additional therapy is largely supportive. Broad-spectrum antimicrobial coverage is indicated. Anabolic steroids and androgens promote hematopoiesis, but their efficacy in people with aplastic anemia is poor. The response of horses is unknown. Whole blood, platelet, or granulocyte transfusions should be reserved for life-threatening anemia, severe bleeding, or severe neutropenia. Although only a few cases of aplastic anemia have been reported in horses, the prognosis is generally poor.

MYELOPHTHISIC DISEASE

Myelophthisic anemia occurs when the normal bone marrow habitat is infiltrated by abnormal tissue. Primary myeloproliferative diseases (see p. 513) and secondary neoplastic invasion of the bone marrow, metastasis, result in proliferation of abnormal cells at the expense of normal hematopoiesis. Typically, a decrease in all marrow-derived elements results in peripheral pancytopenia. Because the life span of platelets and leukocytes is shorter than that of RBCs, clinical signs of thrombocytopenia or infection typically precede those of anemia.

The diagnosis of myelophthisic anemia requires bone marrow evaluation to demonstrate neoplastic cells and evidence of inadequate erythropoiesis. Treatment of myelophthisic anemia is only palliative, since primary hematopoietic neoplasia or neoplastic metastases to bone marrow are considered invariably fatal in horses.

Supplemental Readings

Berggren, P. C.: Aplastic anemia in a horse. J. Am. Vet. Med. Assoc., 179:1400, 1981.
Harvey, J. W., Asquith, R. L., Sussman, W. A., and Kivipelto, J.: Serum ferritin, serum iron, and erythrocyte values in foals. Am. J. Vet. Res., 48:1348, 1987.
Lavoie, J. P., Morris, D. D., Zinkl, J. G., Lloyd, K., and Divers, T. J.: Pancytopenia caused by bone marrow aplasia in a horse. J. Am. Vet. Med Assoc., 191:1462, 1987.
Morris, D. D.: Review of anemia of horses: Part II. Pathophysiologic mechanisms, specific diseases and treatment. Equine Pract., 11:34, 1989.
Weiss, D. J., and Krehbiel, J. D.: Studies of the pathogenesis of anemia of inflammation: Erythrocyte survival. Am. J. Vet. Res., 44:1830, 1983.

Hemolytic Anemia
Michelle M. Henry, ATHENS, GEORGIA

Hemolytic anemia may be acute or chronic, intravascular or extravascular. Most causes of red blood cell (RBC) destruction result in extravascular hemolysis. However, intravascular and extravascular hemolysis often occur simultaneously. Hemolytic anemia in horses may be immune mediated, oxidant induced, secondary to blood parasites, or associated with microangiopathy.

IMMUNE-MEDIATED HEMOLYTIC ANEMIA

Immune-mediated hemolytic anemia occurs when antibodies are bound to the surface of erythrocytes. Primary immune-mediated hemolytic anemia or true autoimmune hemolytic anemia occurs when antibodies are formed specifically against normal RBC surface antigens. Secondary immune-mediated hemolytic anemia occurs via antibodies that are aimed at elements coating the surface of RBCs. Because both forms of immune-mediated hemolytic anemia are indistinguishable clinically and are treated similarly, primary autoimmune hemolytic anemia and secondary immune-mediated hemolytic anemia will be discussed together.

Acquired autoimmune hemolytic anemia is probably quite rare, although isoimmune hemolytic anemia occurs in approximately 1 per cent of foals (neonatal isoerythrolysis), as well as after incompatible blood transfusions. Neonatal isoerythrolysis results when a mare produces antibodies directed against a foal's RBC antigen that she does not possess. Because there is essentially no transplacental antibody exchange during gestation, the foal is born normal and signs of hemolysis become apparent subsequent to the absorption of colostrum that contains anti-foal erythrocyte antibodies. The pathogenesis, clinical signs, diagnosis, and treatment of neonatal isoerythrolysis are described in detail on page 430.

Secondary immune-mediated hemolytic anemia is due to an immune response directed against elements coating erythrocytes that indirectly results in erythrocyte destruction. Possible sources of antigens that may coat erythrocytes include bacteria, viruses, parasites, neoplasms, chemical exposure, and drugs. Fortunately, such misdirected immune responses are uncommon. A well-known example of secondary immune-mediated hemolytic anemia in horses occurs subsequent to infection by the equine infectious anemia (EIA) virus. Because of the importance of EIA, it is discussed separately below. Neoplasia (particularly lymphosarcoma), protein-losing enteropathy, bacterial and viral infections, purpura hemorrhagica, and penicillin administration have been reported to cause secondary immune-mediated hemolytic anemia in horses.

CLINICAL SIGNS

The clinical signs of immune-mediated hemolytic anemia depend on the location, extent, and rapidity of RBC destruction. Antibodies from the IgG class are most commonly involved and usually result in extravascular erythrocyte destruction in the mononuclear phagocyte system via macrophage IgG Fc receptors. Antibodies from the IgM class are more efficient at fixing complement, which typically results in intravascular hemolysis. Icterus is often accompanied by clinical signs of anemic hypoxemia, including pallor, weakness, tachycardia, and tachypnea. Because hemolysis is usually extravascular, hemoglobinemia is uncommon.

In addition to anemia and hyperbilirubinemia, mature neutrophilia may be present. Examination of the peripheral blood may reveal anisocytosis, spherocytes, or siderocytes. Spherocytes, small, hyperchromic RBCs, are remnants of partial erythrophagocytosis. Siderocytes are hemosiderin-laden monocytes that have phagocytosed RBCs.

The most specific test for immune-mediated hemolytic anemia is the direct Coombs test using patient RBCs and a reagent containing anti-equine immunoglobulin. A positive test (agglutination) indicates that the erythrocytes are coated with immunoglobulin, complement, or both. Because the end point of the test is agglutination, autoagglutinated blood should not be tested. Rouleaux formation may be confused with autoagglutination but is distinguishable by dilution of the blood with saline (see p. 490). Available equine Coombs reagents have limited reactivity for different immunoglobulin classes and the Coombs test is frequently negative following a severe acute hemolytic episode (coated RBCs are destroyed in vivo) or recent corticosteroid therapy. The test is also temperature sensitive and erroneous results can occur if it is performed at an inappropriate temperature for the involved immunoglobulin. Because of these difficulties, a negative result on Coombs test does not preclude the diagnosis of immune-mediated hemolytic anemia.

THERAPY

Therapy must address all possible causes of immune-mediated hemolytic anemia. Any drugs should be discontinued. If bacterial infection is suspected, antimicrobial therapy should be continued with drugs from a chemically unrelated class.

If RBC destruction is severe (packed cell volume [PCV] less than 10 per cent), a blood transfusion may be necessary; however, compatible donors are often difficult to identify. Despite the etiology, corticosteroid therapy is generally indicated to decrease phagocytosis of antibody-coated RBCs by the mononuclear phagocyte system. Dexamethasone (0.005 to 0.2 mg per kg given intravenously [IV] or intramuscularly [IM] every 24 hours) should be used for severe acute cases. Once the PCV stabilizes, the dose of corticosteroid can be gradually tapered, usually by 5 to 10 per cent per day, to the lowest maintenance dosage possible, and preferably to alternate-day therapy. Prednisolone (2 to 3 mg per kg PO or IM every 12 to 24 hours) may be used for less severe cases or following dexamethasone therapy. Because corticosteroids are generally effective treatment for immune-mediated hemolytic anemia, there is little experience with the use of other immunosuppressive drugs in large animals.

Renal hypoxemia should be monitored by serial evaluation of serum creatinine levels. If the cause of the immune-mediated hemolytic anemia is not apparent, diagnostic efforts should be turned toward identification of occult infection or neoplasia once the patient has stabilized. Determination of the etiology not only assists in proper therapy to eliminate the source of antigenic stimulation, but also may determine the prognosis and feasibility of long-term therapy.

EQUINE INFECTIOUS ANEMIA

Equine infectious anemia (EIA) is a worldwide contagious disease of Equidae that is spread by blood-feeding arthropods. The etiological agent is a retrovirus that is closely related to the human immunodeficiency virus. Retroviruses have a single-stranded RNA genome and reverse transcriptase, an enzyme that allows the retrovirus to make complementary DNA to its own RNA genome. Once manufactured, the complementary DNA is inserted into the infected host cell's DNA genome, thus allowing synthesis of the proteins essential for viral replication. Once infected, horses remain viremic and lifelong carriers. The clinical signs of EIA wane when host-neutralizing antibodies restrain viral replication. Although neutralizing antibodies diminish overt clinical signs of disease, they are not capable of completely eliminating the virus. Persistent viral replication in the host results in emergence of novel antigenic strains of EIA and recrudescence of clinical signs. It is believed that viral replication occurs first in local phagocytic cells at the site of invasion. Release of virus from these cells results in viremia and dissemination to all parts of the body. Subsequent cell invasion with viral replication appears to have a predilection for cells of the mononuclear phagocyte lineage. It is hypothesized that infection of monocytes and macrophages, which are resistant to cytopathic effects of other closely related retroviruses, may provide a vehicle for viral persistence and dissemination.

Natural transmission of the EIA virus is primarily by hematophagous insects, but any transfer of blood from an infected to uninfected horse can result in dissemination of the disease. Tabanids, or horseflies, are the most effective natural vectors of EIA because of their feeding habits and their large mouth parts. If an insect's blood meal is interrupted, the likelihood of EIA transmission increases. Because of the pain associated with horsefly bites, interrupted feeding is likely. A single interrupted horsefly bite is sufficient for disease transmission. Because of the prevalence of insect vectors, the prevalence of EIA is high in the southern and eastern United States. Acutely ill horses are more infectious, owing to the severe viremia.

Transmission of EIA can occur transplacentally if the degree of viremia during gestation is great enough. An EIA virus carrier mare may either abort or deliver an infected or uninfected foal. Only approximately 10 per cent of foals delivered from carrier mares are viremic at birth and remain lifelong carriers. Because of the presence of maternal antibodies in colostrum, foals born to carrier mares will themselves be antibody positive at 24 hours of age. If the foal is also viremic at birth, neutralizing antibody titers will persist. Maternally acquired passive antibody should be undetectable by 6 months of age.

CLINICAL SIGNS

Acute clinical signs of EIA are usually associated with first exposure to the virus, although carriers may develop acute clinical disease with subsequent emergence of a new antigenic viral strain. Acute disease usually occurs 7 to 30 days following exposure and is characterized by depression, fever, and petechial hemorrhages. This acute stage is generally transient and may even go undetected but is often followed by recurring illness characterized by fever, edema, anemia, icterus, depression, and progressive weight loss. Most recurrences occur within 1 year of infection. The severity and frequency of the recurring clinical episodes usually decline with time. The bouts of illness may last a few days to several months. Mortality is uncommon, but may occur during an acute flare-up.

Most of the clinical signs of EIA are referable to the host's immune and inflammatory response to the viral infection. Fever, hemorrhages, and edema are thought to be associated with massive viral replication and destruction of vascular integrity subsequent to hypersensitivity vasculitis. Anemia is the result of immune-mediated hemolytic anemia associated with the attachment of viral particles to erythrocytes. Complement activation and opsonization of the virus-coated RBCs is enhanced by the presence of EIA-specific antibodies; the coated erythrocytes are then phagocytized by the mononuclear phagocyte system, resulting in icterus. The inappropriate bone marrow response typical of chronic infection exacerbates the severity of hemolytic anemia. The severity of the anemia depends on the stage of the disease but typically worsens with each clinical exacerbation. The PCV may return to normal between exacerbations.

DIAGNOSIS

Laboratory evidence of EIA virus infection is nonspecific for the disease. In addition to anemia and hyperbilirubinemia, mild thrombocytopenia, neutropenia, lymphocytosis, and monocytosis may occur. Examination of a peripheral blood smear during clinical exacerbations may reveal siderocytes. During periods of clinical quiescence, laboratory evidence of EIA may be limited to nonregenerative anemia and hypergammaglobulinemia from chronic viral antigenic stimulation.

Chronic EIA should be considered in any equid with a history of recurrent bouts of fever, anorexia, icterus, edema, anemia, and progressive weight loss. The most accurate and sensitive test for EIA is the serum agar gel immunodiffusion test, which detects neutralizing antibodies to the p26 viral core protein (Coggins test). These neutralizing antibodies persist for life, despite the emergence of new antigenic variants during serial replication in a carrier animal. False positive results on the Coggins test occur in foals that have acquired colostral antibodies from carrier mares. Passively acquired antibodies are usually lost by 6 to 9 months of age. Foals that were viremic at birth remain positive after 9 months of age. False negative titers occur in acute EIA (less than 45 days) when there has not been sufficient time for antibody production, and in approximately 5 per cent of horses with chronic EIA, especially inapparent carriers. To overcome erroneous results, repeat testing is recommended.

At necropsy, splenomegaly, hepatomegaly, and lymphadenopathy are seen. There is widespread lymphocytic infiltration and proliferation of mononuclear phagocytes. Immune complex deposition may result in glomerulonephritis, though typically not severe enough to cause clinical signs.

THERAPY AND PREVENTION

There is no effective means of eliminating the EIA virus from an infected horse. Treatment with IV fluids or blood transfusion is palliative. There is no vaccine available for EIA, so that prevention is aimed at identification and quarantine of infected animals. Any infected equid is capable of disease transmission, though this is most likely to occur during clinical episodes. Vector control may reduce transmission, though this is not as effective as geographic isolation of infected horses. Studies on horsefly behavior indicate that a 200-yard quarantine zone is effective in eliminating vector spread.

Frequent testing and quarantine or euthanasia of Coggins-positive horses is the most successful method of eradication. Although a national eradication program has not been established and intrastate regulations vary considerably (see Appendix III, p. 829), the interstate transport of infected horses is prohibited.

OXIDANT-INDUCED HEMOLYTIC ANEMIA

During the normal oxygenation of hemoglobin, an electron may be loosely donated from iron, converting it from the ferrous (Fe^{++}) to the ferric form (Fe^{+++}). When oxygen is released from hemoglobin, the electron is returned to the iron, and the ferrous form is resumed. If, however, the oxygen "escapes" with the electron, hemoglobin is left with iron in the ferric state, forming methemoglobin. Methemoglobin is incapable of binding oxygen, but under normal conditions there is constant reduction of methemoglobin via nicotinamide adenine dinucleotide phosphate and glutathione reducing pathways. Methemoglobinemia results from either congenital abnormalities of the metabolic processes involved with methemoglobin reduction, abnormal hemoglobin that resists enzymatic reduction, or toxic oxidation of the ferrous iron in hemoglobin. The latter mechanism is most commonly associated with methemoglobinemia in horses and results from the excessive ingestion of nitrites or wilted red maple leaves (*Acer rubrum*). Methemoglobinemia alone does not result in hemolysis. Some types of oxidant stress to erythrocytes cause the formation of disulfide bonds in sulfhydryl groups in the protein portion of hemoglobin. These disulfide bonds cause irreversible denaturation and precipitation of hemoglobin, resulting in the formation of spherical, refractile Heinz bodies. The Heinz bodies attach to the erythrocyte cell membrane, rendering the cell more susceptible to osmotic damage or removal by the mononuclear phagocyte system. Toxicoses with phenothiazine, onions (*Allium* spp.), or wilted red maple leaves result in Heinz body hemolytic anemia in horses.

CLINICAL SIGNS

The clinical signs of oxidant-induced hemolytic anemia depend primarily on the amount of oxidant ingested. Methemoglobinemia results in a characteristic chocolate-brown discoloration of the blood and a gray or bronze appearance of the mucous membranes. RBC destruction causes hemoglobinemia, icterus, and clinical signs of acute hypoxia. The urine is almost always discolored and may appear port wine colored or brownish black. The severe hypoxemia induced by the formation of methemoglobin or hemolysis may cause neurological signs such as dementia, ataxia, and blindness. Rapid deterioration may result in sudden death.

Red maple trees are found throughout the southern and northeastern portions of the United States. Clinical signs are apparent within 3 to 4 days of ingestion of a toxic quantity of leaves. The oxidant in red maple leaves is unknown. Clinical signs of wild onion or phenothiazine toxicity are apparent within 1 week. The toxic oxidant in wild onions is *n*-propyl disulfide; that in phenothiazine anthelmintics is phenothiazine disulfide.

DIAGNOSIS

The diagnosis of oxidant-induced hemolytic anemia depends on documentation of exposure to phenothiazine-containing anthelmintics, wild onions or wilted red maple leaves, characteristic clinical signs, and the presence of Heinz bodies on a blood smear. Only red maple leaves that have wilted are toxic, so that exposure is more common in the fall months. Nitrate toxicity is uncommon in horses, unlike cattle, because the equine colonic flora is less efficient than rumenal bacteria in metabolizing nitrate contained in plants to nitrite.

Heinz bodies can be demonstrated cytologically with new methylene blue stain. Because RBCs containing Heinz bodies are destroyed intravascularly or are removed by the spleen, absence of Heinz bodies does not preclude the diagnosis. The concentration of blood methemoglobin may be quantitated spectrometrically at 630 nm. Normal values for methemoglobin are less than 1 per cent, and levels above 65 per cent are fatal. Due to the nephrotoxic effects of hemoglobin combined with severe hypoxemia, acute renal failure may develop, resulting in azotemia and electrolyte derangements. Urinalysis typically reveals proteinuria and pigment-containing tubular casts.

THERAPY

Therapy is independent of the etiological agent, although identification of the cause is important to prevent further exposure. Chemotherapy with reducing agents such as methylene blue to reverse the ferric iron to ferrous iron in methemoglobin is relatively ineffective in horses and may actually enhance Heinz body formation. Corticosteroid therapy may decrease the phagocytosis of damaged RBCs; however, hypoxemia will persist since methemoglobin and Heinz body–containing erythrocytes are still incapable of carrying oxygen.

Therapy is mainly supportive and is dictated by the degree of anemia and severity of hypoxemia. In severe cases (PCV less than 10 per cent), a whole blood transfusion may be warranted (see p. 517). IV fluid therapy is generally necessary to ensure adequate renal perfusion and to correct electrolyte derangements. Renal function should be closely monitored and overzealous fluid therapy should be avoided as it may exacerbate the anemia by dilution. Simultaneous dopamine administration (3 to 5 μg per kg per minute) with fluid therapy may be beneficial in improving renal perfusion. Stress and unnecessary diagnostic procedures should obviously be avoided in these patients. Early administration of cathartics may reduce absorption of the toxic oxidants from the intestine of exposed individuals (see p. 346).

BLOOD PARASITES

EQUINE PIROPLASMOSIS

Equine piroplasmosis (babesiosis) is caused by the hemoprotozoan parasites *Babesia caballi* and *Babesia equi*. *Babesia caballi* has a worldwide distribution, including Europe, Asia, Africa, and Central, South, and North America. In the United States, *B. caballi* is endemic to Florida and Texas. *Babesia equi* has a more limited but similar distribution as *B. caballi*. It is rarely reported in the United States.

Babesia caballi is transmitted across the ovary by the one-host tropical horse tick, *Dermacentor nitens*. The tick host for *B. equi* in the United States has not been identified. Although the primary mode of transmission is by ticks, babesiosis can potentially be transmitted by other blood-sucking vectors or mechanically by unsanitary veterinary practices. The incubation period spans from 5 to 30 days.

Clinical Signs

Clinical signs of acute babesiosis include depression, fever, anorexia, icteric mucous membranes, ecchymotic hemorrhages, and edema of the extremities and ventral abdomen. Because parasitized erythrocytes are removed from the peripheral blood by the mononuclear phagocyte system, hemoglobinemia and hemoglobinuria are infrequent clinical signs. Death can occur within 24 to 48 hours, and mortality in acute outbreaks may be high. *Babesia equi* is considered to be more virulent than *B. caballi*. Horses raised in endemic areas are generally carriers of *Babesia* but rarely show clinical signs. The carrier stage may be established in foals while they are protected by passive maternal antibodies to *Babesia*. As maternal immunity wanes, active immunity develops gradually during constant exposure to the organism (premunity). Although premunity generally prevents clinical disease, these apparent carriers can develop signs of acute babesiosis when stressed.

Diagnosis

Babesiosis should be suspected in horses with typical clinical signs in endemic areas. The differential diagnosis of babesiosis includes other causes of hemolytic anemia, purpura hemorrhagica, and equine viral arteritis. A definitive diagnosis of babesiosis depends on demonstration of the organism in Giemsa- or Wright-stained blood smears or serology. Since parasitemia precedes fever, and parasitized RBCs are rapidly removed by the mononuclear phagocyte system, failure to demonstrate infested RBCs does not preclude a diagnosis. The complement fixation test for parasite antibodies is a more reliable diagnostic method and may be positive within 5 days after infection.

Therapy and Prevention

Babesia caballi can effectively be eliminated with imidocarb diproprionate° at a dosage of 2 mg per kg IM once daily for two treatments. Side effects of the drug include colic, salivation, diarrhea, and mild myositis at the injection site. Even at higher doses, imidocarb is only approximately 50 per cent effective in eliminating *B. equi*. Buparvaquone† is approximately 80 per cent effective in the treatment of acute clinical signs caused by *B. equi* but will not eliminate the carrier state. Buparvaquone is administered IV as a single dose (4 to 6 mg per kg.). Eradication of the carrier state should be aimed at elimination of the host and identification and isolation of carrier horses. A negative complement fixation titer is required of all horses entering the United States from endemic areas. Following treatment, horses may remain seropositive for 6 weeks to 8 months.

EQUINE EHRLICHIOSIS

Equine ehrlichiosis is caused by the rickettsial organism, *Ehrlichia equi*. Ehrlichiosis is endemic in the foothills of northern California, but sporadic cases have been reported in Colorado, Illinois, Florida, Washington, Pennsylvania, and New Jersey. The disease is most common in late fall, winter, and spring. Although the exact mode of transmission is unknown, equine ehrlichiosis is most likely spread by infected ticks. The incubation period ranges from 1 to 9 days.

Clinical Signs

The clinical signs vary according to the age of the horse. Signs are vague in horses less than 1 year old, with fever often the only clinical sign. Horses 1 to 3 years old develop fever, depression, limb edema, icterus, and ataxia. Horses over 3 years old appear to be most severely affected and may have mucosal petechiation, severely edematous limbs, and reluctance to move, in addition to the above signs.

Diagnosis

Diagnosis of equine ehrlichiosis is based on demonstration of the characteristic *E. equi* morulae in neutrophils and eosinophils with Giemsa or Wright's stain of peripheral blood smears. Serology (indirect fluorescent antibody test) can add support to a tentative diagnosis. Other hematological findings may include mild to moderate anemia, thrombocytopenia, and leukopenia.

Therapy

The mortality from equine ehrlichiosis is low and the prognosis is excellent with appropriate supportive care. The organism is sensitive to oxytetracycline (7 mg per kg IV every 24 hours) and therapy should be continued for 5 to 7 days to prevent relapses. Postinfection immunity persists for at least 2 years.

MICROANGIOPATHIC HEMOLYTIC ANEMIA

Microangiopathic anemia is caused by damage to erythrocytes as they circulate through abnormal vasculature. The damaged RBCs are morphologically characterized by an irregular shape and are called schistocytes. Microangiopathic hemolytic anemia is commonly secondary to microvascular thrombosis caused by disseminated intravascular coagulation, acute fulminant hepatic failure, glomerulonephritis (hemolytic-uremic syndrome), or hypersensitivity vasculitis. Microangiopathic anemia can also result when RBCs circulate through tortuous vessels or areas of turbulent flow caused by hemangiosarcoma or arteriovenous shunts.

°Burroughs Wellcome, Research Triangle Park, NC
†Coopers Animal Health, Berkhamstead, England

MISCELLANEOUS CAUSES OF HEMOLYTIC ANEMIA

Miscellaneous causes of hemolysis include chronic heavy metal toxicosis, dimethyl sulfoxide, and bacterial and snake venom lecithinases. Although rare in horses, chronic consumption of heavy metals such as lead, arsenic, and copper (see p. 363) or of some nonmetal elements such as selenium (see *Current Therapy in Equine Medicine 2*, p. 670) may cause hemolysis by disruption of the erythrocyte cell membrane structure. The severity of the clinical signs and anemia is dictated by the degree and rate of exposure. Because of its hydrophilic nature, dimethyl sulfoxide may cause hemolysis if given undiluted (in excess of 10 per cent) IV. Certain bacteria such as *Clostridium perfringens*, *Staphylococcus aureus*, and *Leptospira interrogans* are capable of producing lecithinases that alter RBC membranes, resulting in hemolysis. Finally, snake venoms such as rattlesnake, copperhead, and water moccasin venoms also contain phospholipases that disrupt the RBC membrane, leading to hemolysis.

Supplemental Readings

Blue, J. T., Dinsmore, R. P., and Anderson, K. L.: Immune-mediated hemolytic anemia induced by penicillin in horses. Cornell Vet., 77:263, 1987.

Clabough, D. L.: Review of equine infectious anemia. *In:* Proceedings of the American College of Veterinary Internal Medicine, 1989, pp. 562–565.

Mair, T. S., Taylor, F. G. R., and Hillyer, M. H.: Autoimmune hemolytic anemia in eight horses. Vet. Rec., *126*:51, 1990.

Madigan, J. E., and Gribble, D.: Equine ehrlichiosis in northern California: 49 cases (1968–1981). J. Am. Vet. Med. Assoc., *190*:445, 1987.

Morris, C. F., Robertson, J. L., Mann, P. C., Clark, S., and Divers, T. J.: Hemolytic uremic-like syndrome in two horses. J. Am. Vet. Med. Assoc., *191*:1453, 1987.

Tennant, B., Dill, S. G., Glickman, L. T., Mirro, E. J., King, J. M., Polak, D. M., Smith, M. C., and Kradel, D. C.: Acute hemolytic anemia, methemoglobinemia, and Heinz body formation associated with ingestion of red maple leaves by horses. J. Am. Vet. Med. Assoc., *179*:143, 1981.

Hemophilia

Ted A. Broome, GAINESVILLE, FLORIDA

Hemophilia A, the only form of hemophilia that has been identified in horses, is an inheritable disorder of the intrinsic coagulation pathway that results specifically from a deficiency in factor VIII coagulant activity (VIII:C). Factor VIII deficiency is inherited as an X-linked recessive trait by male offspring of clinically normal female carriers. The disease has been described in Thoroughbreds, Standardbreds, Arabians, and Quarter Horses, as well as in humans and several other animal species.

CLINICAL SIGNS AND DIAGNOSIS

Clinical signs of hemophilia are usually seen in colts from 3 days to 6 months of age, but there is one reported case of the disease in a 3-year-old Thoroughbred gelding. Affected horses have a bleeding diathesis characterized by large-vessel hemorrhage. The most common physical findings are hemarthroses and intramuscular or subcutaneous hematomas. The hemarthrosis may involve multiple joints; lameness is not necessarily present. Signs of abdominal pain, depression, or dyspnea may occur as a result of hemorrhage into body cavities. Epistaxis and hemoptysis are uncommon. There is an increased propensity to bleed following minor trauma or surgical procedures, which may rarely lead to fatal hemorrhagic shock. Intracranial hemorrhage is the most common cause of death in people with hemophilia A.

The diagnosis is based on laboratory evaluation of hemostatic function. Affected horses have a prolonged activated partial thromboplastin time (APTT) but a normal prothrombin time (unlike what is seen in warfarin toxicosis). Primary bleeding time, plasma fibrinogen, and platelet count are normal, ruling out disseminated intravascular coagulation and other causes for thrombocytopenia. The prolonged APTT can be corrected by addition of plasma from a normal horse. The diagnosis of hemophilia A is confirmed by the specific assay for factor VIII:C activity in plasma. Citrated plasma from the affected horse along with citrated plasma from a normal control horse should be submitted.* He-

---

*Comparative Hematology Labs., New York State Department of Health, Wadsworth Center for Labs. and Research, Albany, NY

mophiliacs usually have plasma factor VIII:C activity less than or equal to 20 per cent of normal concentration.

THERAPY

There is no cure for hemophilia. Repeated treatment is necessary to sustain life. Therapy is only palliative and is usually impractical in horses, owing to the recurrent nature of the disease, the progressively debilitating course, and the fact that the problem is heritable. Equine hemophiliacs can be treated during bleeding episodes with fresh plasma administered at a dose of 15 to 20 ml per kg initially followed by 7 to 10 ml per kg every 16 hours for 3 to 5 days. Cryoprecipitate or factor VIII concentrates are used to treat human hemophiliacs, but equine cryoprecipitate or factor VIII concentrates are not commercially available. Whole blood can be administered as needed during acute episodes if blood loss is severe. Affected horses should be kept in an environment that will minimize the chances of trauma and subsequent hemorrhage or hematoma formation. Hematomas may be treated with pressure bandages to limit their spread. Horses with hemarthroses should be rested until periarticular swelling subsides.

PREVENTION

Because of the poor prognosis for survival and the impracticality of treatment, attempts should be made to prevent the production of affected foals. Genetic counseling of breeders is important. Hemophiliacs are usually males resulting from the mating of a carrier female to a normal male. When this mating occurs, approximately one half of the male progeny are hemophiliacs and one half of the female progeny are carriers. The production of a hemophiliac female is unlikely since affected males rarely survive to breeding age. Carrier females perpetuate the disease and should be removed from the breeding population to prevent more births of affected foals. When hemophilia has been documented in a foal, the dam must be a carrier and should not be used for breeding. Without a definitive diagnosis, the mare remains only suspect. Factor VIII:C activity is usually 40 to 60 per cent of normal concentration in carrier mares; thus specific assays for factor VIII:C can be used for detection of carriers. The plasma concentration of factor VIII:C activity may be elevated from late gestation until approximately 2 months after foaling, which prevents accurate determination of the carrier state. Suspect mares should not be rebred for at least 60 days post partum and until the plasma factor VIII:C activity can be determined.

Supplemental Readings

Archer, R. K., and Allen, B. V.: True haemophilia in horses. Vet. Rec., 91:655, 1972.
Dodds, W. J.: Inherited hemorrhagic disorders. J. Am. Anim. Hosp. Assoc., 11:366, 1975.
Feldman, B. F., and Giacopuzzi, R. L.: Hemophilia A (factor VIII deficiency) in a colt. Equine Pract., 4:24, 1982.
Henninger, R. W.: Hemophilia A in two related Quarter Horse colts. J. Am. Vet. Med. Assoc., 193:91, 1988.
Mills, J. N., and Bolton, J. R.: Haemophilia A in a 3-year-old thoroughbred horse. Aust. Vet. J., 60:63, 1983.

Warfarin Toxicosis
Ted A. Broome, GAINESVILLE, FLORIDA

Warfarin is a coumarin derivative anticoagulant that has been used for the treatment of navicular disease and venous thrombosis in horses. Even when not overdosed, warfarin can result in toxicosis if administered concurrently with other protein-bound drugs such as phenylbutazone, or with anticoagulants. Warfarin toxicosis is more prevalent in the context of hypoalbuminemia or decreased dietary intake of vitamin K. Ingestion of feedstuffs contaminated with warfarin rodenticides may rarely lead to toxicity. Warfarin alters hemostasis by inhibiting the synthesis of vitamin K–dependent clotting factors II, VII, IX, and X. A deficiency in these clotting factors leads to decreased thrombin formation and subsequently reduced activation of factors VIII, V, and XIII; reduced platelet aggregation; and reduced fibrin generation. Factor VII has the shortest half-life of all vitamin K–dependent clotting factors and factor VII deficiency leads to an abnormality of the extrinsic clotting pathway. The prothrombin time (PT) is an indicator of extrinsic pathway function and is the earliest indicator of warfarin toxicosis.

CLINICAL SIGNS AND DIAGNOSIS

Clinical signs of warfarin toxicosis result from the increased bleeding tendency and may include epistaxis, hematuria, ecchymoses on mucosal surfaces, melena, and anemia. There is often hematoma formation following minor trauma or normal activity and increased hemorrhage following injections, wounds, or surgical procedures. Petechial hemorrhages, indicative of thrombocytopenia or vasculitis, are noticeably absent. A presumptive diagnosis is based on a history of warfarin therapy or possible exposure to contaminated feedstuffs in conjunction with one or more of the clinical signs listed above. A definitive diagnosis of warfarin toxicosis is based on laboratory findings of increased PT with normal platelet count and normal concentrations of fibrinogen and fibrin degradation products. Activated partial thromboplastin time, a measure of the intrinsic coagulation pathway, may become prolonged, but this occurs later in the disease due to the longer half-lives of factors II, IX, and X. Hemorrhage may occur before there is significant prolongation of PT, so that lack of abnormal laboratory findings does not rule out warfarin toxicosis when clinical findings support the diagnosis.

THERAPY

Treatment of warfarin toxicosis is aimed at eliminating the source of warfarin and returning hemostasis to normal. Warfarin therapy is immediately discontinued or contaminated feedstuffs are removed. Vitamin K_1 should be administered at a dose of 0.5 to 1.0 mg per kg subcutaneously every 4 to 6 hours until the PT returns to normal or clinical signs resolve. Treatment may be necessary for several days, owing to the continued absorption of warfarin from the gastrointestinal tract and the time necessary for clotting factor production. The PT should be monitored once daily for at least 3 days after it has reached the normal range to ensure maintenance of hemostasis. When there is severe hemorrhage, transfusions of whole blood equaling 20 to 40 per cent of the estimated deficit should be administered to maintain normal circulating volume and to quickly supply necessary clotting factors. Clotting factors can also be quickly replaced by the administration of fresh plasma at a volume of 15 to 20 ml per kg. Administration should be repeated if the PT again becomes prolonged. The use of fresh plasma is essential, because significant degradation of clotting factors may occur under normal storage conditions. Intravenous administration of vitamin K_1 should be avoided because of the potential side effects of hyperexcitability, sweating, tachypnea, hyperactivity, and ataxia. Vitamin K_3 should not be used because of its poor therapeutic value and potential for severe nephrotoxicity in the horse.

PREVENTION

Since warfarin should not be used in horses with pre-existing clotting disorders or liver dysfunction, a thorough physical examination and laboratory evaluation of hemostatic data and hepatic function should be performed prior to initiating therapy. PT should be monitored sequentially during warfarin therapy as an aid to the prevention of toxicity, especially in the dose adjustment period. PT can be accurately determined in commercial laboratories from citrated whole blood or plasma samples that have been stored at room temperature, provided they are received within 3 days of collection. A sample from a clinically normal control horse should be submitted concomitantly to ensure that results are not erroneous due to extreme variations in temperature during transportation to the laboratory. The dose of warfarin should be adjusted as needed to achieve no greater than a twofold increase in PT, a response that is considered to be an effective measure of warfarin therapy. PT is measured daily as the dose is adjusted and then twice weekly thereafter. Since warfarin is highly protein bound, once the effective dose is achieved, the additional use of protein-bound drugs, especially phenylbutazone, should be avoided. Protein-bound warfarin is inactive; thus displacement by other drugs will provide more free active warfarin. The concurrent use of other anticoagulants, such as heparin, should be avoided. Changes in diet from feedstuff high in vitamin K (alfalfa hay) to diets low in vitamin K (grains and poor-quality hays) should be avoided. If any of these management factors change during warfarin therapy, PT should be monitored more frequently until a steady state is ensured.

Supplemental Readings

Byars, T. D., Greene, C. E., and Kemp, D. T.: Antidotal effect of vitamin K_1 against warfarin-induced anticoagulation in horses. Am. J. Vet. Res., 47:2309, 1986.

Scott, E. A., Byars, T. D., and Lamar, A. M.: Warfarin anticoagulation in the horse. J. Am. Vet. Med. Assoc., 177:1146, 1980.

Scott, E. A., Sandler, G. A., and Byars, T. D.: Warfarin: Effects on anticoagulant, hematologic, and blood enzyme values in normal ponies. Am. J. Vet. Res., 40:142, 1979.

Thijssen, H. H. W., van den Bogaard, A. E., Wetzel, J. M., Maes, J. H. J., and Muller, A. P.: Warfarin pharmacokinetics in the horse. Am J. Vet. Res., 44:1192, 1983.

Vrins, A., Carlson, G., and Feldman, B.: Warfarin: A review with emphasis on its use in the horse. Can. Vet. J., 24:211, 1983.

Disseminated Intravascular Coagulation
Debra Deem Morris, ATHENS, GEORGIA

Disseminated intravascular coagulation (DIC) is a pathological process characterized by widespread fibrin deposition in the microcirculation with subsequent ischemic damage of numerous body tissues. A hemorrhagic diathesis ultimately develops owing to the consumption of platelets, clotting factors, and anticoagulant proteins along with hyperactivity of the fibrinolytic mechanism. DIC is never a primary disorder but represents a secondary complication of some underlying disease. In horses, DIC has been described in association with localized or systemic septic processes; disseminated neoplasia; gastrointestinal (GI) disorders such as strangulating intestinal obstruction, acute colitis, and protein-losing enteropathy; renal disease; and hemolytic anemia. Diffuse activation of the hemostatic system is particularly prevalent in horses with acute GI disorders that cause colic and is a likely initiating factor for laminitis.

PATHOGENESIS

Diseases initiate DIC by two major mechanisms: through generation of excessive procoagulant activity within the blood, or by injuring the vascular endothelium. Procoagulant substances released or generated by diseases that initiate DIC include tissue thromboplastin, phospholipids, adenosine diphosphate (ADP), leukocyte procoagulant activity, platelet-activating factor (PAF), and tumor products that directly activate clotting factors. Endothelial disruption by certain diseases, such as vasculitis, exposes collagen, which may directly activate platelets and factor XII as well as allow tissue thromboplastin to enter the blood. Many diseases act by more than one triggering mechanism, and factors that determine whether DIC develops include the nature and intensity of the procoagulant force, the concentration of natural coagulation inhibitors, and the functional capacity of the mononuclear phagocyte system.

In horses, DIC most frequently occurs secondary to diseases that cause endotoxemia. Gram-negative bacterial endotoxins directly damage vascular endothelium, exposing collagen or allowing tissue thromboplastin release. Factor XII is directly activated by endotoxins, and platelets are stimulated to produce thromboxane A_2 and undergo aggregation and the release reaction. The most important mediators of endotoxin-induced coagulation are released from stimulated leukocytes, macrophages, and endothelial cells. In response to endotoxins, these cells produce a procoagulant activity with actions identical to those of tissue thromboplastin. Neutrophils and other cell types produce a PAF that augments the numerous contributions of platelets to coagulation.

The pathogenic focal point for genesis of DIC is the elaboration of systemic thrombin. In addition to causing proteolytic cleavage of fibrinogen to fibrin monomers, thrombin activates factor XIII to render fibrin more resistant to fibrinolysis, enhances the cofactor activity of factors V and VIII, and induces platelet aggregation. The net result of exaggerated thrombin formation is widespread microcirculatory thrombosis leading to ischemic necrosis of organs. The natural coagulation inhibitors, antithrombin III (AT-III) and protein C, are consumed during DIC, resulting in a greater propensity for thrombosis.

Activation of coagulation stimulates a secondary increase in fibrinolysis, which attempts to prevent the consequences of diffuse microthrombosis. Fibrin has a high affinity for plasminogen as well as tissue plasminogen activator (tPA) and absorbs them during the course of DIC. Plasmin is subsequently formed that degrades fibrin deposits and releases fibrin degradation products to the circulation. Fibrin degradation products contribute greatly to the hemorrhagic manifestations of DIC because they have antithrombin activity, interfere with fibrin monomer polymerization, and cause platelet dysfunction. Systemic fibrinolysis may occur if plasmin is swept into the bloodstream after capillary reperfusion. Plasmin in the peripheral blood contributes to factor consumption by degrading factors V, VIII, XIIa, IX, and XI, and fibrinogen in addition to fibrin.

Any disease associated with endotoxemia has great potential to trigger and perpetuate DIC. In addition to the procoagulant actions of lipopolysaccharide, a plasminogen activator inhibitor is released that impairs fibrinolysis and increases microvascular thrombosis.

The mononuclear phagocyte system plays a vital role in the pathogenesis of DIC, because the tissue-fixed macrophages of the spleen and liver normally remove endotoxins, activated clotting factors, fibrin, and fibrin degradation products from the peripheral circulation. Shock and hypoperfusion of the liver and spleen or diseases associated with excessive tissue debris, such as sepsis and metastatic neoplasia, will reduce the function of the mononuclear phagocyte system and predispose to or perpetuate DIC. The thrombotic events of DIC may eventually cause mononuclear phagocyte system failure and a positive feedback "circular pathophysiology."

CLINICAL SIGNS

Coagulopathy often occurs in a compensated form in horses and is rarely attended by life-threatening hemorrhage; however, microvascular thrombosis and subsequent ischemia of vital tissues leads to organ malfunction, such as renal failure, which contributes to the morbidity and mortality of the primary disease process. Unfortunately, the signs of microvascular thrombosis are less specific and more difficult to recognize than hemorrhage; thus, DIC often is not diagnosed until late in its clinical course.

The kidneys are often affected by DIC and renal ischemia produces acute tubular necrosis, which poses a serious threat to life. Aside from oliguria, renal disease may be manifested by depression and ileus subsequent to azotemia and electrolyte imbalances. GI microthrombosis may induce colic due to submucosal necrosis and superficial ulceration. There may be occult fecal blood loss, but melena is rare unless there is a pre-existing strangulating obstruction or severe colitis. Pulmonary microvascular thrombosis may cause tachypnea and variable hypoxemia. Altered behavior or seizures may follow cerebral microvascular thrombosis, although neurological signs are not specific for or highly indicative of DIC. Microangiopathic hemolysis with subsequent hemoglobinemia and hemoglobinuria is rare.

The equine digit may be a site of predilection for microvascular thrombosis in DIC, and laminitis is the only clinical sequela in some circumstances. Laboratory evidence of DIC has been documented during the developmental phase of experimental equine laminitis. The tendency for thrombosis of major peripheral veins is another prominent manifestation of coagulopathy in horses. Often a jugular vein will undergo complete thrombosis within hours of only a routine blood sampling procedure. Spontaneous thrombosis of smaller cutaneous vessels also occurs. As the thrombotic stimulus continues or intensifies, a tendency for hemorrhage develops, characterized by petechial or ecchymotic hemorrhages on mucosae and sclerae and a tendency to bleed after venipuncture or minor trauma. Spontaneous epistaxis, hyphema, and melena are less common manifestations of DIC. Once there are signs of failure of blood to coagulate, the prognosis is very poor.

Horses with illnesses that produce a low-grade or intermittent procoagulant stimulus may develop a chronic, compensated form of DIC that is attended by few or no clinical signs. Localized sepsis (e.g., lung abscess), neoplasia, protein-losing enteropathy and immune-mediated disorders (e.g., vasculitis and anemia) are common initiating diseases. This compensated state may become imbalanced by stress, concurrent diseases, or worsening of the primary process, resulting in clinically obvious DIC.

LABORATORY FINDINGS

The laboratory reflection of DIC is determined by the balance between coagulation and fibrinolytic forces and by the integrity of the mononuclear phagocyte system at the time of blood sampling. Excessive coagulation is refected in reduced plasma concentrations of platelets, coagulant, and anticoagulant proteins and increased concentrations of coagulant byproducts. Fibrinolysis is indicated by elevated fibrin degradation products or reduced concentrations of fibrinolytic and antifibrinolytic proteins. Clarification of the most frequent laboratory abnormalities in horses with DIC is hindered by lack of a definitive diagnosis. A disseminated coagulopathy is manifested by multiple hemostatic abnormalities, and serial analyses should reveal reduced platelet numbers and a trend toward prolongation of the prothrombin time (PT), activated partial thromboplastin time (APTT), and thrombin time (TT), with a reduction in plasma AT-III levels. Elevated serum fibrin degradation products usually indicate DIC, but levels are often normal in the early or compensated form of the disease. Hypofibrinogenemia is uncommon in DIC of horses because the underlying diseases are usually proinflammatory.

DIAGNOSIS

Clinical signs and the clinical history suggest the possibility of DIC, and laboratory tests are only used to support the diagnosis. There are numerous laboratory tests of hemostasis that may be abnormal during DIC; however, no one test consistently and specifically provides a definitive diagnosis. Because of variable utilization, rates of synthesis, and half-lives of the different hemostatic proteins, abnormality on only one test may be observed on a single sample; therefore, repeated hemostatic testing is advised when DIC is strongly suspected. Multiple laboratory abnormalities that reflect procoagulant consumption or inhibition and enhanced fibrinolysis should be expected. The combination of thrombocytopenia with mild to moderate prolongation of the PT or APTT (or both) strongly suggests DIC. Reduced plasma AT-III levels and increased serum fibrin degradation products further support the diagnosis. Although plasma fibrinogen is rarely reduced, the TT is often prolonged as a result of inhibition by fibrinolytic end products. In subacute or chronic forms of DIC, the concentration of some procoagulants may actually be increased due to their function as acute phase reactants. The clinician should seek laboratory assistance when considering the diagnosis of DIC but should appreciate that the findings are not always helpful.

THERAPY

The only noncontroversial treatment modalities for DIC are directed toward identification and alleviation of the primary disorder, along with general supportive measures to combat shock and maintain tissue perfusion. Intravenous (IV) fluid administration helps to prevent organ dysfunction subsequent to microvascular thrombosis and can correct existing acid–base or electrolyte imbalances. Septic conditions should be treated with appropriate antimicrobial agents, and necrotic tissue and purulent exudate should be removed whenever possible. A horse with a strangulating intestinal obstruction requires immediate surgical intervention to resect nonviable bowel. Flunixin meglumine° at a dosage of 0.25 mg per kg IV three times daily helps mitigate the deleterious effects of endotoxemia. At this dose rate, flunixin has minimal analgesic effects that might mask colic. Corticosteroids are not indicated and may even worsen DIC since they reduce the phagocytic action of the mononuclear phagocyte system, thereby allowing fibrin degradation products to accumulate and potentiating the vasoconstrictor effects of catecholamines.

Once specific or supportive care for the primary disorder has been initiated, a clinical decision must be made as to whether or not these measures will allow spontaneous resolution of DIC without serious sequelae. If the patient has only "laboratory evidence of DIC" without active bleeding or thrombosis, supportive care and treatment of the underlying disease will usually suffice. Petechial hemorrhages or oozing from venipuncture sites also do not necessarily indicate a need for coagulant replacement. However, severe, life-threatening hemorrhage should be treated with fresh plasma (15 to 30 ml per kg IV) to replace utilized coagulant and anticoagulant proteins. Platelet concentrates may be useful if the platelet count falls below 50,000 per μl (see discussion of idiopathic thrombocytopenia, p. 507). Some physicians feel that transfusion without prior heparin administration adds fuel to the fire of thrombosis and will not effectively correct the deficiency state. This may be true when DIC is ongoing; however, if the triggering problem for DIC is improving, anticoagulant therapy is not a prerequisite to factor replacement. The platelet count and coagulation times should be determined at regular intervals during and after replacement therapy. If the platelet count is dropping or coagulation times are becoming longer, heparin therapy may be indicated before further replacement is given.

Heparin has been recommended in the treatment of DIC to inhibit the formulation of microthrombi that precipitate organ failure. Heparin's only anticoagulant effect is to accelerate the inhibitory actions of AT-III, primarily against thrombin and activated factor X. Therefore, the plasma concentration of AT-III must be adequate before heparin will have therapeutic benefit. Some physicians reserve heparin anticoagulation for patients with marked hypofibrinogenemia and hemorrhage not controlled by replacement therapy. The plasma AT-III concentration should

---

°Banamine, Schering Animal Health, Union, NJ

be measured prior to heparin administration and levels must be corrected if they are below the normal range. The infusion of plasma after a given dosage of heparin has had no apparent effect may worsen a hemorrhagic diathesis due to replenished AT-III. Suggested heparin dosages vary widely. A recommended dosage for bleeding that does not respond to plasma therapy is an initial 10 units per kg, followed by 15 units heparin per kg per hour by continuous IV infusion; or an initial loading dose of 30 to 40 units per kg. Once hemorrhage stops, heparin should be discontinued. Because massive defibrination is rare in horses, heparin is not recommended as a routine part of therapy for DIC. It has been estimated that only 5 per cent of human patients benefit from heparin therapy, whereas in the vast majority it is not helpful and can be harmful. Heparin in all species can predispose to hemorrhage, thrombosis, and thrombocytopenia; in horses, it causes anemia and erythrocyte agglutination.

The prognosis for DIC in horses is largely dependent on the nature and severity of the underlying disease and on how early and effectively the latter is treated. Once DIC has progressed to the stage where signs of blood incoagulability predominate, the prognosis is poor.

Supplemental Readings

Johnstone, I. B., and Crane, S.: Hemostatic abnormalities in equine colic. Am. J. Vet. Res., 47:356, 1986.
Marder, V. J., Martin, S. E., Francis, C. W., and Colman, R. W.: Consumptive thrombohemorrhagic disorders. In Colman, R. W., Hirsh, J., Marder, V. J. and Salzman, E. W. (eds.): Hemostasis and Thrombosis: Basic Principles and Clinical Practice, 2nd ed. Philadelphia, J. B. Lippincott, 1987, pp. 975–1015.
Morris, D. D.: Recognition and management of disseminated intravascular coagulation in horses. Vet. Clin. North Am. (Equine Pract.), 4:115, 1988.
Mosher, D. F.: Disorders of blood coagulation. In: Wyngaarden, J. B. and Smith, L. H. (eds.): Cecil Textbook of Medicine, 18th ed. Philadelphia, W. B. Saunders, 1988, pp. 1060–1081.
Weiss, A. W.: Acquired coagulation disorders. In: Corriveau, D. M., and Fritsma, G. A. (eds.): Hemostasis and Thrombosis in the Clinical Laboratory. Philadelphia, J. B. Lippincott, 1988, pp. 169–205.

Idiopathic Thrombocytopenia

Debra Deem Morris, ATHENS, GEORGIA

Thrombocytopenia, a platelet count less than 90,000 per μl, can result from one or a combination of three basic mechanisms: (1) decreased or ineffective platelet production, (2) platelet sequestration in the spleen, and (3) decreased platelet survival. Thrombocytopenia secondary to ineffective thrombocytopoiesis is rare in horses, but it has occurred in association with neoplastic infiltration of the marrow (myelophthisis, e.g., granulocytic leukemia) or aplastic anemia. Bone marrow aplasia may be immune mediated or associated with idiosyncratic drug reactions, cytotoxic agents, or radiation damage. Splenomegaly is accompanied by a mild reduction in the platelet count but is unlikely to result in a hemorrhagic diathesis. Shortened platelet life span is by far the most common cause of thrombocytopenia in horses and is generally a manifestation of disseminated intravascular coagulation (DIC). Systemic vasculitis or sepsis may rarely induce consumptive thrombocytopenia. Idiopathic or immune-mediated platelet destruction often results in equine thrombocytopenia.

PATHOPHYSIOLOGY OF IMMUNE-MEDIATED THROMBOCYTOPENIA

Idiopathic thrombocytopenia in horses may occur secondary to the administration of drugs, bacterial infections, viral diseases, other immunological disorders, or neoplasia. Drugs implicated in the pathogenesis of human idiopathic thrombocytopenia include thiazides, digoxin, gold, aspirin, heparin, quinidine, rifampin, penicillin, sulfas, tetracycline, and erythromycin. Thrombocytopenia has been reported in horses secondary to equine infectious anemia, lymphosarcoma, and autoimmune hemolytic anemia. Most cases of idiopathic thrombocytopenia in horses are primary and no underlying cause is found.

The clinical course and response to therapy in equine idiopathic thrombocytopenia resemble the disease in people and dogs, which is known to be immunologically mediated. Antibodies on the platelet surface result in premature platelet removal from circulation by the mononuclear phagocyte system. The antibody in most cases of idiopathic thrombocytopenia in humans is of the immunoglobulin (Ig) G class, directed against a platelet membrane antigen, and mediates platelet removal principally in the spleen. Complement-mediated platelet injury may induce hepatic platelet destruction in cases in which platelet-associated IgM predominates. The mean life of circulating platelets and the platelet count are inversely proportional to the quantity of platelet-associated IgG and complement components. The platelet membrane antigen to which autoantibody is directed may be evidenced at some stage of megakaryocyte maturation and autoantibodies may cause decreased platelet production, in addition to increased destruction.

In secondary idiopathic thrombocytopenia, the Ig bound to the platelet surface is usually part of an immune complex that is nonspecifically attached to the platelet Fc receptor. Thrombocytopenia generally abates following recovery from the primary disease or drug discontinuation, except in cases of gold hypersensitivity, in which thrombocytopenia may persist for weeks to years due to the slow release of tissue-bound gold. In rare cases, the platelet membrane may be altered by a drug or disease process. This exposes novel antigens that induce a syndrome similar to primary idiopathic thrombocytopenia.

CLINICAL SIGNS

Thrombocytopenia results in diffuse small vessel bleeding characterized by petechial hemorrhages on the oral, nasal, or vaginal mucous membranes and the nictitans or sclerae. Epistaxis, melena, hyphema, and microscopic hematuria may occur. Spontaneous hemorrhage is rare; however, prolonged bleeding from injections or wounds and hematomas following minor trauma is quite common when the platelet count drops below 20,000 per μl. The platelet count at which bleeding occurs seems to be determined by concurrent disease processes. Horses with primary idiopathic thrombocytopenia are usually bright and afebrile and may not bleed despite severely reduced platelet numbers. On the other hand, thrombocytopenic horses with sepsis or neoplasia are particularly susceptible to overt hemorrhage.

LABORATORY FINDINGS

Consistent laboratory abnormalities include severe thrombocytopenia (less than 40,000 per μl), prolonged bleeding time, and abnormal clot retraction. The clotting times and plasma fibrinogen levels are normal. Chronic blood loss may induce anemia and hypoproteinemia. Fibrin degradation products are often mildly increased (10 to 40 μg per ml) due to secondary fibrinolysis. Feces and urine may contain occult blood. In most cases of idiopathic thrombocytopenia, bone marrow examination reveals normal or increased megakaryocyte numbers, although in rare cases megakaryocytes may be reduced.

DIAGNOSIS

Clinical signs of small vessel bleeding and severe thrombocytopenia in the absence of other evidence of coagulation dysfunction constitute the basis for a tentative diagnosis of idiopathic thrombocytopenia. The definitive diagnosis of immune-mediated thrombocytopenia requires demonstration of increased platelet-associated Ig (or C3) or plasma antiplatelet activity. Methods that are used in other species to detect Ig or C3 on platelet membranes have not been adapted to horses. Indirect measurements of plasma antiplatelet activity, such as the platelet factor 3 test, have extremely low sensitivity in both animals and man, in part because the most avid antibodies are platelet bound. Response to corticosteroid therapy is supportive of the diagnosis.

Profound thrombocytopenia in a horse with minimal evidence of hemorrhage should be reevaluated. Spuriously low platelet counts may occur owing to improper blood collection, inadequate amount of anticoagulant, or platelet clumping induced by ethylenediaminetetraacetic acid (EDTA). Although rare, EDTA-induced platelet clumping seems to be a problem in patients with an underlying disorder such as colic, and the phenomenon persists during the course of the illness. In people, platelet clumping in EDTA is due to antibodies that react with platelets only in the presence of EDTA. Pseudothrombocytopenia caused by EDTA is documented if the platelet count is normal in a blood sample anticoagulated with 3.8 per cent sodium citrate.

THERAPY

Administration of drugs must cease. If a medication is absolutely necessary, the chemically most dissimilar substitute should be used. For example, penicillin should not be replaced by ampicillin but perhaps erythromycin. Persistent, life-threatening hemorrhage or hemorrhage into the central nervous system is an indication for transfusion of fresh whole blood (4 to 8 liters in a 500-kg horse), platelet-rich plasma, or platelet concentrate. Platelet-rich blood components may be produced by continuous flow centrifugation thrombocytapheresis using a blood cell separator° (2000 rpm; platelet-rich plasma at 5 ml per min). Three hundred ml of normal platelet-rich plasma yields approximately 8×10^{11} platelets, which increases the platelet count in a 500-kg horse by approximately 30,000 per μl. Platelet-rich plasma can also be produced by centrifugation of fresh blood collected in acid–citrate–dextrose solution, 3 to 5 minutes at 250 $\times$ g. Contact of blood or plasma with glass should be minimized so that platelet adhesion and activation do not occur. Storage of blood or plasma for more than 6 hours, even at 4° C, is attended by rapid loss of hemostatic activity.

Most horses with idiopathic thrombocytopenia improve when treated with glucocorticoids. Beneficial actions of glucocorticoids are to improve capillary integrity, impair mononuclear phagocyte system function, decrease the number and the avidity of macrophage Fc receptors, impair antiplatelet antibody production, impede platelet–antibody interactions, and increase thrombocytopoiesis. Dexamethasone† (0.05 to 0.2 mg per kg given intravenously [IV] once daily) usually results in an elevated platelet count within 4 to 7 days. Beneficial effects may not be totally obvious in laboratory tests for 1 to 3 weeks. Prednisolone‡ or prednisone (1 mg per kg given intramuscularly [IM] twice a day) may be tried, but some horses with idiopathic thrombocytopenia are only initially responsive to dexamethasone. Once the platelet count is above 100,000 per μl, the dose of dexamethasone can be reduced by 0.01 mg per kg daily, with close monitoring of the platelet count for a relapse. When prednisolone is used, administration is reduced to once daily, and subsequently the dosage can be reduced by 0.05 to 0.1 mg per kg per day. Prednisolone and prednisone have approximately 15 per cent the potency of dexamethasone and maintain blood levels half as long. When the dose of IV dexamethasone is less than 0.04 mg per kg per day (less than 0.3 mg per kg per day for prednisolone), oral (PO) dexamethasone or prednisone§ may be substituted at an equivalent dose rate. Corticosteroids should not be discontinued until the platelet count has been normal for at least 5 days. If the period of daily glucocorticoid administration has extended beyond 2 weeks, alternate-morning low-dose therapy (0.01 mg per kg dexamethasone or 0.07 mg per kg prednisolone) should be continued for an additional 10 days. Most horses with idiopathic thrombocytopenia have a good prognosis and usually recover after 10 to 21 days of therapy. This suggests that many cases are secondary, yet the initiating cause is rarely found. Chronic or recurrent idiopathic thrombocytopenia requiring prolonged glucocorticoid therapy has been reported.

Splenectomy has been variably successful for treatment of idiopathic thrombocytopenia in people and dogs that have become refractory to corticosteroids. Splenectomy has been used to treat idiopathic thrombocytopenia in horses, but the long-term outcome remains to be documented. The incidence of postsplenectomy sepsis in people warrants caution using this procedure in horses. Cytotoxic drugs have been moderately successful in treating unresponsive idiopathic thrombocytopenia in people. The vinca alkaloids, vincristine and vinblastine, appear to increase platelet production as well as induce immunosuppression. Vincristine‖ (0.01 to 0.025 mg per kg IV once or every 7 days) combined with glucocorticoids has been useful in treating idiopathic thrombocytopenia in horses that were refractory to corticosteroids alone. Cyclophosphamide¶ (1 to 5 mg per kg PO once daily) is used in people with idiopathic thrombocytopenia, but there is little experience with this drug in horses. Side effects of cytotoxic drugs include severe bone marrow suppression and subsequent increased susceptibility to sepsis. These drugs should be used with extreme caution and only after 7 to 10 days of nonresponse to corticosteroids.

Short-term or complete remission of idiopathic thrombocytopenia has been reported in people given 200 to 1000 mg per kg concentrated Ig daily for 2 to 5 days. Suggested therapeutic mechanisms include blockade of Fc receptor–mediated phagocytosis, steric hindrance to antibody binding, preventing C3 fragment binding, an absolute increase in T suppressor cells, and reduced B cell function. There are no commercially available sources of concentrated equine Ig, but high-dose Ig therapy is theoretically possible using equine plasma° with a known Ig concentration. Although high-dose Ig therapy presents less patient risk than splenectomy or cytotoxic drugs, 80 liters of plasma would be necessary to achieve the total Ig dose

---

°International Business Machines Corp., Cranbury, NJ
†Azium, Schering Animal Health, Union, NJ
‡Meticortelone acetate, Schering, Kenilworth, NJ
§Deltasone, Upjohn, Kalamazoo, MI

‖Oncovin, Eli Lilly, Indianapolis, IN
¶Cytoxan, Bristol-Myers, Evansville, IN
°Hi-Gamm-Equi, Lake Immunogenics, Ontario, NY

for a 500-kg horse. The expense would be significant. Danazol† (2.5 to 10 mg per kg PO daily for 1 to 3 months) has induced remission of idiopathic thrombocytopenia in some people and it may act synergistically with glucocorticoids. There is no experience with the use of this drug to treat idiopathic thrombocytopenia in horses.

Supplemental Readings

Byars, T. D., and Greene, C. E.: Idiopathic thrombocytopenic purpura in the horse. J. Am. Vet. Med. Assoc., 180:1422, 1982.

Gernsheimer, T., Stratton, J., Ballem, P. J., and Slichter, S. J.: Mechanisms of response to treatment in autoimmune thrombocytopenic purpura. N. Engl. J. Med., 320:974, 1989.
Marcus, A. J.: Hemorrhagic disorders: Abnormalities of platelet and vascular function. In Wyngaarden, J. B., and Smith, L. H. (eds.): Cecil Textbook of Medicine, 18th ed. Philadelphia, W. B. Saunders, 1988, pp. 1042–1060.
Morris, D. D., and Whitlock, R. H.: Relapsing idiopathic thrombocytopenia in a horse. Equine Vet. J., 15:73, 1983.
Payne, B. A., and Pierre R. V.: Pseudothrombocytopenia: A laboratory artifact with potentially serious consequences. Mayo Clin. Proc., 59:123, 1984.

†Danocrine, Winthrop Pharmaceuticals, New York, NY

Vasculitis
Debra Deem Morris, ATHENS, GEORGIA

Vasculitis is a general term that refers to inflammation of blood vessels of any size, in any location. Most equine vasculitis syndromes have characteristics of immune-mediated hypersensitivity vasculitis and are secondary to infection, neoplasia, or the administration of medications. Vasculitis is less commonly subsequent to direct vessel wall damage induced by viruses, chemicals, or endotoxins.

Generally, antigens from streptococci, influenza virus, and certain drugs such as quinidine initiate hypersensitivity vasculitis in horses. Immune complex deposition within vessels at areas of increased permeability is widely considered the major pathogenic mechanism for hypersensitivity vasculitis. Immune complexes activate complement, and the released C5a is a strong chemoattractant for neutrophils. Infiltrating neutrophils release proteolytic enzymes that cause vessel wall dysfunction, resulting in edema, hemorrhage, and infarction of supplied tissues. Arterioles and postcapillary venules just beneath the epidermis are typically involved and there is a propensity for lesion formation in the skin of the dependent body portions. Factors that determine which individuals develop hypersensitivity vasculitis are not well understood. The physical characteristics of immune complexes, the rates of immune complex formation and removal by the mononuclear phagocyte system (MPS), and complement disorders are likely important in the pathogenesis.

CLINICAL SIGNS

The clinical manifestations of vasculitis in horses include demarcated areas of dermal and subcutaneous edema, which often progresses to skin infarction, necrosis, exudation, and sloughing. The limbs, ventral abdomen, muzzle, and face are most often affected. The edema is not necessarily symmetrical and is commonly warm and painful to palpation. Mucosal hyperemia, petechial and ecchymotic hemorrhages, and ulceration are the next most common clinical signs. Fever is variable, while tachypnea and tachycardia are more consistent, likely subsequent to pain.

Edema, hemorrhage, and necrosis may rarely occur in the gastrointestinal tract, kidneys, muscles, joints, the respiratory tract, and the central nervous system, with resultant colic, diarrhea, weight loss, azotemia, lameness, dyspnea, ataxia, and so forth. Equine vasculitis is often attended by localized infections such as cellulitis and pneumonia, thrombophlebitis, and laminitis.

LABORATORY FINDINGS

Hematological and serum biochemical findings in horses with vasculitis are not specific and are determined by any underlying disease(s), length of illness, multiplicity of organ involvement, and secondary complications. Chronic inflammation is attended by neutrophilia, mild anemia, hyperglobulinemia, and hyperfibrinogenemia. The platelet count and clotting tests are usually normal.

DIAGNOSIS

A presumptive diagnosis of vasculitis is based on the sudden onset of subcutaneous edema that is not associated with local trauma or infection, hypoproteinemia, pleuritis, peritonitis, or congestive heart failure. The presence of mucosal petechial hemorrhages further substantiates the tentative diagnosis. The definitive diagnosis of vasculitis is made histologically. The most common inflammatory pattern in hypersensitivity vasculitis is neutrophilic infiltration and transmural fibrinoid necrosis of venules, capillaries, and arterioles in the dermis and subcutaneous tissue. Luminal thrombosis and infarction may be present. A very similar histological pattern is observed when vasculitis results from direct microbial invasion of or damage to the vascular wall.

Full-thickness punch biopsies (6 mm) of the skin in an affected area, preserved in 10 per cent formalin, are the appropriate samples for histological examination. Because lesions may have a patchy distribution, multiple biopsies from different sites are optimal. One or more biopsy specimens should be preserved in Michele's transport medium and submitted for direct immunofluorescence analysis to identify immune complexes or complement in vessel walls. Immune complexes survive only transiently and histological lesions may be missed in biopsy specimens; therefore, the diagnosis of vasculitis may be made on clinical grounds with appropriate history and response to therapy.

ETIOLOGY AND CLINICAL SYNDROMES

Characterized cutaneous vasculitis syndromes in horses include equine purpura hemorrhagica, equine viral arteritis, equine infectious anemia (EIA), and equine ehrlichiosis.

Although the etiology remains unproven, equine purpura hemorrhagica, the most common vasculitis in horses, is thought to be an allergic reaction to streptococcal or viral antigens. Typically, respiratory tract infection by *Streptococcus equi* (strangles) precedes clinical signs of equine purpura hemorrhagica by 2 to 4 weeks, and immune complexes containing IgA and the M protein of *Streptococcus equi* have been demonstrated in the sera of affected horses. Respiratory infections by *Streptococcus zooepidemicus* or equine influenza may cause equine purpura hemorrhagica, or the latter may occur when a previously sensitized horse is exposed to other horses with respiratory infections. A very similar syndrome may occur subsequent to drug-induced allergy or, rarely, neoplasia. The diagnosis of equine purpura hemorrhagica is based on history and clinical signs in most cases.

The retrovirus that causes EIA establishes permanent infection and stimulates a continuous immune response that may result in immune-mediated anemia and thrombocytopenia, as well as systemic necrotizing vasculitis. Classical signs of acute EIA include fever, anemia, icterus, petechial hemorrhages, ventral edema, and weight loss. The diagnosis of EIA is confirmed by agar-gel immunodiffusion (Coggins) test for serum antibodies to the virus (see p. 497).

Infection with *Ehrlichia equi*, a rickettsial agent transmitted by ticks, is most common in northern California but has been reported in numerous other states. Clinical signs include fever, depression, anorexia, limb edema, mucosal petechiae, ataxia, and reluctance to move. The diagnosis is based on identification of characteristic cytoplasmic inclusions in granulocytes of affected horses (see p. 500).

The etiological agent of equine viral arteritis, a non-arthropod-borne togavirus, causes vasculitis by direct invasion of and proliferation in blood vessel walls. Infection by the equine viral arteritis virus is more common than clinical disease, although pregnant mares are uniquely susceptible. The virus is usually transmitted via inhalation of infected secretions, such as urine and nasal exudate; however, venereal transmission can occur. Clinical signs of equine viral arteritis include fever, anorexia, serous nasal discharge, lacrimation, and chemosis, in addition to edema of the limbs and ventral abdomen. Pregnant mares infected in the last third of gestation often abort. Diagnosis of equine viral arteritis is based on isolation of the virus from nasopharyngeal swabs or buffy coat cells, or seroconversion within 10 to 14 days of infection. Stallions may become persistent carriers and shedders of the virus (see p. 322).

Poorly defined vasculitis syndromes of uncharacterized etiology and pathogenesis, with unpredictable clinical course and response to therapy, occur. Signs may include alopecia, erythema, hyperkeratosis, and hypopigmentation of the skin, with or without edema and hemorrhages.

THERAPY

Treatment of vasculitis includes removing a known antigenic stimulus, providing supportive care, reducing vessel wall inflammation, and reducing any abnormal immune response. For diseases that are known to be self-limiting (equine viral arteritis, equine ehrlichiosis) or cannot be cured (EIA, neoplasia), therapy is palliative. Severe edema can be minimized with aggressive hydrotherapy and pressure wraps on the distal limbs. Polyionic fluids, given either intravenously (IV) or via nasogastric tube, may be necessary for horses that fail to drink or those that develop sufficient pharyngeal edema to have dysphagia. Severe upper respiratory tract edema and stridor may indicate the need for tracheostomy. Furosemide* (1 mg per kg given intramuscularly [IM] or IV) can be used to institute an initial reduction of edema; however, diuretic therapy should only be used in well-hydrated horses that have access to salt and mineral supplementation. There will be no long-term benefit from furosemide administration, since the edema of vasculitis is inflammatory in nature. Nonsteroidal anti-inflammatory drugs such as phenylbutazone† (2 to 4 mg per kg IV or per os [PO] twice daily) and flunixin meglumine‡ (1 mg per kg IV or PO twice daily) are useful to reduce inflammation and provide analgesia. Antimicrobial therapy is often indicated to reduce the incidence or severity of cellulitis, pneumonia, thrombophlebitis, or other septic sequelae. Skin necrosis on the distal limbs often is followed by the growth of exuberant granulation tissue that may require management by surgical excision, pressure wraps, and even skin grafting.

Vasculitides of uncertain etiology such as equine purpura hemorrhagica may be difficult to treat because the antigenic stimulus remains undefined and is not easily eliminated. Any medication should be discontinued and an underlying infection must be ruled out. Horses with a known streptococcal infection require treatment with penicillin (22,000 IU per kg procaine penicillin G given IM twice daily; or potassium penicillin G given IV every 4 hours) for at least 14 days, and accessible abscesses must be drained. In most cases of equine purpura hemorrhagica, the sensitizing infection has resolved. Clinical evidence suggests that systemic glucocorticoids in addition to supportive care are indicated in the treatment of equine purpura hemorrhagica and idiopathic vasculitis syndromes in horses. The beneficial actions of corticosteroids in vasculitis include a potent anti-inflammatory effect by reducing the release of arachidonic acid and subsequent formation of eisosanoids; reduced immunoglobulin production, which alters the ratio of antigen to antibody in the circulation, rendering immune complexes more soluble or more easily removed by the MPS; and increased release of tissue plasminogen activator, which reduces thromboembolic occlusion of the microvasculature. Dexamethasone* (0.05 to 0.2 mg per kg IV or IM once daily in the morning) should be administered at the dosage necessary to effect significant reduction of edema. Prednisolone† (0.5 to 1 mg per kg IM twice daily) may be substituted for dexamethasone but often is not as effective.

Once edema starts to resolve, the dose of glucocorticoids can be gradually reduced (dexamethasone by 0.01 mg per kg daily) over a period of 7 to 21 days, with close monitoring for exacerbation of clinical signs. When the dose of dexamethasone is below 0.04 mg per kg per day, the drug may be given orally or replaced by oral prednisone‡ at an equivalent dose rate. Generally, prednisolone or prednisone have 15 per cent the potency of dexamethasone and maintain blood levels for half as long. Some cases require 4 to 8 weeks of glucocorticoid therapy, and occasional horses relapse despite continued treatment. Some affected horses will stabilize on a certain dose of steroid but have a recrudescence of signs when the dose is reduced. Too rapid a reduction in dosage or premature discontinuation of glucocorticoid therapy may result in death due to edema of the airways. Any horse that has received pharmacological dosages of glucocorticoids (e.g., more than 0.04 mg per kg dexamethasone daily) for more than 14 days should receive 0.01 mg per kg dexamethasone or equivalent every 48 hours for an additional 10 days to prevent signs of adrenocortical insufficiency.

Antimicrobials are indicated throughout the period of daily glucocorticoid therapy to reduce the incidence of secondary sepsis. The spectrum should be broadened from penicillin if gram-negative organisms are suspected or have been identified.

---

*Lasix 5%, American Hoechst Corp., Somerville, NJ
†Butler Co., Columbus, OH
‡Banamine, Schering-Plough Animal Health, Kenilworth, NJ

*Azium, Schering-Plough Animal Health, Kenilworth, NJ
†Meticortelone acetate, Schering-Plough Animal Health, Kenilworth, NJ
‡Deltasone, Upjohn, Kalamazoo, MI

PROGNOSIS

The prognosis for vasculitis not associated with EIA or neoplasia is fair when therapy starts early and is aggressive. Most horses recover within 3 weeks; however, numerous sequelae often prolong the convalescence. Laminitis and infections such as cellulitis, pneumonia, and colitis are common and seem to be directly correlated with the necessary length of corticosteroid therapy. Some horses with idiopathic vasculitis show incomplete response to therapy and have an unpredictable, poor prognosis.

Supplemental Readings

Madigan, J. E., and Gribble, D.: Equine ehrlichiosis in northern California: 49 cases (1968–1981). J. Am. Vet. Med. Assoc., 190:445, 1987.

Morris, D. D.: Cutaneous vasculitis in horses: 19 cases (1978–1985). J. Am. Vet. Med. Assoc., 191:460, 1987.

Smiley, J. D., and Moore, S. E.: Immune-complex vasculitis: Role of complement and IgG-Fc receptor functions. Am. J. Med. Sci., 298:267, 1989.

Tashjian, R. J.: Transmission and clinical evaluation of an equine infectious anemia herd and their offspring over a 13-year period. J. Am. Vet. Med. Assoc., 184:282, 1984.

Traub-Dargatz, J. L., Ralston, S. L., Collins, J. K., Bennett, D. G., and Timoney, P. J.: Equine viral arteritis. Compend. Cont. Educ. Pract. Vet., 7(9):S450, 1985.

Lymphoproliferative and Myeloproliferative Disorders

Chrysann Collatos, ATHENS, GEORGIA

LYMPHOSARCOMA

Lymphosarcoma is the most common tumor of the equine hematopoietic system. It accounts for 1 to 3 per cent of all equine tumors, but it may be the most common cause of neoplasia-associated deaths in horses. Four classes of equine lymphosarcoma have been described: generalized, alimentary, mediastinal, and cutaneous. However, metastasis of the primary tumor is common, with subsequent multiple organ system involvement and variable, nonspecific clinical signs. No breed or sex predilection is known. Although 50 per cent of reported cases have involved horses 4 to 9 years old, equine lymphosarcoma has been diagnosed in horses ranging in age from 4 months to 22 years. The etiology of lymphosarcoma in horses is unknown.

CLINICAL SIGNS

The signs noted most commonly, regardless of the tumor site(s), are anorexia, weight loss, depression, and ventral edema. Lymphadenopathy, pyrexia, and concurrent infections may be present. Immune-mediated hemolytic anemia and thrombocytopenia occasionally occur, and monoclonal gammopathy and cryoglobulinemia have been reported. Additional clinical signs are related to organ pathology associated with specific tumor location. Deterioration typically is rapid following the onset of clinical signs.

Generalized Form

The most commonly affected tissues, in decreasing order of frequency, are lymph nodes, liver, spleen, intestine, kidney, and lung. Neoplastic lymphocytes may also invade the upper respiratory tract, spinal cord, heart, reproductive organs, brain, and retrobulbar spaces. Clinical signs such as icterus, neurological deficits, upper airway obstruction, tachycardia, or dyspnea reflect specific organ involvement. Lymphadenopathy is common but usually localized, and often is only internal.

Alimentary Form

Diffuse involvement of the small intestine is reported most commonly, although the stomach and large colon may be affected. Discrete masses associated with the gastrointestinal (GI) tract do occur. In the diffuse form, neoplastic cells initially invade the intestinal mucosa, and mesenteric lymph nodes are almost always involved. Metastasis tends to occur late in the course of disease. Diarrhea rarely is present. Weight loss, anorexia, ventral edema, and mild colic predominate. Acute abdominal crisis may follow mechanical obstruction by a neoplastic mass.

Mediastinal Form

Englargement of mediastinal lymph nodes secondary to tumor invasion may compress intrathoracic structures. Associated clinical signs include venous distention with jugular pulses or dyspnea due to pleural effusion or tracheal compression (or both). Signs of lower respiratory disease may be due to pulmonary parenchymal involvement or secondary bacterial infection.

Cutaneous Form

Multifocal, firm subcutaneous nodules without inflammation or alopecia may be present for extended periods prior to the onset of systemic disease. Clinical signs usually are related to tumor metastasis to additional organ systems.

DIAGNOSIS

A definitive diagnosis of lymphosarcoma requires identification of neoplastic lymphocytes in tissue, body cavity effusion, peripheral blood, or bone marrow. Neoplastic cells tend to resemble large, relatively well-differentiated lymphocytes. Nuclear chromatin clumping, prominent nucleoli, and cytoplasmic basophilia may be observed. Neoplastic cells are not commonly detected in the peripheral blood, and the total lymphocyte count is variable but frequently normal. Bone marrow involvement is rare; a single case of primary lymphoid leukemia without an associated tumor mass has been reported.

Because affected tissues are frequently internal and the presence of abnormal lymphocytes in the peripheral blood is uncommon, lymphosarcoma can prove an elusive diagnosis. In addition, the presence of nonspecific clinical signs results in a long list of differential diagnoses that must be ruled out if neoplastic cells cannot be found.

Approximately half of the horses with lymphosarcoma exhibit neutrophilia, hypergammaglobulinemia, and hyperfibrinogenemia. Normocytic, normochromic anemia is common. Hypoalbuminemia is variably present. Chronic inflammatory processes, such as abdominal or thoracic abscessation or verminous infestation, must be ruled out. Palpation per rectum may reveal an abdominal mass or enlarged mesenteric lymph nodes, but these findings are not specific. Equine infectious anemia and purpura hemorrhagica must be considered in horses with peripheral edema, pyrexia, and anemia. Patients with granulomatous enteritis and squamous cell carcinoma may exhibit nonspecific GI signs, including weight loss.

A thorough, systematic approach, beginning with a meticulous physical examination, is central to the successful diagnosis of lymphosarcoma. Repeated rectal examinations, abdominocenteses, and thoracocenteses may be warranted as other diagnoses are eliminated. Cytospin preparations of body cavity effusions should be examined for neoplastic cells. Ultrasonography is useful both for evaluation of internal organs and for guiding biopsies. Whenever possible, excisional biopsy specimens are preferable to fine needle aspirates or needle biopsy specimens. Tissue of interest should be submitted in 10 per cent formalin.

THERAPY

Successful long-term treatment of lymphosarcoma has not been reported in the horse. Transient improvement in signs may be associated with corticosteroid therapy. The mass of tumor burden, the debilitated condition of the patient by the time of diagnosis, and the cost of chemotherapy have precluded therapy for equine lymphosarcoma to date.

MYELOGENOUS LEUKEMIAS

The myelogenous leukemias are distinguished by unregulated proliferation and incomplete differentiation of primitive bone marrow stem cell clones. Leukemias are classified by the histochemical characteristics of the predominant neoplastic cell type present in the bone marrow. In the acute leukemias, poorly differentiated cell types predominate, while more mature myeloid cells accumulate in the chronic leukemias.

Although quite rare in horses, forms of acute and chronic leukemia do occur. Reported cases include acute myelomonocytic, acute monocytic, chronic myelogenous, and eosinophilic leukemia. Affected animals have ranged in age from 10 months to 9 years, with no breed or sex predilection.

CLINICAL SIGNS

The duration of signs prior to diagnosis in horses with myelogenous leukemia ranges from 2 weeks to 4 months. In all reported cases, horses had pitting edema of the hind limbs with or without ventral midline involvement, petechial hemorrhages on mucous membranes, and depression. Other frequently observed signs include pyrexia, weight loss, lymphadenopathy, coagulopathy, and signs of infection, particularly pulmonary infection.

DIAGNOSIS

Suspicion of myelogenous leukemia often arises following the observation of pleomorphic, poorly differentiated leukocytes in a peripheral blood smear. Leukocytosis or leukopenia may be present, frequently accompanied by normocytic normochromic anemia and thrombocytopenia. Definitive diagnosis is made by cytological examination of a bone marrow aspirate. Electron microscopy and special stains to detect specific enzyme activities aid in the classification of the leukemia. Increased serum iron levels and decreased iron-binding capacity reflect a state of bone marrow suppression.

THERAPY

Treatment was attempted in one horse with acute myelomonocytic leukemia. Cytosine arabinoside was administered twice daily for 21 days at a dosage of 10 mg per sq m body surface (0.3 mg per kg). The horse's condition continued to deteriorate despite therapy. Bone marrow aspirates obtained after 21 days of therapy were similar to those evaluated at the time of diagnosis, and the horse was killed 7 days later. The rapid clinical deterioration of horses with leukemia is due to the massive leukemic cell burden already present at the time of diagnosis.

PLASMA CELL MYELOMA

The plasma cell myelomas are myeloproliferative diseases characterized by uncontrolled proliferation of a clone of plasma cells. The product of this cell clone is called a paraprotein or M protein which may be a complete immunoglobulin, a single light chain, or a heavy chain fragment that is not immunologically functional. The conditions are rare in horses, but multiple myeloma, solitary plasma cell tumor, and monoclonal gammopathy have been reported. Multiple myeloma, a primary disease of the marrow, occurs most frequently. Affected animals have ranged in age from 3 months to 22 years. No breed or sex predilection is known. Paraproteins of the IgG(T) class and aggregation immunoglobulin classes have been identified in horses.

CLINICAL SIGNS

Signs associated with plasma cell myeloma are related to organ infiltration by neoplastic cells or to systemic effects of the immunoglobulin produced. Clinical signs in horses include weight loss, anorexia, lameness, neurological deficits, renal disease, bleeding diathesis, and chronic infections.

Lameness and neurological deficits may occur secondary to osteolysis via an osteoclast-activating factor produced by myeloma cells. Direct bony invasion by neoplastic tissue also is possible. Hypercalcemia in combination with glomerular infiltration by paraprotein may contribute to renal disease. Circulating paraproteins can coat platelets and interfere with clotting factors, resulting in bleeding dyscrasias. Bone marrow suppression may result in anemia and thrombocytopenia. Infection is the most common cause of death in affected people. Chronic infections result from decreased production and function of normal immunoglobulins as well as progressive bone marrow obliteration by neoplastic cells.

DIAGNOSIS

The vast majority of horses with nonspecific signs of systemic illness, hyperproteinemia, and anemia are affected by a chronic inflammatory process. Serum protein electrophoresis will identify patients with plasma cell myelomas by the presence of a monoclonal γ-globulin peak. Horses with inflammatory processes generally exhibit a polyclonal hypergammaglobulinemia. A definitive diagnosis of multiple myeloma requires the identification of at least 10 per cent plasma cells in a bone marrow aspirate, in addition to a monoclonal gammopathy.

Horses with suspected plasma cell myeloma should be further evaluated with a complete blood cell (CBC) count, platelet count, serum calcium and creatinine concentrations, urinalysis, and radiography of the long bones and vertebral column. The detection of circulating plasma cells is rare. Typical "punched-out" radiolucencies on skeletal survey radiographs and the presence of proteinuria further support the diagnosis. Bence Jones proteinuria, characterized by a low molecular weight light chain paraprotein in urine, is uncommon in horses.

THERAPY

The treatment of multiple myeloma in humans involves chemotherapy, radiation, and supportive care. The most commonly used chemotherapeutic agents are prednisolone and melphalan, an alkylating agent. Plasmapheresis may be considered if hyperviscosity due to circulating paraproteins causes clinical signs, but this is more common in IgM-mediated disorders.

Melphalan was used in one 20-year-old horse with IgG class multiple myeloma at a rate of 7 mg per sq m (approx. 0.22 mg per kg) once a day orally (PO) for 5 days every 3 weeks. Therapy was continued for 4 months. While no decrease in total protein concentration or improvement in persistent leukopenia was observed, this horse's clinical condition remained stable for 1 year following diagnosis. All other horses reported to have plasma cell myeloma died within 3 months of diagnosis. The median survival of humans and dogs undergoing therapy for multiple myeloma is between 1.5 and 3 years.

Prophylactic antimicrobial therapy is recommended during chemotherapy. The use of intravenous (IV) catheters should be avoided when possible, and strict aseptic technique is recommended during invasive procedures.

ERYTHROCYTOSIS

Erythrocytosis (also termed polycythemia) is a condition defined by the presence of an elevated red blood cell (RBC) count, hemoglobin concentration, and packed cell volume (PCV). Relative erythrocytosis occurs when the packed cell volume is elevated, but total RBC mass remains normal. Dehydration and splenic contraction are the most common causes of relative erythrocytosis in horses. Absolute erythrocytosis, with persistently elevated PCV and RBC mass, is exceptionally rare in horses.

Primary absolute erythrocytosis, or polycythemia vera, is a myeloproliferative disease of erythroid precursors. Increased erythropoietin production causes secondary absolute erythrocytosis, which may be an appropriate response to tissue hypoxia due to cardiac insufficiency, hemoglobinopathy, or residence at high altitude. Alternatively, inappropriately increased erythropoietin production with secondary erythrocytosis may accompany certain neoplastic processes or chronic renal diseases.

Secondary absolute erythrocytosis was definitively diagnosed in a yearling horse with hepatocellular carcinoma by the presence of increased serum and tumor tissue erythropoietin concentrations and persistent erythrocytosis. Erythrocytosis was described in another horse with no detectable underlying disease and normal serum erythropoietin concentration, suggesting a primary condition.

CLINICAL SIGNS

Clinical signs associated with erythrocytosis are either related to the underlying disease process or, more commonly, to the hyperviscosity that accompanies polycythemia. Erythema of mucous membranes, hemorrhage (such as epistaxis and hyphema), neurological signs (such as lethargy and seizures), and cardiopulmonary signs are common.

DIAGNOSIS

Relative erythrocytosis is diagnosed if resolution follows IV administration of fluids. Absolute erythrocytosis does not respond to hydration. Further workup of the cause for absolute erythrocytosis includes a CBC count, arterial blood gas determinations, cardiopulmonary examination, renal and hepatic evaluation, RBC mass quantitation, serum erythropoietin concentration, bone marrow aspirate, hemoglobin-oxygen saturation, and erythrocyte 2,3-diphosphoglycerate (DPG) measurement.

THERAPY

Treatment of absolute erythrocytosis should be directed toward alleviating the underlying disease process. Therapy for clinical signs associated with hyperviscosity consists of phlebotomy and removal of 10 to 20 ml per kg of blood with simultaneous volume replacement with balanced polyionic fluid. The frequency of phlebotomy is based on evaluation of serial measurements of PCV.

Hydroxyurea, which causes reversible bone marrow suppression, has been used in small animals to decrease erythrocyte production. A loading dosage of 30 mg per kg PO once daily for 7 to 10 days is followed by 15 mg per kg PO daily maintenance. CBC and platelet counts should be evaluated periodically to detect leukopenia, thrombocytopenia, or anemia, in which case the drug should be discontinued. Use of hydroxyurea in the horse has not been reported.

Supplemental Readings

Blue J., Perdrizet, J., and Brown, E.: Pulmonary aspergillosis in a horse with myelomonocytic leukemia. J. Am. Vet. Med. Assoc., 190:1562, 1987.

Henry, M., Prasse, K., and White, S.: Hemorrhagic diathesis caused by multiple myeloma in a three-month-old foal. J. Am. Vet. Med. Assoc., 194:392, 1989.

Rebhun, W. C., and Bertone, A.: Equine lymphosarcoma. J. Am. Vet. Med. Assoc., 184:720, 1984.

Roby, K. A. W., Beech, J., Bloom, J. C., and Black, M.: Hepatocellular carcinoma associated with erythrocytosis and hypoglycemia in a yearling filly. J. Am. Vet. Med. Assoc., 196:465, 1990.

Van Den Hoven, R., and Franken, P.: Clinical aspects of lymphosarcoma in the horse: A clinical report of 16 cases. Equine Vet. J., 15:49, 1983.

Blood and Plasma Therapy

Lisa Williamson, ATHENS, GEORGIA

The need to transfuse blood or blood components often arises as an emergency, so the practitioner must be prepared to assess the patient's needs and deliver appropriate therapy. Separation of blood into cellular and plasma components facilitates specific replacement therapy and decreases the risk of adverse reaction in the recipient. Currently, whole blood and plasma are the most commonly transfused blood products in adult horses and foals.

BLOOD TRANSFUSION

Whole blood is indicated to treat life-threatening hemorrhage associated with surgical procedures, accidental trauma, and rupture of major blood vessels. Because the survival time of compatible transfused equine red blood cells (RBCs) is only 2 to 6 days, blood transfusion should be reserved for life-threatening situations. A rapid decline in the packed cell volume (PCV) to below 15 per cent indicates the need for transfusion, especially if the animal's condition has not stabilized or if a significant percentage of RBCs remaining in circulation have abnormal oxygen-carrying capacity. A PCV of less than 12 per cent is life-threatening because the resultant cerebral hypoxia may trigger seizure activity and death. Chronic anemia is better tolerated, but a PCV of less than 10 per cent always warrants transfusion.

The total blood volume is approximately 8 per cent of body weight in kilograms and the plasma volume is approximately 5 per cent. The volume (liters) of donor blood needed to restore a recipient's PCV to approximately 30 per cent can be calculated as follows:

$$\frac{(30 - PCV_R)(0.08\ BW_R)}{PCV_D}$$

where PCV_R and PCV_D are the recipient and donor PCV respectively and BW_R is the recipient's body weight in kilograms. Replacement of one third to one half of this calculated volume is adequate to sustain life if no further blood loss occurs. Concentrated RBCs are more appropriate therapy for cases of compensated anemia, especially when due to hemolysis, because transfusions that exceed 20 per cent of the recipient's blood volume may result in volume overload. RBC transfusions also minimize the amount of foreign proteins administered and reduce the likelihood of transfusion reaction. Equine RBCs settle in plasma within 1 to 2 hours without centrifugation; the RBCs can then be removed by gravity flow or the plasma extracted by suction or compression techniques. It is, however, better to centrifuge the blood, because it facilitates complete separation of cellular and fluid portions of the blood. Ideally, RBCs and plasma should be separated by apheresis and the unwanted portion returned to the donor.

The administration of maternal RBCs can be a life-sustaining measure for foals with neonatal isoerythrolysis. One or more washings of the RBCs in normal (0.9 per cent) saline is recommended in order to remove residual plasma erythrocyte antibodies (alloantibodies). Human hospitals and blood banks will often provide these services to veterinarians on an emergency basis, but inquiries should be made to these facilities prior to need.

Concentrated RBCs can be administered with normal saline via a Y-component administration set* in order to reduce RBC viscosity. Five per cent dextrose and fluids containing ionized calcium (Ringer's, lactated Ringer's, etc.) should not be used for this purpose because they may induce hemolysis and coagulation, respectively.

PLASMA THERAPY

Failure of passive transfer in foals over 24 hours of age is the most common indication for plasma transfusion. Since foals are agammaglobulinemic at birth, those that fail to absorb sufficient colostral immunoglobulins are at risk of developing septicemia. Recent studies indicate that most normal foals have serum IgG concentrations in excess of 800 mg per dl. Concentrations of IgG below 800 mg per dl are insufficient in foals with other risk factors for the development of sepsis. Healthy foals with IgG concentrations between 400 and 800 mg per dl and that are raised in clean, relatively stress-free environments may not require plasma transfusion. As a general rule, foals with complete failure of passive transfer need 2 to 4 liters of intravenous (IV)

---

*Baxter Healthcare Corp., Deerfield, IL

plasma over a 2- to 4-day period. The volume of plasma needed depends on the size of the foal, the degree of hypogammaglobulinemia, the IgG content of the infused plasma, and the health of the foal. One 900-ml bag of plasma (containing 1.0 gm per dl IgG or more) should provide at least 9 gm IgG. Because of individual foal variation in disposition of infused IgG and varying IgG concentrations in the infused plasma, the foal's IgG concentration should be rechecked within 24 hours, and further transfusion performed if necessary. The monitoring of serum IgG is especially critical in septic foals, because degradation and utilization of IgG are accelerated in these patients.

Frozen plasma is commmercially available.[*],[†] Its advantages include (1) known IgG concentration, (2) cell-free preparation, and (3) cost-efficiency in terms of materials, labor, and time. These products can be shipped overnight and stored in conventional freezers ($-20°$ C) for up to 6 months if not subjected to repeated freezing and thawing. At temperatures of $-70°$ C, plasma proteins are stable for at least a year. The only disadvantage of commercial plasma is the lack of IgG specific for pathogens on the foal's farm.

Acquired hypoalbuminemia in horses is another indication for plasma therapy. Significant losses of protein, especially albumin, often accompany inflammatory bowel and glomerular disease. Because albumin contributes 75 per cent of plasma colloidal osmotic pressure, hypoalbuminemia results in overhydration of the interstitium, edema, and exacerbates gastrointestinal (GI) fluid losses. Horses that have peripheral edema and a total plasma protein concentration of less than 4.0 gm per dl need plasma transfusion. Plasma protein concentrations of less than 3.0 gm per dl warrant plasma transfusion regardless of other signs.

The volume (liters) of donor plasma needed to correct a total protein deficit can be estimated as follows:

$$\frac{(70 - PP_R)(0.05\ BW_R)}{PP_D}$$

where PP_R and PP_D are donor and recipient plasma protein concentration (gm/L) respectively and BW_R is the recipient's body weight (kg). The administration of this calculated volume usually results in a lower posttransfusion total protein than expected, because low molecular weight proteins equilibrate with the interstitium, and losses may continue as a result of the underlying disease process. Clinical improvement can often be achieved with partial replacement of the deficit. Repeated plasma transfusions may be needed, so the use of products free of RBCs and alloantibodies is recommended.

When clotting factor replacement is the therapeutic goal, for example in warfarin toxicosis or disseminated intravascular coagulation, fresh or frozen plasma should be administered (6 to 10 ml per kg every 8 hours) until hemostatic data improve. The use of plasma therapy for disseminated intravascular coagulation is controversial, because replenishment of clotting factors may promote further thrombotic insult to vital organs. Fresh plasma should be removed from RBCs within 4 hours of collection, stored at $4°$ C, and administered in the first 24 hours. Fresh frozen plasma must be frozen to $-70°$ C within 6 hours of collection and used within 1 year. Plasma that has been fully or partially thawed and refrozen should be considered devoid of clotting factors.

DONOR SELECTION

At least 30 blood factors, such as erythrocyte antigens and alloantigens, have been identified in horses. These antigens have been grouped into seven blood systems by the International Society for Animal Blood Group Research: A, C, D, K, P, Q, and U. Based on the diversity of various antigenic combinations, there are approximately 400,000 possible equine blood types. Because an equine "universal donor" does not exist, a totally compatible blood transfusion is unlikely. In fact, a single transfusion of cross-matched blood results in alloantibody production in at least 50 per cent of recipients. These induced alloantibodies can be of great consequence if a second transfusion is needed or if the recipient is a brood mare. Mares that receive transfusions should be tested for plasma alloantibodies in the last month of gestation to detect potential cases of neonatal isoerythrolysis, especially if the mare is negative for Aa or Qa.

Naturally arising alloantibodies are rare in horses, with the exception of those against Ca alloantigens. Most horses that lack alloantigen Ca have anti-Ca alloantibodies, regardless of genetic and environmental factors. Alloantibodies to Ca have weak hemolytic/agglutination activity, but the safety of transfusion between Ca-negative donors and Ca-positive recipients has not been determined. Up to one half of Aa-negative horses develop anti-Aa alloantibodies regardless of reproductive history. Because these Aa alloanti-

---

[*]HiGamm Equi, Lake Immunogenics, Ontario, NY
[†]Polymune and Polymune Plus, Veterinary Dynamics, Chino, CA

bodies are potent hemolysins and hemoglutinins, Aa-negative donor horses should be screened at regular intervals for Aa alloantibodies.

Potential blood and plasma donors can be identified within a practice area before the need for these products arises. Donors should be healthy, vaccinated, and negative for equine infectious anemia. The serum of potential donors should be screened for alloantibodies and their alloantigens should be characterized. Mares that have foaled and horses that have received blood- or RBC-contaminated plasma transfusions in the past are excluded as potential blood donors. Because alloantigens Aa and Qa are extremely immunogenic, Aa- and Qa-negative donors that are free of plasma alloantibodies are the best choices for blood donors to recipients of unknown blood type. Due to the high prevalence of these alloantigens, Aa- and Qa-negative donors are difficult to find among breeds of light horses. The risks associated with an initial transfusion of whole blood are minimal. If blood types are unknown, a donor that is genetically similar to the recipient is a natural choice, because RBC alloantigen patterns are generally homologous within light horse breeds, such as Thoroughbreds.

Compatibility testing can be performed to select the most appropriate blood donor prior to a second transfusion or when the need to transfuse is anticipated. Compatibilty testing includes the use of agglutination tests (cross-matching, Coombs antiglobulin test*) and a hemolysin test. Rabbit complement,† which must be absorbed with equine RBCs to remove naturally occurring anti-horse antibodies (Frossman's antibodies), is necessary for the hemolysin test. The laboratories listed at the end of this chapter perform compatibility tests.

An adult horse can safely donate 20 per cent of its circulating blood volume without adverse consequences. Whole blood can be taken every 2 to 4 weeks and plasma every week if the RBCs are returned to the donor. The PCV and plasma proteins of frequently used donors should be monitored before each blood collection to ensure sufficient regeneration of blood constituents since the last use.

BLOOD COLLECTION

Strict asepsis should be observed during the collection, separation, and administration of blood. An area over the donor's jugular vein should be clipped and prepared with three alternating povidone–iodine and alcohol scrubs prior to venipuncture. Blood should be collected via a large-gauge indwelling catheter or nondisposable needle and drawn into a receptacle held below the level of the donor's heart. During collection, the blood container can be gently rocked to ensure adequate mixing with the anticoagulant.

Plastic blood collection bags are superior to glass collection containers because they do not activate platelets or clotting factors, are less subject to breakage, and are less likely to induce RBC damage. Only high-quality blood-grade bags should be used, because some plastics can induce RBC lysis. Blood-grade plastic bags of volumes ranging from 1 to 10 liters with options concerning the length and number of tubes, the size and length of the needle on the tubing, and the number and the type of injection or diaphragm ports on the bags are commercially available.° An anticoagulant can be added to the bag via an injection port and allowed to coat the length of the tubing. Blood can be removed from the donor through the large-gauge needle (10 or 12 gauge) directly into the bag. Because 1 liter of blood weighs approximately 1 kg (2.2 lb), the collection bag can be weighed during and after collection to estimate the volume of blood obtained. Once collection is finished, the tubing should be knotted or clamped and the blood administered through a blood administration set† and filter attached to the bag via the diaphragm port.

ANTICOAGULANTS

Acid–citrate–dextrose (ACD) and sodium citrate are the best anticoagulants for therapeutic blood products. Citrate prevents blood clotting through calcium binding, thereby inhibiting calcium-dependent steps in coagulation. Sodium citrate solution is used primarily for the collection and storage of plasma. The dextrose in ACD provides an energy substrate for RBC glycolysis, so ACD is preferred for transfusion of whole blood or RBCs. Fifteen ml of ACD is needed for every 100 ml of collected blood, and 10 ml of sodium citrate is used for every 90 ml of blood. ACD and 4 per cent sodium citrate are available in 500-ml bags‡ and have a shelf life of 18 months.

Heparin§ (5 to 12.5 units per ml blood) can be

---

*Equine antiglobulin, ICN ImmunoBiologicals, Lisle, IL
†Unabsorbed rabbit complement, Pel Freeze, Rogers, AK

°Metrix Co., Dubuque, IA
†Baxter Healthcare Corp. Deerfield, IL
‡Baxter Healthcare Corp. Deerfield, IL
§Heparin sodium, Elkins-Sinn, Cherry Hill, NJ

used for anticoagulation of blood in an emergency situation, but it has several disadvantages. Excessive administration of heparin can promote or intensify patient hemorrhage. In addition, equine RBCs are agglutinated by heparin, which may have deleterious microcirculatory effects. Heparinized blood cannot be stored and should be used within 2 hours of collection.

BLOOD ADMINISTRATION AND COMPLICATIONS

All blood products must be administered IV through blood administration sets equipped with filters (150 to 225 μm) to remove fibrin and other particulate debris. The rate of transfusion should be slow initially (0.25 ml per kg over 15 minutes) and the patient observed for adverse reactions such as restlessness, tachycardia, tachypnea, dyspnea, and sweating, which dictate that the transfusion be stopped. If no problems are observed, the rate of administration can be increased to 10 to 22 ml per kg per hour. The pulse, respiratory rate, and mucous membrane color should be monitored every 15 minutes so that the transfusion can be stopped if changes occur.

To avoid hypothermia, blood and plasma should be warmed to 37° C prior to transfusion. Excessive heating destroys proteins and can precipitate fibrinogen, so plasma should be thawed and warmed at a consistent temperature (37° to 40° C). Frozen plasma can be wrapped in a disposable plastic bag and submerged in a warm water bath until it reaches the desired temperature.

Dyspnea and coughing may be signs of volume overload, which occurs when the rate of administration or the total volume of transfusate are excessive. Citrate-induced hypocalcemia may occur, which results in tremors, seizures, cardiac arrhythmias, and collapse. In affected horses, transfusion should be stopped and 23 per cent calcium borogluconate° administered slowly IV to effect.

Prior to the administration of blood or its components, the clinician should have epinephrine† (1:1000; 4 to 8 ml per 450 kg SC or IM), flunixin meglumine‡ (1.1 mg per kg IV), and prednisolone sodium succinate§ (0.25 to 1.0 mg per kg slowly IV) readily available in case an adverse reaction occurs. Repeated transfusion should be performed cautiously, especially if more than 4 days have elapsed since the initial transfusion. Compatibility testing is recommended, but even this precautionary measure does not preclude a severe and possibly fatal transfusion reaction.

LABORATORIES THAT PROVIDE EQUINE BLOOD TYPING SERVICES

Serology Laboratory
University of California
Davis, CA 95616
Phone: (916) 752-2211

Stormont Laboratory, Inc.
1237 East Beamer St., Suite D
Woodland, CA 95695
Phone (916) 661-3078

David Colling
Mann Equitest, Inc.
5550 McAdam Road
Missisauga, Ontario L4Z 1P1
CANADA
Phone: (416) 890-2555

Dr. Melba Ketchum
Shelterwood Equine Laboratories
Box 215
Carthage, TX 75633
Phone: (214) 693-6424

Veterinary Laboratory, Inc.
1033 N. Limestone
Lexington, KY
Phone: (606) 252-0415

Supplemental Readings

Bailey, E., Conboy, H. S., and McCarthy, P. F.: Neonatal isoerythrolysis of foals: An update on testing. In: Proceedings of the 33rd Annual Convention of the American Association of Equine Practitioners, 1987, pp. 341–353.

Byars, T. D., and Divers, T. J.: Clinical use of blood transfusions. Cal. Vet., 35:14–16, 1981.

Morris, D. D.: Blood products in large animal medicine: A comparative account of current and future technology. Equine Vet. J., 19:272, 1987.

Morris, P.: Blood transfusions. In: Proceedings of the 27th Annual Convention of the American Association of Equine Practitioners, 1981, pp. 331–338.

Schmotzer, W. B., Riebold, T. W., Porter, S. L., and Blauvelt, S. R.: Time-saving techniques for the collection, storage, and administration of equine blood and plasma. Vet. Med., 80:89–94, 1985.

°Calcium 23% solution, Vedco, Inc., St. Joseph, MO
†Adrenalin chloride solution, Parke-Davis, Division of Warner-Lambert, Morris Plains, NJ
‡Banamine, Schering Animal Health, Union, NJ
§Solu-Delta Cortef, Upjohn, Kalamazoo, MI

Section 12

NEUROLOGICAL DISEASES

Edited by Richard M. DeBowes and Judy H. Cox

Neurological Examination

C. P. Coyne, MANHATTAN, KANSAS

Judy H. Cox, MANHATTAN, KANSAS

Despite significant advances in medical technology, an accurate case history and complete neurological examination remain among the most valuable diagnostic tools available to the equine clinician presented with a horse suffering from a neurological condition. Particular attention must be focused on the use of the horse, its feed and water sources, stall and pasture environments, the season of year during which the problem began, the horse's worming and vaccination history, and other factors that may contribute to neurological problems. Feed and water sources are important because feeds such as sorghum–sudan grass, feed contaminants such as mold on corn, and water contaminants such as botulinus toxin in pond water can cause neurological disease. Some problems, for example viral encephalomyelitis, occur only at certain seasons of the year. Current therapy or feed supplementation should also be established. Particular attention should be paid to administration of drugs such as reserpine, which may be responsible for the signs of neurological disease. Duration of illness, progression of signs, and spectrum of abnormalities should be determined.

GENERAL CLINICAL SIGNS

A thorough neurological examination is essential to determine the neuroanatomical location and possibly the etiology of a neurological dysfunction. The clinician must first thoroughly tabulate all the neurological signs and, by applying a knowledge of neuroanatomy and function, attempt to attribute all observed abnormalities to a single lesion or location. If multiple neurological deficits cannot be explained by a single lesion, the clinician must consider multifocal lesions and the conditions capable of producing such dysfunctions.

It is not the intent of this review to extensively outline various subtle neuroanatomical lesions that can be detected on physical examination. Rather, broad guidelines will be presented for the localization of a lesion within the central nervous system (CNS).

Brain stem dysfunction is manifested by alterations in the function of multiple cranial nerves, by abnormal regulation of vital signs, by changes in awareness, and occasionally by motor or proprioceptive deficits. Nystagmus, strabismus, diminished pupillary light reflexes, vision or hearing loss, abnormal ear or lip posture, difficulty in chewing or swallowing, and deficits in cephalic cutaneous sensation can all indicate cranial nerve dysfunction. Abnormalities of heart rate, respiratory control, and temperature regulation may indicate inability to regulate vital signs.

Cerebral hemisphere lesions may produce depression, seizures, head pressing, circling, impaired motor function, difficulties in proprioception, and vision problems.

Cerebellar dysfunction is characterized by head tremors, nystagmus, generalized incoordination, hypermetria, and spasticity.

Spinal cord dysfunction may cause motor, proprioceptive, or sensation deficits in the limbs and torso. Lower motor neuron deficits within the spinal cord are reflected in loss of muscle tone, incontinence, and eventually denervation atrophy. Unless part of a generalized neurological disease, spinal cord dysfunction is not usually accompanied by signs of brain damage.

CRANIAL NERVES

Evaluation of cranial nerve function should be performed early in the neurological examination (Table 1). A systematic approach is critical to accuracy and should include a meticulous examination of the exterior of the head and bony cranium.

Peripheral lesions must be considered if there is evidence of unilateral dysfunction of a single cranial nerve. It must be emphasized that descending upper motor neuron and ascending sensory tracts may be affected by brain stem disease. Alterations in consciousness, a sign of reticular formation dysfunction, and difficulties in regulation of vital parameters such as temperature, pulse, and respiration may also occur. Lesions at certain anatomical locations within the brain stem can affect the function of multiple cranial nerves (Table 2). Several cranial nerves are involved in the proper function of the eye and surrounding ocular viscera. Pathways involved in visual perception, pupillary light reflex, and menace response are discussed in the chapter on blindness of neurological origin (see p. 573).

Multiple anatomical and functional considerations are involved in evaluating the integrity of the facial nerve. Deficits affecting only the muscles of facial expression indicate selective involvement of peripheral buccal branches distal to the rami of the mandible. Prolonged direct pressure in this region often produces facial nerve neuropraxia, resulting in contralateral deviation of the upper lip. Lesions proximal to the rami of the mandible but distal to the stylohyoid foramen and facial canal affect both the buccal and auriculopalpebral nerve branches. The latter nerve branch provides motor input to the upper eyelids and both motor and sensory supply to the concave surface of the pinna. Slightly more proximal lesions will additionally affect the posterior and internal auricular nerves, which innervate the lateral and caudal aspects of the ipsilateral pinna, resulting in paralysis or diminished neurological function of the ipsilateral pinna, decreased cutaneous sensation of the lateral and caudal pinna, and drooping of the upper eyelid. Involvement of cranial nerve VII within the facial canal and petrous temporal bone will produce all of the above signs, in addition to alterations in lacrimal gland secretion, pupillary constriction, and equilibrium (due to concurrent involvement of cranial nerve VIII). Lesions affecting cranial nerve VII brain stem nuclei are often accompanied by additional neurological signs such as loss of abducens nerve function.

Lesions located at or near the petrous temporal bone can affect sympathetic (ocular) and parasympathetic (lacrimal gland) innervation as well as cranial nerves VII and VIII. Sympathetic innervation to the pupil originates in nuclei within the mesencephalon, descends in spinal cord tracts to the level of T1 to T3, synapses on the dorsal horn, joins the cervical sympathetic trunk, and synapses within the cranial cervical ganglion. The lower motor neurons then traverse the middle ear and synapse on the iris. These neurological pathways are entirely ipsilateral. Dysfunction of these pathways results in Horner's syndrome. It is recognized by drooping of the upper eyelid, lack of mydriasis in a dark environment, and sweating over the head and neck on the ipsilateral side. Clinical conditions capable of producing Horner's syndrome include middle ear infections, T1 to T3 cord lesions (loss of the panniculus reflex also occurs), and space-occupying lesions within the brain stem, which may also affect cranial nerve V function. In horses with postganglionic lesions, topical administration of amphetamine typically fails to produce mydriasis, since an intact lower motor neuron capable of norepinephrine synthesis and release is required, whereas topical administration of phenylephrine produces exaggerated, more rapid mydriasis. Conversely, horses with preganglionic lesions exhibit an exaggerated response to topical amphetamine.

CEREBRAL HEMISPHERES

Disease of the cerebral hemispheres can produce a multitude of signs. Classically, cerebral cortical disease is characterized by depression, head pressing, altered consciousness, seizures, lateral head deviation without a head tilt, blindness, and gait alterations. Circling, also common with vestibular disease, sometimes results from lesions in the frontal lobe or rostral thalamus. Lesions affecting the motor cortex produce contra-

TABLE 1. CRANIAL NERVE FUNCTION

I. Olfactory nerve
   Sensory: Mediates sense of smell.
   Clinical: Assess by blindfolding horse and positioning alfalfa, apples, or grain in close proximity to nasal openings.
II. Ophthalmic nerve
   Sensory: Vision and cornea.
   Clinical: Occasionally injured by expanding pituitary tumors and ocular trauma.
III. Oculomotor nerve
   Motor: Innervates dorsal, ventral, and medial rectus; ventral oblique; extraocular musculature; upper eyelid.
   Autonomic: Parasympathetic to pupil, causing miosis.
   Clinical: Dysfunction with brain stem lesions or ocular trauma.
IV. Trochlear nerve
   Motor: Dorsal oblique; extraocular musculature.
   Clinical: Deficit produces dorsal medial strabismus of the ocular globe.
V. Trigeminal nerve
   Sensory: Innervates cutaneous structures of the face, lacrimal gland, mouth, teeth, and parotid gland.
   Motor: Muscles of mastication.
   Autonomic: Parasympathetic within VII peripherally (VII joins V distal to facial canal), innervating lacrimal gland and orbit.
   Clinical: Occasionally involved in cases of yellow star thistle intoxication and cauda equina syndrome.
VI. Abducens nerve
   Motor: Lateral rectus extraocular musculature and ocular globe retraction.
   Clinical: Dysfunction recognized from medial deviation of the globe and exophthalmus.
VII. Facial nerve
   Sensory: Cranial two thirds of tongue.
   Motor: Muscles of facial expression.
   Clinical: Deficit produces deviation of muzzle toward normal side, drooping of ear, drooping of eyelids and lacrimal gland dysfunction. Damage can be due to trauma, guttural pouch mycosis, yellow star thistle ingestion, or cauda equina syndrome. Occasionally focal epilepsy with facial spasms from either cerebral cortex abnormalities or peripheral nerve irritation.
VIII. Vestibularcochlear nerve
   Sensory: Auditory and equilibrium; integration with higher levels of the brain.
   Clinical: Deficit produces head tilt, circling, and nystagmus (rotary, horizontal, and vertical). Vertical nystagmus not seen with peripheral nerve involvement. Visual compensation can mask deficits. Vestibular deficits accentuated by blindfolding (*Caution:* horses may rear over backward). Lesions can occur with inner ear infections, cauda equina syndrome, and brain stem lesions.
IX. Glossopharyngeal nerve
   Sensory: Caudal one third of tongue, pharynx, and guttural pouch opening.
   Motor: Pharyngeal musculature, tongue, and soft palate.
   Clinical: Dysfunction manifested as dysphagia and may accompany severe guttural pouch disease (along with VII, X, XI, and XII, rabies, botulism, lead intoxication, vitamin E/selenium deficiency).
X. Vagus nerve
   Sensory: Larynx, pharynx, and pulmonary tree.
   Motor: Pulmonary viscera, bronchial smooth muscle, gastrointestinal viscera, soft palate, dynamic function of rima glottis.
   Clinical: Deficits produce dysphagia, tachycardia, mild bronchodilation, gastrointestinal stasis. Diminished peripheral innervation to gastrointestinal viscera may result in compensatory increases in vagal tone and bradycardia. Sometimes affected in guttural pouch disease, rabies, botulism, lead intoxication, vitamin E/selenium deficiency.
XI. Accessory spinal nerve
   Motor: Pharyngeal and scapular musculature.
   Clinical: Deficits produce pharyngeal dysphagia, abnormal gait, or muscle atrophy. Pharyngeal involvement is occasionally present with guttural pouch mycoses, rabies, botulism, lead intoxication, vitamin E/selenium deficiency.
XII. Hypoglossal nerve
   Motor: Tongue (glossal) musculature.
   Clinical: Deficits produce hypotonia and diminished tongue movement. Unilateral involvement results in lateral deviation of the tongue toward the contralateral side. Etiologies include yellow star thistle ingestion and guttural pouch disease. (*Caution:* horses with severe systemic disease and depression may also display tongue hypotonia.)

lateral hemiparesis with minimal alterations in gait. Lesions located in progressively lower regions of the motor neuron tracts as they acquire integrated input from the cerebellum are associated with locomotor and postural dysfunctions of increasing severity. Conscious proprioceptive deficits can occur with contralateral parietal lobe lesions. Occipital lobe or optic radiation lesions can produce blindness characterized by an intact pupillary light reflex and lack

TABLE 2. PATTERNS OF MULTIPLE CRANIAL NERVE INVOLVEMENT

I, II:	Nuclei located in the rostral brain stem.
III, IV:	Nuclei are in close proximity. Peripheral nerves diverge from V, VI, as they exit the brain stem but converge again as they leave the cranial vault through the bony foramen.
III:	Closely associated with red nucleus of the upper motor neuron pathway.
IV:	Closely associated with medial longitudinal fasciculus.
V:	Nuclei are in close association in mesencephalon with sympathetic upper motor neuron input to the eye.
VI, VII:	Abducens nuclei closely associated with nuclei of peripheral nerve VII at level of the cerebellar peduncles.
VII, VIII:	Nuclei in close proximity with one another, as are their peripheral nerves near the petrous temporal bone.
VII, IX, X, XI, XII:	Can be involved with extensive erosion of the caudal lateral aspect of the guttural pouch. In addition to guttural pouch disease, conditions that may produce signs of laryngeal-pharyngeal dysfunction include botulism, lead intoxication, rabies, and yellow star thistle intoxication. Ideally, endoscopic examination should precede challenge feeding tests.
IX, X, XI:	Collectively exit the myelencephalon through the tympano-occipital fissure.
XII:	Closely associated with fourth ventricle and reticular formation. Traverses olivary nucleus of the upper motor neuron tracts.

of cranial nerve deficits. Unilateral cortical lesions produce contralateral blindness without nystagmus and strabismus.

Cerebral edema resulting from acute cranial trauma or severe metabolic dysfunction is frequently characterized by depression and altered consciousness. Blurring of the optic disk margins, papilledema, and altered retinal vascular pattern are often detected on ophthalmic examination. Progressive cerebral edema can produce alterations in cranial nerve function and vital signs through brain stem compression. Serial neurological examinations are mandatory in such cases in order to detect progressive neurological deficits as early as possible. See chapter on brain and spinal cord trauma (p. 535) for further discussion.

Metabolic and toxicologic derangements that can cause altered cerebral function should be ruled out. These include pharmaceutical agents, hypoglycemia, hypocalcemia, acidemia, electrolyte alterations, hepatoencephalopathy, rhabdomyolysis, renal disease, lead intoxication, and locoism. Rabies should be included in the differential diagnosis of any condition with neurological signs suggestive of cerebral involvement.

CEREBELLUM

The cerebellum is largely responsible for coordination and refinement of neuromuscular activity. Typical signs of cerebellar dysfunction include incoordination, head tremors, positional nystagmus, and poor or absent menace response. Cerebellar-associated gait alterations classically manifest as hypermetria, hyperextension, spasticity, and uncoordinated movements. Usually these signs are bilateral and symmetrical without evidence of paresis.

The clinician should be cognizant of the condition referred to as paradoxical vestibular syndrome. Cerebellar lesions near the caudal peduncle or flocculonodular lobules may cause contralateral vestibular head tilt, ataxia and strabismus. Successful localization of this lesion is achieved by recognizing ipsilateral generalized proprioception or upper motor neuron deficits.

SPINAL CORD

In equine neurology, one of the most challenging diagnostic problems is the differentiation of spinal cord disease from conditions affecting the musculoskeletal system. Laminitis, rhabdomyolysis, compressive neuropraxia, moderately advanced degenerative joint disease, and osseous fractures can mimic certain neurological diseases but usually can be identified by thorough physical examination or interpretation of serum or synovial biochemical parameters. Interpretation of more subtle alterations in gait and locomotion is more difficult, and accurate assessment often requires repeated neurological examinations. Such examinations should be performed prior to a lameness examination to avoid subjecting the patient to unnecessary diagnostic peripheral nerve or joint anesthesia.

The clinical signs of spinal cord disease are in general quite distinct from those of diseases affecting the cranial central nervous system. Key features present in even the most subtle cases of spinal cord dysfunction include limb interference, toe dragging, limb circumduction, limb pivoting, ataxia, and paresis. With progressive

TABLE 3. EXAMINATION OF EQUINE SPINAL CORD FUNCTION

1. Assess cutaneous sensation over head, neck, limbs, and torso.
2. Assess muscle atrophy over neck, torso, or limbs.
3. Manipulate neck laterally, ventrally, dorsally, flexed and extended.
4. Evaluate gait on level ground and on an incline:
   a. Walk and trot horse with head and neck in normal, flexed, extended, and elevated positions.
   b. Turn horse in tight circle to the left and right.
5. Assess ability to back up.
6. Crossed placement of pectoral and pelvic limbs.
7. Lateral hop challenge in all four legs.
8. Negotiate sigmoid curve over raised curbs.
9. Perform a lateral sway test at rest and at a walk:
   a. Lateral pulling of tail at a walk (pelvic limbs).
   b. Lateral displacement of body by pushing at shoulders and hindquarters (stationary).
10. Assess muscular tone of tail, anal sphincter, vulva, penis and urethra.

loss of function, lateral recumbency may be noted. Depression, bizarre behavior, and cranial nerve dysfunction usually are not compatible with true primary spinal cord diseases.

A variety of simple procedures can be performed in an attempt to detect lesions affecting the spinal cord (Table 3). Once a gait abnormality has been diagnosed as a neurological deficit, accurate serial neurological examinations are central to establishing the etiology of the disease.

Limb pivoting on the inside limb and circumduction on the outside limb when a horse is turned sharply suggests spinal cord disease. Abnormal lateral hop responses imply a neurological deficit but aid little in localizing the lesion.

Deficient cutaneous sensation or deficient reflexes affecting specific dermatomes over the torso or neck can be of great diagnostic significance; sites of compressive vertebral fractures or abscesses can frequently be localized in this fashion. Cutaneous sensation over the cervical or thoracic regions is also frequently deficient in cases of equine degenerative myelopathy. Disease processes affecting spinal cord segments T1 to T3 usually coexist with Horner's syndrome and panniculus reflex deficits. Increased cutaneous sensation or hyperesthesia may represent irritation or impingement of a peripheral nerve by a space-occupying lesion; either of these signs may also be an early sign of rabies.

Proprioception refers to the conscious and unconscious recognition of the position of the limbs and torso in space. In horses, a proprioceptive defect most frequently results from lesions affecting the spinal cord but may also be associated with lesions of the brain stem, thalamus, or cerebral hemispheres. Subtle, early changes in proprioception can often be detected by examination of gait while the horse travels up and down an incline and negotiates raised obstacles such as curbs. Increased limb abduction, fetlock knuckling, excessive toe dragging, limb interference, delayed or absent correction of malpositioned limbs, and truncal sway are features of proprioceptive deficits. False positive findings can be observed in very obedient horses, and accurate assessment may require serial examinations. Decreased resistance and uncoordinated response to lateral displacement of the torso at the pectoral and pelvic limbs or during the pelvic sway test are also supportive of proprioceptive dysfunction. When the horse is turned in a tight circle, proprioceptive deficits are revealed by circumduction of the outside limb, pivoting on the inside limb, and marked limb interference.

Hypermetria with limb hyperflexion is less pronounced in spinal cord disease than in cerebellar disease. Lesions involving proprioceptive tracts above the level of the thalamus produce contralateral deficits; lesions caudal to the thalamus produce ipsilateral deficits. Lesions affecting unconscious proprioception (e.g., spinocerebellar tracts) usually produce more severe deficits than those involving conscious proprioception (e.g., dorsal funiculi). In the equine cervical spinal cord, axons transmitting unconscious (spinocerebellar) proprioceptive input from the pelvic limbs are more abaxial (i.e., superficial) than axons of pectoral limb origin. As a result, cervical compression produces more prominent signs in pelvic than in pectoral limbs. Loss of motor neuron function and deep pain are not classical features of cervical compressive lesions because axons mediating these functions are located deep within the spinal cord. Deep pain sensation is essentially the last sensory modality to be lost during progressive spinal cord compression.

Motor neuron dysfunction is characterized by alterations in gait initiation, paresis, and posture. Lesions at or below the medulla produce ipsilateral alterations in limb function. Features of unilateral disease include ipsilateral hemiparesis, hemiplegia, spasticity, resistance to limb manipulation, hypertonia, and hyperreflexia. Loss of upper motor neuron input classically produces limb hyperextension, spasticity, and hyperreflexia. Disruption of lower motor neuron function produces hyporeflexia, paresis, paralysis, difficulty in gait initiation, and denervation muscular atrophy. Paresis can sometimes be detected by assessing the ability of individual limbs to support a weight-bearing load. Incoordination is not a classical feature of pure motor neuron deficits.

Assessment of specific neurological abnormalities should allow localization of the lesion(s). Depending on the severity of the lesion, cervical spinal cord lesions can produce variable deficits in proprioception, upper motor neuron function, and deep pain of the pectoral and pelvic limbs. Disruption at cord segments C5 to T2 (brachial plexus) produces variable proprioceptive and lower motor neuron signs in the pectoral limbs, possibly accompanied by pelvic limb proprioceptive and upper motor neuron dysfunction. Thoracolumbar cord lesions are classically recognized by normal pectoral limb function accompanied by proprioceptive and/or upper motor neuron pelvic limb deficits. In such instances, large volumes of urine are retained by the bladder, in part due to loss of upper motor neuron inhibition of pudendal nerve innervation to urethral striated musculature. Reflex micturition develops over time, resulting in almost complete voiding of urine. Lesions affecting cord segments L4 to S3 (pelvic plexus) cause proprioceptive and pelvic limb lower motor neuron deficits. Involvement of sacrococcygeal spinal cord segments results in tail hypotonia, urinary and fecal incontinence, penile paralysis, and diminished vulvar tone. Reflexes that can be used to evaluate specific parts of the spinal cord include the biceps reflex (musculocutaneous nerve, C6 to C8), triceps reflex (radial nerve, C7 to T2), panniculus reflex (lateral thoracic nerve, T1 to T3), and patellar reflex (femoral nerve, L4 to L6).

In the recumbent horse, special efforts must be made to perform as complete an examination as possible. The accuracy of such evaluations is often compromised by inability to fully assess the patient's true physical condition, and abnormalities frequently are not detected. Utilization of a sling in such cases can often be beneficial from a diagnostic and prognostic as well as therapeutic standpoint. Some recumbent horses adapt amazingly well to sling support once they have been brought to their feet and provided with relatively passive lateral support.

ANCILLARY DIAGNOSTIC PROCEDURES

Diagnostic procedures for neurological disease include cerebrospinal fluid (CSF) analysis (discussed in the next chapter), biopsy and histopathology, electroencephalography, electromyography, and myelography. Premortem diagnosis of rabies can occasionally be made through immunohistopathological identification of the virus in tactile hair biopsy specimens. Negative results should be interpreted with caution, since the rabies virus ascends to the level of the spinal cord, cerebellum, and brain stem prior to infiltration of the salivary gland and tactile hair tissue.

The primary indications for electromyography are the detection of muscle disease and alterations in upper and lower motor neuron function. Disease processes characterized by loss of lower motor neuron innervation often result in an absence of normal triphasic waveforms, which are replaced by spontaneous, continuous, biphasic fasciculation (motor unit) and fibrillation (muscle fiber) potentials. Such alterations are often evident by 4 to 7 days after denervation. Typically, these changes are accompanied by positive sharp wave potentials. Classically, a "frying eggs" sound accompanies these waveform alterations. Bizarre high-frequency waveforms may be evident with diseases affecting either muscle or peripheral nerves.

A myelogram provides the opportunity to obtain a definitive neurological diagnosis of a compressive cord lesion. Cervical vertebral instability or stenosis, traumatic vertebral fractures, hematomas, or abscesses can be detected. Myelography can be particularly helpful in the recumbent horse in which a comprehensive neurological examination is not possible but history and clinical parameters suggest spinal cord compression. Equine neurological patients can suffer complications such as compromised neuromuscular coordination when myelography is performed. Since myelography requires general anesthesia, it may be impractical or contraindicated in severely affected patients or horses with a poor prognosis for successful therapeutic intervention. In this context, neurological signs may exacerbate following myelographic procedures involving extensive manipulation of the cervical vertebrae. Owners should be thoroughly informed of potential complications before giving consent for this procedure because of the possibility of further injury and subsequent inability of the horse to stand during recovery from general anesthesia. In an effort to minimize such sequelae, prophylactic administration of nonsteroidal anti-inflammatory agents, corticosteroids, or intravenous dimethyl sulfoxide (diluted to 10 per cent in lactated Ringer's solution or 5 per cent dextrose) is recommended.

To perform the myelogram, a spinal needle is inserted at the atlanto-occipital space and directed toward the lower mandible in the horse in lateral recumbency and with the head flexed (see p. 528 for a description of the technique). Contrast medium should be sterile and passed through a 0.22-μm filter prior to injection. Flow of contrast medium into the cranial vault can be minimized by directing the bevel of the spinal needle caudally, elevating the head and neck on an incline, and injecting at a rate of approximately 5 ml per minute.

Lateral survey radiographs should precede contrast studies; osseous abnormalities may indicate that a myelogram is either unnecessary or contraindicated. Analysis of CSF for cytological evidence of sepsis is considered mandatory prior to injection of contrast medium. Myelography with metrizamide in the presence of CNS sepsis increases the risk of seizures due to a combination of inflammatory disruption of the blood–brain barrier, the hydrophobic character of metrizamide, and inhibition of neuronal glucose metabolism. Prophylactic intravenous administration of glucose can minimize or eliminate seizures precipitated by metrizamide. Seizures are most successfully controlled with diazepam, barbiturates, or chloral hydrate. The newly developed contrast reagents iohexol iopamidol and ionosol iopamidol have much less potential for initiating seizures because of their hydrophilic character, lack of a glucose analogue moiety, and isosmotic formulation.

Supplemental Readings

Allen, J. R., Barbee, D. D., and Crisman, M. V.: Diagnosis of equine pituitary tumor by computed tomography: Part I. Compend. Cont. Educ. Pract. Vet., 10:1103–1106, 1988.

de Lahunta, A. (ed.): Veterinary Neuroanatomy and Clinical Neurology, 2nd ed. Philadelphia, W. B. Saunders, 1983.

Geiser, D. R., Henton, J. R., and Held, J. P.: Typanic bulla, petrous temporal bone and hyoid apparatus disease in horses. Compend. Cont. Educ. Pract. Vet., 10:740–754 1988.

Mayhew, I. G., Brown, C. M., Stowe, H. D., Trapp, A. L., Derksen, F. J., and Clement, S. F.: Equine degenerative myeloencephalopathy: A vitamin E deficiency that may be familial. J. Vet. Intern. Med., 1:45–50, 1987.

Smith, J. M., Cox, J. H., and DeBowes, R. M.: Central nervous system disease in adult horses: Part I. A data base. Compend. Cont. Educ. Pract. Vet., 9:561–569, 1987.

Smith, J. M., DeBowes, R. M., and Cox, J. H.: Central nervous system disease in adult horses: Part II. Differential diagnosis. Compend. Cont. Educ. Pract. Vet., 9:772–780, 1987.

Smith, J. M, DeBowes, R. M., and Cox, J. H.: Central nervous system disease in adult horses: Part III. Differential diagnosis and comparison of common disorders. Compend. Cont. Educ. Pract. Vet., 9:1042–1053, 1987.

Cerebrospinal Fluid Collection and Analysis

C. P. Coyne, MANHATTAN, KANSAS

Cerebrospinal fluid (CSF) analysis is one of the most valuable procedures for the diagnosis of equine neurological disease, particularly disease of viral and bacterial etiology. Unfortunately, CSF analysis may not assist in establishing a specific etiological diagnosis in disorders such as cervical vertebral instability, stenosis, equine degenerative myelopathy, and many cases of equine protozoal myeloencephalitis (EPM). Collection of CSF from either the atlanto-occipital or lumbosacral site is contraindicated in the presence of significant cerebral edema, because death may result from rapid decompression and subsequent herniation of the cerebellum through the foramen magnum. Neurological signs suggestive of cerebral edema are described on page 524. Funduscopic examination can reveal papilloedema, blurring of the optic disk margin, and alterations in the retinal vascular pattern, further indications of cerebral edema.

Prior to CSF collection, the skin is clipped, shaved, and aseptically prepared. Sterile surgical gloves and drapes are mandatory to avoid septic contamination of the central nervous system (CNS). Persons with infectious respiratory diseases should refrain from performing such diagnostic procedures or should wear a surgical mask.

LUMBOSACRAL SITE FOR COLLECTION OF CSF

A large proportion of equine neurological conditions affect the caudal regions of the spinal cord, and collection of CSF from the lumbosacral space is preferred in these cases. Lumbosacral space centesis is technically difficult. The site is located on the dorsal midline and is bisected by a transverse line drawn through the caudal aspects of the tuber coxae. Umbilical tape can aid in locating the approximate site. Additional anatomical landmarks include the dorsal spinal processes of L6 (cranial to the site) and S2 (caudal to the site) along with the tuber sacralae (lateral to the site). The dorsal spinous processes of L7 and S1 usually are only palpable in horses with advanced cachexia. Firm digital pressure often assists in detecting the soft tissue corridor directly over the lumbosacral space. In my experience, this is the most helpful step in locating the lumbosacral site following application of umbilical tape. Ultrasonography can aid in establishing the proper location of the lumbosacral space and is particularly helpful in obese or recumbent equine patients.

Spinal needles with a stylet (18 to 19 gauge, 8 to 10 inches long) should be used. Following aseptic skin preparation and surgical draping, a local anesthetic agent is infiltrated at the site and a stab incision is made through the skin with a size 15 surgical blade. A 14-gauge, ½-inch needle is inserted at the site of the stab incision and the spinal needle is passed through its lumen. This optional procedure decreases skin drag on the spinal needle, thereby enhancing detection of penetration of the dorsal vertebral ligament. The spinal needle should be advanced in a strictly vertical plane (when viewed both laterally and caudally).

Successful collection of CSF from horses in lateral recumbency is particularly difficult. Usually such patients have a slightly tilted pelvis. Recognition of this feature is important so that the spinal needle may be advanced in a plane perpendicular to the tilted pelvis (i.e., with a slight upward direction to the needle).

When a "popping" sensation or sudden decrease in resistance is perceived, advancement of the spinal needle is stopped and the stylet is removed to check for the presence of spinal fluid. Gentle aspiration or inducing an increase in CSF pressure by occluding the jugular veins frequently allows collection of CSF when the bevel of the needle is slightly obstructed with tissue. If CSF is not obtained, the stylet is reinserted and the spinal needle rotated 90 degrees and checked again. The cycle is repeated until a full 360-degree arc is completed. If fluid is still not obtained, the needle is advanced further, provided there is no contact with bone. It should be remembered that the tip of the needle may aspirate meninges or may be embedded within the caudal spinal cord, preventing CSF collection. In the latter instance, fluid can be obtained on penetration of the ventral spinal cord surface. Neurological deficits are rarely caused by such minor traumatic insults at this level of the caudal CNS.

Ideally, CSF pressures should be measured and should be less than 400 mm H_2O. A Quackenstendt procedure is also performed to identify inappropriate CSF flow within the vertebral column. This test entails measurement of CSF pressure before and after jugular vein occlusion. Optimal diagnostic information is obtained if the procedure is performed so as to yield a kinetic pressure profile over time at both the atlanto-occipital and lumbosacral sites. Slow or nonexistent elevations in CSF pressure during the Quackenstendt test imply diminished patency of CSF flow within the vertebral column, suggesting an obstruction. Such an abnormality at both the atlanto-occipital and lumbosacral locations implies the presence of an obstructive lesion within the cranium. Conversely, an abnormal Quackenstendt test at the lumbosacral site implies the presence of an obstructive lesion within the cervical or thoracolumbar vertebrae.

Collection of CSF is more convenient if the fluid is aspirated from the hub of the spinal needle using a hypodermic needle and syringe or if a short intravenous (IV) extension set is used as a connection between the spinal needle and the syringe. On completion of the procedure the spinal needle should be withdrawn with the central stylet in place in order to avoid septic contamination.

ATLANTO-OCCIPITAL SITE COLLECTION OF CSF

Collection of CSF from the atlanto-occipital site requires general anesthesia and aseptic preparation of the collection site. The most appropriate site is located on the midline at a point approximately 1 inch (2.5 cm) rostral to a line drawn transversely through the cranial border of the wings of the atlas. An additional anatomical landmark is the occipital protuberance located on the midline cranial to the atlas. The horse's head and neck are flexed and the spinal needle is advanced with the tip of the needle directed toward the lower mandible and the bevel facing caudad. This approach avoids entry through the foramen magnum and penetration of the cerebellum. Usually an obvious decrease in resistance or a slight "popping" sensation is appreciated after penetrating the dorsal intervertebral ligament. Fluid is collected as described for the lumbosacral site.

CEREBROSPINAL FLUID ANALYSIS

Initial evaluation of CSF should include determination of color and clarity. Spectrophotometry, with water used as a control, can serve as an objective means of assessing clarity. Xanthochromia is generally considered to reflect previous hemorrhagic contamination of the subarachnoid space. It may be present in a variety of disease processes, including trauma, EPM, visceral larva migrans (VLM), and especially equine herpesvirus 1 (EHV-1) infection.

Total protein concentration, in addition to the content of albumin and immunoglobulin, is included in the standard analysis of CSF samples. Marked elevations in CSF albumin imply leakage of plasma constituents across a compromised blood–brain barrier. Immunoglobulin is traditionally quantified using the Pandy (phenol) and Nonne Apel (ammonium sulfate) methods. Increased CSF immunoglobulin may occur either from leakage of serum protein across a compromised blood–brain barrier or from intrathecal immune responses. Occurrence of the latter can be detected by calculating increases in the immunoglobulin index using the following equation: (CSF IgG/serum IgG)/(CSF albumin/serum albumin). The normal value of the immunoglobulin index will vary among laboratories. Equine diseases that are frequently accompanied by elevations in CSF immunoglobulin include bacterial meningitis, viral encephalitides, EHV-1, EPM, cauda equina syndrome, and lymphosarcoma. Elevations in CSF protein are a common but inconsistent finding in horses with EPM. Bacterial meningitis usually produces the greatest increase in total protein (more than 100 mg per dl) and immunoglobulin (Pandy or Nonne Apelt score of 2 to 4). Such CSF samples may foam. In the neurological form of EHV-1, antibody titers may be markedly elevated by the time the clinical signs of rear limb ataxia, tail hypotonia, and incontinence are evident.

Cytological evaluation of CSF is most accurate if cytocentrifugation is used to concentrate cell populations. Somewhat comparable results can be achieved using flotation techniques employing simple cylindrical chambers. Normal CSF nucleated cell counts are approximately 2 to 4 per μl, and there is an almost total absence of neutrophils. A hallmark of bacterial meningitis is an elevation in CSF neutrophil count to more than 100 per μl. Increases in CSF neutrophil numbers of a lesser magnitude can also occur in cases of CNS necrosis, neoplasia, and parenchymal disease. In instances of subsurface abscessation within neural parenchymal tissue, CSF neutrophil numbers are often surprisingly low. It should be emphasized that alphaviruses (togaviridae) responsible for eastern and Venezuelan equine encephalitides induce a prominent CSF neutrophilia during the first 2 to 3 days of the disease. Eosinophilia within the CSF suggests the possibility of VLM, especially if accompanied by asymmetrical or multifocal neurological signs.

Mononuclear and lymphocytic infiltration of the CSF in the horse is most frequent in the viral encephalitides. Mononuclear cell increases (more than 50 per cent) occur 2 to 3 days after the initial clinical onset of eastern and Venezuelan equine encephalitis and are a constant feature of western equine encephalitis. All horses thought to have a viral encephalitis should be evaluated for elevations in blood ammonia, hepatic enzymes, fractionated bilirubin, and bile acids in an effort to rule out hepatoencephalopathy. Elevations in CSF mononuclear cells are inconsistently present in horses affected by EPM. Pleocytosis is occasionally seen in the neurological form of EHV-1.

Red blood cells (RBCs) in CSF samples are a relatively common occurrence and may be due to a disease process or be iatrogenically induced. RBCs are reportedly somewhat unstable in CSF and remain intact for less than 4 minutes. Erythrophagocytosis and xanthochromia in CSF samples evaluated within 30 minutes of collection imply the presence of noniatrogenic hemorrhage. Platelets are seen only in instances of acute pathological, traumatic, or iatrogenically induced hemorrhage. Although somewhat controversial, general guidelines have been proposed to adjust for peripheral blood contamination of CSF. An increase of 1 WBC should occur for every 500 RBCs present. An increase of more than 1 WBC per 500 RBCs indicates the possible presence of a CSF neutrophilia irrespective of contamination with peripheral whole blood.

Occasionally, virus isolation can be performed on CSF samples for diagnostic purposes. In horses with EHV-1, viral organisms are usually no longer in the CSF in adequate concentrations to be successfully harvested, but isolation of herpesvirus from CSF and peripheral mononuclear cells should be attempted. In rabies patients, viral particles can be identified with electron microscopy and fluorescent antibody assays. However, such diagnostic attempts are a potential health hazard to medical and technical personnel. The success of such diagnostic approaches to viral identification can be markedly improved with the use of initial antisera treatment to harvest and concentrate organisms.

Measurement of enzymes in CSF can be of benefit in detecting the presence of neurological abnormalities. Enzymes that can be of some value include aspartate aminotransferase (AST or SGOT), lactic dehydrogenase (LDH), and creatine kinases (CK). Elevations in CSF LDH may indicate CNS damage. Isoenzymes LDH_2 and LDH_3 are lymphocyte-associated, and LDH_4 and LDH_5 are neutrophil-associated. If the blood brain barrier is intact, an increase in CSF CK_1 levels is generally interpreted as an indicator of demyelination. In general, CK_1 levels are greater in equine protozoal myelitis and equine degenerative myeloencephalopathy than in wobblers.

Sodium concentrations are normally slightly below (5 to 10 mEq per L) and chloride concentrations slightly greater (5 to 10 mEq per L) than concurrent serum concentrations. Alterations in concentrations can occur following disruption of the blood–brain barrier and in cases of tissue necrosis. European warm blood horses with preparturient hypocalcemia usually have subnormal CSF calcium levels. Glucose concentrations in the CSF are approximately 80 per cent of those in the intravascular compartment and may decrease drastically during episodes of bacterial meningitis.

More advanced methods of analyzing CSF have been described. Horses with cauda equina neuritis have been shown to have elevations in CSF P2-myelin. Recent reports have described CSF elevations in a polypeptide protein referred to as S-100 in various equine neurological diseases. Three different isotypes of this protein can be found in the CSF. In my laboratory, SDS-polyacrylamide gel electrophoresis (SDS-PAGE) in conjunction with sensitive staining techniques has been applied in an attempt to analyze CSF samples in a more detailed fashion. It is hoped that such efforts may provide an avenue for more objective differentiation between neurological conditions such as cervical instability or stenosis with marginal alterations on the myelogram and equine degenerative myelopathy. This is very similar in concept to increases in several distinct protein and lipoprotein fractions in CSF collected from human patients with a variety of neurological conditions.

Supplemental Readings

de Lahunta, A.: Veterinary Neuroanatomy and Clinical Neurology, 2nd ed. Philadelphia, W. B. Saunders, 1983, pp. 227–228.

Freeman, K. P., Brewer, B., and Slusher, S. H.: Membrane filter preparations of cerebrospinal fluid from normal horses and horses with selected neurologic diseases. Compend. Cont. Educ. Pract. Vet., 11:1100–1109, 1989.

Jackson, T. A., Osburn, B. I., and Cordy, D. R., et al.: Equine herpes virus I infections of horses: Studies on the experimentally induced neurologic disease. Am J. Vet. Res, 38:709–719, 1977.

Mayhew, I. G., and MacKay, R. J.: The nervous system. In Mansmann, R. A., McAllister, E. S. (eds.): Equine Medicine and Surgery, 3rd ed. Santa Barbara, American Veterinary Publications, 1982, pp 1184–1188.

Common Malformations and Congenital Abnormalities of the Central Nervous System

Richard M. DeBowes, MANHATTAN, KANSAS
Lisa Gift, MANHATTAN, KANSAS

Congenital malformations of the equine skull, spine, and central nervous system (CNS) are relatively uncommon but potentially serious in nature. Timely initiation of medical and surgical therapy is necessary if clinicians are to have any opportunity to successfully obtund the severity of these conditions. The outcome in each case is determined by the type and magnitude of disease process and by the medical technology available for appropriate clinical management.

HYDROCEPHALUS

Hydrocephalus results from an accumulation of cerebrospinal fluid (CSF) within or around the brain. In horses, this condition is more commonly congenital than acquired. The cranium of affected foals is dome shaped as a result of increased intracranial pressure (ICP) generated by the accumulation of CSF either within the ventricles or surrounding the brain (Fig. 1). Excessive doming of the anterior and lateral cranium is associated commonly with gross malformation of the fetus and can result in dystocia and perinatal death.

The etiology of hydrocephalus in horses remains unclear. In other species, vitamin A deficiency, viral infection, and autosomal recessive mode of inheritance have been identified as contributing factors. In foals, hydrocephalus results

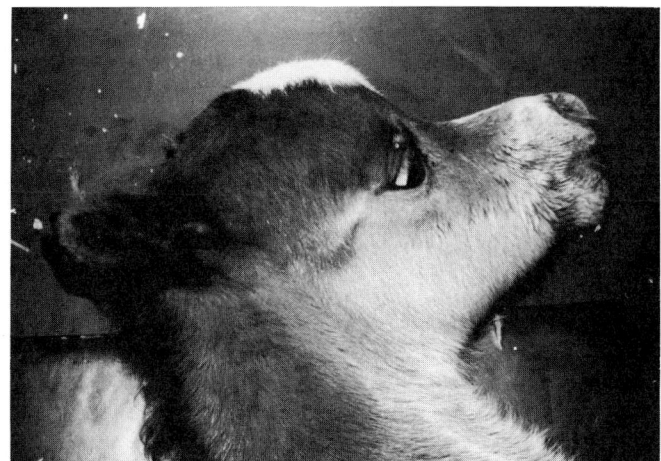

Figure 1. Hydrocephalus is easily recognized from the presence of a dome-shaped calvarium.

most commonly from an anatomical or functional impairment of CSF drainage.

Hydrocephalus is readily suspected from the appearance of a grossly malformed skull. Although a variety of neurological deficits may be noted, none are pathognomonic. Some affected foals appear normal behaviorally and neurologically. When neurological signs are present, they are usually referable to a dysfunction of the cerebral hemispheres. Typically, depression, dementia, or convulsion will be observed. Signs of brain stem involvement are occasionally present as well. Exophthalmos and ventrolateral strabismus are common signs of brain stem dysfunction in affected foals. The clinical diagnosis is supported with plain film radiography and confirmed by cerebral ultrasonography, pneumoencephalography, or lateral ventriculography.

Therapeutic options for the management of hydrocephalus are limited. Medical therapy is usually directed toward stabilizing the patient, controlling seizures, and minimizing exacerbation of the neurological deficits. The administration of corticosteroids has been suggested for reducing CSF production and ICP. It is believed by some that this therapy will temporarily delay the progressive clinical deterioration. Evidence supporting corticosteroid use for this purpose is lacking. Ventriculoatrial shunts have been employed in dogs and humans for surgical management of internal hydrocephalus. Excessive CSF can be shunted to the atria, jugular veins, or pleural or peritoneal cavities for systemic resorption. Shunt diversion of excessive CSF in foals has met with mixed success.

OCCIPITO-ATLANTOAXIAL MALFORMATION

Occipito-atlantoaxial malformation is a disease of light horses that is reported most commonly in animals of the Arabian bloodline. The condition is thought to be familial and is inherited as an autosomal recessive trait. The disease is marked by severe malformation of the occipital condyles, atlas, and axis. The spinal canal is frequently stenotic. In some cases the occipito-atlantal articulation is absent or ankylosed. Malformation and hypoplasia of the dens are common features of this condition.

These malformations produce a variety of clinical signs, most of which result from the rostral cervical spinal cord compression. Clinical signs are present at birth or become evident within the first few weeks to months of life. Truncal ataxia is common. Often, severely affected foals are unable to rise. The head and neck may be carried in an extended position. Further extension of the neck to permit nursing can exacerbate clinical signs and cause the severely affected foal to collapse. Manipulation of the craniovertebral junction can produce an audible click. Conversely, joint motion may be nonexistent in individuals with excessive malformation. Most foals with neurological signs of paresis and ataxia deteriorate with advancing age. Mild cases may be clinically inapparent until adulthood, when significant clinical signs become evident.

The diagnosis of occipito-atlantoaxial malformation should be suspected from typical history and the clinical signs. The diagnosis is confirmed by radiographic demonstration of the various bony malformations (Fig. 2). Prospective candidates for surgical therapy should be evaluated with myelography to establish the anatomical extent and magnitude of spinal cord compression. Medical treatment is generally not efficacious. Dorsal decompressive laminectomy can be performed over the area of spinal cord compression. Patients with mild neurological deficits that undergo surgery early may stabilize or improve. In

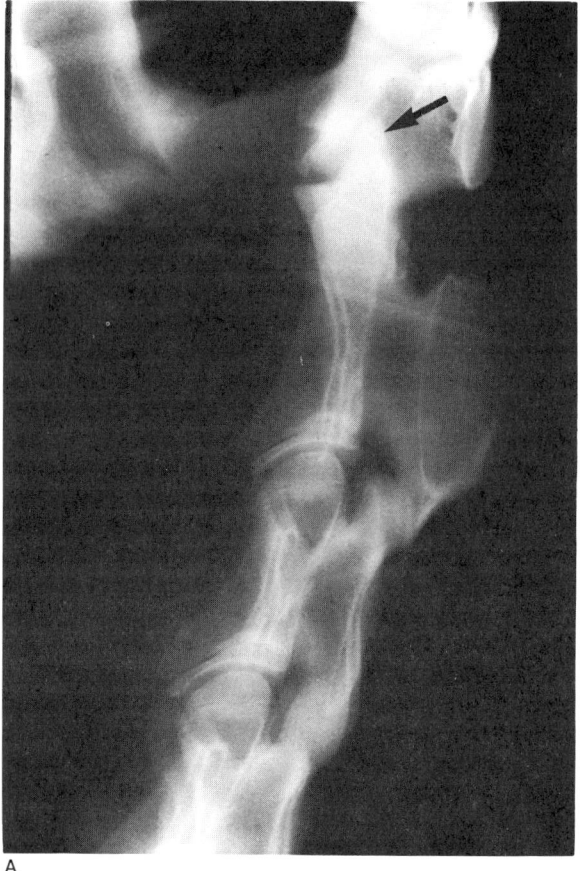 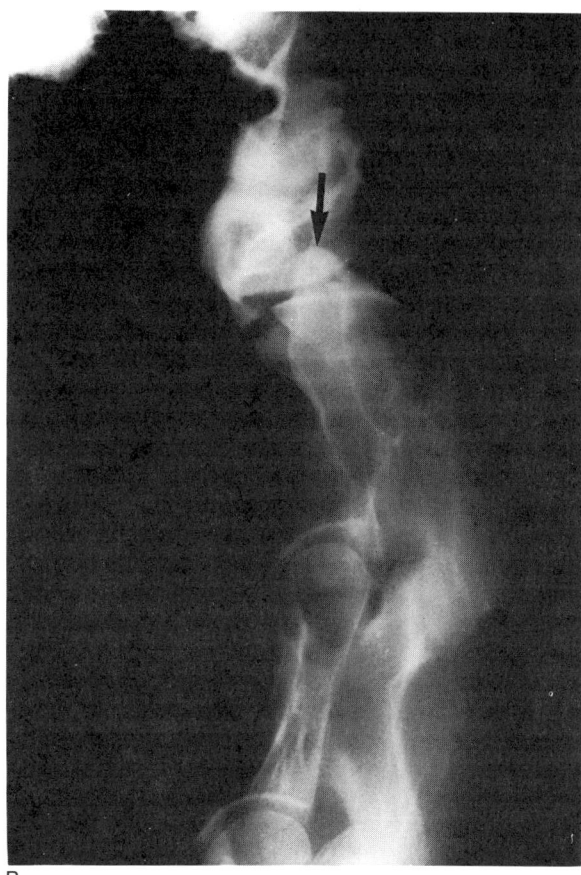

Figure 2. Normal (*A, C*) and malformed (*B, D*) occipito-atlantoaxial relationships are demonstrated on lateral and dorsoventral radiographic projections. *Arrows* identify the normal and malformed odontoid processes.

our experience, foals with advanced clinical signs of some duration are unlikely to improve significantly following surgery.

CERVICAL VERTEBRAL MALFORMATION

Cervical vertebral malformation refers to the relatively common group of functional (dynamic) or anatomical (static) compressive lesions of the equine cervical spinal cord that produce cervical compressive myelopathy. These compressive lesions typically result from either cervical vertebral instability or cervical vertebral malformation. Cervical vertebral instability is a condition in which the spinal cord is dynamically compressed as a result of hyperflexion or hyperextension of malarticulating cervical vertebrae. Positioning of the cervical spine in a normal or neutral position alleviates most or all of the spinal cord compression. Although the entire cervical spine is at risk, these lesions are found most often between the third and fourth cervical vertebrae. The clinical experience of several investigators suggests that these vertebral malarticulations are the result of developmental orthopedic diseases, most probably a form of osteochondrosis (see pages 105 and 462).

Cervical vertebral malformation is a static anatomical lesion in which the spinal canal is stenotic. The condition typically results from improper development of the vertebral body and dorsal laminae. In most cases, spinal cord compression is not affected by cervical spinal manipulation. Lesions may be oberved anywhere along the cervical spine but are most common between the fifth, sixth, and seventh cervical vertebrae.

Cervical myelopathy is a disease of young horses that produces signs of truncal ataxia, weakness, spasticity, and dysmetria. Although congenital malformations do occur, most affected individuals first exhibit clinical signs of the disease between 6 months and 4 years of age. The onset is usually insidious, but many cases are identified shortly after a traumatic injury. Presumably these deficits are noticed because of the increased scrutiny of the horse by the handler following an injury. This condition is diagnosed

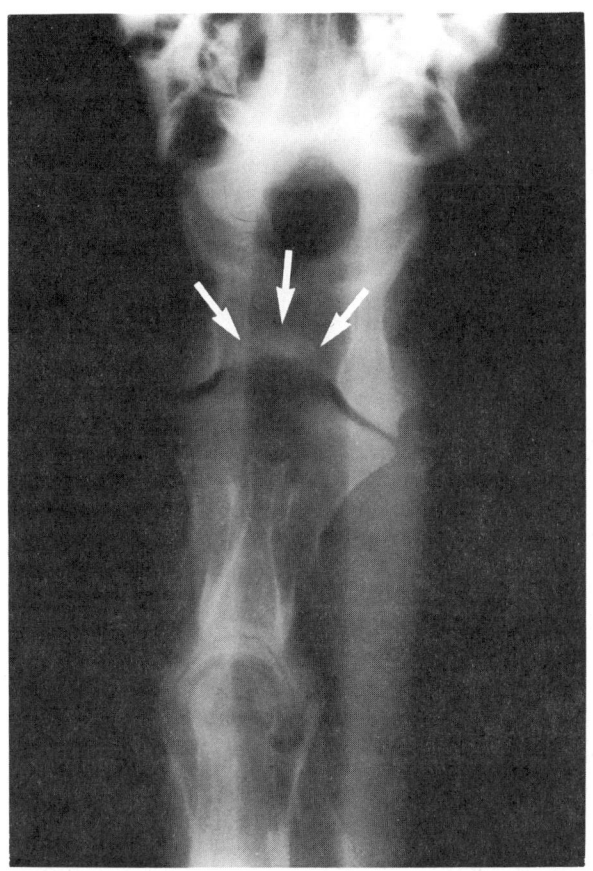 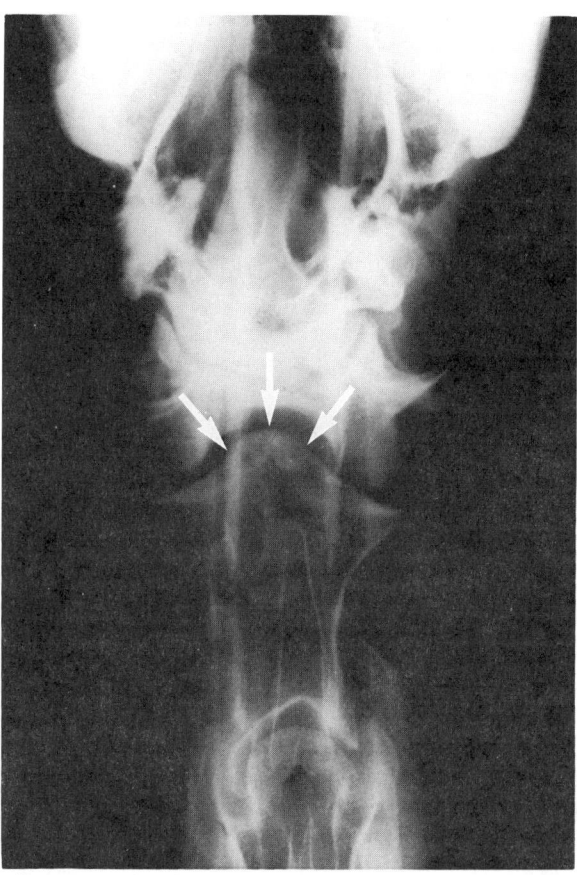

Figure 2. Continued

predominantly among the light breeds of horse and affects males more commonly than females.

Clinical signs may be present in all four limbs. The pelvic limbs are affected to a greater degree than the pectoral limbs when the lesions are located in the rostral cervical region. Horses with caudal cervical spinal cord lesions often exhibit neurological deficits of nearly similar magnitude in both forelimbs and hind limbs. Presumably, caudal cervical compression results in an increased involvement of the brachial intumescence. Clinical signs typically progress over time, accompanied by clinical and neurological deterioration. Although in untreated patients the deterioration may stabilize at some level of impairment, most eventually are no longer functionally useful.

A diagnosis of cervical vertebral instability or malformation is suspected from the history, physical findings, and neurological examination. CSF evaluation should be performed as part of a complete neurological workup; however, the results are typically of little value in making a definitive diagnosis of cervical compressive myelopathy. At present, contrast agent–enhanced myelography is the only definitive method for confirming the diagnosis. Plain film radiography alone will not permit an accurate diagnosis of vertebral instability unless severe subluxation is present. Although compressive myelopathy can be suspected from a reduced sagittal spinal canal diameter, only myelography provides definitive evidence of spinal cord compression. Marked narrowing of both dorsal and ventral columns of contrast agent is required for myelographic documentation of cervical compressive myelopathy (Fig. 3). Narrowing of the ventral dye column alone is not considered diagnostic. A complete myelographic examination of the cervical spine should be performed because of the common occurrence of multifocal lesions.

The treatment of cervical compressive myelopathy varies with the specific pathogenesis. Medical therapy, palliative at best, is directed toward minimizing spinal cord injury and inflammation. Nonsteroidal anti-inflammatory drugs (phenylbutazone,° 4 mg per kg per os [PO] twice

---

°Butazolidin, Vedco, St. Joseph, MO

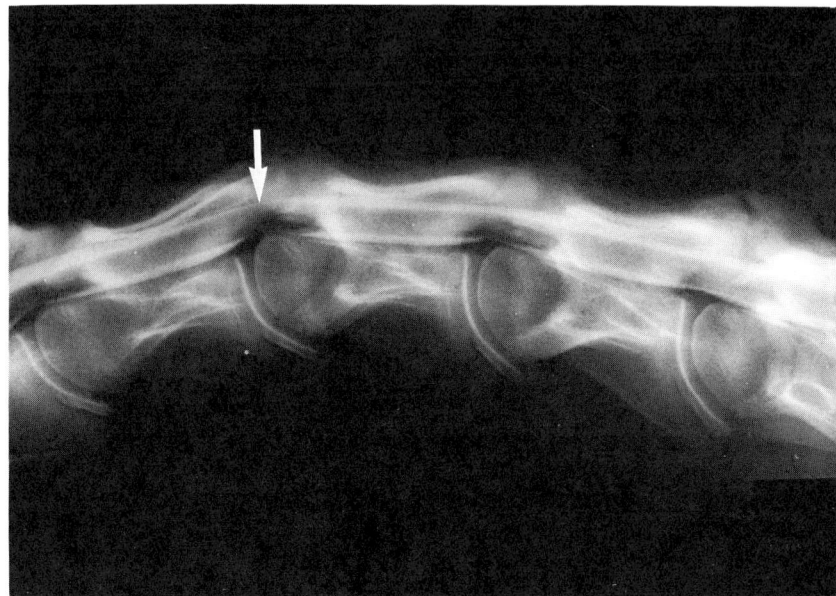

Figure 3. Narrowing of dorsal (arrow) and ventral dye columns is evident at the C3–C4 juncture on this myelographic study of a horse with cervical compressive myelopathy.

a day), corticosteroids (dexamethasone,† 0.1 mg per kg), and dimethyl sulfoxide‡ (1.0 gm per kg intravenously [IV] twice a day) can provide transient improvement; however, the condition usually returns following withdrawal of treatment. Surgical stabilization of malarticulating vertebrae by interbody fusion is clinically effective in managing most cases of instability and selected cases of malformation. Interbody fusion entails removal of the intervertebral fibrocartilaginous disk and insertion of an autogenous cancellous bone graft. A stainless steel bone cage containing the bone graft is inserted between the involved vertebrae to produce an interbody fusion. For management of static or anatomical spinal cord compression (malformation), a decompressive modified Funkquist type B laminectomy is indicated. The dorsal laminae of the offending vertebrae are removed through a dorsal midline approach. Although technically more difficult than interbody fusion, this procedure is moderately successful in alleviating focal spinal cord compression.

The prognosis for horses with cervical compressive myelopathy is guarded. Several factors affect the ultimate outcome of surgical treatment. Generally, younger patients, those 6 to 18 months old, have a better outcome than older horses. Horses with a brief course of clinical disease tend to respond to surgical therapy better than chronically affected horses. Horses with minimal neurological dysfunction tend to recover more completely than those that are severely affected. Recumbent horses with acute traumatic compressive myelopathy secondary to acute fracture or severe subluxation injuries have a poor prognosis for recovery. In general, patients with mild to moderate compressive spinal cord disease of relative brief duration (less than 3 months) can be expected to improve to some degree after surgical treatment.

CEREBELLAR ABIOTROPHY

Cerebellar abiotrophy is a congenital neurological condition of the equine neonate that is most commonly diagnosed in Arabian foals. Although viral infections have been incriminated in other species, efforts to identify a similar cause in horses have been unrewarding. Despite a lack of definitive evidence, the frequency of cerebellar abiotrophy among Arabian horses and Gottland ponies and the apparent increase in incidence within specific bloodlines of Arabian horses make it likely that the condition is inherited.

The cerebellum of affected individuals is grossly normal in size and shape, but Purkinje cells are inadequate in number and distribution to permit the normal functional interrelationships of the granular and molecular layers of the cerebellum. Within the thalamus, mineralized neuronal cell bodies have been identified rostral

---

†Azium, Schering Corp., Kenilworth, NJ
‡Domoso, Syntex Animal Health, Des Moines, IA

to the interthalamic adhesion. These degenerative cells are usually surrounded by limited accumulations of glial cells. Although the relevance of this finding is unknown, it appears unique to horses with cerebellar abiotrophy and may reflect the degenerative nature of this condition.

The clinical signs of cerebellar abiotrophy are readily attributable to cerebellar deficits. Typical signs include cranial intention tremor, spasticity, dysmetria, and ataxia. The intention tremors are noticed most commonly when affected horses purposefully attempt a coordinated action such as grasping feedstuffs. At the walk and trot, the forelimbs can appear hyperextended, producing a gait that has some resemblance to goose-stepping. There is no evidence of muscular weakness. Although most cranial nerves appear to function normally, many foals fail to exhibit a normal menace reflex. Presumably this is the result of disruption in the course of neuronal tracts from the occipital cortex through the cerebellum and into the facial nucleus. Affected horses generally do not have nystagmus, strabismus, or head tilt unless blindfolded. Application of a blindfold usually causes the affected foal to hold its head and neck in unusual positions. Presumably this is the result of acute deprivation of visual cues that are normally used to partially compensate for cerebellar deficits.

The diagnosis of cerebellar abiotrophy is suspected from the classical signalment, history, and physical examination findings. The presence of an intention tremor in a young foal of Arabian breeding is particularly incriminating. Radiography is of no value in the diagnosis of cerebellar abiotrophy. Electroencephalography of affected horses reveals abrupt multichannel changes in wave frequency. These aberrations, although not pathognomonic, can support a diagnosis of cerebellar abiotrophy. The definitive diagnosis rests on histological examination.

No medical or surgical treatment is currently available for cerebellar abiotrophy. The degenerative nature and apparent reduction in Purkinje cell mass suggest that the damage is irreparable. Nevertheless, some affected horses appear to learn to compensate for cerebellar lesions by using visual clues and other sensory inputs. Many horses that were mildly or moderately affected as foals appear to function normally as adults.

Supplemental Readings

DeBowes, R. M., Leipold, H. W., and Turner-Beatty, M.: Cerebellar abiotrophy. Vet. Clin. North Am. (Equine Pract.) 3:345, 1987.

de Lahunta, A.: Large animal spinal cord disease. In de Lahunta, A. (ed.): Veterinary Neuroanatomy and Clinical Neurology, 2nd ed. Philadelphia, W. B. Saunders, 1983, pp. 215–237.

Foreman, J. H., Reed, S. M., Rantanen, N. W., DeBowes, R. M., and Wagner, P. C.: Congenital internal hydrocephalus in a quarter horse foal. J. Equine Vet. Sci., 3:154, 1983.

Wagner, P. C.: Cervical vertebral malformation. In Robinson, N. E. (ed.): Current Therapy in Equine Medicine 2. Philadelphia, W. B. Saunders, 1987, pp. 355–359.

Trauma of the Brain and Spinal Cord

Richard M. DeBowes, MANHATTAN, KANSAS
Lisa Gift, MANHATTAN, KANSAS

Traumatic injury to the central nervous system (CNS) is a common occurrence in horses and should always be a consideration when evaluating equine patients for neurologic deficits. Clinical signs range from mild to severe, depending on the location and magnitude of the injury, and over time can increase or decrease in severity. For this reason, traumatic CNS injuries should be viewed as potentially devastating, and affected horses should undergo thorough evaluation and aggressive therapeutic intervention. Reevaluation should be performed at regular intervals to identify early evidence of progressive neurological deterioration.

The pathophysiology of CNS injury is complex and not completely understood. Traditionally, neurological trauma has been categorized as the result of concussion, contusion, compression, laceration, or hemorrhage. Regardless of the cause, at least two major forms of tissue damage can develop following traumatic injury. Acute disruption of the neural tissues will occur as a result of direct physical injury. Although usually attributed to trauma associated with fractures and subluxations, the examiner should realize that acute acceleration and deceleration (cranial) and tractional (spinal) injuries can produce neurological lesions of equivalent severity. Generally, the magnitude of clinical dysfunction is proportional to the degree of compression, traction, or crushing involved. Injuries associated with functional or anatomical transection of central nervous tissues are catastrophic (Fig. 1) and commonly produce signs of severe dysfunction necessitating euthanasia.

Latent or delayed changes that result from vascular damage are less obvious. Ischemia secondary to vascular disruption or small vessel thrombosis can lead to the generation and release of free radicals, prostaglandins, and numerous vasoactive compounds, some of which function as tissue destructive factors. As inflammatory mediators accumulate, the cerebral edema progresses, reducing vascular perfusion of the affected tissues. Hemorrhage and extravasation of plasma also accentuate the development of edema and compound the vascular compromise.

When edema develops, brain or cord swelling will occur to the extent permitted by the confines of the skull or spinal canal. Continued swelling can result in herniation of neural tissue beneath the tentorium cerebelli or through natural foramina or fracture lines. This produces further injury, exacerbating local ischemia and increasing the severity of the lesion. Within the spinal cord, impact injuries can result in vascular tears leading to hemorrhage and edema. With increasing severity, impact trauma will result in cavitation of both gray and white matter tracts. Heavily myelinated tracts are more susceptible to deterioration following compression injury than smaller fibers or unmyelinated tracts. For this reason, proprioception is lost initially after compressive injury, followed by loss of voluntary motor activity and loss of superficial and deep pain perception.

There is some evidence that the release of endogenous opioid compounds from damaged nervous tissue may increase the magnitude of neurological deficits. Increased amounts of dynorphin, an endorphin-like substance, have been identified at the site of spinal cord injuries. Further, the intrathecal administration of endorphin-like substances has produced neurological injury in clinically normal animals. For this reason, opiate antagonists are presently being evaluated for management of spinal cord injury. Although early results appear promising, experience with equine neural injuries is lacking and the treatment of equine neural injuries with opiate antagonists is not advised.

CRANIAL TRAUMA

Cranial trauma can result from collisions, penetrating wounds, or falls, particularly falls in which the horse rears over backward, striking its occipital or parietal bones. The latter can produce direct injury to neural parenchyma deep to the point of impact (Fig. 2) or indirectly by displacement of basioccipital and basisphenoid

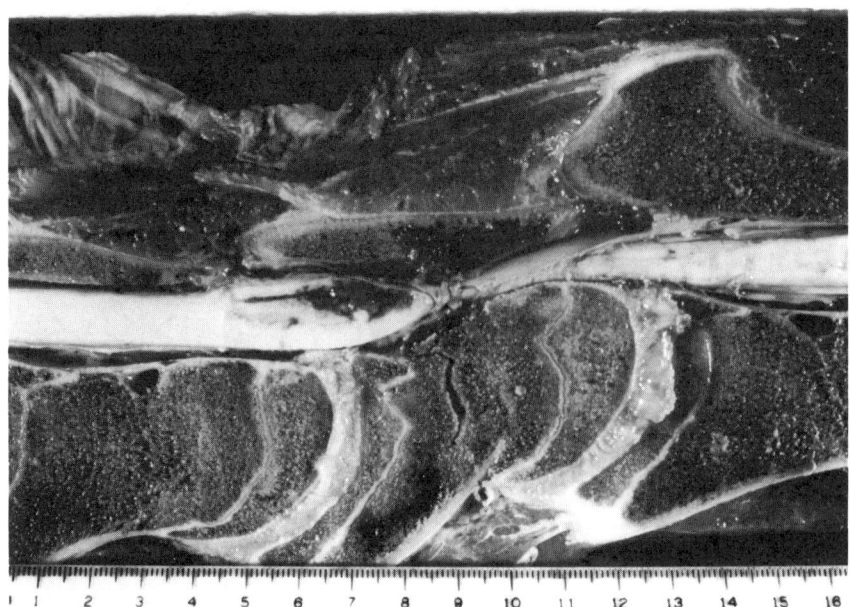

Figure 1. Minimally displaced fracture of C3 with anatomical transection of the cord.

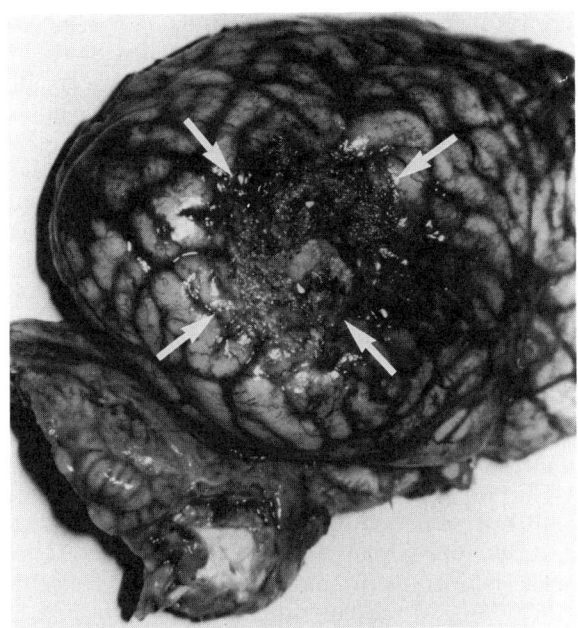

Figure 2. Cerebral parenchymal damage *(arrows)* resulting from a Mullan type III fracture of the temporal bone.

bones into the overlying brain stem. The diagnosis and treatment of cranial trauma are facilitated by an accurate history and thorough physical examination. A detailed description of the injurious event will assist the examiner in directing attention to the area of impact trauma. The examiner should evaluate the patient for intercurrent problems of hemorrhage, cardiovascular collapse, or respiratory distress. The presence of altered respiratory patterns suggests the existence of a severe brain stem injury. Patients with cranial trauma should be stabilized medically before the examiner proceeds with advanced neurological evaluations.

Horses with cranial trauma should be evaluated for mentation, cranial nerve deficits, and alterations in respiratory pattern, heart rate, and motor function. It is essential to reevaluate these parameters regularly to identify progression, deterioration, or improvement in neurological status.

Mentation is evaluated by observation of the patient for evidence of depression, stupor, or coma. Injury to any part of the cranial CNS can produce depression. Clinical depression can progress to stupor or coma following increases in intracranial pressure (ICP) or injuries to the cerebrum or midbrain. Cranial nerve deficits may provide evidence of the location and magnitude of intracranial pathology. Cranial nerve deficits are readily observed when they affect ocular function and position or deglutition. Patients should be examined for evidence of miosis, mydriasis, anisocoria, nystagmus, strabismus, and blindness. Unresponsive bilateral mydriasis is typically a poor prognostic sign associated with midbrain lesions.

Changes in respiratory and heart rates are often associated with brain stem injury. Progressive changes in the rate and character of ventilation can result from increases in ICP or herniation of the brain stem through the foramen magnum.

Motor signs are variable. However, lesions of the midbrain and brain stem are commonly accompanied by hemiplegia, tetraplegia, or ataxia. Lesions of the cerebellum typically result in some degree of ataxia or hypermetria. Tremor is less common following cerebellar trauma.

Struggling or violent horses are difficult and potentially dangerous to examine. Sedation, although generally undesirable, is often required to permit careful examination. The use of phenothiazines is discouraged because of the increased potential for convulsive activity. Xylazine* (0.1 mg per kg given intravenously [IV]) can be administered for mild sedation and restraint without serious complication. In patients suspected of intracranial hemorrhage, the use of xylazine or any sedative that produces a transient bout of hypertension is discouraged.

Convulsions must be controlled prior to evaluation. Diazepam† (10 to 30 mg IV) is generally sufficient to control convulsions in a foal. Larger doses (approaching 200 mg total) may be necessary for adult horses.

THERAPY

The treatment of cranial trauma is directed toward controlling shock, brain edema, and ICP. Dexamethasone‡ (0.1 to 0.2 mg per kg IV two to three times a day) has been used to control inflammation and neural edema. Steroids are most beneficial when administered early in the course of the disease and any clinical improvement is observed typically within 12 to 24 hours. Unfortunately, some risk of laminitis accompanies any use of systemic steroids in horses. Nevertheless, the potential consequences of severe untreated cranial trauma make the short-term use of dexamethasone an acceptable risk.

Mannitol§ (1.0 gm per kg IV) or anhydrous glycerin‖ (1 gm per kg per os [PO]) can also be used to reduce edema and ICP. Clinical results

---

*Rompun, Mobay Corp., Animal Health Division, Shawnee, KS
†Valium, Hoffmann-LaRoche, Nutley, NJ
‡Azium, Schering Corp., Kenilworth, NJ
§Mannitol 25%, Luitpold Pharmaceuticals, Shirley, NY
‖Glycerol 99.5%, Humco Labs., Texarkana, TX

are usually evident within a few hours following treatment. These medications may be repeated every 8 to 12 hours but should not be continued without careful monitoring of hydration. Previous reports and clinical experiences vary regarding the efficacy of these drugs. The use of these compounds or hypertonic IV fluids may be contraindicated if substantial intracranial hemorrhage is suspected. Intracranial accumulations of hypertonic solutions can result in additional accumulations of tissue fluid within the extravascular compartment as a result of osmotic forces.

Although not presently approved for IV use in horses, treatment with dimethyl sulfoxide° (DMSO) appears to have value in managing CNS injury. A powerful anti-inflammatory agent and diuretic, DMSO is administered IV as a 10 to 20 per cent solution of medical grade, 90 per cent stock solution, in 5 per cent dextrose. Doses of 1 gm per kg IV twice a day for 3 days, followed by once daily administration for an additional 3 days, have produced variable success. Rapid administration of DMSO can result in hemolysis or ataxia, particularly when solutions are improperly diluted. As with all osmotic diuretics, hydration must be maintained. Volume-contracted patients or those with compromised kidney function should not be treated with DMSO without concurrent fluid therapy.

Broad-spectrum antibiotics are indicated when an open fracture of the cranium is present. Open fracture should be suspected when hemorrhage from the external auditory canal or nasal passages is observed. Trimethoprim–sulfadiazine† combinations (30 mg per kg PO twice a day) are appropriate initial prophylactic therapy until CSF cytology and culture results are available.

Surgical therapy is limited to cases that would benefit substantially from fracture reduction or intracranial decompression. Patients with Mullan type II or III cranial fractures that encroach on and lacerate the meninges (type II) or impinge directly on the brain parenchyma (type III) are candidates for fracture reduction, hemostasis, decompression, and repair. Patients with progressive neurological deterioration despite appropriate medical therapy are potential candidates for surgical decompression. Referral to a surgical practice with adequate staff and instrumentation is recommended.

SPINAL CORD TRAUMA

Evaluation of the spinal cord trauma patient should be performed after the horse's medical condition has been stabilized. Efforts to support ventilation, control hemorrhage, and treat shock are of paramount importance following spinal cord injury. A careful, systematic physical examination is required to localize the neurological lesion anatomically. If the patient is standing, posture and gait are evaluated first. Typically, spinal trauma patients able to ambulate are ataxic. More commonly, the spinal trauma patient is recumbent and unable to rise. In these situations, it should be determined whether the patient can rise in response to stimulation. Caution must be exercised to avoid cord damage by exacerbating a spinal fracture injury. For this reason, efforts to stimulate the horse to move or stand should be conservative.

Careful examination of the patient for visual or palpable evidence of spinal asymmetry can suggest the approximate location of the lesion. If the horse is able to lift only its head, the lesion is most likely in the rostral cervical region (C1 to C3) (Fig. 3). Elevation of the head and neck only suggests a posterior cervical lesion (C4 to C7). Many of these patients appear to experience discomfort when moving the head and neck. Horses able to right themselves and dog-sit most likely have a lesion posterior to the second thoracic vertebra. These patients may also have a hyporeflexic panniculus and evidence of sweating posterior to the lesion. The Schiff–Sherrington syndrome is observed infrequently in horses.

Evaluation of reflexes is of questionable value when horses have been recumbent for protracted periods and is most informative when performed on the upper limb of laterally recumbent patients. Withdrawal reflexes for the forelimbs (C6 to T2) and hind limbs (L5 to S3) and patellar tendon reflexes (L4 to L5) are readily tested and interpreted. As in other species, lower motor neuron injury is associated with hyporeflexia, areflexia, and hypotonia. Upper

°Domoso 90%, Syntex Animal Health, Des Moines, IA
†Tribrissen 960, Cooper's Animal Health, Kansas City, KS

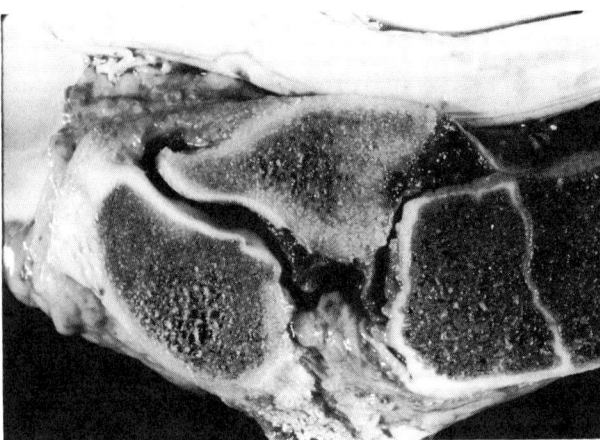

Figure 3. Displaced fracture of the odontoid process associated with spinal cord compression and tetraplegia.

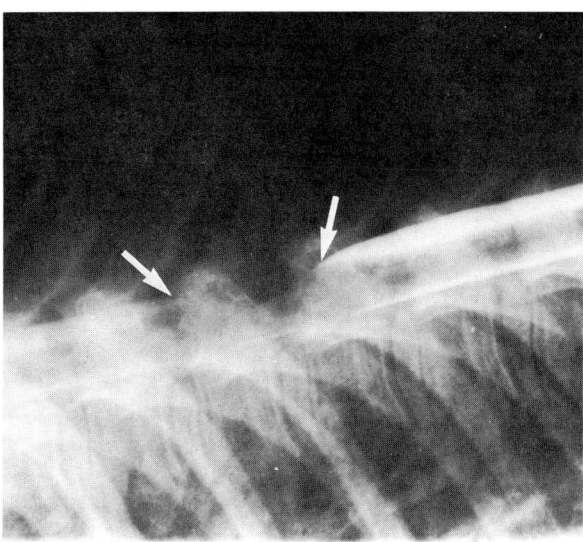

Figure 4. Compressive lesion *(arrows)* associated with a fracture of the dorsal laminae of T10. Concurrent atlanto-occipital and lumbosacral myelography demonstrated the magnitude and extent of cord compression.

motor neuron injury is associated with normal to hyperactive reflexes. When evaluating withdrawal reflexes, it is important to assess patient perception of noxious stimuli in order to evaluate the integrity of the ascending sensory tracts.

The diagnosis of spinal trauma can be augmented by radiographic, myelographic, electrodiagnostic, and clinicopathological methods. Some large animal referral veterinary hospitals have access to computed tomography. When evaluating radiographs of injured patients, the examiner must remember that the magnitude of spinal derangement present in the imaging study can be quite different from the original degree of spinal subluxation or fracture displacement. It can be quite difficult to appreciate the true extent of the injury from a radiograph alone. For this reason, myelography can be useful in defining the degree of cord compression or swelling present at the time of examination (Fig. 4). Imaging studies must always be interpreted in conjunction with the results of the neurological examination. Clinicopathological evaluation of CSF from spinal trauma patients can appear normal. More frequently, xanthochromia, red blood cells, and elevated total protein levels are present. Occasionally, increased creatine kinase levels may be detected, suggesting some degree of demyelination. Infrequently, it may be impossible to collect CSF as a result of spinal block.

THERAPY

The medical treatment of spinal cord injury is similar to that described for cranial trauma. Administration of steroids, diuretics, and hypertonic agents to control edema as previously described is appropriate. For the recumbent patient, the nursing requirements are dramatically increased. Measures to control decubital sores and urine scalding, reduce muscle compression, enhance circulation and ventilation, provide fluid and nutritional support, and maintain gastrointestinal motility must be implemented.

Patients with spinal fracture or subluxation that results in demonstrable vertebral instability or spinal cord compression are candidates for surgical therapy. Techniques for dorsal decompressive laminectomy or ventral interbody fusion may be applied independently or simultaneously to decompress and stabilize lesions of the vertebral column. The prognosis for spinal trauma patients requiring surgical intervention is guarded at best. Usually, patients with anatomical or functional transection of the spinal cord cranial to the lumbosacral plexus are candidates for euthanasia.

Supplemental Readings

DeBowes, R. M., Grant, B. D., Bagby, G. W., et al.: Cervical vertebral interbody fusion in the horse: A comparative study of bovine xenografts and autografts supported by stainless steel baskets. Am J. Vet. Res., 45:191, 1984.

Mayhew, I. G: Neurologic evaluation. In Mayhew, I. G.: Large Animal Neurology: A Handbook for Veterinary Clinicians. Philadelphia, Lea & Febiger, 1989, pp. 15–18.

Mayhew, I. G., de Lahunta, A., Withlock, R. H. et al.: Spinal cord disease in the horse. Cornell Vet., 68(suppl. 6): 1978.

Nixon, A. J., and Stashak, T. S.: Dorsal laminectomy in the horse: I. Review of the literature and description of a new procedure. Vet. Surg., 12:172, 1983.

Wagner, P. C., Bagby, G. W., Grant, B. D., et al.: Surgical stabilization of the equine cervical spine. Vet. Surg., 8:7, 1979.

Tetanus

Rebecca McConnico, RALEIGH, NORTH CAROLINA

Clostridium tetani, a gram-positive, anaerobic, spore-forming bacillus, produces a potent exotoxin that, when liberated in tissues, can cause spasticity and tetany of skeletal muscle. The bacterium is a common inhabitant of the intestinal tract of humans and animals and is abundant in soil. The horse has a much higher susceptibility to the tetanus exotoxin than other domestic animals. This factor, along with its predilection for acquiring lacerations, hoof injuries, and various other wounds, makes the horse a prime candidate for acquiring tetanus.

The three components of the *C. tetani* exotoxin are tetanospasmin, tetanolysin, and nonspasmogenic toxin. Tetanospasmin causes characteristic clinical signs of tetany by preventing the release of the inhibitory transmitter glycine, thereby blocking postsynaptic inhibition of the spinal motor neurons. A second proposed effect of tetanospasmin is blockage of transmission at the myoneural junction. The toxin is inactivated by gastric secretions, is poorly absorbed through mucous membranes, and is resistant to heat. Tetanolysin is an oxygen-labile, hemolytic, antiphagocytic substance that enhances the multiplication of anaerobic bacteria by increasing tissue necrosis. Nonspasmogenic toxin is poorly understood but is thought to produce paralysis. The exotoxin is liberated by cell lysis and carried to the central nervous system (CNS) hematogenously, then moves retrograde in the axons of the peripheral neurons. The migration occurs through both motor and sensory nerves. Once in the spinal cord, the toxin ascends to the brain.

CLINICAL SIGNS

The incubation period, which is determined by the proximity of the wound to the CNS, ranges from 3 days to several weeks, although clinical signs usually become apparent within 7 to 14 days following entry of the organism. The shorter the incubation period, the more serious is the clinical disease. Generalized tetanus begins with spasms and paralysis of voluntary muscles. The masseter muscle is the most commonly affected muscle, with progression to muscles of the neck, trunk, and limbs. Prolapse of the membrana nictitans, eyelid retraction, erect ear carriage, and flared nostrils are classical signs. A sawhorse stance and difficulty walking are common. The animal is usually reluctant to feed from the ground, and saliva often drips from its mouth. Attempts to eat and drink may result in regurgitation of food and water through the nose. Fever can be concurrent with severe muscle rigidity. Convulsions may be precipitated by external stimuli. Consciousness is generally not affected, but the animal's demeanor may be abnormal and unpredictable. Sympathetic stimulation is reflected in vasoconstriction, profuse sweating, hypertension, tachycardia, and death. Additional signs that may confuse diagnosis are gastrointestinal (GI) impaction, colic, urine retention, opisthotonos, hyperesthesia, and dyspnea. Secondary complications include laminitis, aspiration pneumonia due to paralysis of the laryngeal and pharyngeal region, and decubital ulceration, pulmonary disease, and myositis following prolonged recumbency. Clinical signs may be apparent for up to 6 weeks. Muscle spasms may persist for weeks or months, then disappear without any aftereffects. Death is usually a result of respiratory compromise.

THERAPY

Treatment goals include elimination of infection, toxin interception, control of neuromuscular derangements, and supportive nursing care. If there is any doubt about the vaccination history, tetanus toxoid should be administered at the same time as the antitoxin injection but in a separate location. The suggested minimal beneficial dose of antitoxin is 100 U per kg administered intramuscularly (IM), subcutaneously (SC), or intravenously (IV) every 3 to 5 days. Tetanus antitoxin administered by these routes is ineffective in neutralizing toxin in the CNS because it does not cross the blood–brain barrier.

Intrathecal administration of the tetanus antitoxin has been reported to be effective in horses and humans. This procedure requires general anesthesia. Anesthesia can be induced with the combination of glyceryl guaiacolate and followed by a short-acting barbiturate and halothane for maintenance. Ketamine is contraindicated because of its dissociative effects, which cause muscle rigidity. The technique for cisternal puncture is described on page 528. Fifty ml of spinal fluid (30 ml in a foal) is slowly withdrawn and an equal amount of tetanus antitoxin is injected back into the subarachnoid space. Rapid improvement and stabilization of signs should occur after recovery from anesthesia.

Penicillin (22,000 IU per kg IV four times a day or IM twice a day) is the antimicrobial of choice, although tetracycline may be substituted in penicillin-sensitive horses. Antimicrobial therapy should be continued for a minimum of 7 days even if clinical signs are no longer apparent. Wounds should be debrided and lavaged with hydrogen peroxide solution and left open for drainage. It may be useful to infiltrate the wound with antitoxin or penicillin.

Neuromuscular control is accomplished through the use of tranquilizers, hypnotics, sedatives, general anesthesia, or combinations of these, depending on the severity of the signs. Chlorpromazine (1 mg per kg IM twice a day) or acetylpromazine (0.05 mg per kg IM twice a day) is effective. Muscle relaxants such as pancuronium, d-tubocurarine, or succinylcholine will alleviate the severe muscle contractions of tetany but will also cause paralysis of respiratory muscles. Because ventilatory support must be provided when these drugs are used, muscle relaxants are not given to adult animals.

Supportive care is of the utmost importance and should include housing the animal in a dark, quiet stall and minimizing external stimuli. Cotton may be placed in the animal's ears to minimize noise. Padded walls and thick bedding will help prevent injuries. Hydration status and serum electrolyte levels need to be closely monitored since fluid loss and metabolic imbalances can be quite profound. IV fluid therapy may be required if the animal fails to eat or drink. A small-diameter nasogastric tube is useful for administering fluid, electrolytes, and gruels. Nasogastric intubation may be difficult due to pharyngeal paralysis and may even provoke muscle spasms due to the stimulus of the procedure. Equipment for emergency tracheostomy should be readily available.

Prolonged recumbency may warrant the use of a sling or bales of hay to maintain the animal in standing position or sternal recumbency. Urinary catheters, frequent manual fecal evacuation, and routine hygiene will enhance patient comfort. In cases of respiratory muscle paralysis, continuous ventilatory support is required. Extreme cases require 'round-the-clock, intensive monitoring. Secondary complications include aspiration pneumonia, pulmonary congestion, bronchopneumonia, pulmonary emboli, and pleuritis and are highly likely.

PREVENTION

Tetanus prophylaxis should be incorporated into all equine health maintenance programs (see page 37). Vaccination of brood mares 1 month prior to parturition is recommended for optimum passive transfer of tetanus antibodies. Foals should be vaccinated with toxoid at 10 to 12 weeks of age, followed by a booster 3 to 4 weeks later and a third vaccination at 6 months. Administration of tetanus antitoxin to foals that have failure of passive transfer of immunity provides protection for approximately 3 months. Annual tetanus toxoid vaccinations are recommended for adult horses.

Supplemental Readings

Ansari, M. M., and Matros, L. E.: Tetanus. Compend. Cont. Educ. Pract. Vet., 4:S473–S478, 1982.

Jansen, B. C., and Knoetze, P. C.: The immune response of horses to tetanus toxoid. Onderstepoort J. Vet. Res., 46:211–216, 1979.

Liefman, C. E.: Combined active-passive immunisation of horses against tetanus. Aust. Vet. J., 56:119–122, 1980.

Liu, I. K. M., Brown, S. L., Kuo, J., Neeley, D. P., and Feeley, J. C.: Duration of maternally derived immunity to tetanus and response in newborn foals given tetanus antitoxin. Am. J. Vet. Res., 43:2019–2022, 1982.

Botulism

Pamela A. Pintchuk, DAVIS, CALIFORNIA

Botulism is caused by the exotoxin of *Clostridium botulinum,* an anaerobic gram-positive, spore-forming, rod-shaped bacterium. The toxin is the most potent biological toxin known, causing neuromuscular weakness progressing to paralysis.

C. botulinum is found principally in the soil. Eight types have been identified (A, B, Ca, Cb, D, E, F, and G) and are differentiated based on the production of antigenically different toxins. All *C. botulinum* toxins have similar pharmacological actions. Types A, B, and C are the most common in North America, with variable regional distributions. *C. botulinum* was found in 18.5 per cent of soil samples in the United States. Type A is most often found west of the Rocky Mountains, type B in Kentucky and the mid-Atlantic states, and type C in Florida. Recently type C has been documented as a cause of botulism in horses in southern California.

Botulinum neurotoxin is secreted by the bacterium during growth and sporulation. The anaerobic organism grows best in neutral or alkaline environments and is inhibited in environments with a pH of 4.5 or less. Toxin production occurs most frequently in decaying vegetable matter or animal carcasses. Improperly ensiled haylage and silage with high moisture content and inadequate acidification (pH greater than 4.5) provide optimal conditions for growth and toxin production. Animal carcasses containing *C. botulinum* spores and toxin may be baled into hay and made into pellets or cubes that are then ingested. The mechanism of action of all types of botulinum toxin is the same. This potent neurotoxin impairs transmission of nerve impulses at all peripheral cholinergic junctions. Recent work suggests that the toxin interferes with exocytosis of acetylcholine vesicles, preventing release of the transmitter. The resulting weakness and paralysis reflect the toxin dose and are exacerbated by muscular activity.

Three types of botulinal intoxication are described: forage poisoning (ingestion of preformed toxin), toxicoinfectious botulism (ingestion of spores and subsequent toxin production in the gastrointestinal tract), and wound botulism (vegetation of spores in wounds). Most adult cases of botulism follow ingestion of preformed toxin in contaminated feedstuffs. Type B and type C botulinal toxins have been isolated in cases of forage poisoning. Toxicoinfectious botulism occurs in foals and is associated with the "shaker foal" syndrome; most cases are thought to be associated with type B botulinal toxin. Wound botulism (type B) has recently been reported as a sequel to castration in a horse.

CLINICAL SIGNS

FOALS

Toxicoinfectious botulism affects foals from 2 weeks to 8 months of age. Foals show signs of progressive symmetric motor paralysis and are often found in lateral recumbency unable to rise. Occasional foals are found dead. Dysphagia is common, with milk spilling from the mouth when nursing is attempted. Affected foals have a stilted gait and generalized muscle tremors, giving rise to the term "shaker foals." Foals have difficulty rising and may collapse after 4 to 5 minutes of standing. Ptosis, mydriasis, decreased tail tone, and constipation are frequently seen. Aspiration pneumonia can be a complication due to inability to swallow normally. Death is caused by respiratory paralysis. Mortality may exceed 90 per cent.

ADULT HORSES

Botulism in adult horses is commonly known as "forage poisoning." The incubation period varies from 24 hours to 7 days. Onset of clinical signs can be acute, with the animal displaying severe paresis, recumbency, and respiratory distress. Other cases may be slower in onset, with gradual progression over several days. Affected horses exhibit muscle tremors and weakness. Dysphagia may be the first sign recognized, with spilling of water and feed from the mouth and the presence of feed material in the nares. Appetite is usually normal although the animal may be unable to ingest feed and water. Aspiration pneumonia can be a resulting complication. Loss of tail and tongue tone is often observed. Ptosis and mydriasis with sluggish pupillary light responses are frequently seen. In horses that remain standing, the gait is stiff and stilted with short, choppy strides. Stumbling may occur. Ataxia is not a feature and should be differentiated from weakness. Muscular activity and exercise may exacerbate the clinical signs, resulting in increased muscle tremors or collapse. Urinary retention and dribbling may be seen. Constipation, bladder distention, and ileus may occur in advanced cases of paralysis and recumbency. Death occurs from paralysis of the respiratory muscles. Agonal movements are minimal.

DIAGNOSIS

The presumptive diagnosis is based on history and clinical signs. The differential diagnosis should include diseases causing dysphagia and muscle tremors in addition to generalized muscular weakness. Relevant conditions include pharyngeal or esophageal obstruction or ulceration, yellow star thistle poisoning, guttural pouch mycosis, equine protozoal encephalomyelitis, and rabies. Nutritional muscular dystrophy, white muscle disease, septicemia, polyarthritis, and hypoglycemia should be considered in foals. Hypocalcemia must be ruled out in lactating mares. Hyperkalemic periodic paralysis should be considered in heavily muscled stock-type horses.

Hematological and serum biochemical values are usually within normal limits or reflect stress. Necropsy findings are unremarkable. Gastric ulcers and necrotic foci in the liver are sometimes noted in foals and may be suspect sites of infection with C. botulinum. Cerebrospinal fluid analysis is normal. Markedly abnormal clinicopathological findings in bodily fluids should alert the clinician to a disease other than botulism.

The definitive diagnosis is based on identification of botulinum toxin in the serum, gastrointestinal contents, or feedstuffs. Mouse inoculation is the diagnostic method of choice. Toxin can be isolated from the feces of 10 per cent of affected foals. Due to the extraordinary sensitivity of the horse to minute amounts of toxin, attempts to isolate toxin are unsuccessful. Circulating toxin is rapidly bound to peripheral cholinergic nerve receptors, reducing the amount of toxin available for assay. Feces from affected animals should be cultured for *C. botulinum* spores. Spores can be found in the feces of 20 to 30 per cent of affected adults and approximately 80 per cent of "shaker foals." Normal nonexposed horses rarely harbor the organism.

Electrophysiological testing is used extensively in humans to diagnose botulism and has been reported in horses and cattle. Repetitive nerve stimulation in affected humans produces a decremental response in the evoked muscle action potential at low rates of stimulation (2 Hz) and an incremental response at high rates (50 Hz). Variation in results can be considerable.

THERAPY AND PROGNOSIS

The rapidity of onset and the severity of signs depend on the toxin dose. Horses and foals in which signs progress rapidly to respiratory distress and recumbency in less than 48 hours have a very poor prognosis. Animals that develop weakness, muscle tremor, and dysphagia gradually over several days may not develop paralysis and respiratory distress. The latter cases have a better prognosis, although weeks may be required before neuromuscular function and recovery of normal strength is complete.

Therapy is directed toward neutralizing the circulating toxin; other treatment is supportive. Polyvalent antitoxin should be administered to neutralize any circulating toxin not yet bound in synaptic terminals. Antitoxin does not neutralize bound toxin. Administration of antitoxin in the early stages prior to involuntary recumbency can increase the survival rate to greater than 70 per cent. Treatment with antitoxin may be prohibitively expensive in some cases. The recommended dose of equine origin polyvalent antitoxin (100 to 150 IU per ml) is 200 ml for a foal and 500 ml for an adult horse, administered IV or IM. Passively administered antitoxin should be protective for up to 60 days. To obtain antitoxin, inquiries should be made to the University of Pennsylvania.

Supportive treatment includes conscientious nursing care and provision of appropriate nutrition, fluids, and electrolytes to animals unable to swallow (see p. 724). Muscular activity exacerbates weakness and should be restricted. Affected horses should be provided with deeply bedded stalls to prevent the formation of decubital sores from prolonged recumbency. Any decubital lesions should be treated with topical antiseptic dressings and heavily padded to prevent further injury. Frequent turning from side to side is critical in preventing severe decubitus and pulmonary dysfunction.

Nutritional needs should be met by either enteral or IV administration in horses unable to swallow. Parenteral nutritional therapy is expensive and may be prohibitively costly in adults and many foals. All solutions and infusion sets must be sterile and care must be taken to avoid contamination of fluid systems with bacteria. Catheter placement must be sterile, maintained diligently with clean dressings, and monitored frequently for signs of catheter-associated sepsis or thrombophlebitis. Catheters should be changed every 3 days, alternating to the opposite jugular vein each time. Enteral nutrition can be supplied to the dysphagic or recumbent horse by administration of a slurry via nasogastric tube. The tube can be passed several times a day for feeding or maintained in place by suturing it to the nares and securing it with tape. Adults can be maintained on a slurry of water, electrolytes, dextrose, dehydrated alfalfa meal, and dehydrated cottage cheese. Horses capable of normal food intake should be fed diets that will maintain a soft stool. Mineral oil should be administered periodically to prevent constipation and impaction. Foals unable to nurse from the dam should be fed mare's milk or milk replacer through an indwelling nasogastric tube. Small amounts should be fed at frequent intervals to prevent gastric distention or aspiration of milk. All horses fed by nasogastric tube should be maintained in a sternal position during and after feeding to prevent esophageal reflux of feed and secondary pulmonary aspiration. Ileus is frequently present, and gastric decompression should be maintained by nasogastric tube when needed.

Antibiotics are not effective in eliminating *C. botulinum* from the intestinal tract in cases of toxicoinfectious botulism. Oral administration of penicillin is contraindicated, since it may increase toxin release from intestinal vegetative forms of the bacterium. Because the source of infection with *C. botulinum* is rarely known, IV administration of sodium or potassium penicillin is often indicated (22,000 to 44,000 IU per kg four times daily). Antibiotic treatment is also indicated for specific secondary complications such as aspiration pneumonia. Antibiotics that have been associated with neuromuscular weakness are contraindicated, including procaine penicillin, the aminoglycosides, and tetracycline. Oral magnesium cathartics should be avoided, since these may also contribute to neuromuscular weakness.

Treatment with other drugs such as neostigmine, guanidine hydrochloride, 3-aminopyridine, and 3,4-diaminopyridine has produced equivocal results, and these medications may be contraindicated because they deplete the neuromuscular junction of acetylcholine. Muscular activity should be prevented for the same reason. Xylazine and diazepam are useful sedatives for control of horses and foals that struggle in recumbency. Mechanical ventilatory support of horses and foals with respiratory paralysis has met with limited success but may be considered in selected cases (see p. 478).

CONTROL

Clostridium botulinum type B toxoid is available for use in horses in the United States.° In endemic areas, foals can be protected from "shaker foal" syndrome by vaccination of the mares prior to foaling. Initially, mares should be vaccinated three times during gestation, 1 month apart, with the third dose administered 2 to 4 weeks before parturition. Mares should be revaccinated annually with a single booster injection 2 to 4 weeks before parturition. The product is not currently labeled for vaccination of foals. Currently, no toxoid against type C is approved and labeled for use in horses. A *C. botulinum* type C toxoid† is available but is approved for use in mink only. No multivalent vaccine is available at this time.

Supplemental Readings

Kao, I., Drachman, D. B., and Price, D. L.: Botulinum toxin: Mechanism of presynaptic blockade. Science, *193*:1256–1258, 1976.

Smith, M. O.: Botulism (shaker foals; forage poisoning). *In* Smith, B. P. (ed.): Large Animal Internal Medicine. St. Louis, C. V. Mosby, 1990, pp. 1033–1036.

Swerczek, T. W.: Toxicoinfectious botulism in foals and adult horses. J. Am. Vet. Med. Assoc., *176*:218–220, 1980.

Whitlock, R. H., and Messick, J. B.: Foal botulism (shaker foal syndrome): Clinical signs, diagnosis, treatment and prevention. *In:* Proceedings of the American Association of Equine Practitioners, 1987, pp. 359–366.

Whitlock, R. H.: Botulism in large animals. *In:* Proceedings of the 8th American College of Veterinary Internal Medicine Forum, 1990, pp. 681–684.

°Bot Tox-B, Neogen Biologics Corp., Lansing, MI
†United Vaccine, Madison, WI

Rabies

Judy H. Cox, MANHATTAN, KANSAS

The incidence of equine rabies is low; only 38 positive cases were recorded in the United States in 1988. However, equine rabies is of major importance because of the infectious nature of the disease, the potential for exposure of a number of persons to a single rabid horse, and because the presenting signs are extremely variable and nonspecific. For these reasons, rabies should be considered in any horse with a rapidly progressive illness that includes neurological signs.

The enveloped rabies virus, a lyssavirus, is a member of the family Rhabdoviridae. Monoclonal antibody techniques have shown antigenic differences in rabies virus isolates from different wildlife hosts and geographic areas. Using these techniques, the probable source of the virus has been determined in some cases, but this is not currently a routine practice. The virus is distributed worldwide with the exception of some island countries and the Scandinavian peninsula. Horses are moderately susceptible to the virus and, in North America, are most likely to be exposed by the bite of a rabid wild animal. Skunks, foxes, raccoons, and insectivorous bats are the most common reservoirs of the virus in North America. Exposure via salivary contamination of a wound or by aerosol, ingestion, or transplacental transfer is unlikely in horses.

The virus is relatively fragile and is killed by most disinfectants (including 70 per cent isopropyl alcohol, povidone–iodine, quaternary ammonium compounds, formalin, halogens, anionic detergents, and others), ultraviolet light, and heat. The virus dies in dried saliva within hours and will die in a carcass within 24 hours at 20° C. However, the virus survives longer at colder temperatures, living for days in refrigerated carcasses. Although there are no documented cases of human rabies due to exposure to a rabid horse, veterinarians should be vigilant in handling suspect horses.

PATHOGENESIS

Following bite inoculation of the horse, the virus usually replicates locally in myocytes for a variable period. The virus then spreads centripetally along peripheral nerves, again for a variable length of time, depending on the animal's age, the distance from the inoculation site to the central nervous system (CNS), and the degree of innervation of the area of inoculation. Once the virus enters the spinal cord or brain stem it ascends bilaterally and rapidly to the forebrain. Lower motor neuron damage occurring during viral transit may result in an ascending paralysis. Following replication in the CNS, the virus spreads centrifugally along peripheral nerves, including those of the autonomic nervous system, to other body tissues. There is some evidence, such as bilateral sciatic nerve involvement without significant brain involvement, that the virus may not behave classically in all horses.

CLINICAL SIGNS

A wide variety of presenting signs have been documented, and the disease is frequently initially misdiagnosed. Initial complaints have included intermittent fever, lethargy, anorexia, lameness, ataxia, paresis, hyperesthesia, hyperactivity, extraocular muscle spasms, blindness, abdominal pain (colic), urinary incontinence, and anuria. The incubation period averages 2 to 9 weeks but may possibly be as long as 15 months. The disease usually progresses rapidly with a short course ending in death as early as 12 hours after onset, but more typically in 3 to 5 days. In one case, the horse lived for at least 10 days with progressive clinical signs.

While some horses exhibit intermittent or continuous signs of aggressive behavior, affected horses are more typically depressed or stuporous. Obscure lameness and posterior ataxia are relatively common early signs. Varying degrees of hyperesthesia are present in a significant percentage of cases, as is intermittent fever. Some horses are anorectic or refuse to drink, but hydrophobia is not a frequent sign. Occasional horses exhibit ptyalism or bruxism.

Horses exhibiting aggressive signs may attack humans, animals, or inanimate objects. Occasionally self-mutilation of a particular site on the body occurs; it has been speculated that this behavior represents a neuritis at the site of viral entry.

Most horses worsen rapidly, proceeding to sternal or lateral recumbency, followed by paddling, convulsions, or coma. Rabid horses may continue to eat and drink until shortly before death.

DIAGNOSIS

Definitive antemortem diagnosis of rabies is difficult, since clinical signs alone are rarely diagnostic. Complete blood counts, serum biochemical analyses, and cerebrospinal fluid (CSF) evaluations are nondiagnostic. Because of the human health hazard, CSF examination should be avoided if there is a high suspicion of rabies.

Several antemortem tests are available, but the results are often negative until late in the course of the disease. Fluorescent rabies antibody examination of a skin biopsy specimen containing several tactile hairs may confirm a diagnosis of rabies in some cases. A full-thickness skin specimen containing several tactile hairs should be surgically excised from the muzzle area and submitted chilled to the laboratory. A positive result is diagnostic, but a negative result does not exclude the possibility of rabies. If initial test results are negative, resubmission may be indicated in several days if the neurological signs continue to worsen. Fluorescent rabies antibody examination of corneal impression smears is interpreted in the same way as a skin biopsy. Serology can be performed on serum or CSF. Serum titers may reflect previous vaccination or past exposures as well as current exposure; CSF titers do not increase after vaccination. Unfortunately, CSF titers usually do not become positive until clinical signs have been present for at least 7 to 10 days. Serum and CSF titers should be compared to ensure that the CSF titer is not due to protein leakage from contamination during collection or from an inflammatory process that allows disruption of the blood–brain barrier. Virus isolation can be performed on saliva; results may not be available soon enough to be of benefit in diagnosis but may be useful retrospectively.

The postmortem diagnosis of rabies is classically made from examination of the brain, but a recent report documents two cases of equine rabies in which a fluorescent rabies antibody test of the hippocampus was negative or equivocal and similar examination of spinal cord or large peripheral nerves was positive. I have also had a case in which fluorescent rabies antibody assay of the brain was equivocal, but fluorescent rabies antibody assay of the cervical spinal cord was strongly positive. Therefore, fluorescent rabies antibody testing of sections of the spinal cord as well as the brain may be indicated, especially in horses with clinical signs referable to a spinal cord lesion. These tissues should be submitted chilled (not frozen) to an approved diagnostic laboratory. The fluorescent rabies antibody test is rapid and highly accurate. Confirmation by mouse inoculation may also be performed. Histological examination for the presence of characteristic intracytoplasmic inclusion bodies (Negri bodies) is less accurate.

PROPHYLAXIS

Because rabies is considered invariably fatal in the horse, no treatment is available, and horses positively diagnosed with rabies should be euthanized immediately. Unfortunately, since the clinical signs of rabies often are not distinctive enough to rule out a number of other neurological diseases, it is usually necessary to treat the horse supportively while other potential diagnoses are eliminated or until progression of clinical signs occurs.

Rabies should always be considered in horses with a rapidly progressive course that includes neurological abnormalities, and precautions must be taken to avoid unnecessary human exposure. The affected horse should be isolated and persons handling the animal should wear rubber gloves. Preferably, all persons providing medical care to the horse should be immunized prior to exposure. All laboratory samples should be clearly identified as originating from a rabies suspect. Persons performing a necropsy examination should be especially careful, and the use of a power saw or an ax in removing CNS tissue is not recommended; aerosolization of rabies virus is more likely. When rabies is first suspected, a list should be made of all persons that had contact with the horse in the recent past; if a definitive diagnosis is obtained before or after death, all exposed persons should be contacted and promptly referred to a physician for advice on postexposure treatment.

Three killed-cell culture-adapted rabies virus vaccines are currently approved by the U.S. Department of Agriculture (USDA) for rabies prophylaxis in horses 3 months and older.* A single annual vaccination is required. It is not considered justified from either the public health or economic aspect to vaccinate all horses; however, vaccination is justified for horses with significant real or sentimental value, horses in areas of epizootic wildlife rabies, and horses in close contact with humans.

Horses currently vaccinated with a USDA-approved vaccine that are bitten by a rabid animal should be revaccinated promptly and kept under observation for 90 days. A serum sample may be collected from an exposed, vaccinated horse within a few days of exposure, prior to revaccination, and submitted to the laboratory to determine the horse's titer at the time of exposure; a titer of 1:5 is considered protective. Currently, the Department of Veterinary Diagnosis at Kan-

---

*Rabguard-TC, Norden Laboratories, Lincoln, NE; Imrab, Pitman-Moore, Mundelein, IL; Rabvac 3, Solvay Animal Health, Mendota Heights, MN

sas State University, Manhattan, KS, is the only laboratory in the United States that determines rabies titers.

It is recommended that unvaccinated horses with a known exposure to rabies be euthanized or slaughtered immediately. If the owner chooses to keep an exposed horse, the animal should be kept under observation for 6 months. Postexposure vaccination of previously unvaccinated horses is not recommended.

Supplemental Readings

Meyer, E. E., Morris, P. G., Elcock, L. H., and Weil, J.: Hindlimb hyperesthesia associated with rabies in two horses. J. Am. Vet. Med. Assoc., 188:629–632, 1986.

Martin, M. L., and Sedmak, P. A.: Rabies. Part I. Epidemiology, Pathogenesis, and Diagnosis. Compend. Contin. Educ. Pract. Vet., 5:521–528, 1983.

Sedmak, P. A., and Martin, M. L.: Rabies. Part II. Prophylaxis and Control. Compend. Contin. Educ. Pract. Vet., 6:49–58, 1984.

Togaviral Encephalitides: Alphavirus (Eastern and Western) Equine Encephalitis

Joseph J. Bertone, COLUMBUS, OHIO

Several insect-borne viruses of the family Togaviridae, subcategories *Alphavirus* and *Flavivirus*, have been associated with encephalitis in horses. The encephalitic conditions associated with these viruses have similar clinical presentations but disparate epizootic features. Members of the *Flavivirus* spp. are sporadically associated with encephalitis in the United States; *Alphavirus* spp. tend to be more virulent and more commonly associated with disease in the United States and include eastern (EEE), western (WEE), and Venezuelan (VEE) equine encephalitis (p. 765).

The EEE, WEE, and VEE viruses are small, enveloped RNA viruses that are structurally similar but antigenically distinct. There are four subtypes of VEE virus. Type I, variants A, B, and C, are associated with disease and epidemics. There are only minor chemical differences in the subtypes of WEE and EEE.

EPIZOOTIOLOGY

In general, the development of equine and human epidemics associated with EEE, WEE, and VEE viruses requires sufficient quantities of reservoir animals, infected intermediate hosts, insect vectors, and adjacent populations of susceptible horses and persons.

With minor exceptions, the Togaviridae persist by asymptomatically infecting wild animals (sylvatic hosts) such as birds, small mammals, and reptiles. By an unknown mechanism, the viruses persist in reservoir hosts without inducing clinical disease. The viruses survive during the nonvector season in sylvatic populations. There appears to be some specificity of the viruses for specific vectors. This relationship is tenuous, but vector distribution may, to some degree, explain the viral distribution. The vectors for EEE virus include *Culiseta melanura* and *Aedes* spp. The vectors for WEE virus include *Culex tarsalis* and *Dermacentor andersoni*. In Florida, WEE virus persists continuously in *Culiseta melanura*. That mosquito is confined to freshwater swamps and waterways and is rarely found in areas of high horse population.

Disease associated with EEE and WEE viruses is generally restricted to the western hemisphere and occurs in temperate to desert climates. In general, each virus and each incidence of associated equine disease have characteristic distributions. Disease distribution (Fig. 1) is restricted, compared with the distribution of asymptomatic horses and sylvatic hosts. For example, clinical disease associated with VEE virus was only identified in the southern United States in 1971, but asymptomatic horses with significant titers for VEE virus (type II) are regularly identified in Florida. The WEE virus is identified in reservoir avian hosts in the eastern United States, but clinical disease is rarely identified in that region.

Vectors transmit viral particles between sylvatic hosts when taking a blood meal. If the virus is able to penetrate the insect gut, it may multiply and subsequently be shed in oral secretions. If the blood meal contains adequate viral parti-

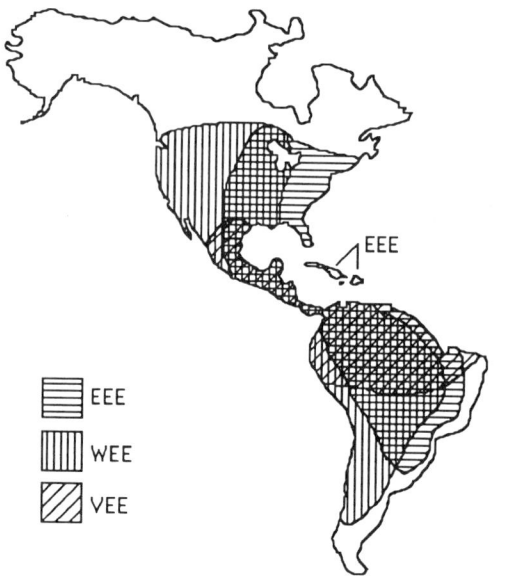

Figure 1. Predominant distribution of disease associated with *Alphavirus spp* equine encephalitis.

cles, the multiplicative cycle may not be required. In most instances, the mosquito remains infected for life.

The diseases occur most commonly during the height of the vector season. In temperate climates, the greatest number of cases occurs between June and November. In warm climates, where the vector season is longer, the disease problem is more continuous. Circulating virus concentrations often are too low for transmission of EEE virus from infected horses to humans, mosquitoes, and other animals. Human disease is most likely associated with insect vector contact and often coincides with or is preceded by equine epizootics. However, in the acute stages of equine disease a transient, substantial viremia does occur. Therefore, if vector density is high, an acutely infected horse could be a transient amplifier of EEE virus.

Both persons and horses are terminal hosts for WEE virus. Human cases of WEE viral disease, associated with vector contact, occur yearly. High numbers of equine cases indicate heavy sylvatic concentrations of virus but not a potential source of infection for humans. Generally, increased numbers of horse cases precede cases in humans by 2 to 5 weeks. Therefore, horses serve as sentinels for humans in a given area.

With any of the alphaviral equine encephalitides, sufficient viral particles for infection may be present in central nervous tissues, and in the case of VEE, precautions should be taken during necropsy examinations of suspect cases. Strict mosquito control in affected areas is necessary to prevent both human and equine cases, and all equine cases should be reported to state health officials. Cases of VEE must be reported in the United States; other measures of disease control may be instituted by public health officials.

PATHOGENESIS

After the viruses are inoculated, they multiply in muscle, enter the lymphatic circulation, and localize in lymph nodes. The virus replicates in macrophages and neutrophils and is subsequently shed in small numbers. Many of the viral particles are cleared at this time. If clearance mechanisms are successful, no further clinical signs develop, but neutralizing antibodies will be produced. If viral elimination is not complete, the remaining viruses infect endothelial cells and concentrate in highly vascular organs, such as the liver and spleen. Viral replication in these organs is subsequently associated with high concentrations of cirulating virus. The second viremic period is often associated with early clinical signs of disease. Infection of the central nervous system (CNS) occurs within 3 to 5 days.

CLINICAL SIGNS

Acute clinical signs of EEE and WEE are nonspecific and include fever, mild to severe pyrexia, anorexia, and stiffness. After an experimental dose of EEE and WEE viruses, there is a 1- to 3-week incubation period. The incubation period is often shorter with EEE than WEE. Transient early signs of the diseases are frequently undetected and often include fever and mild depression. Acute signs may last for up to 5 days. Many cases of WEE do not progress beyond this point. With EEE, progression is more common. In progressive cases the fever may rise and fall sporadically. Cerebral signs can develop at any time but often do not occur until a few days after infection. Acute cerebral signs range from compulsive walking, depression, and somnolence to hyperesthesia, aggression, and excitability. Some horses may become frenzied after any sensory stimulation. Often conscious proprioceptive deficits are evident in the early stages. With progression, signs become less disparate and more consistent between EEE and WEE. Later signs include head pressing, compulsive walking, blindness, circling, head tilt, and facial and appendicular muscle fasciculations. Paralysis of the pharynx, larynx, and tongue is common. Death is often preceded by recumbency for 2 to 7 days. Survivors show a gradual improvement of function over weeks to months.

Clinical signs of VEE are described on page 765.

DIAGNOSIS

The presumptive diagnosis is based on clinical findings and the presence of associated epidemiological features. Serological and necropsy evaluation provide a definitive determination. Viral infections are usually identified by complement fixation, hemagglutination inhibition, and cross-serum neutralization assays. A combination of these techniques increases the likelihood of a positive diagnosis. Although a fourfold rise in antibody titers in convalescent sera is commonly recommended for diagnosis, a rise in titer may not always be detected. Viral antibodies are commonly present by 24 hours after the initial viremia and their presence often precedes clinical encephalitis. Antibody concentration increases rapidly and then decreases over 6 months. The initial sample is often taken when encephalitic signs are present and peak titers may already have been reached; the second sample may have a decreased titer as compared to the initial sample. Colostral antibodies may interfere with serodiagnosis in foals. Antibody titers to VEE, WEE, and EEE viruses in the sera of 2- to 8-day-old foals are similar to those in the dams. The serum half-life of maternal antibodies in foals is approximately 20 days.

The cerebrospinal fluid (CSF) changes associated with togaviral infections are similar to those of other viral encephalitides and include increased cellularity (50 to 400 mononuclear cells per μl) and protein concentration (100 to 200 mg per dl). The virus may be isolated from the CSF of horses with acute infections.

Animals that die or are euthanized should be necropsied and gross and histological examinations performed with special reference to the CNS. The brain and spinal cord often have a normal gross appearance, but vascular congestion and discoloration of the CNS can be found in some cases. Histological findings include nonseptic mononuclear cell and neutrophilic inflammation. Lesions are found in the cerebral cortex, thalamus, and hypothalamus. Specific lesions include marked perivascular cuffing with mononuclear and neutrophilic cell infiltration, gliosis, neuronal degeneration, and mononuclear cell meningeal inflammation.

The differential diagnosis of EEE, WEE, or VEE should include other conditions associated with diffuse or multifocal neurological deficits such as other togaviral encephalitides, trauma, hepatoencephalopathy, rabies, mycotoxic encephalomalacia, bacterial meningoencephalitis, equine protozoal myeloencephalitis, and verminous encephalitis.

THERAPY

There is no effective, specific treatment for the viral encephalitides. Treatment is primarily supportive. Nonsteroidal anti-inflammatory drugs (phenylbutazone, 4 mg per kg every 12 hours; flunixin meglumine, 1 mg per kg every 12 to 24 hours) are used to control pyrexia, inflammation, and discomfort. Dimethyl sulfoxide (1 gm per kg in 20 per cent solution given intravenously) may help control inflammation and provide some analgesia and mild sedation. The use of corticosteroids is controversial since beneficial effects are short term and there is an increased risk of secondary bacterial infections. Convulsions can be controlled by the use of pentobarbital, diazepam, phenobarbital, or phenytoin. If horses develop secondary bacterial infections, appropriate antibiotic therapy should be employed.

Hydration should be monitored and balanced fluid solutions administered orally or intravenously as needed. Other supportive care includes dietary supplementation. Laxatives should be administered to minimize the risk of gastrointestinal impaction. If anorexia persists for more than 48 hours, enteral or parenteral supplementation should be employed. Commercial formulations can be used. For the short term, suspensions of soaked pelleted feeds can be administered orally. Protection from self-induced trauma includes protective leg wraps and head protection. All animals should be bedded heavily. If the horse is recumbent, attempts should be made to provide support in a sling.

PROGNOSIS

Complete recovery from the neurological deficits associated with these viruses is rare. Animals that have recovered from EEE often have residual neurological deficits that commonly include ataxia, depression, and abnormal behavior. Neurological sequelae are similar, but less common, in horses that recover from WEE. For horses that develop neurological signs, the mortality rate for EEE is 75 to 100 per cent, for WEE it is 20 to 50 per cent, and for VEE it is 40 to 80 per cent. Horses that recover seem to be variably protected for up to 2 years after infection, but it is probably wise to assume that no protection is afforded by infection. Horses with VEE can be persistently viremic and are quarantined for 3 weeks after complete recovery.

PREVENTION

Prevention of togaviral encephalitides is directed toward reducing the concentration of insect vectors and implementing vaccination programs. Insecticides and repellents should be used when possible and practical. Standing water should be eliminated, if possible. In endemic areas or during an outbreak, environmental insecticide application and screened stalls may be implemented.

Most vaccines are formalin-inactivated viruses of chick tissue culture origin. Vaccination of susceptible horse populations with monovalent, divalent, or trivalent vaccines containing EEE, WEE, or VEE virus should be employed. There is increased specific antibody production to all viruses when trivalent vaccines are administered. Antibodies formed against WEE or EEE virus afford limited protection against VEE virus. If VEE vaccine is given, all three should be administered simultaneously. The response to VEE vaccination alone is diminished in horses previously vaccinated against WEE and EEE. Annual vaccination should be completed in late spring or several months prior to the beginning of the encephalitis season. Adequate titers appear to last for 6 to 8 months. In areas where the mosquito season is prolonged or continuous, biannual or triannual vaccination is suggested. Vaccination of susceptible horses in the face of an outbreak is recommended. If vaccinated horses develop disease, the affected individuals are often very young or old.

Vaccination of mares 1 month prior to foaling will enhance colostral antibody concentrations. Antibody concentrations in foals born to immunized mares appear by 3 hours after colostrum is fed and persist for 6 to 7 months. Vaccination may begin at any age, but foals that are vaccinated early should be revaccinated at 6 months and 1 year to ensure adequate protection.

Supplemental Readings

Barber, T. L., Walton, T. E., Lewis, K. J.: Efficacy of trivalent inactivated encephalomyelitis virus vaccine in horses. Am. J. Vet. Res., 39:621, 1978.
Byrne, R. J.: The control of eastern and western arboviral encephalomyelitis of horses. In: 3rd International Conference on Equine Infectious Diseases. Basel, S. Karger, 1972, p. 115.
Calisher, C. H., Emerson, J. K., and Muth, D. J. et al: Serodiagnosis of western encephalitis virus infections: Relationships of antibody titer and test to observed onset of clinical illness. J. Am. Vet. Med. Assoc. 183:438, 1983.
Ferguson, J. A., Reeves, W. C., and Hardy, J. L.: Antibody studies in ponies vaccinated with Venezuelan equine encephalomyelitis (strain tc-83) and other alphavirus vaccines. Am. J. Vet. Res., 38:425, 1977.
Gibbs, E. P. J.: Equine viral encephalitis. Equine Vet. J., 8:66, 1976.
Kissling, R. E.: Venezuelan equine encephalitis. Adv. Vet. Sci., 11:65, 1967.
Walton, T. E., and Johnson, K. M.: Epizootiology of Venezuelan equine encephalomyelitis in the Americas. J. Am. Vet. Med. Assoc., 161:1509, 1972.

Equine Herpes Myeloencephalopathy

Gregg Kortz, DAVIS, CALIFORNIA

As early as 1949 Manninger reported neurological signs associated with equine herpesvirus 1 (EHV-1) infection. Cases of EHV-1–induced neurological signs have since been reported from several countries, including Australia, Denmark, Germany, Norway, the United States, and the United Kingdom. EHV-1 neurological disease is characterized primarily by signs of spinal cord involvement, with varying degrees of ataxia and paresis. Abnormalities of the cauda equina and brain stem are frequently identified. Although the disease is generally sporadic, both single cases and epizootics have been reported at breeding farms, racetracks, and training stables. Stallions, geldings, pregnant and nonpregnant mares, and foals may develop neurological signs associated with EHV-1 infections.

CLINICAL SIGNS

An incubation period of 4 to 14 days is typical, and exposure to other horses with fever, upper respiratory infection, or abortion may be reported in the history. Proximity to or direct contact with mules or donkeys was implicated in herpes myeloencephalitis in two epizootics.

Clinical signs are variable and depend on the extent and location of the neuraxis involved. The typical clinical presentation is one of acute onset that sometimes progresses rapidly over 24 to 48 hours, followed by stabilization. The ataxia and paraparesis are usually symmetrical. The thoracic limbs can be involved but usually to a lesser extent than the pelvic limbs. Signs referable to the cauda equina include urinary bladder paralysis, anal sphincter paresis with fecal retention, penile prolapse, and repeated erections. Sensory deficits in the perineum and tail head area can occur. Less frequently, vestibular involvement and facial, tongue, and pharyngeal weakness are encountered. The affected horse may be febrile, cough, and have a nasal discharge. Occasionally subcutaneous edema of the distal limbs and scrotal edema in males accompanies the onset of clinical signs. Mares rarely abort during the course of the neurological disease.

DIAGNOSIS

Hematological and biochemical evaluation of the affected animal is usually unremarkable. During the febrile period the horse may be leukopenic, lymphopenic, and thrombocytopenic. The cerebrospinal fluid (CSF) demonstrates an albuminocytological dissociation and is often xanthochromic due to the action of the enzyme heme oxygenase, which converts heme to bilirubin, the major pigment accounting for the xanthochromia. The total protein content in the CSF is characteristically elevated to a level of 100 to 300 mg per dl. Recent interest in CSF EHV-1 antibodies is noteworthy. Because of the proposed pathogenesis of EHV-1 infection, the presence of EHV-1 antibodies in CSF can be compared to that in serum at the time of sampling. A higher CSF titer suggests intrathecal production; serum contamination is suspected when the CSF titer is equal to or less than the serum titer. The use of newer diagnostic techniques in CSF analysis, IgG index, and albumin quotient determinations may prove helpful. Currently, the most reliable diagnostic aid is paired serum samples obtained 2 to 3 weeks apart that show a threefold to fourfold increase in serum-neutralizing or complement fixing antibody titer.

The histological abnormalities in EHV-1 infection have been well characterized. Lesions include vasculitis, endothelial necrosis, and thrombosis and are most prominent in the small arterioles. The majority of affected blood vessels supply the ventral and lateral white matter tracts. Perivascular cuffing with necrosis of the vessel walls has been identified. The resulting ischemia from the vasculitis and thrombosis produces white and gray matter malacia. Hemorrhage may be seen in association with the ischemic changes. Although most prominent in the central nervous system (CNS), the vasculitis is diffuse and can be seen in extraneural sites such as the nasal mucosa and pulmonary and endometrial tissues. Repeated attempts at isolating the virus from the nervous system of affected horses has been inconsistent and usually unrewarding.

Unlike herpesvirus infections in other species, EHV-1 infection in the horse is endotheliotropic rather than neurotropic. Experimental studies have shown that the virus is transported to the neural tissues in infected leukocytes. The infected leukocytes may result from primary infection, reinfection, or possibly reactivation of the EHV-1 virus. Viral antigen, IgG, and complement have all been detected in the arteriolar wall of several confirmed EHV-1 cases, suggesting that the pathogenesis of the neurological signs in EHV-1 infection is an immune-mediated, Arthus-type reaction, affecting small to medium-sized arterioles, particularly those in the CNS.

THERAPY

Treatment of equine herpes myeloencephalopathy is predominantly supportive. The level of care is determined by the degree of neurological deficits present. Mildly affected horses usually eat and drink normally. Severely ataxic horses should be confined to an area with easy access to food and water. Adequate bedding should be provided if prolonged recumbency is anticipated. The area should be large enough for personnel to manage and treat the animal safely. Nursing care is a major determining factor in the overall prognosis when extended recumbency occurs. See page 543 for detailed descriptions of the care of recumbent horses.

Antibiotic therapy is generally not required unless the horse develops abrasions, pneumonia, or deep pressure sores due to the imposed recumbency. If these occur, broad-spectrum antibiotics are instituted. Corticosteroid therapy has been advocated because of the evidence that the vasculitis is immune mediated. In the acute phase, dexamethasone, 0.05 to 0.1 mg per kg given intramuscularly twice a day for 1 to 3 days, as clinical signs dictate, is recommended. Corticosteroids must be used with caution, as they can be immunosuppressive and exacerbate a viral or secondary bacterial infection. Dimethyl sulfoxide (DMSO) (0.5 to 1 gm per kg in a 10 to 20 per cent solution once a day, up to three doses) is commonly used in horses suspected of CNS trauma or inflammatory conditions. In some cases the animal will receive both medications. However, available data are not conclusive that DMSO alone or in combination with steroids is superior to steroids alone. Because the condition usually improves and controlled studies are lacking, the response to different treatment modalities is difficult to judge objectively. The prognosis is generally good for animals that do not become recumbent, and improvement is usually seen over several days, although complete recovery may take months. Horses that are unable to stand have a much poorer prognosis, even with excellent nursing care. These animals will take longer to recover and may have permanent neurological deficits.

PREVENTION

There are currently no vaccines available for the prevention of the neurological form of EHV-1 infection. Outbreaks of equine respiratory tract infection due to EHV-1 subtype 1 should not be regarded as self-limiting and of minor clinical significance, since these infections can lead to serious complications involving the neuraxis. Therefore, the following guidelines have been advocated for the containment and prevention of spread of EHV-1 infection. Infected horses and their contacts should be isolated from other horses. Caretakers should schedule handling of affected horses after other horses on the farm. Disposable gloves and protective clothing should be worn while working with affected animals. No new entries or departures from the premises should be allowed for 21 days following recovery of the last clinical case. It is important to isolate and type the causative agent in suspicious respiratory disease outbreaks, since the management procedures and risk for subsequent development of CNS disease differ significantly according to the subtype of EHV-1 involved.

Vaccination or revaccination of all unexposed horses on the property to create an immune barrier to infection at the respiratory mucosa is recommended for prevention of CNS disease. Vaccination of contact horses that are likely to have been exposed to the virus has not yet been assessed thoroughly; because of the proposed immune-mediated pathogenesis of this disease, vaccination of these animals cannot be recommended at this time. The population of horses at risk for serious EHV-1–related disease, and therefore candidates for a vaccination program, is no longer limited to pregnant brood mares. It includes all horses in frequent contact with other horses at tracks, shows, and boarding facilities. It is also important to monitor the level of EHV-1–related CNS disease and the strains causing this disorder. New strains of EHV-1 with different genetic and biological properties can emerge over a short time and become clinically important.

Supplemental Readings

Allen, G. P., and Bryans, J. T.: Molecular epizootiology, pathogenesis, and prophylaxis of equine herpesvirus-1 infections. Prog. Vet. Microbiol. Immunol., 2:78–144, 1986.

Edington, N., Bridges, C. G., and Patel, J. R.: Endothelial cell infection and thrombosis in paralysis caused by equid herpesvirus-1: Equine stroke. Arch. Virol., 90:111, 1986.

Kohn, C. W., and Fenner, W. R.: Equine herpes myeloencephalopathy. Vet. Clin. North Am. (Equine Pract.), 3:405–419, 1987.

Mayhew, I. G.: Large Animal Neurology: A Handbook for Veterinary Clinicians. Philadelphia, Lea & Febiger, 1989, pp. 272–274.

Bacterial Meningitis and Cerebral Abscesses

Jonathan H. Foreman, URBANA, ILLINOIS

Bacterial meningitis in the horse is a rare but devastating neurological disease. The diagnosis is difficult to make because of the nonspecific, diffuse nature of the neurological signs, yet early diagnosis is critical if there is to be any chance of controlling the infection.

Neonates are more commonly affected because of their poor immune status at birth. Any foal with partial or complete failure of passive transfer is at risk for the development of neonatal septicemia and, as a result, meningitis. The blood–brain barrier in other species is quite permeable in the immediate postnatal period. This increased permeability may make the neonate more susceptible to bacteria entering the meninges and the central nervous system (CNS).

Horses older than neonates develop meningitis as a result of direct extension of localized infections. Cerebral abscesses due to *Streptococcus equi* infections ("bastard strangles") often result in intracranial meningitis in weanling and yearling horses. Surgery for tail-docking or setting may be complicated by ascending meningitis in the cauda equina region. Similarly, ascending meningitis may occur after anesthetic blocking of the ventral tail region to reduce active tail motion during showing. Viral and fungal meningitis are rare but have been reported in horses.

DIAGNOSIS

Neurological signs are nonspecific because meningitis is usually a diffuse process involving more than one portion of the CNS. Neonates with failure of passive transfer, septicemia, and acute onset of diffuse neurological signs should be considered as meningitis suspects. Older horses with signs of intracranial disease and a history of strangles exposure or with pelvic limb signs and a history of tail blocking or surgery should have meningitis included in the differential diagnosis.

The definitive diagnostic test is analysis of cerebrospinal fluid (CSF), preferably taken from the site (atlanto-occipital or lumbosacral) closest to the lesion. Elevated white blood cell count and protein content, an increase in the per centage of neutrophils, and the presence of bacteria confirm a diagnosis of meningitis.

THERAPY

Treatment is directed toward controlling the bacterial infection. Ideally, the choice of antibiotics should be made based on culture and sensitivity data. While waiting for culture results, however, it is essential that the horse be treated with an antibiotic with high CNS activity. Antibiotics considered to penetrate into the CNS include culfonamides, chloramphenicol, third-generation cephalosporins, isoniazid, and pyrimethamine. The latter two have a limited spectrum of antibacterial activity.

Chloramphenicol (10 to 25 mg per kg per os [PO] four times daily) is highly effective but requires frequent administration and can cause dangerous side effects in persons exposed during its use. Sulfonamides potentiated with trimethoprim are bactericidal, affordable, and may be administered intravenously (IV) or PO (30 mg sulfa per kg twice a day). Excellent results with cefotaxime sodium* (80 mg per kg IV three to four times a day) have been reported in two neonatal foals with meningitis. Ceftiofur sodium† (0.5 mg per kg once or twice a day) is a more affordable third-generation cephalosporin that may in the future prove to have high efficacy in the CNS. The use of high doses of penicillin (20,000 to 50,000 IU per kg IV four times a day or IM twice a day) has been advocated for the aggressive treatment of cerebral abscesses due to bastard strangles.

Corticosteroids are generally considered to be contraindicated in CNS infections. Mannitol (0.25 mg per kg IV in a 20 per cent solution) can effectively reduce CNS edema within 30 minutes and may be repeated at 4- to 6-hour intervals for up to 24 hours. Dimethyl sulfoxide (DMSO) has antiedema, diuretic, anti-inflammatory, and antibacterial effects. It is frequently administered IV (1 gm per kg in a 10 per cent solution) once daily for three treatments, followed by every other day for three more treatments. Kinetic studies have shown, however, that twice daily administration may be necessary to maintain blood levels. Side effects include hemolysis if DMSO is given too rapidly or in too concentrated a solution, and a pungent aroma when the compound is exhaled by the patient.

Immediate control of seizures in neonates can be achieved with diazepam (0.1 mg per kg IV). Phenobarbital (10 mg per kg IV or 0.5 to 2.0 mg per kg PO twice daily or to effect) can be used for longer term control. To prevent phenobarbital toxicity, serum levels should be kept below 50 ng per ml.

Successful surgical drainage of a cerebral abscess has been described in a yearling Quarter Horse, but the filly was destroyed 2 months later due to laminitis.

Foals should be maintained on foal beds kept near but not in the mares' stalls. Recumbent patients with meningitis must be turned frequently and must be adequately padded to prevent the development of skin pressure sores. Fluid and acid–base status should be monitored and balanced. Adequate protein and calorie intake must be maintained. Attempts must be made to control concurrent problems such as self-induced trauma, corneal ulcers, gastric ulcers, pneumonia, diarrhea, septic joints, and other complications of septicemia.

---

*Claforan, Hoechst-Roussel, Somerville, NJ
†Naxcel, Upjohn, Kalamazoo, MI

Supplemental Readings

Allen, J. R., Barbee, D. D., Boulton, C. R., Major, M. D., Crisman, M. V., and Murnane, R. D.: Brain abscess in a horse: Diagnosis by computerized tomography and successful surgical treatment. Equine Vet. J., *19*:552, 1987.

Foreman, J. H., and Santschi, E. M.: Equine bacterial meningitis: Part II. Compend. Cont. Educ. Pract. Vet., *11*:640, 1989.

Morris, D. D., Rutkowski, J., and Lloyd, K. C. K.: Therapy in two cases of neonatal foal septicemia and meningitis with cefotaxime sodium. Equine Vet. J., *19*:151, 1987.

Santschi, E. M., and Foreman, J. H.: Equine bacterial meningitis: Part I. Compend. Cont. Educ. Pract. Vet., *11*:479, 1989.

Protozoal Myeloencephalitis

Kathleen Yvorchuk, MANHATTAN, KANSAS

Equine protozoal myeloencephalitis includes diseases once referred to as segmental myelitis, focal or segmental myelitis–encephalitis, and toxoplasma-like myeloencephalitis. Equine protozoal myeloencephalitis is classically described as a multifocal, nonsuppurative, necrotizing, inflammatory neurological disorder, currently considered to be caused by a protozoan sharing characteristics with the sporozoa of the *Sarcocystis* genus. Though this disorder most frequently affects the spinal cord, brain involvement has also been observed. Equine protozoal myeloencephalitis has been reported in California, Florida, Pennsylvania, Ohio, Illinois, Kentucky, New York, Oklahoma, Texas, Maryland, Saskatchewan, Ontario (Canada), and southern Brazil. It probably occurs throughout most of North America.

CLINICAL SIGNS

Because the lesions are multifocal, occurring anywhere within the central nervous system (CNS), presenting clinical signs are highly variable. The most consistent signs include frequent falling or stumbling that progresses rapidly to severe ataxia or recumbency, and long-standing vague lamenesses. These lamenesses, which cannot be localized and are refractory to accepted modes of therapy, often progress to more obvious neurological involvement. Acute head tilt is one of the most frequently observed forms of cranial involvement. Because equine protozoal myeloencephalitis involves both white and gray matter, severe weakness and muscle atrophy are important clinical features of this disease. Multifocal areas of inflammation also imply asymmetry. Thus, equine protozoal myeloencephalitis should be the major entity in the differential diagnosis when a horse presents with progressive asymmetrical neurological dysfunction in which weakness, ataxia, and muscle wasting are evident.

Though no sex predilection has been described, breed predilections do appear to be a factor, as Thoroughbreds and Standardbreds tend to be affected more frequently. It has been suggested that this may be due to environmental factors rather than to actual breed differences. A recent retrospective report determined that affected animals range from 2 months to 19 years old. However, more than 60 per cent of horses were 4 years old or younger and approximately 33 per cent were 2 years old or younger. Cases appear as isolated incidents, although multiple cases may occur in the same location over several years. Outbreaks are not observed. The possibility of genetic predispostion has been raised, based on the occurrence of equine protozoal myeloencephalitis in two full siblings within the same year.

PATHOLOGY

Significant lesions are confined to the CNS. Lesions appear grossly as dark red hemorrhagic foci or brown malacic (softened) areas, depending on the severity of the lesion. These foci can be observed in either white or gray matter of the spinal cord or brain. Malacic foci have been reported as 1.0 to 1.5 cm in diameter. Histopathological lesions include vacuolization and degeneration with swelling of axons. Inflammatory changes are confined to malacic areas and primarily surround blood vessels. Predominant infiltrative cell types consist of lymphocytes and large mononuclear cells, although neutrophils and plasma cells have been observed. Some authors report the consistent presence of eosinophils, but cell numbers observed are variable.

Protozoal organisms have been detected at postmortem examination in approximately 50 per cent of untreated animals with characteristic lesions. Organisms appearing as closely packed ovoid bodies or in rosette formation are usually located in pericytes of capillaries and at times within macrophages or neutrophils, but they can also be found within and around axons. Organisms are usually located extracellularly and often require a thorough search of areas with lesions for detection.

DIAGNOSIS

Although typical clinical signs can be helpful, no specific tests are available to direct an antemortem diagnosis of equine protozoal myeloencephalitis. It is therefore a diagnosis of exclusion and can only be confirmed at necropsy. Abnormal cerebrospinal fluid (CSF) is often the most contributory diagnostic aid. It has been reported that mononuclear pleocytosis is only observed in approximately 20 to 30 per cent of cases. The CSF of affected individuals may exhibit mild to moderate elevations in white blood cells, mostly small lymphocytes and large mononuclear cells. Although eosinophils are observed histopathologically, they are rarely seen in the CSF. Acute cases may be accompanied by mild xanthochromia. Mild elevations in protein levels (90 to 150 mg per dl) are reported inconsistently. Ancillary diagnostic aids such as electromyography may be helpful in determining the presence, extent, and localization of lower motor neuron involvement. Response to therapy is an aid in diagnosing equine protozoal myeloencephalitis.

In support of the theory that *Toxoplasma* or *Toxoplasma*-related organisms are not the causative agents of equine protozoal myeloencephalitis, serum *Toxoplasma* titers have usually been negative. Elevations in *Sarcocystis* titers have been reported, though their significance and diagnostic implications are as yet uncertain.

The differential diagnoses include bacterial, parasitic, and viral encephalitides, myelitides, trauma, polyneuritis equi, cervical vertebral instability or malformation, and neurotoxicosis. Clinical signs, history, and progression of the disease should help distinguish these disorders.

THERAPY

Minimal information is available regarding successful treatment of equine protozoal myeloencephalitis, but clinical experience indicates that attempts have been rewarding. Therapy is extrapolated from the use of antifolate drugs in experimental and human protozoal conditions. The treatment is based on the use of pyrimethamine* (0.25 mg per kg given per os [PO] twice daily for 3 days, followed by 0.25 mg per kg once daily for 27 days) and trimethoprim–sulfadiazine† (15 mg per kg total dose PO twice daily for 1 month). Since these drugs potentially reduce folic acid production of host cells, it is recommended that animals be monitored regularly for cytopenia (neutropenia, thrombocytopenia, anemia) and receive folinic acid supplementation as required. In my experience this supplementation has not been necessary.

In severe or acute cases, the inflammatory component of this disease is very active and extensive and justifies the use of specific anti-inflammatory therapy. Most frequently used is a short course of IV dimethyl sulfoxide (DMSO),‡ 1 gm per kg mixed as a 10 to 20 per cent solution with 5 per cent dextrose or lactated Ringer's solution given once daily for 3 to 5 days. This can be extended by continued administration every other day for three to five more treatments. Phenylbutazone may be administered (5 mg per kg per day PO), though care should be taken to ensure adequate hydration. In very severe, recumbent, rapidly deteriorating cases, glucocorticoids may be given, although most authors tend to avoid their use as they have been demonstrated to allow expression of toxoplasmosis in experimental animals and man. Clinically, glucocorticoids appear to be associated with clinical deterioration in some cases. Pyrimethamine is not licensed for use in horses, and the parenteral administration of DMSO is an extralabel use.

The duration of therapy for equine protozoal myeloencephalitis is uncertain. A minimal therapeutic regimen usually lasts for 30 days. Some horses respond rapidly, but most require a few weeks before improvement can be noted. Therapy is aimed at arresting the condition. If no improvement is seen after the first course of therapy, there is often no advantage to further treatment. However, if the horse's condition and owner's compliance allow, therapy should be continued for another 30 days, as response may occur. If amelioration is observed after the initial month of treatment, another 30 days can result in further improvement. Some affected horses have shown clinical resolution; others recover partially and are left with residual deficits. If de-

---

*Daraprim, Burroughs Wellcome Co., Research Triangle Park, NC
†Tribrissen, Coopers Animal Health, Inc., Mundelein, IL
‡Domoso, Diamond Labs., Des Moines, IA

terioration continues despite treatment, the horse must be humanely destroyed. Termination of therapy is sometimes associated with recurrence of clinical signs. The duration of required treatment to achieve an acceptable static state is variable; treatment frequently must be continued for 2 to 3 months.

Animals that are tentatively diagnosed in life as having equine protozoal myeloencephalitis and are treated with antifolates demonstrate reduced numbers of organisms at post-mortem histopathological examination, thus substantiating the use of these drugs and their effectiveness at destroying organisms within the CNS.

Supplemental Readings

Beech, J.: Equine protozoan encephalomyelitis. Vet. Med. (Small Anim. Clin.), 69:1562, 1974.
Beech, J., and Dodd, D. C.: Toxoplasma-like encephalomyelitis in the horse. Vet. Pathol., 11:87, 1974.
Divers, T. J.: Equine protozoal myeloencephalitis. J. Vet. Intern. Med., 15:231, 1988.
Dubey, J. P. et al.: Equine encephalomyelitis due to a protozoan parasite resembling *Toxoplasma gondii*. J. Am. Vet. Med. Assoc., 165:249, 1974.
Fayer, R., Mayhew, I. G., Baird, J. D., et al.: Epidemiology of equine protozoal myeloencephalitis in North America based on histologically confirmed cases. A report. J. Vet. Intern. Med., 4:54, 1990.
Mayhew, I. G., de Lahunta, A., Whitlock, R. H., et al.: Spinal cord disease in the horse. Cornell Vet. 68:Suppl. 6, 1978.
Mayhew, I. G., de Lahunta, A., Whitlock, R. H., and Pollock, R. V. H.: Equine protozoal myeloencephalitis. In: Proceedings of the 22nd Annual Convention of the American Association of Equine Practitioners, 1976, pp. 107–114.
Mayhew, I. G., and Greiner, E. C.: Protozoal diseases. Vet. Clin. North Am. (Equine Pract.), 2:439, 1986.
Simpson, C. F., and Mayhew, I. G.: Evidence for *Sarcocystis* as the etiologic agent of equine protozoal myeloencephalitis. J. Protozool., 27:288, 1980.

Verminous Myelitis
Wendy M. Duckett, RALEIGH, NORTH CAROLINA

Parasites documented as infesting the central nervous system (CNS) of Equidae and resulting in neurological signs are *Halicephalobus (Micronema) deletrix*, *Strongylus vulgaris*, *Hypoderma* spp., *Draschia megastoma*, and *Setaria* spp. Reported cases worldwide tend to be sporadic except in India, where *Setaria* infestation can be enzootic and is called "kumri."

The life cycle of *Halicephalobus deletrix* is unknown. This species is considered a facultative parasite in horses and humans and is not found free-living or considered to be saprophytic, as are other species of *Halicephalobus*. Because of the pattern of granulomatous lesions that can be present in the oral and nasal mucosa, it is speculated that *Halicephalobus deletrix* may enter its host by the hematogenous route. Tissues that can be affected are brain, spinal cord, lungs, nasal and oral cavities, pituitary gland, kidneys, lymph nodes, heart, stomach, liver, and bone. In the horse, the brain, spinal cord, and meninges are the most frequently affected tissues. Once in the CNS the parasites cause malacia, necrosis, granulomatous inflammatory infiltration, meningitis, and vasculitis. Only one author reported seeing free parasites in the vessel lumina, suggesting that the primary mechanism of disease is not embolic.

Strongylus vulgaris has two potential pathogenic mechanisms. This parasite could directly cause necrosis, malacia, and inflammation along a path of aberrant migration or initiate pathology by thromboembolic showers from a thromboarteritis of a great vessel elsewhere in the body to the ipsilateral cerebrum.

Hypoderma instar larvae can inadvertently reach the brain through the foramina of the skull during aberrant life cycle migration. The larvae produce proteolytic enzymes that facilitate tissue migration. Pathogenesis of disease in one case was due to severe CSF hemorrhage when the larva penetrated a vessel.

Draschia megastoma and *Setaria* spp. cause disease during random and aberrant migration through the CNS. The host specificity of *Setaria* spp. is not strict, and *Setaria labiotopapillosa*, the parasite usually found in cattle, has been identified in cases of verminous encephalomyelitis in horses in the United States.

CLINICAL SIGNS AND DIAGNOSIS

In most cases, onset of neurological signs is acute and rapidly progressive over 2 to 6 days. In some cases there has been a history of neurological signs with improvement or resolution of signs before an acute, rapidly fulminating attack.

A definitive diagnosis is not easy to establish ante mortem. There is no age, sex, or breed predilection.

Signs are variable and can include evidence of spinal cord, brain stem, forebrain, cerebellar, upper motor neuron, and lower motor neuron lesions. The pattern is usually asymmetrical and can be focal or multifocal. Severity of signs varies with location and extent of the lesion(s). Specific clinical signs described include ataxia, stumbling, incoordination, depression, head tilt, circling, treading, cranial nerve deficits, visual impairment, seizures, recumbency, and death. A beta-globulinemia has been described but is also seen with other parasitic infestations. There are no characteristic, pathognomonic hematological changes in this disease.

Other findings on examination may support a diagnosis of verminous myelitis. For example, *Halicephalobus* often causes multisystem infections. Oral and nasal granulomas may be present. Renal involvement sometimes occurs and there may be renal impairment or parasites found in the urine. The presence of additional *Hypoderma* larvae subcutaneously might support a diagnosis of aberrant larval migration.

The presence of eosinophils in cerebrospinal fluid (CSF) would be the most significant evidence to support the diagnosis. In actuality, in the cases reported for which CSF analysis was done, the results varied from normal to the presence of eosinophilia, neutrophilia, xanthochromia, hemorrhage and increased protein. Repeating CSF aspirate analyses may be most beneficial. *Halicephalobus* parasites can potentially be seen in the CSF sample.

The differential diagnoses can include virtually any neurological disease seen in horses, including equine protozoal myelitis, trauma, viral encephalidites, cervical vertebral malformation, rabies, and mycotoxic encephalomalacia.

THERAPY

In the event that the supporting diagnostic evidence is not present, a presumptive diagnosis might be made by ruling out other causes. If a definitive diagnosis cannot be ascertained and the animal's condition deteriorates, empirical therapy can be considered. Therapy for a confirmed or presumptive case should include anthelmintic, anti-inflammatory therapy and supportive care. Ivermectin (200 µg per kg per os [PO]) may take up to 2 weeks to kill the parasites. Fenbendazole (50 mg per kg PO once a day for 1 to 3 days), thiabendazole (440 mg per kg PO once a day for 2 days), diethylcarbamazine (50 mg per kg PO once a day for 10 days), and trichlorfon (35 mg per kg PO) have all been recommended. Concomitant anti-inflammatory therapy should be administered. Flunixin meglumine (1.1 mg per kg given intravenously [IV], intramuscularly [IM], or PO twice a day), phenylbutazone (4.4 mg per kg PO once a day), dimethyl sulfoxide (DMSO, 1 gm per kg as a 10 to 20 per cent solution IV once or twice daily for 3 days), or dexamethasone (0.1 to 0.2 mg per kg IV, IM, or PO once daily, alone or in combination with the DMSO) can be given. Dexamethasone should be avoided if protozoal myelitis is in the primary differential diagnosis, because it may exacerbate that condition, or if bacterial infection is suspected. Prolonged dexamethasone administration may precipitate laminitis. Thiamine, vitamin E, and selenium, which are supportive of normal nervous tissue function, may be administered. Other supportive care will depend on the needs of each individual case. Some animals may die or may become so debilitated or unmanageable that euthanasia is necessary; others may recover completely, while others recover with residual signs.

Supplemental Readings

Blunden, A. S., Khalil, J. F., and Webbon, P. M.: *Halicephalobus deletrix* infection in a horse. Equine Vet. J., *19*:255, 1987.

Cho, D. Y., Simpson, R. M., Hodgin, E. C. and Roberts, E. D.: Diagnostic features of *Micronema* infection in horses. *In*: Proceedings of the 28th Annual Meeting of the American Association of Veterinarian Laboratory Diagnosticians, 1985, pp. 31–38.

Frauenfelder, H. C., Kazacos, K. R., and Lichtenfels, J. R.: Cerebrospinal nematodiasis caused by a filariid in a horse. J. Am. Vet. Med. Assoc., *177*:359, 1980.

Hadlow, W. J., Ward, J. K., and Krinsky, W. L.: Intracranial myiasis by *Hypoderma bovis* (Linnaeus) in a horse. Cornell Vet., *67*:272, 1977.

Mayhew, I.G.: Tetraparesis, paraparesis and ataxia of the limbs, and episodic weakness. *In* Mayhew, I.G.: Large Animal Neurology: A Handbook for Veterinary Clinicians. Philadelphia, Lea & Febiger, 1989, pp. 243–334.

Spalding, M.G., Greiner, E. C., and Green, S. L.: *Halicephalobus (Micronema) deletrix* infection in two half-sibling foals. J. Am. Vet. Med. Assoc., *196*:1127, 1990.

Mycotoxic Encephalomalacia

Maria D. Masri, GAINESVILLE, FLORIDA

Mycotoxicosis due to *Fusarium* spp. can present as an acute, severe neurological disorder, a hepatic syndrome, or as acute death. It has been reported as a sporadic cause of death in horses throughout the world. Other terms used for this condition are moldy corn poisoning, blind staggers, leukoencephalitis, foraging disease, corn stalk disease, and epizootic cerebritis. Mycotoxic encephalomalacia is the preferred name because it describes the etiology of the disease (mycotoxins) and the pathological lesions (necrosis of gray and white matter of the brain). Mycotoxic encephalomalacia is caused by an as yet uncharacterized toxin elaborated by the mold *Fusarium* spp., which grows readily on cereal grains, particularly corn. The presence of fusarial mycotoxins in grain is generally an indication that the grain was contaminated prior to harvesting. Mycotoxic encephalomalacia is a seasonal disease, usually occurring from late fall through early spring.

Mycotoxic encephalomalacia can be reproduced using crude isolates from corn inoculated with *Fusarium* spp. However, purified extracts of fusarial toxins have not consistently produced disease. Experimental horses continuously fed moldy corn develop clinical signs after 10 to 90 days. Once clinical signs develop, the course of the disease is short, lasting from several hours to 3 days. The clinical syndrome is highly variable and will depend on the toxin dose, duration of exposure, and host susceptibility. High dosages of toxin induce the hepatic syndrome, while small doses consumed over a longer period of time result in the encephalomalacia syndrome. Different toxins may be responsible for the different syndromes.

CLINICAL SIGNS

The first signs of experimentally induced disease may consist of inappetence and unthriftiness. These are soon followed by evidence of central nervous system (CNS) disease including asymmetrical cranial nerve deficits, behavioral changes varying from depression to mania, and ataxia and weakness followed by recumbency, delirium, coma, and death. No specific pattern of clinical neurological manifestations is typical of mycotoxic encephalomalacia since symmetrical, asymmetrical, focal, or diffuse CNS lesions may be present. Because of extensive brain destruction, few animals survive. During the manifestation of neurological signs, temperature, pulse, or respiratory rate may remain relatively normal. Hemograms reflect stress, while liver function tests and enzymatic activity are abnormal in the majority of the cases. Cerebrospinal fluid (CSF) analysis may reveal abnormalities ranging from neutrophilic pleocytosis to a slight elevation in total protein level, depending on the degree of damage and its location at the time of sampling. Clinical tests have not been useful in diagnosing or monitoring the disease. Some horses have made a slow partial recovery after the acute illness, but it is not known if full recovery has occurred.

NECROPSY FINDINGS

Necropsy findings are diagnostic in naturally occurring and experimentally induced mycotoxic encephalomalacia. Gross lesions characteristic of mycotoxic encephalomalacia include generalized edema of the brain with focal areas of liquefactive necrosis of cerebral white matter. Malacic areas are not confined to subcortical white matter but are visible throughout the cerebral cortex. Microscopically these areas contain rarefaction, perivascular hemorrhage, edema, and cellular infiltrates composed mainly of plasma cells and eosinophils. Satellitosis and neurophagia are commonly seen. Lesions of encephalomalacia have been reported in the cerebral cortex, cerebellum, brain stem, and midbrain. Lesions occur in white and gray matter and range from mild neuronal necrosis with inflammatory infiltrates to severe liquefactive necrosis involving most of the cortical region. Although the pathogenesis of the lesions is unknown, they may result from injury to the vascular endothelium, since initial stages of the lesion consist of areas of marked perivascular edema. The resulting cortical lesions vary with the duration of disease, ranging from macroscopic malacia and cavitations in acute cases to microcirculatory lesions in peracute cases. The livers of affected horses appear grossly normal. Microscopic hepatic lesions are not specific and consist of mild diffuse vacuolization of hepatocytes, focal or periacinal necrosis, and fatty degeneration. In chronic cases the liver is cirrhotic with diffuse fibrosis and infiltration of lymphocytes and histiocytes.

DIAGNOSIS

The primary entities in the differential diagnosis of the neurological form of the disease are hepatoencephalopathy, viral encephalomyelitis (herpesvirus 1; eastern, western, and Venezuelan encephalomyelitis), parasite migration, trauma, equine protozoal encephalomyelitis, parasite migration, and a space-occupying brain abscess or tumor. Differential diagnoses for sudden death and hepatic disease as an individual or herd problem are described on page 253 and 340. Since the toxin causing mycotoxic encephalomalacia has not been identified, with the exception of one case induced by fumonisin B_1 toxin, the definitive diagnosis of this disease is based on the demonstration of characteristic histopathological lesions involving the CNS. Feeding trials with feed implicated in the outbreak can demonstrate toxicity.

The following factors have been commonly noted in reported outbreaks of mycotoxic encephalomalacia:

1. Most affected horses were fed some form of corn-based ration for at least 2 weeks. Fatality was variable, but horses confined to stalls or paddocks without access to other feedstuffs had a higher incidence of disease, and larger, more aggressive animals in group-fed horses were more commonly affected.
2. Colonies of *Fusarium* spp. were consistently grown from the suspect corn.
3. Clinical signs included either sudden death, an acute afebrile neurological syndrome, or hepatic syndrome. Hemograms and biochemical profiles usually were not helpful unless hepatic damage was present.

In summary, a single case of mycotoxic encephalomalacia is difficult to diagnose ante mortem. CSF evaluation may be useful in making an antemortem diagnosis and enables differentiation from hepatoencephalopathy. The diagnosis becomes much more obvious retrospectively or during a confirmed outbreak. Therapy is supportive (see p. 378).

Supplemental Readings

Brownie, C. F., and Cullen, J.: Characterization of experimentally induced equine leukoencephalomalacia (ELEM) in ponies (Equus Caballus): Preliminary report. Vet. Hum. Toxicol., 29:34, 1987.

Marasas, W. F. O., Kellerman, T. S., Gelderblom, W. C. A., Coetzer, J. A. W., Thiel, P. G., and Van Der Lugt, J. J.: Leukoencephalomalacia in a horse induced by fumonisin B_1 isolated from *Fusarium moniliforme*. Onderstepoort J. Vet. Res., 55:197, 1988.

Masri, M. D., Olcott, B. M., Nicholson, S. S., McClure, J. J., Schmidth, S. P., Freestone, J. F., and Kornagay, W. R.: Clinical, epidemiologic and pathologic evaluation of an outbreak of mycotoxic encephalomalacia in South Louisiana horses. *In*: Proceedings of the 33rd Annual Convention of the American Association of Equine Practitioners, 1987, pp. 367–374.

Mirocha, C. J., Abbas, H. K., and Vesonder, R. F.: Absence of trichothecenes in toxigenic isolates of *Fusarium moniliforme*. J. Applied Environ. Microbiol. 56:520, 1990.

Wilson, B. J., Marronpot, R. R., and Hildebrandt, P. K.: Equine leukoencephalomalacia. J. Am. Vet. Med. Assoc., 163:1293, 1973.

Degenerative Myeloencephalopathy

Linda L. Blythe, CORVALLIS, OREGON

A. Morrie Craig, CORVALLIS, OREGON

Equine degenerative myeloencephalopathy is an idiopathic, diffuse, degenerative disease of the spinal cord and selected parts of the brain in young horses that results in gait deficits. Since equine degenerative myeloencephalopathy was first described in 1977, it has become recognized as one of the major causes of ataxia in young horses in the United States. The reported prevalence of the disease varies throughout the United States. In the initial 1978 survey of 100 "wobblers" in New York state in 1978, 24 per cent of horses had this disease. A more recent histopathological study of 287 ataxic horses in New York state placed the incidence at 49 per cent. On the West Coast, there appears to be a lesser incidence of disease, with Oregon reporting a 22 per cent incidence of confirmed diagnoses of equine degenerative myeloencephalopathy in 280 wobblers. While not proven, development of the disease appears to be associated with an increased dependence on hay or pelleted feed in areas where horses do not have regular access to pasture. In an epidemiological survey, dirt lot confinement and exposure to either insecticides or wood preservatives were identified as risk factors associated with a higher incidence of equine degenerative myeloencephalopathy. A familial predisposition has been identified in Standardbreds, Appaloosas, Morgans, Arabians, Peruvian Pasos, Thoroughbreds, and Norwegian Fjord horses.

CLINICAL SIGNS

The onset of this disease is most commonly insidious and progressive, although some owners report an acute onset. Horses less than 3 years old are at risk. The first indication of the disease in horses between 4 and 8 months of age is often a clumsiness that progresses to varying degrees of sensory and motor ataxia. Gait deficits consist of symmetrical ataxia, paresis, and hypometria affecting all four limbs. The degree of involvement can vary from minor deficits in the thoracic limbs with markedly affected pelvic limbs to equal severity in all four limbs. Although the disease is progressive, quadriplegia rarely develops, and clinical signs appear to plateau once the animal matures. In some animals, especially in the latter stages of the disease, decreased focal cervical, cervicofacial, cutaneous trunci, and slap test reflexes can be demonstrated. Hyporeflexia of the cutaneous trunci reflex reflects dysfunction primarily of the thoracic segments of the spinal cord. When present, this abnormality can help differentiate this disease from cervical stenotic myelopathy, since equine degenerative myeloencephalopathy is a diffuse disease involving the entire spinal cord, while cervical stenotic myelopathy is a focal compressive lesion of the cervical spinal cord.

DIAGNOSIS

There is no definitive premortem method for diagnosis of equine degenerative myeloencephalopathy, although the index of suspicion should be high if there has been a familial history of this disease or if signs of hyporeflexia are present. Young horses that present with acute signs of ataxia need radiographic evaluation to rule out traumatic, congenital, or developmental (cervical stenotic myelopathy) bony diseases, and a cerebrospinal fluid (CSF) analysis to attempt to rule out possible equine protozoal myelopathy, myelitis, and the neurological form of equine rhinopneumonitis. In equine degenerative myeloencephalopathy, elevated CSF creatine kinase values may be seen, reflecting current nervous tissue damage. However, this abnormality is not specific for this disease. In cases with long-standing neurological deficits, it is more difficult to ascertain cause, beyond ruling out bony lesions radiographically.

Definitive diagnosis of equine degenerative myeloencephalopathy requires demonstration of the histopathological lesions of neuroaxonal dystrophy in the cuneate, lateral cuneate, and gracilis nuclei of the medulla oblongata and diffusely throughout the spinal cord. In the latter case, the lesions are often most prominent in the thoracic spinal cord. Histopathological abnormalities consist of eosinophilic spheroids, asterogliosis, loss of neurons in a number of the sensory relay nuclei, and lipofuscinosis.

The etiology of equine degenerative myeloencephalopathy remains obscure. The pathological features of this disease are similar to those of a number of hereditary, nutritional, and toxic diseases. However, accumulating evidence supports vitamin E as a factor in the pathogenesis of this disease. Supportive data consist of (1) a neuropathology similar to induced vitamin E deficiencies in experimental animals and documented clinical cases of human vitamin E deficiency syndromes, (2) consistently low serum vitamin E values in a number of horses with the disease, (3) a reduction in incidence of equine degenerative myeloencephalopathy from 40 per cent to zero with vitamin E supplementation of offspring of families of horses with known equine degenerative myeloencephalopathy, and (4) an improvement in clinical signs in horses with equine degenerative myeloencephalopathy given massive doses (6000 IU per day) of vitamin E. Plasma α-tocopherol values have been serially monitored in foals sired by a stallion with equine degenerative myeloencephalopathy from a family of Appaloosa horses with a high incidence of the disease. The α-tocopherol values were similar to those in control foals during the neonatal period. However, from 6 weeks to 10 months of age the plasma α-tocopherol levels in foals sired by a stallion with equine degenerative myeloencephalopathy were significantly lower than in control foals, and eight of the nine foals in the former category developed clinically detectable ataxia during this period. The mechanism for the low plasma α-tocopherol levels in these horses is unknown. Oral vitamin E absorption tests have ruled out gastrointestinal malabsorption as a cause.

Single serum or plasma α-tocopherol values cannot be used as a definitive diagnostic test for equine degenerative myeloencephalopathy. Serum α-tocopherol values vary by 12 per cent (range, 7 to 17 per cent) over several hours. Due to this variation throughout the day, and to the narrow difference between normal and deficient α-tocopherol values in horses, an animal can be considered deficient (less than 1.5 μg per ml) or normal (more than 2.0 μg per ml) on the same day. In addition, a plasma α-tocopherol value measured at the time of ataxia may not reflect the antioxidant status at the time the horse developed the disease. Measurement of α-tocopherol levels does have value in herd situations if deficiencies of the vitamin are suspected due to lack of pasture, long-term use of pelleted feed, or increased antioxidant stress due to high levels of polyunsaturated fats in the diet.

THERAPY

Massive vitamin E therapy has resulted in improvement in clinical signs with optimum recovery seen in horses in which the disease was recognized in the early stages, less than 12 months of age. Current recommendations for treatment are *d,l*-α-tocopherol acetate* at 6000 IU per day per 250 to 500 kg body weight, mixed with 30 ml of vegetable oil and 1 quart of mixed grain. Improvement can be seen within 2 to 3 weeks, with continued progress over the next 6 months to 1 year. Prophylactically, oral administration of vitamin E at 1500 to 2000 IU per day to foals from equine degenerative myeloencephalopathy–affected lines has been shown to prevent the development of clinical ataxia.

Supplemental Readings

Beech, J., and Haskins, M.: Genetic studies of neuroaxonal dystrophy in the Morgan. Am. J. Vet. Res., 48:109, 1987.
Blythe, L. L., Craig, A. M., Lassen, E. D., et al.: Serially determined plasma α-tocopherol concentrations and results of oral vitamin E absorption test in clinically normal horses and in horses with degenerative myeloencephalopathy. Amer. J. Vet. Res., 52:908, 1991.
Blythe, L. L., Craig, A. M., Lassen, E. D., et al.: Vitamin E deficiency as a causative factor in equine degenerative myeloencephalopathy. Vitamin E: Biochemistry and Health Implications. Ann. NY Acad. Sci., 570:415, 1989.
Blythe L. L., Hultgren, B. D., Craig, A. M., et al.: Clinical, viral, and genetic evaluation of equine degenerative myeloencephalopathy in a family of Appaloosos. J. Am. Vet. Med. Assoc. 198:1005, 1991.
Craig, A. M., Blythe, L. L., Lassen, E. D., et al.: Variations of serum vitamin E, cholesterol, and total serum lipid concentrations in horses during a 72-hour period. Am. J. Vet. Res., 50:1527, 1989.
Dill, S. G., Corrca, M. T., Erb, H. N., et al.: Factors associated with the development of equine degenerative myeloencephalopathy. Amer. J. Vet. Res., 51:1300, 1990.
Dill, S. G., Kallfelz, F. A., de Lahunta, A., et al.: Serum vitamin E and blood glutathione peroxidase values of horses with degenerative myeloencephalopathy. Am. J. Vet. Res., 50:166, 1989.
Mayhew, I. G.: Large Animal Neurology. Philadelphia, Lea & Febiger, 1989, pp. 243–334.
Mayhew, I. G., Brown, C. M., Stowe, H. D., et al.: Equine degenerative myeloencephalopathy: A vitamin E deficiency that may be familial. J. Vet. Intern. Med., 1:45, 1987.

---

*Rovimix 20, Hoffman-LaRoche, Nutley, NJ

Seizures and Narcolepsy

Frank M. Andrews, KNOXVILLE, TENNESSEE
Hilary K. Matthews, KNOXVILLE, TENNESSEE

SEIZURES

A seizure is a clinical manifestation of rapid excessive electrical discharges from the cerebral cortex that result in involuntary alterations of motor activity, consciousness, autonomic functions, or sensation. A seizure is sometimes referred to as a fit, attack, stroke, convulsions, or epilepsy. However, seizure refers to a specific clinical event, regardless of the etiology or morphology, whereas epilepsy refers to recurring seizures with nonprogressive intracranial alterations that may be genetic or acquired. Inherited epilepsy probably does not occur in horses. Convulsions, on the other hand, are seizures accompanied by tonic–clonic muscle activity and loss of consciousness.

Seizure in horses may be categorized as partial or generalized, based on clinical signs. A partial seizure involves a discrete area of the cerebral cortex and results in localized clinical signs, such as facial or limb twitching, compulsive running in a circle, or self-mutilation. A partial seizure may be observed after cervical myelography, anesthesia, or cranial trauma and may spread throughout the cortex and produce a secondary generalized seizure. A generalized seizure involves the entire cerebral cortex and whole body musculature and results in generalized tonic–clonic muscle activity, with loss of consciousness. Generalized seizures are the most common form of seizures observed in adult horses and foals.

ETIOLOGY AND PATHOGENESIS

Adult horses have a high seizure threshold. Severe brain damage must occur before adult horses have a seizure. Foals, on the other hand, have a lower seizure threshold and are more susceptible to conditions causing seizures. Seizures may be caused by either intracranial or extracranial factors (Table 1 and 2). The most common causes of seizures in foals under 2 weeks of age are neonatal maladjustment syndrome, trauma, and bacterial meningitis (see Table 1). The most common causes of seizures in foals less than 1 year old are trauma and in Arabian foals idiopathic epilepsy. The most common causes of seizures in horses more than 1 year old are brain trauma, hepatoencephalopathy, and toxicity (see Table 2). Tumor, especially pituitary adenoma, can cause seizures and blindness in horses more than 7 years old.

The pathophysiological mechanisms of seizure are not thoroughly known, but several factors are thought to play a role. These include an increase in excitatory neural transmitters (acetylcholine), a decrease in inhibitory neural transmitters (γ-aminobutyric acid, GABA), an alteration of neural transmitter receptor sites, or a derangement in internal cellular metabolism. A decrease in inhibitory neurons and inhibitory neurotransmitters can lead to uncontrolled spread of electrical activity over the cerebral cortex. Once a critical mass of neurons has fired, a generalized seizure is precipitated. Head trauma and decreased cerebral blood supply can result in cerebral cortical hypoxia, which may result in necrosis of inhibitory neurons. Cerebral inhibitory neurons are more sensitive to hypoxia than excitatory neurons. Phenobarbital and pentobarbital potentiate inhibitory neural transmitters, such as GABA, and block hypoxic seizure foci. Also, systemic electrolyte abnormalities may disturb excitatory neuron homeostasis and lead to spontaneous, excessive action potentials. Spontaneous action potentials can spread to other parts of the cerebral cortex, causing a generalized seizure. Phenytoin prevents sodium influxes into the neuron and desensitizes hyperexcitable neurons and prevents seizure formation.

CLINICAL SIGNS AND DIAGNOSIS

A wide spectrum of clinical signs is produced by seizure activity, depending on the area and extent of cerebral cortex involved. In partial seizure, asymmetrical twitching of a limb, facial twitching, excessive chewing, compulsive running, and self-mutilation may be seen. A localized seizure can develop into a generalized seizure.

In a generalized seizure, three distinct clinical periods can be observed: just prior to the seizure (aura), horses may exhibit anxiety and anxiousness; during the seizure (ictus), horses may become recumbent and unconscious and have symmetrical clonic muscle contractions (contraction and relaxation of muscles occurring in rapid succession), followed by symmetrical tonic muscle contraction (for example, continuous unremitting muscle contractions). Horses with seizures may also show deviation of eyeballs, dilated pupils, ptyalism, trismus or jaw clamping, opisthotonos, lordosis or kyphosis, violent paddling movements of limbs, uncontrolled urination and defecation, and excessive sweating. A generalized seizure can last from 5 to 60 seconds. After the seizure (postictus phase) there can be depression and blindness for hours to days.

Diagnosis of the underlying cause of a seizure is based on history, clinical signs, and ancillary diagnostic tests (see Tables 1 and 2). In all paroxysmal, involuntary neurological events, seizures should be considered first unless proven otherwise. Careful questioning of the owner can reveal information about the event, the time of day, the relationship to feeding, unusual environmental circumstances such as thunderstorms or fireworks occurring on the date of the seizure, housing, recent trauma, febrile episodes, exposure to drugs or toxins, recent behavioral changes, and seizure history of the dam, sire, and other siblings. It is important to rule out other conditions that mimic seizures, including painful conditions such as colic, limb fractures, and exertional myopathy, hyperkalemic periodic paralysis (see p. 117), and syncope. In these conditions horses do not lose consciousness but remain bright and alert.

Narcolepsy and cataplexy can be confused with seizures. Most narcoleptic horses (except for some ponies) remain standing with the head hanging close to the ground. If recumbency occurs, loss of muscle tone and rapid eye movement (REM) sleep may follow. Cardiac arrhythmia or severe murmurs are supportive of syncope. Auscultation of the heart can determine the presence of severe murmurs, and electrocardiography (ECG) can help determine the presence of arrhythmias. Icteric mucous mem-

TABLE 1. KNOWN AND SUSPECTED CAUSES OF SEIZURES IN HORSES LESS THAN 1 YEAR OLD

Classification	Differential Diagnosis — Extracranial	Differential Diagnosis — Intracranial	Diagnostic Aids*
Congenital anomalies		Hydrocephalus	1, 2, 3, 4, 5, 6, 8, 11
		Hydranencephaly	
		Benign epilepsy	2, 3, 4, 8, 11
Metabolic	Hypoxia		
	Hyponatremia		
	Hypoglycemia		
	Hyperkalemia		
Toxic	Organophosphates	Moldy corn	2, 3, 4, 5, 6, 9, 10, 11
	Strychnine	Locoweed	
	Metaldehyde		
Trauma		Brain trauma	2, 3, 4, 5, 6, 8, 10, 11
		Lightning strike	
Vascular		Neonatal maladjustment syndrome (vascular accidents)	2, 3, 4, 5, 6
Infectious	Septicemia	Bacterial meningitis	2, 3, 4, 5, 6, 7, 8, 9, 11
	Endotoxemia	Cerebral abscesses	
	Fever	Rabies	
	Tetanus	Viral encephalitis	
	Botulism		

*Diagnostic aids: 1 = breed, 2 = onset, 3 = clinical course, 4 = physical examination, 5 = neurological examination, 6 = clinical pathology/CSF analysis, 7 = serology, 8 = radiology (computerized tomography, ultrasound, radiography), 9 = toxicology, 10 = electrodiagnostics (EEG, EMG), 11 = pathology.

TABLE 2. KNOWN AND SUSPECTED CAUSES OF SEIZURES IN HORSES GREATER THAN 1 YEAR OLD

Classification	Differential Diagnosis — Extracranial	Differential Diagnosis — Intracranial	Diagnostic Aids*
Metabolic	Hepatoencephalopathy		2, 3, 4, 5, 6, 11
	Hypomagnesemia		
	Hypocalcemia		
	Uremia		
	Hyperlipidemia		
Toxic	Organophosphates	Moldy corn	2, 3, 4, 5, 6, 9, 11
	Strychnine	Locoweed	
	Metaldehyde	Braken fern	
		Lead, arsenic, mercury	
		Rye grass	
Traumatic		Brain trauma	2, 3, 4, 5, 6, 8, 10
Vascular		*Strongylus vulgaris*	11, 2, 3, 4, 5, 6, 11
		Cerebral thromboembolism	
		Intracarotid injection	
Tumor		Neoplasia	2, 3, 4, 5, 6, 8, 10, 11
		Hemarthroma	
		Cholesterol granuloma	
Infectious		Cerebral abscess	1, 3, 4, 5, 6, 7, 8, 12, 13
		Rabies	
		Tetanus	
		Arbovirus encephalitis	
		Mycotic *Cryptococcus*	
		Protozoal myelitis	

*Diagnostic aids: 1 = breed, 2 = onset, 3 = clinical course, 4 = physical examination, 5 = neurological examination, 6 = clinical pathology/CSF analysis, 7 = serology, 8 = radiology (computerized tomography, ultrasound, radiography), 9 = toxicology, 10 = electrodiagnostics (EEG, EMG), 11 = pathology.

branes may be seen in horses with hepatoencephalopathy, and diarrhea may be seen in horses after toxin ingestion.

A complete neurological examination will determine the presence of other neurological signs. The neurological examination should be performed during the interictal period, because examination during the postictal period (24 to 48 hours after seizure) often reveals depression, weakness, blindness, and crossed extensor reflex and may lead to incorrect anatomical localization of lesions.

Cerebrospinal fluid (CSF) from the cisterna magna may be helpful in determining the cause of seizures. Increased CSF protein, red blood cell count, white blood cell (WBC) count, and abnormal differential WBC count are indicative of inflammatory processes in the CNS. Increased CSF lactic acid concentration may occur in horses with cerebral abscess.

Skull radiographs can help determine the presence of skull fractures. Bone scan may reveal nondisplaced skull fractures. A fundic examination may reveal papillary edema, detached retina, or active inflammation that can suggest trauma or an infectious etiology. Electroencephalography and computed tomography can be helpful in localizing and determining a cause for seizure in horses. If an underlying cause for the seizure cannot be found, then a diagnosis of idiopathic epilepsy can be made.

Therapy

Treatment of horses having seizures must be based on medical considerations, client considerations, owner preference and compliance, and the long-term expense of medication. Initial anticonvulsant therapy should be based on frequency and severity of the horse's seizures. Anticonvulsant therapy is indicated for status epilepticus (rare in adult horses, uncommon in foals); one seizure occurring every 2 months; clusters of seizures occurring more than three to four times per year; or several multiple seizures occurring over 1 to 3 days. Also, foals with idiopathic epilepsy that have several seizures over 1 to 3 days may require short-term (1 to 3 months) anticonvulsant therapy. The chronic use of anticonvulsants in horses is rare. Therapy guidelines are listed in Table 3. The drug doses required for maintenance therapy should be decreased slowly to determine if continued therapy is needed. The goal of anticonvulsant therapy is to reduce the frequency, duration, and severity of seizures without producing intolerable side effects. The complete elimination of seizures may not be possible. Each horse must be treated as an individual and the treatment dosages and frequency tailored to fit the patient. The best initial therapeutic agents for seizures in horses are diazepam and phenobarbital sodium.

Adult horses and foals with seizures may also benefit from the anti-flammatory actions of DMSO (1 gm per kg) given IV as a 10 per cent solution in lactated Ringer's solution or 5 per cent dextrose. Corticosteroids stabilize neuronal membranes and decrease seizure foci and may be effective initially as anticonvulsant therapy. Corticosteroids and DMSO are synergistic.

Drugs that are contraindicated in horses with seizures include acetylpromazine, xylazine, and ketamine. Acetylpromazine lowers the seizure

TABLE 3. ANTICONVULSANT DRUGS USED TO TREAT SEIZURE DISORDERS IN HORSES

Regimen	Drug	50-kg Foal Dose	450-kg Horse Dose
Initial therapy (including status epilepticus)	Diazepam	5–20 mg IV	25–100 mg IV
	Pentobarbital	150–1000 mg IV	To effect
	Phenobarbital	250–1000 mg IV	2–5 gm IV
	Phenytoin	50–250 mg IV or PO q. 4 h.	—
	Primidone	1–2 gm PO	—
	Chloral hydrate ($\pm$ MgSO$_4$, barbiturate)	3–10 gm IV	15–60 gm IV
	Xylazine°	25–100 mg IV or IM	300–1000 mg IV or IM
	Guaifenesin ($\pm$ barbiturate)	To effect	40–60 gm IV
	Carbamazepine	250–500 mg PO	
	Triaziline	1 gm PO	
Maintenance therapy	Phenobarbital	100–500 mg PO b.i.d.	1–5 gm PO b.i.d.
	Phenytoin	50–250 mg PO b.i.d.	50–1000 mg PO t.i.d. (low therapeutic index)
	Primidone	1 gm PO s.i.d. or b.i.d.	

°Should be used only in the emergency situation until an appropriate anticonvulsant agent can be started.
Adapted from Table 6-1 in: Mayhew, I.G., Large Animal Neurology; A Handbook for Veterinary Clinicians. Philadelphia, Lea & Febiger, 1989, p. 116.

threshold. Xylazine decreases cerebral blood flow and increases intracranial pressure, which can exacerbate cerebral hypoxia and worsen seizures. However, it may be necessary to give xylazine in an emergency situation until a more appropriate drug is available. Ketamine may exacerbate seizures by increasing cerebral blood flow, oxygen consumption, and intracranial pressure.

NARCOLEPSY

Narcolepsy is a rare incurable sleep disorder of the CNS characterized by uncontrolled episodes of loss of muscle tone (cataplexy) and sleep. The disease has been reported in Suffolk and Shetland foals ("fainting disease"), Welsh ponies, a Miniature horse, Thoroughbreds, Quarter Horses, Morgans, Appaloosas, and Standardbreds. A familial occurrence is thought to exist in affected Suffolk and Shetland pony foals.

The four components of narcolepsy seen in humans include excessive daytime sleepiness associated with short periods of REM sleep, cataplexy, hypnagogic hallucinations, and sleep paralysis. Cataplexy (sudden collapse with complete inhibition of skeletal muscle tone) is seen most often in horses with narcolepsy. Respiratory and cardiac muscles are spared.

In narcolepsy–cataplexy, a biochemical abnormality in the sleep–wake centers of the brain stem is thought to exist. A decreased concentration or decreased turnover of serotonin (mediator of slow-wave sleep), dopamine, and norepinephrine (mediator of REM) may be responsible for the condition.

Cataleptic episodes can be precipitated by petting, stroking the head and neck, hosing with water after exercise, leading out of a stall, initiation of eating or drinking, and stall rest. Exercise does not appear to precipitate cataleptic episodes.

Onset of narcolepsy–cataplexy normally occurs by 6 months of age, but adult-onset cases have been reported. A predictable pattern of duration and frequency of cataleptic attacks is generally set within the first 1 to 2 weeks following the initial onset of the disease.

Clinical Signs

Clinical signs of narcolepsy vary from mild muscle weakness to complete collapse. Adult horses can drop their heads, buckle at the knees, and stumble. If forced to walk, the horse may be ataxic; ponies are more likely to become recumbent. Horses and ponies that collapse can show absent spinal reflexes and REM sleep. Occasional sudden contraction of a limb or trunk muscle can occur, resulting in a spasmodic motion. Episodes can last from a few seconds to 10 minutes. Eye and facial responses, cardiovascular function, and respiratory function are maintained during the attack. Horses can be aroused from the attack with varying degrees of difficulty, and most recover and rise quietly without incident. Affected horses are neurologically normal between attacks.

Diagnosis

The diagnosis of narcolepsy is based on history, clinical signs, pharmacological testing, and the absence of other diseases. A complete blood cell count and serum biochemical profile can rule out underlying systemic and metabolic abnormalities. The CSF is normal in affected horses. Electroencephalography and needle electromyography during an attack may reveal fast waves of REM sleep and the absence of postinsertional activity of resting muscle, respectively.

A provocative test is useful in diagnosing narcolepsy–cataplexy in horses. Physostigmine salicylate, an anticholinesterase drug (0.06 to 0.08 mg per kg by slow IV infusion), precipitates a cataplectic attack within 3 to 10 minutes in affected horses. This compound crosses the blood–brain barrier. Careful monitoring of the horse after physostigmine administration is necessary because its cholinergic effects may cause colic, bronchospasm, and bradycardia.

Atropine sulfate, a muscarinic blocker (0.04 to 0.08 mg per kg IV), reduces the severity of cataleptic attacks within minutes after IV administration and can prevent their recurrence for 3.5 to 30 hours. Horses given atropine sulfate must be monitored for signs of ileus and colic.

Neostigmine, a cholinesterase inhibitor, does not cross the blood–brain barrier and therefore has no effect on cataleptic attacks. However, neostigmine provocation may help rule out conditions causing muscle weakness, such as myasthenia-like syndromes and botulism. Horses with muscle weakness will show increased muscle tone and a favorable response to neostigmine.

Differential Diagnoses

Acute collapse without warning is characteristic of syncope. Atrial fibrillation, ruptured chordae tendineae, myocardial infarction, myocardial fibrosis, aortic endocarditis, and pericarditis have been associated with syncope in horses. Cerebral hypoxia can occur in these conditions and lead to coma, with or without signs of cardiac failure. Seizures should also be considered. Botulism ("shaker foal" syndrome, forage poisoning), myasthenia-like syndrome, postanesthetic neuromyopathy, exertional rhabdomyolysis, and metabolic causes of collapse such as hyperthermia, shock, hypoglycemia, hypocalcemia, hypokalemia, hyperkalemia, endotoxemia, anaphylaxis, and snake bite should also be considered. Hyperkalemic periodic paralysis in young male Quarter Horses may strongly resemble narcolepsy.

A cataleptic state may be induced in neonatal foals by excessive whole body restraint. This response is thought to be an inherent in utero mechanism that prevents violent movements, especially during parturition.

THERAPY AND PROGNOSIS

Imipramine, a tricyclic antidepressant drug used to control narcolepsy and cataplexy, blocks the uptake of serotonin and norepinephrine and decreases REM sleep. Imipramine can be used at 0.55 mg per kg IV or 1.5 mg per kg PO, three times a day. Oral administration is reported to produce inconsistent results. Atropine sulfate can provide relief from acute attacks for up to 30 hours, but its use must be weighed against its adverse gastrointestinal side effects.

The prognosis for narcolepsy–cataplexy is variable. Some newborn Thoroughbreds and Miniature horses may have several attacks yet recover fully. In Shetland and Suffolk ponies, the disease may persist throughout life, as is true with the adult-onset form. In horses 1 to 3 years old, several episodes may occur without permanent consequence.

Supplemental Readings

Collatos, C.: Seizures in foals: Pathophysiology, evaluation, and treatment. Compend. Cont. Educ. Pract. Vet., 12:393–400, 1990.
de Lahunta, A.: Veterinary Neuroanatomy and Clinical Neurology, 2nd ed. Philadelphia, W. B. Saunders, 1983, pp. 88–89, 326–343.
Mayhew, I. G.: Large Animal Neurology: A Handbook for Veterinary Clinicians. Philadelphia, Lea & Febiger, 1989, pp. 113–125, 133–139.
Mayhew, I. G.: Seizure disorders. In Robinson, N. E. (ed.): Current Therapy in Equine Medicine. Philadelphia, W. B. Saunders, 1983, pp. 344–349.
Sweeny, C. R., and Hansen, T. O.: Narcolepsy and epilepsy. In Robinson, N. E. (ed.): Current Therapy in Equine Medicine 2. Philadelphia, W. B. Saunders, 1987, pp. 349–353.

Hypocalcemic Tetany

Gary W. Brandt, MANHATTAN, KANSAS

Equine hypocalcemic tetany (eclampsia, transit tetany) is still reported, although the incidence has declined since the draft horse era. Hypocalcemic tetany occurs in mares in midgestation, within 2 weeks of the end of gestation, 10 to 86 days post partum, and 1 to 2 days after weaning. Historically, postpartum day 10 and 1 to 2 days after weaning are the times of greatest prevalence, but unconfirmed hypocalcemia has been described as early as 2 hours post partum. Hypocalcemic tetany has also been reported in foals, stallions, geldings, and mares exposed to the stresses of gastrointestinal disorders, endurance events, prolonged transport, estrus, malnutrition, and confinement accompanied by a high grain intake. Idiopathic hypocalcemic tetany has been reported in nonlactating, nontransported Equidae.

Hypocalcemic tetany can occur as a result of lactational demands, alkalemic conditions, urea poisoning, hepatitis, blister beetle toxicosis, pancreatic atrophy, and stress-induced corticosteroid release as well as idiopathically. Alkalosis may be metabolic or respiratory in origin and originates from or accompanies the hypokalemia that follows anorexia or excessive sweating; the hypochloremia associated with profuse gastric reflux, intestinal stasis, or sweating; the hyperventilation that occurs during exposure to hot humid environments, strenuous exercise, or severe pain such as that observed with laminitis; and exogenous bicarbonate therapy. Tetany has been associated with malignant hyperthermia, oxalate toxicity, chronic liver disease, malabsorption syndromes, cadmium toxicosis, renal disease, exertional rhabdomyolysis, postoperative myopathy, and heat stroke.

The pathophysiology is related to deficits in the calcium pool. Lack of calcium intake, high milk production, fecal and urinary calcium loss, excess utilization, and decreased calcium solubility can independently or collectively produce a hypocalcemic state. The hyperirritability of peripheral nerves that results in neurological signs may be associated directly with hypocalcemia or may be due to alkalosis or hypokalemia. Hypokalemia and hypochloremia usually initiate neuromuscular signs indirectly, through a negative influence on the calcium pool. Both electrolyte abnormalities can initiate an alkalemic state, which decreases calcium solubility and significantly decreases ionized calcium concentration. The total calcium pool is depleted by severe stress. Serum calcium levels decline as a result of calcium loss through sweating and endogenous glucocorticoid release. The latter decreases calcium absorption by the small intestine and increases renal excretion of calcium and potassium ions.

CLINICAL SIGNS

Hypocalcemic tetany refers to the neurological component of a complex metabolic deficiency. Tonic spasms are only one facet of the clinical symptomatology of hypocalcemia. Signs may include decreased sensory awareness, depression or anxiety, abnormal facial expressions that occasionally resemble a sardonic grin, rear limb ataxia, stiffness of gait with occasional goose-stepping in the pelvic limbs, elevation of the tail head, muscle fasciculations or tremors of the temporal, masseter, triceps, shoulder, or back regions, trismus, twitching and trembling of the abdominal and lateral thoracic musculature, generalized muscular tension, tachypnea (40 to 100 breaths per minute) with flared nostrils, laryngospasm, dyspnea, dysphagia, salivation, inability to chew and swallow (difficulty in stomach tube passage has been reported), bruxism, profuse sweating, tachycardia (60 to 120 bpm), cardiac arrhythmias, synchronous diaphragmatic flutter, and cyanosis. Pupillary light reflexes are normal. Body temperature is normal to highly elevated. Urination and defecation diminish. Rectal palpation occasionally reveals a distended urinary bladder. An increase in small intestinal sounds and absence of cecal and large colon sounds can be observed. Handling, but not noise, may precipitate increased tetany. If the clinical syndrome progresses and is untreated, the horse becomes recumbent within 24 hours, tetanic convulsions develop, and death occurs 48 hours after onset of the clinical signs. Clinical signs of hypocalcemia are most readily recognized when total serum calcium levels approximate 4–6 mg/dl. In general, signs are directly related to the level of calcium deficiency. Increased excitability is observed if calcium levels remain above 8 mg per dl, tetanic spasms and slight incoordination may occur at serum calcium concentrations of 5 to 8 mg per dl, and recumbency and stupor may occur at concentrations below 5 mg per dl. However, a serum calcium concentration of 3.8 mg per dl has been reported in a mare exhibiting only depression.

Alterations in serum magnesium and phosphorus levels have been observed in association with signs of hypocalcemia in the horse. Hypo- or hypermagnesemia and hypo- or hyperphosphatemia have all been observed with hypocalcemia. Although the role of magnesium in the syndrome is unclear, magnesium concentrations ranging from 0.9 to 1.9 mg per dl (normal, 2.5 mg per dl) have been reported in horses manifesting signs of hypocalcemic tetany.

DIAGNOSIS

The diagnosis is based on a clinical history of predisposing conditions, clinical signs, and concentrations of serum calcium less than 8 mg per dl and of magnesium less than 1.9 mg per dl. Recognition of hypocalcemia is important because of its acute course and potentially fatal outcome. Entities in the differential diagnosis include tetanus, myositis, laminitis, colic, seizures, botulism, viral encephalitis, and other electrolyte imbalances.

Normal serum calcium levels range from 10.3 to 12.5 mg per dl, with normal serum magnesium levels approximately 2.5 mg per dl. In evaluating calcium concentrations, the practitioner should note the form of calcium reported. The extracellular level is a suitable measure of total calcium distribution, since the amount of intracellular calcium is minute in comparison. Extracellular calcium is divided into two fractions: nondiffusible, which is protein bound, and diffusible, which is complexed (citrate, carbonate, phosphate) or ionic. Only ionized calcium diffuses across capillary membranes and is responsible for neuromuscular stability. In normal horses, the ionized calcium fraction is approximately 50 per cent of total plasma calcium. In the assessment of hypocalcemic disease, the ionized fraction should be evaluated, because it will determine clinical symptomatology. This is of paramount importance when one is considering the metabolic influences previously described. For example, since alkalosis decreases the solubility of calcium salts, signs of hypocalcemic tetany could coexist with a normal total serum calcium concentration but an elevated protein-bound fraction and a subnormal ionized calcium fraction. Similarly, the protein-bound calcium fraction is lower in hypoproteinemia, especially hypoalbuminemia. This could result in a reduced

TABLE 1. CONCENTRATION OF CALCIUM IN VARIOUS COMMERICAL PREPARATIONS

Form of Calcium Compound	Concentration of Calcium Compound (gm/100 ml)	Calcium in Compound (%)	Elemental Calcium*† (mg/ml)	Elemental Calcium‡ (mEq/ml)
Calcium gluconate	23.00	9.30	21.39	1.07
	10.00	9.30	9.30	0.47
	18.08§	9.30	16.80	0.84
	23.62‖	9.30	22.00	1.10
	18.08¶	9.30	16.80	0.84
	23.62#	9.30	22.00	1.10
Calcium borogluconate	26.00°°	8.35	21.70	1.09
Calcium chloride	5.00	27.20	13.60	0.68
	10.00	27.20	27.20	1.36

*Elemental Ca (mg/ml) = $\dfrac{\text{Ca compound concentration (gm/100ml)} \times \text{Ca in compound (\%)}}{10}$.

†To convert Ca (mg/ml) to Ca (mEq/ml), multiply by 0.05
‡To convert Ca (mEq/ml) to Ca (mg/ml), multiply by 20
§Cal-Dextro No. 2 (calcium, dextrose, phosphorus, magnesium).
‖Cal-Dextro Special (calcium, dextrose, phosphorus, magnesium).
¶Cal-Dextro K (calcium, dextrose, potassium).
#Cal-Dextro C (calcium, dextrose).
°°Norcalciphos (calcium, dextrose, phosphorus, magnesium).

total serum calcium with a normal ionized calcium level. Therefore, a hypoproteinemic horse could have a normal ionized calcium fraction, low protein-bound fraction, and low total serum calcium level and be clinically normal.

THERAPY

Treatment consists of slow intravenous (IV) administration of a calcium solution with simultaneous auscultation of the heart. The expected cardiovascular response is an increase in intensity of the heart sounds. Slowing of the heart rate (bradycardia) or a change in rhythm is an indication to suspend IV treatment at once. Complete recovery after initial therapy may require several hours to days, and retreatment may be necessary. The veterinarian should be familiar with the various calcium preparations available, because concentrations of elemental calcium differ (Table 1). The dosage should be based on the availability of elemental calcium rather than the amount of total calcium salt. However, a formula for calculating the actual calcium replacement is difficult to derive because of the fluctuating metabolic influences that govern calcium ion concentrations. Treatment usually entails IV administration of standard calcium solutions that also contain magnesium and phosphate salts, such as are used for cattle. The literature cites an empirical dosage of 500 ml of these solutions, given slowly IV and repeated if necessary. Initial dosages of 55 ml per 100 kg have also been reported. The solutions may be given by slow IV infusion or, preferably, diluted in an isotonic solution, such as lactated Ringer's solution, saline, or 5 per cent dextrose, at 90 to 150 ml calcium solution per liter. Dilution allows more rapid administration with minimal chance of cardiotoxicity. Administration of diluted calcium solutions at flow rates of 3 liters per hour is reported to be safe. Dilution in 5 per cent sodium bicarbonate solutions is not recommended because of precipitation of calcium salts. An early sign of recovery is the voiding of large volumes of urine. Most authorities do not recommend removing foals from lactating mares but do recommend addition of a high-calcium feed (alfalfa) to the mare's diet.

Prevention of hypocalcemic tetany in horses includes feeding according to current work load, anticipated stresses, and milk production. Extensive long-term feeding of mineral additives containing calcium or leguminous roughage parturiently or during training may predispose a horse to hypocalcemic tetany once calcium depletion occurs from any of the aforementioned causes. In contrast, a lower calcium diet during the prestress period avoids excessive gastrointestinal absorption of calcium. This prepares the parturient mare or equine athlete to react to a hypocalcemic challenge by activation of a sensitized parathormone/osteoclastic pool and mobilization of bone for calcium homeostasis.

Supplemental Readings

Baird, J. D.: Lactation tetany (eclampsia) in a shetland pony mare. Aust. Vet. J., 47:402, 1971.
Brewer, B. D.: Disorders of equine calcium metabolism. Compend. Cont. Educ. Pract. Vet., 4:S244, 1982.
Coffman, J. R.: Acute hypocalcemia in horses. Mod. Vet. Pract., 54:61, 1973.
McAllister, E. S.: Hypocalcemia in two horses. J. Equine Med. Surg., 1: 230–233, 1977.
McKee, T. J., and Kimble, W. B.: Eclampsia in a horse. Mississippi Vet. J., 13, 1987.

Polyneuritis Equi

Kathleen Yvorchuk, MANHATTAN, KANSAS

Polyneuritis equi is a neural inflammatory disease of suspected immune-mediated origin. Commonly referred to as neuritis of the cauda equina, it bears close pathological resemblance to Guillain–Barré syndrome in humans and its experimental counterpart, experimental allergic neuritis in rodents. Polyneuritis equi primarily affects adult horses, though one report concerned a 17-month-old saddlebred filly. No sex or breed predilections are described. Classically, most clinical signs are referable to nerve roots of the cauda equina.

CLINICAL SIGNS

Two forms of this disease are most consistently described. In the acute form cranial or perineal hyperesthesia (or both) is initially observed. The latter manifests clinically as tail rubbing and chewing. The chronic form follows the acute phase or may be the initial presentation. The classical signs of gradual and progressive paralysis of the tail, bladder, and rectum develop in the chronic form. The signs may be accompanied by hind limb ataxia with possible muscle atrophy, depending on the extent and severity of the nerve involvement. Neurological deterioration will frequently progress to a certain level and subsequently remain static. Progression to complete recumbency is not a usual feature of this disorder. Clinical findings reflect lower motor neuron involvement of the caudal spinal cord. Observations include tail weakness or paralysis, anal dilation and diminished or absent anal reflex (hypotonia or atonia), fecal retention, and urinary incontinence. Lower motor neuron paralysis of the bladder manifests as a dilated atonic bladder accompanied by urethral relaxation. Though there is absence of voluntary micturition and the bladder is distended, there is minimal resistance to manual evacuation. Geldings and stallions can have a relaxed, protruding penis with reduced skin sensation (due to the penis's common sensory nerve supply with the perineum). The sheath and prepuce typically maintain sensory input as their innervation arises from a different location.

Neurological deficits also often involve the head area. Although sacrococcygeal dysfunction has been noted occurring alone, simple cranial nerve involvement has not been described. Clinical signs of head tilt and unilateral facial paralysis are most frequently noted; these may occur transiently and can change sides. The most commonly involved cranial nerves are the facial, trigeminal, and vestibulocochlear nerves. Reports of deficits of nerves II, III, IV, VI, IX, X, and XII have also been described. Sacral and lumbar neurological involvement is typically bilateral and symmetrical, as opposed to cranial nerve involvement, which is often unilateral.

PATHOLOGY

Macroscopic examination of severely affected areas discloses granulomatous inflammation, possibly with microabcesses, localized mainly to the level of the extradural nerve roots. The inflammatory reaction may be of such intensity that the fibrous material covering the nerves can involve meninges and result in adhesions with the meninges and occasionally the vertebral periosteum. Characteristically, lesions of cranial nerves are less severe than those of the cauda equina. Swelling, edema, petechiae, and hemorrhage of cranial nerves may be observed.

Microscopic examination has classically shown changes in extradural nerve roots with some extension to intradural roots. Recently a report described primary intradural nerve root abnormalities with some involvement of the autonomic nervous system. Individual nerve fibers are affected apparently randomly, with affected nerves in close proximity to completely normal fibers. Thickening of the epi-, endo-, and perineurium results in separation of nerve bundles. Infiltration of inflammatory cells (lymphocytes, plasma cells, macrophages, eosinophils, giant cells, and rarely neutrophils) contributes to the thickening around affected nerves. Axonal degeneration and demyelination are the major recognized features of the histopathology of polyneuritis equi. These occur concurrently with infiltration and inflammation of varying degrees. Some areas demonstrate mild regenerative changes. As the condition progresses, proliferation of perineurium results in eventual obliteration by fibrous tissue.

DIAGNOSIS

The specific etiology of polyneuritis equi remains unknown, although migrating helminth larvae and infectious bacterial, mycotic, and viral organisms have been proposed. The most accepted hypothesis suggests the involvement of allergic-type responses, possibly associated with prior viral respiratory disease, as is seen in Guillain–Barré syndrome in man. Both direct viral infection, such as with equine herpesvirus 1 or adenovirus 1, equine viral arteritis, or subsequent immunogenic responses are thought to result in neural lesions. Some authors suggest an association with previous hemolytic streptococcal infections, or possibly subsequent autoimmune phenomena. When compared to Guillain–Barré syndrome and experimental allergic neuritis, lesions observed in cases of polyneuritis equi are most indicative of a combination of inflammatory and immune-mediated reactions. In experimental allergic neuritis, which is created by injections of antigens isolated from peripheral nerve tissues (basically myelin protein P2), animals subsequently develop anti-P2 antibodies.

Recently, radioimmunoassay and ELISA detection of anti-P2 bovine or equine myelin protein antibodies has been successful in some cases of horses affected with polyneuritis equi. However, similar antibodies were also detected in horses diagnosed with herpesvirus paresis. These findings support the assay of anti-P2 antibodies as a diagnostic aid for polyneuritis equi, although the specificity of positive results is questionable. Anti-P2 antibodies may simply indicate destruction of myelin resulting from neuropathies of various etiologies.

Currently, diagnosis of polyneuritis equi basically relies on history, clinical signs, and progression of the disease. Frequently the diagnosis is only confirmed at necropsy. Complete blood cell counts usually indicate the presence of chronic, low-grade inflammatory responses (mature neutrophilia, mild to moderate anemia, and hyperfibrinogenemia) reflective of the neurological disease process and secondary chronic cystitis. Cerebrospinal fluid analysis can be helpful when abnormal; most typically moderate protein elevations are observed (reported as 70 to 300 mg per dl) with possible increased white blood cell counts (usually due to elevated lymphocyte numbers).

THERAPY

Treatment of affected individuals is palliative, since no specific etiology is known. Supportive therapy, such as broad-spectrum antibiotics and manual rectal and bladder evacuation or urinary catheterization, are recommended for secondary problems. Because of the postulated immune-mediated and known inflammatory components of the disorder, corticosteroid therapy should be considered. Although corticosteroids may temporarily decrease inflammatory responses and possibly reduce or arrest ongoing immunogenic responses, the benefits have been limited. One report described short-term amelioration (for approximately 1 month) subsequent to the use of dexamethasone, but clinical signs recurred within 1 year. Most cases have been terminal due to the presence of persistent irreversible neurological deficits.

Supplemental Readings

Beech, J.: Neuritis of the cauda equina. In: Proceedings of the 22nd Annual Convention of the American Association of Equine Practitioners, 1976, pp.75–76.

Cummings, J. F., deLahunta, A., and Timoney, J. F.: Neuritis of the cauda equina, a chronic idiopathic polyradiculoneuritis in the horse. Acta Neuropathol., 46:17, 1979.

Fordyce, P. S., Edington, N., Bridges, G. C., et al.: Use of an ELISA in the differential diagnosis of cauda equina neuritis and other equine neuropathies. Equine Vet. J., 19:55, 1987.

Held, J. P., Vanhooser, S., Prater, P. and Blackford, T. J.: Impotence in a stallion with neuritis of the cauda equina: A case report. J. Equine Vet. Sci., 9:67, 1989.

Kadlubowski, M., and Ingram, P. L.: Circulating antibodies to the neurotogenic myelin protein, P2, in neuritis of the cauda equina of the horse. Nature, 293:299, 1981.

Klingeborn, B., Dinter, Z., and Hughes, R. A. C.: Antibody to neurotogenic myelin protein P2 in equine paresis due to herpesvirus 1. Zentralblatt, Vet. Med. B, 30:137, 1983.

Rousseaux, C. G., Futcher, K. G., Clark, E. G., and Naylor, J. M.: Cauda equina neuritis: A chronic idiopathic polyneuritis in two horses. Can. Vet. J., 25:214, 1984.

Wright, J. A., Fordyce, P., and Edington, N.: Neuritis of the cauda equina in the horse. J. Comp. Pathol., 97:667, 1987.

Yvorchuk-St.Jean, K.: Neuritis of the cauda equina. Vet. Clin. North Amer. (Equine Pract.), 3:421, 1987.

Neuromuscular Disorders

Judy Cox, MANHATTAN, KANSAS

MYOTONIA

Equine myotonia, a skeletal muscle disorder characterized by a long period of continuous, involuntary contraction after stimulation or voluntary motion, has not been accurately classified into a type. Some features of both myotonia congenita and myotonia dystrophica (as defined in humans) are present in the same or different horses. Clinical signs are usually noticed before 6 months of age. The mode of inheritance in horses is unknown.

Equine myotonia primarily affects the extensor muscles of the limbs and is characterized by a stiff gait and firm muscles. The pelvic limbs are more severely affected, and focal enlargement of the proximal caudal thigh muscles occurs. Percussion of affected muscles causes formation of "dimples" that persist for a minute or more. Affected muscles are firm and tense on palpation and do not relax fully when the horse is at rest. Some foals have difficulty rising from recumbency. Clinical signs are usually worst when the horse travels after resting; affected horses often improve when turned out continuously and worsen when kept in stalls.

On electromyography, a continuous series of repetitive, waxing and waning, motor unit action potentials (myotonic discharges) are found. Histological findings include marked variation in size and shape of muscle fibers; clusters of a single muscle fiber type are seen on histochemical staining. Increases in connective tissue, acute degeneration of fibers, atrophy of fibers, central nuclei, and ring bands have all been found.

In some horses, signs ameliorate slightly with age and horses can be used for breeding. Most animals stabilize by age 6 to 7 months, but progressive worsening can occur. There is currently no treatment for affected horses.

STRINGHALT

Stringhalt is characterized by an abrupt onset of continuous (with every stride) or intermittent hyperflexion of one or both hind limbs during motion. Hyperflexion may be mild or severe enough that the rear fetlock strikes the abdomen with each stride; very severely affected horses may "bunny-hop" in the rear limbs or be unable to rise voluntarily when recumbent. Signs are most obvious when the horse is turned or backed and may worsen in cold weather. In some horses, signs are worse following rest and resolve with exercise. If the forelimbs are also involved, stumbling and toe scuffing are seen, due to either limited flexion or knuckling of the carpus. The condition is seen primarily in the light horse breeds.

The cause is poorly understood and may be due to a sensory neuropathy, a myopathy, or a spinal cord lesion. A distal axonal degeneration selectively involving large myelinated nerve fibers has been identified in an Australian outbreak of stringhalt. In order of decreasing severity, the long left recurrent laryngeal nerve, the right recurrent laryngeal nerve, the hind limb peripheral nerves, and the forelimb peripheral nerves were affected, with neurogenic atrophy of muscles innervated by affected nerves. Lathyrism can cause similar clinical signs. Consumption of *Lathyrus sativus* (chickling pea), *L. sativus* (wild winter pea), or related species can cause a distal axonopathy. The toxic principal is a neuroexcitatory amino acid, β-N-oxalylamino-L-alanine. In addition to hypermetria and hyperreflexia, other signs such as proprioceptive deficits, flaccid tail and anus, and loss of bladder control may be present.

The diagnosis is based strictly on clinical appearance. Mild cases must be differentiated from upward fixation of the patella and equine protozoal myeloencephalitis. Some cases of stringhalt improve with time; lateral digital tenectomy may or may not result in improvement.

A potentially different stringhalt syndrome occurs in Australia and New Zealand. Australian stringhalt occurs sporadically in summer and autumn in horses at pasture. Consumption of *Hypochaeris radicata* (flatweed) or unidentified mycotoxins is a possible etiology. In one outbreak, *Taraxacum officinale* (dandelion), a close relative of flatweed, was abundant in the pasture. Horses are unilaterally or bilaterally affected. Local muscle atrophy is a usual accompaniment. Electromyographic abnormalities have been identified in the long digital extensor muscle; peroneal nerve conduction velocity and repetitive nerve stimulation are abnormal. Most affected horses develop some degree of laryngeal asynchrony or hemiplegia. Spontaneous recovery occurs in 6 to 12 months. There is no treatment except removal from the pasture. A similar outbreak was reported in California.

SHIVERS

Shivers affects only draft horses and onset can occur at any age. Bilateral muscle fasciculations and tremors ("shivering") occur in the muscles of the pelvis, pelvic limbs, and tail. Signs usually worsen when the horse is backed, and sudden jerky extensor movements of the tail may occur. When backing, severely affected horses hyperflex a limb and abduct it, with the limb remaining in this position and trembling. Usually the tail elevates and trembles simultaneously. Signs subside in a few seconds but recur if the horse is backed again. Fibrillation potentials have been seen on electromyography. The forelimbs are less often affected, but carpal elevation and abduction is reported. Signs may progress slowly, remain static, or improve after a prolonged period of rest. The cause is unknown. No treatment has been described.

POSTANESTHETIC MYONEUROPATHY

Postanesthetic lameness, which may be myogenic, neurogenic, or a combination (myoneuropathy), occurs most often in well-conditioned, large, heavy horses following general anesthesia of 2 hours or longer. It may be the most common life-threatening complication of equine anesthesia. Two syndromes occur: a painful form dominated by myopathy, and a relatively nonpainful form affecting function, in which a neuropathy is suspected. The pathogenesis is probably complex; systemic hypotension during anesthesia, anaerobic glycolysis and lactic acid overproduction, pressure-induced or ischemic neuropathy, tissue reperfusion with oxidant injury, and compartment pressure elevation have all been suggested as causes. The incidence increases when significant hemorrhage occurs before or during anesthesia. Occasional horses exhibit a myasthenic syndrome, and a malignant hyperthermia-like syndrome has been suspected in some cases.

Localized or generalized muscle involvement may occur. Horses anesthetized in lateral recumbency usually have dependent muscle involvement, with the forelimbs frequently affected; the triceps is most commonly involved, but the pectoral, brachiocephalic, deltoid, and rib cage muscles may also be involved. Following anesthesia in dorsal recumbency, the gluteal and longissimus dorsi muscles are most commonly affected, but the adductor muscles (adductor, pectineus, gracilis, and possibly vastus medialis) may also be affected. In addition, nondependent muscle groups are sometimes affected.

Clinical signs include a prolonged recovery period and paresis or plegia of one or more limbs following anesthesia. Pain, swelling, induration, and obvious plaques of affected muscle groups may or may not be apparent. Neuropraxia, especially of the radial or peroneal nerves, may be present. If muscle pain is present, affected horses sweat and may have tachycardia and tachypnea, and exhibit violent behavior during recovery; self-trauma may necessitate euthanasia for humane reasons. Myoglobinuria may be present and serum muscle enzyme activities are significantly elevated.

Recumbent horses should be kept in the sternal position or supported in a sling as much of the time as possible. Liberal quantities of oral (PO) or intravenous (IV) fluids are indicated to induce diuresis and reduce myoglobin-induced renal damage. Electrolyte imbalances should be corrected. Analgesia should be provided, keeping in mind the potential toxicity of nonsteroidal anti-inflammatory drugs if hydration is inadequate. Intractable horses should be sedated. Low doses of phenothiazine derivative tranquilizers also combat vasospasm and increase the arterial blood supply to affected muscle masses. The administration of dimethyl sulfoxide IV (1 gm per kg, diluted to 10 to 20 per cent in 5 per cent dextrose solution) may diminish oxidant-induced injury. Dantrolene sodium (2 to 4 mg per kg IV or 10 mg per kg PO) has been recommended to reduce excessive calcium release within muscle cells. The half-life of this drug is short in horses, and these dosages will only provide an adequate blood level for 2 hours. Good nursing care is essential and includes massage, warm water hydrotherapy, protective bandages on the lower limbs, and nutritional support. Most horses show clinical improvement within 24 to 48 hours, although occasionally animals fail to recover and are euthanized because of intractable pain and prolonged recumbency.

Preventative measures include proper padding, elevation of the upper thoracic and pelvic limb, positioning the dependent thoracic limb in a forward position, adequate fluid support to prevent hypotension, maintaining a light plane of anesthesia, and minimizing total anesthetic time. A prophylactic dose of 10 mg per kg of dantrolene sodium 1 hour prior to general anesthesia has been advocated.

Occasional cases of flaccid paralysis (postanesthetic myasthenic syndrome) may occur following general anesthesia. A diffuse neuromuscular blockade occurs. The use of animoglycosides or tetracyclines in combination with halothane anesthesia may be contributing factors. Treatment involves general supportive care. Neostigmine and calcium salt administration has been advocated.

HYPERKALEMIC PERIODIC PARALYSIS

Hyperkalemic periodic paralysis is a condition of the stock breeds characterized by intermittent episodes of muscular weakness and fasciculations accompanied by a transient elevation in serum potassium, as described on page 117.

Supplemental Readings

Hodgson, D.R.: Diseases of muscle. In Colahan, P. T., Mayhew, I. G., Merritt, A. M., and Moore, J. N. (eds.): Equine Medicine and Surgery, 4th ed. Goleta, CA, American Veterinary Publ, 1991, pp. 1317–1330.

MacKay, R. J., and Mayhew, I. G.: Diseases of the peripheral (spinal) nerves. In Colahan, P. T., Mayhew, I. G., Merritt, A. M., and Moore, J. N. (eds.): Equine Medicine and Surgery, 4th ed. Goleta, CA, American Veterinary Pub., 1991, pp. 826–832.

Pemberton, D. H., and Caple, I. W.: Australian stringhalt in horses. Vet. Annu., 20:167–171, 1980.

Neurological Causes of Blindness

Sarah Maxwell, MANHATTAN, KANSAS

Blindness or decreased visual acuity may be the result of opacification of ocular structures (corneal scarring, marked aqueous flare, cataracts, or vitritis) or it may be the result of neurological dysfunction, the focus of this article. The neural portions of the visual system include the retina, optic nerve, optic chiasma, optic tracts, lateral geniculate bodies (located in the thalamus), optic radiations, and the visual cortex (in the occipital lobe of the cerebrum). Eighty-five to 90 percent of the optic nerve fibers decussate at the chiasm in the horse.

CLINICAL SIGNS AND DIAGNOSIS

The detection or localization of subtle lesions in neural portions of the visual system may be difficult but is aided by historical information. In addition to collecting a general history, including diet, environment, and medications, the clinician should ascertain whether the horse has had any known cranial trauma, episodes of severe hemorrhage, recent systemic illness, or any signs suggestive of neurological dysfunction. Information regarding the horse's vision should also be collected from the owner, including onset of problems, how the animal functions in its regular and new environments, behavioral or postural changes, and whether the animal performs better in light or dim conditions.

Vision is assessed in a number of ways, each requiring some subjective evaluation and fraught with its own limitations. These include the menace response, with care taken not to touch the cilia or stimulate the corneal reflex by air currents, and tracking or evaluating response to a moving object. Maze testing can be performed by covering one eye and leading the animal through a room with large objects in both bright and dim settings. Care should be taken when covering the "good" eye or turning down the lights on a night-blind animal because the animal's behavior may be unpredictable.

The ophthalmological examination should be performed with a bright light source in a room that can be dimly lit. Pupil size and presence of anisocoria should be noted in both light and dim conditions. Evaluation of both direct and consensual pupillary light reflexes is essential. Assessment of the consensual pupillary light reflex may be facilitated by having an assistant illuminate one eye while the clinican observes the opposite pupil for a response. Both speed and degree of pupillary constriction should be noted. Knowledge of vision and pupil light reflexes along with other neurological signs such as cranial nerve deficits, gait disturbances, and attitude can help localize the lesion in the central nervous system (CNS). The nuclei for the efferent portion of the pupillary light reflex are located in the midbrain; thus, normal pupillary light reflexes indicate that the system is intact to the level of the diencephalon. Sight and an abnormal pupil light reflex point to a lesion in the efferent nerves to the pupil. The supplemental readings listed should be consulted for further information.

Retina and optic nerve lesions produce similar clinical signs. Complete unilateral lesions will produce a blind ipsilateral eye with no direct or consensual pupillary light reflex. Vision and pupillary light reflexes of the contralateral eye should be normal. Due to crossover at the efferent side of the pupillary light reflex, the affected pupil will not be widely dilated in room light, although a mild anisocoria may be present. Bilateral retinal and optic nerve lesions appear clinically similar to a lesion at the optic chiasm. Pupils are widely dilated and nonresponsive and the animal is totally blind. Retinal diseases accompanied by funduscopic changes are described on page 608.

NIGHT BLINDNESS

If the animal's vision is decreased in dim light and the retina appears normal funduscopically, night blindness should be considered. Stationary night blindness is most common in the Appaloosa, in which a recessive mode of inheritance is suspected. This disease is congenital and nonprogressive. The definitive diagnosis rests on electroretinography. Night blindness has also been produced experimentally in horses maintained on diets deficient in vitamin A for over 1 year. Serum vitamin A levels can be evaluated if the animal's diet is suggestive of deficiency. Dietary supplementation may restore night vision in cases of hypovitaminosis A.

OPTIC NERVE DISORDERS

Optic nerve hypoplasia is a well-documented congenital defect. If hypoplasia is present bilaterally, the foal will appear blind from birth and have dilated, poorly responsive pupils. A unilateral defect may go unnoticed until the animal is older and then may be difficult to clinically differentiate from optic nerve atrophy even though histological differences exist.

Optic nerve diseases are varied and are often grouped together as "optic neuritis," although optic neuropathy may be a better term. These diseases can be further subclassified into those that involve the optic papilla, and therefore may be diagnosed on funduscopic examination, and those that involve the retrobulbar optic nerve ("the animal sees nothing and the doctor sees nothing").

Funduscopic changes occur in exudative optic neuritis, a bilateral disease characterized by diminishing vision and pupillary light reflexes in horses. Proliferative gray to yellow, ovoid lesions protrude from the optic papilla into the vitreous humor. Retinal hemorrhage and vitritis may be noted near the optic disk preceding or accompanying the proliferative lesions. This disease has been described following episodes of severe hemorrhage, especially prolonged epistaxis or hemorrhage post castration, trauma or systemic illness, and has been postulated to result from disturbed ocular circulation. Aggressive anti-inflammatory therapy can be initiated, but the prognosis for return of vision is poor. Exudative optic neuritis should be differentiated from proliferative optic neuritis, in which a unilateral, proliferative growth is found on the optic papilla. It is seen in older horses and does not affect vision or pupillary light reflexes.

Diseases producing a retrobulbar optic neuritis include (1) orbital inflammation, orbital neoplasia, or optic nerve tumors, which tend to be unilateral and may affect the optic nerve by compression or inflammation; and (2) ischemia, which tends to be bilateral in cases of severe hemorrhage and decreased blood pressure, and unilateral or bilateral in cases of thrombosis, embolism, vascular spasm, or decreased venous return. Retrobulbar optic neuritis may also be the result of infectious viral diseases affecting the optic nerve, such as eastern equine encephalitis or Borna disease. Therapy should be directed at the underlying etiology and reducing inflammation.

Traumatic lesions of the optic nerve or chiasma are not uncommon and may produce unilateral or bilateral blindness. Lesions vary from orbital inflammation affecting the optic nerve to rupture of the optic nerve axons. The latter is associated with posterior movement of the brain or chiasmal hemorrhage as a result of fracture of the basisphenoid bone. Aggressive treatment should be initiated immediately and includes systemic corticosteroids and nonsteroidal anti-inflammatory drugs (NSAIDs). Dimethyl sulfoxide may also be administered intravenously (IV) over 30 minutes (1 gm per kg body weight diluted in an equal volume of 5 per cent dextrose in water). Improvement is expected in the first 72 hours. If no changes are noted after 7 days, a poor prognosis is warranted. After 30 days, there may be evidence of optic nerve atrophy such as a pale optic disk and decreased retinal vasculature. Optic nerve atrophy (evidenced by a pale disk and decreased retinal vasculature) is the end-stage of a number of processes, including optic neuropathy and trauma. If the horse is examined later in the course of the disease, it may be impossible to determine the underlying etiology.

OTHER CAUSES OF BLINDNESS

Pituitary tumors are an uncommon cause of blindness in horses but may affect the visual system by expansion and compression on the chiasma, by infiltration, or by interference with blood supply. Associated signs of polyuria, polydypsia, and coat abnormalities will help point to this disorder.

Lesions of the lateral geniculate body, optic radiations, or visual cortex are manifested by decreased vision in the contralateral eye and normal pupillary light reflexes. Concomitant signs of CNS disease would be expected and can help localize the lesion. Causes include brain abscess associated with strangles, verminous granulomas, and neoplasia. Several diseases, including viral, bacterial, protozoal, parasitic, or fungal encephalomyelitis, intoxication, hypoxemia, hydrocephalus, leukoencephalomalacia, hepatic encephalopathy, or herniation of the posterior cerebrum under the osseous tentorium, can cause CNS lesions resulting in total blindness and normal pupillary light reflexes (unless the midbrain is also affected). A neurological examination and cerebrospinal fluid (CSF) tap are indicated in cases of blindness of central origin. Neoplastic processes may produce an elevation in CSF pressure and occasionally one may collect a sample containing neoplastic cells. Evaluating total and differential white blood cell count in the CSF, along with serology and culture, will aid in the diagnosis of an infectious process. Aggressive NSAID therapy may be initiated with systemic antibiotics if an infectious agent is suspected. If the underlying etiology is not infectious, steroids may also be used.

Client education regarding limitations of a visually impaired horse is imperative. The clinician must accurately assess the extent of vision loss and predict long-term visual prognosis so that the client can determine what functions the horse may still serve.

Supplemental Readings

de Lahunta, A., and Cummings, J. F.: Neuro-ophthalmological lesions as a cause of visual deficit in dogs and horses. J. Am. Vet. Med. Assoc., 150:994, 1967.
English, R. V.: Diagnosis of vision loss in small animals. Kal Kan Forum, 1988, pp. 9–15.
Lavach, J. D.: Large Animal Ophthalmology, Vol. 1. St. Louis, C. V. Mosby, 1990, pp. 209–224.
Platt, H., Barnett, K. C., Barry, D. R., and Bell, A. S. W.: Degenerative lesions of the optic nerve in Equidae. Equine Vet. J. Suppl. 2:91–97, 1983.
Slatter, D.: Fundamentals of Veterinary Ophthalmology, 2nd ed. Philadelphia, W. B. Saunders, 1990, pp. 587–661.

Vestibular Disease

Jana M. Smith, CLOVIS, CALIFORNIA

The vestibular system maintains the animal's balance and orientation in its environment, both at rest and in motion. It is composed of the paired receptor organs (semicircular canals, utricle, and saccule), vestibular nerves, and vestibular nuclei. Vestibular efferent projections to the brain stem, reticular formation, cerebellum, and spinal cord coordinate eye, limb, and trunk movements with changes in head position. Due to their close proximity, the facial nerves and nuclei are frequently involved by diseases affecting the vestibular system.

ETIOLOGY

Head trauma and otitis media and interna are the most common causes of vestibular disease in horses. Head trauma is frequent in foals and young horses during early training, where rearing over backward and striking the poll may fracture the basisphenoid-basioccipital region. Acute vestibular signs result, with or without signs of facial nerve and central involvement. Trauma of the cranium or temporal region in adult horses may occur as a result of falls, collisions, or inflicted blows to the skull. Large lesions typically result from such injuries and vestibular signs may be less important than other central neurological deficits.

In adult horses, chronic infection of the middle ear is thought to lead to osteitis of the tympanic bulla and stylohyoid bone, progressing to fusion of the temporohyoid joint. Mechanical stresses induced by swallowing, vocalizing, and head and neck movements can cause an acute skull fracture involving the temporal, hyoid, or basilar bones. Traumatic inflammation of the vestibular and facial nerves results, producing an acute severe vestibular disease with facial nerve signs.

Other causes of asymmetrical vestibular disease include equine protozoal myeloencephalitis, aberrant migrating parasites, polyneuritis equi, and space-occupying masses. Diffuse brain diseases, including the viral encephalitides and hepatoencephalopathy, may produce vestibular signs in addition to symmetrical signs of central nervous system disease. Ototoxicity from aminoglycosides has been reported in horses, with irreversible degeneration of vestibular and auditory receptors. Lightning strike has been incriminated in cases of unilateral vestibular disease. A transient idiopathic acute vestibular syndrome without other signs has been reported in adult horses; immune-mediated and viral labyrinthitis are proposed causes.

CLINICAL SIGNS

Destruction, inflammation, or dysfunction of vestibular pathways produce clinical signs that vary with lesion location. Unilateral peripheral vestibular disease is commonly observed and is characterized by loss of balance, asymmetrical ataxia without loss of strength, and head tilt. The horse may stagger, lean, circle, or drift sideways when walking. Voluntary head shaking or blindfolding the horse may aggravate the ataxia or cause the horse to fall. A head tilt is usually present, with the more ventral ear and eye on the affected side and the muzzle pointed away from the lesion. The head may be turned toward the affected side and the horse frequently adopts a base-wide stance. A spontaneous nystagmus may be elicited by flexing the neck laterally or elevating the head. Strabismus may be observed as ventral or ventrolateral deviation of the eye on the affected side. With severe vestibular dysfunction the horse may be recumbent and unable to rise. Rolling may occur; if quiescent, the horse will usually lie on the affected side. Violent efforts to rise or right itself may be mistaken for cerebral involvement or seizures.

Clinical signs of facial nerve involvement frequently accompany vestibular disease and include muzzle deviation, decreased nostril flare, buccal impaction of food, ptosis, ear droop, and inability to close the eyelids. Decreased tear production, keratitis, corneal ulcers, or Horner's syndrome may occur due to damage to adjacent parasympathetic or sympathetic fibers. Head shaking, ear rubbing or sensitivity, and chomping motions may be observed in horses with otitis media and interna days to weeks prior to vestibular signs, while dysphagia frequently accompanies the acute onset of neurological signs.

In peripheral vestibular disease, the horse is cognizant of the position of its limbs and postural reactions and muscular strength are normal. Central vestibular disorders cause generalized proprioceptive deficits and mild paresis. The trunk may be flexed laterally, appearing concave on the affected side, and mild hypertonia and hyperreflexia of the contralateral limbs may be noted. Depression and other cranial nerve signs are further indications of central disorders. Paradoxical vestibular signs, with a head tilt and ataxia opposite the lesion, may occur with certain cerebellomedullary lesions. Bilateral peripheral vestibular disease with complete loss of function is uncommon; clinical signs are symmetrical ataxia with wide swaying motions of the head and trunk and lack of nystagmus.

DIAGNOSIS

Diagnosis of a vestibular problem is largely based on a thorough physical and neurological examination. Definitive diagnosis of skull fractures or chronic otitis media and interna is achieved by radiography. Precise ventrodorsal radiographs under anesthesia are required for accurate diagnosis of ossifying otitis; the subsequent temporal or stylohyoid fracture is infrequently identified. A transtympanic membrane tap of the middle ear may be performed under anesthesia, but interpretation of culture and cytology results is complicated by the interval between the onset of bacterial otitis and fracture development. Cerebrospinal fluid (CSF) cytology and culture are helpful in the diagnosis of traumatic or inflammatory disease. Hematology, serum biochemistry, or serology may assist the diagnosis of infectious and metabolic disease. External ear cultures and guttural pouch endoscopy and culture may identify bacterial extension from the middle ear. Computed tomography, where available, may identify space-occupying masses such as abscesses or tumors.

THERAPY

Acute trauma cases should be treated for central nervous system (CNS) edema and inflammation. Dexamethasone (0.1 to 0.15 mg per kg) may be administered intravenously (IV) every 8 to 12 hours for the first 24 to 48 hours. Most trauma cases stabilize within this time period. The potential for steroid-induced laminitis is greater with higher doses and repeated treatments. Osmotic diuretics such as dimethyl sulfoxide (DMSO) or mannitol are frequently beneficial in CNS edema; DMSO also has anti-inflammatory activity and scavenges superoxide radicals. DMSO (0.5 to 1.0 gm per kg IV) may be administered as a 10 to 20 per cent solution in saline, lactated Ringer's solution, or 5 per cent dextrose solution and given every 8 to 12 hours for 1 to 3 days. Mannitol (0.25 gm per kg as a 20 per cent solution) may be administered by slow IV infusion once or twice within the first 24 hours; however, it is contraindicated in the presence of cerebral hemorrhage. Antimicrobial therapy is indicated when disruption of the blood–brain barrier is suspected or hemorrhage or CSF is observed in the external ear. Sedation of a violently struggling patient with diazepam (100 to 200 mg for an adult horse and 10 to 25 mg IV for a foal) or xylazine (0.2 to 1.0 mg per kg IV or IM) may be necessary; however, the hypotensive tendencies of xylazine should be considered in cases of severe CNS trauma or shock.

Otitis media and interna cases should be treated with antibiotics and nonsteroidal anti-inflammatory agents for 30 days. Potentiated sulfonamides (trimethoprim–sulfadiazine, 30 mg per kg twice a day) are broad-spectrum, inexpensive antimicrobials with CNS penetrance and are a reasonable choice when specific culture and sensitivity results are lacking. The prognosis for recovery is fair to good when CNS signs are limited to the vestibular system; however, residual vestibular or facial signs may persist.

Treatment of other causes of vestibular disease are addressed elsewhere in the text. Idiopathic vestibular syndrome appears to resolve completely irrespective of therapy; however, since definitive diagnosis cannot be made, conclusive statements are not possible.

Supplemental Readings

Blythe, L. L.: Otitis media and interna in the horse: Its relationship to head tossing and skull fractures. In: Proceedings of the 7th Annual Forum of the American College of Veterinary Internal Medicine, 1989, pp. 1015–1018.

de Lahunta, A.: Vestibular system-Special proprioception. In: Veterinary Neuroanatomy and Clinical Neurology, 2nd ed. Philadelphia, W. B. Saunders, 1983, pp. 238–254.

Mayhew I. G.: Head tilt, circling, nystagmus, and other signs of vestibular abnormalities. In Mayhew, I. G. (ed.): Large Animal Neurology: A Handbook for Veterinary Clinicians. Philadelphia, Lea & Febiger, 1989, pp. 179–192.

Watrous, B. J.: Head tilt in horses. Vet. Clin. North Am. (Equine Pract.), 3:353, 1987.

Peripheral Neuropathies

Simon J. Wheeler, RALEIGH, NORTH CAROLINA

Methods of evaluating the peripheral nervous system include an assessment of the history and clinical signs, physical examination, neurological examination, and diagnostic tests including radiography, electrophysiology, blood and cerebrospinal fluid (CSF) analysis, and biopsy of nerve and muscle. Because of the limited information available from the history, the owner's subjective analysis of the condition, and the neurological examination, there is much to be gained from ancillary diagnostic aids in evaluating the equine peripheral nervous system. When available, electromyography and nerve conduction studies can provide useful diagnostic information in suspected cases of peripheral neuropathy. The following discussion summarizes the clinical signs of some of the more common peripheral neuropathies of the horse. More extensive details of therapy can be found in *Current Therapy in Equine Medicine 2*, page 384.

CRANIAL NERVES

The cranial nerves are affected by lesions at various sites along their course both within the central nervous system (CNS) and in the peripheral nerves themselves. CNS disorders are characterized by multiple cranial nerve deficits accompanied by signs of central dysfunction such as changes in behavior or temperament, ataxia, paresis, and proprioceptive loss.

TRIGEMINAL NERVE

The trigeminal nerve is motor to the muscles of mastication via the mandibular branch and is sensory to the head. Lesions of the mandibular branch of the trigeminal nerve lead to neurogenic atrophy of the muscles of mastication. Unilateral lesions may have little effect on jaw function, although the jaw may deviate away from the affected side. Bilateral lesions cause drooping of the jaw with inability to close the mouth. Sensory losses over the face may be recognized by loss of the palpebral reflex, but it must be remembered that the facial nerve must be normal for this reflex to function. Conscious perception of pain is assessed by pinching the skin with forceps or by stimulating the nasal septum. There are several reported cases of trigeminal paralysis due to neoplastic infiltration. Cauda equina neu-

Facial Nerve

The facial nerve innervates the muscles of facial expression, is secretomotor to the lacrimal gland, and sensory to the rostral part of the tongue. Facial nerve paralysis produces a spectrum of clinical signs. Traumatic lesions to the buccal branches of the facial nerve may occur as a result of direct trauma or following a period of lateral recumbency. Here signs are restricted to the lips, the eye and ear being spared as the lesion is distal to the branches to these structures. There is paresis of the muscles of facial expression and a deviation of the muzzle away from the affected side.

Lesions more proximal on the nerve near its exit from the stylomastoid foramen involve the branches to the eyelid and ear. Lesions within the facial canal may involve the branch to the lacrimal gland, leading to reduced tear production. Paralysis of the eyelids and a deficit in tear film may result in exposure keratitis. The facial nerve may be involved in cauda equina neuritis, and neoplastic involvement has been described. Facial nerve paralysis occurs in association with other cranial nerve abnormalities, particularly those of the vestibulocochlear nerve, leading to vestibular syndrome.

Vestibulocochlear Nerve

Vestibular disease is seen with or without facial paralysis. Vestibular syndrome is characterized by a head tilt, ataxia, circling, dysmetria and nystagmus. Vestibular syndrome has been described in trauma, temporal bone fractures, otitis media, diseases of the temporohyoid joint, neoplasia, and cauda equina neuritis. Radiography is useful to diagnose trauma and otitis media and should be performed whenever there are signs of facial or vestibulocochlear nerve injury.

Cochlear Nerve

Cochlear nerve deficits leading to deafness, especially if unilateral, are difficult to detect clinically in the horse. The advent of brain stem auditory evoked response testing has made assessment of the auditory pathways possible.

Glossopharyngeal and Vagus Nerves

Diseases of the glossopharyngeal and vagus nerves produce pharyngeal and laryngeal dysfunction. Guttural pouch disorders can involve these nerves and lead to dysphagia, pharyngeal paralysis, laryngeal hemiplegia, Horner's syndrome, and soft palate disorders.

Idiopathic laryngeal hemiplegia, first described by a farrier named Gibson in 1722, has received more attention than any other equine peripheral neuropathy. There is a progressive distal loss of myelinated fibers with demyelination, remyelination, and occasional wallerian type degeneration in both left and right recurrent laryngeal nerves. These changes, observed even in horses that are not clinically affected, may represent an axonal transport defect and be part of a generalized polyneuropathy. Bilateral laryngeal paralysis has been described following treatment with the anthelmintic haloxon and with haloxon-contaminated mineral oil.

Limb Nerves

Disorders of the limb nerves often result in locomotor disturbances. *Suprascapular nerve* paralysis occurs with reasonable frequency, causing neurogenic atrophy of the supraspinatus and infraspinatus muscles. If muscle atrophy has been present for a long period, fibrosis and contracture may result. In a study of suprascapular nerve from affected and clinically normal horses, both the affected and some of the unaffected horses had evidence of a chronic demyelinating neuropathy in the nerve, most severe at the point of reflection of the nerve around the cranial border of the scapula. This underlying neuropathy may make the nerve more sensitive to trauma. The clinical syndrome resulting from suprascapular paralysis is known as "sweeny." The shoulder is abducted during walking, and there is atrophy of the muscles over the scapula. Surgical treatment by suprascapular notch resection to decompress the nerve may be beneficial (see *Current Therapy in Equine Medicine 2*, page 385).

Femoral nerve paralysis has been described following general anesthesia. The condition is rare and the prognosis for recovery variable. Nerve root lesions of the fourth and fifth lumbar nerves can also lead to signs of femoral paralysis, and neoplastic and inflammatory causes have been implicated. Because the femoral nerve supplies the quadriceps femoris muscles, femoral paralysis results in inability to extend the stifle. The tarsus and digit are flexed and the horse cannot bear weight. Intermittent luxation of the patellae has also been attributed to pathological changes in the peripheral nerves of the hind limb.

Neurogenic atrophy of the gluteal muscles is seen with neoplastic or inflammatory involvement of the *gluteal nerves*, equine protozoal myelitis being a frequent cause in the United States.

CAUDA EQUINA NEURITIS

Horses with cauda equina neuritis initially demonstrate hyperesthesia of the tail and perineum, followed by paralysis of the tail, anus, and vulva. Urinary incontinence and fecal retention occur and there are cranial nerve abnormalities, particularly affecting nerves VII and VIII. The pathological changes include inflammation and degeneration of axons and myelin. Although clinical signs may be restricted to the tail and perineum, microscopic evidence of pathological change is more widespread. The etiology of the condition is unknown. Diagnosis of this condition is assisted by detection of circulating antibody to P2 myelin protein (see p. 569).

STRINGHALT

Stringhalt, a condition characterized by exaggerated flexion of the hind limbs, may occur sporadically or in outbreaks of Australian stringhalt. In Australian stringhalt, the distal axonopathy that affects various nerves is accompanied by neurogenic atrophy of muscles. A toxic etiology is suspected as the disease is associated with ingestion of the plant *Hypochaeris radicata*. Some of the sporadic cases do not have lesions in the peripheral nerves and the etiology in these horses is unknown (see p. 571).

Supplemental Readings

Cummings, J. P., deLahunta, A., and Timoney, J. F.: Neuritis of the cauda equina: A chronic polyradiculoneuritis in the horse. Acta Neuropathol. (Berl.), 46:17, 1979.

de Lahunta, A.: Veterinary Neuroanatomy and Clinical Neurology. Philadelphia, W. B. Saunders, 1983.

Dyson, S., Taylor, P., and Whitwell, K.: Femoral paralysis after general anaesthesia. Equine Vet. J., 20:376, 1988.

Fordyce, P. S., Edington, N., Bridges, G. C., Wright, J. A., and Edwards, G. B.: Use of an ELISA in the differential diagnosis of cauda equina neuritis and other equine neuropathies. Equine Vet. J., 19:55, 1987.

Huntington, P. J., Jeffcott, L. B., Friend, S. C. E., Luff, A. R., Finkelstein, D. I., and Flynn, R. J.: Australian stringhalt: Epidemiological, clinical and neurological investigations. Equine Vet. J., 21:266, 1989.

Marshall, A. E., Byars, T. D., Whitlock, R. H., and George, L. W.: Brainstem auditory evoked response in the diagnosis of inner ear injury in the horse. J. Am. Vet. Med. Assoc., 178:282, 1981.

Mayhew, I. G.: Large Animal Neurology: A Handbook for Veterinary Clinicians. Philadelphia, Lea & Febiger, 1989.

Mitchell, W. M.: Intermittent luxation of the patellae in a hunter. Vet. Rec., 61:352, 1949.

Power, H. T. Watrous, B. J., and de Lahunta, A.: Facial and vestibulocochlear nerve disease in six horses. J. Am. Vet. Med. Assoc., 183:1076, 1983.

Wheeler, S. J.: Effect of age on sensory nerve conduction velocity in the horse. Res. Vet. Sci., 48:141, 1990.

Wheeler, S. J., and Plummer, J. M.: Age-related changes in the fibre composition of equine peripheral nerve. J. Neurol. Sci., 90:53, 1989

Tail Alterations in Show Horses

Steven B. Colter, FORT COLLINS, COLORADO

Since the American Quarter Horse Association (AQHA) began enforcing rules barring tail alteration in the show ring, equine veterinarians have been asked to evaluate the tail function of show horses, frequently as part of the prepurchase examination. This has caused concern among veterinarians, because many have never seen a tail that has been altered and they are unaware of alteration techniques used. This chapter discusses normal tail function, techniques known to have been used to alter tail function, and clinical signs seen as a result of the alterations.

Tail alterations are not allowed in AQHA events and are grounds for severe disciplinary action. The horse's registration papers are stamped "ineligible for participation in AQHA approved events." The owner must then prove that the horse has returned to normal before it can be reinstated. All Quarter Horses born after 1 January 1990 must have normal tail function and appearance to participate in shows, regardless of the cause of abnormalities. These rules make it imperative that veterinarians examine tail function and appearance very carefully. If the veterinarian studies normal function and uses the following techniques, the examination can lead to an accurate assessment.

NORMAL TAIL FUNCTION

The normal tail function of a horse is taken for granted by most people working with horses (including veterinarians) but is actually much more complex and coordinated than usually assumed. The ability to swat flies in a lateral motion does not prove that the horse has normal tail function. A horse without alteration elevates its tail above the horizontal plane (and in most cases raises the tail in a rooster tail-like fashion) when the anus is gently massaged. All unaltered animals have supple, symmetrical, uninterrupted musculature over the length of the tail. The tails of unaltered animals can be moved in all directions with no asymmetrical limitation of movement and can readily be pressed ventrally to contact the anus. No surgical scars or other signs of physical alteration are present. When electromyograms (EMGs) are performed on unaltered horse's tails and both involuntary and voluntary activity is evaluated, the findings are consistent with normal motor unit function.

SURGICAL ALTERATION

The method of tail alteration that was most popular before enforcement began was a surgical procedure to alter the lifting function of the tail. The sacrocaudalis medialis and sacrocaudalis lateralis muscles were cut surgically by making a small incision on the ventrolateral aspect of the tail at the junction with the body. A teat bistoury was introduced through the incision and under the muscles in a craniomedial direction. The bistoury was then turned and the muscles severed. This was done bilaterally and symmetrically and resulted in inability of the horse to lift its tail, which achieved the desired effect of a tail that was not arched, not wringing, and more relaxed in appearance.

The surgical procedure described above causes a loss of lifting function that gradually returns as the muscles scar and heal. The surgical incisions leave very small visible scars but also leave a palpable depression or dimple in the muscles under the scars at the junction of the tail with the body. These are usually located at the 3 o'clock and 9 o'clock position when the tail is viewed from the rear of the horse. There are also bilateral depressions in the dorsal muscles from the junction of the tail with the body craniomedially to the midline where the muscles were severed. When the horse is stimulated to raise its tail by anal massage, the muscles tend to "bunch up" cranial to the grooves. Muscles cranial and caudal to the surgical lesion are normal in appearance. EMG findings are normal except for changes compatible with muscle fibrosis in the grooves described above.

CHEMICAL ALTERATION

When horses with surgically altered tails were barred from competition, chemical methods of alteration of tail function became popular. The method most commonly employed involved the use of 95 per cent ethanol to perform paravertebral nerve blocks. Alcohol has also been administered epidurally for the same purpose. These methods of alteration cause the dropped, relaxed tail look without surgical scarring and deformation.

Paralysis, paresis, and muscle atrophy are the major clinical signs of denervation. Chronic denervation may also lead to fibrosis of muscle fibers, which can restrict movement. Denervation also causes abnormal electrical activity of muscle that can be detected with EMG. Diseased or damaged muscle will also result in abnormal electrical activity on EMG.

All of the above clinical signs are seen in varying degrees in horses that have had chemical alterations of the tail. The animals cannot lift their tails to horizontal and the tail does not arch. In many cases the arc of the tail is concave, resembling a dog's tail. When some of these horses are stimulated to lift the tail, it consistently deviates to one side due to muscle asymmetry resulting from the alteration. Some animals have enough atrophy and fibrosis that the tail cannot be flexed ventrally to contact the anus. Other restrictions of movement may prevent the tail moving to one side or the other. The tail may be consistently deviated to one side due to the asymmetrical atrophy or secondary complications of the chemical alteration, such as abscessation.

ELECTROMYOGRAPHIC CHANGES WITH TAIL ALTERATIONS

The EMG signs are consistent with denervation and muscle damage. Abnormal spontaneous, induced, and voluntary activity can be found to varying degrees in affected animals, depending on the time elapsed since the alteration procedure and whether or not complications have occurred. Spontaneous activity (fibrillation potentials) occur in most affected horses for up to 8 months after the alteration. However, in one case, spontaneous activity in the muscles of the tail was present 32 months after an alcohol blocking. Abnormal induced activity, such as positive sharp waves, parallels the spontaneous activity, i.e., most animals examined 8 months or later after alteration have no detectable abnormal induced activity except for a decrease in insertional potentials. EMG abnormalities observed 8 months or more after alteration are generally limited to decreased insertional activity and decreased amplitude and density of the motor unit action potentials in the affected areas of the tail muscle. When the motor activity is monitored as the animals are stimulated to raise their tails, the interference pattern of motor unit action potentials in the affected areas of the tail is less dense and shows a decreased amplitude when compared with the interference pattern seen in normal muscle in the tail of the same animal (cranial and caudal to the affected area). These findings are consistent with chronic denervation or chronic fibrosis due to complications of the block such as muscle damage and abscessation.

EXAMINATION TECHNIQUE

The examination for the presence of tail alterations should be thorough and meticulous. The horse should be walked and the carriage of the tail observed for movement restriction, lack of lifting ability (especially when turning), obvious deformities, and the character of motion (Is there a reverse arc? Is the tail only moved side to side?). Walking the horse over an obstacle can be helpful, because most horses lift their tails when they step up or over obstacles; horses with alterations often cannot lift the tail. After observing the animal when walking, the examiner should visually inspect the tail for the presence of scars, grooves, dimples, muscle asymmetry, muscle atrophy, hair color change, and limitations of movement. The tail should then be palpated to detect dimples, scars, muscle tone and mass, muscle atrophy, limitations in movement, grooves in the dorsal muscles, and evidence of osseous abnormalities. The horse should be stimulated to raise the tail by gently massaging the anus. The first 6 to 10 inches of the tail should rise straight and above the horizontal. The arc of the tail should form an arch, much like a rooster tail. If the tail does not rise past the horizontal or consistently deviates to one side, one should consider the tail function abnormal, especially if other abnormalities are found. "Bunching" of the dorsal muscles should be watched for during lifting, as it is common in surgically altered animals.

EMG examination is important and is used in the official inspection at AQHA shows. Standard methods and principles are used. The tail is cleaned and scrubbed with a suitable preparation and the underside of the tail is also cleaned with alcohol. A bipolar surface electrode (Teca Rigid Plastic Mount No. 6030-1) is placed on the ventral side of the tail and held in place with a Velcro strap that goes around the tail. The active electrode is a 37-mm teflon-coated monopolar needle (Teca MG37). The dorsal muscles of the tail are explored at sites 4 inches above the beginning of the long tail hairs, below the beginning of the long tail hairs, and in an area from the beginning of the long tail hairs craniad for about 3 inches. The areas cranial and most caudal are the areas that are usually normal in chemically altered tails. If grooves that are typical of surgical alteration are present, they should also be explored. All areas explored are checked for insertional activity, spontaneous activity, abnormal induced activity (positive sharp waves, bizarre high frequency waves), and abnormal voluntary activity (decrease in density and amplitude of motor units in the interference pattern). The areas above and below the alteration site serve as normal comparisons for that animal. All areas are checked for voluntary activity by stimulating the tail lifting by anal massage during EMG examination. This protocol has been very effective in detecting tail alterations in horses with known histories of previous tail alteration and is the protocal used in AQHA-sanctioned horse shows.

Supplemental Readings

Colter, S. B.: Electromyographic detection and evaluation of tail alterations in show ring horses. *In:* Proceedings of the 6th Annual Veterinarian Medical Forum, ACVIM, 1988, pp. 421–423.

Goodgold, J., and Eberstein, A.: Electrodiagnosis of Neuromuscular Disease. Baltimore, Williams & Wilkins Co., 1972.

Section 13

OCULAR DISEASES

Edited by Mary B. Glaze

Ocular Discharge

Cecil P. Moore, COLUMBIA, MISSOURI

Ocular discharge is a primary sign of eye disease and is often the owner's main complaint. Ocular discharges may be serous (watery), catarrhal (mucoid), mucopurulent, or hemorrhagic. Serous discharge usually indicates milder forms of eye disease while mucopurulent or hemorrhagic discharges indicate more serious ocular disorders. In general, greater amounts of discharge occur with more serious disease. The volume and type of discharge noted initially with an ocular problem will frequently change as the disease progresses or as the clinical course changes.

Epiphora, spillage of tears (serous discharge) from the medial canthus, may result in facial wetting. Epiphora may occur from excessive secretion of tears or from obstruction of the nasolacrimal excretory ducts with subsequent overflow of tears. Mucoid ocular discharge may be observed concurrently with epiphora in mild or acute ocular surface infections. Mucopurulent exudate is typical of bacterial and fungal infections. Mucopurulent discharge in the absence of ocular inflammation suggests infection of the nasolacrimal ducts or nasolacrimal sac (dacryocystitis) with reflux of exudate from the lacrimal puncta. Hemorrhagic discharge usually indicates acute ocular trauma, although conjunctival ulceration from infection or neoplasia may also result in bleeding. Possible causes of various types of ocular discharge are summarized in Table 1.

EXAMINATION PROCEDURES

Available instruments should include a focused light source such as a 3.5-V halogen light with transilluminator, magnifying loupes, and thumb forceps with shallow serrations. Necessary diagnostic supplies are sterile fluorescein dye strips, tear test strips, culture swabs, physiologic saline solution, and topical anesthetic (0.5 per cent proparacaine). For nasolacrimal irrigation, polyethylene tubing (No. 5 French) should also be available.

Initial examination includes a general inspection and neuroophthalmological assessment. Since neurological deficits may influence tear production and distribution, an evaluation of the integrity of cranial nerves associated with ocular functions is important. This includes a rapid assessment of the animal's ability to perceive tactile stimuli to the periocular and ocular surfaces, blink effectively, and move the eyes normally. Signs of ocular pain, such as blepharospasm or photophobia, should be noted.

After the initial inspection, the examiner must determine if ocular cultures or tear measurements are needed, because these procedures should be completed prior to further manipulations and before instillation of topical pharmacological agents. Depending on the history, clinical signs, and the duration and severity of the ocular discharge, either viral, bacterial, or fungal

TABLE 1. CAUSES OF OCULAR DISCHARGE IN THE HORSE

Epiphora (serous discharge)
  Reflex tearing/irritation
    Eyelid diseases
      Cilia disorders: distichia, ectopic cilia, trichiasis
      Conformational abnormalities: entropion, ectropion
    Mild or acute conjunctivitis
      Allergic conjunctivitis
      Early phase of primary or secondary conjunctivitis (many possible causes; see under Mucopurulent Discharge—Severe or chronic conjunctivitis, below)
    Foreign material/aerosol irritation
    Acute ulcerative keratitis
    Uveitis
    Dermoid
  Insufficiency of nasolacrimal drainage
    Congenital: absence of nasolacrimal duct, lack of nasal opening, multiple openings, punctal atresia
    Acquired: dacryocystitis, nasolacrimal foreign body, scarring of puncta, maxillary fracture, nasal tumor, sinusitis

Mucopurulent discharge
  Severe or chronic conjunctivitis
    Infectious
      Viral: viral arteritis, adenovirus, equine herpesvirus, influenza
      Bacterial: *Streptoccus, Moraxella, Rhodococcus, Pseudomonas, Leptospira,* coliforms
      Mycotic: candidiasis, cryptococcosis, histoplasmosis, sporotrichosis
    Parasites: *Habronema, Thelazia, Onchocerca*
  Dacryocystitis
  Complicated ulcerative keratitis
    Infectious
    Collagenase
  Keratoconjunctivitis sicca
    Periocular trauma
    Facial nerve palsy
    Idiopathic
  Orbital disease/exophthalmos
    Trauma
    Cellulitis
    Tumor
  Foreign bodies in the conjunctiva or orbit
  Surface masses such as tumors and granulomas

Hemorrhagic discharge
  Acute trauma
    Blunt or penetrating trauma, conjunctival or eyelid laceration, ruptured globe
    Severe ulcerative conjunctivitis, chemical irritation
  Neoplasia: ulcerated or necrotic lesion, such as squamous cell carcinoma
  Infectious keratitis with uveal prolapse

---

cultures may be indicated. A sample is taken for culture by applying to the conjunctiva or cornea a sterile swab moistened with saline, enrichment broth, or the appropriate transport media.

Examination of the nasolacrimal system includes evaluation of both secretory and excretory components. In cases of ocular dishcarge, it is critical to differentiate conditions that increase secretion, such as corneal ulceration or anterior uveitis, from those that preclude normal tear drainage, such as congenital or acquired obstructions. Schirmer tear test strips may be used to quantify the volume of aqueous tear secretion. In horses, it is sufficient to measure the amount of wetting in 30 seconds (normal is greater than 20 mm). To examine the excretory component of the nasolacrimal system, the upper and lower puncta and nasal openings are identified and examined for patency and the presence of exudates.

In suspected cases of nasolacrimal obstruction, the application of fluorescein stain to the ocular surface will aid in assessing nasolacrimal patency. Passage of dye from the nasal opening of the nasolacrimal duct within 5 minutes confirms patency. Retrograde irrigation of the nasolacrimal duct, which entails inserting a flexible tubing (No. 5 French) and flushing with physiologic saline solution, may be necessary to differentiate excretory insufficiency from excessive secretions.

Detailed evaluation of extraocular structures includes evaluation of the conjunctiva for chemosis, hyperemia, focal swellings, follicles, adhesions, and masses. Following topical anesthesia and manipulation with blunt-tipped, slightly serrated thumb forceps, both surfaces of the third eyelid should be thoroughly examined for follicles, masses, or foreign material. Cytological evaluation of ocular surface scrapings or aspirates of masses may provide a definitive diagnosis for inflammatory and neoplastic ocular diseases. The cornea is inspected for irregularities, opacities, vascularization, and pigmentation. Fluorescein dye instillation will determine if corneal ulceration is present. Intraocular structures should also be examined to rule out uveitis as a cause of ocular discharge.

COMMON CAUSES AND THERAPY

Ocular Discharge in Foals

Epiphora in foals is usually caused by entropion or congenital abnormalities of the nasolacrimal ducts. When eyelids turn inward against the eye, lashes or cutaneous hairs come in contact with the ocular surface and may cause extreme irritation, including conjunctivitis, keratitis, pain (squinting), and reflex lacrimation. Developmental defects or malformations of the nasolacrimal duct, such as agenesis or atresia of the duct system, often account for ineffectual outflow of tears in young horses.

Entropion

Premature or dehydrated foals are often enophthalmic and, therefore, predisposed to entropion. Painful primary ocular diseases may cause severe blepharospasm, which initiates a cycle of pain and spastic entropion. Conformational entropion, although less common than other types, has been observed in closely line-bred foals, suggesting a hereditary cause.

Mild cases of entropion may be treated several times daily with topical lubricant ointments to relieve irritation of the corneal surface. Lubricants may constitute the sole treatment in some cases, although it is frequently necessary to temporarily evert the eyelid margins with cutaneous sutures. This procedure is referred to as eyelid tacking. Following local or general anesthesia, nonabsorbable 3-0 suture is placed perpendicular to the lid margin and tacked to the periocular skin over the rim of the orbit in a vertical mattress pattern. Several sutures may be needed to correct the inversion. After eyelid tacking, a topical antibiotic lubricant ointment is applied to the eye(s) three to four times daily. Everting sutures are left in place for 2 to 3 weeks and should prevent further blepharospasm and allow healing of the ocular surface during this period.

Severe or chronic entropion may require surgical correction. The most common blepharoplastic procedure involves an elliptical skin excision (Hotz–Celsus procedure). An arrowhead modification of this procedure may be necessary in some cases.

Dysgenesis of the Nasolacrimal Duct

Maldevelopment of the nasolacrimal duct system usually involves defects in the distal portion of the duct where it normally exits into the ventral floor of the nostril. In affected foals, epiphora is usually noticed during the first few months of life. Epiphora may be misinterpreted as reflex tearing. An important clinical feature of nasolacrimal malformation is that the eye is normal on the affected side. However, in some cases of congenital obstruction secondary infection occurs and reflux of exudate may result in concurrent blepharoconjunctivitis.

The nature of the ocular discharge in the setting of nasolacrimal obstruction reflects the presence or absence of infection within the duct system. Whether congenital or acquired, simple nonseptic obstructions are characterized by epiphora (serous fluid). Occlusions with concurrent sepsis result in mucopurulent reflux from the eye or drainage from the nostril on the affected side (or both). Treatment of nasolacrimal disease is described below.

OCULAR DISCHARGE IN ADULT HORSES

In adult horses, serous ocular discharge is usually a direct result of reflex lacrimation. Reflex lacrimation and the associated overabundance of tears may occur as a pain response from surface irritants such as a conjunctival foreign body, from ocular surface or intraocular inflammation, or from acute trauma. Epiphora is generally the earliest sign of conjunctivitis, ulcerative keratitis, or anterior uveitis. When epiphora is noted in such cases, careful visual and manipulative examination for foreign bodies under the third eyelid and between the bulbar and palpebral conjunctivae is imperative. Conjunctivitis and nasolacrimal insufficiency are considered in more detail below. Table 1 lists other possible causes of the various types of ocular discharge observed in the horse.

Conjunctivitis

Bacterial conjunctivitis in the horse is usually secondary to frictional or environmental irritants, trauma, or systemic infectious disease, and manifests as hyperemia with mucopurulent exudate. Plant foreign bodies and surfaces masses, such as squamous cell tumors, will also commonly be accompanied by associated bacterial infections. A variety of aerobic opportunists and pathogens (e.g., *Staphylococcus* spp., *Streptococcus* spp., *Pseudomonas* spp., coliform organisms) may cause secondary conjunctival infections. Although less common than secondary infections, *Moraxella* spp. may cause a primary conjunctivitis accompanied by excoriation of the eyelid margins and canthal region.

Treatment of bacterial conjunctivitis consists of removing or treating the primary cause, such as foreign body, dermoid, or neoplastic mass, and applying topical antibiotic ointment to the affected eye(s) three times daily for 7 to 10 days. Either gentamicin or a triple antibiotic combination is generally quite effective in treating bacterial infections. In nonresponsive cases or if the conjunctivitis is associated with ulcerative keratitis, scrapings should be obtained for culture and sensitivity testing. Topical corticosteroids may be useful if the conjunctivitis is characterized by severe inflammation. However, corticosteroids, are most prudently used when the primary cause has been identified and eradicated. Since ulcerative keratitis is a contraindication to topical corticosteroid use, the owner must be alerted to discontinue the topical corticosteroid immediately if the clinical signs worsen or if suspicion arises that a corneal ulcer may have developed subsequent to topical corticosteroid administration.

Other infectious causes of conjunctivitis include respiratory viruses, such as rhinopneumonitis, influenza, adenovirus, and viral arteritis. The eyes should be examined carefully to rule out other possible concurrent ocular disease. Treatment consists primarily of supportive therapy for the systemic illness. Although the conjunctivitis is usually self-limiting, topical broad-spectrum antibiotic ointment may be applied three times daily to control secondary bacterial conjunctivitis.

Parasitic causes of conjunctivitis in the horse include habronemiasis, which is the most common and the most clinically significant. *Thelazia* and *Onchocerca* may also cause conjunctivitis; however, these parasites have low pathogenicity and the inflammatory response is usually subclinical. *Habronema* conjunctivitis is characterized by focal raised, rough conjunctival granulomas with intralesional inspissated or mineralized exudates. *Habronema* lesions may occur on the anterior aspect of the third eyelid or on the bulbar or palpebral conjunctiva. Clinical signs are variable depending on the location and size of granulomas and whether mineralized exudates are present.

The diagnosis of habronemiasis is based on seasonal occurrence (summer and early fall), the clinical appearance of the lesions, and cytological or histological findings of eosinophilic granuloma. Treatment usually consists of a combination of a systemic larvicide (ivermectin), surgical debulking of lesions, and local anti-inflammatory therapy consisting of topical and intralesional corticosterids.

Nasolacrimal Insufficiency

Acquired nasolacrimal obstructions may result from infections or foreign bodies within the duct system, facial trauma, nasal tumors, sinusitis, or rhinitis, which may occlude some portion of the duct system. Previously undiagnosed congenital defects may also cause persistent ocular discharge in adult animals. Diagnosis of the specific cause of nasolacrimal obstruction usually depends on a combination of close inspection of openings, irrigation, percussion of sinuses, dental examination, radiography, and biopsy. When attempts to irrigate the nasolacrimal duct are unsuccessful, cannulation and insertion of a retention catheter is attempted. If this is unsuccessful, contrast radiography is useful in identifying the site of occlusion or rupture.

Treatment of nasolacrimal obstruction entails removing the initiating cause, if feasible, establishing patency of the duct system, placing a retention catheter into the duct, and treating with topical or systemic antimicrobial and anti-inflammatory medications. A canine male urinary catheter (No. 5 French) or polyethylene tubing (size 160) is inserted in the duct either from the dorsal

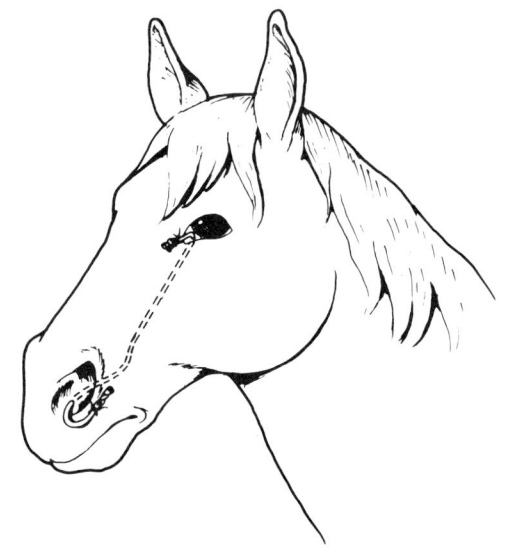

Figure 1. Placement of nasolacrimal catheter. After the tubing is inserted into the nasolacrimal duct, each end of the tubing is secured to the adjacent skin with 3-0 nonabsorbable suture.

eyelid punctum or from the nasal punctum. After successful catheterization, the ends are sutured to the skin near the medial canthus and muzzle, respectively (Fig. 1), and the tubing is left in place for 2 to 3 weeks. Topical antibiotic–corticosteroid solution is placed in the eye three to four times daily until the tubing is removed. In cases of suppurative dacryocystitis, systemic antibiotics (selection based on culture and sensitivity results) are administered for 7 days.

Since anomalies of the nasolacrimal duct in foals most frequently involve an imperforate nasal punctum, the skin over the imperforate area is simply incised and a retention catheter inserted. Acquired obstructions may be considerably more challenging to treat. Of acquired causes, infectious or foreign body dacryocystitis (in the absence of osteomyelitis) and periodontitis are among the more readily treated. Traumatic maxillary fracture involving the duct may preclude catheterization of the duct and correction of the nasolacrimal insufficiency. When potentially life-threatening diseases such as osteomyelitis or neoplasia are diagnosed, nasolacrimal insufficiency becomes a secondary concern and treatment of the nasolacrimal obstruction is postponed, if possible, until the outcome of the primary disease is determined.

Supplemental Readings

Latimer, C. A., and Wyman, M.: Atresia of the nasolacrimal duct in 3 horses. J. Am. Vet. Med. Assoc., *184*:989–992, 1984.

Latimer, C. A., Wyman, M., Diesem, C. D., and Burt, J. K.: Radiographic and gross anatomy of the nasolacrimal duct of the horse. Am. J. Vet. Res., 45:451–458, 1984.

Lavach, D.: Large Animal Ophthalmology. Vol. I. St. Louis, C. V. Mosby, 1990.

Senk, G. W.: Ocular discharge in young horses. In Robinson, N. E. (ed.): Current Therapy in Equine Medicine. Philadelphia, W. B. Saunders, 1983, pp. 305–388.

Slatter, D. H.: Fundamentals of Veterinary Ophthalmology, 2nd ed. Philadelphia, W. B. Saunders, 1990.

Ocular Injuries
David A. Wilkie, COLUMBUS, OHIO

The equine eye is often subject to severe traumatic injury, perhaps the result of its prominent position in the head. Traumatic injuries are divided according to the tissues involved and the severity of the injury. Contusions damage underlying tissues, but the overlying tissue is intact; penetrating injuries abrade or partially cut the tissue; and perforating injuries cut tissues completely. Regardless of the nature of the injury, a few basic rules are applicable to the examination and treatment of all horses that have sustained ocular trauma (Tables 1 and 2).

ORBIT

The horse has a complete bony orbital rim comprised of the frontal, lacrimal, zygomatic, and temporal bones. The caudolateral and ventral walls of the equine orbit are fascia. The zygomatic arch and the supraorbital process of the frontal bone and the medial orbital wall are most susceptible to injury. Damage to these areas can involve the supraorbital foramen and its associated nerve or the osseous portion of the nasolacrimal system, respectively.

The diagnosis of an orbital fracture is based on history, clinical signs (Table 3), and radiographs. Radiographic evaluation of the equine orbit is technically difficult and often unrewarding. Oblique views, highlighting the area of greatest concern, are usually required. Care must be taken to evaluate the frontal, maxillary and sphenopalatine paranasal sinuses, especially when subcutaneous emphysema is present.

Traumatic fractures of the orbit are often associated with concomitant injury of the globe and adnexa. Complete ophthalmic examination is essential. This includes assessment of vision (menace response, maze testing), pupillary light reflex, fluorescein staining for the presence of a corneal ulcer, examination of the anterior chamber for hyphema or anterior uveitis, fundic examination evaluating the retina and optic nerve, assessment of globe and eyelid mobility, and nasolacrimal irrigation. If ocular damage precludes examination of the posterior segment, ocular ultrasonography is advised.

Blunt trauma to the orbit can result in breakdown of the fibrous orbital septum and subsequent herniation of orbital fat. Clinically this is a nonpainful swelling that appears at the time of or following orbital trauma. It is best treated by surgical removal or replacement of the herniated portion of the orbital fat pad and attempted surgical repair of the rent in the septum.

Traumatic proptosis is rare in the horse because of the complete bony orbital rim. Proptosis of the globe indicates severe head trauma, and thorough physical and neurological examinations are necessary. If the optic nerve and extraocular muscles are intact, a proptosed globe should be replaced under general anesthesia. Once the globe is replaced, a temporary tarsorrhaphy is performed to protect the eye until the swelling subsides. Systemic antibiotics and anti-inflammatory drugs are indicated to control postoperative complications.

Treatment of orbital trauma in the acute phase includes systemic anti-inflammatory therapy, systemic antibiotics, especially if a paranasal sinus is involved, and cold compresses. The anti-inflammatory drug of choice is systemic flunixin meglumine° (1.0 mg per kg in divided doses twice a day). Local therapy is required for the management of corneal exposure, ulceration, and anterior uveitis. If eyelid movement is impaired, either as the result of neurological dysfunction or as the result of eyelid swelling, the cornea must be protected from exposure and dessication with a topical, sterile ophthalmic lubricant applied as frequently as possible, or in the more severe cases with a temporary tarsorrhaphy. Topical broad-spectrum antibiotics are indicated in horses with corneal ulceration, and

---

°Banamine, Schering Corp., Kenilworth, NJ

TABLE 1. INITIAL EXAMINATION PROCEDURES FOR A TRAUMATIC OCULAR EMERGENCY

1. Review history for duration of condition, cause, and medication administered.
2. Perform complete physical examination to assess associated injuries.
3. Assess vision using the response to menace test and maze testing.
4. Perform sedation and eyelid nerve blocks as required for examination.
5. Palpate the orbital rim for crepitus, fractures, and emphysema.
6. Examine eyelids for contusions and laceration. Evert eyelids and membrana nictitans to examine for foreign bodies.
7. Gently retract eyelids and examine the cornea and globe. Apply fluorescein stain to all corneas suspected of sustaining trauma. If lacerations are present, note their depth and extent.
8. Note the pupil size and compare it with the opposite pupil. Assess the pupillary light reflex.
9. Inspect for hyphema.
10. Evaluate for the presence of lens luxation.
11. Perform a fundic examination. Examine the optic disc for size, color, and shape. Look for retinal hemorrhage or detachment.
12. Irrigate the nasolacrimal system if there is soft tissue or bony involvement of the medial canthus.
13. Avoid doing harm. Refer the horse to a specialist if you do not feel confident repairing the injury.

TABLE 2. MEASURES TO AVOID WHEN TREATING OCULAR INJURIES

1. Avoid dispensing topical anesthetics for superficial pain. These delay healing and their effect decreases with each administration. Their use is appropriate to aid in the examination of a painful eye.
2. Avoid topical corticosteroids if the diagnosis is uncertain, if the corneal epithelium is damaged, or if corneal infection is present.
3. Avoid topical ointments if penetrating trauma is present. The ointment may enter the anterior chamber, where it will incite inflammation.

TABLE 3. CLINICAL SIGNS OF ORBITAL FRACTURES

Swelling
Pain
Crepitus
Epistaxis
Asymmetry
Subcutaneous emphysema
Exophthalmos
Globe entrapment

---

atropine is used to relieve the discomfort associated with anterior uveitis (Table 4).

Although facial and orbital fractures in horses will often heal without surgery, they may do so in a manner that results in deformity and interferes with the normal function of the eye and adnexa. Therefore, surgical correction may be indicated, especially for displaced fractures. Fractures that extend into a paranasal sinus must be considered as open fractures as these sinuses contain resident bacterial and fungal flora. Early repair is associated with a more favorable cosmetic result as skull fractures consolidate rapidly and the resulting fibrous callus may interfere with surgical reduction. Generous skin flaps in the surgical approach are advised as fractures are often more extensive than initially thought. Excessive periosteal dissection should be avoided.

EYELIDS

Eyelid trauma includes both contusions and lacerations. Commonly associated with eyelid trauma are corneal abrasions and anterior uve-

TABLE 4. COMMONLY USED OPHTHALMIC MEDICATIONS

Category/Drug	Indication	Dosing Interval
Topical		
Antibiotics		
Gentamicin	Corneal ulceration	q. 2–6 h.
Neomycin/bacitracin/polymixin B	Corneal ulceration	q. 2–6 h.
Antifungals		
Natamycin°	Corneal ulceration with suspected fungal keratitis	q. 2–4 h.
Miconazole IV 1%	Corenal ulceration with suspected fungal keratitis	q. 2–4 h.
Parasympatholytics		
Tropicamide 1%	Diagnostic agent to dilate the pupil	Single dose
Atropine 1%	Therapeutic agent to dilate the pupil long term	1–4 times a day
Systemic		
Anti-inflammatory		
Flunixin meglumine	Extraocular or intraocular inflammation	0.5 mg/kg b.i.d. PO, IM, IV
Phenylbutazone	Extraocular or intraocular inflammation	2-4 mg/kg b.i.d. PO

°Natacyn, 5% natamycin, Alcon Labs, Forth Worth, TX

itis. Eyelid contusions often result in blepharedema and hemorrhage. Although this does not require therapy, recovery can be hastened by using systemic flunixin meglumine, cold compresses in the acute phase, and warm compresses beginning the day after the injury.

Eyelid lacerations are more serious and usually require immediate therapy. The vascular supply to the eyelid is extensive, and many apparently avascular segments of eyelid will recover following repair (Fig. 1). If possible, primary wound closure is preferred (Table 5). The eyelid surface and adjacent tissues are disinfected with a 1:50 dilution of povidone–iodine solution. Tissue debridement should be minimized, and under no circumstances should a pedicle of eyelid be amputated. If the laceration is near the medial canthus, the nasolacrimal system must be evaluated and repaired if damaged.

Lacerated eyelids are sutured in a two-layer closure, ensuring accurate anatomical apposition of the wound edges and eyelid margin. Minor repairs can be performed with sedation and local nerve blocks, but serious injuries may require general anesthesia. The deeper, conjunctival layer is sutured first with 4-0 to 6-0 absorbable polyglactin 910 suture° placed in a horizontal mattress pattern beginning away from and working toward the eyelid margin. Care is taken to avoid penetrating the conjunctiva so that the suture does not contact the cornea. The skin is closed with 4-0 to 6-0 nonabsorbable suture. The eyelid margin is the most important portion of the wound repair and is closed first. I prefer to use a cruciate suture pattern at the eyelid margin and a simple interrupted pattern for the remainder of the skin closure. Medical therapy includes systemic antibiotics for 5 to 7 days, tetanus toxoid, and flunixin meglumine if inflammation and swelling are a problem. Topical medication is not required for eyelid injuries unless there is associated corneal or anterior segment damage. If the blink response is impaired, the cornea should be protected with topical lubricants applied as often as possible.

GLOBE

Regardless of the type of injury to the globe, an attempt should be made to ascertain and eliminate the etiology.

ANTERIOR UVEITIS

The problem most frequently seen in association with trauma to the globe is anterior uveitis. This inflammatory response of the iris and ciliary body may be a direct result of the trauma, a consequence of intraocular penetration, or the result of an axonal reflex seen in eyes with corneal ulceration. The management of anterior uveitis is reviewed elsewhere in this volume (see p. 592).

CORNEA

Treatment of a traumatic corneal ulcer is not different from treatment for other forms of corneal ulceration (see p. 596).

Corneal edema, if not associated with a corneal ulcer, is the result of corneal endothelial damage. Blunt injuries can result in displacement of the corneal endothelium from the posterior surface of the cornea. This results in full-thickness, diffuse corneal edema, which may gravitate to the ventral cornea with time. Although there is no specific treatment, topical hyperosmotic agents such as 5 per cent NaCl ointment† applied topically every 4 to 6 hours may

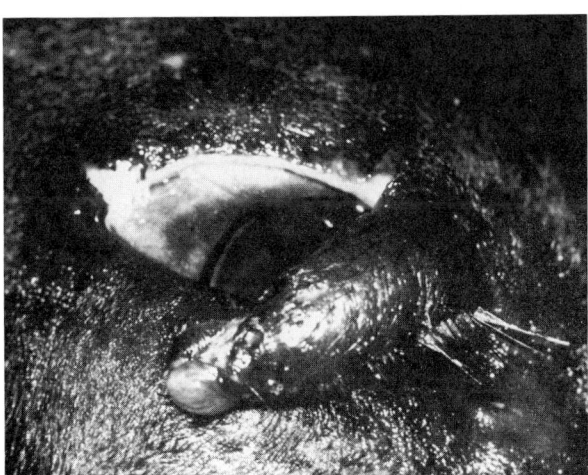

Figure 1. Traumatic laceration of the superior eyelid resulting in a pedicle of eyelid attached only at the medial canthus. (Courtesy of Dr. Milton Wyman.)

TABLE 5. TENETS OF EYELID REPAIR

1. Treat promptly.
2. Irrigate copiously to remove debris.
3. Debride a minimum of tissue.
4. Never amputate a pedicle of eyelid.
5. Close in two layers, beginning with the deeper layer.
6. Choose the smallest suture possible.
7. Restore the eyelid margin anatomically and functionally.
8. Prevent self-trauma following surgery.
9. Control swelling with compresses and anti-inflammatory drugs.
10. Administer systemic antibiotics to prevent infection.

°Vicryl, polyglactin 910, Ethicon Inc., Somerville, NJ
†Muro-128, 5% NaCl, Bausch & Lomb, Rochester, NY

decrease the severity of the edema. In my opinion, this has only minimal efficacy. The compromised, edematous cornea is at risk of ulceration and topical corticosteroids should be avoided. With time the corneal endothelium may reattach or adjacent endothelial cells may hypertrophy, resulting in a decrease in the corneal edema.

RUPTURE OF THE FIBROUS TUNIC
(Cornea and Sclera)

Blunt trauma, whether contusive, penetrating, or perforating, generally results in more severe ocular damage than injury from a sharp object. Once the extent of the damage has been ascertained, treatment is directed toward repairing the rent, reestablishing the anterior chamber, preventing infection, and decreasing inflammation and pain. Removal of a penetrating object is best done at the time of repair. If the horse is referred for consultation and treatment, self-trauma during transport can be prevented using sedation or protective devices such as cradles.

Tetanus toxoid is administered prior to repair. The aqueous humor and any retained foreign object should be cultured for aerobic bacteria and fungi. If the iris is protruding but appears viable and minimally contaminated, it is replaced. Otherwise, the unhealthy portion of the iris is amputated. A ruptured lens should be removed; lens protein is antigenic and may stimulate severe anterior uveitis. The cornea is repaired with partial-thickness, simple interrupted 6-0 to 7-0 absorbable sutures. The anterior chamber is reformed with a balanced salt solution or lactated Ringer's solution. Conjunctival grafts can be used to promote rapid corneal vascularization. Following surgery, topical broad-spectrum antibiotics are administered every 2 to 4 hours, topical atropine is applied as needed, and systemic antibiotics and flunixin meglumine are also administered. If topical treatment is difficult, a subpalpebral lavage delivery system should be placed to ensure delivery of medication (see *Current Therapy in Equine Medicine 2*, pp. 436–439). The prognosis is guarded.

In contrast to sharp perforating injuries, blunt trauma results in a rapid increase in intraocular pressure, an explosive rupture from the inside outward, and expulsion of the intraocular contents (Fig. 2). The rent in the fibrous tunic is often large and irregular, and portions of the cornea or sclera may be lost. The typical wound originates at the limbus and extends forward into the cornea and posteriorly into the sclera. If the posterior portion of the eye ruptures, the horse presents with hyphema and decreased intraocular pressure, and ocular ultrasonography may be necessary for accurate diagnosis.

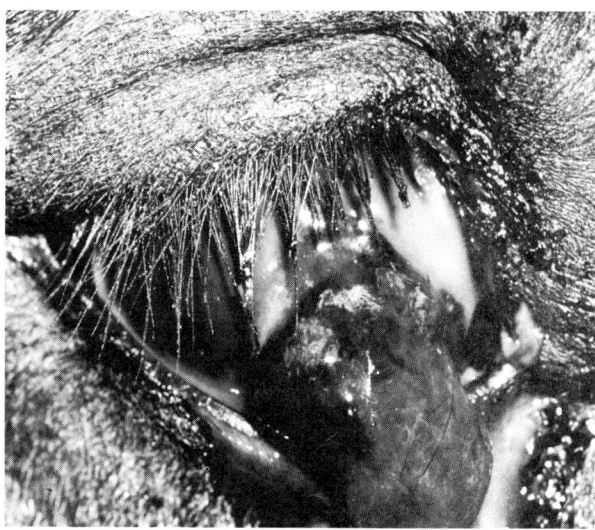

Figure 2. Blunt trauma to the globe has resulted in explosive perforation with expulsion of the internal contents of the eye. The anterior uvea (black) and associated hemorrhage are seen protruding through the rent in the cornea. Ocular ultrasonography revealed no lens within the globe.

Repair of these explosive ruptures is difficult and the treatment of choice may be enucleation. If cosmetic repair is important, an intraocular silicone prosthesis can be used in some patients if there is sufficient tissue left to close the fibrous tunic. This procedure should be performed as soon as possible after injury. If the injury is chronic and atrophy of the globe has occurred, placement of an intraocular prosthesis is not possible. The only cosmetic alternative in these horses is an orbital prosthesis, which is expensive, time-consuming, and requires frequent maintenance on the part of the owner.

HYPHEMA

Not all hyphema is the result of ocular trauma. Consideration must be given to systemic diseases that result in clotting disorders or intraocular inflammation.

If the hyphema is complete and precludes the evaluation of intraocular structures, ocular ultrasonography is indicated to assess the lens position, retina, and posterior eyewall. The greatest resolution in ocular ultrasonography is achieved with a 7.5-MHz or, preferably, a 10-MHz probe. The probe can be placed directly on the cornea, or imaging can be performed through the eyelid or an offset device. Provided no other intraocular damage is seen, hyphema will resolve often without significant sequelae. Potential sequelae of severe trauma include cataract, posterior synechia, glaucoma, and blindness (Fig. 3).

When hyphema results from a traumatic event, concurrent anterior uveitis is usually pres-

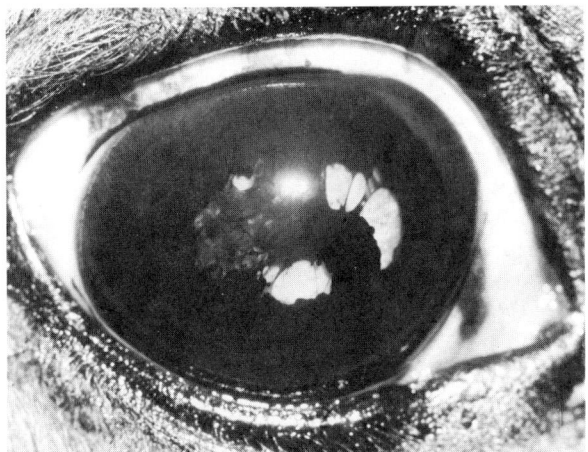

Figure 3. As sequelae to ocular trauma and the resultant anterior uveitis, a complete mature cataract and posterior synechiae are present. No menace response was present in this eye.

ent. Although hyphema does not usually require therapy, the associated anterior uveitis is treated with topical atropine and systemic flunixin meglumine. If there is no corneal ulcer associated with the hyphema, topical corticosteroids may also be administered. Resolution of hyphema may require 7 to 21 days and the horse should not be exercised during this time to decrease the incidence of rebleeding. Surgical intervention to remove the hyphema is rarely, if ever, indicated.

OPTIC NERVE

Trauma to the head of the horse has been associated with acute unilateral or bilateral blindness. The pupil in the affected eye will be dilated, but the remainder of the ophthalmic examination may be normal initially. Occasionally, retinal hemorrhage and papilledema are present. Fundic examination several weeks later reveals optic nerve pallor, indicating atrophy (Fig 4). The cause of this lesion is hypothesized to be stretching of the optic nerve or trauma from bony fractures adjacent to the optic nerve. A small number of affected horses may benefit from systemic anti-inflammatory therapy in the acute phase. However, the prognosis is guarded and treatment is usually unrewarding.

CONCLUSION

If a horse has sustained traumatic injury, the practitioner must examine the entire eye, associated structures, and perform a complete physical examination. Adequate restraint and sedation must be used to avoid further trauma to the eye. Rapid assessment and repair of the damage

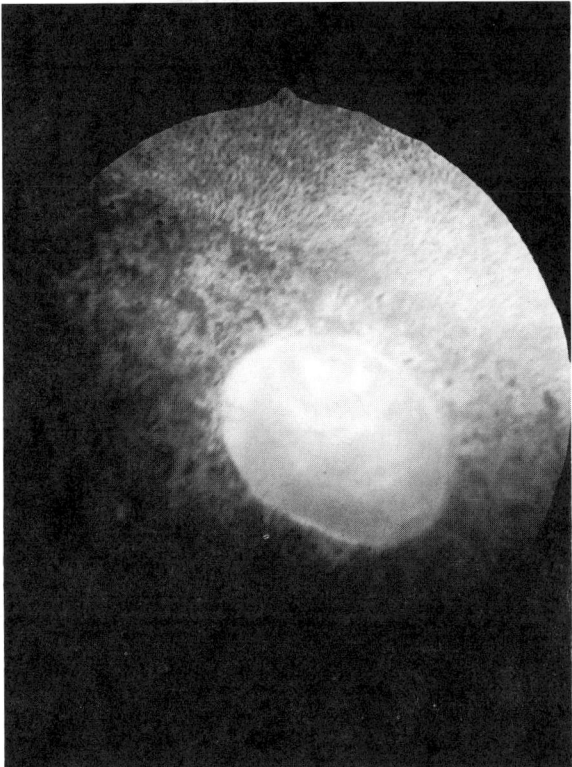

Figure 4. One month following head trauma and acute blindness in this eye, the optic nerve appears pale, with atrophy of the retinal blood vessels and foci of peripapillary depigmentation. (Courtesy of Dr. E. Dan Wolf.)

will yield the best cosmetic and functional results. Instrumentation and sutures appropriate to the eye should be used. Topical and systemic medications are selected to treat inflammation and pain and prevent infection. The owners or caretakers must be able to apply the topical medications prescribed. A subpalpebral lavage system may be used if the owners are unable to treat the eye topically. The eye must be evaluated frequently following injury. The practitioner should treat only those problems that he or she is capable of repairing and should refer more severe injuries.

Supplemental Readings

Brooks, D. E., and Wolf, E. D.: Ocular trauma in the horse. Equine Vet. J. Suppl., 2:141, 1983.

Lavach, J. D.: Large Animal Ophthalmology. St. Louis, C. V. Mosby, 1990.

Munger, R. J.: Equine ophthalmic emergencies. Vet. Clin. North Amer: Large Anim. Pract. 6: 467–487, 1984.

Turner, L. M., Whitley, R. D., and Hager, D.: Management of ocular trauma in horses: Part 2. Orbit, eyelids, uvea, lens, retina, and optic nerve. Mod. Vet. Pract., 67:341, 1986.

Whitley, R. D., and Turner, L. M.: Management of ocular trauma in horses: Part 1. Cornea and sclera. Mod. Vet. Pract., 67:233, 1986.

Anterior Uveitis

Michael Davidson, RALEIGH, NORTH CAROLINA

Anterior uveitis and the chronic intraocular sequelae from recurrent uveitis are reportedly the leading causes of blindness in horses around the world. Equine uveitis occurs in acute and, more commonly, recurrent forms, each having a different prognosis and often necessitating different therapeutic strategies.

CLINICAL SIGNS

Acute uveitis is associated with blunt and penetrating ocular trauma, corneal and scleral ulceration, intraocular neoplasia, intraocular onchocerciasis, and any number of systemic infectious diseases capable of inciting septicemia, endotoxemia, exotoxemia, and immune complex formation. Clinical findings of acute anterior uveitis vary depending on severity and may include conjunctival and scleral vessel prominence, miosis, blepharospasm, corneal edema, and hypotony. Aqueous flare or turbidity is perhaps the most consistent and sensitive clinical sign of anterior uveitis. More severe disruption of the blood–aqueous barrier is characterized in order of severity by fibrinous exudate in the anterior chamber, hypopyon, or hyphema.

A series of complex and poorly defined immunologically mediated events occurs within the ocular tissues following acute anterior uveitis. The immunological response often leads to chronic, recurrent episodes of unilateral or bilateral intraocular inflammation. It is in the chronic stage that clinical evaluation is most commonly sought and medical treatment is first initiated. Clinical findings consistent with chronic uveitis include corneal fibrosis, posterior synechiae, altered pupillary shape, pigment deposition on the anterior lens capsule, varying degrees of cataract formation, lens luxation and phthisis bulbi. Secondary glaucoma with enlargement of the globe is a rare sequela. Retinal detachment and peripapillary retinal degeneration may also occur as a result of concurrent posterior uveitis.

Equine recurrent uveitis (ERU) is characterized by repeated episodes of intraocular inflammation, punctuated by variable periods of clinical quiescence. Inflammation often increases in severity with each recurrence. The resulting opacification of the ocular media, pupillary dysfunction, retinal degeneration, and phthisis bulbi account for the vision loss associated with recurrent uveitis in the horse.

While a number of etiological agents have been incriminated in the pathogenesis of ERU, only two agents, *Leptospira interrogans* and the microfilaria of *Onchocerca cervicalis*, have been clinically and experimentally confirmed to be associated with an undefined percentage of cases. Only rarely, however, is an etiological diagnosis apparent in horses with recurrent uveitis, even after exhaustive diagnostic evaluation. This likely reflects both the chronic stage at which medical care is sought for these animals and the fact that the initiating event or agent has been supplanted by immunologically mediated phenomena.

PROGNOSIS

Horses with acute anterior uveitis have a prognosis for vision commensurate with the causative factors and the severity of the uveitis. For example, uveitis associated with mild blunt trauma or superficial corneal ulceration often resolves without overt ocular changes following therapy. All animals with acute uveitis, however, should be considered at risk for developing chronic recurrent uveitis. Whereas horses with recurrent uveitis have a guarded to poor long-term prognosis for vision, those animals treated aggressively during the initial bouts of uveitis and those treated diligently during subsequent episodes appear to have a somewhat more favorable outcome.

THERAPY

Topically and systemically administered anti-inflammatory agents and topically administered mydriatics or cycloplegics are indicated for acute uveitis when the underlying etiology is being addressed concurrently. Chronic, recurrent idiopathic uveitis is treated similarly during the active stages of the disease when clinical signs are evident, and treatment should continue several weeks past cessation of active inflammation. The frequency of systemically administered anti-inflammatory therapy is dictated by the severity of the intraocular inflammation. Ointments are less difficult to administer and are generally preferred over topical solutions or suspensions if treatment by the owner is anticipated. However, solutions or suspensions can generally be administered without difficulty by placing several drops in a tuberculin syringe without a needle, opening the palpebral fissure, and applying the medication to the corneal surface. The owner's ability to medicate the animal should always be assured prior to discharging the patient, as the powerful eyelid muscles of the horse, particularly one with a painful eye, often make topical therapy difficult. Should the horse's temperament not allow topical administration, or if therapy is required more than three to four times daily, placement of a subpalpebral lavage catheter system is strongly recommended. Subconjunctival administration of anti-inflammatory agents, repeated as necessary, should be considered in cases where frequent topical administration is not possible (see *Current Therapy in Equine Medicine 2*, pp. 436–439).

TOPICAL ANTI-INFLAMMATORY THERAPY

Topically administered corticosteroids are the most critical therapeutic component in horses with uveitis in which corneal ulceration is not concurrently present. Therapeutic failure in horses with uveitis often follows use of a topical corticosteroid that is of insufficient potency (i.e., hydrocortisone or cortisone) or, more commonly, use of a preparation that does not penetrate the cornea adequately. High-quality, soluble topical corticosteroids that are of sufficient potency and concentration and achieve adequate intracameral levels include 1 per cent prednisolone acetate suspension,[*] 0.1 per cent dexamethasone phosphate[†] or sodium phosphate ointment,[‡] and 0.1 per cent dexamethasone suspension.[§] Although these specific topical preparations are often more expensive and may require dispensing through a pharmacist, use of many of the common veterinary ophthalmic preparations invites both ineffective response and prolonged administration. Application three to four times daily for mild uveitis and up to eight to ten times daily for severe or immediate vision-threatening uveitis is indicated. Subconjunctival triamcinolone[||] (40 mg per ml, 0.25 ml) is used when necessary and may be repeated every 2 to 4 days. Because topical corticosteroid use is contraindicated in the presence of corneal ulceration, careful examination and fluorescein dye evaluation should routinely be performed in horses prior to its administration.

Topical antibiotics or preparations containing both corticosteroids and antibiotics are not indicated for the treatment of equine uveitis. Unnecessary use of topical antibiotics may provide a milieu for fungal overgrowth and may shift the normal bacterial flora of the ocular surface from a gram-positive to a gram-negative population.

A recently introduced topical nonsteroidal agent, 0.1 per cent flurbiprofen,[¶] given three to six times daily, is a useful adjunctive therapy with topical corticosteroids for horses with severe or recalcitrant anterior uveitis. Topical steroidal and nonsteroidal anti-inflammatory compounds have a synergistic effect in suppressing intraocular inflammation. The latter are particularly useful in horses with corneal ulceration and uveitis, where topical corticosteroid use is of concern.

MYDRIATIC/CYCLOPLEGIC THERAPY

Topically administered 1 per cent atropine is also necessary in horses with anterior uveitis. Its mydriatic effect prevents posterior synechiae formation while its cycloplegic action blocks painful ciliary muscle spasm. The frequency of administration is dictated by the severity of the uveitis. Animals with mild uveitis require only once or twice daily therapy, but those with severe inflammation may require application at 2- to 3-hour intervals. Atropine is administered until the pupil dilates; dilation is then maintained by application from once every other day to twice daily. For patients failing to respond by mydriasis after 24 to 48 hours, a limited course (1 to 2 days) of 4 per cent atropine may be attempted. Ten per cent phenylephrine administered concurrently may also aid in pupillary dilation but has no effect on ciliary body spasm. Varying degrees of gastrointestinal (GI) stasis may occasionally be encountered with very frequent atropine administration or use of concentrated forms (4 per cent), and horses receiving this therapy should be monitored. However, overt colic requiring medical intervention appears to be extremely rare following even four to six times daily 1 per cent atropine administration. In almost all cases, the benefits and necessity of topical atropine administration in horses with uveitis greatly outweigh the risk of GI side effects. Horses with moderate to extreme mydriasis may experience discomfort in bright sunlight and should be stabled or kept in a shaded area.

SYSTEMIC ANTI-INFLAMMATORY THERAPY

For all but the mildest forms of equine anterior uveitis, a course of systemic anti-inflammatory

---

[*] Pred Forte, Allergan, Irving, CA
[†] Decadron, Merck, Sharpe & Dohme, West Point, PA
[‡] Maxidex ointment, Alcon, Fort Worth, TX
[§] Maxidex suspension, Alcon, Fort Worth, TX
[||] Kenalog-40, Squibb, Princeton, NJ

[¶] Ocufen, Allergan, Irving, CA

therapy is also indicated. Flunixin meglumine (1 mg per kg given intravenously or orally twice a day) and oral phenylbutazone (2 mg per kg twice a day) appear to be equally efficacious. The potential GI side effects limit the duration of use of both of these drugs to 5 to 7 days for flunixin meglumine and 10 to 14 days for phenylbutazone. For unrelenting anterior uveitis, a 5-day course of oral prednisolone (0.5 mg per kg twice a day) in lieu of nonsteroidal agents may be beneficial. Because of the potential for systemic side effects, systemic corticosteroids are generally reserved for patients with severe, recalcitrant anterior uveitis.

SYSTEMIC ANTIBIOTIC THERAPY

Systemically administered antibiotics are of no benefit in the management of recurrent uveitis in horses unless a concurrent systemic bacterial infection has been identified. Although several different serovars of *Leptospira interrogans* have been identified as important in the pathogenesis of an undefined per centage of cases of ERU, the resultant uveitis typically occurs months to years after the initial bacteremia, when antibiotic therapy would be of benefit.

OTHER THERAPY

Uveitis associated with *Onchocerca* is usually suggested by the presence of other ocular findings compatible with parasite migration: sclerosing or punctate keratitis, lymphoid follicles in the conjunctiva, or vitiligo of the temporal conjunctiva. Although elimination of the microfilariae is recommended, inflammation should first be controlled with topical and systemic corticosteroid therapy.

Chronically painful and irreversibly blind eyes that are unresponsive to medical therapy may be treated by placement of an intraocular silicone prosthesis or surgical removal of the globe.

Supplemental Readings

Cook, C. S., Peiffer, R. L., and Harling, D. E.: Equine recurrent uveitis. Equine Vet. J. Suppl., 2:57–60, 1983.
Lavach, J. D., Roberts, S. M., and Severin, G. A.: Current concepts in equine ocular therapeutics. Vet. Clin. North Am.: Large Anim. Pract. 6:435–449, 1984.
Lees, P., and Higgins, A. J.: Clinical pharmacology and therapeutic uses of non-steroidal anti-inflammatory drugs in the horse. Equine Vet. J., 17:83–96, 1985.
O'Connor, G. R.: Basic mechanisms responsible for the initiation and recurrence of uveitis. Am. J. Ophthalmol., 96:577–599, 1983.

Corneal Stromal Abscesses

Mary B. Glaze, BATON ROUGE, LOUISIANA

The corneal stromal abscess is an uncommon yet noteworthy ocular disease in the horse. The disorder is capable of producing severe keratitis and uveitis and is often misdiagnosed as one of these more familiar clinical entities. Its management is complicated by an insular location within the avascular stroma, which serves as a barrier to pharmacological agents and endogenous immunological defenses.

Breaching of the corneal epithelium is the first in a series of events leading to corneal stromal abscessation. A small object such as a piece of straw penetrates the corneal epithelium and inoculates its deeper layers with surface flora. Rapid reepithelialization of the small surface defect traps the infectious organisms within the stroma. The intact epithelium and the avascular stroma form effective barriers against both endogenous and exogenous antimicrobials. As the microorganisms multiply in this protected position, microbial toxins and inflammatory mediators accumulate within the stroma and damage the surrounding cornea and adjacent uvea.

CLINICAL SIGNS

The horse's initial discomfort following the penetrating corneal injury diminishes as the epithelial defect heals within a couple of days. If veterinary care is sought at this early stage, a focal area of corneal edema may be seen but the lesion will seldom retain fluorescein dye. With progression of the infection, the horse again begins to squint and tear. The abscess develops an off-white to yellow color as inflammatory cells invade the area. The corneal edema intensifies and blood vessels invade the cornea, extending from the limbus toward the abscess. The depth of the abscess determines the character of the corneal vessels: superficial lesions are associated with treelike vessels, while deeper abscesses stimulate a compact wave of fine vessels originating from the deep ciliary vasculature. Generalized corneal edema, circumferential corneal vascularization, aqueous turbidity, and miosis signal the onset of anterior uveitis. The severity of the uveitis is often the limiting factor in achieving a visual eye.

DIAGNOSIS

A history of corneal injury followed by the appearance of a focal off-white to yellow lesion in the corneal stroma is highly suggestive of stromal abscessation. Samples for bacterial and fungal culture may be obtained from superficial abscesses by debriding the overlying epithelium and swabbing the affected stromal surface with a sterile, moistened cotton swab. Deeper abscesses are inaccessible unless the overlying stroma is removed. Invasive techniques such as biopsy risk weakening an already compromised cornea but may be indicated if empirical antimicrobial therapy has failed to halt the progression of the abscess over a period of several days. If the abscessed area is accessible, cytological evaluation of corneal scrapings is also recommended following application of a topical anesthetic. Gram stains of scrapings should be used as a basis for initial antimicrobial therapy.

THERAPY

After samples have been obtained for culture and cytology, treatment should be started immediately. The Gram-stain characteristics of organisms should be considered when selecting an antimicrobial, at least until the results of specific antibacterial sensitivity tests are available. Gentamicin is effective against most gram-negative isolates, although a recent report suggests that amikacin is a better empirical agent against gram-negative organisms in the horse. Gentamicin ophthalmic solution° can be fortified for topical use by adding to the dispensing bottle 50 mg of the injectable formulation. Injectable amikacin† may be diluted to a 5 per cent solution and applied directly to the eye. Ophthalmic preparations of chloramphenicol or erythromycin‡ are effective in gram-positive infections. Studies suggest that cephalothin is slightly more effective than chloramphenicol in the treatment of staphylococcal and streptococcal infections but is

TABLE 1. ANTIBIOTIC DOSES FOR SUBCONJUNCTIVAL INJECTION

Antibiotic	Dose
Amikacin	75–100 mg
Ampicillin	50 mg
Carbenicillin	200 mg
Cephalothin	100 mg
Chloramphenicol succinate	50–100 mg
Erythromycin	20–40 mg
Gentamicin	10–40 mg
Methicillin	100 mg
Tobramycin	10–30 mg

probably better suited to subconjunctival injection than topical application. The appropriate antimicrobial solution or ointment should be applied at least six times daily. Subconjunctival antibiotic injections are also recommended daily for the first 3 to 4 days (Table 1). The easiest site for injection is beneath the superotemporal *bulbar* conjunctiva. Endophthalmitis secondary to corneal abscessation is an indication for systemic antibiotics such as ampicillin or trimethoprim–sulfa.

If fungal elements are identified in corneal scrapings, miconazole§ or natamycin‖ should be applied topically at least six times daily. Miconazole is formulated for intravenous administration but is well tolerated topically. Although the natamycin is designed for topical use, its cost is almost four times that of miconazole.

Concurrent uveitis must also be treated. Topical 1 per cent atropine solution or ointment should be applied several times daily to dilate the pupil. The frequency of application can then be reduced to the level necessary to maintain dilation. Overzealous atropinization may reduce gastrointestinal motility. In severe uveitis, systemic nonsteroidal anti-inflammatory agents such as flunixin meglumine may also be needed to control inflammation. Topical corticosteroids are contraindicated in the early management of corneal abscesses.

PROGNOSIS

The time necessary for healing ranges from 1 to 4 weeks and is influenced by the size of the corneal abscess. Corneal vessels surround and invade the lesion; granulation tissue eventually replaces the abscess. Topical corticosteroids should not be used to discourage this early vascular response. Vessels will often disappear with-

---

°Gentocin, Schering Corp., Kenilworth, NJ
†Amiglyde-V, Ft. Dodge Labs., Ft. Dodge, IA
‡Ilotycin, Dista Products, Indianapolis, IN

§Monistat IV, Janssen Pharmaceuticals, Piscataway, NJ
‖Natacyn, Alcon Labs., Fort Worth, TX

out treatment within 2 to 4 weeks of healing. Residual vascularization 4 weeks after resolution of the abscess may be treated with a topical ophthalmic corticosteroid preparation applied two to three times daily. Most eyes will have residual scarring, the severity of which is often linked to the size and chronicity of the abscess. The impact on vision is determined by the scar's location and density.

Intractable intraocular inflammation or infection can develop in mismanaged cases as infectious agents or their toxins enter the anterior chamber. Enucleation is generally recommended in cases of endophthalmitis or panophthalmitis.

Corneal stromal abscessation should be ruled out in all cases of refractory keratitis and uveitis.

Abscesses must also be differentiated from nonulcerative keratouveitis, a recently reported equine disorder characterized by steroid-responsive perilimbal stromal infiltration and iridocyclitis.

Supplemental Readings

Brooks, D. E., Millichamp, N. J., Peterson, M. G., Laratta, L. J., Morgan, R. V., and Dziezyc, J.: Nonulcerative keratouveitis in five horses. J. Am. Vet. Med. Assoc., 196:1985, 1990.
Moore, C. P., Fales, W. H., Whittington, P., and Bauer, L.: Bacterial and fungal isolates from equidae with ulcerative keratitis. J. Am. Vet. Med. Assoc., 182:600, 1983.
Rebhun, W. C.: Corneal stromal abscesses in the horse. J. Am. Vet. Med. Assoc., 181:677, 1982.

Corneal Ulceration
Cecil P. Moore, COLUMBIA, MISSOURI

Corneal ulcers are usually due to trauma. With superficial ulceration only the epithelium is lost. Squinting, photophobia, and lacrimation are observed clinically. On closer examination the corneal surface usually appears slightly irregular and mildly edematous. Application of fluorescein solution to the eye delineates the ulcerated area. Healing of epithelial defects normally occurs rapidly by migration and mitosis of epithelial cells. Depending on the total area involved, an epithelial defect may heal in 2 to 8 days without scar formation.

Regrettably, corneal ulcerations frequently involve the stroma, which is slower to heal than the epithelium. Stromal defects present more readily visible changes in corneal contour, variable degrees of opacification, and moderate to severe ocular pain with reflex pupillary constriction. Healing usually occurs after inflammatory cell infiltration, dissolution of damaged stroma by degradative enzymes, neovascularization, and reformation of collagen. Focal or diffuse ulcerations in which the entire corneal stroma has been lost, leaving only Descemet's membrane and the endothelium to prevent aqueous loss, are termed *descemetoceles.* Repair of Descemet's membrane requires regeneration by endothelium. The corneal endothelium has limited potential for healing and repair occurs primarily by sliding of cells rather than by mitosis.

An accurate and carefully acquired history provides useful information to formulate the initial therapeutic plan. Frequently after the initial corneal trauma, opportunistic microorganisms, enzymatic degradation of the corneal stroma, mechanical irritants, corneal desiccation, and inappropriate therapy may delay and complicate healing. Corneal penetration by plant foreign material suggests the inoculation of fungi into the corneal stroma. Topical corticosteroids account for a high incidence of mycotic keratitis, while resistant bacterial organisms commonly follow unsuccessful treatment with topical antibiotics. A rapidly progressive keratopathy with degradation of the corneal stroma indicates excessive enzymatic activity. *Pseudomonas* organisms and certain genera of fungi such as *Aspergillus* may produce collagenase. When combined with enzymes from degranulating inflammatory cells and proliferating fibrocytes, collagenase results in rapid destruction of corneal tissue.

THERAPY

Diagnostic and therapeutic measures for ulcerative keratitis depend on the history and the extent of the ulcer. Acute, focal, superficial ulcers may be treated empirically with topical broad-spectrum antibiotics such as gentamicin, chloromycetin, or triple antibiotics (neomycin, bacitracin, and polymixin B). Ointments are preferred when treating uncomplicated ulcers be-

TABLE 1. INITIAL LOCAL ANTIBIOTIC THERAPY OF CORNEAL ULCERS

Organism(s)	Local Antibiotic	
	Subconjunctival (may be repeated in 24 hr)	Topical (every 1 to 4 hr)
Gram-positive cocci	Methicillin (50 mg), cefazolin (50 mg) or ampicillin (50 mg)	Triple antibiotic or chloromycetin
Gram-negative rod	Gentamicin (20–25 mg)	Gentamicin or tobramycin
Gram-negative cocci	Penicillin G (250,000 IU)	Triple antibiotic or tetracycline
Mixed bacteria	Gentamicin (20–25 mg) and methicillin (50 mg) or appropriate substitute	Triple antibiotic or gentamicin
Fungi	Miconazole (10 mg)	Miconazole or natamycin

Based on Gram staining characteristics of bacteria observed on cytological examination.

cause of their prolonged contact time. Antibiotic ointment applied three or four times daily and topical 1 per cent atropine ointment applied to effect pupillary dilation will usually allow rapid healing of an uncomplicated traumatic ulcer.

Complicated corneal ulcers are generally subacute, infected, and progressive, with varying degrees of keratomalacia and neovascularization. Aggressive diagnostic and therapeutic measures are necessary. Corneal cultures and scrapings are essential to determine the presence of opportunistic microorganisms. Following tranquilization and eyelid anesthesia, a sterile cotton or Dacron swab moistened with transport medium is applied to the margin of the ulcer and submitted to the laboratory for aerobic bacterial culture. Topical anesthetic is applied to desensitize the cornea and a scraping of the ulcer margin is obtained for cytology and fungus culture. For a corneal scraping, some affected corneal stroma dislodged for cytological analysis is most reliable for locating and identifying fungi. Corneal scrapings are placed on glass slides for Wright's and Gram stains. A small specimen of tissue is placed on Sabouraud's medium for fungus culture.

Initial therapy for complicated ulcers entails aggressive antimicrobial therapy on the basis of history, clinical findings, and results of cytology (Table 1). Results of bacterial culture and susceptibility tests may indicate that therapy should be modified at 48 to 72 hours. If gram-negative rods are identified cytologically, gentamicin° (20 mg) or carbenicillin (100 mg) is injected subconjunctivally. When gram-positive organisms are observed, cefazolin† (50 mg), chloromycetin (40 mg), methicillin‡ (5 mg), or ampicillin (50 mg) may be injected subconjunctivally. The relatively rare identification of gram-negative occi requires pencillin G§ subconjunctivally (250,000 units). When two or more bacteria are present, methicillin (or appropriate substitute) and gentamicin may be used simultaneously subconjunctivally if injected at different sites. When fungal elements are present or suspected, miconazole‖ (10 mg) is adminstered subconjunctivally.

Following initial subconjunctival injections, topical antimicrobial solutions should be applied at a minimum of every 2 hours or ointments every 4 hours. Hourly application of solutions may be necessary in rapidly progressive cases of *Pseudomonas* or *Aspergillus* keratitis or in cases of very deep ulcers of unknown cause. Antibacterial solutions available commercially for topical administration include gentamicin,° chloromycetin,† triple antibiotic solution,‡ and tobramycin.§ Other solutions may be formulated using sterile injectable preparations with artificial tear diluents. Antibiotic ointments commercially available include gentamicin, chloromycetin, triple antibiotic, erythromycin, tobramycin, and tetracycline.‖ Commercially prepared antifungals are limited to natamycin,¶ which is available as a 5 per cent suspension. Although not approved for use in the eye, miconazole 1 per cent solution may be used topically and appears to be safe and effective in treating fungal keratitis. Topical dermatological creams containing miconazole have also been used in the eye for 2 to 3 weeks without complications.

In addition to eliminating infectious agents, other goals of therapy are removing mechanical irritants, preventing further enzymatic destruction of the cornea, relieving pain and concurrent uveitis, ensuring adequate moisture to the eye,

---

°Gentocin (Injectable), Schering Corp., Kenilworth, NJ
†Kefzol, Eli Lilly & Co., Indianapolis, IN
‡Staphcillin, Bristol Labs., Syracuse, NY
§Penicillin G potassium, E. R. Squibb, Princeton, NJ

‖Monistat IV, Janssen Pharmaceutica Inc., New Brunswick, NJ
°Gentocin Ophthalmic, Schering Corp., Kenilworth, NJ
†Chloroptic, Allergan Pharmaceuticals, Irvine, CA
‡Neosporin, Burroughs Wellcome Co., Research Triangle Park, NC
§Tobrex, Alcon Labs., Forth Worth, TX
‖Achromycin, Lederle Labs., Wayne, NJ
¶Natacyn, Alcon Labs., Forth Worth, TX

and providing surgical support of the cornea in cases of deep ulcerations.

Therapy for rapidly progressive infected ulcers with extensive keratomalacia in which causative agents have not ben identified, consists of the topical application of an antibiotic, an antifungal, a cycloplegic, and an anticollagenase preparation. Therapy must be initially intensive and often prolonged. Miconazole (10 mg per ml), gentamicin solution (3 mg per ml) and 1 per cent ophthalmic atropine and 5 per cent acetylcysteine have been successfully applied sequentially every 1 to 2 hours. Alternate therapy might include tobramycin substituted for gentamicin and natamycin suspension in place of miconazole solution. Although natamycin is generally quite effective, it is considerably more expensive.

A subpalpebral or nasolacrimal infusion tube may greatly enhance the administration of liquid drugs. After 48 to 72 hours, therapy may be modified according to the results of bacterial culture and sensitivity tests. Common opportunistic bacterial isolates include streptococci, staphylococci, *Pseudomonas*, and coliform organisms. As the ulcer begins to heal, frequency of topical solutions may be reduced to every 3 to 4 hours. If destruction of the cornea is controlled and healing is indicated by reepithelialization and neovascularization, gentamicin and atropine ophthalmic ointments and miconazole dermatological cream may be substituted for solutions. Ointments are applied four times daily for an additional 2 weeks and if acetylcysteine solution was administered, it may be discontinued.

Superficial and deep corneal neovascularization occurs in many cases of infectious keratitis. This normal healing response should not be inhibited by corticosteroids until the affected area has completely vascularized and epithelialized as evidenced by a lack of retention of fluorescein stain. Frequently this requires 3 to 4 weeks. Following complete healing, topical corticosteroid antibiotic combinations will hasten the regression of the fibrovascular infiltrates. The degree of scarring is directly related to the degree of initial corneal involvement and may vary from transient focal superficial scarring to diffuse deep stromal scarring that may be permanent or, at best, remodels slowly with some clearing over several years.

In cases of severe keratomalacia or descemetocele formation surgical intervention may be indicated. A temporary tarsorrhaphy or a third eyelid flap may be used as a short-term emergency measure to keep the eye moist and to support and protect it until more definitive surgical repair can be attempted. A temporary tarsorrhaphy is recommended before transporting an animal with a deep corneal ulceration or corneal staphyloma. Two horizontal mattress sutures of 0 Supramid or silk are usually adequate.

Third eyelid flaps are difficult to perform successfully in the horse. Three to four horizontal mattress sutures are generally necessary. These are placed through the upper eyelid with deep bites into connective tissue on the anterior side of the third eyelid. The use of upper eyelid stints will prevent the suture from cutting into the eyelid. The most common complication is the suture pulling through the third eyelid conjunctiva. Third eyelid flaps have been used to support healing in cases of granulating staphylomas with protrusion of tissue beyond the normal corneal curvature.

Focal perforated ulcers may be sutured with 6-0 to 7-0 Dexon, Vicryl, or silk if the ulcer margins are healthy enough to support the suture. Principles of surgical repair of the cornea are discussed on p. 589. Deep, nonvascularizing ulcers or descemetoceles may be treated with conjunctival flaps. Whether a simple advancement flap, a pedicle flap, a bridge flap, or a 360-degree flap, the conjunctiva is meticulously dissected free from the underlying bulbar connective tissue. A properly dissected conjunctival flap should be quite thin and nearly transparent. Opaque thick flaps result when epibulbar connective tissue (Tenon's layer) is dissected with the conjunctiva. Conjunctival flaps provide support for the weakened cornea and serve as a source of nutrition and fibrocytes to the healing cornea. Large corneal defects may be repaired by performing a corneal-limbal-conjunctival transposition or full-thickness corneal graft. Detailed discussion of these surgical procedures is beyond the scope of this chapter.

Soft, hydrophilic contact lenses have been used in equine ulcerative keratitis to support and protect the cornea and to reduce the pain associated with an ulceration. When presoaked in antimicrobial solutions, lenses may provide a constant perfusion of medications to infected corneal tissue. Although therapeutic soft contact lenses for horses have become more readily available in recent years, the cost of the lenses and variations in surface curvature of equine corneas have limited their widespread use.

Providing additional moisture to the ulcerated eye is usually not necessary because profuse lacrimation characterizes most cases. If facial nerve paralysis accompanies ocular trauma, atony of the orbicularis oculi muscle and the inability to blink may cause neuroparalytic keratitis. Characteristically the inferior central cornea dries and diffusely ulcerates, necessitating tear supplementation, application of lubricant ointments, or a temporary tarsorrhaphy. Motor innervation to the palpebral muscles often returns in such cases within 4 to 6 weeks.

Inapparent, persistent mechanical irritants may cause recurrent corneal ulceration. Frictional irritants include masses, foreign bodies of the bulbar surface of the third eyelid, distichiasis, ectopic cilia, and chalazia. Masses or foreign bodies may involve the eyelid margin or palpebral conjunctiva. Irregularities of the eyelid margin, such as notching or scarring of the eyelid, and misdirected eyelid hairs from previous injury must not be overlooked as possible causes of corneal irritation. A thorough systematic external ocular examination, performed with a bright focal light and magnifying source in a darkened area, is essential in every case of ulcerative keratitis.

INDOLENT ULCERS

Chronic nonhealing ulcers characterized by epithelial undermining or lack of neovascularization are not common but present a therapeutic challenge. Differential diagnoses for indolent ulcers include viral keratitis, resistant bacterial keratitis, mycotic keratitis, drug-induced keratopathy (as from phenylephrine), low-grade frictional irritant, and tear film deficiency. One type of indolent ulcer is a static superficial stromal ulcer, which over a period of several weeks or months does not vascularize or epithelialize. A second type is a superficial epithelial ulcer with undermining around its rim. Therapy may include debridement of undermined epithelium with a dry cotton swab or superficial keratectomy if a static stromal ulceration is present. Cautery with 7 per cent tincture of iodine may remove devitalized tissue and stimulate neovascularization. Empirically, hypertonic solutions or ointments may be used to allow local dehydration of the epithelium and encourage attachment to its underlying basement membrane. Hydrophilic soft contact lenses used as a physiologic bandage encourages adherence of the epithelium while protecting the cornea. Lubricant antibacterial ointments may be helpful to sterilize the ulcer and reduce frictional rubbing from the third eyelid or eyelid margins. More extensive surgical procedures such as conjunctival flaps might be considered, particularly with an indolent stromal ulcer. The use of topical corticosteroids in treating indolent ulcers in horses is controversial at this time and is not recommended.

Supplemental Readings

Barnett, K. C., Rossdale, P. D., and Wade, J. F. (eds.): Equine Ophthalmology Supplement, Equine Vet. J., Suppl 10, September 1990.
Davidson, M. G.: Equine Opthalmology. In Gelatt, K. N. (ed.): Veterinary Opthalmology 2nd ed. Philadelphia, Lea & Febiger, 1991.
Dziezyc, J., and Millichamp, N.J.: Infectious ocular diseases. In Smith B. P. (ed): Large Animal Internal Medicine. St. Louis, C. V. Mosby, 1990, pp 1215–1236.
Moore, C. P. (ed.): Large Animal Ophthalmology. Vet. Clin. North Am. (Large Anim. Pract.), 6, No. 3, November, 1984.

Punctate Keratitis

Thomas R. Miller, GAINESVILLE, FLORIDA

Punctate keratitis in the horse is one manifestation of superficial keratopathy. The condition may occur singularly or in conjunction with superficial lacelike opacities, diffuse superficial corneal opacity, or corneal ulceration. There is no known age or breed predisposition, although the disease may be more common in mules than in horses.

In man, the pattern of the lesion is suggestive of but generally not specific for its etiology. Certainly this is true in the horse. Superficial keratopathy may result from a number of causes including infection, immune-mediated disease, corneal drying resulting from exposure or tear film abnormalities, mechanical abrasion, or chemical injury, including adverse reactions to topical medications.

Punctate keratitis with multiple superficial corneal opacities is suggestive of viral keratitis. The various viral agents associated with keratitis in the horse include equine adenovirus, equine herpesvirus 1 (EHV-1), and equine herpesvirus

2 (EHV-2, cytomegalovirus). The diagnosis of viral keratitis is often based on concurrent signs of systemic disease.

CLINICAL SIGNS

Affected horses may have clinical signs of keratitis, with blepharospasm and excessive tearing and photophobia, or may be asymptomatic. Lesions may vary from epithelial stippling (orange-peel appearance) to fine punctate epithelial or subepithelial opacities, or coarse, more granular-appearing opacities (Fig. 1). Larger, 5- to 10-mm lesions appear as dark foci with surrounding corneal edema.

DIAGNOSIS

Punctate keratitis lesions are frequently subtle. Recognition may require focal illumination of the cornea with the horse in a dark stall. Magnification is also helpful. The lesions have variable fluorescein uptake and may stain intensely, faintly, or not at all. The use of rose bengal solution may help to identify epithelial changes; the devitalized cells stain an intense red. Topical anesthetics often produce a rapid change in corneal epithelium; evaluation for superficial keratopathy should be performed prior to the administration of these agents.

Cases of adenovirus keratitis usually have a primary conjunctivitis and a secondary low-grade keratitis. Diagnosis can be confirmed through the demonstration of intranuclear inclusion bodies in conjunctival scrapings stained with Giemsa stain. Cases of herpetic keratitis may be more difficult to confirm. A positive serum antibody titer is not diagnostic for either EHV-1 or EHV-2, due to the ubiquitous nature of these viruses. Demonstration of a higher titer in affected horses than in nonaffected stablemates may be of value. Similarly, positive viral isolation is not conclusive evidence, again because of the frequency with which these viruses occur in the normal population. Response to specific antiviral therapy may be the best confirmation of the diagnosis.

THERAPY

Topical antiviral agents may be indicated for viral keratitis. Treatment of equine viral keratitis with idoxuridine, desoxyuridine, and trifluridine has been reported. Trifluridine* is possibly the best choice because of its ability to penetrate the cornea. Treatment is administered every 2 hours during the day, up to nine times daily, until corneal ulcers have healed. The frequency of administration is then reduced to four times daily for another week. Idoxuridine† is useful for superficial (epithelial) infections but its usefulness when there is stromal involvement is limited by its poor penetration. Treatment should be given four to six times daily and continued for 1 week after the keratitis has resolved. With either drug, therapy should be reevaluated if no response is evident within the first week of treatment. Although concurrent corticosteroid therapy may cause a failure in therapy with idoxuridine, trifluridine generally has no loss in efficacy when used concurrently with corticosteroids. This may be important in cases where corticosteroids are prescribed to control clinical signs. Horses with stromal involvement may especially benefit from corticosteroid therapy.

Recommendations for the symptomatic treatment of punctate keratitis have generally consisted of antibiotics and corticosteroids applied topically. This will often lead to resolution of the clinical signs, although signs may recur after treatment is discontinued. However, corticosteroid therapy in the absence of antiviral therapy may lead to exacerbation of a viral infection and may predispose the horse to recurrence of the infection. Cases with corneal ulceration should not receive corticosteroids topically.

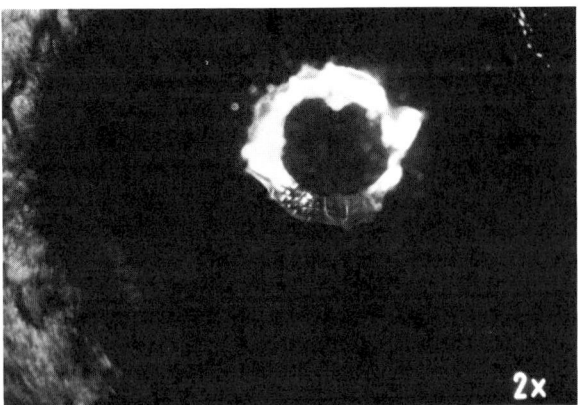

Figure 1. Coarse granular subepithelial corneal infiltrates in a horse with suspected EHV-2 keratitis (original magnification ×2). Large central circular area is ring flash artifact.

---

*Viroptic 1% solution, Burroughs Wellcome Co., Research Triangle Park, NC
†Herplex 0.1% solution, Allergan Pharmaceuticals, Irvine, CA; Stoxil 0.1% solution or ointment, Smith, Kline & French Labs., Philadelphia, PA

Supplemental Readings

Lavach, J. D.: The Handbook of Equine Ophthalmology. Fort Collins, Giddings Studio Publishing, 1987.
Matthews, A. G., and Handscombe, M. C.: Superficial keratitis in the horse: Treatment with the antiviral drug idoxuridine. Equine Vet. J. Suppl., 2:29, 1983.
Miller, T. R., Gaskin, J. M., Whitley, R. D., and Wittcoff, M. L.: Herpetic keratitis in a horse. Equine Vet. J. Suppl. 10:15, 1990.
Riis, R. C.: Equine ophthalmology. In Gelatt, K. N. (ed.): Textbook of Veterinary Ophthalmology. Philadelphia, Lea & Febiger, 1981, p. 569.
Thein, P.: The association of EHV-2 infection with keratitis, and research on the occurrence of equine coital exanthema (EHV-3) of horses in Germany. In Bryans, J. T., and Gerber, H. (eds.): Equine Infectious Diseases IV. Princeton, NJ, Veterinary Publications, 1978.

Cataracts

Joan Dziezyc, COLLEGE STATION, TEXAS
Nicholas J. Millichamp, COLLEGE STATION, TEXAS

Cataracts are an optical opacity in the lens that are seen fairly commonly in the horse. The opacity can range from minute spots that do not interfere with vision to total opacification of the lens and blindness in that eye. Because the horse uses monocular vision extensively, even a unilateral cataract can cause a performance horse to be incapacitated.

Cataracts can be divided into two categories: congenital and acquired. A congenital cataract is first noted at birth and can be unilateral or bilateral. Hereditary congenital cataracts have been reported in the Belgian and Morgan breeds. However, anecdotal accounts from veterinary ophthalmologists suggest a hereditary basis in other breeds. Certainly one must be suspicious of a hereditary disease in any case of bilateral congenital cataracts, especially if one parent is similarly affected. Other problems may be associated with congenital cataracts; we have seen microphthalmos associated with congenital cataracts in an Appaloosa and three Quarter Horse foals.

There are numerous causes of acquired cataracts described in many species. In the horse, the two main causes of acquired cataracts are trauma and equine recurrent uveitis (periodic ophthalmia, moon blindness). Traumatic cataracts can be seen following either blunt or perforating trauma. In equine recurrent uveitis, cataracts are seen with other signs of uveitis such as corneal edema, posterior synechiae, darkened iris, lens luxation, chorioretinal degeneration (butterfly lesions), or retinal detachment.

THERAPY

The only treatment for cataracts is surgical removal. Cataract removal in horses is not performed frequently, partly because of the expense, partly because of the potential postoperative complications. However, cataract removal in a horse can be successful and turn an unproductive horse into one that is again useful.

The candidate for cataract surgery must be chosen carefully. Foals with congenital cataracts should ideally have no other ocular defects, although we have successfully performed cataract surgery in foals with mild microphthalmos. Foals should probably be operated on as soon as possible to allow the visual pathway in the brain to develop. In humans and cats, visual deprivation at a young age will not allow the normal central visual pathway to develop, and blindness is permanent. We may be doing a disservice to clients by waiting until foals are weaned before performing cataract surgery.

In horses with acquired cataracts, the presence of equine recurrent uveitis is a contraindication for cataract surgery. Horses with traumatic cataracts can have the cataracts successfully removed if the eye is no longer inflamed and the pupil can be well dilated.

Phacofragmentation in our experience is the best method of cataract removal in the horse. This method uses ultrasound to break up the lens and aspirate the particles from the eye. We use a modified lithotriptor* to break up the lens, attached to a phacofragmentor aspiration unit† to perform the aspiration. We cannot use a phacofragmentor designed for humans because the needles are too short. The needle is inserted into a small incision made at the limbus under a limbal-based conjunctival flap, or near the limbus in

---

*Fibrasonics Lithotriptor, Fibrasonics, Chicago, IL
†Model 8000 (V) Cavitron/Kellman Phaco-Emulsifier Aspirator, Cooper Vision, Irvine, CA

a clear cornea. The eye is kept inflated throughout surgery by infusing lactated Ringer's solution through a 20-gauge needle inserted into the anterior chamber through the limbus. The advantages of phacofragmentation over conventional surgery include the complete removal of all lens material, the speed of completion, and preservation of the anterior chamber during surgery. These factors add up to far less inflammation after surgery and a better prognosis for a visual eye.

Postoperative uveitis is the major complication seen in all eyes after cataract surgery. Uveitis can cause corneal edema, glaucoma, posterior synechiae, fibropupillary membranes, and endophthalmitis. Corneal ulcers associated with the incision site are common. Late complications include retinal detachments, glaucoma, and chronic uveitis.

Even with phacofragmentation, the prognosis for equine cataract patients is guarded after surgery. If postoperative inflammation becomes uncontrollable, complications can easily result in blindness. We perform cataract surgery only in horses with cataracts that prevent them from being useful.

We do not have a definitive answer for the question of how well the animal will see after cataract surgery, but we have had some encouraging results. We have performed cataract surgery in several adult performance horses (roping horse, cutting horse, polo pony), all of which were having problems working after developing a cataract. After surgery all owners reported that their horses were working well and most felt the horses were working as well as they had prior to the onset of the cataract.

Supplemental Readings

Beech, J., Aguirre, G., and Cross, S.: Congenital nuclear cataracts in the Morgan horse. J. Am. Vet. Med. Assoc., 184:1363, 1984.
Whitley, R. D., Meek, L. A.: Cataract surgery in horses. Compend. Cont. Educ. Pract. Vet., 11:1396, 1989.
Whitley, R. D.,: Moore, C. P., and Slone, D. E.: Cataract surgery in the horse: A review. Equine Vet. J. Suppl. 2:127, 1983.

Glaucoma

Dennis E. Brooks, GAINESVILLE, FLORIDA

Glaucoma is an elevation in intraocular pressure that is detrimental to normal ocular function. The abnormal rise in intraocular pressure is caused by an obstruction to the outflow of aqueous humor and eventually results in optic nerve damage and blindness.

Glaucoma is reported to be a rare ocular condition in the horse, but its actual incidence may be much higher. The early ocular signs are subtle, with many horse owners unaware that veterinary care is needed. The more widespread use of electronic applanation tonometers to measure intraocular pressure is revealing a previously misdiagnosed and unique disease. As more equine-oriented veterinarians obtain appropriate tonometric instrumentation to detect elevated intraocular pressure in the horse, the true incidence of equine glaucoma will be revealed.

Aqueous humor is produced in the ciliary body, where the enzyme carbonic anhydrase plays an important role in the energy-dependent phase of production. Aqueous humor passes through the dual ciliary epithelium into the small posterior chamber, then through the pupil into the large anterior chamber. Conventional drainage from the anterior chamber occurs through the iridocorneal angle, but extensive alternative pathways also exist in the horse. Aqueous humor may pass through the supraciliary and suprachoroidal spaces to be absorbed into the scleral vessels or may be absorbed directly into the iridal vessels. The prominence of these unconventional pathways may explain the low incidence of overt glaucoma following the intraocular inflammation and scarring of the iridocorneal angle that characterize equine recurrent uveitis.

ETIOLOGY

Glaucoma is caused by an impairment to aqueous humor outflow. This blockage can occur at the pupil, the surface of the iris, or the iridocorneal angle. Glaucoma may be primary, that is, not associated with any detectable ocular or systemic condition. Primary glaucoma has a bilateral, hereditary potential and may be related to biochemical abnormalities within the iridocorneal angle. Elevations in intraocular pressure may also occur secondary to other ocular disease processes, such as iridocyclitis, lens disease, or intraocular neoplasia. Congenital glaucoma due to malformation of the iridocorneal angle is also reported in many species.

Anecdotal reports of primary glaucoma exist in the horse, although secondary glaucoma associated with intraocular inflammation is reported by some ophthalmologists to be the most common cause of equine glaucoma. In many cases, however, a convincing link between uveitis and glaucoma is difficult to make. Obstruction of the trabecular meshworks with inflammatory cells and debris, resulting in decreased flow of aqueous humor via the iridocorneal angle, or the formation of pre-iridal fibrovascular membranes, resulting in reduced drainage via iridal vessels, may increase intraocular pressure in the horse. Secondary glaucoma due to intraocular neoplasia is rare in the horse, although intraocular melanomas causing secondary glaucoma have been seen. Congenital glaucoma due to maldevelopment of the trabecular meshworks or iris hypoplasia is reported in the horse.

CLINICAL SIGNS

Horses with glaucoma are most easily classified into those with early disease signs and those with late-onset or chronic signs. Early glaucoma has been reported in the Quarter Horse, Tennessee Walking Horse, Thoroughbred, Arabian, Welsh pony, American Saddlebred, warm bloods, and Appaloosa breeds.

The clinical signs of early glaucoma include generalized corneal edema, deep linear corneal band opacities, and, in a few cases, a fixed, dilated pupil. Prominent scleral vessels are rarely seen early in the disease, and the affected eye is seldom painful or blind. The corneal edema may dissipate with the use of topically applied corticosteroids, suggesting that equine glaucoma may indeed have an inflammatory component. The intraocular pressure does not decrease in response to the topical corticosteroids.

The linear corneal band opacities are a consistent feature of early equine glaucoma. The opacities extend from limbus to limbus, may branch, and histologically represent thin areas of Descemet's membrane. These bands are also found in normal horses and in the buphthalmic (enlarged) globes of horses with chronic glaucoma. The presence of these linear corneal opacities in normal-sized, normotensive equine globes is confusing and may represent a congenital corneal defect.

Chronic glaucoma in the horse is characterized by corneal edema and vascularization, buphthalmos, blindness due to optic nerve atrophy, and pain in some cases. An ulcerative exposure keratitis may develop. The intraocular pressure will eventually decrease in buphthalmic globes as the ciliary body atrophies.

DIAGNOSIS

The normal range of intraocular pressure of the horse measured by applanation tonometry varies from 16 to 32 mm Hg and averages 24 mm Hg. The intraocular pressure of the two eyes in the same individual should be within approximately 5 mm Hg. Applanation tonometry is the most convenient and accurate means of measuring intraocular pressure in the horse. Digital tonometry is occasionally useful in detecting large intraocular pressure elevations but is worthless in detecting the subtle elevations in intraocular pressure found in early equine glaucoma, when therapy is undoubtedly most beneficial. A portable applanation tonometer* is available and has been found to be accurate for the horse. The Schiotz indentation tonometer cannot be routinely used in the horse. An auriculopalpebral nerve block (see *Current Therapy in Equine Medicine 2*, p. 429) should be done prior to intraocular pressure measurement to prevent artificially high intraocular pressure readings caused by excessive pressure on the eyelids during tonometry.

The mydriatic provocative test is valuable in predicting potential elevations in intraocular pressure in the horse. The intraocular pressure is measured before and 15 minutes after instillation of one drop of 0.5 per cent tropicamide† in the eye. Little change should occur in normal eyes, but elevations of 10 to 20 mm Hg will occur in equine eyes with compromised or narrowed iridocorneal drainage angles.

THERAPY

Therapy for equine glaucoma is in its trial stages. The goals of therapy are to preserve vision and minimize discomfort. Glaucoma may be treated medically (Table 1) or surgically. Therapy is directed at decreasing the intraocular pressure by reducing production or increasing outflow of aqueous humor. It is a difficult disease

---

*Tonopen, Oculab, Glendale, CA
†Mydriacyl, Alcon Labs., Fort Worth, TX

TABLE 1. TOPICALLY APPLIED MEDICATIONS FOR GLAUCOMA

Drug	Frequency of Application
0.5% timolol maleate solution	b.i.d.
0.25% demecarium bromide solution	b.i.d.
0.03% echothiophate iodide solution	b.i.d.
4% pilocarpine HCl gel	b.i.d. to q.i.d.

to manage in the horse and vision is unlikely to be preserved unless the condition is detected early. Glaucoma is particularly aggressive and difficult to control in the Appaloosa.

Outflow should be increased with topically applied demecarium bromide and aqueous production should be reduced with a β-adrenergic blocker, timolol maleate.° Demecarium bromide,† phospholine iodide,‡ and pilocarpine§ increase outflow by causing contraction of the ciliary muscle. These agents will also exacerbate iridocyclitis and should be used carefully if uveitis is present. Topically applied corticosteroids and sodium flurbiprofen‖ are indicated if intraocular inflammation is present. Atropine will increase outflow through iridal vessels in many species but is contraindicated in the horse as it will rapidly increase the intraocular pressure in horses with compromised drainage angles.

Systemically administered carbonic anhydrase inhibitors are too expensive to use in the horse but should be applied topically when they become available commercially. Systemic nonsteroidal anti-inflammatories, such as phenylbutazone or flunixin meglumine, may be beneficial in horses with glaucoma secondary to uveitis.

Surgical therapy for glaucoma in the horse is directed toward reducing production of aqueous humor by damaging the ciliary body with nitrous oxide (cyclocryotherapy) or laser energy (cyclophotocoagulation). Cyclophotocoagulation has the best potential for preserving vision in glaucomatous eyes if the glaucoma is detected early. Chronically painful and blind buphthalmic globes should be enucleated or have an intrascleral prosthesis implanted.

Supplemental Readings

Barnett, K. C., Cottrell, B. D., Paterson, B. W., and Ricketts, S. W.: Buphthalmos in a thoroughbred foal. Equine Vet. J., 20:132, 1988.
Lavach, J. D.: The Handbook of Equine Ophthalmology. Fort Collins, CO, Giddings Publishing, 1987.
Samuelson, D., Smith, P., and Brooks, D.: Morphologic features of the aqueous humor drainage pathways in horses. Am. J. Vet. Res., 50:720, 1989.
Smith, P., Samuelson, D., and Brooks, D.: Aqueous drainage paths in the equine eye: Scanning electron microscopy of corrosion cast. J. Morphol., 198:33, 1988.
Smith, P. J., Samuelson, D. A., Brooks, D. E., and Whitley, R. D.: Unconventional aqueous humor outflow of microspheres perfused into the equine eye. Am. J. Vet. Res., 47:2445, 1986.
Wilcock, B. P., Brooks, D. E., and Latimer, C. A.: Glaucoma in horses. Vet. Pathol., Vet Puthol. 28: 74, 1991.

Acknowledgments

The author acknowledges the helpful insights on equine glaucoma provided by Drs. Paul Dice, Claire Latimer, Tom Miller, Joe Wolfer, Ken Abrams, Sam Vainisi, and Charles Martin.

°Timoptic, Merck, Sharp & Dohme, West Point, PA
†Humorsol, Merck, Sharp & Dohme, West Point, PA
‡Phospholine iodide, Ayerst Labs., New York, NY
§Pilopine HS, Alcon Labs., Fort Worth, TX
‖Ocufen 0.03%, Allergan Optical, Irvine, CA

Ocular Neoplasia

J. Daniel Lavach, FOUNTAIN VALLEY, CALIFORNIA

Ocular and periocular tumors can cause disfigurement, blindness, and death. A diagnosis of an ocular neoplasm may be cause to classify a horse as temporarily or permanently unsound, depending on the tumor type and interference with vision. The clinician must proceed in a logical sequence to obtain an accurate diagnosis for the client. This will allow the owner to be informed of the treatment protocols and the expected prognosis.

The initial examination of a patient with any tumor should include three segments, and findings should be noted in the patient's record. First, the tumor should be characterized as to size and shape, mobility or immobility, consistency, pigmentation or lack of pigmentation, areas of ulceration, number of sites affected, appearance of the periocular tissues, and appearance of the affected eye by comparison with the opposite eye.

In the second part of the examination the examiner looks for metastatic disease by palpating the regional lymph nodes and salivary glands. Metastases may cause filling of the supraorbital fossa or may be observed in the oral cavity. They may also invade the sinuses, causing loss of resonance. Endoscopy and ultrasonography may help to locate metastases.

Third, the examiner obtains impressions for cytological examination and biopsy specimens for histopathological study. The definitive diagnosis of a neoplastic disease and selection of the most effective mode of therapy usually depends on a pathologist's findings.

SQUAMOUS CELL CARCINOMA

Squamous cell carcinoma is the most common tumor of the equine eye and adnexa. Some cases are caused by solar irradiation damage to epithelial cells. Horses lacking pigment in the eyelids and along the margin of the third eyelid are more likely to sustain solar injury than pigmented horses. Other factors that cause chronic irritation, such as windy and dusty environments, can be contributing stimuli for tumor formation. Draft horse breeds have a higher risk for developing squamous cell carcinoma than other breeds. Squamous cell carcinoma can occur at any age, but most affected horses are more than 9 years old.

Squamous cell carcinomas often originate at sites of transition from one type of epithelium to another. The limbus is an area of a transition from conjunctival to corneal epithelium. The mucocutaneous junction along the eyelid margin is another common site for squamous cell carcinoma. The anterior surface of the third eyelid has an epithelial transition area where verrucous types of squamous cell carcinoma occur. In addition, the free margin of the third eyelid is a common site for squamous cell carcinoma, especially if it lacks pigment. The tumor can also originate in a sinus and invade the orbit.

Squamous cell carcincomas in the eyelid are usually erosive and ulcerative. Untreated or uncontrolled tumors will invade the deeper soft tissues and bones of the orbit. Local destruction is significant, and metastases can occur to the lymph nodes of the head, neck, and thorax. Tumors arising from the third eyelid are either erosive or proliferative. They can invade the gland of the third eyelid and then spread into the orbit. Limbal tumors are usually proliferative initially but will invade the globe if not controlled.

THERAPY

Many treatments are available for squamous cell carcinoma. Complete surgical excision is curative and is recommended whenever it can be done without causing loss of function and extraordinary disfigurement. Most tumors are radiosensitive, and various irradiation sources, including radioactive gold, iridium, cesium, and cobalt, can be implanted to destroy the tumor when the tumor is diffuse and cannot be excised. Beta irradiation is an excellent adjunct following superficial keratectomy for removal of a corneal or conjunctival tumor. Liquid nitrogen delivered as a spray or through stainless steel probes to cancerous surfaces is a very effective cryogen. Tissue temperatures should reach $-25°$ C, and a double freeze-thaw cycle is recommended for maximal tumor destruction. Cryotreatments can cause temporary skin depigmentation and permanent poliosis of hair or eyelashes. Eyelids that undergo repeated treatments may contract from collagen shrinkage, and surgical treatment for blepharophimosis may be necessary for severely affected patients. Hyperthermia is an effective treatment for superficial tumors. The effective penetration with surface probes is limited to 4 mm. Penetrating probes can be inserted into deeper tumor sites, but their effectiveness is limited to a small zone around the probe tip, and this treatment is not feasible with larger tumors.

Carbon dioxide laser removal of squamous cell carcinomas represents the newest method for treatment of surface tumors. The tumor can be excised or vaporized by varying the delivery of the laser energy to the site. It can be applied to eyelid, third eyelid, conjunctival, and corneal tumors. Laser treatments leave an open wound with a charred appearance, but patient discomfort following surgery is usually minimal. Laser treatments of eyelid sites usually result in a dry eschar that sloughs, leaving a granulating surface until epithelialization is complete. Corneal, limbal, and conjunctival sites heal quickly, and the postoperative inflammatory reaction is minimal. Complete healing occurs within 2 months of treatment. Other types of lasers such as the holmium-doped yttrium-aluminum-garnet (THC:YAG) laser are being adapted for use through fiber-optic delivery probes. The lasers offer another effective mode for treating squamous cell carcinoma. Clinical trials using combinations of lasers and photodynamic chemicals are encouraging, but their use is still experimental at this time.

The prognosis for a horse with a squamous cell carcinoma is guarded. Although most surface tumors can be eradicated, some tumors are refractory to all treatments and are relentless in their growth and destruction. Occasionally a tumor will worsen following treatment. Clients are advised that this tumor growth represents a breakdown in the local immune system. Once a horse develops a squamous cell carcinoma, it is predisposed to further tumor development. Most affected horses will acquire squamous cell carcinoma in other sites within 2 years of the initial tumor diagnosis.

EQUINE SARCOID

Equine sarcoid is the second most commonly diagnosed tumor affecting the eyelids of the horse. It is probably caused by a virus, which explains its occurrence in younger horses. The average age of an affected horse is 4 years. Sarcoids can develop as firm nodules or as verrucose warty growths. Either type can ulcerate and become infected. An eyelid sarcoid can invade the orbit.

Sarcoids are refractory to many types of treatment. Recurrences are very common following surgical excision. Nevertheless, local excision or treatment with cryotherapy, hyperthermia, and irradiation can result in complete destruction of the tumor.

Immunotherapy has been a very reliable method for treating periocular sarcoids. The site is injected with cell wall extracts of Bacillus Calmette–Guerin (BCG) in oil. A total dose of 1 ml per sq cm is administered through a 25-gauge needle until tumor saturation is complete. The treatment is repeated at 3-week intervals until the tumor has been eradicated. An average of four treatments is usually required, but occasional patients require additional injections. Each treatment is accompanied by an active inflammatory reaction, which can include ulceration with tumor necrosis. The local immune system is responsible for this action, and it is a favorable prognostic sign for an intense reaction to occur following the administration of BCG. Treatments with live BCG organisms or whole organisms have been associated with anaphylactic reactions and death. The cell wall preparations rarely cause any adverse reactions, but the clinician should administer intravenous corticosteroids if a generalized hypersensitivity occurs. Unfortunately, sarcoids occuring on other body sites seem to be less susceptible to immunotherapy.

Carbon dioxide laser removal is excellent for verrucous sarcoids. The tumor and a surrounding zone of normal skin can be quickly vaporized by the laser. Follow-up care is minimal and healing proceeds beneath an eschar that is sloughed after several days. Epithelialization is usually completed within 2 months of surgery, and scarring is minimal. Long-term studies evaluating the effectiveness of laser removal have not been reported, but limited experience suggests that it is an excellent treatment modality.

EYELID MELANOMAS

Eyelid melanomas are most common in gray horses, and Arabian horses acquire eyelid melanomas more often than other horses. Older horses are at a greater risk than young horses for developing a melanoma. Most eyelid melanomas begin as a darkening of the tissue with some tissue thickening. Ulceration and erosions are not usually features of this type of tumor, which can occur singly or simultaneously at multiple sites. The tumor may be squamous or wartlike. Eyelid melanomas are usually a local disease with little tendency to metastasize, but tumors that invade the conjunctiva are more malignant. Treatment is not always warranted. Horses with slow-growing tumors that are not stimulating local tissue reaction or patient discomfort may be observed and left untreated. If the melanoma is growing rapidly or causing patient discomfort, it can be treated. Various treatment modalities have been applied to eyelid melanomas, including local excision, cryosurgery, hyperthermia, and carbon dioxide laser vaporization. Melanomas are often resistant to irradiation therapy. Recently, melanomas have been treated with H_2-histamine blocking agents. This chemotherapeutic approach to tumor control needs further evaluation before specific recommendations can be presented.

Horses often acquire more tumors along the eyelids. The owners should be advised that melanoma development will continue to be a problem for the affected patient.

MAST CELL TUMOR/*HABRONEMA* GRANULOMA

Mast cell tumors are uncommon eyelid tumors that may be smooth and covered by normal skin or may be ulcerated. The tumor may be diffuse throughout the eyelid or a discrete nodule. Mast cell tumors are difficult to eradicate and often recur following excision and other treatments. Local injections of depot corticosteroids have caused tumor regression. Cryotherapy has been applied to a tumor and caused complete remission during a 2-year follow-up period. Mast cell tumors are occasionally sensitive to radiation, and irradiation can be recommended if other treatments are not possible or have failed. Laser ablation may be possible for discrete tumors but would not be appropriate for diffuse tumors in the eyelid since too much tissue destruction would be necessary to eradicate the tumor.

Mast cells are commonly encountered surrounding *Habronema* granulomas. Their presence often confuses the diagnosis, and a mast cell tumor may be reported instead of the correct diagnosis of habronemiasis. The clinician should inform the pathologist of the presence of *Habronema* and this differential diagnosis when biopsy specimens are submitted for examination.

Habronema is common in certain geographic areas, and its presence varies from year to year, depending on local climatic factors. The granulomatous reaction from larvae can persist for months following actual infection. The parasite can invade the eyelids, conjunctiva, and nasolacrimal system. The local immunological reaction can simulate squamous cell carcinomas in addition to mast cell tumors.

INTRAOCULAR MELANOMA

The most common primary intraocular tumor is the melanoma. The tumor arises from the uveal tract, usually the base of the iris and ciliary body region. Tumors often grow slowly, displacing the contents of the globe. The aqueous humor can be filled with cells and pigment desquamating from the tumor. Glaucoma results from invasion of the filtration angle by the tumor, from obstruction of the outflow channels by cellular material in the aqueous humor, or by iridal displacement causing drainage angle closure. Small, discrete intraocular melanomas are potentially amenable to surgical excision. If the tumor cannot be completely excised, the site can be treated by application of a cryoprobe over the base of the tumor following debulking of the iridal mass. Lasers offer another potential method for treatment of small melanomas. The neodymium:YAG laser operating in a continuous wave (thermal mode) can be applied transsclerally over the tumor. The laser energy causes coagulation of the tissues and destroys the tumor. THC:YAG laser energy can be delivered into the globe through a 26-gauge needle. Both of these lasers will cause destruction of the tumor and may stimulate the local immune system to eradicate remaining tumor cells. This laser application in horses has not been reported. Large tumors cannot be treated, and the eye should be enucleated to reduce the chances of extraocular tumor growth. Melanomas tend to spread slowly out the vascular channels and along the optic nerve. Patient death is usually the result of extensive orbit involvement or tumor in the cranial vault.

LYMPHOSARCOMA

Lymphosarcoma is generally considered a systemic neoplastic disease. Most affected horses do not have ocular signs, but a horse with lymphosarcoma can have a variety of manifestations, including involvement of the orbit, eyelids, conjunctivae, third eyelid, or globe. Lymphosarcoma of the orbit or gland of the third eyelid can fill the orbit and displace the globe. Eyelid saturation with tumor cells can prevent eye opening. One or both eyes may be affected.

Intraocular lymphosarcoma is usually manifested as a uveitis with hyphema. The cornea is usually edematous. The aqueous humor contains varying amounts of blood and fibrin, and the iris is thickened and congested with tumor cells. The fundus may be spared, but the view of the fundus may be obscured by the anterior segment changes. One eye may be affected initially, but in most patients with ocular changes intraocular abnormalities will eventually occur in both eyes.

The intraocular and periocular manifestations of lymphosarcoma usually respond to local and systemic administration of corticosteroids. Other chemotherapeutic agents may prolong the patient's life, but it is a fatal neoplastic disease.

Benign lymphoid proliferation within the orbit can be confused with lymphosarcoma. The affected eye becomes more exophthalmic until corneal exposure causes clinical disease. It can cause blindness from injury to the optic nerve. The diagnosis of benign lymphoid proliferation is difficult to make. Aspiration of the orbit for cytology specimens and biopsy specimens can provide nondiagnostic or confusing results. It is generally a unilateral local disease that does not cause any signs of discomfort. No treatments are helpful, but the disease may be cured once the orbit is eviscerated.

TUMORS OF THE ORBIT

Primary tumors of the orbit are uncommon and pose a diagnostic challenge. The clinical signs can include exophthalmos, displaced globe, prominent third eyelid, restricted eye movement, and blindness with mydriasis. The ophthalmic examination may be noncontributory, or the optic nerve and fundus may be invaded by the neoplasm. Mass lesions against the globe may cause a visible indentation into the eye. This is usually evident during the ophthalmoscopic examination.

The examiner can palpate beneath the eyelids for any evidence of a local mass. Aspiration of the orbit and examination of cytological specimens can be informative. Eosinophils are suggestive of parasitic invasion, and local injection of corticosteroids may be beneficial. Additional special diagnostic testing includes radiography and ultrasonography. Computed tomography is very helpful if available.

The diagnosis may remain elusive despite complete examination and specialized testing. Blind eyes with exposure keratitis should be enucleated and the orbit explored for the etiology. All tissues should be submitted for histopathological examination. Eyes with vision should be examined on a regular basis for changes that might aid in the diagnosis.

Squamous cell carcinoma can extend from a primary site in a sinus into the orbit and cause exophthalmos. Sinus mucoceles can cause exophthalmos. Their surgical debulking by removal from the sinus will temporarily reduce the exophthalmos, but the disease can recur. Chondroma rodens can be debulked and treated with irradiation. Mast cell tumors, lymphosarcoma, lipoma, hemangiosarcoma, and nerve sheath tumors have all been diagnosed as causes of exophthalmos. Most diagnoses are made following enucleation. The patient's prognosis depends on the final diagnosis.

Supplemental Readings

Lavach, J. D.: Large Animal Ophthalmology. St. Louis, C. V. Mosby, 1990.
Nasisse, M. P., and Davidson, M. G.: Laser therapy in veterinary ophthalmology: Perspective and potential. Semin. Vet. Med. Surg., 3:52, 1988.
Palmer, S. E.: Carbon dioxide laser removal of a verrucous sarcoid from the ear of a horse. J. Am. Vet. Med. Assoc., 195:1125, 1989.

Visual Impairment
Kerry L. Ketring, CINCINNATI, OHIO

Acute onset of bilateral total blindness in the horse is relatively easy to identify. The animal bumps into objects in a familiar environment and is unable to perform previously accomplished tasks. The horse may hold the eyelids wide open, appear nervous, and be easily startled when quietly approached and touched.

A horse with unilateral total blindness may spook when approached from the blind side, resist loading from the affected side, and tilt the head so that the normal eye is more forward. Riders report difficulty in keeping the horse's head aligned when taking jumps.

The horse that slowly loses vision in one or both eyes is not as easily identified. In its own environment and when performing a task for which is has already been trained, a horse can function well with severely limited vision. The loss of vision may not be apparent until the horse's environment or function changes.

In addition to these observations from owners, several pertinent questions should be asked. Is vision worse at night or in bright light? Thoroughbreds and Morgans with nuclear cataracts have a greater visual deficit in bright light, while Appaloosas with congenital stationary night blindness have greater difficulty in the dark. Is there a history of recurring ocular discharge or conjunctivitis? If so, visual impairment may reflect damage to the optic nerve and retina resulting from equine recurrent uveitis. Is there a history of severe blood loss or trauma to the globe or skull? Damage to the optic nerve and retina may not be clinically apparent until some time after these injuries. Has the horse been recently dewormed? Chorioretinitis has been reported following anthelmintic administration. Has upper respiratory disease or septicemia been diagnosed? Both could result in chorioretinitis. A similar medical history should be obtained for the mare with a visually impaired foal.

ASSESSMENT OF VISION

Conventional methods of visual testing in the horse are crude and interpretation of results is often subjective. The practitioner should avoid telling a client that a horse has 20 or 50 per cent normal vision. There is no way to determine the quality of vision so precisely.

The horse should be tested in a spacious, unfamiliar area with as few external distractions as possible. The animal is first observed as it is led around the obstacle-free area on a loose lead. Binocular vision is then tested by the examiner's making a menacing gesture with a twitch or broom handle from 3 to 5 feet in front of the horse. If the horse fails to respond, it may be necessary to strike the twitch firmly on the side of the neck and then threaten the horse a second time to evaluate its response. The menace response of each eye should then be determined, which may require that the eyes be alternately blindfolded. A horse that responds to a menace following pharmacological dilation of the pupil cannot be totally blind. Another simple test gauges the horse's response to cotton balls tossed in its visual field. Ideally, all visual testing should be repeated in dim light.

An obstacle course can be devised using bales of straw. Although the test does assess vision for stationary objects, the added risk of injury to the horse and handler may not be justified.

Pupillary Light Response

It is necessary to have a darkened area to correctly evaluate pupillary light response. A bright focal light source such as a new penlight (with fresh batteries) or a Finoff transilluminator on a direct ophthalmoscope handle are good choices.

Both pupils should dilate maximally and uniformly in the dark-adapted animal. Failure to do so may indicate previous or concurrent anterior uveitis. Posterior involvement in equine recurrent uveitis can account for vision deficits and total blindness.

The direct pupillary light response in a normal horse is brisk, but the consensual response in the unstimulated eye is sluggish compared to that in small animals. It is often necessary to have a second observer evaluate the unstimulated eye.

The presence of a pupillary light response does not indicate vision. Central lesions in the visual cortex, recent retinal detachments, and mature cataracts can all result in total blindness accompanied by a normal pupillary light response. It is also possible to have significant damage to the retina and optic nerve that spares the pupillary light response but is sufficient to cause a visual deficit.

The most common cause of a negative pupillary light response in a normal eye with vision is prior topical application of atropine sulfate. One application can keep the pupil in a noninflamed eye dilated for up to 4 weeks. These horses will have a normal consensual pupillary light response if only one eye was treated.

Ophthalmoscopy

Since ophthalmoscopy and the anatomy of the fundus have been reviewed in previous editions of *Current Therapy in Equine Medicine* (see *Current Therapy in Equine Medicine 2*, p. 427), only one aspect of this technique will be included as it relates specifically to the evaluation of the blind or visually handicapped eye.

Following chemical dilation of the pupil with 1 per cent tropicamide, the tapetal reflection should be evaluated. This is done with the direct ophthalmoscope set at zero diopters, the scope positioned firmly against the examiner's brow, and the light directed into the eye from a distance of 2 to 3 feet. A uniform yellow, blue-green, or red reflection should be observed. Any opacity in the cornea, aqueous, lens or vitreous will obscure a portion of the reflection and create a dark area in the tapetal reflex. If a tapetal reflection is observed in a totally blind eye, a lesion of the retina or optic nerve is likely.

BLINDNESS IN THE FOAL

Congenital bilateral blindness in the foal is uncommon but when present is associated with a searching nystagmus. Even in normal foals, the menace response and pupillary light responses may be poor in the very young animal.

Cataracts are the most common cause of congenital blindness in the foal. Blindness in foals less than 1 week of age has also been described without ophthalmoscopic lesions. Some of the foals have been born prematurely. As they age, vision improves and ocular reflexes normalize. The cause of this visual deficit has not been defined. The finding is not associated with the neonatal maladjustment syndrome since the foals show no other clinical abnormalities and the "blindness" is transient.

Optic nerve hypoplasia has been identified in the horse as a unilateral or bilateral condition. The optic disc may appear normal in size but is pale gray and void of retinal vessels.

Retinal dysplasia resulting in retinal detachments has also been reported. In these cases, the detached retina can be seen as a gray irregular veil floating in the vitreous. The optic disc is often pale and the tapetum appears hyperreflective. There is no treatment for congenital retinal detachments of this nature.

Retinal dysplasia and optic nerve hypoplasia may occur with other ocular defects such as microphthalmia, cataracts, lens subluxation, and corneal opacities. A tapetal reflex in a blind eye should alert the examiner to the retinal and optic nerve disease in addition to the more obvious corneal and lens changes.

Upper respiratory tract infection or septicemia in the mare during gestation or neonatal septicemia in the foal have the potential to damage the foal's retina. When active, these defects appear as gray, circular lesions in the nontapetal area. When inactive, they appear as depigmented areas with deeply pigmented centers, commonly referred to as "bullethole" lesions. Larger comma-shaped and bar-shaped lesions may also be found, along with linear areas of tapetal hyperreflectivity. The lesions are usually coincidental findings on soundness examinations and seldom affect vision.

Blunt trauma to the globe is common in the foal and may be responsible for the neuroretinopathies of unknown etiology reported in the young horse. Injury may result from a kick by the mare or other foals or by accidental self-trauma. Injured eyes are often treated initially for a corneal ulcer or anterior uveitis, without regard for the concurrent retinal damage. Animals have been evaluated for vision loss several weeks or months following a history of such trauma. Ophthalmoscopic findings include preretinal and subretinal hemorrhage, peripapillary retinal atrophy, focal areas of abnormal pigment in the tapetum, pallor of the optic disc, and decreased retinal vessel number and caliber. This posttraumatic atrophy may be avoided if the fundus is examined at the time of trauma. Systemic corticosteroids should be instituted soon after the injury to be effective, but the prognosis is guarded. Topical agents are of no benefit in the management of retinal disease.

CHORIORETINITIS

The most common cause of chorioretinitis in the horse is associated with equine recurrent uveitis. In most severe cases of chorioretinitis, the optic nerve is secondarily involved. The most remarkable fundic lesions are found in the peripapillary region and in the nontapetal retina. Gray streaks radiating from the optic disc in a sunburst pattern represent perivascular infiltrates and elevations of the retina. Circular gray lesions, larger comma-shaped defects, or bar-shaped lesions may also be seen in the nontapetal area. Vermiform areas of abnormal pigmentation may extend from the nontapetum into the tapetal retina. Larger areas of serous retinal elevation may be seen. In severe cases, the detached retina may be seen floating immediately behind the lens. All of these findings are frequently obscured by the inflammation of the vitreous and anterior uvea. The treatment of equine recurrent uveitis is outlined on page 592. Any horse with equine recurrent uveitis has a poor prognosis for long-term vision in the affected eye; the opposite eye is also in jeopardy.

Septicemia, upper respiratory diseases, onchocerciasis, leptospirosis, and toxoplasmosis have all been incriminated as causes of chorioretinitis. Fundic lesions in these diseases are similar to those previously described; the causative agent cannot be determined by ophthalmoscopic examination alone. The diagnosis is often presumptive and is based on clinical findings and serology.

A distinct chorioretinitis has been reported that causes severe vision loss in one or both eyes. The only lesion appears as a horizontal band of multifocal gray or depigmented areas below the optic disc. Vascular infarction has been proposed as the cause.

CHORIORETINAL SCARS

In the nontapetal area, inactive chorioretinitis appears as depigmented foci with darkly pigmented centers. Abnormal pigmentation and hyperreflectivity may occur in the tapetal fundus. Multiple confluent hyperpigmented and depigmented foci adjacent to the optic disc have been described as "butterfly" lesions and may have a relationship to equine recurrent uveitis. Vision is seldom altered by these lesions alone.

OPTIC NEURITIS

The most common cause of optic neuritis in the horse is associated with equine recurrent uveitis, since all cases of severe chorioretinitis can ultimately involve the optic nerve. The inflamed optic disc appears pink with indistinct margins; the normal fasciculations of the optic nerve are obscured.

Exudative optic neuritis causes acute blindness. The severely inflamed optic nerve will also have raised nodules projecting into the vitreous. Peripapillary hemorrhage is commonly found. The etiology is unknown and response to therapy is poor.

Blunt trauma to the globe or orbit can result in optic neuritis characterized by a hyperemic disc with hemorrhages within the nerve and nerve fiber layer of the retina. The latter appear small and linear due to compression by the nerve fibers. There may also be large areas of intraretinal hemorrhage.

All cases of active chorioretinitis and optic neuritis should be treated with systemic nonsteroidal anti-inflammatory drugs. Systemic corticosteroids may also be used concurrently if an infectious etiology has been ruled out. In severe cases, dimethyl sulfoxide (DMSO) may be administered intravenously at a dosage of 1.0 gm per kg body weight, diluted with an equal volume of 5 per cent dextrose.

OPTIC NERVE ATROPHY

All previously described etiologies of optic neuritis can result in optic nerve atrophy. The chalk-white disc will be devoid of retinal vessels. Extensive peripapillary retinal atrophy will also be present.

Atrophy of the optic nerve has also been reported in primary and secondary glaucoma. Documentation of elevated intraocular pressure would be needed for definitive diagnosis.

Two scenarios have been reported that result in acute bilateral blindness. Profound blood loss, as from epistaxis or prolonged bleeding following castration, and severe trauma to the skull, as when a horse falls backward and strikes the poll, have resulted in bilateral optic nerve and peripapillary retinal atrophy. The precise mechanism of injury to the nerve has not been defined. Aggressive treatment instituted within hours of the traumatic incident has failed to prevent blindness.

ADVICE TO OWNERS

Because it is not possible to accurately quantify a horse's vision as a percentage of normal (e.g., 50 per cent normal vision), the terms totally blind, functionally blind, functionally visual, and normally sighted are best used to describe a horse's vision. Categorization is based on vision testing, ocular examination findings, the function and temperament of the animal, and the experience of the rider. It must be understood that the quality of vision necessary for racing, jumping, trail riding, or breeding varies considerably. The examiner must therefore make a subjective judgment as to whether vision is adequate for the horse to perform the desired function with the desired rider. A visually impaired horse could be described as functionally blind or functionally visual, depending on the task it is expected to perform. A visual handicap is less acceptable as the level of performance rises or the experience of the rider diminishes. Finally, any horse with less than normal vision may startle easily, threatening its own safety as well as that of the rider.

Supplemental Readings

Barnett, K. C., Rossdale, P. D., and Wade, J. F. (eds): Equine Vet. J. (Equine Ophthalmol. Suppl.), Suppl. 2, 1983.
Glaze, M. B.: Examination of the eye. In Robinson, N. E. (ed): Current Therapy in Equine Medicine 2. Philadelphia, W. B. Saunders, 1987, pp. 427–433.
Lavach, J. D.: The Handbook of Equine Ophthalmology. Fort Collins, CO, Giddings Studio Publishing, 1987.
Rebhun, W. C.: Diseases of the retina and optic nerve. In Robinson, N. E. (ed): Current Therapy in Equine Medicine 2. Philadelphia, W. B. Saunders, 1987, pp. 458–460.

Section 14

URINARY TRACT DISEASE

Edited by Thomas J. Divers

Obstruction and Rupture of the Urinary Tract

Troy S. Ford, COLLEGE STATION, TEXAS

Obstructive disease of the urinary tract in the horse is an uncommon but potentially serious disorder. Urolithiasis, the most prevalent form of obstructive disease, can occur at any location in the urinary tract, but the bladder is the most common. Less common areas include the kidney, ureter, and urethra. Infrequently, the urinary tract becomes obstructed by neoplasia, inflammatory or granulomatous disease, or a cicatrix caused by trauma or surgery.

The presenting signs are highly variable and depend on the anatomical location of the obstruction. Signs can range from acute and persistent abdominal pain to general unthriftiness. Rupture of the bladder, although more common in neonates, can occur in older horses, primarily from prolonged obstruction of the urethra.

The etiology of uroliths is largely unknown. Because crystals of calcium carbonate and mucoproteinaceous material are a normal component of equine urine, it is difficult to formulate an explanation of calculus formation based solely on the presence of these materials. Possibly, desquamated epithelial cells or mucous collections may serve as the nidus for urolith formation. Crystallization and precipitation may then occur in the presence of a high mineral content and alkaline pH in normal equine urine.

Primarily two types of uroliths develop in the horse. One form is moderately friable, yellow, and frequently spiculated. The second type is a firm concretion that is hard and resistant to fragmentation. Although generally smooth and white, they also may be spiculated. Both types are primarily composed of calcium carbonate in various hydrated forms, with the occasional addition of phosphate, magnesium, and ammonium.

NEPHROLITHIASIS AND URETEROLITHIASIS

The prevalence of renal and ureteral calculi is quite low. Horses generally are asymptomatic or exhibit vague clinical signs that may include weight loss, poor performance, decreased appetite, hematuria, lumbar pain, or hind limb lameness. Signs of chronic azotemia, such as oral ulcerations, excessive dental tartar, and melena, may be present. Laboratory analysis of serum often indicates renal failure.

Diagnosis is generally made by rectal examination and ultrasonography. Palpation per rectum of a urolith or dilated ureter is physically possible when a calculus is lodged in the mid- to distal ureter. Percutaneous or transrectal ultrasonography of the kidney is necessary to confirm the presence of a nephrolith, determine the size of the left and right kidney, and estimate the extent of renal fibrosis. If a calculus is found in one kidney or ureter, strong consideration should be given to the possibility that the disease has also occurred in the contralateral kidney.

The patency of the proximal urinary tract may be evaluated by cystoscopic evaluation of the ureteral openings with a flexible fiber-optic endoscope in either sex, or with a rigid fiber-optic endoscope in females. The ureters of clinically normal horses empty urine from the ureteral openings in pulsatile fashion at a frequency of approximately one to two discharges per minute. Failure to observe this occurrence from a ureteral opening suggests a proximal urinary tract obstruction.

Therapy

Unfortunately, there appears to be no early indication of obstructive disease of the proximal urinary tract, which makes early detection and treatment before the onset of renal failure difficult. Determining the presence and extent of renal disease by renal biopsy and measurements of glomerular filtration rate is of paramount importance before surgical removal of the stone is considered, since bilateral involvement seems to be the rule. Once signs of chronic renal failure are present, surgical treatment may prolong life, but long-term recovery is unlikely.

Ureteral calculi have been retrieved by ureterolithectomy through a ventral celiotomy; however, visualization and access by this method are limited. Temporary placement of a ureteral stent following ureterolithectomy, with or without closure of the ureteral incision, has been used successfully to ensure patency of the ureter. Ureteral calculi have also been retrieved by passing a basket stone dislodger* through a vestibulourethral approach, guided by digital manipulation per rectum. A calculus must be approximately 2 cm or less in diameter and lodged within 30 cm of the trigone to be successfully retrieved by this method.

Calculi located within the kidney and the proximal ureter are removed by nephrotomy or nephrectomy. The kidney and proximal ureter are accessed through a lateral retroperitoneal approach. The procedure is described in surgical texts.

CYSTIC CALCULI

The most common form of urolithiasis is cystic calculi. Males are clinically affected more frequently than females, in part because of anatomical differences between the male and female urethra. The male urethra is long and narrow, particularly at the level of the ischial arch, whereas the short, wide, female urethra is easily distensible and permits passage of a calculus. Typical signs of cystic calculi include dysuria, stranguria, and pollakiuria. Hematuria is often evident, particularly after exercise or at the end of urination. The horse often maintains a prolonged urinary stance and the male protrudes its penis. Signs of restlessness, grunting, or tenesmus may also be noted during attempted urination. A cystic calculus is readily diagnosed on rectal examination and palpation of a firm, oval, possibly spiculated mass within the bladder. Additional information can be obtained by ultrasonographic and cystoscopic examination. Direct visualization of the lumen of the bladder with a cystoscope allows assessment of the mucosa and the ureteral openings and determination of the number, shape, and texture of the calculi.

Therapy

Cystic calculi can be managed with a variety of surgical procedures. The choice of surgical approach is dictated by the sex and physical condition of the horse, the size of the calculus, and the surgeon's preference. In the male, an ischial urethrotomy can be performed under epidural anesthesia in the standing horse. Identification of the urethra during urethrostomy is greatly enhanced by prior placement of a urinary catheter in the urethra. Once the urethra is entered, the pelvic urethra is dilated to admit a lithotrite or grasping forceps into the bladder. The surgeon's free hand is passed into the horse's rectum to guide the forceps to the calculus. A small calculus can be removed intact, whereas larger calculi must be broken apart with a lithotrite. Fragmentation produces multiple small pieces of calculi that must be removed by a grasping instrument or by lavage and siphonage. Unremoved pieces could subsequently serve as a nidus for further calculus formation or produce a urethral obstruction.

In the mare, cystic calculi can be removed under epidural anesthesia in the standing horse. The short distensible urethra is dilated by the surgeon's gloved fingers until a lithotrite or grasping forceps can be introduced into the blad-

---

*Dormia Stone Dislodger, V. Mueller Co., Division of American Hospital Supply Co., Chicago, IL

der. A dorsal urethrotomy (sphincterotomy) can be used to provide a wider exit. Following removal of the calculus, the bladder is copiously lavaged and siphoned to remove remaining fragments. If a sphincterotomy was performed the incision is reapposed.

An alternate approach for removal of a cystic calculus, particularly for a large or hard calculus, is laparocystotomy. The procedure is performed with the horse under general anesthesia and positioned in dorsal recumbency. A ventral celiotomy of the caudal abdomen permits access to the bladder. Firm and steady traction is needed to access the bladder near the surgical field for cystotomy and calculus removal. Prior to closure, the bladder is lavaged and siphoned to remove any remaining fragments.

URETHRAL CALCULI

Obstructive urethral calculi occur almost exclusively in the male. The long, narrow urethra of the male is more likely to become obstructed than the short, wide, distensible urethra of the female. The calculus commonly lodges in the pelvic portion of the urethra near the ischial arch or distal portion of the urethra. Typically the affected male horse maintains a urinary stance with its penis protruded. Blood may be present at the urethral orifice. Tenesmus, restlessness, and abdominal pain are often evident. Unless ruptured, the bladder is often distended and taut. The level of the obstructing calculus can be determined by palpation per rectum or percutaneously along the course of the urethra, or by passage of a urinary catheter or fiber-optic endoscope. Complete or protracted urethral obstruction is likely to progress to rupture of the bladder, uroperitoneum, and peritonitis. The ability to void urine does not completely rule out the possibility of a ruptured bladder. Usually a peritoneal fluid creatinine concentration greater than serum creatinine concentration by a ratio of 2:1 or more is diagnostic of a ruptured bladder.

Therapy

A calculus that lodges at the distal urethra can be manually expressed or removed with a grasping instrument with the horse sedated or anesthetized. A calculus lodged distal to the ischial arch that cannot be dislodged by these methods is removed through an incision on the median raphe directly over the calculus. This is generally performed with the horse anesthetized and positioned in dorsal recumbency. The incision can be sutured or left to heal by secondary intention.

A calculus that lodges proximal to the ischial arch can be removed with the horse standing under local or epidural anesthesia. An ischial urethrostomy similar to that previously described is performed. The calculus is located by passage of a urinary catheter or instrument. The calculus is dislodged by cautiously dilating the urethra with fluid and grasping the calculus with an instrument, or is crushed with a lithotrite. The urethra can be ruptured during the course of manipulation, particularly if the urethral wall is compromised. Formation of a cicatrix at the site of the obstructing calculus or, less likely, at the site of the urethrostomy can occur and produce a postoperative urethral obstruction.

Management of a ruptured bladder that has occurred secondary to a urethral obstruction can be assessed by cystoscopic evaluation of the bladder following removal of the obstructing calculus. Horses with small or dorsal rents in the bladder and that retain the ability to void urine are usually managed conservatively. Large or ventral rents require surgical closure of the tear, accessed by ventral celiotomy. Management of ruptured bladder in the foal is discussed in *Current Therapy in Equine Medicine 2*, page 717.

Aftercare

Antibiotic therapy is often justified following surgical correction of urolithiasis when preoperative urinary cultures reveal the presence of bacterial infection. The choice of antimicrobial drug is dictated by in vitro sensitivity testing, and predicted concentrations of drug that can be obtained in the urine. The use of urinary acidifiers (ammonium chloride, 20 to 520 mg per kg per day, given orally) to prevent precipitation of calcium carbonate in alkaline urine has also been suggested, but its effectiveness has been questioned.

Supplemental Readings

DeBowes, R. B., Nyrop, K. A., and Boulton, C. H.: Cystic calculi in the horse. Compend. Cont. Educ. Pract. Vet., 6:S268, 1984.

DeBowes, R. M.: Surgical management of urolithiasis. Vet Clin. North Am. (Large Anim. Pract.), 4:461, 1988.

Ehnen, S. J., Divers, T. J., Gillette, D., and Reef, V.B.: Obstructive nephrolithiasis and ureterolithiasis associated with chronic renal failure: Eight cases (1981–1987). J. Am. Vet. Med. Assoc., 197:249, 1990.

Macharg, M. A., Foerner, J. J., Phillips, T. N., and Barclay, W. P.: Two methods for the treatment of ureterolithiasis in a mare. J. Vet. Surg., 13:95, 1984.

Trotter, G. W., Bennett, D. G., Behm, R. J.: Urethral calculi in five horses. J. Vet. Surg., 10:159, 1981.

Walker, D. F., Vaughan, J. T.: Surgery of the urinary tract. *In* Walker, D. F., and Vaughan, J. T. (eds.): Bovine and Equine Urogenital Surgery, 2nd ed. Philadelphia, Lea & Febiger, 1980, pp. 59–68.

Cystitis and Pyelonephritis

Mary Gardiner Boy, KENNETT SQUARE, PENNSYLVANIA

CYSTITIS

The urinary bladder is resistant to infection because the flow of urine removes and dilutes bacteria in the bladder. In addition, the normal bacterial flora competitively binds epithelial receptor sites to prevent pathogen adherence, produces bacteriocidins that interfere with pathogen metabolism, and preferentially consumes essential nutrients. Local secretory immunoglobulins in the urinary tract may also play a role in host defense. Extremes of urinary pH, osmolality, and the high urea content of concentrated urine as well as other unknown substances can inhibit bacterial growth.

Cystitis is uncommon in horses. It most often occurs secondary to conditions that cause urine stasis or that injure the bladder or urethra. A common cause is an ascending bacterial infection; rarely, a descending, hematogenously established pyelonephritis may result in cystitis. The shorter length of the female urethra is thought to be responsible for the higher prevalence of cystitis in females than in males. Conditions predisposing to cystitis include trauma sustained at parturition, neurological dysfunction of the bladder and urethra, physical obstructions to urination, and cystic calculi.

Paralysis or paresis of the bladder may occur in diseases such as equine herpesvirus 1 (EHV-1) infection, neuritis of the cauda equina, Sudan sorghum toxicity and fractures, osteomyelitis, or neoplasia of the lower lumbar, sacral, or upper coccygeal vertebrae that affects neurological control of the bladder.

Mares in late pregnancy may be unable to completely empty the bladder, owing to their gravid state, and trauma sustained during parturition can contribute to urethral and bladder irritation and possible dysfunction, predisposing the animal to cystitis. Obstruction of urine outflow by vaginal scars, polyploid masses, and a vaginal fibrosarcoma have been reported. There are also reports of cystitis secondary to urethral obstruction in males caused by inadvertent penile amputation at castration and by squamous cell carcinoma of the penis.

Long-term repeated urinary catheterization can also predispose to the development of bladder infections. Both the physical trauma to the urethra and bladder and the potential introduction of pathogens are predisposing factors that may arise with catheterization.

Bacterial organisms most commonly associated with cystitis in the horse include *Escherichia coli*, *Proteus mirabilis*, *Enterobacter* spp., *Klebsiella* spp., *Pseudomonas* spp., *Staphylococcus* spp., *Streptococcus* spp., and *Corynebacterium* spp. *Candida* has been seen as a cause of cystitis in neonatal foals receiving prolonged antibiotic therapy. The wide variety of bacterial pathogens that may be involved should be considered in the diagnosis and subsequent choice of an antimicrobial agent.

CLINICAL SIGNS

Clinical signs result from the urethritis that accompanies cystitis, causing pain and stimulating urination. The signs include frequent urination, passing of small amounts of urine at a time, tenesmus, dribbling of urine (pollakiuria), and urine scalding. Males may demonstrate variable degrees of penile relaxation. Urination may be accompanied by grunting, and the horse may remain in position to urinate for a prolonged period following the act of urination. Systemic signs of infection, fever, depression, and anorexia may be seen in severe cases. Urine may be normal in appearance or may be grossly turbid or discolored by blood. Many cases of cystitis in horses are chronic, and the bladder wall may feel thickened on palpation per rectum. On cystoscopy, the bladder mucosa may appear roughened and irritated and erosions may be present. Horses with a neurogenic cause of urine stasis and subsequent cystitis may have a large, distended, flaccid bladder and frequently exhibit other neurological deficits such as hind limb ataxia and weakness.

LABORATORY EVALUATION

The urine may be visually normal or abnormal. A strong ammonia smell may be present due to bacterial breakdown of urea. The urine of neonatal foals with cystitis caused by *Candida* characteristically has a thick, cheesy appearance. It is not unusual to require microscopic examination of the urine to confirm the diagnosis of cystitis. Free catch samples are adequate for determination of the presence of red blood cells, white blood cells, desquamated epithelial cells, and debris but are unacceptable for bacteriological examination. Samples to be submitted for bacteriological analysis should be collected aseptically by urinary catheterization. The sample should be collected prior to institution of antimicrobial therapy. Quantitative colony counts provide the most accurate reflection of the bacterial population in the bladder. Determination of the minimum inhibitory concentration (MIC) of the antimicrobial agent is helpful in selecting the most appropriate agent.

THERAPY

The therapeutic goal is elimination of pathogenic bacteria using an effective antimicrobial agent. Because cystitis is most often a secondary disease, treatment of the primary problem is a major factor in effective therapy. In mild cases, removal of the predisposing cause may allow resolution of the cystitis through normal defense mechanisms. In other cases aggressive antimicrobial therapy is required to control or eliminate the underlying disease.

Factors affecting the choice of an antimicrobial agent include the sensitivity pattern of the pathogens, excretion of the antimicrobial and its activity in urine, ease of administration, cost, and potential side effects. Identification and sensitivity testing of the bacteria involved are of utmost importance in selecting an antimicrobial agent because of the wide variety of bacteria that might be involved. Some common antimicrobial agents used in the treatment of equine urinary tract infection are trimethoprim–sulfadiazine, gentamicin, amikacin, and penicillin. Cystitis caused by *Candida* in foals may resolve following discontinuation of broad-spectrum antibiotics. In some cases, *Candida* infections may become systemic and the organism can be isolated from blood and joints. Agents that have been employed in the treatment of systemic candidiasis in foals include fluconazole, amphotericin B, ketoconazole, and rifampin.

Equine cystitis is frequently chronic and requires a month or more of sustained antimicrobial therapy. Colony counts performed on urine during the course of treatment and 2 to 6 weeks after treatment is discontinued are useful in evaluating treatment efficacy. In more acute disease, treatment for 7 to 14 days may be effective. Bacteria may persist within a thickened bladder wall, particularly in chronic cases, and relapse is not uncommon.

Ancillary therapy includes irrigation of the bladder with a nonirritating solution such as isotonic fluids. This may be useful at the start of treatment if a large amount of sediment and debris has accumulated in the bladder. However, it may be difficult to adequately empty the bladder of debris. Urinary acidifiers may have bacteriostatic effects in the urine and may potentiate the effects of some antimicrobial agents. Systemically affected horses may require supportive care such as intravenous (IV) or oral fluids to maintain adequate hydration and urine flow. Horses with bladder paresis or paralysis may be managed by manual expression of urine from the bladder or repeat urinary catheterization. Indwelling soft Foley catheters may be used, although their presence may predispose to the development of infection. Pharmacological manipulation with a combination of cholinergic and sympatholytic agents may be effective in restoring the animal's ability to void urine. Bethanechol (0.025 mg per kg IV three or four times a day) and phenoxybenzamine (1 mg per kg IV three times a day) have been employed with some success in the management of horses with EHV-1 infection and neuritis of the cauda equina.

PYELONEPHRITIS

Pyelonephritis, an inflammation of the renal parenchyma, calyces, and pelvis due to bacterial infection, is rare in the horse. Urine stasis or lower urinary tract infection and an ascending infection most commonly cause pyelonephritis, although hematogenous seeding of the kidney with bacteria may occur.

Pyelonephritis may be unilateral or bilateral. The renal papillae and medulla are most often involved, although the infection may extend to the cortex. Embolic pyelonephritis more often shows a cortical distribution. The bacteria involved in pyelonephritis are the same as those found in cystitis.

CLINICAL FINDINGS

Horses may present with signs of chronic systemic disease, including fever, depression, inappetence, and weight loss. Cystitis, dysuria, strangury, and pollakiuria may be seen. As with cystitis alone, the urine may be either grossly normal or abnormal. Rectal examination may reveal enlargement or irregularity of the renal shape and distended ureters may be detected. The bladder may have a thickened wall. Cystoscopy may be useful in determining unilateral or bilateral involvement. In foals and other small equids, IV pyelography may be useful in determining unilateral or bilateral involvement and the extent of renal and ureter involvement. Ultrasonography of the kidney and proximal ureters, performed percutaneously or per rectum, also provides valuable information regarding the extent of involvement of the upper urinary tract as well as the presence of urolithiasis.

LABORATORY FINDINGS

Urinalysis will often reveal the presence of white blood cells, red blood cells, epithelial cells, and bacteria. Urine should be collected aseptically by catheterization for bacteriological analysis and antimicrobial sensitivity testing. Horses with pyelonephritis are more likely to have changes in hematological and metabolic laboratory parameters than horses with cystitis. In chronic cases, anemia, hyperfibrinogenemia, and leukocytosis may be evident. When renal function has been compromised, elevations in blood urea nitrogen and creatinine levels, and electrolyte derangements occur.

THERAPY

Chronic severe unilateral pyelonephritis is best managed by nephrectomy in combination with antimicrobial therapy. Intensive therapy is indicated in cases of pyelonephritis. Gram staining of urine may be helpful in the initial choice of an antimicrobial agent while awaiting results of bacteriological analysis of the urine. The choice of antimicrobial agents is based on the pH of the urine, the excretion and activity of the drug in the urine, and the MIC of the drug. The ability to achieve high levels of antimicrobial agent in the renal parenchyma tissue is an important factor in eliminating bacteria sequestered there. The antimicrobial agents useful in the treatment of cystitis may also be used in healing equine pyelonephritis. Pyelonephritis, particularly chronic cases, may be difficult to treat and response to medical therapy may be poor. Animals with impaired renal function will need fluid therapy to establish normal urine output and to resolve the azotemia. Because of the insidious onset and chronic course, prognosis is poor.

Supplemental Readings

Blood, D. C., Radostitis, O. M., Henderson, J. A.: Diseases of the urinary system. In: Veterinary Medicine: A Textbook of the Disease of Cattle, Sheep, Pigs, Goats and Horses, 6th ed. London, Bailliere Tindall, 1983, pp. 348–367.
Divers, T. J.: Urinary tract—Horse, cow. In Johnston, D. E. (ed.): The Bristol Veterinary Handbook of Antimicrobial Therapy. Syracuse, NY, Bristol Laboratories, 1982, pp. 84–91.
Divers, T. J., Byars, T. D., Murch, O., and Sigel, C. W.: Experimental induction of *Proteus mirabilis* cystitis in the pony and evaluation of therapy with trimethoprim-sulfadiazine. Am. J. Vet. Res., 42:1203–1205, 1981.
Hodgson, D. R.: Cystitis and pyelonephritis. In Robinson, N. E. (ed): Current Therapy in Equine Medicine 2. Philadelphia, W. B. Saunders, 1987, pp. 708–712.
Johnson, P. J., Goetz, T. E., Baker, G. J., and Foreman, J. H.: Treatment of two mares with obstructive (vaginal) urinary outflow incontinence. J. Am. Vet. Med. Assoc., 191:973–975, 1987.
Markel, M. D., Wheat, J. D., and Jones, K.: Genital neoplasms treated by en bloc resection and penile retroversion in horses: 10 cases (1977–1986). J. Am. Vet. Med. Assoc., 192:396–400, 1988.
Roberts, M. C.: Ascending urinary tract infections in ponies. Aust. Vet. J., 55:191–193, 1979.
Sloet Van Oldruitenborgh-Oosterbaan, M. M., and Kalsbeek, H. C.: Ureteropyelonephritis in a Friesian mare. Vet. Rec., 122:609–610, 1988.

Urinary Incontinence
E. Susan Clark, ATHENS, GEORGIA

Urinary incontinence, although not particularly common in horses, poses a diagnostic and therapeutic challenge. The loss of voluntary control of micturition may result from neurogenic or nonneurogenic causes. Nonneurogenic causes of urinary incontinence that have been reported in horses include cystitis, urolithiasis, ectopic ureters, and estrogen-responsive urinary incontinence. Each of these is characterized by urinary incontinence and an absence of other neurological signs. Cystitis, urolithiasis, and bladder tumors (see pp. 616, 613, and 623, respectively) are the most common causes. Ectopic ureters have been identified in very young animals, and estrogen-responsive incontinence has been rarely documented in aged mares. This discussion concentrates on neurogenic causes of urinary incontinence.

ETIOLOGY

Urinary incontinence due to upper motor neuron disease is rarely observed in horses. Because ataxia and recumbency preclude normal posturing during micturition, horses with upper motor neuron disease may have altered micturition behavior without damage to the spinal tracts responsible for upper motor neuron control of micturition.

The most common neurological causes of urinary incontinence in horses are neuritis of the cauda equina, equine herpesvirus 1 (EHV-1) myeloencephalitis, and sorghum ataxia cystitis. Less commonly, trauma, osteomyelitis, equine protozoal myelitis, neoplasia, and other lesions of the caudal lumbar, sacral, and cranial coccygeal vertebral column or spinal cord may lead to micturition disorders. Cerebral lesions occasionally lead to incontinence. All of the above conditions produce signs of urinary incontinence typical of damage to lower motor neurons. Analgesia, hypalgesia, or hyperalgesia of the perineum; paralysis of the tail, penis, vulva, rectum, and anal sphincter; pelvic limb weakness; and atrophy of the pelvic limb musculature are often observed in conjunction with urinary incontinence. Signs of brain stem disease may also be present in horses with EHV-1 myeloencephalopathy and cauda equina neuritis.

It is hypothesized that neuritis of the cauda equina is due to an inflammatory reaction of unknown etiology involving nerve roots and peripheral nerves, especially of the sacrococcygeal and cranial nerves. The disease is slowly progressive and ultimately euthanasia is necessary.

Sorghum ataxia cystitis is associated with ingestion of plants of the *Sorghum* genus. Focal axonal degeneration and demyelination result from intoxication with hydrocyanic acid or another toxic substance in the grass. Although horses may improve after removal of the grass, signs will not totally resolve.

EHV-1 myeloencephalitis (see p. 550) causes vasculitis in the central nervous system. Pelvic limb ataxia is the most consistent sign; however, forelimb ataxia and cranial nerve deficits also occur. Urinary incontinence characterized by bladder paralysis (lower motor neuron) and excessive urethral resistance frequently occurs. Anal sphincter paralysis, perineal analgesia, and vulvar and penile paralysis occur uncommonly. Many animals with this condition improve and totally recover.

Lesions of the spinal tracts are the most common causes of neurogenic micturition disorders in horses. In some cases the causative neurological disease is permanent and progressive, rendering management of the incontinence impractical. In contrast, normal micturition may return in animals with reversible neurological diseases. Because complete recovery may require several weeks, temporary pharmacological management of the urinary incontinence is sometimes useful. Effective management depends on accurate evaluation of detrusor and sphincter function. Observation of micturition behavior and rectal examination are necessary parts of this evaluation. Cystometrograms and urethral pressure profiles have been used in the evaluation of a few incontinent horses. A complete neurological examination and, in some cases, cerebrospinal fluid analysis may help in the differential diagnosis of diseases that cause urinary incontinence. Because bacterial cystitis often occurs secondary to urine retention, urinalysis and urine culture should be performed.

CLINICAL SIGNS

Clinical signs of urinary incontinence are characterized by intermittent or continuous dribbling of small volumes of urine. Exercise and coughing may increase abdominal pressure and lead to urine spurting. In the presence of upper motor neuron lesions (cranial to sacral segments), rectal examination reveals variable bladder size and marked resistance to bladder evacuation. Urine dribbling is inconstant. Reflex bladder may develop in one to a few weeks. Lower motor neuron lesions result in an atonic, distended bladder. There is usually little resistance to manual evacuation of the bladder. Anal tone and perineal reflexes are usually absent in equids with lower motor neuron disorders.

MICTURITION TESTING

The cystometrogram and urethral pressure profile allow more specific evaluation of detrusor and urethral function when upper or lower motor neuron disease is the cause of incontinence. To obtain the cystometrogram, a urinary catheter is inserted into the bladder. The catheter is connected to a pressure transducer and an infusion pump via a three-way stopcock. Either air, sterile saline, or carbon dioxide is pumped into the bladder. As the bladder is filled, vesical pressure is recorded and when the threshold volume is reached, the micturition reflex occurs. Normally, the maximal contraction pressure is 60 to 120 cm H_2O. Decreased maximal contraction pressure could indicate paralysis of the detrusor muscle consistent with a lower motor neuron lesion. In addition, dysfunction of the detrusor muscle may result from excessive or prolonged distention.

The urethral pressure profile may also be valuable in evaluation of incontinence. A catheter is placed at the urethral sphincter and continuously infused with saline or carbon dioxide. The catheter is then withdrawn at a constant speed through the urethra. The maximal urethral pressure is 49.1 ± 19.4 cm H_2O. In horses with upper motor neuron disease, urethral resistance is usually increased and pressures are higher. Generally, lower motor neuron bladder paralysis results in urethral relaxation and lower pressures. In some cases of lower motor neuron disease, however, sympathetic activation of α-adrenergic receptors causes increased resistance to bladder evacuation.

THERAPY

There is no specific treatment for neuritis of the cauda equina, sorghum ataxia cystitis, or EHV-1 myeloencephalitis. Corticosteroids and other anti-inflammatory drugs are sometimes administered to horses with EHV-1 myeloencephalopathy (see p. 550). Other conditions such as bladder tumors, cystitis, calculi, and ectopic ureters should receive therapy appropriate for these conditions. In older mares with incontinence that cannot be related to specific neurogenic or nonneurogenic diseases, estradiol therapy (0.004 to 0.008 mg per kg given intramuscularly every other day) may be attempted.

The primary goal of treatment of urinary incontinence caused by neurological diseases is to assist micturition until neurological function returns. The bladder should be emptied by manual compression via rectal examination three to four times daily. Pharmacological manipulation may be beneficial to improve bladder function until neurological function is restored. Cholinergic agents are used to increase intravesical pressure. Bethanechol (0.025 to 0.075 mg per kg given subcutaneously every 8 hours) is the cholinergic agent of choice for detrusor atony. The dosage is variable and should be titrated for each patient. Salivation, abdominal pain, and lacrimation are rare side effects. Excessive resistance at the urethral sphincter may be decreased with α-adrenergic receptor blocking agents. Phenoxybenzamine (0.7 mg per kg given orally every 6 hours) is the drug used most often.

Supplemental Readings

Clark, E. S.: Cystometrography and urethral pressure profiles in healthy horse and pony mares. Am. J. Vet. Res. 48:552–555, 1987.
Madison, J. B. Estrogen-responsive urinary incontinence in an aged pony mare. Comp. Cont. Ed. Pract. Vet. 6:S390–S392, 1984.
McClure, J. J.: Paralytic Bladder. In Robinson, N. E., ed.: Current Therapy in Equine Medicine, 2nd ed. Philadelphia, Pa., W. B. Saunders, Co. 1987.

Polyuria
Robert H. Whitlock, KENNETT SQUARE, PENNSYLVANIA

Polyuria may result from either water or solute diuresis. In water diuresis, the urine specific gravity and urine osmolality are less than plasma (specific gravity less than 1.008, osmolality less than 280 mOsm) as a result of diabetes insipidus, nephrogenic diabetes insipidus, or psychogenic polydipsia. In solute diuresis, the urine specific gravity and osmolality are similar to plasma valves (1.008 to 1.012; 270 to 290 mOsm) as a result of solute load exceeding the tubular resorption mechanisms, for example, glucosuria in diabetes mellitus or tubular nephropathy. The diagnostic ruleouts for polyuria are listed in Table 1.

Primary diabetes insipidus results from decreased release of antidiuretic hormone (ADH) from the neurohypophysis. Release of ADH is controlled by many factors, but blood volume and plasma osmolality are most important. ADH is produced in the supraoptic and paraventricular nuclei of the hypothalamus and stored in the posterior pituitary. The most common cause of decreased ADH release in horses is enlargement of the pars intermedia from a pituitary tumor (secondary diabetes insipidus). Rare cases of primary idiopathic diabetes insipidus have been reported.

CLINICAL SIGNS

The primary signs noted by an owner include profuse polyuria and pronounced polydipsia. When sufficient water is not available, extreme thirst may cause abnormal behavior such as restlessness and drinking urine. The urine specific gravity is 1.008 or less, usually closer to 1.001. Polyuria should not be confused with pollakiuria

TABLE 1. DIFFERENTIAL DIAGNOSIS OF POLYURIA/POLYDIPSIA

Solute load related
   Diabetes mellitus
   Hyperadrenocortocoidism (Cushing's disease)
   Primary renal glycosuria
   Psychogenic salt consumption
Non-solute load related
   Diabetes insipidus
   Psychogenic diabetes insipidus
   Nephrogenic diabetes insipidus
   Pituitary diabetes insipidus
   Hyperaldosteronism (Addison's disease)
   Chronic renal disease

(frequent passage of urine with normal total volume). Pollakiuria is commonly seen in mares in estrus, or in horses with cystic calculi or cystitis. Although relatively rare, psychogenic polydipsia with resultant polyuria has been reported in horses. Affected animals consume extraordinary volumes of water and void vast quantities of very dilute urine.

The normal adult horse (weighing 530 kg) fed alfalfa hay and with access to water has an average urinary output of 15.6 liters per day with a mean specific gravity of 1.028 and osmolality of 1.040 mOsm per kg.

DIAGNOSIS

In chronic renal disease a two-thirds loss of functioning nephrons may result in polyuria but with fixation of urine specific gravity near the plasma specific gravity (1.008 to 1.012). If more than three fourths of the nephrons are nonfunctional, azotemia would be expected; thus, fixed specific gravity urine without azotemia occurs in the narrow window when inadequate nephrons are available to concentrate urine but homeostatic mechanisms compensate to excrete nitrogenous wastes, preventing azotemia. If the urine specific gravity is less than 1.008, nonsolute causes of polyuria should be considered.

Primary diabetes insipidus occurs in patients unable to synthesize or secrete adequate quantities of the antidiuretic hormone vasopressin. Vasopressin permits passive resorption of water from the collecting ducts of the nephron into the hypertonic medullary interstitium. The glomerular filtrate in the ascending loop of Henle is hypotonic (100 mOsm per kg), and without the specific action of ADH the glomerular filtrate is not able to be concentrated. A very dilute urine is produced and the horse is unable to conserve water during times of increased plasma osmolality (dehydration). In cases of diabetes insipidus, water deprivation will not result in an increased urine specific gravity or urine osmolality greater than plasma osmolality, but exogenous ADH should increase urine osmolality by 50 to 800 per cent. Partial ADH deficiency may also occur. The urine specific gravity in these horses would be expected to be very low (1.000 to 1.007), which helps differentiate the condition from chronic renal failure, in which the urine specific gravity is closer to 1.010.

In nephrogenic diabetes insipidus the renal tubules are nonresponsive to endogenous or exogenous ADH. Osmoregulatory mechanisms are normal, with ADH secretion occurring in response to increased plasma osmolality (dehydration). Both water deprivation and parenterally administered ADH do not increase urine osmolality. This defect may occur as a result of tubular immaturity or may be acquired with renal disease, drug intoxications, prolonged corticosteroid therapy, and metabolic disorders, including renal amyloidosis, hypokalemia, and hypercalcemia.

Psychogenic polydipsia or compulsive water drinking is rare in horses and is considered to be a mental disorder in humans. In chronic cases, the physiological mechanism may be further confused by the loss of ions in the renal medulla, reducing the solute concentration gradient (medullary washout), thus making it more difficult to distinguish psychogenic polydipsia from diabetes insipidus or nephrogenic diabetes insipidus. However, if the urine is maximally dilute (specific gravity of 1.001), psychogenic diabetes insipidus is likely.

Polyuria associated with an increased solute load is relatively easy to distinguish from other causes of polyuria. Persistent polyuria with heavy glucosuria is a consistent feature of hyperadrenocorticism (Cushing's disease), diabetes mellitus, and renal tubular glucosuria. In cases of psychogenic salt consumption, a good history is invaluable, along with an assessment of fractional sodium clearance.

WATER DEPRIVATION TESTS

Water deprivation is the first diagnostic approach to differentiate diabetes insipidus, nephrogenic diabetes insipidus and psychogenic polydipsia. The deprivation test stimulates release of endogenous ADH in response to increasing plasma osmolality due to restricted water intake. Since water deprivation can be life-threatening in animals with severe polyuria, the patient's clinical status needs to be monitored closely, including vital signs and mentation. If the horse is azotemic, the test is contraindicated. If the patient is not dehydrated, remove all access to water and catheterize the bladder to determine baseline urine specific gravity and urine osmolality, which should be compared to plasma osmolality. It is sound practice to include two to three control animals of the same size in the same test to make adequate comparisons that normalize the results for diet, temperature, and environmental conditions. At the conclusion of the test, water should be offered in small incremental amounts rather than by immediate free access. If allowed free access, horses often drink 60 to 70 per cent of their deficit within 30 to 60 minutes, which can lead to other complications such as colic.

Two approaches to the water deprivation test are possible. The first approach is to catheterize the bladder every 2 hours to monitor the urine specific gravity following removal of the water source. The patient and control horses' body weight, packed cell volume, total plasma protein (TPP), plasma osmolality, and blood ADH level should be monitored each time a urine sample is obtained. Maximal urine concentration is reached when less than a 5 per cent increase in urine osmolality occurs between 2-hour sampling. The second approach is to evaluate the urine and plasma osmolality at 24-hour intervals for a minimum of 48 hours and a maximum of 72 hours, provided there is no evidence of azotemia or other serious clinical problems prior to the test.

Near maximum urine specific gravity (1.050 ± 0.004) and urine osmolality (1648 ± 169 mOsm) can be achieved in most adult horses after 48 to 60 hours of water deprivation. Maximum urine specific gravity occurs following body weight loss of 12 to 15 per cent, which is often not reflected in a concurrent increase in packed cell volume but coincides with a moderate increase in TPP of approximately 1.2 gm per dl.

During the water deprivation test, plasma samples should be saved to determine plasma ADH concentration in comparison with that of the control horses. Normal concentrations of vasopressin are reported to be 1.5 ± 0.36 pg per ml and increase to 4.3 ± 1.12 pg per ml after 24 hours of water deprivation, during which time the plasma osmolality increases by 9 mOsm. The values for patients with diabetes insipidus should be substantially lower than those of the controls.

If the patient's urine becomes concentrated, psychogenic polydipsia is the most likely diagnosis. However, failure to concentrate urine leaves all three disorders as possible since medullary washout may obviate the countercurrent mechanism in psychogenic polydipsia, with the result that the patient is unable to adequately concentrate the urine.

ADH RESPONSE TEST

ADH in the form of pitressin tannate (40 to 80 units in oil) should be administered intramuscularly. Water intake and urine output should be monitored every 1 to 2 hours for 24 to 36 hours. If the condition is responsive to exogenous ADH, water consumption and urine output should decrease, with a concomitant increase in urine osmolality. A 24- to 48-hour baseline for comparison is strongly recommended. The response to ADH may last from 24 to 48 hours.

ADH in the form of vasopressin is administered intravenously. Urine and plasma osmolality are measured at 2-hour intervals. If the urine osmolality increases to 1.025 or more, diabetes insipidus is present. No change indicates nephrogenic diabetes insipidus, providing medullary washout of solutes has not occurred.

THERAPY

Treatment of primary diabetes insipidus should include exogenous ADH, i.e., pitressin tannate in oil given intramuscularly. This should decrease water consumption and increase concentration of urine for at least 24 hours. However, in the absence of renal disease, polyuria is most likely due to a pituitary tumor (Cushing's disease) in the older horse.

Supplemental Readings

Breukink, H., Van Wegen, P., and Schotman, A. J. H.: Idiopathic diabetes insipidus in a Welsh pony. Equine Vet. J., 15:284–287, 1983.
Brobst, D. F., and Bayly, W. M.: Responses of horses to a water deprivation test. J. Equine Vet. Sci., 2:51–56, 1982.
Buntain, B. J., and Coffman, J. R.: Polyuria and polydipsia in a horse induced by psychogenic salt consumption. Equine Vet. J., 13:266–268, 1981.
Falk, J. L.: Conditions producing psychogenic polydipsia in animals. Ann. N.Y. Acad. Sci., 157:569–589, 1969.
Genetzky, R. M., Loparc, F. V., and Ledet, A. E.: Clinical pathologic alterations in horses during a water deprivation test. Am. J. Vet. Res., 48:1007–1011, 1987.
Horvath, C., Ames, T., Metz, A., and Larson, V. L.: Adreno corticotropin-containing neoplastic cells in pars intermedia adenoma in a horse. J. Am. Vet. Med. Assoc., 192:367–371, 1988.
Houpt, K. A.: Thirst in horses: Physiological and psychological causes. Equine Pract., 9:28–30, 1987.
Houpt, K. A., Thornton, S. N., and Allen, W. R.: Vasopressin in dehydrated and rehydrated ponies. Physiol. Behav., 45:659–661, 1989.
Lage, A. L.: Nephrogenic diabetes insipidus in a dog. J. Am. Vet. Med. Assoc., 163:251–253, 1973.
Rumbaugh, G. E., Carlson G. P., and Harold, D.: Urinary production in the healthy horse and in horses deprived of feed and water. Am. J. Vet. Res., 43:735–737, 1982.
Sufit, E., Houpt, K. A., and Sweeting, M.: Physiological stimuli of thirst and drinking patterns in ponies. Equine Vet. J., 17:12–16, 1985.

Urinary Tract Neoplasia

Thomas J. Divers, ITHACA, NEW YORK

Primary neoplasia of the equine kidney is rare. The most common neoplasia is renal cell carcinoma, which is sporadically found in middle-aged or older horses. Tumors of the urinary bladder of the horse are even less common than tumors of the kidney, with the most common being a squamous cell carcinoma. A transitional cell carcinoma and a fibromatous polyp have been reported. All reported bladder tumors have been in horses more than 10 years old.

CLINICAL SIGNS AND DIAGNOSIS

The main clinical signs of a renal tumor are depression, anorexia, weight loss and hematuria. A palpable mass can often be detected on rectal palpation. Mucous membranes appear pale if the horse is anemic as a result of hematuria. Tumors usually involve only one kidney, so that renal failure and uremia are rare. Abdominal pain and diarrhea are probably the result of perirenal invasions by the neoplasm and widespread metastasis. The lungs, regional lymph nodes, and liver are most frequently involved by metastasis.

A tentative diagnosis can be based on clinical signs (especially if hematuria is present) and rectal examination findings. Ultrasound examination using a 3.5- or 5-MHz sector scanner is useful to determine the extent of renal and perirenal involvement. Neoplastic cells are occasionally found in the peritoneal fluid but have not been reported in the urine.

The clinical signs of bladder neoplasia are hematuria, pollakiuria, and weight loss. The tumor, usually easily palpated during rectal examination, is not as hard as a cystic calculus. It must be distinguished from the amorphous debris that accumulates in some horses with bladder paresis. Ultrasound examination per rectum may help distinguish among neoplasia, calculus, and amorphous debris. Definitive diagnosis can be made by biopsy of the mass during cystoscopic visualization. Metastasis occurs by local extension into the peritoneal cavity, via the lymphatics to iliac and sublumbar lymph nodes, or hematogenously to the lungs and other organs.

THERAPY

Treatment of renal tumors is rarely if ever attempted, although unilateral nephrectomy would be possible if early detection occurred. Successful long-term therapy of bladder tumors has not been reported. In one horse the neoplasm was removed from the bladder but the animal died 2 months later of abdominal adhesions and colic. 5-Fluorouracil° (100 mg in 50 ml of saline) for 4 days was used intracystically in treating one horse, but the neoplasm had spread beyond the bladder, which prevented an accurate assessment of the therapy.

Supplemental Readings

Fischer, A. T., Spier, S., Carlson, G. P., and Hackett, R. P.: Neoplasia of the equine urinary bladder as a cause of hematuria. J. Am. Vet. Med. Assoc., *186*:1294–1296, 1985.
West, H. J., Kelly, D. F., and Ritchie, H. E.: Renal carcinomatosis in a horse. Equine Vet. J., *19*:548–551, 1987.

°Fluorouracil, Roche Lab., Nutley, NJ

Acute Renal Failure

Thomas J. Divers, ITHACA, NEW YORK

Acute renal failure is characterized by a sudden decline in glomerular filtration rate (GFR) to the extent that clinical signs of uremia are observed. Hemodynamic, toxic, septic, and obstructive causes of acute renal failure have been identified.

Hemodynamic causes of acute renal failure are perhaps the most frequent in horses. Any condition that predisposes to hypotension or release of endogenous pressor agents may initiate hemodynamically mediated acute renal failure. The most common predisposing causes of this vasomotor nephropathy in the horse are acute diarrhea, disseminated intravascular coagulation (DIC), myositis, hemorrhagic crisis, heart failure, abdominal pain, and bacterial toxemia (for example, septic metritis). Bacterial toxins, consumptive coagulopathy, vasoactive amines, and hemodynamic alterations may all be involved in the pathogenesis. Acute tubular necrosis is the most pronounced microscopic finding. Severe renal cortical necrosis has also been described in association with presumed endotoxemia.

A hemolytic-uremic-like syndrome with acute glomerular lesions has also been described in the horse. Horses with this syndrome are usually oliguric or anuric. Intravascular hemolysis accompanies the acute renal failure.

Causes of nephrotoxic acute renal failure in the horse include aminoglycosides, vitamin K_3, heavy metals, mycotoxins, acorns, vitamin D, and phenylbutazone. Aminoglycoside nephrotoxicity is the most common of these and is most often observed when a predisposing condition has caused a prior decrease in GFR. Dehydration caused by excess fluid loss, for example diarrhea or inadequate intake of fluids, is the most common predisposing cause. Premature foals or foals less than 3 days old also seem quite susceptible, perhaps more a result of their potential for dramatic fluid shifts than because of any underdevelopment of nephron function.

CLINICAL SIGNS

The predominant clinical signs of acute renal failure are depression and anorexia. Less frequently noted clinical signs include brick-red mucous membranes, spontaneous hemorrhage, dysuria, discolored urine, edema, laminitis, diarrhea, seizures, and mild colic. Rectal examination may reveal an enlarged and edematous-feeling left kidney in about 50 per cent of horses with acute renal failure.

DIAGNOSIS

The diagnosis of acute renal failure in the horse is based on the history, clinical findings, laboratory findings, ultrasonography, and microscopy of kidney tissue. The most frequent electrolyte abnormalities include hyponatremia, hypochloremia, variable potassium levels depending on the acuteness of the disease, and variable calcium concentrations, with hypocalcemia being more common than hypercalcemia. Virtually all horses with acute renal failure are azotemic and most have urine osmolality close to the isosthenuric range (1.008 to 1.020). This combination of azotemia and low urine specific gravity is the most commonly used laboratory test for confirmation of renal failure. Abnormal fractional excretion of sodium and phosphate and enzymuria, while not vital in the diagnosis of acute renal failure, may be of some help in detecting renal disease prior to failure. Much has been written of the measurement of urinary enzymes and their use in detecting early renal disease produced by nephrotoxins. Enzyme levels increase after the administration of certain drugs, but some enzymes provide too sensitive a test and may result in unnecessary withdrawal of a needed therapeutic agent.

A renal biopsy is indicated in horses with acute renal failure only if the etiology is unknown or prognostic information is needed. The prognostic information gained from a renal biopsy in horses with acute renal failure may not be meaningful unless electron microscopy is available. The biopsy is best performed after ultrasonography of the right kidney.

THERAPY

Initial therapy for acute renal failure of any cause should consist of replacement of fluid deficits and correction of any electrolyte and acid–base abnormalities. Serum concentrations of sodium, chloride, potassium, and bicarbonate should be monitored daily and corrected as needed. Sodium and chloride replacement is often required in horses with polyuric acute renal failure. Bicarbonate therapy is more likely to be required as treatment for the predisposing cause of the acute renal failure than for the acute renal failure itself; many horses with acute renal failure have normal plasma bicarbonate concentrations. The serum potassium concentration in horses with acute renal failure is often normal and, except in the case of postrenal diseases caused by obstruction or urinary tract rupture, therapy intended to lower the serum potassium level is usually not needed. It is usually not necessary to correct the hypocalcemia that is often present in horses with acute renal failure.

After volume and electrolyte deficits have been corrected, an attempt should be made to determine if the acute renal failure is oliguric or polyuric, because fluid and sodium replacement in oliguric renal failure must be monitored carefully by daily measurement of body weight and monitoring of intravascular volume expansion by measurement of packed cell volume (PCV), total plasma protein concentrations, and central venous pressure, or by measurement of fluid input compared to fluid output. There is no convenient method of collecting all the urine voided in foals and mares, but this may be easily accomplished in the adult male horse with a urine collection device strapped around the abdomen. In mares, urine is collected by means of an indwelling Foley catheter emptying into a urine collection bag. Venous pressure is most easily monitored with an intravenous (IV) catheter placed through the jugular vein into the anterior vena cava and connected to a manometer held level with the right atrium. Normal central venous pressure is less than 8 cm H_2O.

Fluid and electrolyte replacement may be followed by an IV solution of 20 per cent mannitol (0.25 to 1.0 gm per kg) and the administration of furosemide (1.0 mg per kg every 2 hours) in horses with oliguric renal failure. The efficacy of furosemide, if any, may depend on administration early in the course of acute renal failure with the hope of increasing renal blood flow and glomerular filtration and tubular flow. Dopamine (3 to 5 μg per kg per minute) in 5 per cent dextrose can be given IV with furosemide in patients with anuric or severely oliguric acute renal failure in an attempt to improve renal blood flow and urinary output. Blood pressure should be monitored and must not become abnormally high during this infusion.

The majority of horses with acute renal failure resulting from acute tubular necrosis are more likely to be nonoliguric than oliguric after replacement of volume deficits and therefore require only 0.9 per cent isotonic NaCl or balanced-electrolyte fluids to cause a marked decrease in serum creatinine concentration. Horses with nonoliguric acute renal failure should be given 40 to 80 ml per kg per day of IV fluids until there is a precipitous drop in serum creatinine. Continuation with 10 to 20 ml per kg per day may then be required for a number of days until the creatinine concentration has returned to a normal or steady-state values and the horse is eating and drinking adequately. Serum creatinine should be measured again 2 to 4 days after fluid therapy is discontinued. Mannitol, furosemide, and dopamine are not necessary in most nonoliguric cases. If sedation for pain or anxiety is necessary, xylazine (0.4 to 0.8 mg to kg IV) may be used if IV fluid volume and blood pressure are near normal. Xylazine causes an increased urine production in normal horses. The addition of 50 to 100 gm of dextrose per liter of fluids will provide some needed calories to anorexic horses.

The administration of cyclooxygenase inhibitors may be important in treating the cause of hemodynamically mediated acute renal failure. They may help maintain a near normal mean arterial blood pressure when used early in horses with endotoxemia, but may also decrease intrarenal blood flow. If cyclooxygenase inhibitors are needed for the predisposing disease, for example sepsis, they are best used in low dosages (one-fifth to one-third normal dosage) in animals with acute renal failure resulting from hemodynamic causes, and only after correction of prerenal factors. At this dosage, the cyclooxygenase inhibitors may decrease thromboxane production without inhibiting urinary prostaglandin production. The treatment of coagulopathies associated with renal failure has not been sufficiently investigated in the horse to provide objective treatment data beyond those recommended for generalized DIC (see p. 504).

An important aspect of the treatment of nephrotoxic acute renal failure is to remove the nephrotoxic agent and/or correct the predisposing condition. Recovery from aminoglycoside toxicity can occur without withdrawal of the drug if the interval between treatments is lengthened to correlate with the rise in serum creatinine concentration and if predisposing causes, for example dehydration, are corrected. This should not be practiced unless the drug is absolutely necessary in treating an infectious condition.

Most horses with aminoglycoside or vitamin K nephrotoxicity are nonoliguric. In these patients, fluid therapy should be continued until the serum creatinine concentration has returned to steady-state values. The serum creatinine concentration should be monitored during aminoglycoside therapy and for 2 days after this therapy is discontinued since renal disease may progress to failure even after drug administration has been discontinued.

The use of hemodialysis has been reported in one horse with myoglobinuric acute renal failure. Peritoneal dialysis has been attempted in a few horses with nephrotoxic-induced acute renal failure; omental plugging of the catheter has limited its success in foals. Hemo- or peritoneal dialysis would most likely benefit horses with early nephrotoxic acute renal failure. Dialysis may be warranted in horses with aminoglycoside-induced acute renal failure if they remain oliguric and if plasma concentrations of the drug are greater than 1.5 μg per ml after the discontinuation of therapy. Electrolytes should be closely monitored during any dialysis therapy.

Lactated Ringer's solution with 1.5 per cent dextrose warmed to above body temperature may be used for peritoneal dialysis. If there are no cardiopulmonary abnormalities, up to 40 ml per kg of the dialysis fluid can be administered intraperitoneally. After 30 minutes, the initial fluid should be removed and fresh fluid instilled. At least 70 per cent of the dialysis fluid must be recovered in order to continue with the procedure.

PROGNOSIS

The prognosis for acute renal failure in the horse can be provided after identifying the cause, the duration of the renal disease, and determination of the amount of urine production (oliguric or nonoliguric). Acute renal failure due to nephrotoxic causes, with the exception of heavy metals, usually has the best prognosis. Horses with aminoglycoside and vitamin K_3 nephrotoxicity are usually polyuric. Although the condition persists for several days and serum creatinine concentrations are often greater than 10 mg per dl, these horses, with appropriate therapy, usually have a very favorable prognosis. Those with oliguria have a very poor prognosis despite dialysis.

The prognosis for hemodynamically mediated acute renal failure is the most variable. If the predisposing factors such as diarrhea, sepsis, hemorrhagic episodes, and myositis are controlled, the prognosis for complete recovery is usually fair to good. Except for renal cortical necrosis, the predominant damage to the kidney from vasomotor nephropathy is usually tubular, and recovery can be expected if the basement membrane has remained intact and appropriate early therapy is provided. Horses that show no clinical improvement of the predisposing factors after appropriate therapy or those with oliguria have a guarded to poor prognosis.

Regardless of the cause, the duration of illness prior to the beginning of fluid and solute therapy is of the utmost importance. Early therapy may prevent the further development of acute renal failure to a state that is no longer reversible by routine medical therapy. Horses that have been experiencing acute renal failure for several days without treatment may develop irreversible nephron damage, a decrease in functional nephron number, and suffer from chronic renal disease and failure despite the institution of intensive therapy. In the majority of cases, the serum creatinine concentration will stabilize or even decrease after 24 hours of fluid therapy. However, the initial decline in serum creatinine concentration may reflect only a reconstituting or an expanding of body fluid volume. Only with a progressive decline in serum creatinine concentration over several days does the prognosis become favorable. Horses with marked renal enlargement or perirenal edema based on rectal or ultrasound examination appear to have a worse prognosis than those without such findings. Secondary complications of diarrhea, laminitis, hemolysis, and encephalitic signs are not uncommon in horses with acute renal failure, and, if severe, lessen the chance of survival.

Supplemental Readings

Bayly, W. M., Brobst, D. F., Elfers, R. S., and Reed, S. M.: Serum and urinary biochemistry and enzyme changes in ponies with acute renal failure. Cornell Vet., 76:306, 1986.

Divers, T. J., Whitlock, R. H., Crowell, W. A., et al.: Acute renal failure in six horses resulting from hemodynamic causes. Equine Vet. J., 19:178, 1987.

MacKay, J., French, T. W., Nguyen, H. T., and Mayhew, I. G.: Effects of large doses of phenylbutazone administration to horses. Am. J. Vet. Res., 44:774, 1983.

Markel, M. D., Dyer, R. M., and Hattel, A. L.: Acute renal failure associated with application of mercuric blister in a horse. J. Am. Vet. Med. Assoc., 185:92, 1984.

Morris, C. F., Robertson, J. L., Mann, P. C., Clark, S., and Divers, T. J.: Hemolytic uremic syndrome in two horses. J. Am. Vet. Med. Assoc., 191:1453, 1987.

Rebhun, W. C., Tennant, B. C., Dill, S. G., and King, J. M.: Vitamin K3 induced renal toxicosis in the horse. J. Am. Vet. Med. Assoc., 184:1237, 1984.

Riviere, J. E., Traver, D. S., and Coppoc, G. L.: Gentamicin toxic nephropathy in horses with disseminated bacterial infection. J. Am. Vet. Med. Assoc., 180:648, 1980.

Renal Tubular Acidosis

Yves Rossier, ST-HYACINTHE, QUEBEC

Renal tubular acidosis is characterized by abnormal renal tubular function. The condition typically results in metabolic acidosis with hyperchloremia. Substantial renal insufficiency is usually absent. Several types of renal tubular acidosis have been described in humans. Proximal tubular acidosis (type II) occurs when the proximal tubules are unable to adequately reabsorb urinary bicarbonate, resulting in excessive urinary losses of bicarbonate. As hydrogen ions are normally secreted when bicarbonate is reabsorbed, acidosis results. However, as the kidney does not lose its ability to acidify urine in the distal tubules, the degree of acidosis may be limited. Distal renal tubular acidosis (type I) occurs when the distal tubules are unable to excrete enough hydrogen ions, resulting in inability to maximally acidify urine. Another form of renal tubular acidosis (type IV) described in humans entails inadequate secretion of both potassium and hydrogen ions by the distal tubule.

Distal renal tubular acidosis (type I) and proximal renal tubular acidosis (type II) have been described in the horse. Type IV has not been described. Types I and II renal tubular acidosis may be primary or secondary, depending on whether another systemic disease is associated with the illness. Secondary renal tubular acidosis may be found in association with diarrhea and renal disease in horses.

CLINICAL SIGNS AND DIAGNOSIS

Horses with renal tubular acidosis may present with clinical signs of depression, weight loss, weakness, anorexia, or mild chronic abdominal pain. Physical examination is usually unremarkable other than the poor body condition.

Hyperchloremic metabolic acidosis without clinical signs associated with other causes of metabolic acidosis, such as gastrointestinal disease, renal failure, tying up, acid administration, and so forth, is highly suggestive of renal tubular acidosis. The serum chloride concentration may reach 120 mEq per L, while the blood pH and the plasma bicarbonate concentration may be as low as 7.0 and 10.0 mEq per L, respectively. Some horses may be hypokalemic. Most horses also have an alkaline urine despite the severe metabolic acidosis. It must be remembered that herbivores normally have an alkaline urine.

Further diagnostic tests include urine specific gravity, urine osmolarity, and water consumption to rule out other renal diseases. Urine acidification in response to oral NH_4Cl loading has been used to document cases of renal tubular acidosis in humans, dogs, and horses. Administration of 0.1 gm of NH_4Cl per kg body weight in 6 liters of water by nasogastric tube is followed by urine pH measurements every hour for 6 hours. Bladder catheterization, emptying of the bladder, and subsequent sample collection are necessary. Normal horses show a significant decrease in urinary pH to 6.5 at 4 hours, whereas horses with renal tubular acidosis will show minimal urinary pH change. The magnitude of the acidification is less than in humans or dogs, in which a urinary pH of less than 5.5 is considered to be a normal response to the above test. The test should not be performed if the animal is acidemic (arterial pH less than 7.38).

TREATMENT

The main therapeutic goal is correction of the electrolyte and acid–base abnormalities. The bicarbonate deficit may be calculated using the formula:

$$0.3 \text{ or } 0.4 \times (BW \text{ kg}) \times (Base \text{ deficit})$$

The deficit may be corrected by intravenous (IV) administration of isotonic bicarbonate or by polyionic replacement fluid administration supplemented with bicarbonate. Half the calculated deficit should be administered rapidly, the other half given more slowly (over 24 to 36 hours). Once the blood pH and the base deficit values have been corrected, oral bicarbonate administration (150 gm orally twice per day) may be necessary for maintenance purposes.

Once the acidosis has been corrected, potassium supplementation is also usually necessary because of the intracellular potassium shift. Initially, potassium chloride administered IV should not exceed 100 to 150 mEq per hour in the adult horse. Oral potassium supplementation (40 gm KCl per 4 to 6 liters of water via nasogastric tube two or three times a day) can also be used. Once appetite resumes, potassium supplementation may not be necessary, as hay contains high potassium concentrations.

Some horses have recovered spontaneously; others have required long-term bicarbonate supplementation (50 to 75 gm of bicarbonate in the feed twice per day for up to 20 to 28 months).

Supplemental Readings

Hansen, T. O.: Renal tubular acidosis in a mare. Compend. Cont. Educ. Pract. Vet., 8:864, 1986.

Polzin, D., Osborne, C., and O'Brien, T.: Renal tubular acidosis. In Ettinger, S. J. (ed.): Textbook of Veterinary Internal Medicine 3rd ed. Philadelphia, W. B. Saunders, 1989, pp. 2026–2027.

Rocher, L. L., and Tannen, R. L.: The clinical spectrum of renal tubular acidosis. Annu. Rev. Med., 37:319–331, 1986.

Trotter, G. W., Miller, T., Parks, A., and Arden, W.: Type II renal tubular acidosis in a mare. J. Am. Vet. Med. Assoc., 188:1050–1051, 1986.

Ziemer, E. L., Parker, H. R., Carlson, G. P., and Smith, B. P.: Clinical features and treatment of renal tubular acidosis in two horses. J. Am. Vet. Med. Assoc., 190:294–296, 1987.

Ziemer, E. L., Parker, H. R., Carlson, G. P., Smith, B. P., and Ishizaki, G.: Renal tubular acidosis in two horses: Diagnostic studies. J. Am. Vet. Med. Assoc., 190:289–293, 1987.

Chronic Renal Failure

Robert H. Whitlock, KENNETT SQUARE, PENNSYLVANIA

Chronic progressive renal failure is most often associated with extensive loss of nephron function. Systemic signs such as weight loss, anorexia, or poor physical condition are rarely associated with renal disease unless more than 75 per cent of renal function is lost. Examples of these uncommon diseases are septic nephritis, pyelonephritis, and renal neoplasia. Chronic renal failure may be subdivided in two broad clinicopathological classifications: glomerular disease and tubulo-interstitial disease. However, since the nephron is a single functioning unit, disease processes affecting glomeruli will secondarily affect the tubule, and vice versa; the end result is loss of nephron function. Histologically it is often difficult to determine if the original lesion was glomerular or tubular. The collective literature on equine kidney disease suggests that glomerular lesions predominate as the cause of chronic renal failure. Generally, horses with chronic renal failure are over 5 years of age. If the horse is less than 5 years old, renal hypoplasia is more likely than renal failure.

Renal disease with a progressive nephron loss leads to a decrease in glomerular filtration rate (GFR). With the reduction in GFR, protein metabolic byproducts, including urea and creatinine, are retained, giving rise to the clinical syndrome of uremia. Other metabolic byproducts may be retained or preferentially excreted, contributing to the multisystemic disease state, uremia. Electrolytes, including sodium, chloride, and phosphorus, which are normally reabsorbed by the tubular epithelium are excreted in the urine in chronic renal failure, resulting in decreased serum or plasma concentrations. Polyuric horses with chronic renal failure often have increased concentrations of sodium, chloride, and phosphorus in the urine. Other ions such as calcium, magnesium, potassium, and hydrogen may be retained during chronic progressive renal failure, leading to the syndrome of acidosis, hyperkalemia, and hypercalcemia. Progressive nephron loss results in decreased ability to concentrate urine, leading to polyuria and secondary polydipsia. With progression of the disease the animal is often unable to compensate for the polyuria with polydipsia and is predisposed to dehydration and hypovolemia. If unrecognized, this critical clinical situation leads to a continued decline in GFR and eventual death.

Acid–base values are variable in horses with chronic renal failure. Most horses are normal or only mildly acidemic in the early phases of the disease. However, as the disease progresses and becomes more severe, with a further decrease in GFR there is a greater tendency to develop metabolic acidosis. Occasionally some horses will become hypochloremic, predisposing them to metabolic alkalosis. Progressive uremia often results in gradually decreased hematopoiesis leading to a mild anemia (packed cell volume = 20 to 30 per cent). Occasionally horses will develop oral ulceration in the center of the tongue and along the buccal surfaces. A uremic odor to the breath and excessive dental tartar are common findings in the more advanced stages of chronic progressive renal failure. Obese horses are predisposed to developing hyperlipidemia as the uremia interferes with peripheral removal of triglyceride.

ETIOLOGY

By the time most cases of progressive renal failure are clinically recognized, the cause is almost impossible to determine. A number of conditions and disease processes may predispose to the development of chronic progressive renal failure. These conditions include aminoglycoside antibiotic administration, vitamin K administration, heavy metal administration (especially mercury), intravascular hemolysis releasing free hemoglobin, severe muscle necrosis with release of myoglobin, and immune-mediated glomerular diseases. An excellent history from the owner is needed to elicit potential exposure to a specific nephrotoxin that may predispose to the development of chronic renal failure. Chronic renal failure in young horses may be secondary to equine infectious anemia or streptococcal infections. Other pathological causes include amyloidosis, congenital abnormalities such as polycystic kidneys and renal hypoplasia, obstructive nephropathy, pyelonephritis, and, rarely, neurologic diseases that interfere with normal bladder function.

CLINICAL SIGNS

Unexplained chronic weight loss with partial anorexia and depression is the most frequent clinical sign associated with chronic renal failure. Other clinical signs include polyuria; laminitis; dysuria; strangury; fever; oral, mucosal, and tongue erosions or ulcers; excess dental tartar; and abnormally dark manure. If the horse is hypoproteinemic, ventral subcutaneous edema extending to distal extremities is a common but inconsistent finding that may occur prior to the onset of azotemia. Polyuria and polydipsia are frequent signs of chronic progressive renal failure but, like oral ulceration or a fetid mouth odor, often remain undetected by the owner. A complete physical examination should include rectal examination to determine the size, shape, and consistency of the left kidney and both ureters. It is not possible to palpate the right kidney except in unusual circumstances. In many types of chronic renal disease the palpable left kidney is smaller than normal but non-painful. In cases of ureteral obstruction, enlargement of the ureter may be due to pyelonephritis, lymphosarcoma, renal carcinoma, or ureterolithiasis. Renal enlargement may occur in horses with renal carcinoma, polycystic kidney disease, and in unusual cases of chronic pyelonephritis.

DIAGNOSIS

The most frequent blood chemistry abnormalities include azotemia with increased creatinine and blood urea nitrogen (BUN) concentrations. However, in horses with a normal appetite and water intake, these abnormalities may be relatively modest. In horses with renal decompensation, the severity of the uremia may be more readily apparent with creatinine concentrations exceeding 10 to 15 mg per dl. Hypercalcemia (greater than 13 mg per dl) with hypophosphatemia is a classic and unique sign of equine renal failure. Horses on a high calcium ration are more prone to develop hypercalcemia, which may occur with either acute or chronic renal failure. The anemia, if present, is usually moderate in horses with chronic progressive renal failure. The plasma protein concentration is quite variable in chronic progressive renal failure but commonly is low (less than 6.0 gm per dl), often in the range of 4 to 5 gm per dl if dependent edema is present and or in the presence of moderate to heavy proteinuria. The plasma protein concentration may be markedly elevated (up to 10 gm per dl) in horses with chronic inflammatory diseases such as pyelonephritis. Nonspecific yet characteristic clinicopathological changes include hypercholesterolemia, hyperlipidemia, hyponatremia, hypochloremia, hypoglycemia, hyperkalemia, and typically metabolic acidosis or alkalosis if the horse is sufficiently hypochloremic.

Horses with chronic renal failure are usually isothenuric (specific gravity range: 1.008 to 1.014); however, with a heavy proteinuria the specific gravity may exceed 1.014 yet may still be compatible with chronic progressive renal failure. The normal urine specific gravity must be interpreted with due consideration of the horse's hydration status. Severely dehydrated animals may have higher urine specific gravity if adequate renal reserve is present. However, isothenuria with dehydration is indicative of serious loss of renal function. The presence of cellular or hyaline casts is more suggestive of acute renal disease than of chronic progressive renal failure. However, numerous leukocytes and bacteria are expected in chronic pyelonephritis, one cause of chronic progressive renal failure. Horses with renal carcinoma often have gross or microscopic hematuria, which on rare occasions has been associated with renal failure.

Inulin clearance is the reference standard for determining GFR but is not readily measured by practitioners. Sodium sulfanilate clearance provides a reasonable alternative but mildly underestimates the values obtained by inulin clearance testing since serum chromogens may falsely increase the concentration of sulfanilate.

Both BUN and serum creatinine concentration are insensitive indices of reduced GRF until nearly 75 per cent of the glomeruli are nonfunctional, then both are sensitive to further reductions in GFR. The serum creatinine concentration is the most reliable index of GFR for the practitioner; values of 10 to 12 mg per dl represent significant reductions in renal function and a guarded prognosis. Values above 16 to 18 mg indicate a grave prognosis. Marked elevations in creatinine usually accompany anion gap values greater than 15 mEq per L; both correlate with a poorer prognosis.

Further assessment of renal failure should include ultrasonography to evaluate renal size (e.g., a smaller kidney than normal), to find evidence of a stone in the renal calyces, or to detect a mass suggestive of a neoplasm. Ultrasonographically, kidneys with chronic progressive renal failure are smaller than normal. There is poor differentiation of the cortex and medulla, often with increased echogenicity of the collecting tubules, most likely due to mineralization. Renal calculi are recognized from their location in the renal pelvis or calyces and from their nearly complete acoustic shadow over the deeper tissues. Renal biopsy should be performed only if the degree of renal failure is uncertain and it is necessary to attempt an etiological diagnosis. Rarely will the biopsy results enhance the therapeutic approach.

THERAPY

Therapy is primarily supportive since it is rarely possible to restore nephron function in horses with chronic progressive renal failure. In some horses with mild renal decompensation there may be an acute component caused by inflammation, drug usage, or obstruction of the urinary tract. Correction of these clinical problems may allow a modest increase in renal function to ameliorate the clinical signs of renal failure. Horses with chronic pyelonephritis should be treated with antibiotics that follow microbiological sensitivity patterns, are concentrated in the urine, and are effective at that urine pH. Trimethoprim–sulfa is often the most appropriate antimicrobial combination. Nephrotomy to remove obstructing calculi in the renal pelvis and proximal ureter should be considered in horses with confirmed calculi but only after full evaluation of residual renal function.

Horses with chronic renal failure, especially hypercalcemic animals, benefit from lowered calcium intake. This is best accomplished by providing a grass hay diet with grain comprised primarily of oats and corn. If the patient is hypoproteinemic, protein supplements of linseed or soybean meal should be recommended. Legume forages should not be fed because of the high calcium content. Patients with plasma protein concentrations less than 4.5 gm per dl and with prominent edema often benefit from plasma transfusions. Three to five liters of plasma given intravenously will increase the blood plasma given protein concentration by 1.0 gm per dl in a 500-kg horse and help restore the oncotic pressure to relieve the edema.

Supportive medical care should also include oral or parenteral fluid therapy to promote diuresis, thus reducing the accumulated load of uremic metabolic byproducts. Repeated nasogastric intubation and administration of a balanced electrolyte solution containing 2 per cent glucose may be adequate to promote diuresis and reduce the azotemia. However, parenteral isotonic fluids specifically designed to correct the existing metabolic derangements are preferable if the economics warrant and the facilities are available. Upwards of 30 to 80 liters per day may be required for 5 to 7 days to reduce the creatinine concentration to normal levels. Once the azotemia is corrected the clinician needs to assess whether the horse can maintain food and water intake with minimal increase in serum creatinine. If the serum creatinine cannot be maintained, a more critical assessment needs to be made regarding possible restoration of renal function or at least compensation for azotemia by increasing oral fluid intake. In a small proportion of patients it may be possible to stabilize the patient for a number of weeks, until foaling for example. The final prognosis for progressive chronic renal failure is often grave, but the clinician must weigh all the available evidence before recommending euthanasia.

Supplemental Readings

Bertone, J. J., Traub-Dargatz, J. L., Fettman, M. J., Wilke, L., Wrigley, R. H., Jaenke, R., and Paulsen, M. E.: Monitoring the progression of chronic renal failure in a horse with polycystic kidney disease: Use of the reciprocal of serum creatinine concentration and sodium sulfanilate clearance half-time. J. Am. Vet. Med. Assoc., 191:565–568, 1987.
Divers, T. J.: Chronic renal failure in horses. Compend. Cont. Educ. Pract. Vet., 5:5310–5317, 1983.
Ehnen, S. J., Divers, T. J., Gillette, D., and Reef, V. B.: Obstructive nephrolithiasis and ureterolithiasis associated with chronic renal failure in horses: eight cases (1981–1987). J. Am. Vet. Med. Assoc., 197:249-253, 1990.
Kohn, C. W., and Chew, D. J.: Laboratory diagnosis and characterization of renal disease in horses. Vet. Clin. North Am. (Equine Pract.), 35:585–615, 1987.
Ralston, S. L.: Clinical nutrition of adult horses. Vet. Clin. North Am., 6:339–354, 1990.

Rantanen, N. W.: Diseases of the kidney. Vet. Clin. North Am. (Equine Pract.) 2:89–103, 1986.

Riviere, J. E., Traver, D. S., and Coppoc, G. L.: Gentamicin toxic nephropathy in horses with disseminated bacterial infection. J. Am. Vet. Med. Assoc., *180*:648–651, 1982.

Tennant, B., Bettleheim, P., Kaneko, J. J.: Paradoxical hypercalcemia and hypophosphatemia associated with chronic renal failure in horses. J. Am. Vet. Med. Assoc., *180*:630–634, 1982.

Tennant, B. C., Kaneko, J. J., Lowe, J. E., et al.: Chronic renal failure in the horse. *In:* Proceedings of the 24th Annual Convention of the American Association of Equine Practitioners, 1978, pp. 293–298.

Section 15

REPRODUCTION

Edited by Gordon L. Woods

Sexual Behavior Dysfunction in Mares

Sue M. McDonnell, KENNETT SQUARE, PENNSYLVANIA

The equine mare is infamous among the domestic species for "normal peculiarities" of reproductive physiology and behavior. Although many instances of problematic reproductive behavior in mares represent normal variations in estrus cyclicity and seasonality, some cases do represent abnormal behavior and need special evaluation and management. The veterinarian's role in this regard includes (1) understanding and communicating to clients the unique reproductive physiology and behavior of the mare, with suggestions for efficient management, and (2) detecting the unusual behavior that may represent a true behavioral problem or underlying pathology.

The greatest challenge in the behavioral evaluation of horses may be sorting out the history. Commonly the facts are nested within complex, often anthropomorphic, interpretative narratives. Terms such as "psychic heat," "nymphomania," "homosexual," or "outlaw," while used freely among horse owners, managers, and veterinarians, can convey an array of widely different meanings. Although there are specific clusters of behavioral responses that might quite loosely be referred to with such terms, their use in general can be confusing. For example, the term "aggressive" may be applied to several different types of behavior, such as strongly proceptive or solicitous estrus, male-type sexual behavior (teasing, herding, mounting), failure to stand for breeding, or interfemale aggression (bossiness at the feed bunk). Therefore, in evaluating reproductive behavior, it is most efficient to describe specific behavioral responses rather than accept a general descriptive term. Video recordings of the horse exhibiting the undesirable behavior are invaluable in identifying the specific problem. When the specific behavioral complaints are identified, the practitioner frequently finds a much simpler problem fitting into one of the following general categories.

ABNORMAL ESTRUS

FAILURE TO SHOW ESTRUS

Some mares fail to show estrus during the ovulatory season. In a small proportion, a tightly closed cervix and the presence of a corpus luteum suggest that a persistent corpus luteum is responsible for failure to show estrus and ovulate. In most of these mares, lysis of the corpus luteum will permit resumption of normal cyclical ovulation and estrus. The majority of mares that fail to show estrus during the ovulatory season, however, are actually cycling, as indicated by palpable cyclic follicular and cervical changes. Critical information on the steroid levels in such mares is lacking, but the interovulatory interval is usually normal, suggesting that steroid levels are normal. These cycling mares may "break down" after prolonged or creative teasing. Some mares will show estrus to one stallion and not another; others show markedly different behavior in different teasing situations. In general, such mares will more readily signal estrus if teased in an unrestrained as opposed to haltered situation. For example, a mare that does not show typical estrus with conventional in-hand or stall teasing may reliably signal estrus if placed in a paddock with the stallion presented at the fence line or pastured in a neighboring paddock. This situation expands the possible behavioral signals of estrus to some of the more subtle yet reliable indicators of sexual interest, notably approaching or lingering near the stallion. The teasing necessary for some mares may take considerable time and effort and therefore may not be practical. Managers of large brood mare populations often find it more efficient to place all "no show" mares on schedules of regular transrectal ovarian palpation and ultrasonography of the reproductive organs.

Less commonly, exposure to steroids may be responsible for failure to show estrus among mares with normal ovaries. Recently retired racing or performance mares that have received androgenic anabolic steroids often do not show normal estrus, even when the ovaries appear to be undergoing normal cyclic changes. Experimental findings confirm that at near recommended doses, boldenone undecylenate suppresses estrus without altering ovarian activity. At higher doses boldenone undecylenate also suppresses ovarian activity. However, even when ovarian activity resumes after treatment has been withdrawn, estrous behavior remains suppressed. Failure to show estrus despite normal ovarian activity may also occur in mares in early stages of hormone-secreting ovarian tumors (granulosa cell tumors).

FAILURE TO STAND FOR BREEDING

Some mares show estrus when teased but refuse to stand for breeding. They appear anxious as the stallion approaches, particularly if the stallion is aggressive or loud. Some "explode" when the stallion mounts. Many such mares reportedly become worse when restrained. Examination of the reproductive organs and endocrine profiles do not provide a ready explanation for the behavior. Observations of free-running wild and domestic horses suggest that under natural field breeding conditions, mares may show mild estrus for many days before actual breeding occurs. Stallions may mount many times during this period, as though testing the receptivity of the mare. Mares sometimes walk or run away from the stallion as he mounts. But explosively repulsive reactions of mares are not common under field breeding conditions. In the domestic situation, it is reasonable to expect that many such problems result from or are aggravated by management factors, including improper time for breeding, inadequate socialization of the mare during development, or fear induced by restraint during breeding. In some cases this behavior seems complicated by the presence of a foal at side during breeding. These explanations have not been systematically studied.

EXCESSIVE OR INAPPROPRIATE ESTRUS

A common complaint regarding mare behavior is too frequent, too intense, or inappropriate estrous behavior. These problems for the most part fall into one of six different groups.

Prolonged or Frequent Irregular Estrus

Prior to the first ovulation of the breeding season, most mares experience either a prolonged continuous or a split estrous period. For most mares this transition period consists of several days in estrus, a few days out, and then back in, with no definite pattern. This behavioral phenomenon is probably related to the waves of follicular growth that occur before the first ovulation of the season. Although most mares begin seasonal cyclic ovulation between March and May in the northern hemisphere, some mares do not commence seasonal cyclicity until June. Treatment regimens designed to synchronize ovulation among transitional mares with active ovaries have proved a relatively efficient method of managing mares during the transitional period. Prolonged or frequent irregular estrus also occurs outside the transitional period and may be traceable to ovarian granulosa cell tumors, although more often granulosa cell tumors are associated with failure to show estrus and/or male-type behavior. Finally, a small number of mares for unknown reasons show a mild estrus or an absence of diestrus when teased, in this respect resembling ovariectomized mares. These same mares show normal-intensity estrus in association with ovulation. The reproductive management problem underscores the importance of familiarity with the individual mare's response to teasing.

Short Cycles

Some mares reported to be "always in heat" in fact are experiencing estrus of normal length, but at a greater than normal frequency. Short ovarian cycles, that is, interovulatory intervals of 10 to 12 days, do occur in mares, but the actual estrous periods are usually of normal duration and the diestrous period is shortened. One of the most likely causes of short ovulatory cycles is chronic or recurring endometritis. Although fertilization may be normal, early pregnancy loss occurs, possibly in association with demise of the corpus luteum or abnormal conceptus–endometrium interaction.

Winter Estrus

Although ovarian function in most mares is quiescent during winter, some continue to cycle regularly throughout the year. Estrus during winter is a potential problem in mares with estrus-related performance problems.

Estrus During Pregnancy

It is relatively rare for a mare to show estrus for a prolonged period during pregnancy or after the first expected estrus following breeding. Since progesterone is an effective suppressor of estrus in mares, estrus during pregnancy is an unusual phenomenon that cannot be readily explained. There is some evidence that estrus during pregnancy is associated with low progesterone levels. Recent research suggests that mares carrying female foals are more likely to show estrus during pregnancy than those carrying male foals.

Extremely Intense Estrus

Mares vary considerably in the intensity of estrus. For example, some mares reliably show estrus in response to other mares or even to people. These mares, although usually the breeding farm manager's delight, often are a problem during training or performance. Most mares can be controlled with normal discipline and training under show or performance conditions, but extreme cases will show estrus even under saddle. Treatment with progestogens may effectively suppress estrus.

Other Behaviors Resembling Estrus

Some mares exhibit a submissive cowering and urine-squirting behavioral sequence that is easily mistaken for estrus. In addition, some mares in pain tend to frequently lift the tail, also sometimes mistaken for estrus. If such mares are teased daily with a stallion through one or more estrous cycles, their true estrus, distinct from the submissive behavior, can usually be differentiated. Clitoral winking, full urination, and breeding posture are usually not elements of the behavior, associated with pain. Another distinguishing aspect is that submissive cowering and urination can be elicited by any threatening situation, e.g., other mares or people, while estrous posture and urination are usually more pronounced in response to a stallion.

ESTROUS CYCLE–RELATED PERFORMANCE PROBLEMS

A relatively common complaint of trainers and riders is variable performance or trainability of mares related to the estrous cycle. In addition to undesirable estrus in performance situations, complaints include periods of deterioration, either mild or marked, in performance or temperament associated with a particular stage of the ovarian cycle. Some mares are hyperexcitable and difficult to handle at certain stages of the cycle. Some appear particularly sensitive to weight or manipulation that might affect the area of the ovaries during the periovulatory period of the cycle. Cases of coliclike discomfort associated with ovulation have been reported. In some cases the problem behavior is associated with the diestrous phase of the cycle, but in most it is associated with estrus or ovulation. The riders and trainers may report that the mare experiences abnormally frequent or long estrous periods. In a number of cases such behavior has been associated with short cycles.

Performance and training problems are part of the complex array of human–animal interactions that are difficult to evaluate objectively. The history of the problem and the various corrective measures that have been attempted may be difficult to elicit. However, in several cases we have systematically evaluated sexual behavior, performance behavior, general handling behavior, ovarian activity, and steroid hormones over two or more cycles. Significant changes in temperament, trainability, and tractability can occur in association with apparently normal ovarian cycles and estrus. In most instances estrus was associated with changes in temperament and tractability, that resulted in less desirable performance. However, in two recent cases the problem behavior was associated with diestrus.

The underlying reasons for cycle-related performance problems are incompletely understood and therapeutic recommendations are limited. After careful observation of the problem behavior and endocrine and physical examination to rule out pathological conditions requiring attention, one might consider progesterone therapy for mares whose problems are associated with estrus. Either progesterone in oil or any of several synthetic progestin preparations have been used. There seems to be considerable individual mare variation in the behavioral response to different products and doses. During estrus, human chorionic gonadotropin can be used to hasten ovulation (see p. 637). For mares whose problem behavior is associated with diestrus, repeated short cycling with prostaglandin may be useful (see p.

638). Long-acting tranquilizers have also proved useful in a number of cases. Ovariectomy remains a controversial treatment for cases of estrous cycle–related performance problems.

STALLIONLIKE BEHAVIOR

Male sexual behavior responses are not a normal part of mare behavior. For example, while it is normal for cows to mount other cows, it is unusual for mares to mount other horses. Any persistent male-typical behavior, such as posture and gait, vocalization pattern, herding, teasing, elimination-marking behavior, copulatory responses, or intermale aggression, in a mare should be viewed as abnormal. Such behavior suggests the presence, at one time or another, of abnormally high androgen levels. The two most common sources of androgen associated with stallionlike behavior in mares are exogenous steroids, such as testosterone, estrogen, or androgenic anabolic steroids, and ovarian tumors. Stallionlike behavior often persists for weeks to months after the source of androgen has been removed and measurable circulating androgens have returned to normal mare levels. However, the intensity of male-type behavior usually subsides within a few weeks after removal of androgen.

In some cases, stallionlike behavior has emerged during pregnancy. In the few cases seen in our clinic, the abnormal behavior was first noticed during the fourth or fifth month of gestation, continued until parturition, then ceased. Total plasma androgens are normally elevated during the middle trimester in mares as a result of fetal–placental steroid activity. These steroids are usually in a bound form and are not associated with behavioral or conformational masculinization. So the stallionlike behavior in the occasional mare is difficult to explain. Owners find male-type behavior especially disturbing in pregnant mares. Such mares may actively herd and mount other mares and, if separated from mares, may run fence lines or otherwise become disturbed by mares just as stallions do. Behavior usually returns to normal following parturition. We have also encountered pregnant mares with stallionlike behavior in which a granulosa cell tumor was found and believed to be responsible for the androgenization.

In our experience, mares with levels of androgens of exogenous or endogenous origin greater than 0.1 ng per ml in our assay system usually exhibit male-type behavior. Not all of the anabolic steroid preparations currently used in horses are routinely detectable in the common radioimmunoassay systems in use in referral laboratories.

ABERRANT MATERNAL BEHAVIOR

A rare yet urgent reproductive behavior problem in mares is inadequate or abnormal mothering behavior. There appear to be several types and degrees of aberrant response to a foal, ranging from apparent discomfort during nursing or fear of the foal to frank rejection or savage attack of the foal. Problems are more common in primiparous mares and tend to recur in the same mare. The abnormal behavior usually occurs immediately after parturition but may emerge after one or several days of normal behavior. The etiology of such behavior as well as the most efficient course of intervention or therapy for the various types of problem continue to be subjects of controversy. Options for immediate management of aberrant maternal behavior include restraint of the mare and temporary or permanent transfer of the foal to a nurse mare. Physical restraint of the mare in a nursing chute seems to work better than tranquilization (see *Current Therapy in Equine Medicine 2*, pages 126–128). Phenothiazine-based tranquilizers, reserpine (up to 4 mg), and benzodiazepine derivatives have been used, but precautions must be taken to avoid adverse effects on the nursing foal.

Another maternal behavior problem is excessive aggression toward humans or other animals, seemingly related to extreme protectiveness of the foal. Occasionally the mare may injure her foal while rushing to interpose herself between the foal and the approaching party. The intensity of such protectiveness typically subsides within a few days but may persist through weaning in some mares. Management aimed at avoiding evoking protectiveness when the foal is in a position where it might be trampled, coupled with deliberate training of the mare to accept necessary intruders, usually is adequate. Injuries to the foal may be less apt to occur if the mare and foal are housed in a large stall or paddock rather than in a small stall.

Supplemental Readings

Asa, C. S.: Sexual behavior of mares. *In* Crowell-Davis, S., and Houpt, K. (eds.): Vet. Clin. North Am. (Equine Pract.), 3(2):519–534, 1986.

Asa, C. S., Goldfoot, D. A., and Ginther, O. J.: Assessment of the sexual behavior of pregnant mares. Horm. Behav. 17:405–413, 1983.

Cox, J. H., and DeBowes, R. M.: Colic-like discomfort associated with ovulation in two mares. J. Am. Vet. Med. Assoc., *191*:1451–1452, 1987.

Crowell-Davis, S. L., and Houpt, K. A.: Maternal behavior. Vet. Clin. North Am. (Equine Pract.), 3(2):557–551, 1986.
Freeman, D. E., and Hinrichs, K.: Granulosa cell tumor. In White, N. A., and Moore, J. N. (eds.): Current Practice of Equine Surgery. Philadelphia, J. B. Lippincott, 1990.
Ginther, O. J.: Reproductive Biology of the Mare: Basic and Applied Aspects. Cross Plains, Wis., Equiservices, 1979.
Ginther, O. J., Garcia, M. C., Bergfelt, D. R., Leith, G. S., and Scraba, S. T.: Embryonic loss in mares: Pregnancy rate, and length of interovulatory progesterone concentrations, intervals associated with loss during days 11 to 15. Theriogenology, 24:409–417, 1985.
Loy, R. G., Pemstein, R., O'Canna, D., and Douglas, R. H.: Control of ovulation in cycling mares with ovarian steroids and prostaglandin. Theriogenology, 15:191–199, 1981.
McDonnell, S. M., Garcia, M. C., Blanchard, T. L., and Kenney, R. M.: Evaluation of androgenized mares as an estrus detection aid. Theriogenology, 26:261–266, 1986.
Palmer, E.: Reproductive management of mares without detection of estrus. J. Reprod. Fertil., 27(Suppl.):263–270, 1979.

Embryo Transfer

Katrin Hinrichs, NORTH GRAFTON, MASSACHUSETTS

The process of embryo transfer (ET) consists of collecting an embryo from the uterus of one mare (the donor mare) and transferring it to the uterus of another mare (the recipient mare) for gestation to term. The major reasons for performing ET are donor mare infertility, resulting in inability to carry a foal to term; physical problems in the donor mare such as laminitis or pelvic trauma that prevent the mare from carrying or delivering a foal normally; the desire to maintain the donor mare in competition while still obtaining foals from her; and the desire for increased productivity from a given mare (obtaining more than one foal per year). Clients should familiarize themselves with the regulations of their breed associations regarding registry of ET progeny.

The basic procedures performed in ET are synchronization of ovulation between the donor and recipient mares (this may be avoided by use of ovariectomized recipient mares), breeding of the donor mare, flushing of the donor mare's uterus for embryo recovery on day 7 after ovulation, and transfer of the recovered embryo to the uterus of the recipient mare. Expected success rates using donor mares of normal fertility are a 50 to 70 per cent embryo recovery rate per cycle and a 50 to 70 per cent pregnancy rate after transfer, leading to an overall efficiency of one pregnancy for every two to four cycles.

THE DONOR MARE

The reproductive status of the donor mare has an important effect on the success of ET. While infertility is a major reason to perform ET, the success rates with infertile donor mares are low. One commercial ET group recently reported embryo recovery rates of 61 per cent, pregnancy rates after transfer of 69 per cent, and embryo loss rates of 12 per cent for maiden donor mares. In infertile donor mares the rates were 29, 49, and 34 per cent, respectively. Rates were calculated for over 600 cycles. Stallion fertility may also have an effect on embryo recovery rates.

The donor mare should receive a complete breeding soundness examination consisting of a history, physical examination, palpation and ultrasonography per rectum, vaginal speculum examination, digital palpation of the cervix, and culture and biopsy of the endometrium. Treatable problems such as cervical lacerations or endometritis should be corrected prior to using the mare for ET. Donor mares should be examined by ultrasonography daily during estrus to determine the size and number of preovulatory follicles present. Donor mares with more than one preovulatory follicle should be treated with human chorionic gonadotropin (hCG), 2000 IU given intravenously (IV), when the follicles are greater than 33 mm in diameter, to ensure that they ovulate at approximately the same time (36 to 48 hours after hCG administration). This will reduce the chance that embryos of greatly disparate size are recovered at the time of embryo recovery. Breeding is done as if the mare were being bred for a conventional pregnancy; however, ultrasonography is essential to determine the exact day of ovulation, on which the day of embryo recovery is based. The day that ovulation is detected is designated day 0.

Donor mares with endometritis must be managed intensively. Mares with susceptible uteri may tend to become reinfected after every breeding and after every embryo recovery attempt. In addition to conventional therapy for endometritis, more aggressive measures may be taken with embryo donors. The uterus may be lavaged and infused with antibiotics after ovulation. The embryo enters the uterus on day 5 or 6 after ovulation, and there is evidence that flushing the uterus with an embryo-compatible medium (see p. 639) as late as day 4 does not interfere with later pregnancy. In mares that never appear to clear of uterine infection, the uterus may be lavaged with saline on days 0 through 4, then flushed for embryo recovery, using embryo recovery medium, on days 5, 6, and 7. One complication of this technique in some mares is that the cervix becomes soft after lavage and may cease being competent enough to hold the embryo in the uterus. Although it is possible to recover embryos in a flush that also yields pus, the success rate with such embryos is low.

THE RECIPIENT MARE

The selection and management of the recipient mare is one of the most important aspects of successful ET. Recipient mares should be between 3 and 10 years of age, with no history of reproductive problems. The recipient mare should be approximately the same size as the donor. While foaling mares have been shown to have normal pregnancy rates after ET, we prefer maiden mares, to ensure that the uterus has not been manipulated previously. The recipient mare should receive a complete breeding soundness examination; mares with any abnormalities should be rejected. Only mares with category I uteri on endometrial biopsy should be used as recipients.

Synchronization of Ovulation

The recipient mare should ovulate 1 day before to 3 days after the donor mare ovulates. If a large recipient mare herd is available, mares that have ovulated at the appropriate time may be selected from the herd. If small numbers of recipients are used, the time of ovulation of the donor and recipient mares must be synchronized. Good synchronization is achieved using progesterone in oil, 150 mg, and estradiol-17β in oil (not estradiol cypionate), 10 mg given intramuscularly (IM), daily for 10 days, with 10 mg prostaglandin $F_{2\alpha}$ ($PGF_{2\alpha}$) also administered IM on day 10. Recipient mares should be started on the regimen 2 days after the donor, to ensure that they do not ovulate before the donor does. After day 10, all mares should be examined by ultrasound daily to detect ovulation. Around 85 per cent of mares ovulate 9 to 13 days after the $PGF_{2\alpha}$ injection. To aid synchronization, ovulation may be speeded in the donor or recipient by administration of hCG after the follicle has reached 33 mm in diameter. Two recipients should be synchronized for each donor and the recipient with the best synchronization is chosen at the time of transfer; in addition, both recipients may be needed if the mare ovulates two follicles. Recipients that ovulate more than 3 days after the donor may have better pregnancy rates if progesterone (300 mg IM) or altrenogest (22 mg per os [PO]) is administered to the recipient starting on the day of ovulation. The progestin may be discontinued when the corpus luteum is fully functional (about 5 days after ovulation).

Ovariectomized Recipients

Ovariectomized, progesterone-treated mares have a pregnancy rate following ET equal to that of intact recipients. Use of ovariectomized mares eliminates the need for synchronization and for examination of recipient mares to detect ovulation. Recipients should be ovariectomized at least 21 days before ET. The ovariectomized recipient is untreated until donor ovulation is detected (day 0). Starting on day 2, the ovariectomized recipient is given progesterone in oil, 300 mg per day IM. If an embryo is not recovered from the donor mare, progesterone is discontinued and the recipient is untreated for 7 to 10 days before being used for a subsequent transfer. Although estrogen administration is not necessary, normal pregnancy rates after ET have been reported in ovariectomized mares treated with up to 10 mg estradiol-17β or estradiol cypionate daily for up to 10 days before onset of progesterone administration. Ovariectomized mares that have not received hormones for a long period (a year or more) may have a lowered pregnancy rate after ET. However, such mares treated with estrogen and progesterone for a period of 10 to 14 days (followed by a period of no treatment) have subsequently been used successfully as recipients.

Following ET, ovariectomized recipients are continued on progesterone daily until day 100 of gestation, after which placental progesterone is sufficient to maintain pregnancy. Ovariectomized recipient mares have normal parturition, lactation, and maternal behavior and may successfully be used again as embryo recipients after foaling.

EMBRYO RECOVERY

Embryo recovery is usually performed on day 7 or 8 after ovulation. Embryo recovery rates on day 6 are reported to be lower than those on day 7 or later, and pregnancy rates decrease when embryos are transferred after day 8. We perform all embryo recoveries on day 7 to ensure that the embryo is small. If the donor mare ovulates two follicles asynchronously, the embryo flush is performed on day 7 or 8 after the first ovulation; thus, a day 7 or day 8 embryo and a younger embryo may be recovered. Use of hCG during breeding as outlined above should eliminate the chance of having embryos more than 2 days apart in age.

Modified Dulbecco's phosphate-buffered saline (DPBS) is used for embryo recovery. If tissue culture quality (i.e., double-distilled, deionized) water is available, DPBS may be mixed from prepackaged dry solutes.* Good quality water may be obtained using a commercial water purification system,† but the initial quality of the water used is important. If tissue culture quality water is not available, liquid DPBS should be purchased.‡ Ten ml neonatal calf serum,§ and 60,000 IU penicillin, and 60,000 μg streptomycin‖ are added to each liter of DPBS. While three 1-liter flushes are usually performed for embryo recovery, some groups have achieved good embryo recovery rates using only 500 to 250 ml of medium for each flush. About 150 ml of medium is reserved before flushing, for rinsing cylinders and preparing transfer medium after embryo collection. It is important that all manipulations during media preparation, embryo collection, and embryo transfer be performed using syringes made entirely of plastic¶ without a black rubber tip on the plunger, which may be embryotoxic.

For embryo recovery, we use a customized, 150-cm-long silicone catheter[1] with the air inlet at 80 cm. This catheter may be autoclaved, and the extra length eliminates the need for junctions. The mare is restrained in stocks with the tail wrapped and tied to the side. The perineum is scrubbed and rinsed three times with a povidone–iodine scrub and then dried. The operator dons a clean rectal sleeve and sterile surgical gloves. Using a small amount of sterile, water-soluble lubricant,[2] the operator passes the catheter manually through the vagina and cervix and into the uterine body. The cuff is then inflated with 30 to 40 cc of air, and the catheter is pulled caudad until the cuff is snug against the internal cervical os.

One liter of the flush medium is infused by gravity flow into the uterus, using a rubber adapter that fits over the neck of the bottle and connects with the end of the catheter. The medium may be used at room temperature or warmed, but must not be over body temperature. While some ET groups massage the uterus per rectum during embryo recovery, we prefer not to do this because of the potential for fecal contamination. The fluid is drained from the uterus by gravity flow into a 1-liter graduated cylinder; 95 per cent of the infused fluid should be recovered. If fluid recovery is slow, the catheter tip may be moved craniad or caudad to contact fluid pockets. Oxytocin (20 to 40 IU IV) works well to expel fluid from the uterus, but because its effect on the embryo has not been determined, it should be used only if necessary. In 1989, we modified the recovery technique to include a wait of 3 minutes before draining the fluid from the uterus. Using this 3-minute technique, we had an embryo recovery rate in normal mares of 21/20 (105 per cent, including three sets of twins), recovering embryos from 18 of 20 mares flushed. Although some ET groups use an embryo filter‡ to collect the embryo from the recovered fluid, we feel that an in-line filter reduces the rate of outflow and may increase the trauma to the embryo.

After the three uterine flushes have been performed, the donor mare is given PGF, 10 mg IM. This is done both to short-cycle the mare in preparation for the next embryo recovery attempt and to reduce the chance of endometritis due to organisms introduced into the uterus during flushing.

EMBRYO IDENTIFICATION AND TRANSFER

The fluid in the graduated cylinders is allowed to settle for 10 minutes. All but the bottom 50 ml of fluid is then siphoned from each cylinder. The siphoned fluid is passed through an embryo filter, in the rare case that the embryo has not yet settled to the bottom and may be in the siphoned fluid. The bottom 50 ml of fluid is poured into a sterile plastic Petri dish. The cylinder is rinsed three times with a small amount of the reserved medium, and the rinse is also poured into a Petri dish. When this has been done for all three cylinders and the embryo filter, the Petri dishes are examined using a dissection microscope at 10 to 25×. If embryos 6 days or younger are expected, the higher power should be used. At 7 days, embryos may still be enclosed in a zona

---

*Dulbecco's PBS packets, Gibco Labs., Grand Island, NY
†Water purification systems, Fisher Scientific Co., Pittsburgh, PA
‡Dulbecco's PBS media, Gibco Labs., Grand Island, NY
§Neonatal calf serum, Gibco Labs., Grand Island, NY
‖Penicillin-streptomycin, Gibco Labs., Grand Island, NY
¶Air-Tite syringes, Air-Tite of Virginia, Inc., Virginia Beach, VA
[1] Equine uterine flushing catheter, Bivona, Inc., Gary, IN
[2] HR Sterile Lube, A. J. Buck, Cockeysville, MD

‡Emcon filter, Em-Tex Supply Co., Gran Prairie, TX

pellucida, or may be seen as expanding blastocysts. Identifying characteristics of embryos that may be used by the inexperienced searcher are the presence of the thick, clear, smooth zona pellucida surrounding smaller embryos; and the smoothly cellular, translucent, spherical blastocyst, surrounded by a thin capsule, of larger embryos.

When the embryo is located, it should be transferred using a sterile, fire-polished 1-ml glass pipette into a small (35-mm) sterile Petri dish containing transfer medium. The transfer medium is prepared by adding 1 ml of neonatal calf serum to 9 ml of reserved flush medium in a syringe, and is sterilized by passing it through a 0.2-μm filter attached to the syringe.* The embryo is washed by transferring it at least two more times to new dishes of transfer medium. If the flush contained pus (i.e., the flush was cloudy), the embryo should be washed ten times.

As soon as the embryo is washed, it may be transferred; it should be transferred within 3 hours of collection. Most ET groups now use transcervical transfer, achieving pregnancy rates of 65 to 75 per cent with embryos from normal mares. However, pregnancy rates after transcervical ET are dependent on the skill of the technician, and a few laboratories still report lower pregnancy rates with transcervical than with surgical ET.

For transcervical transfer, the recipient should be restrained and the perineum scrubbed as described above for the donor. The operator dons a clean rectal sleeve and a pair of sterile surgical gloves and attaches a sterile insemination pipette to a sterile 10-ml syringe. Four ml of air is drawn into the syringe and the tip of the pipette is placed in the Petri dish containing the embryo. The pipette is loaded in approximately 0.5-ml increments (about 1-inch lengths along the pipette) in the following sequence: medium, air, medium, air, medium containing the embryo, air, medium, air. When the contents of the pipette are expressed into the uterus, these will come out in the reverse order. The pocket of fluid and air at the end of the pipette prevents embryo loss during cannulation of the cervix; the pockets after the embryo assure that it is washed from the pipette.

For transfer, the operator uses a small amount of sterile lubricant and passes the pipette manually into the vagina. The cervix is cannulated with the finger and the pipette is slipped gently beside the finger through the cervix and into the uterus until it hits resistance. The finger is removed from the cervix and the hand compresses the cervix around the pipette while the contents of the syringe are expressed. The pipette is then gently withdrawn. Some ET groups use sterile sheaths over the pipette to minimize contamination of the uterus; however, since the sheath and finger still cannulate the cervix, it is doubtful whether this achieves its purpose. Whereas embryo guns such as those used in cattle may also be used in the horse, there is no strong evidence that they increase pregnancy rates. Administration of antibiotics, anti-inflammatories, or progestins to recipient mares at the time of transfer has not been shown to increase pregnancy rates. The recipient may be examined by ultrasonography as early as 4 days after transfer, when the embryo is 11 days old.

FUTURE DIRECTIONS

Embryo freezing is still not widely used in the horse, because embryos larger than day 6 have poor viability after thawing. However, embryos have been successfully cooled in CO_2-gassed Hams F-10 and stored for up to 24 hours in semen transport containers, allowing time for shipment to an ET facility; initial results with this technique have been excellent.

Exciting work has recently been reported on methods for oocyte manipulation. In 1987, workers in Colorado achieved a pregnancy by transfer of a mature oocyte to the oviduct of a bred recipient mare (GIFT; gamete intrafallopian transfer). Successful in vitro fertilization of equine oocytes was first reported by French workers in 1989, and successful in vitro maturation was reported by workers in England in 1989. In our laboratory in 1989 we obtained embryos from immature oocytes that had been transferred to the preovulatory follicles of recipient mares. Techniques of oocyte manipulation and transfer hold great promise for infertile mares for which ET is not possible. This is certain to be an area of intense interest for future research and clinical development.

Supplemental Readings

Allen, W. R., Antczak, D. F., and Wade, J. F. (eds.) Equine Embryo Transfer: II. Equine Vet. J. Suppl., 8, 1989.

Hinrichs, K.: A simple technique that may improve the rate of embryo recovery on uterine flushing in mares. Theriogenology, 33:937, 1990.

Hinrichs, K.: Use of ovariectomized mares as embryo transfer recipients. Proc. Soc. Theriogenol. 1986, pp. 107–110.

McKinnon, A. O., Squires, E. L., Voss, J. L., and Cook, V. M.: Equine embryo transfer. Compend. Cont. Educ. Pract. Vet., 10(3):343, 1988.

Sertich, P. L.: Transcervical embryo transfer in performance mares. J. Am. Vet. Med. Assoc., 195:940, 1989.

---

*Acrodisc disposable filters, versapor nylon, Gelman Sciences, Ann Arbor, MI

Persistent Estrus: Fact or Fiction?

Patricia L. Sertich, KENNETT SQUARE, PENNSYLVANIA

Estrus is the recurrent sexual receptivity to a stallion associated with ovulation. Normal behavioral responses in estrus include interest in the stallion, elevation of the tail, repeated eversion of the vulvar lips ("winking"), abduction of the hind legs, and urination ("breaking down") in the presence of the stallion. The occurrence, intensity, and frequency of these specific responses vary from mare to mare, and normal mares may display none of them ("silent ovulation"). Very often mares are referred for evaluation of what is subjectively described as "persistent estrus." Some of these mares may have abnormalities of the reproductive tract and aberrations of the estrous cycle, but often what is deemed to be undesired behavior is in fact normal or, if abnormal, has little or nothing to do with the estrous cycle. Accordingly, before proceeding with extensive examination and testing, it is important to ascertain exactly what specific bothersome behaviors occur and when they occur in relation to the reproductive cycle.

CLINICAL EVALUATION

Mares are referred with a variable set of complaints, including frequent and excessive urination, erratic performance or temperament associated with stage of the estrous cycle, intense estrous reponses that hinder performance, and frequent or constant estrus. Clinical evaluation of these cases requires a complete history that includes specific details of the behavior and the surrounding circumstances. It is not uncommon for disobedience, resistance, or aggression to be erroneously attributed to estrus. If an unusual, contradictory, or incomplete history is provided, one can systematically chart the specific behavior and time of each occurrence over a 3-week period to determine whether a cyclic pattern exists.

A general physical examination, including a musculoskeletal evaluation, may be performed to rule out the presence of a nonreproductive medical abnormality. A complete examination of the reproductive tract will reveal most obvious reproductive abnormalities. Ideally, especially in cases of reported changes in temperament throughout the estrous cycle, ovarian activity should be monitored on a frequent schedule (every other day) by palpation and ultrasonography per rectum for at least one normal interovulatory period (21 days). The mare should also be teased aggressively by a stallion at least every other day and her specific reactions recorded when she is in diestrus as well as estrus. If the mare's performance appears to be affected by stages of the cycle, performance should be evaluated daily or every other day. The most unbiased results can be expected if the observer of performance does not know the results of the daily reproductive examinations. Plasma progesterone concentrations may be helpful in confirming ovarian status. A 12- to 24-hour video monitoring of undisturbed stall behavior is valuable in determining general temperament or unusual behaviors.

CLINICAL FINDINGS AND DIAGNOSIS

NORMAL BEHAVIOR

Some cases presented as persistent estrus may actually represent normal behavior associated with different phases of the reproductive cycle. Anestrous mares with no follicular activity are usually passive but may be receptive to a stallion. Anestrus may be due to seasonal ovarian inactivity related to the short photoperiod that occurs in winter. Mares that are anestrous due to severe health problems or old mares whose ovaries have ceased to function normally may be receptive to a stallion. Although these behaviors are physiological, they can usually be suppressed by administration of progestagens. Progesterone, 150 mg per day given intramuscularly (IM) or altrenogest°, 0.044 mg per kg per day given orally, will usually suppress estrus.

During the transitional phase of the breeding season, mares often have intermittent and irregular periods of estrus. Multiple large follicles may be present on the ovaries, but fail to ovulate due to insufficient concentrations of luteinizing hormone (LH) during the transition period. Once an LH surge is present, ovulation will occur and estrus ceases. Anovulatory mares with irregular periods of estrus can be managed

---

°Regumate, Hoechst-Roussel Agri-Vet Co., North Somerville, NJ

through this transitional period by administering a combination of progesterone (150 mg) and estradiol (10 mg) IM for 10 to 15 days. During treatment, estrus and follicular activity are inhibited. Following cessation of treatment, normal estrus and ovulation will ensue.

Finally, the occasional gregarious mare will be mistakenly perceived as persistently in estrus. While she will be the first mare to the tease rail and will demand the stallion's full attention, careful evaluation of her specific responses will reveal social interaction (vocalization, nose-to-nose contact, physical proximity) rather than sexual receptivity. If followed throughout an entire ovulatory cycle, this mare will show normal sexual behavior, distinct from general social behavior, near ovulation. This phenomenon emphasizes the need for a teasing program based on specific behavior responses rather than a generalized, extemporaneous judgment.

UROGENITAL PROBLEMS

Frequent urination due to a urogenital problem such as cystitis, urethritis, vaginitis due to pneumovagina or iatrogenic irritation, or urethral mass may be mistaken for persistent estrus. Correction of the urogenital tract problem can eliminate the signs (see p. 616).

TUMORS

Estrogen-secreting ovarian tumors can produce undesirable behaviors in mares. The most common tumor affecting the equine ovary is the granulosa cell tumor, which has been associated with three types of behavior, depending on the steroids produced: diestrous behavior, due to elevated concentrations of progesterone; constant estrus ("nymphomania"), due theoretically to elevated concentrations of estrogen; and stallion-like behavior, due to elevated concentrations of androgens. In approximately 50 per cent of cases, plasma testosterone concentrations are elevated. There may also be no detectable elevation in steroid hormone concentrations. Provisional diagnosis of a granulosa cell tumor is supported by clinical findings including infertility, acyclicity, and possibly abnormal behavior. Ultrasonography may reveal irregular multicystic areas on the ovary. One ovary will be enlarged and have no palpable ovulation fossa while the opposite ovary will be small and inactive. In the past, the small, inactive condition of the opposite ovary was attributed to the presence of high circulating levels of ovarian steroids exerting negative feedback on the hypothalamus and pituitary; however, in some cases there are no detectable elevations in progesterone or estrogen. It has recently been found that granulosa cell tumor cells have the genetic capacity to produce inhibin. It is postulated that inhibin may prevent the growth of normal follicles on the opposite ovary. Definitive diagnosis requires histological evaluation of the tumor. Therapy includes surgical removal of the tumor. The opposite ovary will usually resume follicular activity in 3 to 18 months.

MALE-TYPE BEHAVIOR

In some mares, careful evaluation of specific behavioral responses reveals that the problem behavior is actually male-type behavior. This can result from testosterone-producing tumors or exogenous androgenic compounds. Management of these mares requires removal of the androgen source. However, the male-type behavior may persist for months after androgen withdrawal (see p. 636).

LAMENESS OR DISCOMFORT

Examination may reveal that the mare is lame. Soreness in the back has been attributed to "sore ovaries." Hock problems with related back soreness, common in dressage and harness horses, may lead to behavior that is interpreted as reproductive discomfort. Treatment of the lameness may alleviate the behavioral signs.

INSUFFICIENT TRAINING OR CONDITIONING

In many cases, neither a relationship to the reproductive cycle nor physiological reproductive or other physical abnormalities can be found. The behavior problem may represent resistance due either to lack of training or to insufficient physical condition to perform the desired task. Unfortunately, this is the least popular diagnosis with owners.

Supplemental Readings

Ginther, O. J.: Sexual behavior and characteristics of the ovulatory season. In: Reproductive Biology of the Mare. Ann Arbor, Mich., McNaughton and Gunn, Inc., 1979, pp. 59–72, 136.

Piquette, G. N., Sertich, P. L., Kenney, R. M., Yamto, M., and Hsueh, A. J. W.: Equine granulosa-theca cell tumors express inhibin alpha and beta A-subunit mRNAS and proteins. Biol. Reprod., 43:1050, 1990.

Sertich, P. L., Hamir, A. N., Orsini, P., and Kenney, R. M.: Paraurethral lipoma in a mare associated with frequent urination. Equine Vet. Educ., 2:121–122, 1990.

Taylor, T. B., Pemstein, R., and Loy, R. G.: Control of ovulation in mares in the early breeding season with ovarian steroids and prostaglandin. J. Reprod. Fertil. Suppl., 32:219–224, 1982.

Age-Related Ovulatory Dysfunction

Dirk K. Vanderwall, MOSCOW, IDAHO
Gordon L. Woods, MOSCOW, IDAHO

After age 12 years, mares experience decreasing fertility with increasing age. This decrease in fertility is exemplified by a 28 per cent lower foaling rate for mares more than 13 years old in comparison with mares aged 2 to 11 years. Fertilization rates are high but detected pregnancy rates are low for aged mares, indicating that embryonic death is one factor in the age-related decrease in fertility. Most embryonic deaths occur prior to the time of routine pregnancy detection; many aged mares that are determined to be nonpregnant may have experienced embryonic death. Because of embryonic death, aged mares usually require breeding on multiple estrous cycles in order to establish a pregnancy that results in a live foal. Another age-related cause of decreased fertility in the mare is ovulatory dysfunction. We have observed delayed initiation of the ovulatory season and failure of ovulation in aged mares, which, together with embryonic death, cause decreased fertility.

DELAYED OVULATION

Under natural photoperiod, mares more than 19 years old experience their first ovulation of the year 2 weeks later than mares less than 13 years old. The average first ovulation of the year is April 24 for young mares and May 8 for aged mares. This 2-week delay in initiation of ovulation for aged mares represents a 10 per cent loss (2 weeks of 20 weeks) in the effective length of the operational breeding season (February 15 to July 1). Therefore, aged mares, which because of embryonic death require more breeding opportunities, may have fewer estrous cycles during the breeding season.

Artificial light, which is used routinely on commercial breeding farms to hasten the onset of the ovulatory season, may be provided to increase the number of estrous cycles that aged mares have during the breeding season. Approximately 60 to 90 days of artificial light are necessary to stimulate ovulatory activity in the mare; therefore, lighting should be initiated between November 15 and December 15. Incandescent or fluorescent light that provides enough illumination to read a newspaper at every point in a stall will stimulate ovarian activity. One 200-watt incandescent bulb per stall is adequate. Natural light can be supplemented with artificial light to provide a continuous 16-hour period of light (natural and artificial) per day from the time treatment is initiated, or artificial light can be added in a stepwise manner (increase ½ to 1 hour each week) until 16 hours of light per day is reached.

Aged mares should begin the breeding season in good body condition. Henneke et al. documented that mares in good body condition ovulate earlier in the year than thin mares. To maintain good body condition, aged mares may require individual management, including grain supplementation, special dental care, intensive foot care, and elimination of social stress within the herd. Social stress from younger, more vigorous mares may interfere with an aged mare's ability to obtain feed or her ability to obtain shelter during inclement weather.

FAILURE OF OVULATION

Some aged mares do not ovulate. We observed that 7 of 19 mares (37 per cent) more than 24 years old did not ovulate during the ovulatory season. Some of the aged mares exhibited estrous behavior resembling that of seasonally anovulatory mares. Estrous behavior in seasonally anovulatory mares is thought to be stimulated by steroid hormones produced by the adrenal glands; therefore, it is likely that the same mechanism causes estrous behavior in aged anovulatory mares. If aged mares are to be mated based on estrous behavior alone, ovulation failure should be ruled out as a cause of infertility.

Aged anovulatory mares are clinically similar to seasonally anovulatory mares. The ovaries of an aged anovulatory mare are small and firm with either no follicles or a few small follicles (less than 15 mm in diameter). The cervix and uterus are flaccid, and vaginal mucous membranes are pale and dry. The serum progesterone concentration is less than 1 ng per ml. Uterine biopsy discloses endometrial gland atrophy. There is currently no treatment for age-related anovulation in the mare. Some aged mares with small, firm ovaries devoid of follicles at the start of the breeding season will eventually develop normal follicular activity and ovulate. Therefore, repeated examinations are necessary to document complete failure of ovulation. Further research is needed to determine the underlying causes of delayed ovulation and ovulation failure in aged mares.

Supplemental Readings

Ball, B. A., Little, T. V., Weber, J. A., and Woods, G. L.: Survival of day-4 embryos from young, normal mares and aged, subfertile mares after transfer to normal recipient mares. J. Reprod. Fertil., 85:187, 1989.

Ginther, O. J.: Reproductive Biology of the Mare: Basic and Applied Aspects. Cross Plaines, Wis., Equiservices, 1979.

Henneke, D. R., Potter, G. D., and Kreider, J. L.: Body condition during pregnancy and lactation and reproductive efficiency of mares. Theriogenology, 21:897, 1984.

Vanderwall, D. K., and Woods, G. L.: Age-related subfertility in the mare. In: Proceedings of the 36th Annual Convention of the American Association of Equine Practitioners, pp. 85–89, 1990.

Embryonic Loss

Barry A. Ball, ITHACA, NEW YORK

Embryonic loss is a major factor in subfertility and reduced reproductive efficiency in mares. Although a better understanding of the magnitude of embryonic loss in mares has been gained, there is only limited understanding of the causes of such loss. Much of the available information is derived by extrapolation from other species and from observations in clinical cases. Because early pregnancy in the mare is unique in a number of aspects, such extrapolations may be inappropriate.

INCIDENCE

To estimate the magnitude of embryonic loss in mares, the fertilization rate must be known. The fertilization rate is over 90 per cent in fertile mares and 81 to 92 per cent in subfertile mares. Fertilization failure, therefore, accounts for a relatively small proportion of infertility cases when breeding management and stallion fertility are optimal. Embryonic loss, however, accounts for a major portion of reproductive inefficiency. Embryonic loss can occur before or after pregnancy is confirmed by ultrasonography or rectal palpation (days 10 to 14). The incidence of embryonic loss between fertilization and day 14 is 9 per cent for young, fertile mares and greater than 60 per cent for aged, subfertile mares. A significant proportion of embryonic losses in subfertile mares appear to occur before the embryo reaches the uterus on days 5 to 6. These losses are confirmed by the low recovery of embryos from the uterus on days 6 to 8 despite the relatively high fertilization rate in these mares.

Field study estimates of the incidence of embryonic loss vary depending on the method of pregnancy determination, the interval of detection, and the population of animals under study. The embryonic loss rate between day 11 and day 40 or 50 is approximately 10 per cent in fertile mares, higher in subfertile mares. The incidence of embryonic loss from fertilization through approximately day 40 is about 20 per cent in fertile mares and above 70 per cent in subfertile mares (Fig. 1).

DIAGNOSIS

The ultrasonographic morphology of the embryo and uterus from spontaneous and induced embryonic losses (Fig. 2) provides some information on detection of impending embryonic loss. Many spontaneous embryonic losses between days 11 and 20 are unaccompanied by ultrasonographic changes. Changes that may indicate impending embryonic loss include (1) accumulation of intraluminal uterine fluid, (2) an irregular shape to the embryonic vesicle, (3) prolonged mobility of the vesicle, (4) an undersized vesicle, (5) loss of the embryonic heartbeat, (6) dislodgment of the vesicle with loss of fluid, and (7) edema of the endometrial folds.

In some horses with pending embryonic loss, small collections of free fluid, possibly inflammatory exudate, may be observed in the uterine lumen. Poorly defined margins or irregularity of the embryonic vesicle may be noted prior to embryonic loss between days 11 and 20. However, changes in vesicle shape can also occur normally

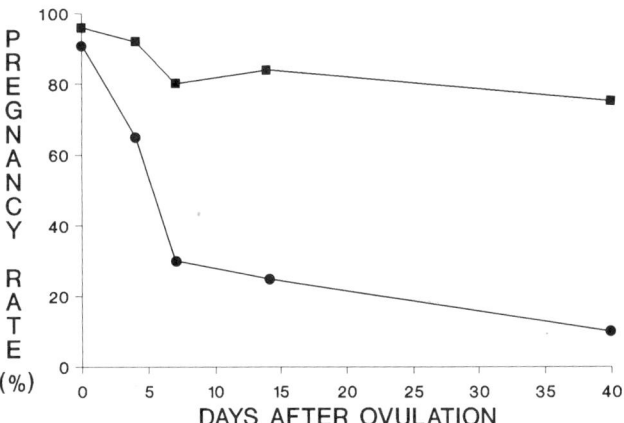

Figure 1. Pregnancy rates for fertile (■) and subfertile mares (●) through day 40 after ovulation. Data points are combined from several studies.

by days 17 to 19. Prolonged mobility of the embryonic vesicle beyond day 17 has been observed in a few cases of spontaneous embryonic loss. In these cases, the embryonic vesicle fails to become fixed at the base of one of the uterine horns. Edema of the endometrial folds may be imaged as progesterone concentrations decrease in pregnant mares that have undergone luteolysis.

Although a high per centage (62 to 78 per cent) of undersized vesicles (more than 1 or 2 SDs below the mean diameter of embryos of the same age) are lost by day 25, many continue to grow at a relatively normal rate until loss occurs. In contrast to undersized vesicles, oversized vesicles are not associated with increased embryonic loss. Further information on the ultrasonographic morphology of embryonic losses has been gained by inducing loss with prostaglandin $F_{2\alpha}$ ($PGF_{2\alpha}$). Mares given 5 mg $PGF_{2\alpha}$ on day 12 lose their embryos approximately 7 days later. In these mares, failure of fixation of the vesicle, a loss of uterine tone, and separation of the yolk sac membrane from the endometrium are noted. After administration of $PGF_{2\alpha}$ on day 30, the interval to loss of the conceptus averages 8.5 days. In these mares, the vesicle dislodges from the base of the uterine horn and often moves into the uterine body. Motion of the embryo's heart ceases approximately 3 days after administration of $PGF_{2\alpha}$. There is prominent edema of the endometrial folds prior to loss. The loss of the conceptus following $PGF_{2\alpha}$ administration on day 30 is characterized by a gradual decrease in fluid behind a closed cervix; the conceptus remnant is expelled when the mare returns to estrus.

RECOVERY AND EVALUATION OF EMBRYOS

Nonsurgical embryo recovery from the uterus of mares between days 6 and 10 is used in equine ET. Evaluation of embryos from mares with a history of embryonic loss may hold some diagnostic benefits. A cloudy or turbid effluent accompanying the embryo usually indicates an active endometritis. Embryos recovered from the uterus of subfertile mares on day 7 or day 8 are smaller and have more morphological defects than embryos from fertile mares. Some embryos from subfertile mares are degenerate and contain fungal elements.

ENDOCRINOLOGY

Monitoring serum or plasma progesterone concentrations has been suggested as a method to predict impending embryonic loss. Although progesterone concentrations vary during pregnancy and between animals, concentrations below 4 ng per ml over 2 consecutive days can indicate impending embryonic loss, and there is a high rate of embryonic loss in mares with progesterone concentrations under 2 ng per ml. Maintenance of pregnancy in ovariectomized, progesterone-treated, embryo-recipient mares requires progesterone concentrations above 2.5 ng per ml. The effective use of progesterone data requires rapid reporting of test results. Altrenogest can be administered if low progesterone levels are suspected. It will not interfere with the progesterone assay. Identification of a low progesterone concentration does not, however, indicate whether the cause is related to inappropriate luteolysis, luteal insufficiency, or failure of maternal recognition of pregnancy.

Estrone sulfate can be used to assess fetal viability, but there are no other readily available assays to assess the equine conceptus during the embryonic period. Estrone sulfate levels in maternal blood decrease when the fetus dies. Assays for early pregnancy factor (EPF) in the mare indicate that it may be possible to use a blood-based test to assess the pregnancy status of mares as early as day 7; however, the rosette-inhibition assay used to detect EPF is difficult to perform and is not widely available.

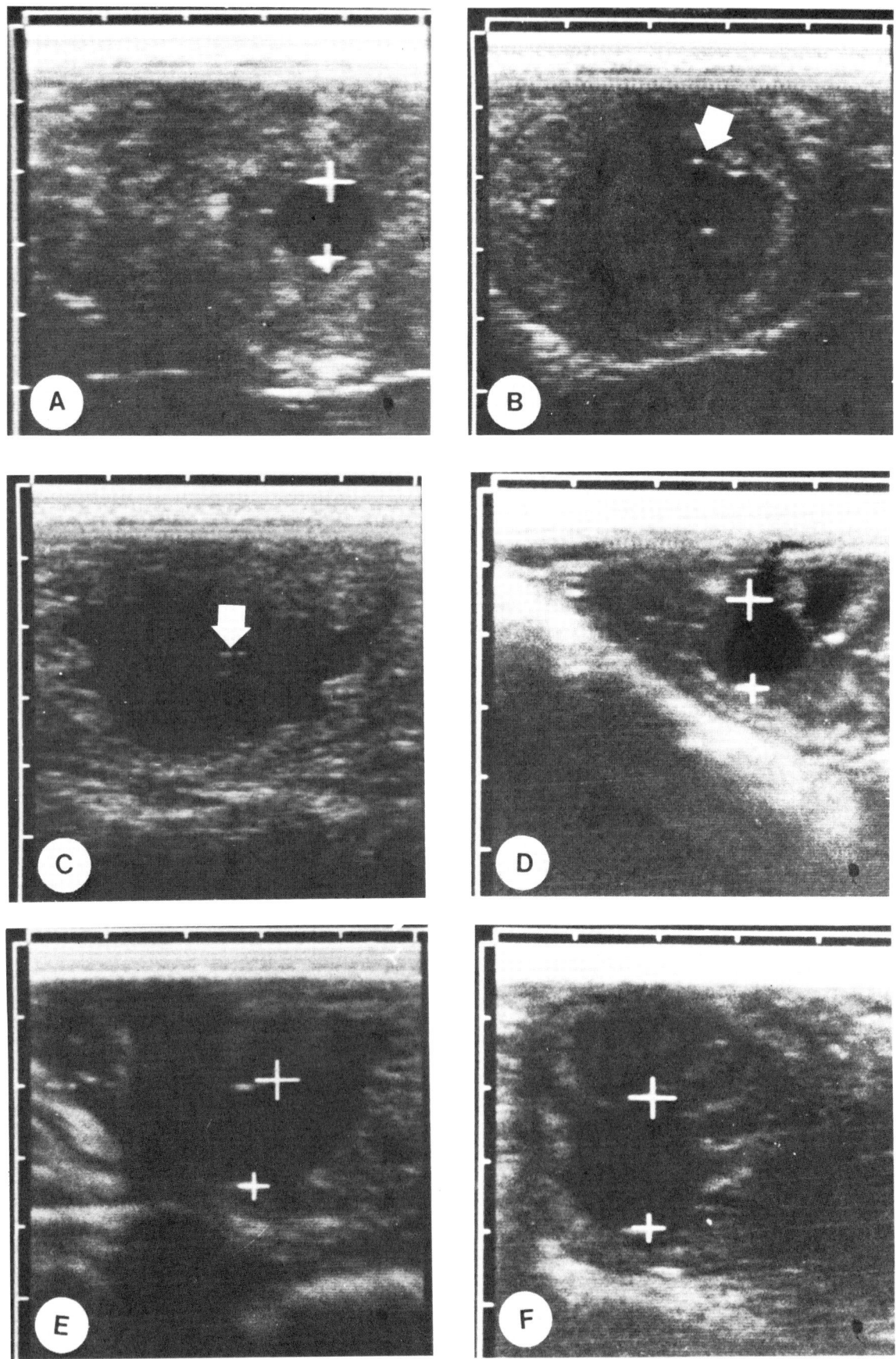

Figure 2. See legend on opposite page.

PREVENTION, MANAGEMENT, AND THERAPY

No single therapeutic or management scheme is likely to prevent embryonic loss, because there are a multitude of causes. Even with careful evaluation, the cause of many spontaneous embryonic losses remains undiagnosed. Mares must be identified as soon as possible after embryo loss occurs. This requires weekly or biweekly examination between days 14 and 40 in order to identify mares that have undergone embryonic loss. These mares may then be mated or inseminated again before the breeding season is over. Use of ultrasonography for early pregnancy diagnosis greatly aids accurate detection of pregnancy as well as detection of embryonic loss. Endometrial cytology, microbiology, and histopathology may be useful in identifying mares in which endometritis may have contributed to embryonic loss (see *Current Therapy in Equine Medicine 2*, p. 503). Endometrial biopsy will indicate the ability of a mare to carry a pregnancy to term. Mares with significant periglandular fibrosis have a high rate of early fetal loss.

Prevention of embryonic loss requires the evaluation of mating practices. The long duration of estrus, the extended longevity of stallion sperm in the mare's reproductive tract, and the maintenance of sexual receptivity after ovulation allow male and female gametes to age before fertilization. Aging of the ovum after ovulation can significantly increase the incidence of polyspermic fertilization and subsequent embryonic loss. Mating 12 or more hours after ovulation results in a higher embryonic loss rate than mating before ovulation. Timing of insemination or mating is therefore an important consideration in routine reproductive management of the mare.

Much attention has been placed on the use of exogenous progesterone to prevent or treat impending embryonic loss because progesterone is critical for pregnancy maintenance in mares. Controversy exists regarding the merits of exogenous progesterone therapy as well as dosage regimens and duration of therapy. Many dosage regimens do not effectively elevate or maintain serum progesterone concentrations. Progesterone in oil, 200 to 300 mg given intramuscularly once daily, 1000 mg of repositol progesterone given every 4 days, 11 to 44 mg of altrenogest* given orally (PO) once daily have all been used to maintain pregnancy in ovariectomized recipient mares. Altrenogest does not appear to suppress endogenous progesterone secretion and provides a convenient method of oral supplementation of progesterone. Clitoral enlargement has been reported in fillies born to dams treated with altrenogest. The introduction of controlled-release formulations of progesterone, however, holds promise for administration of progesterone every 10 to 14 days instead of daily as with currently available products.

The duration of progestin therapy has also been debated. Most benefits of exogenous progesterone therapy are probably realized during the first 3 to 4 months of pregnancy, because placental production of progesterone is adequate to maintain pregnancy after days 50 to 70. Serum progesterone levels normally decline after days 120 to 150, and other forms of progesterone (pregnanes) become important later in pregnancy. However, withdrawal of supplemental progesterone therapy during midgestation may leave the clinician open to criticism if the mare subsequently aborts, even though the abortion may be unrelated to progesterone withdrawal.

Nonsteroidal anti-inflammatory drugs, such as flunixin meglumine, have been used to block $PGF_{2\alpha}$-mediated luteolysis and subsequent embryonic loss in mares with experimentally induced endotoxemia. Chronic therapy with flunixin meglumine† (1.1 mg per kg per day from day 10 to day 60) has also been used to prevent luteolysis in a mare with repeated embryonic loss that was apparently related to chronic uterine inflammation. However, the safety of chronic flunixin meglumine therapy during early pregnancy in the mare has not been extensively tested, and long-term progestin therapy may be equally as effective in preventing embryonic loss.

---

*Regumate, Hoechst-Roussel Agri-Vet Co., Somerville, NJ
†Banamine, Schering Animal Health, Union, NJ

Figure 2. Ultrasonographic appearance of the uterus and embryonic vesicle after intrauterine inoculation with *Candida parapsilosis*. Each division along the left and top margins represents 10 mm. (*A*) Day 12 embryonic vesicle (between calipers) in the uterine body 1 day after inoculation. (*B*) Day 13 embryonic vesicle *(arrow)* located within an accumulation of fluid in the right uterine horn 2 days after inoculation. (*C*) Fluid accumulation and free-floating debris *(arrow)* in the uterine body 3 days after inoculation. (*D*) Day 12 embryonic vesicle located in the uterine body 1 day after inoculation. Note edematous endometrial folds around the vesicle. (*E*) Day 14 embryonic vesicle (between calipers). Note edematous endometrial folds and small accumulation of fluid adjacent to the vesicle. (*F*) Day 14 embryonic vesicle (between calipers) in the left uterine horn 1 day after inoculation. (From Ball, B. A.: Embryonic loss in mares: Incidence, possible causes, and diagnostic considerations. Vet. Clin. North Am. (Equine Pract.) 4:263, 1988. Reproduced by permission.)

Supplemental Readings

Adams, G. P., Kastelic, J. P., Bergfelt, D. R., and Ginther, O. J.: Effect of uterine inflammation and ultrasonically detected uterine pathology on fertility in the mare. J. Reprod. Fertil. Suppl., 35:445, 1987.

Ball, B. A., Little, T. V., Hillman, R. B., and Woods, G. L.: Pregnancy rates at days 2 and 14 and estimated embryonic loss rates prior to day 14 in normal and subfertile mares. Theriogenology, 26:611, 1986.

Ball, B. A., Little, T. V., Weber, J. A., and Woods, G. L.: Viability of day-4 embryos from young, normal mares and aged, subfertile mares after transfer to normal recipient mares. J. Reprod. Fertil., 85:187, 1989.

Daels, P. F., Stabenfeldt, G. H., Kindahl, H., and Hughes, J. P.: Prostaglandin release and luteolysis associated with physiological and pathological conditions of the reproductive cycles of the mare: A review. Equine Vet. J. Suppl., 8:29, 1989.

Darenius, K., Fredriksson, G., and Kindahl, H.: Allyl trenbolone and flunixin meglumine treatment of mares with repeated embryonic loss. Equine Vet. J. Suppl., 8:35, 1989.

Ginther, O. J.: Reproductive Biology of the Mare: Basic and Applied Aspects. Cross Plains, Wis., Equiservices, 1979.

Ginther, O. J.: Ultrasonic imaging and reproductive events in the mare. Cross Plains, Wis., Equiservices, 1986.

Kenney, R. M.: Cyclic and pathologic changes of the mare endometrium as detected by biopsy, with a note on early embryonic death. J. Am. Vet. Med. Assoc., 172:241, 1978.

McKinnon, A. O., Squires, E. L., Carnevale, E. M., and Hermenet, M. J.: Ovariectomized steroid-treated mares as embryo transfer recipients and as a model to study the role of progestins in pregnancy maintenance. Theriogenology, 29:1055, 1988.

Woods, G. L., Hillman, R. B., and Schlafter, D. H.: Recovery and evaluation of embryos from normal and infertile mares. Cornell Vet., 76:386, 1986.

Ultrasonographic Examination of the Mare's Reproductive Tract

Gregg P. Adams, MADISON, WISCONSIN

Transrectal ultrasonography (US) has proved to be an extremely valuable diagnostic tool for the evaluation of the reproductive system in many species. The mare is particularly well suited for this imaging technique because of the uterine anatomy and the size and location of ovarian structures. In addition, the relatively large size and spherical morphology of the early conceptus facilitate early pregnancy detection with US.

Initially, the use of US scanners for reproductive tract examination was limited to early pregnancy detection, but as the technology improved, it became apparent that diagnostic US had a much broader potential. A tremendous amount of information can be gained from even a single scan. Ovarian follicles and corpora lutea are easily distinguished, counted, and measured. Detection of double ovulations and twin conceptuses is possible. The early, immature corpus luteum can be distinguished from a mature or atretic corpus luteum. The uterus and endometrial folds have distinctively different image characteristics at different stages of the estrous cycle. In addition, US is ideal for the detection of embryonic loss, pathological intrauterine fluid collections, and uterine cysts. Diagnostic US, therefore, can be used for breeding management, detection of ovulation, detection and management of twins, monitoring postpartum involution, and detection and management of ovarian and uterine abnormalities. It can also be used to determine if a filly has reached puberty or if a mare has entered the ovulatory season. The following is a discussion of the use of transrectal diagnostic US for evaluating the reproductive organs during the estrous cycle and pregnancy and for diagnosing reproductive tract abnormalities in the mare.

PRINCIPLES OF ULTRASONIC IMAGING

Current US instruments for use in the mare are B-mode, real-time scanners equipped with a 3.5-, 5.0-, or 7.5-MHz linear array or sector transducer. *B-mode* refers to *brightness modality*, where the image is a two-dimensional display of dots of varying brightness. *Real-time* refers to a live or moving display of echoes recorded instantly and continuously, analogous to the continuous image production of a cinema.

Diagnostic US uses high-frequency sound waves, measured in megahertz (1 MHz = 1 million sound waves per second), to produce images of soft tissues and organs. The production and behavior of audible sound waves (20 to 20,000 Hz), such as those produced by beating a drum, are analogous to US waves produced by electrical stimulation of piezoelectric crystals. Vibration of the drum head causes alternate compression and rarefaction of air molecules on either side of it, thereby emitting waves that are transduced by the eardrum and perceived as audible sound. Piezoelectric crystals in US transducers vibrate at a characteristic ultrasonic frequency when electrically stimulated and, like the drumhead, cause alternate compression and rarefaction of tissue molecules. The crystals in the transducer emit a thin (i.e., 2 mm) "curtain" of sound waves, and depending on the density and characteristics of the tissue, sound waves are either transmitted (nonechogenic) or reflected (echogenic). The transducer is connected to the console by a cable comprised of many wires connecting individual crystals to both a pulser and a receiver (Fig. 1). Electrical stimulation is episodically turned on and off by the pulser to allow the crystals to vibrate and emit sound waves and then to "listen" for reflected sound waves (echoes) that again cause the crystals to vibrate. The vibration caused by the echo is transduced into electrical impulses that are sent to the receiver, amplified, and converted to a moving real-time image on a television screen. Hence, this process is called *pulse-echo diagnostic ultrasonography*. The proportion of sound waves reflected is represented on the US image by shades of gray vary-

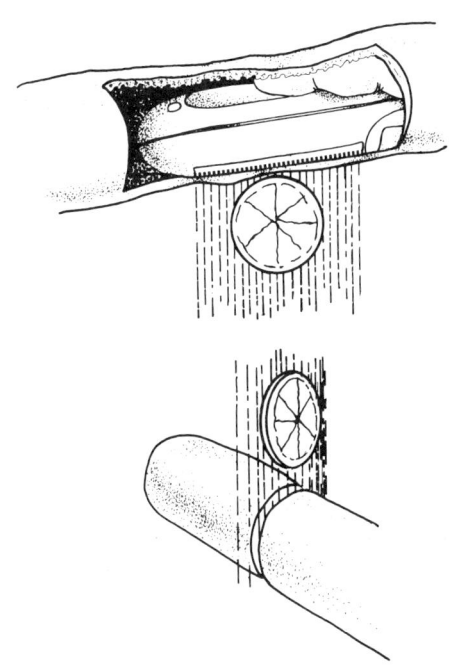

Figure 2. Ultrasound beam from a hand-held intrarectal transducer acoustically samples a cross-section of uterine horn.

ing from black to white. Fluid-filled structures such as follicles and embryonic vesicles are nonechogenic and produce a dark or black image. Tissues of increasing density (uterus, corpus luteum, bone) have increasing echogenicity so that the image varies from dark gray to white. Accordingly, this process has also been referred to as *gray-scale diagnostic ultrasonography*. Analogous to the way in which a knife can be used to section a piece of tissue, the US beam acoustically sections a slice of the tissue through which it passes (Fig. 2).

TRANSDUCERS

There are three major types of US transducers: linear array, convex array, and sector transducer. Linear array transducers have a row of piezoelectric crystals embedded side-by-side along the length of the probe. Sequential stimulation along this array produces a rectangular image, the horizontal length of which corresponds with the length of the row of crystals (e.g., 5 cm). The beam is usually oriented along the longitudinal axis of the mare during intrarectal use; therefore, the uterine body is imaged in sagittal section and the uterine horns in transverse section. Linear array transducers are the most common type for transrectal use in the mare because the rectum provides a long flat surface that accommodates this type of probe.

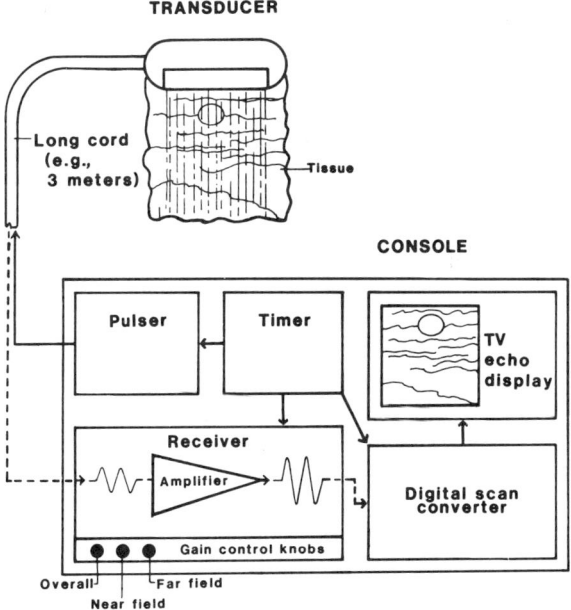

Figure 1. Components of an ultrasound scanner with a linear array transducer. (From Ginther, O. J.: Ultrasonic Imaging and Reproductive Events in the Mare. Cross Plains, Wis., Equiservices, 1986, p. 36. Reproduced by permission.)

Sector transducers produce a sound beam and hence an image that is triangular or pie-shaped because sound waves radiate from a single point. Depending on the orientation of the transducer, the beam plane may be parallel or perpendicular to the longitudinal axis of the mare when inserted into the rectum. The sector transducer provides the advantage of scanning through "confined windows" where a long flat surface is not available (e.g., intercostal spaces). Because of the proximity of the genitalia to the rectum, however, images of the genitalia are often confined to the narrow apex of the pie-shaped image during transrectal use. Except for more elaborate and expensive machines, most US consoles cannot accommodate both linear array and sector transducers.

Convex array transducers are a recent advance in US technology and represent a compromise between linear array and sector transducers. Crystals in convex array transducers are arranged like those in linear array transducers, but the transducer face is convexly curved instead of flat. Hence, sound waves are emitted in a radial fashion, creating somewhat of a pie-shaped image but one with a broader apex. Since the sound waves and the image are created in the same fashion as with linear array transducers, the same console can accommodate either a convex or a linear array transducer. This innovation provides more flexibility in the application of diagnostic US for examination of the reproductive system and other body systems of large and small animals.

The minimum size of a structure that can be imaged (resolution) and the clarity of the image are a function of the resolving power of the transducer and the quality of the scanner. Higher frequency transducers (e.g., 5 or 7.5 MHz) provide greater resolution than low-frequency transducers (e.g., 3.5 MHz). For example, a 3.5-MHz transducer can effectively image a 6-mm follicle and a newly formed corpus luteum; however, a 5-MHz transducer can image a 2-mm follicle and the corpus luteum throughout its functional life. High resolution, however, is gained at the expense of penetrating ability. Great penetration is generally not needed during intrarectal use because the transducer is in close proximity to the reproductive organs; the tissues of interest are usually no farther than 6 cm from the transducer surface. A 5- or 7.5-MHz transducer is the instrument of choice for most transrectal reproductive examinations in the mare; however, for imaging the uterus during advanced stages of pregnancy or the early postpartum period, a 3.5-MHz transducer is more appropriate.

METHOD OF EXAMINATION

Restraint and preparation of the mare, and the procedure for transrectal US, are similar to those for transrectal palpation. However, the importance of subdued lighting cannot be overemphasized for viewing the US image on the television monitor. An electrical outlet free from electronic interference must be available and the scanner should be positioned near the operator at approximately eye level. Good contact between the transducer and the rectal mucosa is essential; feces or air between the transducer and mucosa will block the sound waves and obliterate the image. As in any examination it is important to establish a standardized procedure to avoid mistakes of oversight.

ULTRASONIC APPEARANCE OF THE OVARIES

FOLLICLES

Structures in the equine ovary are excellent for US imaging because they are large and readily accessible by the transrectal route. Follicles appear as roughly spherical, well-circumscribed black (nonechogenic) structures on the US image. Irregular shapes are attributable to compression by an adjacent follicle, corpus luteum, or ovarian stroma. Determination of the size and shape of follicles, particularly with respect to the appearance of a corpus luteum and the endometrium, provides the clinician with considerable diagnostic information regarding the stage of the estrous cycle.

Transrectal US has made possible detailed studies of the dynamics of follicular populations in mares. Results support the hypothesis that follicular growth occurs in waves and that most mares have only one wave per estrous cycle; however, more recent data show that a minority of mares have two-wave cycles. Growth of a cohort of follicles larger than 15 mm in diameter is evident by days 8 to 10 (day 0 = day of ovulation) and is maximum by about day 15. By individual follicle mapping, it has been shown that the follicle destined to ovulate, the dominant follicle, is detectable as a member of the cohort by day 6, and within a few days it becomes the largest follicle. Although the dominant follicle continues to grow until ovulation, the remaining follicles in the cohort start to regress after approximately day 15.

IMPENDING OVULATION

Because of the need for criteria that can be used to determine the optimum time to breed, studies designed specifically to examine the US-detectable attributes of preovulatory follicles in mares have been conducted. Results have shown that significant changes occur in follicle diameter, follicle shape, and thickness of the follicle wall as ovulation approaches. Follicle diameter can be measured far more accurately by US than by palpation. To estimate follicle diameter, measurements are taken of the largest cross-sectional image; in nonspherical follicles the average of two measurements made perpendicular to each other is used. The dominant follicle increases in diameter at a rate of approximately 3 mm per day until the day before ovulation, at which time the mean diameter is approximately 45 mm. Season and multiple ovulations affect maximum diameter of the ovulatory follicle. Mean diameter is largest in May (48 mm) and smallest in July (40 mm), and is smaller in double ovulators (bilateral, 40 mm; unilateral, 35 mm). Of 181 single ovulations monitored in two studies, none of the follicles ovulated before reaching 35 mm, compared with 11 of 24 (46 per cent) double preovulatory follicles that ovulated before reaching 35 mm. Follicle diameter is the most useful predictor of impending ovulation in the mare. During the period from day −7 to day −1, 85 per cent of follicles exhibit a pronounced change in shape from spherical to nonspherical (pear-shaped or conical) (Fig. 3). Although no significant changes occur in the echogenicity of the follicular wall or fluid, the thickness of the follicle wall increases as ovulation approaches.

OVULATION

Ovulation has been studied by frequent and sometimes continuous US observation. Two extremes of follicular fluid evacuation have been described, one in which evacuation occurs in less than 1 minute and the other in which evacuation occurs gradually over 4 minutes. Regardless of whether initial fluid loss is fast or slow, 96 per cent of fluid is evacuated within 6 minutes. Even without knowledge that a large follicle had been present, ovulation can usually be diagnosed by US detection of an ovulation site on the day of occurrence and subsequently can be confirmed by visualization of a corpus luteum. The ovulation site appears on US as an area of increased echogenicity in the ovary, representing the apposition of the collapsed follicle walls. Often a

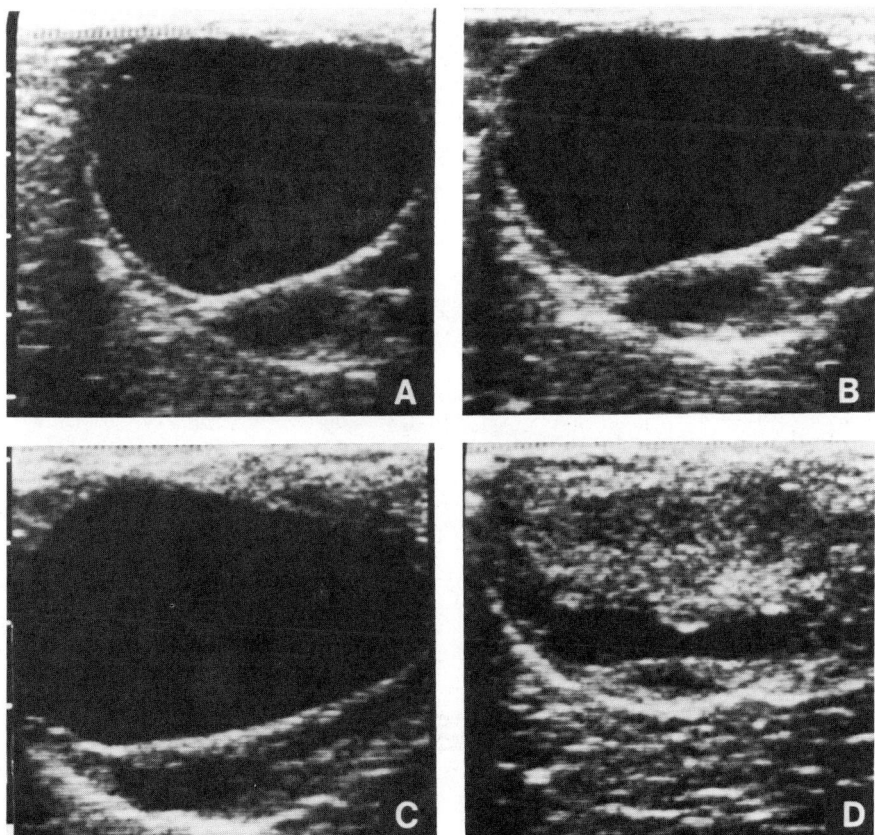

Figure 3. Shape change in the preovulatory follicle before ovulation. Images taken at the following times before the end of ovulation: 5 hours and 17 minutes (A), 2 hours and 17 minutes (B), 23 minutes (C), and at completion of evacuation. (D) (From Ginther, O. J.: Vet. Clin. North Am. (Equine Pract.), 4:197–213, 1988. Images recorded by D. T. Townson. Reproduced by permission.)

portion of the apposed walls is separated by a small slitlike pocket of antral fluid that has not yet been completely evacuated.

Corpus Luteum

The corpus luteum can be identified for an average of 17 days starting on the day of ovulation using a 5-MHz transducer and a good-quality scanner. Two distinct luteal morphologies have been described on US. Approximately 50 per cent of corpora lutea develop a central fluid-filled nonechogenic area, whereas the remaining 50 per cent are uniformly echogenic (luteinized) (Fig. 4). The central nonechogenic areas represent the accumulation of blood and the formation of a clot that begins on day 0 or 1 and continues to enlarge until day 2 or 3. The clot varies considerably in size but becomes progressively more organized and decreases in size as luteinization ensues. The development of a central area is not associated with an altered interovulatory interval or plasma progesterone concentration. During the 3 or 4 days after ovulation the luteinizing portion of the developing corpus luteum is intensely echogenic (bright white) in the mare. Hyperechogenicity is also sometimes seen during luteal regression, probably due to increasing density of the gland. The corpus luteum cannot be reliably detected by rectal palpation after the first few days post ovulation, and progesterone assays are not convenient for immediate evaluation. A major advantage afforded by US is the consistent and immediate detection and evaluation of the corpus luteum.

UTERUS AND CERVIX

The uterus is a major target organ for ovarian hormones, and changes in the character of the uterus reflect the dynamics of ovarian steroid output. During estrus (follicular phase), under the prevailing influence of estrogen, the tubular genitalia imbibe water, mucous secretion and

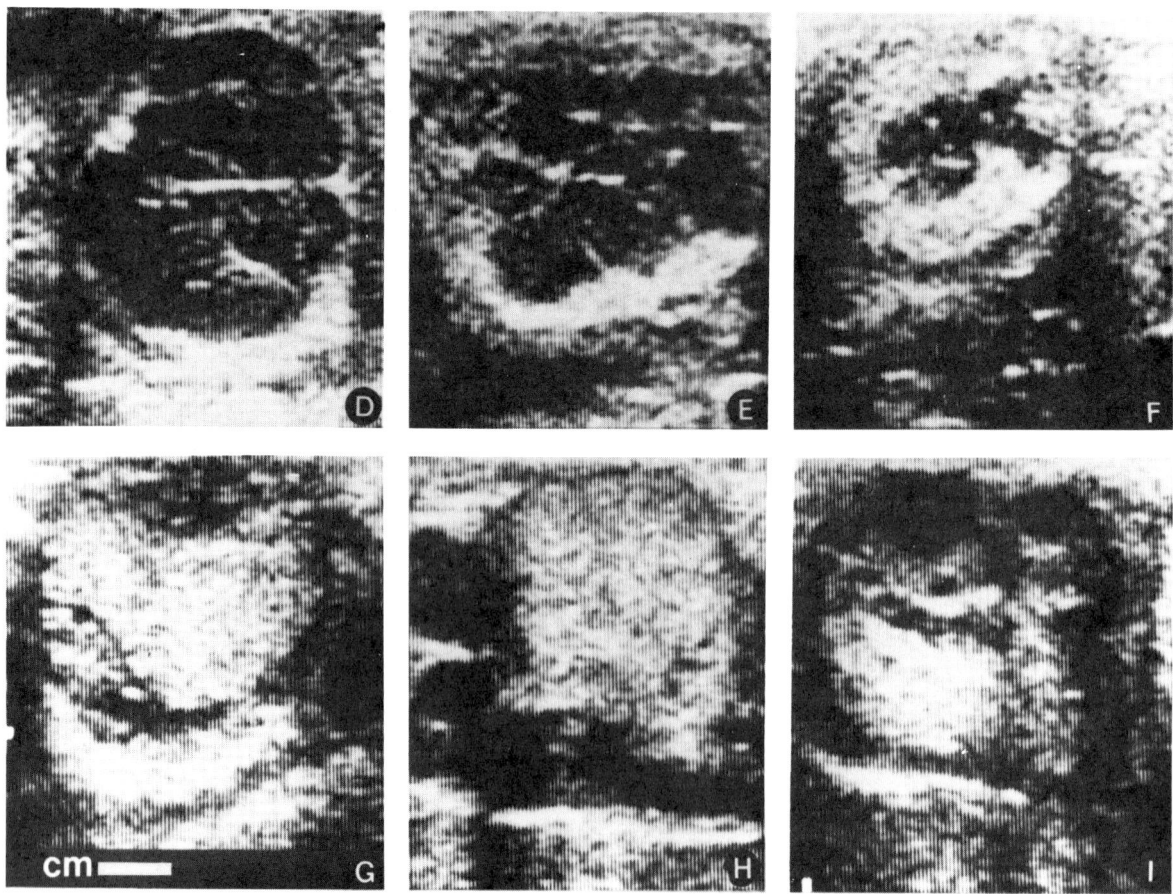

Figure 4. Two types of ultrasonographically detectable luteal morphology. Images are of developing, mature, and regressing (left to right, respectively) corpora lutea. The top three images show central nonechogenic areas; the bottom three images are uniformly echogenic. (Modified from Ginther, O. J.: Ultrasonic Imaging and Reproductive Events in the Mare. Cross Plains, Wis., Equiservices, 1986, p. 162. Reproduced by permission.)

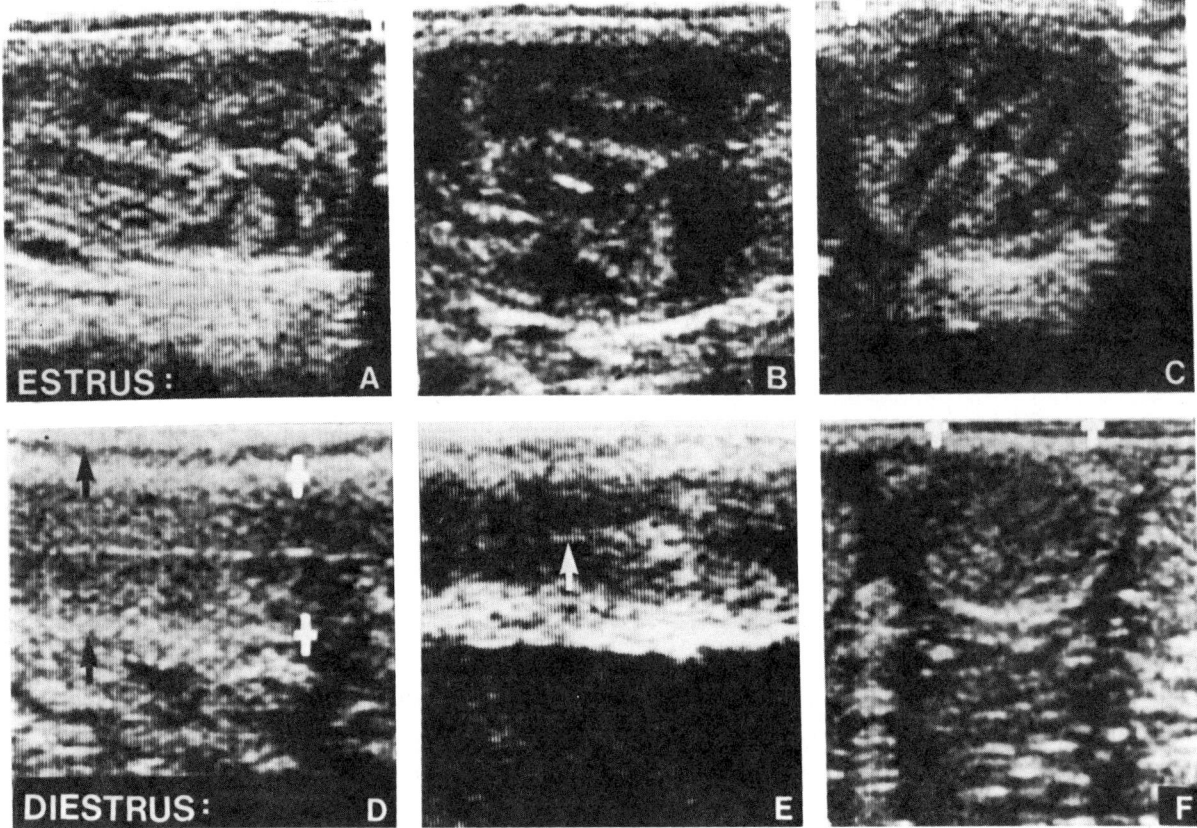

Figure 5. Ultrasonograms of the uterine body (*A, B, D, E*) and uterine horns (*C, F*) during estrus and diestrus. *Black arrows* mark the dorsal and ventral borders of the uterus; *white arrow* indicates luminal "white line." (Modified from Ginther, O. J.: Ultrasonic Imaging and Reproductive Events in the Mare. Cross Plains, Wis., Equiservices, 1986, p. 178. Reproduced by permission.)

blood circulation increase, and the longitudinal mucosal folds of the endometrium and endocervix hypertrophy. The effects of estrogen dominance are clearly visible on US. Edema of the endometrial folds during estrus gives the uterus a characteristic heterogeneous echotexture characterized by alternating areas of hyperechogenicity and hypoechogenicity. The convergence of folds at the center of the lumen gives the appearance of a spoked wheel when the uterine horn is viewed on US in cross-section (Fig. 5). During diestrus (luteal phase), under the prevailing influence of progesterone, the tubular genitalia do not imbibe water, mucous secretion decreases, and endometrial and endocervical folds are small. Individual endometrial folds are less distinct or not discernible on US during diestrus, resulting in a characteristic homogeneous uterine echotexture. A luminal "white line" is frequently seen on longitudinal views of the uterine body during diestrus and has been attributed to the apposition of longitudinal folds at the lumen, causing a relative increase in the number of tissue reflectors oriented parallel to the face of the transducer (specular echoes). Changes in endometrial echotexture, scored from 1 (folds not apparent) to 4 (folds most prominent), and uterine horn diameter throughout one estrous cycle are shown in Figure 6. Changes in the two are highly correlated; endometrial echotexture score and horn diameter were minimal during diestrus, maximal during estrus, and decreasing by the time of ovulation.

During estrus the cervix is indistinct on US and difficult to differentiate from the caudal uterine body. The cervix is less echogenic during estrus than during diestrus as a result of estrogen-induced edema. During diestrus the dense, nonedematous fibrous connective tissue of the cervix results in a more clearly defined, hyperechogenic appearance on US.

PREGNANCY

SINGLETONS

Early fascination with the US appearance of pregnancy in the mare resulted in much initial research devoted to early pregnancy diagnosis, embryo and fetal development, embryonic loss,

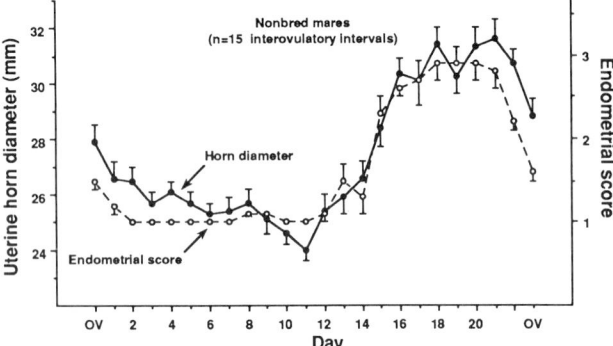

Figure 6. Uterine horn diameter and endometrial echotexture score (see text) for nonbred mares during the estrous cycle. (From Griffin, P. G., and Ginther, O. J.: Am. J. Vet. Res., *52:* 298, 1991. Reproduced by permission.)

detection of twins, and photographic documentation. Such interest may be attributable to several factors: (1) the large, spherical (easily detectable) form of the early equine conceptus, (2) the fascination of viewing live conceptuses (heartbeat, fetal movements), (3) the suitability of the equine uterus for transrectal US, and (4) the intensive veterinary involvement in breeding and pregnancy management in the horse industry.

Studies by experienced examiners using a 5-MHz linear array transducer and high-quality scanners demonstrated that the embryonic vesicle was first detectable on days 9 to 11 (day 0 = ovulation) when it reached 3 to 5 mm in diameter. The vesicle was first detected by day 9 in about 10 per cent of mares, by day 10 in 70 per cent, and by day 11 in 98 per cent. Perhaps the embryonic vesicle could be detected a day earlier with a 7.5-MHz transducer, but this possibility has not been investigated. Detection by day 8 may have important implications for embryo transfer.

Research utilizing US imaging has demonstrated that the equine embryonic vesicle constantly interacts with the uterus in a dynamic, physical fashion. These interactions include (1) embryo mobility (movement of the embryonic vesicle throughout the length of the uterine lumen many times per day on days 9 to 15), (2) fixation (cessation of mobility on day 16), and (3) orientation (rotation of the vesicle on days 16 to 20 so that the embryonic pole is on the ventral aspect of the vesicle). Because of early embryo mobility, the vesicle may be found anywhere within the uterine lumen from the day of first detection (days 9 to 11) through day 15. Thereafter the vesicle becomes fixed in the caudal portion of one of the horns. As the time of fixation approaches, the rate of embryo mobility (number of location changes over time) increases, and the time spent in the uterine body (vs. horns) decreases. Characteristic size and shape changes of the embryonic vesicle, as well as morphological changes in the embryo proper, can be used as indicators of the stage of pregnancy. Figure 7 shows the changes in cross-sectional height of the embryonic vesicle, which are useful for estimating the day of pregnancy. Age can be estimated with 95 per cent accuracy within ±1.5 days for 6- to 23-mm vesicles, and within ±4 days for 27- to 56-mm vesicles. On the S-shaped portion of the curve (days 16 to 28) the cross-sectional height does not change enough to be an adequate indicator of age. During this stage and later, profound morphological changes occur that facilitate age determination. On days 9 to 15, the vesicles are spherical and produce a nonechogenic, circumscribed image resulting from the enclosed collection of yolk sac fluid. By day 18, the vesicles tend to have a triangular form with the apex oriented dorsally. The embryo proper is detectable by about day 20 on the ventral aspect of the vesicle. The allantoic sac is usually well defined by day 24 beneath the embryo. The allantoic sac enlarges and the yolk sac recedes over days 24 to 33 so that the embryo and the echogenic line separating the two sacs move toward the dorsal aspect of the vesicle (Fig. 8). Useful morphological indicators of day

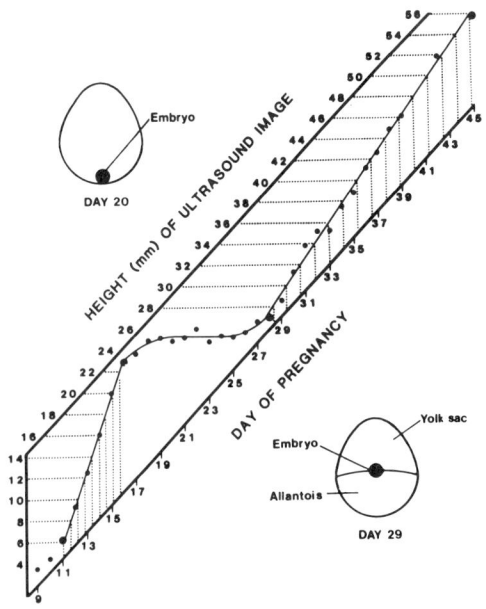

Figure 7. Changes in height of the embryonic vesicle in cross-section from day 9 to day 45 (day 0 = ovulation). (From Ginther, O. J.: Ultrasonic Imaging and Reproductive Events in the Mare. Cross Plains, Wis., Equiservices, 1986, p. 221. Reproduced by permission.)

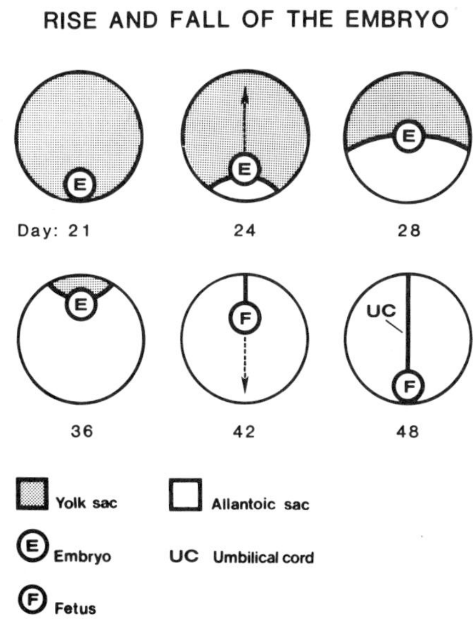

RISE AND FALL OF THE EMBRYO

Figure 8. Representation of changes in morphological appearance of the equine conceptus from day 21 to day 48 (day 0 = ovulation) as detected by transrectal ultrasonography. (From Ginther, O. J.: Ultrasonic Imaging and Reproductive Events in the Mare. Cross Plains, Wis., Equiservices, 1986, p. 22. Reproduced by permission.)

of pregnancy include the first detection of the embryo proper at the ventral pole, the proportion of the vesicle that consists of yolk sac versus allantoic sac during ascent of the embryo, and the descent of the fetus as indicated by the length of the umbilical cord.

Transrectal US imaging of equine fetal anatomy beyond day 50 has not been extensively studied. Studies of the anatomy of the genital tubercle on US have documented that transrectal US can be used to diagnose fetal sex in horses between days 59 and 68 (see page 660). Recent US studies between days 69 and 81 of pregnancy have shown that the early equine fetus is extremely mobile within the allantoic fluid and changes its location, recumbency, and presentation within the uterus several times per hour. The eye orbits of the fetus are often accessible to imaging performed via the transrectal route during later stages of pregnancy, and measurement of the orbits may have predictive significance in estimating fetal age. Transabdominal US has also been used after 100 days' gestation to monitor fetal orientation and viability.

TWINS

The detection and management of twin embryos is an important and anxiety-ridden facet of equine reproduction. US scanners have contributed greatly to our understanding of twinning in the mare and have provided the practitioner with superb diagnostic and management approaches. A review of the subject of equine twins is presented on page 657; only a brief summary is offered here.

Twin embryos undergo intrauterine mobility and fixation similar to singletons. However, in mares with twins an additional factor plays a role during fixation (day 16): fixation of one vesicle may serve to trap and therefore contribute to fixation of the other. Fixation occurs unilaterally (both in one horn) more often (70 per cent) than one would expect by chance alone.

There is a wide disparity between the incidence of double ovulation and the incidence of twin births. Most of this disparity may be accounted for by the embryo reduction mechanism. Embryo reduction is the natural elimination of excess embryonic vesicles so that only one viable vesicle enters the fetal stage (survives beyond day 40). Nearly all embryo reductions occur after fixation, between days 17 and 40, and the incidence is profoundly increased when the vesicles become fixed unilaterally rather than bilaterally. As a result of this and other observations, the "deprivation hypothesis" has been proposed to account for embryo reduction. The hypothesis states that one vesicle of a twin set is deprived of adequate embryonal–maternal exchange, and therefore regresses, when it becomes oriented so that a major portion of its three-walled area (vascularized area) is apposed to the wall of the adjacent vesicle rather than the endometrium.

Two US-aided approaches may be considered for correcting twin embryos: initial pregnancy examination during the mobility phase, with correction of all detected twin sets *(prefixation correction)*, and initial examination after fixation but before day 25, with correction of bilateral twin sets *(postfixation correction)*.

Prefixation correction entails compressing the uterine horn transrectally between finger and thumb caudal to the selected vesicle and moving the hand toward the tip of the horn. The vesicle may rupture in place, during movement up the horn, or upon being trapped at the tip of the horn. If the vesicles are in contact, the operator can wait for an hour or a day until the vesicles separate due to the mobility phenomenon, or an attempt can be made to separate them by gentle massage. The vesicles are easier to rupture when large (days 13 to 15; 12 to 18 mm) than when small (days 11 and 12; 6 to 9 mm). For this reason, the mobility-phase pregnancy examination should be done late (days 13 to 15). Prefixation manual reduction is highly effective. Data indicate that the probability that the remaining embryonic vesicle will develop normally and enter the fetal stage is equivalent to the probability that a singleton of corresponding age will enter the fetal stage.

Postfixation correction is readily accomplished in bilateral twin sets by digital compression of one of the embryonic locations or bulges. The success rate for manual reduction of bilateral fixation, when done by day 25, is equivalent to the success rate for prefixation manual reduction. A disadvantage of postfixation reduction is that unilaterally fixed vesicles are difficult to correct; this disadvantage must be weighed against the probability of natural reduction. Manual reduction of unilaterally fixed twins is often tedious, time-consuming, and frustrating, especially a day or two after fixation, when the twin set has assumed a compressed, irregular shape. In addition, if the initial examination is done during days 17 to 19, when vesicles are compressed and irregular, twin unilaterally fixed vesicles will occasionally be missed.

REPRODUCTIVE TRACT ABNORMALITIES

Transrectal US is useful not only for monitoring normal reproductive events but also for diagnosing and managing reproductive abnormalities. The following is a discussion of ovarian and uterine pathological conditions that are detectable on US.

Ovaries

Ovarian irregularities and pathological changes detectable on US include double ovulation, ovulation failure, hemorrhagic follicles, quiet ovulation (silent estrus), diestrous ovulations, prolonged maintenance of the corpus luteum, ovarian tumors, and cystic periovarian structures.

Double ovulations occur in 8 to 25 per cent of ovulatory periods, depending on the breed and familial background of horses in a particular area. Thoroughbreds and draft mares have the highest rate, Standardbreds an intermediate rate, and Quarter Horses, Appaloosas, and ponies the lowest rate of double ovulations. As previously mentioned, follicles ovulate at a smaller diameter in double versus single ovulations (double unilateral, 35 mm; double bilateral, 40 mm; single, 45 mm). This is an important consideration in deciding when to have the mare bred.

In a recent US study, ovulation failure during the ovulatory season was reported to be 4.7 per cent and all apparent anovulations involved filling of the follicle with blood (hemorrhagic anovulatory follicles). The blood clots over time and produces a characteristic trabecular network of fibrin detectable with US. These hematomas occasionally become extremely large (more than 10 cm) but gradually regress over one or more of the following estrous cycles. Other than ovulation failure at the time of occurrence, these structures apparently do not alter subsequent ovarian function. Hemorrhagic anovulatory follicles need to be studied in more detail, but they may represent the phenomenon known as "autumn follicles." Cystic ovarian disease comparable to that described in cattle has not been documented as an entity in mares.

In an early study the incidence of diestrous ovulations was reported to be 24 per cent. Recent US studies have reported the incidence to be 4 to 6 per cent. The condition known as spontaneous persistence of the corpus luteum has been reported to occur in up to 25 per cent of ovulatory periods but was not detected in a recent US study of 69 interovulatory intervals. In this regard, confusion has resulted in the use of terms such as persistence of the corpus luteum, prolonged diestrus, persistent luteal activity, and pseudopregnancy.

Prolonged luteal activity can be due to persistence of an individual corpus luteum or to the sequential development of luteal glands, each of which may have a normal life span. Luteal tissue can originate from an unovulated follicle or from an ovulation during the follicular phase (primary corpus luteum) or luteal phase (secondary corpus luteum). In the absence of critical monitoring (e.g., by US) of the primary corpus luteum, the prolonged activity could be erroneously attributed to persistence of the primary corpus luteum. Although persistence of an individual corpus luteum can occur in association with severe endometrial damage resulting in loss of the uterine luteolytic mechanism, spontaneous (no known uterine pathology) persistence of the primary corpus luteum should not be accepted as a clinical entity on the basis of available reports.

Although not critically examined by US, granulosa cell tumors appear as large (15 to 20 cm or more) multiloculated cystic structures that obliterate the normal architecture of the ovary. Periovarian cysts can be detected with US, but, depending on their size and proximity to the ovary, they may be confused with an ovarian follicle. Digital palpation may help differentiate these structures.

Uterus

Pathological changes of the uterus detectable on US include uterine cysts, intrauterine fluid collections, and fetal debris. Uterine cysts as small as 3 mm in diameter can be detected; some reach a size of 10 cm or more. Uterine cysts may occur singly or in multiloculated clusters in one or more areas of the uterine body and horns. In one study, there appeared to be a quantitative effect of uterine cysts on infertility. Pregnancy rate tended to be lower only for mares severely affected by uterine cysts. It was emphasized, however, that age must be considered in attempts to attribute infertility to uterine cysts since these structures are more common in older mares. In the same study, fluid collections within the uterine lumen, especially during diestrus, were indicative of endometritis. Mares with diestrous intrauterine fluid collections had cytological (endometrial swab) and histological (endometrial biopsy) evidence of an inflammatory process and had abbreviated interovulatory intervals associated with a premature decrease in progesterone. Mares with diestrous intrauterine fluid collections during the previous estrous cycle had a lower pregnancy rate and a higher embryonic loss rate than unaffected mares. US is a powerful tool for studying embryonic loss in the mare because of early detectability of the conceptus. Fetal death and the subsequent disposition of fetal debris can also be easily monitored. Dense tissues such as fetal cartilage and bone are excellent reflectors and show up clearly on US scans. Fetal bones may remain in the uterus for an indefinite time (1 year or more) and render the mare infertile until removed. The bones may be difficult to remove by flushing because some apparently become embedded in the endometrium. Extraction by grasping with the fingers or with an instrument may be successful. On one occasion, a fetal bone was removed with a uterine biopsy instrument while guiding it onto the bone by transrectal US.

CONCLUSION

The technique of transrectal US and the interpretation of findings require training and experience. Transrectal US is not necessarily any easier or more difficult than transrectal palpation; it requires a thorough understanding of the mare's anatomy and physiology. Digital palpation is not required for routine examination of the reproductive organs if a scanner is available unless tactile information such as tone or consistency is needed. Most clinicians prefer to scan the reproductive tract prior to palpation to visualize it in the undisturbed state and to determine luminal content and pregnancy status.

Supplemental Readings

Adams, G. P., Kastelic, J. P., Bergfelt, D. R., and Ginther, O. J.: Effect of uterine inflammation and ultrasonically-detected uterine pathology on fertility in the mare. J. Reprod. Fertil. Suppl., 35:445–454, 1987.

Ginther, O. J.: Ultrasonic Imaging and Reproductive Events in the Mare. Cross Plains, Wis., Equiservices, 1986.

Ginther, O. J.: Ultrasonic imaging of equine ovarian follicles and corpora lutea. Vet. Clin. North Am. (Equine Pract.), 4:197–213, 1988.

Ginther, O. J., and Pierson, R. A.: Regular and irregular characteristics of ovulation and the interovulatory interval in mares. Equine Vet. Sci., 9:4–12, 1989.

Griffin, P. G., and Ginther, O. J.: Uterine and fetal dynamics during early pregnancy in mares. Am. J. Vet. Res., 52: 298, 1991.

McKinnon, A. O., Squires, E. L., Carnevale, E. M., Harrison, L. A., Frantz, D. D., McChesney, A. E., and Shideler, R. K.: Diagnostic ultrasonography of uterine pathology in the mare. *In:* Proceedings of the 33rd Annual Convention of the American Association of Equine Practitioners, New Orleans, 1987, pp. 605–622.

Pierson, R. A., and Ginther, O. J.: Follicular population dynamics during the estrous cycle of the mare. Anim. Reprod. Sci., *14*:219–231, 1987.

Pierson, R. A., Kastelic, J. P., and Ginther, O. J.: Basic principles and techniques for transrectal ultrasonography in cattle and horses. Theriogenology, 29:3–20, 1988.

Management of Twin Pregnancy

A. L. Hallowell, AUBURN, WASHINGTON
Gordon L. Woods, MOSCOW, IDAHO

A program to minimize the number of twin pregnancies should be cost-effective; should not decrease the mare's overall pregnancy rate; should, during the same season, enable the rebreeding of mares that lose their pregnancies; and should prevent the abortion or birth of weak or dead twin foals. We recommend that all mares be bred, whether they have single or multiple preovulatory follicles; that all breeds or types of mares with a high prevalence of multiple ovulations be examined for twins, whether single or multiple ovulations are detected; and that mares with twin embryos (less than 40 days) be treated to prevent the development of twin fetuses (more than 40 days).

BREEDING

Mares with multiple preovulatory follicles should be bred since mares with multiple ovulations have high pregnancy rates. Programs to eliminate twins by restricting the breeding of mares with multiple preovulatory follicles are not successful since the incidence of twins is not decreased and the overall pregnancy rate may decrease.

EXAMINATION FOR TWINS

Twins originate from multiple ovulations; therefore, it is not cost-effective to perform examinations for twins on mares that have a low rate of multiple ovulations (e.g., pony mares). In contrast, Thoroughbred or draft mares, which have a high rate of multiple ovulations, should routinely be examined for twins. Under field conditions, the majority of twin fetuses occur in mares in which only one ovulation has been detected; therefore, regardless of the number of ovulations detected, all mares with a high rate of multiple ovulations should be examined for twins. Misdiagnosis of multiple ovulations likely occurs under field conditions because either double ovarian follicles occur in adjacent ovulation sites in the same ovary and are detected as one ovulation or because a first ovulation is diagnosed, ovulation detection is discontinued, and a second ovulation subsequently occurs. Utilization of ultrasonography (US) to detect and confirm ovulation should decrease the incidence of misdiagnosis of multiple ovulations. We recommend that the first routine examination for twins be performed at 13 to 15 days post ovulation, when the embryo is still mobile.

The examination should be thorough and systematic. It should be completed by an operator who understands the developmental morphology of the equine embryo and its US imaging appearance. A high-quality US scanner with a 5-MHZ linear array transducer is preferred to identify twin embryos. The number of ovulations can be estimated by using US to scan and count the corpora lutea on the mare's ovaries.

Operator inexperience, improper US instruments, adjacent twin embryos, fractious or improperly restrained mares, rapid examinations, and endometrial cysts are possible reasons why twin embryos are misdiagnosed. Operators should study a textbook that accurately describes the US morphology of the equine embryo. Knowledge of the expected size and morphology of the equine embryo is essential for accurately interpreting the US images.

Adjacent twin embryos may be difficult to differentiate as two separate embryos. Their combined diameter will be larger than the expected diameter of a similarly aged single embryo; they may be separated by a bright dorsoventral line that represents their adjacent membranes; and there may be a cleavage between the two embryonic vesicles. If adjacent twin embryos are suspected, reexamination of the mare for twins by day 29 post ovulation is recommended. In the case of misdiagnosis, there is still consolation in the fact that many adjacent twin embryos reduce to one surviving embryo by day 40 post ovulation. Fortunately, nonadjacent twin embryos, which usually do not reduce to one surviving embryo by day 40 post ovulation, are easier to diagnose than adjacent twin embryos.

Endometrial cysts, which occur primarily in aged mares, are another reason for misdiagnosis of twin embryos. These cysts, like embryonic vesicles, are fluid-filled. The cysts may be the same size and shape as embryonic vesicles. Careful recording of the location, size, and shape of endometrial cysts at the beginning of the breeding season or shortly after ovulation will help to differentiate between endometrial cysts and embryonic vesicles on subsequent examinations. If multiple fluid-filled structures are detected, the size, shape, and location of the structures should be recorded and the mare reexamined in 3 to 4 days. If the structures do not change in size or shape and they do not develop into an embryo proper with a heartbeat, they are likely to be endometrial cysts. The embryo proper and heartbeat are accurately identified by day 28. We recommend the routine video recording of all US examinations, as video recording is a simple and economical procedure that becomes a permanent record of each scan.

THERAPY

Mares should be routinely examined three times for twins. The first examination is done prior to the expected detection of embryos so that the location of endometrial cysts can be carefully recorded. The second is done on day 13 to 15 after ovulation and the third by day 29. Table 1 gives the observations on days 13 to 15 and on day 29 and the recommended treatments. When two nonadjacent embryos are clearly evident, the smallest conceptus can be crushed by

TABLE 1. TREATMENT OF TWIN PREGNANCIES DETECTED AT DAYS 13 to 15 AND BY DAY 29 OF GESTATION.

Day	Observation	Recommendation
13 to 15	One embryo	Reexamine on day 29
	Two nonadjacent embryos	Crush smallest conceptus
	Two adjacent embryos	Reexamine on day 29
29	Two nonadjacent embryos	Crush one embryo
	Adjacent twin embryos	Abort with prostaglandin $F_{2\alpha}$ if sufficient time to rebreed, or allow pregnancy to proceed and hope only one embryo will survive

compressing it ventrocaudally against the pelvis or crushing it between one's fingers and thumb. One must be certain that one of the fluid-filled structures is not an endometrial cyst. Antiprostaglandins and progesterone therapy are not recommended in conjunction with the crushing technique since use of these products has not increased the success of the procedure.

Mares with twin fetuses (more than 40 days post ovulation) are difficult to manage, since the endometrial cups have become established, the probability of spontaneous fetal reduction is low, and the success rate of manually eliminating only one fetus is quite low. It is believed that if the mare aborts the fetuses after the endometrial cups are established, she will not recycle for rebreeding until after day 120, when the endometrial cups regress. The incidence of spontaneous reduction of one fetus is low for twin fetuses that are either adjacent as embryos and fail to reduce or that are nonadjacent as embryos and first establish membrane-to-membrane contact as fetuses. Killing one fetus by manual crushing usually results in the death of both fetuses.

When considering the possible options for treating mares with twin fetuses, it is important to consider the effect that abortion or birth of twins will have on the mare's chances of becoming pregnant during the subsequent breeding season. Since the number of available days in a breeding season is limited, one should consider how many days of the subsequent breeding season will be lost due to a full-term pregnancy. For example, if parturition is expected to occur in late May, the likelihood of that mare becoming pregnant during the season in which she foals is quite low. Also, the fertility of the mare may be decreased following the abortion or birth of twins. Therefore, it may be economically prudent to abort a mare with twin fetuses and have a better opportunity for a pregnancy during the next season.

One plausible approach to managing twin fetuses is to monitor the pregnancy by transrectal US until approximately midpregnancy in the hope that only one fetus will spontaneously die. The accuracy of monitoring fetuses by transrectal US decreases as the size of the conceptus increases. A 3.5-MHZ instead of a 5.0-MHZ transducer might be beneficial, since the lower frequency transducer has a greater depth of field. Electrocardiography has also been used to accurately detect twin fetuses.

If both fetuses survive to midpregnancy, one might consider aborting the mare with prostaglandin $F_{2\alpha}$ and beginning the subsequent breeding season with a nonpregnant mare. An alternative treatment for midgestation twin fetuses is to insert a needle into the heart of one fetus under US guidance and inject it with a potassium chloride solution. If both fetuses fail to survive this procedure, the mare would begin the subsequent breeding season as a nonpregnant mare.

Additional research is required to understand fetal twins and the effect of twin abortions or births on the mare's subsequent fertility. Just as the recently acquired knowledge of twin embryo interactions now enables the logical management of twin embryos, additional knowledge of twin fetuses will enable the logical management of twin fetuses.

Supplemental Readings

Ginther, O. J.: Ultrasonic Imaging and Reproductive Events in the Mare. Cross Plains, Wis., Equiservices, 1986.

Ginther, O. J.: The nature of embryo reduction in mares with twin conceptuses: Deprivation hypothesis. Am. J. Vet. Res., 50:45–53, 1989.

Hallowell, A. L., and Woods, G. L., Roberts, C. J.: Termination of twin gestation by blastocyst crush in the mare. Equine Vet. J., 15:40–42, 1983.

Jeffcott, L. B., and Whitwell, K. E.: Twinning as a cause of fetal and neonatal loss in the Thoroughbred mare. J. Comp. Pathol., 83:91, 1973.

Parkes, R. D., and Colles, C. M.: Fetal electrocardiography in the mare as a practical aid to diagnosing singleton and twin pregnancy. Vet. Rec., 100:25–26, 1977.

Pascoe, R. R.: Methods for the treatments of twin pregnancy in the mare. Equine Vet. J., 15:40–42, 1983.

Pascoe, D. R., Pascoe, R. R., Hughes, J. P., et al: Management of twin conceptuses by manual embryonic reduction: Comparison of two techniques and three hormonal treatments (abstract). Am. J. Vet. Res. 48:1594,1987.

Rantanen, N. W., and Kencaid, B.: Ultrasound guided fetal cardiac puncture: A method of twin reduction in the mare. In: Proceedings of the Annual Convention of the American Association of Equine Practitioners, 1988, pp 173-180.

Simpson, R. E., Greenwood, S., Ricketts, S. W., Rossdale, P. D., Sandersen, M., and Allen, W. R.: Use of ultrasound echography for early diagnosis of single and twin pregnancy in the mare. J. Reprod. Fertil., Suppl. 32, 1982.

Diagnosis of Fetal Gender by Ultrasonography

Sandra S. Curran, MADISON, WISCONSIN

The ultrasonographic (US) appearance of external genitalia has been used to determine fetal gender in humans and cattle. In humans, the scrotum and labia are detected with a high degree of accuracy after 140 days of gestation. In cattle, the scrotum and mammary glands have been imaged with US 73 to 120 days after insemination. Transrectal US identification and location of the genital tubercle is a highly accurate method for determining gender in horses 59 to 68 days after ovulation.

The genital tubercle is the embryonic structure that differentiates into the penis in males and the clitoris in females (Fig. 1). During differentiation the anogenital distance (distance from the anus to the genital tubercle) increases greatly in the male but not in the female (Fig. 2). The genital tubercle changes in relative location from its initial position between the rear limbs to the proximity of the umbilical cord in the male and the tail in the female.

US imaging of the equine fetus is performed using a real-time B-mode diagnostic scanner equipped with a 5-MHz linear array transrectal transducer. The following conditions optimize the potential for diagnosis: (1) use of a high-quality scanner, (2) subdued external light, (3) scanner screen in close proximity and at eye level, and (4) horses that tolerate rectal examinations with minimal movement. The three sequential views that can be used include cross-sectional, frontal (a plane perpendicular to the dorsoventral middle of the fetus), and sagittal (a plane parallel to the dorsoventral midline).

Cross-sectional views are most useful for routine purposes because of ease of orientation of

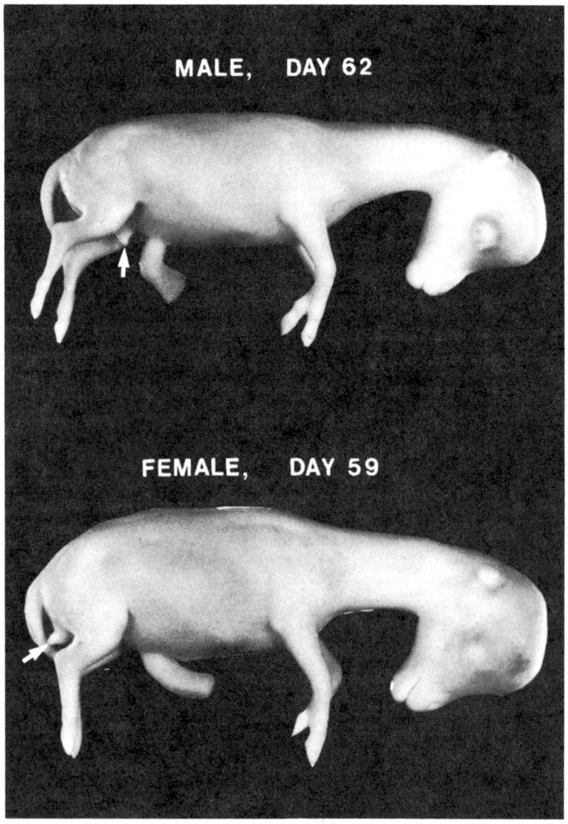

Figure 1. Location and appearance of the genital tubercle *(arrow)* in individual male and female equine fetuses. (From Curran, S., and Ginther, O. J.: J. Equine Vet. Sci., *9*:77, 1989. Reproduced by permission.)

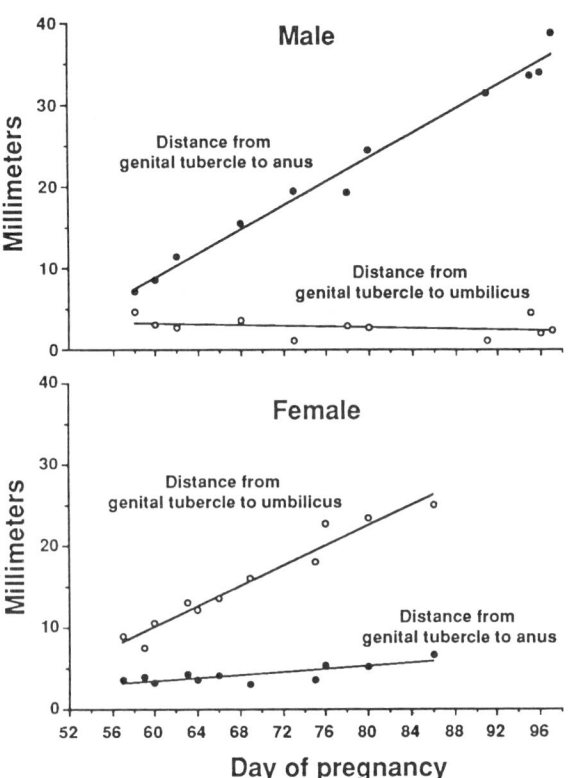

Figure 2. Distances from genital tubercle to anus and umbilicus in horse fetuses. Prepared from tabulated data of Curran and Ginther, 1989.

the transducer across the fetus and identification of the bilobed morphology of the genital tubercle. Fetal examination should begin at a landmark, such as the head or beating heart, and move caudad through the umbilical area, abdomen, rear limbs, and tail area. The scans should concentrate on the area of the umbilical cord and tail. A slightly oblique cross-section involving the rear limbs, tail, and perineal area is useful for identifing the genital tubercle in the female. It is crucial to identify reference structures when determining the location of the genital tubercle.

Frontal views are sometimes useful in determining the location of the genital tubercle relative to the umbilical cord, rear limbs, and tail. However, orienting the transducer and achieving a consistent imaging plane are more difficult than for cross-sectional views. Fetal landmarks are more easily identified on sagittal views, but identification of the genital tubercle is more difficult. The US morphology of the genital tubercle is similar in male and female fetuses (Fig. 3). The tubercle is hyperechogenic and usually bilobed. Each lobe is elongated and oval-shaped. Sometimes the cranial ends of the two lobes are in close contact, forming a V-shaped structure. This distinct bilobed appearance and location along the ventral body wall enable differentiation of the tubercle from other echogenic structures. When first detected, the tubercle is approximately 2 mm in length and width. On average, the tubercle begins to increase slightly in width and greatly in length after approximately day 50. A trilobed form begins to appear in some male and female fetuses by approximately day 80 after ovulation (Fig. 4). In older male fetuses, the penis and prepuce (former genital tubercle) is seen as three parallel echogenic lines just caudal to the umbilical cord.

In one study of 26 riding-type mares, US diagnoses of fetal gender were made every other day from day 35 or 36 (after ovulation) until fetal removal on days 41 to 97. End points were determination of gender; length and width of the genital tubercle, with degree of certainty scored from 1 to 4 (1 = gender not determinable; 2, 3, and 4 = gender determined with minimal, intermediate, and maximal certainty); and determination of the location of the genital tubercle, scored from 1 to 5 (1 = area of the umbilical

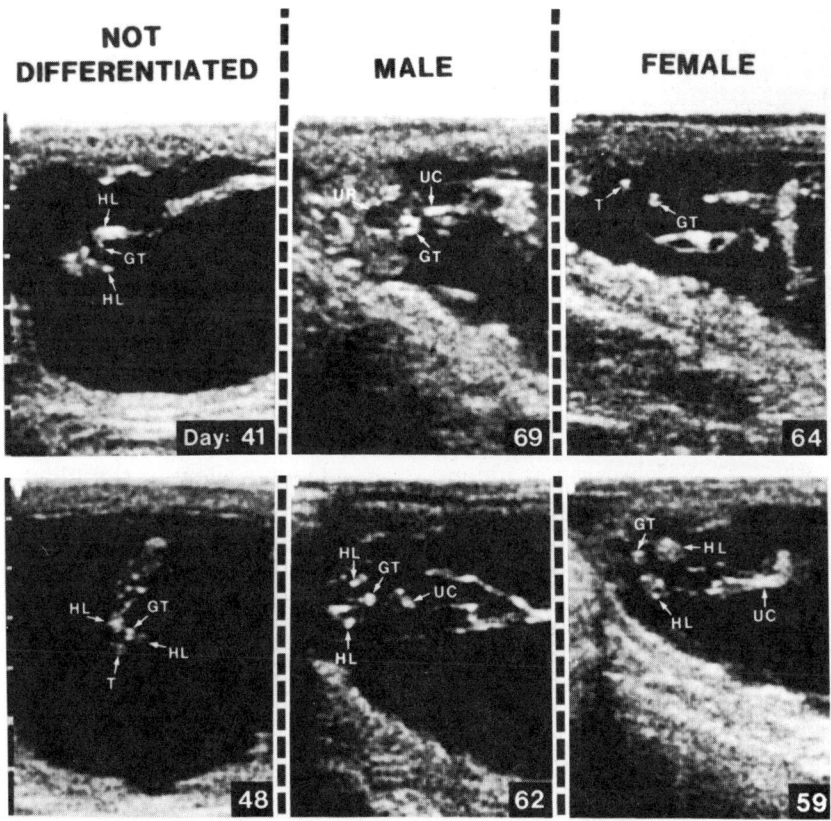

Figure 3. Ultrasonic images of the genital tubercle and associated structures in undifferentiated, male, and female fetuses. Images in the upper row are cross-sectional views, images in the lower row are frontal views. Day of pregnancy is shown in the lower right corner of each image. GT = genital tubercle, HL = hind limbs, T = tail, UC = umbilical cord, UR = urachus (From Curran, S., and Ginther, O. J.: J. Equine Vet. Sci., 9:77, 1989. Reproduced by permission.)

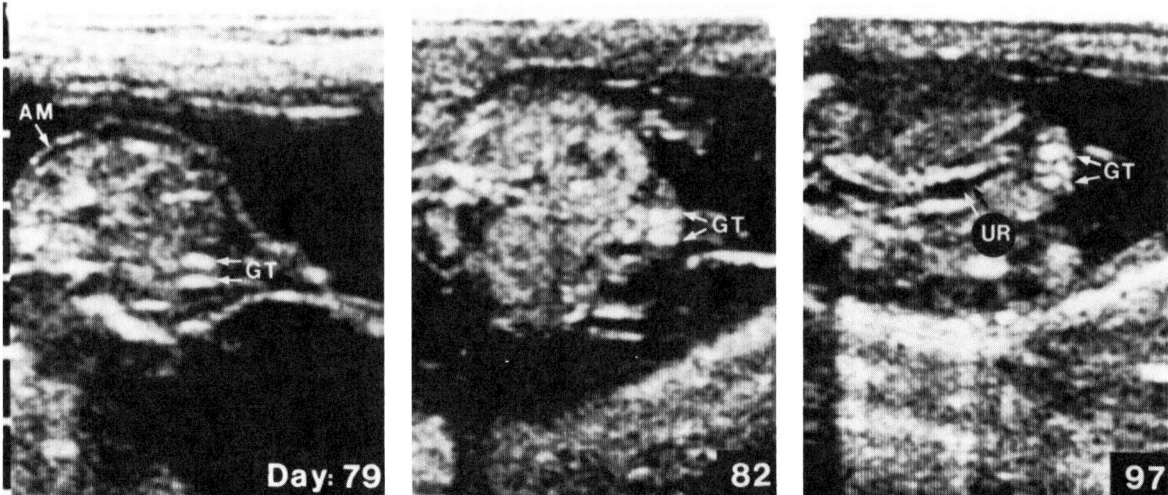

Figure 4. Trilobular genital tubercle or penis in older male fetuses. The tubercle is distinctly bilobular on day 79, beginning to form a third lobe between the two outer lobes by day 82, and has a distinct trilobular or three-layered appearance by day 97. Images are in cross-section, except for the image on the right, which is an oblique view. AM = amnion, GT = genital tubercle, UR = urachus. (From Curran, S., and Ginther, O. J.: J. Equine Vet. Sci., 9:77, 1989. Reproduced by permission.)

cord, 2 = intermediate between the umbilical cord and rear limbs, 3 = on the midline between the rear limbs, 4 = area between the rear limbs and tail, 5 = close proximity to the tail). A certainty score of 2 was assigned when the views were inadequate to clearly identify and locate the genital tubercle. A score of 3 was assigned when either the area near the umbilical cord or near the tail was thoroughly examined (and the genital tubercle identified), but both areas could not be viewed completely or the location score was not yet a 1 or 5. A certainty score of 4 was reserved for adequate examination of both the areas of the tail and the umbilical cord and when the genital tubercle was identified and location determined. The accuracy of the US diagnosis of fetal gender was determined from the location of the genital tubercle relative to the tail and umbilical cord on removed fetuses.

The apparent genital tubercle was not identifiable on US prior to day 36. There was a gradual increase in the per centage of identifications up to days 53 to 54, at which time the tubercle was identified in all fetuses and remained consistently identifiable through day 68. Between days 69 and 97, the tubercle was not found in 8 to 33 per cent of the fetuses (Fig. 5). Failures to identify the genital tubercle prior to day 53 were primarily due to the small size of the fetus. Failures after day 68 were primarily due to the fetus being deeply situated in the mare and not adequately accessible, even with ballottement.

The genital tubercle was initially positioned between the rear limbs (score of 3). Beginning on days 49 to 50, scores of 2 and 4 were recorded. Day 58 was the first day on which a score of 1 (near the umbilicus, male) or 5 (near the tail, female) was recorded in any fetus. Thereafter the number of scores 1 and 5 gradually increased (see Fig. 5). The mean day on which the tubercle was immediately caudal to the umbilical cord (male) was day 62, and in the proximity of the tail (female), day 64.

Fetal gender was recorded as male when the genital tubercle was immediately caudal to the abdominal attachment of the umbilical cord and female when the tubercle was in close proximity to the tail. Therefore, gender was considered not diagnosable with US before day 48 (certainty score of 1; see Fig. 5). By days 59 to 60, a certainty score of 3 or 4 (intermediate or maximal) was reached in all of the 20 fetuses not yet removed. After day 70, certainty scores began to fluctuate, due primarily to difficulty in obtaining an adequate view in the older fetuses (see Fig. 5).

The diagnosis of gender was correct for 138 of 143 (97 per cent) of diagnoses of male fetuses and 92 of 92 (100 per cent) of diagnoses of female fetuses. The errors occurred in the first few horses examined and were therefore attributed to operator inexperience.

A second study included the same end points but with a single examination of each of 85 riding-type horses and pony mares. Fetal age ranged from 50 to 99 days after ovulation. Gender was not determinable in ten fetuses (three male, four female, and three undifferentiated fetuses; Table 1). Errors in diagnosis of gender were made at certainty level 2 (one of six female

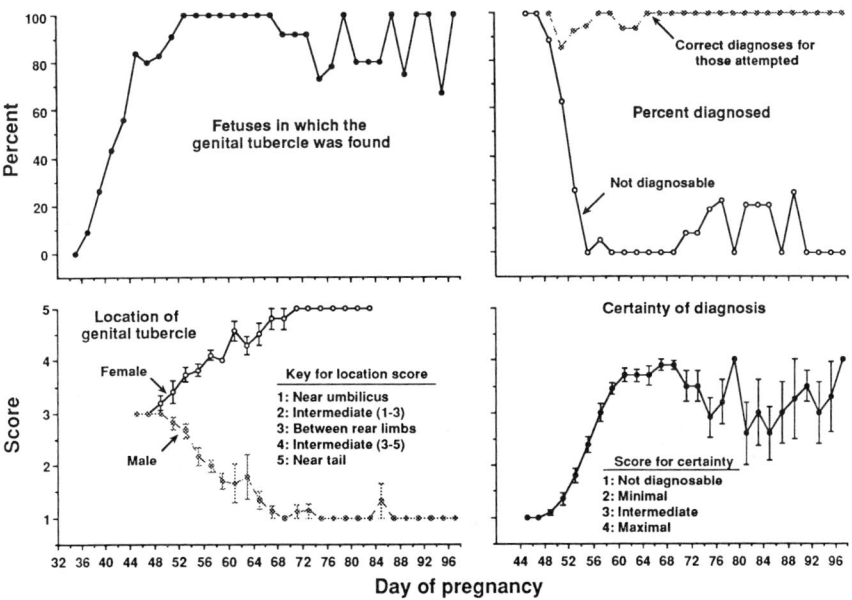

Figure 5. Results of US imaging–based diagnosis of fetal gender by location of the genital tubercle in 26 riding-type horse mares, primarily Quarter Horses. (Adapted from Curran S., and Ginther, O. J.: Equine Vet. Sci., 9:77, 1989. Reproduced by permission.)

fetuses) and at certainty level 3 (one of ten male fetuses). At certainty levels 3.5 and 4, all 23 male and 21 female fetuses were correctly diagnosed. In total, gender was determinable in 75 of 85 examinations (88 per cent). When gender was determinable (certainty level 2 or greater), gender was correctly diagnosed in 73 of 75 fetuses (97 per cent). Reasons for inability to determine gender included (1) abdominal straining, leading to concerns about rectal tears (days 58, 59, 65, and 68), (2) extreme movement of the mare or fetus (day 57), and (3) fetus too deeply situated in the mare (days 70 and 82). The average time required for reaching a gender determination (after removal of feces) was 1 minute, 17 seconds (range, 15 seconds to 4 minutes).

In conclusion, US imaging–based identification and location of the genital tubercle is a highly accurate means of determining fetal gender in the horse. The optimal days for gender diagnosis are days 59 to 68. During this time, the fetus is most accessible and the genital tubercle identifiable and assignable to a location characteristic of either male or female.

Considerable experience is required. Learning the technique requires viewing large numbers of fetuses to learn manipulation of the probe and identification of the fetal structures. Risks for this procedure are the same as for any transrectal procedure, including rectal tears. A direct risk to the fetus does not seem likely. The advantages are speed, the potential for extreme accuracy, and the level of certainty that can be recorded with each diagnosis. The technique can be done under most barn conditions.

Supplemental Readings

Curran, S., and Ginther, O. J.: Diagnosis of equine fetal sex by location of the genital tubercle. J. Equine Vet. Sci., 9:77, 1989.

Curran, S., Kastelic, J. P., and Ginther, O. J.: Determining sex

TABLE 1. RELATIONSHIPS BETWEEN CORRECT DIAGNOSES AND CERTAINTY LEVELS FOR DIAGNOSIS OF FETAL GENDER IN HORSE AND PONY MARES

Certainty Level*	Number of Correct Diagnoses			
	Male Fetus	Female Fetus	Undifferentiated Fetus	Total
1	0/3	0/4	0/3	0/10 (0%)
2	3/3	5/6	—	8/9 (89%)
3	9/10	12/12	—	21/22 (95%)
3.5	4/4	5/5	—	9/9 (100%)
4	19/19	16/16	—	35/35 (100%)

*Certainty scored from 1 (not determinable) to 4 (maximum confidence).

of the bovine fetus by ultrasonic assessment of the relative location of the genital tubercle. Anim. Reprod. Sci., 19:217, 1989.

Elejalde, B. R., de Elejalde, M. M., and Heitman, T.: Visualization of the fetal genitalia by ultrasonography: A review of literature and analysis of its accuracy and ethical implications. J. Ultrasound Med., 4:633, 1985.

Muller, E., and Wittkowski, G.: Visualization of male and female characteristics of bovine fetuses by real-time ultrasonics. Theriogenology, 22:571, 1986.

Wideman, D., Dorn, C. G., and Kraemer, D. C.: Sex detection of the bovine fetus using linear array real-time ultrasonography (abstract). Theriogenology, 31:272, 1989.

Prefoaling Management of the Mare and Induction of Parturition

William B. Ley, BLACKSBURG, VIRGINIA

PREFOALING MANAGEMENT

Preventive medical care of the mare and preparation for foaling vary by locality, disease incidence, and intensity of management on each individual farm. All mares should be immunized against equine herpesvirus-1, equine influenza, encephalomyelitis, and tetanus; immunization against salmonellosis, botulism, Potomac horse fever, and equine viral arteritis may be indicated by local disease patterns. Since the foal is dependent on colostral transfer for its initial immunoglobulins (IgG, IgA, and IgM), preimmunization of the mare either actively by vaccine administration or passively by exposure to the foaling environment 4 to 6 weeks in advance of parturition is recommended (see p. 422). Administration of a broad-spectrum anthelmintic at this same time (or during the immediate postpartum period) reduces the shedding of fecal parasitic ova and transmammary transfer of *Strongyloides westeri* larvae (see p. 53). A bank of good-quality colostrum should be established on large brood mare farms or by veterinary practices that attend many foalings per year. Four to 12 ounces (120 to 360 ml) of colostrum may be obtained from postparturient mares after their foals have been allowed to suckle vigorously for the first 4 to 6 hours. This colostrum should be filtered, batched, and frozen ($-20°$ C) in 16-ounce (500-ml) aliquots. Immunoglobulin content should be measured by either specific gravity or single radial immunodiffusion assay. Good-quality colostrum has a specific gravity greater than 1.06. The minimum IgG concentration necessary to support adequate passive transfer of immunity has been reported to range from 1,000 to 3,000 mg per dl; foals should receive 2 to 4 liters of good-quality colostrum during the first 6 to 8 hours post partum.

Mares suspected of having been immunologically sensitized against the foal's antigenic blood type should be screened for anti-red cell antibodies (Aa and Qa blood groups) 30 days prior to foaling (see end of chapter and p. 431). A jugular venous blood sample (10 ml) in acid–citrate–dextrose (ACD) anticoagulant and a serum sample should be submitted to one of the laboratories listed at the end of this chapter. If the test is positive, the mare should be attended at parturition and the foal prevented from consuming her colostrum. Colostrum from a nonsensitized mare should be given to the foal. The foal can be returned to nurse freely from its dam after 18 to 24 hours and after the mare has been milked out. A field screening test for colostrum has been developed that shows good correlation with the standard hemolytic assay recommended for colostrum screening in the laboratory (see Bailey et al; 1987).

Mares on which the Caslick's vulvoplasty has been performed should be closely monitored for signs of foaling. Those that are likely to foal unattended should have the vulva opened 5 to 7 days in advance of their expected foaling date. Mares that will foal with an attendant present or are induced should be opened early in stage 2 of labor.

The nutritional requirements for the mare during the last trimester of gestation increase according to the demands placed on her body's metabolism by fetal growth. In the last 3 months of gestation, fetal growth is almost linear. Mean fetal weight increases progressively from 150

TABLE 1. NUTRIENT CONCENTRATIONS IN TOTAL DIETS FOR PREGNANT MARES IN COMPARISON WITH MAINTENANCE REQUIREMENTS IN THE MATURE HORSE

Nutrient	Mature Horse Maintenance	Pregnant Mare		
		9 mo.	10 mo.	11 mo.
Digestible energy, Mcal/kg°	2.00	2.25	2.25	2.40
Crude protein, %†	8.0	10.0	10.0	10.6
Calcium, %†	0.24	0.43	0.43	0.45
Phosphorus, %†	0.17	0.32	0.32	0.34
Vitamin A, IU/kg	1830	3710	3650	3650
Vitamin D, IU/kg	300	600	600	600
Vitamin E, IU/kg	50	80	80	80

From Nutrient Requirement of Horses, 5th rev. ed. Washington, D.C., National Academy Press, 1989.
°Values are per kg feed and assume concentrate contains 3.3 Mcal/kg and hay contains 2.0 Mcal/kg dry matter.
†Per cent on a dry matter basis

days to term, but the weight vs. age curve is steepest from 200 days to term. Mares in late gestation should consume 1.0 to 1.5 per cent of their body weight as forage and 0.5 to 1.0 per cent as concentrate. Table 1 compares nutrient requirements of pregnant mares and maintenance requirements of mature horses. Microsmineral requirements are not different from those of the mature nonpregnant horse. Body condition score is a clinical tool to evaluate the efficacy of the feeding program in meeting the brood mare's demands. Nutritional management of the brood mare should ensure above-average (score of 6 on a scale of 1 to 10) body condition. Mares foaling in better than average body condition conceive early in the postpartum period, have a high conception rate, and maintain their pregnancies beyond 90 days of gestation. Obese mares do not have increased foaling difficulties but produce small birth weight foals with an increased tendency to develop angular limb deformities.

READINESS FOR BIRTH

The concept of fetal "readiness for birth" is the phenomenon whereby each individual has its own inherent gestational length that may or may not correspond to the expected mean gestational length of the species. Foals born spontaneously between 300 and 320 days of gestation (320 and 360 days are the normal limits in the Thoroughbred for optimal survival with normal birth weight) have a reasonable chance of survival; however, mares induced to foal between 300 and 320 days more often than not produce nonviable foals. Clinical experience also supports this theory: mares induced to foal after a known gestational length of 330 days will occasionally produce foals with signs of immaturity or dysmaturity, and these foals may also be nonviable.

The fetal maturational events occurring during the last days of gestation accompany a series of interrelated changes in maternal organ systems, most notably the mammary gland. There is a rise in mammary blood flow, a fall in the sodium to potassium ratio in prepartum mammary secretions, and sudden increases in mammary secretion levels of calcium and citrate. The maturation of the hypothalamic–pituitary–adrenal system of the fetus plays a key role in these changes. Rising fetal adrenocorticosteroid levels are associated with completion of fetal lung maturation, production of alveolar surfactant, maturation of the gastrointestinal tract, increased storage of hepatic glycogen, and activation of various enzyme systems. Full-term foals have high plasma cortisol concentrations in the early neonatal period, indicating enhanced adrenal activity before delivery; by contrast, premature or nonviable foals show minimal plasma cortisol levels after delivery. Although it has yet to be demonstrated that a significant rise in cortisol is directly associated with onset of parturition in the mare (as it has in other species), it is plausible to assume that such is the case. The rising cortisol levels in maternal and fetal plasma and in placental fluids near term alter the metabolism of progesterone, leading to increased myometrial activity and sensitivity. With uterine sensitivity enhanced, the opportunity exists to establish the onset of stage 2 labor more readily by use of myometrial agonists such as $PGF_{2\alpha}$ and oxytocin.

Changes in mammary secretions, especially calcium and magnesium (total hardness), are associated with fetal readiness for birth. There is good correlation between the results of laboratory methods and field testing kits (water hardness and calcium carbonate test strips or colorimetric titration tests°,†,‡,§) for measurement of milk calcium and magnesium. These methods indicate the fetus's approaching readiness for birth but do not accurately indicate actual parturition time. The probability that a mare will foal within 24 hours after first reaching 250 ppm total hardness (calcium + magnesium) in diluted (1 part mammary secretion to 6 parts distilled water) mammary secretion samples is reported to range for 53 to 79 per cent. The interval from first reaching 250 ppm total hardness to foaling ranges from 12 to 54 hours. When changes in calcium alone are evaluated, all mares foal when calcium exceeds 10 mmol per L in undiluted mammary secretion and over 50 per cent foal within 48 hours of first attaining this concentration (mean mammary secretion calcium at birth for all mares is 18.3 mmol per L). In comparison, a field test kit measuring calcium carbonate (ppm) in diluted mammary secretions (1:6) reports that 88 per cent of mares foal within 24 hours of first attaining 200 ppm, and 94 per cent of all mares that foal reach this threshold value (mean mammary secretion calcium carbonate at birth for all mares is 298 ppm). Differences in techniques make comparisons difficult, but measurements of calcium changes alone in prepartum mammary secretions are less variable than measurements of total hardness. None of these tests predict parturition time accurately but will indicate when a mare is not ready to foal. No mares foal spontaneously when calcium is less than 10 mmol per L; the average interval to foaling is 3.6 nights when values are below this threshold. Of note, abnormal electrolyte values in prepartum mammary secretions, such as elevations in calcium or total hardness weeks prior to the expected parturition date, are associated with premature parturition and stillbirths. These tests are at present a clinical tool of some assistance to evaluate the mare's approaching readiness for birth, but as with most biological tests, large variations can be expected to occur.

Frequent (two to three times daily) monitoring of rectal temperature, when used with other signs of impending readiness for birth, may be a useful adjunct to determine day of parturition. A decrease in core body temperature occurs with the onset of stage 1 labor and is indicated by a decrease in rectal temperature (0.1° C; 0.2° F) within 24 hours of parturition. Circadian rectal temperature changes make it difficult to spot the temperature changes unless rectal temperature is measured frequently.

PARTURITION

Parturition includes a prepartum preparatory phase and first, second, and third stages of labor. The preparatory signs are variable but include relaxation of sacrosciatic ligaments, elongation and relaxation of vulval lips, udder enlargement, and secretion of small amounts of a honey-colored colostrum that often dries and accumulates on the teat orifices (waxing). These events may occur as much as 2 to 4 weeks to as little as 1 to 2 days before the onset of labor. The first stage of labor is somewhat under the voluntary control of the mare. External signs include inappetence, restlessness, pacing, a raised tail, dripping of colostrum from teats, and mild to moderate sweating. The onset of the second stage of labor is marked by rupture of the chorioallantoic membrane and release of allantoic fluid (breaking water). This is a much more active stage and cannot be readily stopped or reversed by either the mare or iatrogenic intervention. The white, glistening surface of the amnion should be presented through the vulval lips, followed by both forefeet and nose of the foal at the level of the carpi (anterior dorsosacral presentation). Delivery of the foal should be complete within 20 to 40 minutes following the onset of stage 2 labor. If a delay is noted or if the fetal limbs or nose are not presented in timely fashion, aseptic investigation of the problem is warranted (see *Current Therapy in Equine Medicine 2*, p. 537). Premature separation of the placenta can occur spontaneously during this stage and is recognized by presentation of the reddish, velvety surface of the chorion through the vulval lips in advance of the amnion. The chorion should be ruptured immediately by sharp or blunt incision and fetal delivery assisted to diminish the effects of fetal hypoxemia that is imminent as the chorioallantois detaches from the maternal endometrium. The third stage of labor commences once delivery of the foal is complete but is not over until the fetoplacental membranes have been expelled. The postpartum period (1 to 12 hours after delivery) is often accompanied by mild to moderate signs of colic as the uterus undergoes very active involutionary contractions. These should be differentiated from other causes of postpartum pain, including uterine intramural or mesometrial hemorrhage, obstipation of the small or large colon, rupture of the cecum or

---

°Sofchek Water Hardness Test Strip, Environmental Test Systems, Elkhart, IN
†Predict-A-Foal Mare Foaling Predictor Kit, Animal Healthcare Products, Vernon, CA
‡Titrets Calcium Hardness Test Kits, CHEMetrics, Calverton, VA
§Merckoquant Water Hardness Test Strip, E. Merck, Darmstadt, Germany

large colon, uterine or vaginal rupture, and tenesmus due to peritonitis or bowel herniation through a rupture site.

INDUCTION OF PARTURITION

Extensive reviews of methods for induction of parturition in the mare have been published. Although induction of parturition is a routine procedure on some farms, complications are frequently encountered. Criteria for selection of candidates for induction include a minimum known gestational length of 330 days, udder enlargement and filling with colostrum, relaxation of sacrosciatic ligaments and vulval lips, and relaxation of the cervix. To further judge fetal readiness for birth, mammary secretion electrolyte changes and rectal body temperature should also be monitored. Mares that fulfill all of the above criteria may still occasionally produce foals with signs of dysmaturity or prematurity when induced to foal on an elective basis. A review of the indications for induction of parturition in the mare is provided in *Current Therapy in Equine Medicine 2*, page 533.

The greatest success in induction of foaling is achieved with the administration of either oxytocin or prostaglandins. Oxytocin has long been used, with both safe and disastrous results. Dose and routes of administration have varied (e.g., 20 to 100 IU given intramuscularly [IM], 2.5 to 10 IU given as an intravenous [IV] bolus, 120 IU in 1 liter of saline given by IV drip to effect). Smaller doses (2.5 to 5.0 IU) given by frequent IV bolus (every 20 minutes) provide a physiological response and fewer untoward complications such as hyperstimulation of myometrial contractions, induction of myometrial spasms, premature placental separation, and malpresentation. Oxytocin administration can induce parturition in mares as early as 300 days of gestation, thereby producing premature or nonviable foals.

The prostanoid dinoprost tromethamine* (7.5 to 10 mg IM) can induce parturition in the mare prior to 330 days of gestation, when the fetus is premature and nonviable. Fluprostenol† (250 μg IM) can induce parturition within 0.5 to 3 hours of administration, but its safety and efficacy have been questioned. However, unlike oxytocin and dinoprost, fluprostenol is unlikely to induce the birth of nonviable, premature foals. Fenprostalene‡ produces no adverse local or systemic reactions when used in mares selected for induction of foaling based on the above defined criteria. The dose of fenprostalene is 0.5 mg per mare administered subcutaneously, followed by a repeat dose in 2 hours. Stage 2 of labor begins within 3.5 to 4.5 hours following the first injection. The time to foaling can be shortened by administration of small IV doses of oxytocin (2.5 IU every 20 minutes to effect) 20 to 30 minutes following the second fenprostalene injection.

It has not been determined which uterotonic agent (i.e., oxytocin or prostaglandin) is responsible for initiating spontaneous foaling in the mare. In spontaneously foaling mares, release of oxytocin precedes detection of prostanoids by only minutes. Induction of parturition with oxytocin or prostaglandins will lead to physiological birth of the foal. The differences in success rates are related to the degree of accuracy in predicting fetal readiness for birth prior to induction and controlling the dose response to minimize excessive myometrial stimulation that might compromise oxygen delivery to the foal prior to delivery.

U.S. LABORATORIES THAT PERFORM BLOOD TYPING

Serology Laboratory
College of Veterinary Medicine
University of California at Davis
Davis, CA 95616
(916) 752-2211

Equine Blood-Typing Research Lab.
Department of Veterinary Science
University of Kentucky
Lexington, KY 40546
(606) 257-3022

Stormont Laboratories
1237 E. Beamer St., Suite D
Woodland, CA 95695
(916) 661-3078

Shelterwood Equine Lab.
Box 215
Carthage, TX 75633
(214) 693-6424

Supplemental Readings

Adams-Brendemuehl, C., and Pipers, F.: Antepartum evaluations of the equine fetus. J. Reprod. Fertil. Suppl., 35:565, 1987.
Bailey, E., Conboy, H. S., and McCarthy, P. F.: Neonatal isoerythrolysis in foals: An update on testing. In: Proceedings of the 33rd Annual Convention of the American Association of Equine Practitioners, 1987, pp. 341–350.

---

*Prostin F₂ Alpha, Upjohn Co., Kalamazoo, MI
†Equimate, Haver-Lockhart, Shawnee, KS
‡Bovilene, Syntex Agribusiness, Des Moines, IA

Bazer, F., and First, N.: Pregnancy and parturition. J. Anim. Sci., 57 (suppl.2):425, 1983.
Haluska, G., and Wilkins, K.: Predictive utility of pre-partum temperature changes in the mare. Equine Vet. J., 2:116, 1989.
Hillman, R. B.: Induction of parturition. In Robinson, N. E. (ed.): Current Therapy in Equine Medicine 2. Philadelphia, W. B. Saunders, 1987, pp. 533–537.
Ley, W. B., Hoffman, J., Crisman, M. V., Meacham, T. N., Sullivan, T. L., and Kiracofe, R.: Daytime foaling management of the mare: 2. Induction of parturition. J. Equine Vet. Sci., 9:95, 1989.
Ley, W. B., Hoffman, J., Meacham, T. N., Sullivan, T. L., Kiracofe, R., and Wilson, M. H.: Daytime foaling management of the mare: 1. Prefoaling mammary secretions testing. J. Equine Vet. Sci., 9:88, 1989.
Ousey, J., Delclaux, M., and Rossdale, P. D.: Evaluation of three strip tests for measuring electrolytes in mares' prepartum mammary secretions and for predicting parturition. Equine Vet. J., 21:196, 1989.
Renton, J.: Parturition in the mare. Practice, 6:19, 1984.
Rossdale, P. D., and Silver, M.: The concept of readiness for birth. J. Reprod. Fertil. Suppl., 32:507, 1982.

Sexual Behavior Dysfunction in Stallions

Sue M. McDonnell, KENNETT SQUARE, PENNSYLVANIA

Sexual behavior problems in the stallion include several distinct types of dysfunction. Successful treatment, whether by traditional behavior modification or by pharmacological manipulation, usually depends on diagnosis of the specific dysfunctions involved. The following discussion of behavioral problems, evaluation, and therapy is organized according to the common types of sexual behavior dysfunction in stallions.

LOW LIBIDO

Probably the most common type of behavioral dysfunction in stallions involves inadequate sexual interest and arousal. The problem is most typically seen in young or inexperienced stallions. Listed in Table 1 are some of the behavioral characteristics common among slow-starting novice breeding stallions. Many of the problems appear to be related to inexperience or to a history of active discouragement of sexual behavior during training or performance. Slow-starting stallions typically show remarkable improvement after the first successful copulation. Therefore, the training program should include whatever is necessary to assist the stallion toward the first ejaculation. Young, inexperienced stallions usually show remarkably rapid improvement with simple repeated exposure with minimal restraint and plenty of gentle, patient encouragement. For example, manual stimulation of the penis or application of an artificial vagina can be useful in encouraging a stallion that is reluctant to mount. The stimulus mare often seems more important to inexperienced than to experienced stallions. A selection of mares showing strong natural estrus is often useful. Interestingly, frisky, even feisty, mares often elicit the desired stallionlike response sooner than will a quiet mare. One of the oldest and most reliable methods is to turn the slow-starting stallion out to pasture with one or more mares.

Some young slow-starting stallions have low levels of circulating androgens. Many of these are young, recently retired racing stallions and just off anabolic steroids. We have found that gonadotropin-releasing hormone (GnRH) treatment (50 μg given subcutaneously 2 hours and again 1 hour before breeding), which usually leads to increased androgen levels within 1 hour after administration, improves sexual interest and arousal.

Novice stallions that appear fearful or anxious in the breeding situation often improve with antianxiety medication. Signs of anxiety include vigilant alertness, distractibility, attention to handlers more than to the mare, and frequent loss of erection. Diazepam (0.05 mg per kg given slowly intravenously 5 to 7 minutes before breeding) sometimes leads to sudden improvement in sexual interest in such stallions.

Managers often find slow-starting stallions frustrating to work with. Unfortunately, it is during this critical time that impatience and mishandling may complicate and prolong sexual behavior dysfunction. Unnecessary punishment should be avoided. The veterinarian can best help by offering the advice that many stallions with exemplary adult breeding behavior started out as slow or "shy" breeders. Our research and clinical ex-

TABLE 1. BEHAVIORAL CHARACTERISTICS COMMON TO SLOW-STARTING NOVICE STALLIONS

1. Little or no interest in mare
2. Sexually "shy" in presence of handlers
3. Juvenile, playful, or submissive responses, e.g., jaw champing, rubbing head against side of mare, or prolonged nuzzling of udder; may even allow the mare to investigate genitals
4. Approach–avoidance responses, e.g., interest at a distance, but anxious when near mare; initial brief burst of interest; hyperdistractibility; discontinuous behavioral sequences; anxious, fearful expression; slow and intermittent erection
5. Awkward precopulatory and copulatory responses, e.g., mounts from the side or head of the mare, mounts without erection, mounts without insertion or thrusting, withdraws before ejaculation, or slow to dismount after ejaculation
6. Prolonged bouts of repetitive single elements of precopulatory behavior, e.g., mouthing the tail, nipping the withers, licking the hocks
7. Marked preference or aversion for particular mares, handlers, or breeding location
8. Hypersensitive to correction or punishment

perience suggests that about 5 to 10 per cent of stallions show some difficulty when first breeding. While most such stallions improve to normal levels of sexual arousal and response within 1 to 5 days of traditional retraining, some require weeks. Most cases resolve on the farm and do not require a specialized behavior modification facility or pharmacological aids.

Although mostly a problem of novice breeders, inadequate libido is also seen in experienced breeding stallions. Some individuals show an annual pattern of problems similar to those of the slow-starting stallion. They may be slow to start the breeding season each spring or, more commonly, may each year experience periods of low libido near the end of a breeding season. Stallions with semen-related fertility problems that result in an increased number of mares to be bred near the end of the season tend to develop aberrant behavior. Some show a gradually diminishing level of arousal and response, others suddenly refuse to breed. These stallions are referred to as stale or sour. Listed in Table 2 are

TABLE 2. BEHAVIORAL CHARACTERISTICS COMMON TO SOUR OR STALE BREEDING STALLIONS

1. Sour attitude, e.g., pinned ears; may lunge at mare with lowered head; bites rather than nips mare
2. Little vocalization
3. Slow to achieve or regain erection
4. May appear to be in pain
5. Preferences or aversions for particular mares, handlers, or breeding locations

some characteristics common to such stallions. Although poor condition or pain may in some instances be identified as a contributing factor, often the diminished libido appears to have no physical explanation. A sudden reduction in libido can also occur in experienced stallions in association with mishandling or a specific negative experience related to breeding. These stallions may appear anxious or simply disinterested rather than sour. Lowered libido in an experienced stallion usually resolves with time off from breeding or changes in the breeding routine. Diazepam or the GnRH treatments described for slow-starting novice stallions may aid in the return of normal libido.

A change in environment may have positive or negative effects on the sexual behavior of stallions. In experimental situations, most normal breeding stallions show minor though measurable reduction in sexual arousal and response when the breeding location is changed. Some experienced stallions, particularly those that appear dependent on the established breeding routine, may suffer more serious, yet usually temporary, diminished sexual response in association with changes in environment or management. On the other hand, stallions with low libido may show more arousal when moved to a novel environment.

COPULATORY OR EJACULATORY DYSFUNCTION

Some stallions that experience normal sexual arousal fail to ejaculate. These stallions generally fit into one of two distinct categories. One type, referred to here as copulatory dysfunction, appears to involve deficiencies in mounting, insertion, coupling, or thrusting. The second type, referred to here as ejaculatory dysfunction, involves specifically a disturbance in the emission or ejaculation processes. Precopulatory and copulatory behavior appears normal, but emission or ejaculation does not occur. Tables 3 and 4 list some characteristics of each of these problems. Although theoretically distinct, the two categories are not always easy to distinguish.

TABLE 3. BEHAVIORAL CHARACTERISTICS COMMON TO STALLIONS WITH COPULATORY DYSFUNCTION

1. May have difficulty mounting, especially repeatedly
2. Difficulty inserting or maintaining insertion
3. Poor coupling, with shallow or irregular thrusts
4. Waves of two to three thrusts, with pauses
5. May appear to be in pain

TABLE 4. BEHAVIORAL CHARACTERISTICS ASSOCIATED WITH EJACULATORY DYSFUNCTION

1. Typically no arousal problems, at least for initial period of dysfunction, e.g., readily achieves and maintains erection
2. Readily and repeatedly mounts, inserts, and thrusts; will continue beyond the typical six to nine thrusts required for ejaculation
3. Sometimes squeals and dismounts just as ejaculation appears imminent
4. May exhibit signs of ejaculation with no semen; may produce copious amount of presperm fluid.

After long periods of specific ejaculatory dysfunction, the stallion may become frustrated and fail to mount and thrust with normal vigor.

In most cases of copulatory dysfunction, a physical problem that would explain copulatory difficulty can be identified. Copulatory dysfunction in stallions has been seen in association with potentially painful limb and back problems, pleuritis, aortoiliac thrombosis, neurological deficits, painful testicular conditions, urethritis, and penile lesions. A fairly simple cause of copulatory dysfunction is abrasions on the medial aspect of the carpus incurred during mounting, particularly of a dummy mare. Factors related to an artificial vagina can also lead to reluctance to mount, couple, and thrust or to failure to ejaculate. Some stallions appear extremely finicky about the conditions of an artificial vagina, and slight changes in temperature or pressure result in inadequate coupling or thrusting, or failure to ejaculate. Finally, some stallions show this pattern following a negative experience during breeding. These stallions will mount, but thrust half-heartedly, and may fail to ejaculate.

Many stallions return to normal copulatory function with alleviation or accommodation of the physical problems or pain. Improvement is often remarkable with 10 days to 2 weeks of phenylbutazone treatment. Rearrangement of the breeding situation to reduce pain or stress on affected limbs, such as altering the height or angle of the mare or dummy, can be helpful. For most horses, thrusting can also be enhanced by applying warm compresses and manual stimulation to the base of the penis. Similarly, an artificial vagina with increased temperature and pressure often elicits better coupling and thrusting. Measures taken to increase arousal at the time of mounting can also improve copulatory function. Toward this end, we have found prolonged teasing before mounting and treatment with GnRH to be useful.

Treatment of specific ejaculatory failure includes a variety of neuromyotropic regimens aimed at enhancing smooth muscle contraction. The Klug regimen involves intramuscular injection of 0.01 mg per kg of L-norepinephrine 15 minutes before breeding, followed by 0.015 mg per kg of the β-adrenergic antagonist carazolol 10 minutes before breeding. We have found that a low oral dose of the dibenzazepine imipramine (100 to 600 mg twice a day in grain for minimun of 2 weeks) enhances ejaculatory function. In addition, xylazine, an α-adrenergic agonist, can be used to induce ejaculation ex copula. A dose of 0.66 mg per kg IV can be given to a stallion standing quietly in the stall to induce ejaculation. We collect the semen in a plastic bag positioned over the prepuce by a girth strap.

Retrograde ejaculation (ejaculation into the bladder) is often suspected when there are visible signs of ejaculation but no semen. This condition, common in men, apparently has not been confirmed in the stallion.

UNRULY AND SAVAGE STALLIONS

Another undesirable behavior in stallions is seemingly uncontrollably high libido. Specific problem behaviors include charging the mare, refusal to stand for washing or examination of the genitals, and wheeling and kicking out at the mare or handler. In our experience most cases result from inadequate or improperly applied discipline. We have recently shown experimentally that almost any stallion can develop unruly, dangerous breeding habits within 2 weeks of improper handling. Fortunately, most can be brought under control again with consistent, firm, judicious handling. We have found the most efficient behavior modification strategy for dangerously unruly stallions is to initially bring the horse under control using an expert stallionaire, and then provide training of the handlers with the horse on the home farm. There is little work on pharmacological aids for training unruly stallions.

In contrast to the more simple unruly behavior is the truly savage, aggressive behavior of some stallions. Often quite well-mannered and easy to handle most of the time, these stallions occasionally savage another horse or a handler. By contrast to unruly stallions, they remain refractory to normal retraining techniques. Specific behaviors include charging with bared teeth and lowered head, sometimes picking the handler up by the shoulder or waist, or attacking with forelimbs. Savage stallions, if kept, usually repeat such episodes. Some have been safely bred under bull stud conditions.

Supplemental Readings

Klug, E.: Ejaculatory failure. In Robinson, N. E. (ed.): Current Therapy in Equine Medicine 2. Philadelphia, W. B. Saunders, 1987, pp. 562–563.

McDonnell, S. M.: Reproductive behavior of the stallion. Vet. Clin. North Am. (Equine Pract.), 3(2):535–555, 1986.

McDonnell, S. M., Garcia, M. C., and Kenney, R. M.: Pharmacological manipulation of stallion sexual behavior. J. Reprod. Fertil. Suppl., 35:45–49, 1987.

McDonnell, S. M., Garcia, M. C., Kenney, R. M., and Van Arsdalen, K. N.: Imipramine-induced erection, masturbation, and ejaculation in male horses. Pharmacol. Biochem. Behav., 27:187–191, 1987.

McDonnell, S. M., and Love, C. C.: Manual stimulation collection of semen from stallions: Training time, sexual behavior, and semen quality. Theriogenology, 33(6):1201–1210, 1990.

McDonnell, S. M., Love, C. C., Reef, V. B., Martin, B., and Kenney, R. M.: Ejaculatory failure in association with aortic-iliac thrombosis in two horses. J. Am. Vet. Med. Assoc., in press.

McDonnell, S. M., Pozor, M. A., Beech, J., and Sweeney, R. W.: Use of manual stimulation on the ground for collection of semen from a neurologic stallion unable to breed by natural service. J. Am. Vet. Med. Assoc., in press.

Stallion Seminal Characteristics and Fertility

David J. Jasko, FORT COLLINS, COLORADO

At present, no one test of semen quality has proved to be a good predictor of fertility, even though investigators have attempted to define relationships between such tests and fertility for several decades. The difficulty in proving the existence of such relationships may be traceable to the difficulty of designing appropriate experiments. Therefore, the prediction of potential fertility in the stallion based on the evaluation of seminal characteristics is derived more from the presumed importance of seminal characteristics than from solid experimental data. This article reviews seminal characteristics thought to be important for the prediction of fertility in the stallion.

The semen studied in a fertility evaluation must be obtained from ejaculates representative of a stallion's current sperm production and quality. Ejaculates obtained with a properly used artificial vagina are the most acceptable for semen evaluation. The proper handling of semen immediately after ejaculation to avoid exposure of semen to the high temperature of the artificial vagina liner and to avoid exposure to cold temperatures during collection in inclement weather is also important.

Following collection, semen samples should be maintained at 37° C or allowed to cool slowly to ambient room temperature and evaluations should be performed in a rapid, efficient, and orderly manner, because many characteristics will change with time. The seminal characteristics that are evaluated during a fertility evaluation are outlined below (Table 1).

APPEARANCE

Fresh stallion semen has a watery, opaque, near-white appearance that will be affected by the concentration of sperm cells in the semen. Semen appears more opaque in samples with a high concentration of sperm cells. A yellow or red tinge should alert the clinician to the possibility of contamination with urine or blood, respectively.

VOLUME

Semen volume alone is thought not to be a good predictor of fertility. Its determination is useful only for calculating the total number of sperm in an ejaculate. The gel fraction of semen, which is produced by the seminal vesicles, is often removed during semen collection with an in-line gel filter or alternatively by passing the ejaculate through a suitable filter, such as a milk filter, and the volume of remaining gel-free semen is measured in any suitable container such as a graduated cylinder. The quick removal of gel, preferably at the time of ejaculation, will prevent mixing of gel and semen and the resulting loss of sperm absorbed into the gel.

SPERM CONCENTRATION

Sperm cell concentration has been correlated with fertility in the stallion and can be deter-

TABLE 1. MEANS AND RANGES FOR STALLION SEMINAL CHARACTERISTICS

Characteristic	Mean	(Range)
Gel-free volume, ml	45	(20–150)
Sperm concentration, 10^6/ml	175	(60–350)
Total sperm/ejaculate, 10^9	9	(2–25)
Seminal pH	7.4	(7.2–7.6)
Motile sperm, %	75	(60–90)
Progressively motile sperm, %	50	(40–90)
Morphologically normal sperm, %	50	(40–85)

mined with a hemacytometer after appropriate dilution. A 1:100 dilution can be made accurately with a disposable dilution system designed for counting platelets and white blood cells.° When a 1:100 dilution is used and all the sperm heads within the 25 large squares of the hemacytometer enumerated (or the total number in five large squares multiplied by 5), this number represents the number of sperm in millions (10^6) per milliliter of semen.

An alternative method is the use of a spectrophotometer† after construction of a standard curve (calibration). A standard curve can be constructed using comparisons between hemocytometry counts and spectrophometry readings. Some universities will construct such standard curves as a service for veterinarians or farm managers. It has been suggested that each spectrophotometer be recalibrated at the beginning of each breeding season. A precalibrated instrument that gives a digital display of stallion sperm cell concentration is available.‡ Any instrument that relies on optical density for the determination of sperm cell concentration can produce erroneous results if the sample contains debris, white blood cells, or red blood cells, as these will affect the optical density of the sample.

TOTAL SPERM

The total number of sperm cells in the ejaculate is calculated from the gel-free volume (ml) and the concentration of sperm cells (10^6 per ml). An attempt must be made to recover all semen from the artificial vagina as accurate determination of the total number of sperm in the ejaculate is an important criterion in the fertility evaluation of a stallion.

°B-D Unopette, Becton-Dickinson, Rutherford, NJ
†Spectronic 20, Bausch & Lomb, Rochester, NY
‡Equine Sperm Cell Counter, Animal Reproduction Systems, Chino, CA

SEMINAL PH

The pH of a semen sample should be determined soon after collection with a standardized pH meter as sperm metabolism will decrease the pH with time. The normal range of seminal pH is 7.2 to 7.6. Semen samples with a high concentration of sperm cells have lower pH values due to the acidic nature of epididymal secretions. A higher pH may be caused by contamination of semen with urine or purulent debris.

SPERM MOTILITY

Differences of opinion exist as to the most appropriate method to determine sperm motility. Viewing unextended, raw semen under the microscope at a magnification of 200× has been advocated. Alternatively, it has been recommended that semen first be extended to prevent agglutination and allow easy viewing of individual sperm cells. There is a tendency to overestimate motility in concentrated samples and thus extension of semen prior to viewing does have an advantage in reducing sperm concentration. Extending samples of some stallions will improve motility and therefore raw samples should also be evaluated. However, some commercially available or home-made extenders may be improperly formulated or handled and may become toxic to sperm. Therefore, if extenders are used, one must still evaluate the raw sample to determine if there has been a beneficial or detrimental effect of the extender on sperm motility.

Regardless of the method used, sperm motility is best visualized with a phase-contrast microscope equipped with a heated stage. The visual estimation of the per centage of progressively motile sperm (those that move progressively across the field) is more critical than the estimation of the per centage of total motile cells, as it is thought that only progressively motile cells are likely to achieve fertilization. The per centage of progressively motile sperm in a semen sample is thought to be the best single criterion of fertility.

In recent years computerized image analysis instruments have been developed to analyze sperm motion. Such instruments provide precise and accurate measurements on motile sperm, including the per centage of motile cells, mean velocity and progressiveness of motile cells, and sophisticated measurements related to flagellar propulsion. The high cost of these instruments precludes their widespread use, but information derived from such analyses may become useful in evaluating stallion fertility. Many universities have acquired such instruments and their expertise with these instruments may add additional valuable information on sperm motion for particular stallions.

LONGEVITY OF MOTILITY

The longevity of progressive motility is often determined for raw or extended semen samples in capped, filled test tubes held in the dark at room temperature. Criteria of normalcy are not standardized; however, the maintenance of 10 per cent progressive motility for 6 hours under the above conditions for raw semen has been advocated as a criterion for a fertile stallion.

With the increased use of cooled, transported, and frozen–thawed semen in some breeds, it may be useful to process an ejaculate of semen and determine the motility at some time after cooling or freeze–thawing to determine the effect of the process on sperm motility. Criteria to judge the fertility of such samples are lacking, and there appears to be large stallion-to-stallion variation in the ability of sperm to survive cooling and freeze–thawing.

SPERM MORPHOLOGY

Stallion sperm morphological features can be determined from unstained, buffered formalin-fixed suspensions with the use of a phase-contrast or differential interference microscope. Such examinations may afford better preservation of sperm morphology but are tedious and time-consuming to perform. More commonly sperm morphology is evaluated in specimens stained with eosin–nigrosin (available from the Society for Theriogenology). Such specimens are easily prepared by mixing a small drop of stain and semen and air drying a smear of the mixture.

At least 200 cells from each ejaculate should be evaluated microscopically ($1000\times$). Sperm morphological features can be classified according to the following scheme: (1) normal sperm, including those with abaxially positioned tails, (2) abnormal heads, (3) detached heads, (4) proximal droplets, (5) distal droplets, (6) abnormal midpieces, and (7) abnormal tails. Which specific abnormalities affect fertility in the stallion are unclear. Presently only the per centage of normal sperm is used as a criterion for fertility; however, certain abnormalities, such as those of the head and midpiece, may be more detrimental to fertility than others.

SEMINAL CHARACTERISTICS AND POTENTIAL FERTILITY

The clinical fertility evaluation of a stallion is based in part on the seminal characteristics determined for two ejaculates collected 1 hour apart from a sexually rested stallion. Seminal characteristics in the second ejaculate are determined in exactly the same way as described previously. The use of two ejaculates allows the clinician to determine the representativeness of the semen samples. For a sexually rested stallion the first and second ejaculate should be of similar volume, the total number of sperm in the second ejaculate should be about half the number in the first, the seminal pH should remain the same or rise slightly in the second ejaculate, and progressive motility and the per centage of morphologically normal sperm should remain the same or be higher in the second ejaculate. If these criteria are not met, the samples may not be representative and interpretation may be misleading.

The final criterion used by the Society for Theriogenology in regard to seminal characteristics for the classification of a stallion as a satisfactory prospective breeder for a full book of mares (40 mares with natural service or 120 mares with artificial insemination) is the potential ability of a stallion to ejaculate at least 1 billion (10^9) morphologically normal, progressively motile sperm in the second ejaculate of each month of the year. This number is determined by the following equation: sperm concentration (10^6) $\times$ semen volume (ml) $\times$ morphologically normal sperm (%) $\times$ progressively motile sperm (%). Since sperm output in the stallion is affected by season, the minimal number of 1 billion morphologically normal, progressively motile sperm cells is used for a stallion that is evaluated during December but is raised to a maximum of at least 2.2 billion morphologically normal, progressively motile sperm in the second ejaculate in the month of June.

This calculation attempts to determine the number of cells that are morphologically normal and progressively motile. However, it may be misleading in some cases to calculate this number by multiplying the per centage of morphologically normal sperm by the per centage of progressively motile cells, as these estimates in fact may be of the same population of sperm cells. That is, the progressively motile cells may be the same cells that are morphologically normal.

Daily sperm output may be an additional criterion for the prediction of fertility in a stallion.

It may also allow the clinician to estimate the largest book of mares for a particular stallion. Daily sperm output can be estimated by the depletion of a stallion's extragonadal sperm reserves with daily semen collections over a week. Further daily semen collections are then used for estimating daily sperm output. Fertility in mares is thought to be maximized with the alternate-day insemination of 500 million progressively motile sperm. With knowledge of a stallion's daily sperm output, the maximum number of daily covers (natural service) can be determined (daily output of progressively motile sperm divided by 500 million), provided that those covers are scheduled evenly throughout the day. For stallions in artificial breeding programs the number of spermatozoa collected (and available for insemination) is maximized by alternate-day collections. Again, the determination of daily or alternate-day sperm output can be useful in determining the appropriateness of a given sized book of mares.

The protocol described above allows the clinician to determine if a stallion qualifies as a satisfactory potential breeder, based on our current knowledge, and provided that the stallion is sound in other respects (has good libido and normal external and internal genitalia, is free of venerally transmitted pathogens and genetic defects). The true relationship of seminal characteristics to fertility may never be accurately determined for the stallion; however, the seminal characteristic presumed to be most highly correlated with fertility is the number of morphologically normal, progressively motile sperm that a stallion can potentially ejaculate.

Supplemental Readings

Kenny, R. M.: Clinical fertility evaluation of the stallion. In: Proceedings of the 21st Annual Convention of the American Association of Equine Practitioners, 1975, pp. 336–355.

Kenny, R. M., Hurtgen, J., Pierson, R., Witherspoon, D., and Simons, J.: Manual for breeding soundness examination of stallions. J. Soc. Theriogenol. 9:3–54, 1983.

Pickett, B. W., Faulkner, L. C., and Sutherland, T. M.: Effect of month and stallion on seminal characteristics and sexual behavior. Anim. Sci., 31:713–728, 1970.

Pickett, B. W., Voss, J. L., and Squires, E.L.: Factors affecting quality and quantity of stallion spermatozoa. Compend. Cont. Educ. Pract. Vet., 5:S259–S267, 1983.

Pickett, B. W., and Voss, J. L.: Reproductive management of the stallion. In: Proceedings of the 18th Annual Convention of the American Association of Equine Practitioners, 1972, pp. 501–531.

Pickett, B. W., Voss, J. L., and Squires, E. L.: Fertility evaluation of the stallion. Compend. Cont. Educ. Pract. Vet., 5:S194–S202, 1983.

Handling of Stallion Semen

Dickson D. Varner, COLLEGE STATION, TEXAS

The stallion has the means to effectively deliver semen to the protective confines of the mare reproductive tract at the time of coitus. For semen evaluation or artificial insemination, man interferes with this delivery process by intercepting ejaculated spermatozoa normally en route to the mare. It therefore becomes mandatory that semen be appropriately handled in this artificial environment so that the fertilizing capacity of the spermatozoa is retained and semen quality, as measured during a fertility examination, is an accurate reflection of that produced by the stallion.

COLLECTION OF SEMEN

Ejaculated semen is collected from stallions for artificial insemination of mares or for assessment of semen quality as part of a fertility examination. In either case it is important that the spermatozoa be protected against injury, beginning with the semen collection process. Numerous factors can result in destruction of spermatozoa, including temperature extremes, excessive light, toxic chemicals, or physical trauma from improper handling. To ensure utmost protection to spermatozoa, semen should be collected using an artificial vagina that has been properly prepared. Most stallions can be readily trained to serve an artificial vagina. The quality of semen collected in a condom is generally quite inferior to that obtained with an artificial vagina.

ARTIFICIAL VAGINAS

Several models of artificial vaginas are commercially available and are listed in Table 1. Each has distinct attributes and limited disadvantages, but all serve their purpose well. Initial cost, maintenance costs, types of accessories, du-

TABLE 1. MODELS AND SOURCES OF EQUINE ARTIFICIAL VAGINAS

Model	Source
Missouri	Nasco 901 Janesville Ave., Ft. Atkinson, WI 53538
C.S.U.	Animal Reproduction Systems 14395 Ramona Ave. Chino, CA 91710
Lane	Lane Manufacturing Co. 2075 S. Valentia Denver, Co 80231
Japanese (Nishikawa)	Scott Medical Supply Co. 459 Ginger Ave. Hayward, CA 94541
Roanoke	Roanoke A.I. Labs. Route 7, Box 230 Roanoke, VA 24018

rability, weight, temperature maintenance, and spermatozoal losses incurred during semen collection should be considered when the purchase of an artificial vagina is contemplated. Homemade artificial vaginas may also be constructed to meet specific needs.

It is imperative that all components of an artificial vagina that come in contact with semen be nontoxic to spermatozoa. Therefore, any reusable items (including semen receptacles and rubber liners) should be properly cleaned and dried prior to use. The use of soaps and disinfectants to clean these parts is discouraged. Thorough rinsing with deionized water is advised. If possible, sterile, nontoxic disposable equipment (e.g., artificial vagina liners or semen receptacles) should be used to avoid contamination of semen with toxic chemicals and to minimize transmission of venereal diseases.

A filter should be installed in the artificial vagina prior to collection of semen. This filter allows the sperm-rich portion of an ejaculate to pass into the semen receptacle but retains the gel fraction. The result is a higher usable sperm harvest, because fewer spermatozoa become trapped within the gel during collection. Newly developed nylon micromesh filters are preferable to conventional polyester matte filters.

Internal temperature of the artificial vagina should not exceed 45° to 48° C at the time of semen collection, since irreversible damage to spermatozoa can result from exposure (even short-term) to temperatures above this level. Only nonspermicidal lubricants should be used to lubricate the interior of the artificial vagina.

OTHER CONSIDERATIONS

Semen is generally collected after allowing the stallion to mount a breeding dummy or a receptive and properly restrained mare. Stallions can also be trained to ejaculate while standing. Prior to collecting semen, the stallion's penis (particularly the distal portion) should be cleansed with water and thoroughly dried. Soaps should be avoided since their use may lead to surface overgrowth with potentially pathogenic bacteria.

Ejaculated semen is promptly transported to the laboratory for evaluation and further processing. During transit, semen should be maintained near body temperature (i.e., 36° to 40° C) and protected from sunlight. If a filter was incorporated into the artificial vagina during semen collection, it is removed promptly to prevent seepage of gel into the gel-free portion of the ejaculate. Upon arrival the semen should be promptly placed in an incubator adjusted to 37° to 38° C, then mixed with an appropriate semen extender.

EVALUATION OF SEMEN

Spermatozoal quality and quantity are assessed soon after collection (see p. 671 for more details). The color and consistency of the ejaculate are noted, with particular attention paid to contamination of the sample with blood, urine, debris, or purulent material. The volume of the gel-free semen is determined using a graduated cylinder to ensure accurate measurement. The spermatozoal concentration is determined using a hemacytometer counting chamber or a spectrophotometer (550-nm wavelength) or densimeter properly calibrated using hemacytometer counts.

Evaluation of spermatozoal motility is considered to be a fundamental laboratory test for assessing the fertilizing capacity of an ejaculate. Since spermatozoal motility is extremely sensitive to environmental conditions, the semen must be protected from injurious agents or conditions prior to analysis. Taking such precautionary steps will help ensure that the motility estimate is representative of that intrinsic to the stallion and not depressed because of artifactual changes. The following basic steps should be observed to minimize environmental damage of spermatozoa prior to analysis: (1) The semen is collected using a properly prepared artificial vagina. (2) Gel-free semen is promptly transported to the laboratory in a warm, light-shielded container, then placed in an incubator maintained at 37° to 38° C. (3) The gel-free semen is mixed with an appropriate prewarmed (37° C) semen extender within 2 minutes after its collection. (4) Spermatozoal motility is examined microscopically within 10 minutes after the semen is combined with a semen extender. (5) All equipment and glassware that comes in contact with the semen is clean, nontoxic, and prewarmed to 37° C.

To further enhance the reliability of motility estimation, the procedure should be done by an experienced person using a properly equipped microscope. A microscope with a built-in stage warmer and phase-contrast optics is preferred.

Several different techniques and instruments have been developed for objective evaluation of spermatozoal motility; however, methods such as time-lapse photomicrography, frame-by-frame playback video micrography, spectrophotometry, or computerized analysis are too tedious or expensive for routine use. Subjective assessment of motility by visual estimation is more practical. This method is generally quite acceptable, provided that personnel are experienced in analysis of spermatozoal motility, a properly equipped microscope is used, and the semen is appropriately diluted with a good-quality semen extender prior to analysis. Dilution of semen to a spermatozoal concentration of 25×10^6 per ml is recommended before analysis of motility. Parameters of measurement generally include the percentage of spermatozoa that are motile, the percentage of spermatozoa that are progressively motile, and spermatozoal velocity (assessed on a scale of 0 to 4). Longevity of spermatozoal motility may also be evaluated, both in raw semen (at room temperature, 20° to 25° C) and extended semen (at room temperature or refrigerated temperature, 4° to 6° C).

The morphology of spermatozoa is typically examined at $1000\times$ magnification. Major morphological defects such as abnormal heads, abnormal midpieces, or proximal cytoplasmic droplets are known to interfere with fertility of stallions. A standard bright-field microscope can be used to examine air-dried, stained semen smears. Visualization of structural detail can be enhanced by viewing unstained spermatozoa as a wet mount, using a microscope with phase-contrast or differential interference optics. Clinicians inexperienced in assessment of spermatozoal morphology are encouraged to submit specimens to a reference laboratory for analysis.

SEMEN EXTENDERS

Semen collected for artificial insemination should always be placed in a semen extender, whether the semen is to be inseminated immediately or preserved. The semen extender enhances spermatozoal survival outside the stallion's genital tract by (1) providing spermatozoa with metabolizable substrates, (2) accommodating spermatozoal pH and osmotic pressure requirements, (3) protecting spermatozoa against cold shock, and (4) eliminating or reducing bacterial growth in the semen through incorporation of antibiotics. Seminal extenders may be purchased commercially or prepared in the laboratory (Table 2). If semen is to be used for insemination soon after collection, it should be mixed with semen extender at a 1:1 to 1:3 ratio. More extensive dilution is recommended if semen is to be stored for a prolonged period prior to insemination.

TABLE 2. COMMONLY USED SEMEN EXTENDERS

Name	Formulation*
Kenney	1. Mix nonfat dry milk solids (2.4 gm) and glucose (4.9 gm) with 92 ml deionized water. 2. Add: (a) crystalline penicillin G (150,000 units) and crystalline streptomycin sulfate (150 mg), or (b) gentamicin sulfate (100 mg) mixed with 2 ml of 7.5% sodium bicarbonate.
Skim milk	1. Heat 100 ml nonfortified skim milk to 92° to 95° C for 10 minutes in a double boiler. Cool. 2. Add polymyxin B sulfate (100,000 units).
Cream gel	1. Dissolve 1.3 gm unflavored Knox gelatin in 10 ml sterile deionized water. Sterilize. 2. Heat Half & Half cream to 92° to 95° C for 2 to 4 minutes in a double boiler. Remove scum from surface. 3. Mix gelatin solution with 90 ml of heated Half & Half cream (100 ml total volume). Cool. 4. Add crystalline penicillin G (100,000 units), streptomycin sulfate (100 mg), and polymyxin B sulfate (20,000 units).

*Many different antibiotics and antibiotic dosages have been used with these basic extenders, incuding penicillin G (1000–1500 units/ml), streptomycin sulfate (1000–1500 μg/ml), polymyxin B sulfate (200–1000 units/ml), gentamicin sulfate (100–1000 μg/ml), amikacin sulfate (100–1000 μg/ml), and ticarcillin (100–1000 μg/ml). Use of gentamicin sulfate or amikacin sulfate generally requires the addition of sodium bicarbonate to adjust the pH of the extender.

ARTIFICIAL INSEMINATION

Artificial insemination is permitted by the vast majority of U.S. breed associations. Only sterile, nontoxic disposable equipment should be used for the procedure. All-plastic syringes* are recommended for artificial insemination since the rubber plunger seals of some syringes contain

---

*Air-Tite, Vineland, NJ

toxic materials that may leach into the semen. All inseminations should be performed using a minimum-contamination technique. With the mare adequately restrained and her tail wrapped and elevated, the area between the base of the tail and the ventral commissure of the vulva is thoroughly scrubbed, rinsed, and dried. Particular attention is given to removal of debris from the caudal vestibule and clitoral fossa. Semen contained within a syringe is deposited into the anterior uterine body through an 18- to 22-inch sterile insemination pipette. A sterile or clean plastic shoulder-length sleeve should be worn when passing the pipette through the cervix to the uterine body where the semen is to be deposited.

Mares are generally inseminated with 250 to 500 × 10^6 progressively motile spermatozoa contained in a semen extender. The volume of the inseminate typically ranges from 5 to 20 cu cm. For maximum pregnancy rates, it is best to inseminate mares within 12 to 24 hours prior to ovulation, although pregnancies have been achieved at a similar rate when mares were inseminated within 12 hours following ovulation. If semen from highly fertile stallions is used, mares may be inseminated 48 to 72 hours prior to ovulation with no depression in pregnancy rate.

PRESERVATION OF SEMEN

Relatively few breed registries in the United States permit the use of a stored (cooled or frozen) or transported semen. Nonetheless, this form of reproductive management is rapidly increasing in popularity among breeders belonging to the more lenient organizations. Semen from fertile stallions can often be stored in the liquid state for 24 hours or longer without a reduction in fertility. To maximize the longevity of spermatozoal viability when stored in this manner, semen should first be mixed with a good-quality semen extender at a high dilution ratio. Best results are obtained when semen is diluted to 25 to 50 × 10^6 per ml prior to storage.

Slowly cooling the extended semen to refrigerator temperature (4° to 6° C) will also maximize spermatozoal survival following storage. Studies to date indicate that the optimal cooling rate is −0.3° C per minute (initial cooling rate). The manner of achieving this cooling rate depends on the volume of extended semen to be stored. For instance, to cool 40 mL of extended semen at this rate, the semen can first be poured into a plastic bag, which is subsequently sealed to prevent leakage. This bag is then lowered into a beaker containing 160 cu cm of 37° C water, followed by placement of the unit in a refrigerator. A commercially available container* can also be used to achieve this cooling rate and at the same time protect the semen if it is to be shipped to another location. Development of this product has made breeding with mail order semen a relatively easy and successful venture for mare owners.

Freezing of horse semen has not been as successful as freezing of dairy bull semen, probably because of biophysical and biochemical differences in the spermatozoa of these two species. The pregnancy rate per cycle in mares bred with frozen–thawed semen is reported to range from 70 to 10 per cent or less. Although the upper level of this range would lead one to suspect that it might be commercially feasible, the pregnancy rate is in the 30 to 40 per cent range for many stallions. Further studies are needed to develop a simple, reliable method for freezing semen from a larger percentage of fertile stallions.

Supplemental Readings

Amann, R. P., and Pickett, B. W.: Principles of cryopreservation and a review of cryopreservation of stallion spermatozoa. J. Equine Vet. Sci., 7:145, 1987.

Jasko, D. J., Lein, D. H., and Foote, R. H.: Determination of the relationship between sperm morphologic classifications and fertility in stallions: 66 cases (1987–1988). J. Am. Vet. Med. Assoc., 197:389, 1990.

Kenney, R. M., Bergman, R. V., Cooper, W.L., and Morse, G. W.: Minimal contamination techniques for breeding mares: Technique and preliminary findings. In: Proceedings of the 21st Annual Convention of the American Assocation of Equine Practitioners, 1975, pp. 327–336.

Kenney, R. M., Hurtgen, J. P., Pierson R., Witherspoon D., and Simons, J.: Manual for Clinical Fertility Evaluation of the Stallions. Hastings, Neb., Society for Theriogenology, 1983.

Pickett, B. W., and Amann, R. P.: Extension and storage of stallion spermatozoa: A review. J. Equine Vet. Sci., 7:289, 1987.

Varner, D. D.: Collection and preservation of stallion spermatozoa. In: Proceedings of the Annual Meeting of the Society of Theriogenology, 1986, pp. 13–33.

---

*Equitainer, Hamilton-Thorn Research, Danvers, MA

Ultrasonographic Evaluation of Accessory Sex Gland Structure and Function in the Stallion

James A. Weber, MOSCOW, IDAHO
Gordon L. Woods, MOSCOW, IDAHO

The accessory sex glands of the stallion include the paired vesicular glands, the paired ampullae of the ductus deferens, the prostate gland, and the paired bulbourethral glands. These glands, which are located on the pelvic floor (Fig. 1), are digitally palpated per rectum as a routine part of the stallion breeding soundness examination. Their soft consistency and thick connective tissue coverings allow only gross changes in glandular structure to be detected by digital palpation. Transrectal ultrasonography (US), which has been used to obtain high-resolution images of the mare's reproductive tract, can also be used to detect subtle changes in the structure of the stallion's accessory sex glands. This discussion reviews the technique used to visualize the accessory sex glands of the stallion and the ultrasonographic appearance and dimensions of these glands at sexual rest, after sexual preparation (teasing), and after ejaculation.

ULTRASONOGRAPHIC TECHNIQUE

We use a B-mode, real-time scanner with a 7.5-MHz linear array transducer to visualize the stallion's accessory sex glands. The stallion is restrained in stocks without sedation and his rectum is cleared of fecal material. The transducer is lubricated with coupling gel, inserted into the rectum to the depth of the examiner's wrist, and oriented so that the US beam is directed ventrally through a gland (see Fig. 1). The size, shape, and fluid content of each gland are determined by scanning over the entire length of the gland. Dense tissue is described as hyperechoic (white), soft tissue as isoechoic (gray), and fluid as hypoechoic (black).

VESICULAR GLANDS

The vesicular glands are located dorsolateral to the bladder. When visualized in longitudinal section (Fig. 2A), their muscular walls are smooth in outline and slightly more hyperechoic than the surrounding viscera. The contents of their lumina (the gel fraction of semen) are hypoechoic when distended with secretions. In sexually rested stallions, each vesicular gland is flattened dorsoventrally and conforms closely to the surrounding structures (bladder, ampullae, digestive tract). The vesicular glands are readily identified when filled with fluid, but they are difficult to distinguish when devoid of fluid. The vesicular gland, when it contains gel, changes from a flattened, elongated shape after sexual rest to a shorter, more rounded shape after teasing (Figs. 2A and B). In stallions that contribute gel to the ejaculate, the vesicular gland lumen decreases in diameter or is not visible after ejaculation (Fig. 2C). The decrease in luminal dimensions after ejaculation is related to the amount of gel in the ejaculate. Stallions whose vesicular glands contain gel do not always contribute it to the ejaculate; in these cases a postejaculation decrease in luminal size does not occur. In stallions that contribute gel to the ejaculate, no changes in vesicular gland wall thickness are detectable after ejaculation; however, the vesicular gland changes in shape from a smooth outline after teasing to an irregular outline after ejaculation (Fig. 2C).

AMPULLAE

The ampullae are located dorsolateral to the bladder and medial to the vesicular glands. When the ampullae are followed in a craniocaudal direction, they converge, pass between the prostatic isthmus and the dorsal surface of the urethra, and taper to excurrent ducts within the lumen of the proximal urethra. When visualized in transverse section (Fig. 3A), the lumen of the ampulla appears as a hypoechoic circle when it contains fluid and as a broken hyperechoic line when it does not contain fluid. The parenchyma of the ampulla is mottled in most stallions. The average echogenicity of the paren-

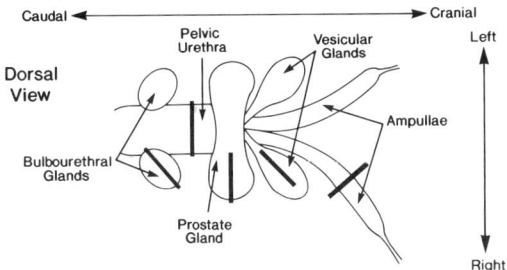

Figure 1. Dorsal view of stallion accessory sex glands. Bars represent the orientation of the ultrasound transducer that was used to produce the ultrasonographic images of each gland.

chyma varies widely among stallions. The ampullary lumen increases in diameter after teasing, then decreases in diameter after ejaculation (Figs. 3B and C). The lumen of the ampulla appears to store fluid when stallions are teased and to release the fluid during ejaculation. No changes in ampullary wall thickness are detectable after teasing or ejaculation.

PROSTATE GLAND

The prostate lobes and isthmus border the dorsal and lateral edges of the pelvic urethra just caudal to the insertion of the ampullae and vesicular glands. The interior of each prostate lobe contains numerous hypoechoic bands that radiate laterally from a single origin near the lateral border of the urethra. These bands are surrounded by homogeneous, isoechoic parenchyma. The prostatic isthmus contains parenchyma interspersed with small hypoechoic pockets. The prostate gland increases in overall size and fluid content after teasing and decreases to sexually rested values after ejaculation (Fig. 4).

BULBOURETHRAL GLANDS

The bulbourethral glands are located dorsolateral to the pelvic urethra near the pelvic outlet. When visualized in longitudinal section, each gland is outlined by a thin hypoechoic border corresponding to the bulboglandularis muscle, which surrounds mottled, isoechoic glandular parenchyma. Small hypoechoic areas are inconsistently observed throughout its parenchyma. The bulbourethral glands increase in overall size and fluid content after teasing and decrease to sexually rested values after ejaculation (Fig. 5). After teasing, fluid is occasionally visible within

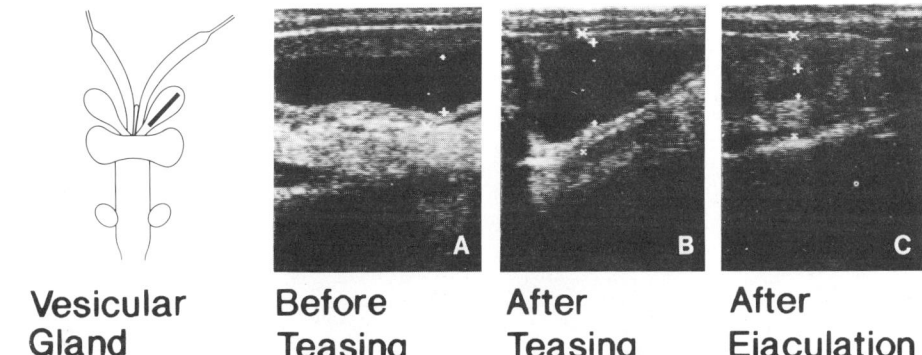

Figure 2. Ultrasonographic images of the vesicular gland: (A) before teasing, (B) after teasing, and (C) after ejaculation.

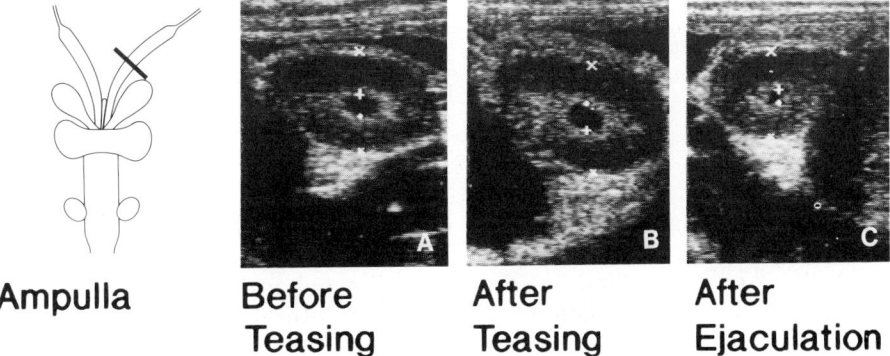

Figure 3. Ultrasonographic images of the ampulla: (A) before teasing, (B) after teasing, and (C) after ejaculation.

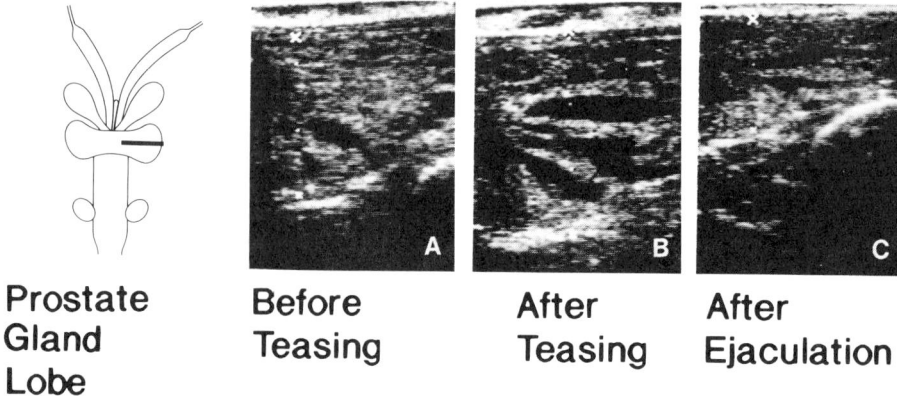

Figure 4. Ultrasonographic images of the prostate lobe: (A) before teasing, (B) after teasing, and (C) after ejaculation.

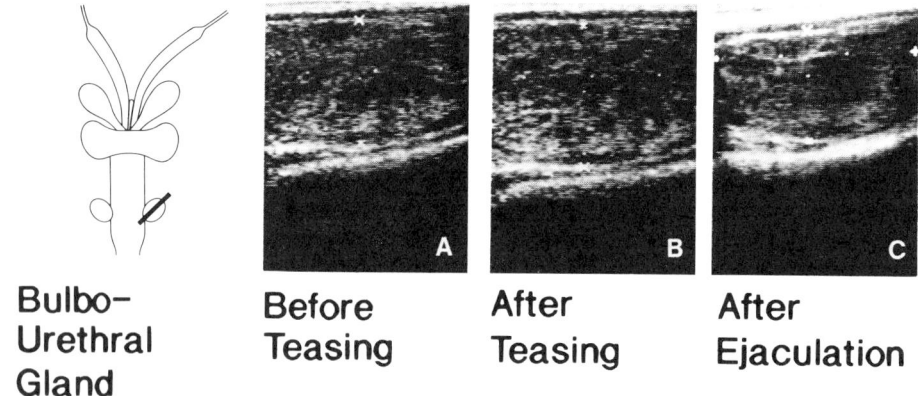

Figure 5. Ultrasonographic images of the bulbourethral gland: (A) before teasing, (B) after teasing, and (C) after ejaculation.

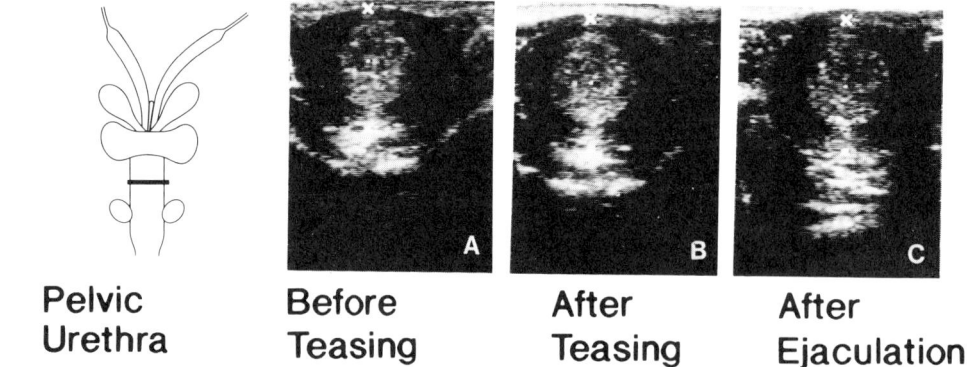

Figure 6. Ultrasonographic images of the pelvic urethra: (A) before teasing, (B) after teasing, and (C) after ejaculation.

the urethral lumen in the vicinity of the bulbourethral gland excurrent ducts. This may be the source of the clear fluid often secreted by sexually stimulated stallions prior to ejaculation.

PELVIC URETHRA

The pelvic urethra appears as a hypoechoic ring (urethralis muscle) surrounding a mottled central circular region (Fig.6). When the proximal urethra is visualized the excurrent ducts of the ampullae and vesicular glands appear as laterally compressed hyperechoic crescents within its central region. The excurrent ducts of the ampullae are located medial to the excurrent ducts of the vesicular glands. No changes in the diameter of the pelvic urethra are detectable after teasing or ejaculation (see Fig. 6).

Supplemental Readings

Little, T. V. and Woods G. L.: Ultrasonography of accessory sex glands in the stallion. J. Reprod. Fertil. Suppl., 35:87–94, 1987.

Weber, J. A., Geary, R. T., and Woods, G. L.: Changes in accessory sex glands of stallions after sexual preparation and ejaculation. J. Am. Vet. Med. Assoc., *196*:1084–1089, 1990.

Section 16

SKIN DISEASES

Edited by Diane Bevier

Skin Biopsies in the Diagnosis of Inflammatory Skin Diseases

Robert W. Dunstan, EAST LANSING, MICHIGAN
Mitchell D. Song, DAVIS, CALIFORNIA

Of all the equine diseases, diseases of the skin are among the most difficult to diagnose and treat. Skin diseases are clearly visible to the client and often are not associated with systemic signs. Fortunately, many skin diseases that are difficult to define on physical examination can be readily diagnosed with a skin biopsy. The skin biopsy is a deceptively simple technique and its successful implementation requires care and attention on the part of the clinician and also the pathologist.

WHEN TO BIOPSY

The decision to perform a skin biopsy can be made only after a thorough history has been obtained, a complete physical examination has been performed, and routine diagnostic procedures such as skin scrapings and Tzank preparations have been evaluated. Although there are no definitive indications for a skin biopsy, in general, biopsy should be considered for any dermatosis that has not responded to rational therapy, cannot be diagnosed with routine diagnostic tests, could potentially be neoplastic, or is severe enough to be associated with systemic illness. Although practitioners generally will try several different therapeutic modalities before considering a skin biopsy, it must be remembered that the more chronic the disease process, the less likely it is that the pathologist will be able to make a useful histological interpretation. Ideally, the biopsy specimen should be obtained within the first 2 to 3 weeks of the onset of the skin lesions. The value of a skin biopsy greatly diminishes if it is used as the last option in establishing a diagnosis.

WHERE AND WHAT TO BIOPSY

The information gleaned from a skin biopsy depends on lesions that depict the primary disease in varying stages of development. Because early, fully developed, and chronic changes may exist concurrently in inflammatory skin diseases, more than one biopsy sample should be routinely submitted. Gross lesions can be divided into primary or secondary lesions. Primary lesions are a direct expression of the disease process and include macules, papules, plaques, nodules, tumors, pustules, wheals, vesicles, and papillomas. Secondary lesions develop as a result of self-trauma or therapy, or simply represent changes associated with resolution of the lesion. They include scales, crusts, comedones, vegetations, fissures, erosions, and ulcerations, as well as zones of lichenification and hyperpigmentation. Primary lesions tend to be more diagnostic on histopathological evaluation than secondary lesions; however, this is not invariably true. As a general guide, the first biopsy specimen should always be from the most representative lesion on the horse, regardless of whether the lesion is primary or secondary. Additional biopsy specimens should be limited to primary lesions, even if they are extremely rare. If an alopecic process is present, biopsy specimens should be taken from the area that is most alopecic, areas that are moderately alopecic, and areas of normally haired skin. This is necessary because alopecic diseases are often extremely difficult to identify histologically. Any area directly over a nerve, blood vessel, joint capsule, or bony prominence should be avoided. If this is not possible, the skin should be stretched away from the site before the sample is taken.

HOW TO BIOPSY

The three most common skin biopsy methods are the punch, wedge, and shave biopsies. The punch biopsy is the easiest to perform and is indicated for routine skin biopsies. A wedge biopsy is never contraindicated and is mandatory for diseases displaying a transitional zone, diseases of the subcutis, and for bullae or large pustules. In veterinary dermatology a shave biopsy is used almost exclusively for exophytic lesions such as warts but may also be used to obtain superficial samples from sites such as the external nares, eyelid, and aural pinna (Table 1).

PUNCH BIOPSY

Once the site has been selected, the area is prepared by clipping the hair. The punch biopsy is not a sterile procedure. The site should not be washed or scrubbed, and care should be taken not to remove crusts, scales, or material adherent to the hair or skin during clipping as histologically diagnostic changes can be removed in the process. After it is clipped, the biopsy site is outlined with an indelible felt tip marker to ensure that the area to be anesthetized is biopsied. After marking, 1 ml of lidocaine or lidocaine with 1:1000 epinephrine (which provides better hemostasis) is injected subcutaneously at the marked site. The injection of lidocaine may be moderately painful to the animal owing to the low pH of the solution. Once the area has been infiltrated, 2 to 5 minutes should be allowed for the onset of anesthesia before proceeding.

A 6-mm or 8-mm Baker's key cutaneous biopsy punch° is recommended. The punch is placed on the skin and rotated in one direction with firm pressure until there is relief of resistance to the punch, which often feels like a "popping" through the skin. This indicates that the

---

°Chester A. Baker Labs., Miami, FL

TABLE 1. EQUINE SKIN BIOPSY TECHNIQUE ACCORDING TO SITE

Site	Technique	Comments
Haired skin	Punch, wedge, or shave	Use wedge biopsy for all lesions that display a transitional zone, or are present in subcutaneous fat, or are bullous or pustular. Reserve shave biopsies for exophytic lesions such as warts.
Chestnut, ergot	Punch or wedge	
External nares	Punch, wedge, or shave	May cause significant hemorrhage. Hemorrhage may be stopped by ligation and application of direct pressure. No suturing is required. Because the nares are a highly innervated region, tranquilization and physical restraint may be needed.
Eyelid	Shave or wedge	No suturing required for shave biopsy. Tranquilization and physical restraint may be necessary.
Ear pinna	Shave or wedge	Do not use epinephrine with lidocaine. Epinephrine may cause vasoconstriction and necrosis of the pinna.
Coronary band	Shave or wedge	No suturing required. May be of value in defining lesions of the hoof wall.
Oral mucosa	Wedge	Biopsy site should be allowed to heal by granulation. Suturing is not necessary.

punch has penetrated the subcutaneous fat. The base of the biopsy is then lifted by gently grasping it with a pair of rat-toothed forceps and the remaining unattached tissue is cut with a pair of iris scissors. In many adult horses, the punch is not long enough to extend into the subcutis. In these cases, the blade should penetrate the skin up to its hub and iris scissors should be used to dissect the base of the biopsy to the subcutaneous fat. All punch biopsies should extend into the subcutaneous fat to ensure first intention healing and to secure adequate material for histopathological evaluation of the entire dermis. To close the biopsy, 2-0 or 3-0 nylon suture can be used in a simple interrupted or cruciate pattern. The horse may be bathed within 2 to 3 days after the biopsy has been taken as long as the biopsy sites are not vigorously scrubbed. The sutures should be removed in 10 days.

WEDGE BIOPSY

Attention should be paid to the orientation of the elliptical incision. Whenever anatomically feasible, the long axis of the biopsy should follow the flow of the hair. For ulcerated lesions, the long axis should extend from the ulcer at one edge to normal skin at the other. The technique for a wedge biopsy is essentially the same as that of a punch biopsy except that the biopsy site is anesthetized in a ring block. A No. 10 or 40 scalpel blade and handle is used to excise an ellipse of tissue. The area is undermined with general operating or Metzenbaum scissors and closed with 2-0 or 3-0 suture.

SHAVE BIOPSY

The raised mass is anesthetized as for a wedge biopsy. The skin is raised as a fold and cut with a scalpel or razor blade parallel to the skin surface. The area left by the incision can be sutured, bandaged, or left to heal if minimal hemorrhage is present.

FIXATION OF THE BIOPSY

Immediately after the punch or wedge biopsy specimen is removed from the horse, it is gently wiped free of hemorrhage and placed dermal side down on a piece of tongue depressor or cardboard. The subcutaneous fat adheres to the surface and prevents artifactual contracture of the biopsy during fixation. The tissue is submerged in a leak- and trauma-resistant vessel containing a minimum of 10 times the volume of formalin to the volume of the mass. Because shave biopsy specimens of exophytic lesions usually do not have subcutaneous fat and adhere poorly to a tongue depressor, they are immersed directly in the formalin. When tissues are to be mailed to or out of cold temperature zones, 10 per cent by volume of 95 per cent ethyl alcohol is added to the formalin to prevent freezing. Freezing results in ice crystal formation in the tissues, which can make the sample uninterpretable.

It is sometimes necessary to define the presence of immunoglobulins in tissues in order to confirm the diagnosis of an autoimmune disease. The laboratory to which the sample is being sent should be contacted to learn how the biopsy specimen should be fixed and if the laboratory will perform this test on equine skin. Most laboratories use an immunofluorescence procedure that requires fixation in Michel's fixative.° Michel's fixative preserves tissue antigenicity but causes severe distortion of tissue morphology and is unsuitable for routine histological evaluation. The fixative does not penetrate tissues as readily as formalin, and to ensure adequate fixation, tissues no larger than one-half of an 8-mm punch biopsy specimen should be placed in a volume of fixative that is 10 times that of the volume of the specimen. Tissues placed in Michel's fixative should not be stored for longer than 3 months.

A number of laboratories use immunoperoxidase procedures to evaluate for the presence of cutaneous immunoglobulins. This procedure is as accurate as immunofluorescence assay and can often be performed on formalin-fixed tissues.

There is a considerable controversy over the value of immunofluorescence assay and immunohistochemistry analysis in the evaluation of immune-mediated dermatoses in veterinary medicine. False positive and false negative results are common. Therefore, these techniques should only be used as confirmatory tests after histopathological evaluation has been completed. An experienced veterinary dermatopathologist can often establish the diagnosis of an immune-mediated skin disease with such a high degree of certainty that immunohistochemical examination is not needed.

WHO SHOULD INTERPRET THE BIOPSY?

To obtain the maximum benefit from the interpretation of a skin biopsy specimen, the clinician must be assured that the laboratory produces good-quality slides and has a pathologist knowledgeable in both clinical and histological aspects

---

°Zeuss Scientific, Raritan, NJ

of equine skin diseases. Although it is difficult for a clinician to assess the quality of unseen histological sections, a key indication is the amount of time used to infiltrate the tissues with paraffin, a procedure known as tissue processing. Because of the density of equine collagen, a processing time of less than 12 hours results in slides with many artifacts that may obscure a subtle lesion. A pathologist with an interest in equine dermatology can be recommended by a member of the American College of Veterinary Dermatology. Alternatively, board-certified pathologists who are members of the American Academy of Veterinary Dermatologists are often well qualified to interpret equine skin biopsies.°

WHAT CAN THE CLINICIAN EXPECT FROM THE PATHOLOGIST?

The skin biopsy is a useful diagnostic aid. Its limitations stem primarily from the fact that although knowledge of the histological features of equine dermatoses has grown markedly over the past decade, many skin diseases of horses remain undefined, poorly defined, or appear to overlap with a number of clinically distinctive disorders. A pathologist's interpretation will necessarily reflect the state of knowledge relative to a disease process. For many diseases, histological evaluation will result in a definitive diagnosis, but for less well-defined diseases, especially allergic, autoimmune, or certain alopecic disorders, a pathologist may only be able to suggest a reasonable diagnosis and advise what further tests may be necessary for confirmation. A close working relationship must exist between clinician and pathologist for optimal results in the histopathological evaluation of equine skin disease.

Supplemental Readings

Dunstan, R. W.: A user's guide to veterinary surgical pathology laboratories, or, why do I still get a diagnosis of chronic dermatitis even when I take a perfect biopsy? Vet. Clin. North Am., 20:1397, 1990.
Haines, D. M., Cooke, E. M., and Clark, E. G.: Avidin-biotin-peroxidase-complex immunohistochemistry to detect immunoglobulin in formalin fixed skin biopsies in canine autoimmune disease. Can. J. Vet. Res., 51:104, 1987.
Ihrke, P. J., and Gross, T. L.: The skin biopsy: Maximizing the benefits. In: Proceedings of the 55th Annual Meeting of the American Animal Hospital Association, 1988, pp. 299–301.
Lever W. F., and Schaumburg-Lever, G.: In Histopathology of the Skin, 3rd ed. Philadelphia, J. B. Lippincott, 1990, pp. 1–2.
Scott, D. W.: Dermatohistopathology. In Large Animal Dermatology. Philadelphia, W. B. Saunders, 1988, pp. 29–30.

°American Academy of Veterinary Dermatology, c/o Dr. Marvin L. Samuelson, Veterinary Teaching Hospital, Texas A & M University, College Station, TX 77843-4457

Nutrition and Skin Diseases
Harold F. Hintz, ITHACA, NEW YORK

An inappropriate supply of almost any essential nutrient can cause undesirable skin conditions in the horse. Some of the nutrients most likely to be involved in skin diseases are discussed below.

ENERGY AND PROTEIN

A lack of energy, either simple or induced by factors such as malabsorption, a heavy parasite load, or lack of protein, can cause an unthrifty appearance and a rough hair coat. Shedding can be prolonged. Protein deprivation can cause morphological changes in the hair such as bulb atrophy and a reduction in bulb diameter.

The use of fat supplements, particularly unsaturated fat, has long been thought to improve coat appearance. The effect of fat is thought to be additional to that of supplying energy. As early as 1917 it was reported that a pound of linseed meal per day was a helpful conditioner for run-down horses with rough hair coats and was excellent in the spring to hasten shedding of the hair and to give bloom and finish to show or sale horses. Some of the beneficial effects may have been due to the protein, but the 5 per cent fat in old process linseed meal was more likely to be the factor. New process linseed meal has only 1.5 per cent fat. Coats that fail to shed and lack luster may improve within 40 to 60 days by adding 2 ounces of vegetable oil to the grain ration daily.

MINERALS

ZINC

Foals fed diets containing 5 mg of zinc per kg of diet develop skin lesions similar to those seen in pigs fed zinc-deficient diets. The lesions are initially characterized by alopecia and superficial flaking of the dried epidermis. The lesions extend progressively upward along the medial and lateral aspects of the legs. Eventually hair is lost and the epidermis flakes from the lateral and ventral surfaces of the abdomen and thorax. In advanced stages of deficiency, areas of skin devoid of hair are covered with dried serous exudate and desquamated epithelium. Microscopic lesions include acanthosis, hyperkeratosis, and parakeratosis. The National Research Council recommends that the diet contain at least 40 mg of zinc per kg of dry matter. Thus, a 500-kg horse needs about 400 to 600 mg of zinc daily.

Several zinc compounds have been used in animal nutrition. Zinc sulfate contains 40.5 per cent zinc and 1 to 1.5 gm per day will supply the total requirement. Zinc oxide contains 80.3 per cent zinc, so 500 to 600 mg daily will supply the total requirement. Zinc methionine complexes have been used for ruminants and it has been suggested that the zinc is readily absorbed. However, I am not aware of any studies with these compounds in horses.

IODINE

Iodine deficiency in the mare can result in weak, hairless foals with goiter. Animals with hypothyroidism may have a rough hair coat. Excessive iodine was reported to cause alopecia in a horse being treated with ethylenediamine-dehydroiodide for dermatophilosis. Free choice feeding of iodized or trace mineralized salt should supply the needed iodine.

COPPER

A deficiency in copper may cause hypochromotricia, because copper is needed for the enzymatic conversion of tyrosine to melanin. In other species copper deficiency causes faulty keratinization of the skin and hair follicle. The National Research Council suggests that the ration of horses contain at least 10 mg of copper per kg of feed (90 per cent dry matter basis).

VITAMINS

VITAMIN A

Either deficiency or excessive intake of vitamin A can cause a rough, dull hair coat. After 20 weeks of excessive vitamin A intake, ponies lose large areas of hair and epidermis. Vitamin A deficiency causes a wide variety of lesions including hyperkeratinization of the skin. The National Research Council suggests that the diets of horses contain 2000 to 3000 IU of vitamin A activity per kg of dry matter. This is equivalent to approximately 20,000 to 50,000 IU of vitamin A per day for a mature horse. According to the National Research Council, the maximum tolerance level is 16,000 IU per kg of dry matter, or about 160,000 to 240,000 IU per day for a mature horse. Horses fed high-quality roughage or commercial grains containing supplemental vitamin A are not likely to develop vitamin A deficiency. A likely candidate for deficiency would be a growing horse fed poor-quality forage, particularly a forage that had been stored for a prolonged period, and grains such as barley or oats, which contain very low levels of vitamin A activity.

VITAMIN E

Vitamin E deficiency has been reported to cause dermatosis in dogs. Acanthosis nigricans in dogs has been successfully treated with oral vitamin E. However, no studies have been reported on the role of vitamin E in dermatosis in horses.

B-COMPLEX VITAMINS

The B-complex vitamins are necessary for a healthy skin. Dermatitis due to deficiencies in thiamine, riboflavin, niacin, pantothenic acid, biotin, or folic acid has been demonstrated in laboratory animals. Biotin supplementation (10 to 15 mg per day) has been recommended for horses with flaky, shell-like hooves, but little is known about the role of B-vitamins in the prevention of skin problems in horses. The National Research Council suggests that B-complex vitamins with the exception of vitamin B_{12} are usually supplied in adequate amounts in good-quality forage. Vitamin B_{12} is synthesized in the large intestine if cobalt is available.

Supplemental Readings

Donoghue, S., Kronfeld, D. K., Berkowitz, S. J., and Copp, R. L.: Vitamin A nutrition of the equine: Growth, serum biochemistry and hematology J. Nutr. *111*:365, 1981.

Fadok, V. A., and Wild, S.: Suspected cutaneous iodism in a horse. J. Am. Vet. Med. Assoc., *183*: 1104–1108, 1983.

Harrington, D. D., Walsh, J., and White, V.: Clinical and pathological findings on horses fed zinc-deficient diets. In: Proceedings of the 3rd Equine Nutrition and Physiology Symposium, 1973, pp. 51–54.

Henry W. A., and Morrison, F. B.: Feed and Feeding, 17th ed. Madison, Wis. Henry Morrison Co., 1917.
National Research Council: Nutrient Requirements of Horses. Washington, D. C., NAS-NRC, 1989.
Slade, L. M.: Blood and tissue chemistry relationship to nutritional status of horses and other animals. Stud Managers Handbook, vol. 16. Clovis, CA, Agriservices Foundation, 1980, p. 193.
Tyznik, W. J.: Energy requirements and sources for the equine. Stud Managers Handbook, vol. 9. Clovis, CA, Agriservices Foundation, 1973, p. 58.

Control of Ectoparasites

Lane Foil, BATON ROUGE, LOUISIANA
Carol Foil, BATON ROUGE, LOUISIANA

The arthropod pests of horses are insects and acarines. The subdivisions of these two groups in this article have been selected relative to management strategy (Table 1), rather than taxonomic relationships. The insecticidal and repellent components currently available in formulated pesticides and general use are listed in Tables 2 and 3. Since the majority of pesticides for equids are available to horse owners, this article will focus on designing integrated management strategies.

INSECTS

The flies (Diptera) are the most ubiquitous pests of equids. The general life cycle of flies includes four stages: egg, larva, pupa, and adult. Flies that are most dependent on vertebrates for energy sources are the easiest to control. For example, larval development is manageable when the larvae are dependent on host tissue or excrement. In some species of flies, such as horn flies, the adults utilize the vertebrate as a primary energy source. However, for many free-living Diptera species, only the adult female feeds on vertebrates and a single blood meal is used as a source of energy for egg production.

TABANIDS, BLACK FLIES, AND BITING MIDGES

In North America, the Tabanidae are represented by deer flies (*Chrysops* spp.), relatively small (6 to 11 mm long), yellow to orange flies with dark body markings, usually with patterned wings; and by horse flies. The term horse fly applies to a diverse group of flies that vary in color, body markings, wing markings, and size (9 to 33 mm). Blood meals are taken at 3- to 4-day intervals during diurnal and crepuscular periods to support egg development. The larvae are generally predators that can be found in a variety of aquatic to semiaquatic habitats and take from 3 months to 2 years to develop. Tabanids have been described as the mechanical vectors of over 35 pathogenic agents of livestock, including equine infectious anemia virus. They are painful biters, causing extreme annoyance and blood loss; local reactions to bites include dermal nodules. Protection from adult female tabanids is the only management for this group. The frequent use of repellents is often most practical. Pastures located well away from wooded areas are preferable. Few tabanid species enter barns, and stabling of animals during peak tabanid activity can help. An electrified insect light trap hung inside barns can be useful when tabanid species that do enter structures are present.

Black flies are relatively small (2 to 5 mm), diurnal pests of horses and man. These flies are best recognized from their humpbacked appearance. Females blood-feed every 3 to 5 days; the larvae develop in moving water, and mass emergence of flies can occur one to several times per year. Population density normally reduces with distance from the larval habitat, but swarms migrating on winds can travel several hundred miles. Extreme annoyance and pruritus can be caused by flies feeding inside the ears and on the head, neck, chest, medial thighs, and abdomen. The ears are the best place to look for these pests; the individual bites cause petechial hemorrhage and bloody crusts. Protection from adult flies is the management strategy. Stabling of horses during peak fly activity periods can be helpful. Individual horses can be protected with ear nets or frequent treatments with repellents. Application of petroleum jelly inside the ears after clipping can also help.

Biting midges are small flies (0.6 to 5.0 mm) and are commonly referred to as "punkies," "no-see-ums," or "sand flies." Two genera, *Culicoides* and *Leptoconops* (valley black gnat), are the major pests of horses in the United States. Females take blood meals at 3- to 4-day inter-

TABLE 1. PRIMARY MANAGEMENT STRATEGIES FOR COMMON EQUINE PESTS

1. Stabling
   Tabanids: Diurnal and crepuscular periods
   Black flies: Diurnal and crepuscular periods
   Biting midges: Under fans, nocturnal and crepuscular periods
2. Exclusion devices
   Black flies: Ear nets
   House flies: Face masks
   Face flies: Face masks
3. Hay and manure management
   Stable flies: Particularly hay in pastures
   House flies: General sanitation
4. Cattle management
   Horn flies: Control pest on natural host
   Face flies: Undisturbed cattle manure requisite for larval development
5. Water management
   Mosquitoes: Only certain species
   Biting midges: Only certain species
6. Source identification and removal
   Straw itch: Normally infested hay
   Blister beetle: Normally products containing alfalfa
7. Restricted grazing or movement
   Chiggers: Erratic distribution in spring or fall
   Ticks: Mowing and understory control also helpful
   Tabanids: Allow horses to escape from wooded areas
   Poultry pests (sticktight and lice): Separate horses from poultry

TABLE 3. GENERAL INSECTICIDE TYPES USED FOR EQUINE PESTS

Insecticides
 Face flies
 Facultative myiasis
 Horn flies
 House flies
 Lice
 Mosquitoes
 Sticktight flea
 Poultry lice
 Ticks

Repellents
 Black flies
 Biting midges
 Chiggers
 Horseflies

Insecticides and repellents
 Biting midges
 Black flies
 Chiggers
 Facultative myiasis
 Mosquitoes
 Stable flies
 Ticks

Premise treatment
 House flies
 Mosquitoes
 Stable flies

Categories may overlap, owing to differences in management systems or life cycles of different species. Pests controlled by systemic treatments, such as mites and lice, and obligate myiasis are discussed elsewhere in this volume (see article by Klei, p 696).

vals. *Leptoconops* larvae develop in sandy or clay–silt soils and emerge as adults following rainy seasons. Depending on species, *Culicoides* larvae develop in aquatic habitats, decaying vegetation, or manure. One or multiple generations may be produced yearly. These flies are most active during crepuscular and nocturnal periods and have an extremely painful bite. *Onchocerca cervicalis* is transmitted by *Culicoides*. Some species induce a seasonal familial hypersensitivity, "sweet itch" or "Queensland itch." Pruritus is often most intense along the base of the mane and tail and over the withers; however, the chest, ventral, and facial areas can be affected. Lesions consist of self-inflicted hair loss, excoriations with crusting, scaling, and eventually hyperkeratosis and thickening of the skin. The onset of pruritus during *Culicoides* feeding periods aids in the diagnosis. Hypersensitive horses can be treated with corticosteroids, but management of sweet itch is based on protection from adult gnats. Stabling of horses during peak feeding times is advisable. Owing to the weak flight capabilities of *Culicoides*, fans, even in open-sided stalls, can provide protection under some conditions. Screened windows impregnated or treated with residual insecticides can also afford

TABLE 2. PESTICIDES RECOMMENDED FOR EXTERNAL PARASITE CONTROL ON HORSES

Residual Insecticides	Other Compounds
Pyrethroids Cypermethrin Fenvalerate Permethrin Resmethrin Tetramethrin S-Bioallethrin Sumethrin Organophosphates Coumaphos Dichlorvos Malathion Tetrachlorvinphos Organochlorines Lindane Methoxychlor	Repellents MGK 326 *di-n-propyl isocinchomeronate* Stabilene: butoxypolypropylene glycol Botanicals Pyrethrins (also insecticidal) Synergists Piperonyl butoxide 5-[[2-(2-butoxyethoxy) ethoxy]methyl]-6-propyl-1,3-benzodioxole MGK 264 *N-octyl bicycloheptene dicarboximide*

Categories may overlap: e.g., some pyrethrins are also insecticidal, and some pyrethroids are repellent. William B. Warner and Roger O. Drummond assisted in compiling this list.

protection. Frequent application of repellents is recommended. Water management recommended for mosquito control may aid in reducing endemic populations of some gnat species.

STABLE FLIES, HORN FLIES, AND MOSQUITOES

The adult stable fly, *Stomoxys calcitrans*, is easily distinguished from the house fly by its characteristic prominent, blood-sucking mouthparts that extend anteriorly. The optimal stable fly larval habitat is hay, silage, or green chop contaminated with urine, water, and manure. Multiple generations are produced per year. Both sexes are blood-feeders and feed primarily on the legs and abdomens of horses. Blood loss and annoyance as well as wheals, crust, cutaneous papules, and nodules have also been associated with stable fly feeding. The stable fly is capable of mechanically transmitting pathogenic agents, including equine infectious anemia virus. Both stable flies and house flies are considered vectors of habronemiasis, "summer sores." Repellents and residual insecticides can be used in stable fly control; materials should be directed primarily toward the legs. Spraying of premises is also recommended. The use of feeders and proper hay disposal can prevent problems for pastured animals.

Horn flies, *Haematobia irritans*, are small (4 mm) obligate parasites of cattle; the entire adult life is essentially spent on the host. Horn fly larvae develop in fresh bovine manure; multiple generations are produced per year. Horses are attacked by horn flies (both sexes are blood-feeders) when they are pastured with or near cattle. Horn flies feed head-down in aggregates, primarily on the shoulders, neck, withers, and abdomen, and may contribute significantly to the commonly observed seasonal ventral midline dermatitis of horses. The salient aspects of horn fly dermatitis are ulcers and crusting. Fly control may be necessary in addition to ivermectin therapy for complete resolution of cutaneous onchocerciasis when horn fly populations are above 25 per horse. Since this pest depends on cattle manure to complete the life cycle and spends the majority of its life on the host, the horn fly is relatively easy to control on horses. The use of residual insecticide sprays on horses at labeled intervals adequately controls horn flies. Separation from cattle or controlling the flies associated with the cattle can reduce the problem.

Female mosquitoes blood-feed every 3 to 4 days. In general, the most active feeding period of mosquitoes is the first 2 hours after sunset. Larvae develop in permanent water sources or in habitats subject to water level fluctuation, including pastures, tree holes, and artificial containers. Multiple generations are produced, and the life cycle can be completed within a week during warm weather. Explosive populations of mosquitoes can cause considerable annoyance. However, the primary impact of mosquitoes on equine populations is the transmission of viruses, in particular western (WEE), eastern (EEE), and Venezuelan (VEE) equine encephalitis (see pp. 547 and 765). Routine vaccination for the encephalitides is recommended. Larval habitat control is frequently beneficial. Chemical control can be in the form of insecticides or surfactants. Water management such as drainage of standing water, frequent drainage of troughs, cleaning of rain gutters, and elimination of manmade containers can greatly reduce mosquito problems. Minnows can help in water sources that cannot be drained. Space sprays and treatment of resting sites (walls) and horses with residual insecticides can help to keep mosquito populations at a moderate level. Frequent application of repellents during peak mosquito outbreaks is often necessary.

HOUSE FLIES AND FACE FLIES

The house fly, *Musca domestica*, and face fly, *M. autumnalis*, can be differentiated by the color on the lateral aspects of the adult abdomen (yellowish in the house fly, black in the female face fly, orange in the male face fly). The face fly larva is yellowish and the pupa is dirty white; the house fly larva is white and the pupa is reddish brown. Face fly larvae mature only in undisturbed cattle manure. House fly larvae develop best in manure but mature in a wide variety of organic debris. Both species can produce multiple generations per year. The face fly and house fly can cause considerable annoyance to horses while feeding on lacrimal secretions. The house fly and the stable fly are vectors of habronemiasis, "summer sores." The house fly has also been incriminated in the transmission of over 60 pathogens of vertebrates. The face fly has been shown to transmit eye worms of the *Thelazia* spp.

For the house fly, larval habitat control is considered of primary importance. Proper disposal of hay and manure should be part of any fly control program. Since undisturbed cattle manure is requisite for face fly reproduction, treatment of proximal cattle can be beneficial. Residual insecticide application on the face and neck can aid in house fly and face fly control. Commercially available fly masks or face masks attached to halters can also reduce eye feeding by flies. Combinations of premise sprays, residual wall, or timed space spray pyrethrin systems, in addition to baits, sticky traps, or electric grids, are often used for adult house fly control. Oral insecticides (larvicides) are also available in the form of feed additives and mineral blocks. However, the success of any strategy is predicated on good sanitation.

MYIASIS

Myiasis is the infestation of tissue by fly larvae. Facultative myiasis can be produced by a variety of fly larvae that routinely develop in carrion, notably *Cochliomyia macellaria* (secondary screwworm), *Phormia regina* (black blow fly) and *Phaenicia* spp. (green or bronze blow flies). The larvae develop in necrotizing skin lesions of horses. Maggot-infested wounds should be thoroughly cleansed and debrided. Treatment with residual insecticides, in addition to supportive treatment, is recommended. Prevention by treatment of wounds with repellents is helpful.

Hypoderma lineatum and *H. bovis* (cattle grubs) are obligate parasites of cattle that occasionally infest horses. Subcutaneous and dermal nodules are found most frequently in the spring and early summer and are most often located dorsally. A characteristic central breathing pore may be found in most lesions. Individual lesions may be resolved surgically, but ivermectin in standard dosages has been reported to control development of *Hypoderma* larvae. Migration of *Hypoderma* larvae can also produce intracranial equine myiasis; clinical signs vary relative to the location and magnitude of larval migration.

Horse bots (*Gasterophilus* spp.) are flies that as adults are superficially beelike in appearance. The life cycle of bot flies takes about 1 year. Eggs are firmly attached to the hairs of horses, and larvae (bots) live inside the horse's mouth for a few weeks, burrowing into the mucous membranes of the lips and tongue, causing transient irritation. The larvae then migrate to the stomach, grow for up to 10 months until being passed in the feces, and pupate in the ground for 1 to 2 months. The asynchronous development and discharge of larvae results in extended periods of oviposition. Stomach bots can cause mechanical blockage, colic, or rupture of the stomach wall and resultant peritonitis. Many of the treatments for internal parasites effectively control stomach bots when routinely administered (see p. 51).

OTHER INSECTS

Lice are normally species-specific ectoparasites of mammals; survival off the host is limited. The chewing lice, most commonly *Bovicola equi*, feed on sloughed epidermal tissues and sebaceous secretions. Chewing lice of poultry can infest horses stabled near poultry. The sucking louse of horses, *Haematopinus asini*, feeds on blood. The life cycle can be completed in 3 weeks, allowing production of multiple generations per year. Lice are first seen on the head, neck, mane, and tail during winter and early spring. The major dermatological problem associated with louse infestation is pruritus with attendant excoriation. Lice are easily controlled by treatment with residual insecticides; ivermectin is extremely effective for controlling the rare sucking louse.

The sticktight flea of poultry firmly attaches to the skin of birds but can also attack horses that are allowed in areas with infested chickens. Local pruritic dermatitis has been associated with foci of sticktight flea attachment in horses. The use of residual insecticides and separation from poultry are recommended.

Blister beetles, in particular *Epicauta* spp., can cause toxicosis in horses. Typically, consumption of alfalfa hay containing blister beetles produces cantharidin toxicosis in horses, which can be fatal. Clinical signs include salivation, oral lesions, colic, and frequent urination. Repeated doses of mineral oil and intravenous fluid therapy are recommended, along with removal of the toxic source.

ACARINES

The life cycle of ticks and mites includes four stages: egg, larva, nymph, and adult. The larvae have six legs; nymphs and adults have eight legs. The discussion of this group will generally progress from the least to the most host-specific.

CHIGGERS, PYEMOTID MITES, AND TICKS

Chiggers (redbugs or harvest mites) are parasitic on vertebrates in the larval stage and free-living in the nymphal and adult stages. Pastured horses or horses on trail rides can contact chigger populations that may be extremely dense. Papular dermatitis with crusting can occur over the entire body, but particularly on the head, neck, chest, and legs. Pyemotid mites (cause of straw, hay, or grain itch) are predators of insects and attack vertebrates that come in contact with infested products. The straw itch mite, *Pyemotes tritici*, which causes dermatitis in man, has been described in an outbreak of equine dermatitis (nonpruritic papular eruptions on the neck and withers). *Pyemotes* mites are not very mobile; therefore, regions of infestation on horses are limited to sites in close contact with infested substrates such as hay. Humans associated with horses may also have typical straw itch mite reactions, such as erythematous pruritic papules, and vesicles. Limiting access to areas of chigger infestation is recommended, but prophylactic treatment with repellents can help. Removal of infested sources will eliminate pyemotid mite problems. Bird and rodent mites can cause intense transient problems when their hosts are depleted. Miller's itch, caused by *Acarus farinae* in oats, has been reported in horses in Europe. Identification of the source is the primary tactic in controlling chigger and itch mite dermatitis.

Ticks are subdivided into the soft ticks (Argasidae) and the hard ticks (Ixodidae). The soft tick that parasitizes horses in the United States is the spinose ear tick *(Otobius megnini)*. Over 14 species of hard ticks have been reported on horses in the United States. The majority of these hard tick species are three-host ticks; i.e., individuals complete engorgement on the host, and detach. The larvae and nymphs molt to the next stage, crawl up structures, and become quiescent until a host approaches. Mating occurs on the host and females detach to oviposit. Ticks are vectors of equine piroplasmosis, *Babesia caballi* and *B. equi*, and borreliosis, *Borrelia burgdorferi*. The vectors of Potomac horse fever, *Ehrlichia risticii*, are undescribed; attempted transmission studies with ticks have been unsuccessful. Tick paralysis is usually associated with *Dermacentor* ticks. Heavy tick burdens can result in general unthriftiness, anemia, and susceptibility to disease. Tick bites can also create sites for myiasis and secondary infection. Limiting grazing to mowed pastures or vegetation modification to eliminate understory can decrease tick problems. The use of repellents or residual insecticides can afford some protection.

HOST-SPECIFIC MITES

Mange mites are uncommon parasites of horses. The sarcoptic mange mite, *Sarcoptes scabei* var. *equi*, is a nearly circular mite with short legs. *Psoroptes* spp., the scab mites, have an oval body shape with legs extending beyond the margins of the body; pedicels are segmented. *Chorioptes equi*, the chorioptic mange mite, is similar to *Psoroptes* in having long legs, but the pedicels are unsegmented. The life cycle of these mites is completed on the host. Sarcoptic mites tunnel into the epidermis. Sarcoptic mange is usually located on the head, neck, and ear. Psoroptic mites live on the skin surface and pierce the skin with mouthparts, feeding on serum and cellular components. Psoroptic mange is initially found at the base of the long hairs of the mane, tail, and forelock. Alopecia and papules are the initial clinical signs. As the disease progresses, a characteristic moist, hemorrhagic crust forms. Chorioptic mites live on the skin surface and feed on skin debris. Chorioptic mange is most often identified in the winter and is the most prevalent. Clinical signs are usually limited to the lower parts of the legs and consist of a scaling, fine papular eruption. Mange mite infestations should be considered contagious; quarantine and treatment of infested animals are recommended. Management of three of the mange mites is discussed on page 697.

Demodex (follicle mites) are host-specific, minute, barrel-shaped mites. The legs are stubby and the abdomen is elongated and transversely striated. Two species have been described as normal residents of the skin of horses. *Demodex caballi* (long, thin body) occurs in the meibomian glands of the eyelids and the pilosebaceous apparatus of the skin of the muzzle. *D. equi* is more widespread; the entire life cycle transpires within hair follicles. Demodicosis, consisting of patchy alopecia and scaling, is rare in horses; it has been associated with debilitating illness or glucocorticoid therapy in some cases. Many acaricides have been used to treat this disease, with questionable results. Application of 0.025 per cent amitraz has been reported to cause severe illness in horses.

Supplemental Readings

Foil, L. D., and Foil, C. S.: Dipteran parasites of horses. Equine Pract., *10*:21–38, 1988.

Foil, L. D., and Foil, C. S.: Parasitic skin diseases of horses. Vet. Clin. North Am. (Equine Pract.), *2*:403–437, 1986.

Greiner, E. C., Fadok, V. A., and Rabin, E. B.: Equine *Culicoides* hypersensitivity in Florida: Biting midges collected in light traps near horses. Med. Vet. Entomol., *2*:129–135, 1988.

Harwood, R. F., and James, M. T.: Entomology in Human and Animal Health, 7th ed. New York, Macmillan, 1979.

McLean, R. G., Calisher, C. H., and Parham, G. L.: Isolation of Cache Valley virus and detection of antibody for selected arboviruses in Michigan horses in 1980. Am. J. Vet. Res., *48*:1039–1041, 1987.

Patton, S., and McCracken, M. D.: The occurrence and effect of *Thelazia* in horses. Equine Pract., *3*:53–57, 1981.

Ray, A. C., Kyle, A. L. G., Murphy, M. J., et al.: Etiologic agents, incidence, and improved diagnostic methods of cantharidin toxicosis in horses. Am. J. Vet. Res., *50*:187–191, 1989.

Culicoides Hypersensitivity

Joy Barbet, TAMPA, FLORIDA

Dermatitis resulting from a hypersensitivity reaction to the bites of any of several species of gnats of the genus *Culicoides* has been identified in horses in many parts of the world. It is the most common allergic skin disease in the horse. It has various common names: "Queensland itch" (Australia), "sweet itch" (England and Ireland), "kasen" (Japan), "dhobie itch" (India), "muck itch" or "summer itch" (North America), and *Sommerekzem* (Germany).

The insects involved are commonly referred to as biting midges, "punkies," or "no-see-ums." They have been improperly called sand flies, a term more accurately used to refer to members of the genera *Phlebotomus* and *Lutzomyia*. *Culicoides* are minute and are distinguished by the patterns of spots on the costal border of the wings. Breeding habitats include the muddy or sandy margins of still or slowly running water (fresh or salt) and damp accumulations of organic vegetable matter such as compost piles, rotting leaves, peaty soils, and manure. Peak activity of adult gnats occurs when there is little or no breeze and temperatures exceed 50° F (9° to 10° C). They generally fly only short distances from their breeding grounds. Most species are crepuscular, preferring to feed at dusk, into the early evening, and again at dawn. Different species of *Culicoides* feed preferentially at different sites on the horse, which may account for some variety in clinical signs. However, the ears, poll, mane, withers, tail head, ventral abdomen, and inguinal region are favored feeding sites.

PATHOGENESIS

Type I hypersensitivity plays a major role in the pathogenesis of *Culicoides* dermatitis in horses. Evidence for a type I hypersensitivity reaction in affected horses includes blood eosinophilia and elevated blood histamine levels at insect feeding times as well as immediate intradermal skin test reactivity to crude extracts of *Culicoides* spp. A reaginic antibody against *Culicoides*-derived antigens has been identified in the serum of affected horses; further analysis has revealed properties similar to human IgE.

Additionally, intradermal skin testing and histopathology provide evidence suggestive of delayed-type hypersensitivity. Some horses fail to exhibit positive immediate intradermal skin test reactions to extracts of *Culicoides* spp. but develop delayed reactions 6 to 48 hours post injection. Some horses exhibit both reactions. Histopathologically, a significant per centage of horses with clinical lesions of *Culicoides* hypersensitivity have dermal lymphohistiocytic perivascular infiltrates in addition to or instead of the dermal perivascular eosinophilic infiltrates classically associated with arthropod hypersensitivity reactions. Lymphohistiocytic perivascular infiltrates are not exclusive to delayed-type hypersensitivity reactions, however, and may be associated with chronic allergic skin disease or with IgE-mediated late-phase (type I hypersensitivity) reactions. The complete nature of the immunological reaction involved remains unclear.

Other factors play a role in the development of the disease. Epidemiological studies of Icelandic ponies demonstrated that adult ponies imported to Sweden from Iceland (where there are no *Culicoides* spp.) were much more likely to develop the disease than were those born in Sweden, where early exposure to *Culicoides* and to colostrum and milk of *Culicoides*- exposed mares would occur simultaneously. The importance of the interrelationship of these two events (early exposure and passive transfer) to the development of the disease has yet to be demonstrated conclusively. However, studies of allergic disease in man and laboratory animals have demonstrated reduced incidences of atopic diseases in young reared on mother's milk versus those fed on formula. Such differences may result from altered maturation of the immune system, particularly the development of T cell subsets in the thymus, in the absence of maternally derived immunity. The onset of clinical signs in the Icelandic ponies also tended to occur within fewer grazing seasons in imported ponies than in the Swedish-bred ponies. Other researchers have observed an apparent familial susceptibility to development of the condition.

HISTORY AND CLINICAL SIGNS

Onset of the disease correlates with the advent of warm weather, worsens throughout the summer months, and subsides with the onset of cool weather leading into winter. One or two seasons of mild disease may precede the development of a condition requiring veterinary attention. Previous management conditions resulting in lack of exposure, such as stabling or dry outdoor environment, may delay onset and progression of the disease in susceptible horses. Therefore, horses of any age may be affected, but cases in animals less than 3 years old are unusual and seldom severe. In tropical and subtropical climates, however, the prolonged insect season may allow sensitization and development of mild clinical disease during the first year of exposure and more rapid worsening thereafter. Usually only a few horses in a herd are affected, but an extremely high level of exposure caused the dermatitis in up to 30 per cent of horses on one farm that was surrounded by swampland.

Severe pruritus is the hallmark of *Culicoides* hypersensitivity and causes the clinical lesions for which a horse is referred to the veterinarian: broken hairs, alopecia, fresh excoriations, crusting, and secondary infection. Owners have reported that horses attempt to drag their abdomens on the ground or straddle tree stumps or similar objects in order to rub those areas. Trees, fences, and barns may be damaged by the incessant rubbing. The pruritus subsides, with healing and hair regrowth, during the winter, only to recur the following spring or summer.

Early lesions are often missed but consist of small papules at the favored feeding sites of the gnat. The predominant area of involvement is related to the particular *Culicoides* species involved. In Florida, three syndromes have been described. The classical (or dorsal) syndrome, orginally described, involves the face, ears, mane, withers, dorsal rump, and tail. A more ventral syndrome, described in Florida, involves the ears, intermandibular space, chest, ventrum, and groin. Many Florida horses have a generalized disease involving both the dorsal and ventral regions.

Facial lesions may vary from alopecia anteroventral to the eyes to excoriations and crusting. Lesions on the ears begin with hair loss on the rims only and can progress to total alopecia of the inside of the pinna, thickening of the pinna, and patchy alopecia and crusting of the external surface of the pinna. In early or mild cases, the mane may show only focal breakage and thinning. More commonly, the skin over the neck and withers becomes thickened, alopecic, crusted, and corrugated. In severe cases the mane and tail, or portions thereof, may be completely rubbed out each season. After several seasons, regrowth may be sparse to nonexistent. There may be crusting and alopecia in the intermandibular space and on the ventral neck. Horizontal "rub lines" with or without alopecia, excoriation, and crusting may be visible on the chest. A ventral midline dermatitis involving much of the ventrum with hair loss, crusting, and sometimes pigmentary changes is occasionally present and must be distinguished from other causes of ventral midline dermatitis. Tail and rump involvement ranges from mild hair breakage at the tail base to severe excoriations of the rump and tail, which can result in development of chronic tail pyoderma.

DIAGNOSIS

Seasonality, severity of the pruritus, location and character of the lesions, and sporadic occurrence in a herd strongly suggest a diagnosis of *Culicoides* hypersensitivity. The differential diagnosis of dorsal pruritus should include sarcoptic and psoroptic mange, pediculosis, other insect-related dermatoses, cutaneous onchocerciasis, dermatophytosis, and other atopic conditions. The differential diagnosis of ventral pruritus includes cutaneous onchocerciasis, horn fly dermatitis, nematode larva dermatitis *(Strongyloides* or *Pelodera)*, other insect bite hypersensitivities, dermatophytosis, and other atopic conditions. The differential diagnosis of tail pruritus usually involves diseases of the tail without concurrent disease of the mane. Regular deworming or treatment with ivermectin effectively rules out onchocerciasis and oxyuriasis and probably eliminates the manges as well.

Skin scrapings and fungal culture are indicated. Biopsy is useful for diagnosing an insect-related allergic dermatitis. It is best to biopsy an affected site that is not secondarily infected, since infection may mask the classical pattern of insect bite hypersensitivity. The usual finding is a superficial and deep perivascular dermatitis with variable mixtures of eosinophils, lymphocytes, and macrophages (histiocytes) considered compatible with insect hypersensitivity.

Intradermal skin testing with multiple antigens including those from insects, dusts, pollens, and feeds may aid in pinpointing the allergen. Although different *Culicoides* spp. cause this disease in different parts of the world, there appears to be cross-reactivity between the salivary antigens among the species. Hypersensitive horses react similarly to intradermal injection of extracts prepared from different species of *Culicoides* from different parts of the world. It is therefore unnecessary to test horses with extracts from several different species of *Culicoides*. Salivary antigens of *Culicoides* spp. are multiple and complex, with at least five allergenic fractions that induce dermal reactivity in affected horses. Normal horses commonly exhibit immediate intradermal skin test reactions, especially during the insect season, and some even have delayed reactions. Therefore, immediate and delayed intradermal skin test reactions should be interpreted in the context of the clinical history and signs and are useful supportive evidence for the clinical diagnosis. Unfortunately, a *Culicoides* spp. extract is not commercially available for diagnostic use. Some veterinary teaching institutions have allergen for research use and offer intradermal skin testing for diagnosis.

THERAPY

Successful management of affected horses is time-consuming and expensive, and in the tropics and subtropics, the management season may last for more than 9 months of the year. Stabling from before dusk until 1 to 2 hours after dawn with daily applications of insecticides and repellents is the most successful treatment. Sometimes three walls and a ceiling provide adequate shelter from the gnats, yet in other locations more thorough protection may be necessary. Fine mesh (32×32) screens may be necessary, as conventional mosquito screens are inadequate. Fans, ceiling or wall mounted, create a breeze that prevents the tiny gnats from flying. Insecticides applied to the screens and time-operated spray mist insecticide systems may be helpful. It is important that this management routine be carried out faithfully, since just one night's exposure can result in up to 3 weeks of itching. Insecticides and repellents must be applied daily or more frequently. The best products are synergized pyrethrins or synthetic pyrethroids. They are available in sprays, gels, wipe-ons, and pour-on formulations. Applications should be primarily directed to the favored feeding sites of the gnat (head and ears, mane and tail, dorsal and ventral midlines, chest and inguinal regions). Attaching cattle ear tags containing fenvalerate to halters or braiding them into the mane and tail should be done with care, if at all, to avoid ocular exposure and subsequent damage by the insecticide. Insect control measures are best started in advance of the season.

Alternatively, moving affected animals to drier locations, sometimes just a few kilometers from the *Culicoides* source, often results in dramatic improvement. Alteration of larval habitat by diking, draining, or flooding reduces populations. Elimination of such wetlands may not be feasible or may not be allowed for environmental reasons.

Other treatments for this dermatitis are merely palliative and often ineffective if exposure to the insects is not reduced. Although quite effective initially and useful for early treatment, glucocorticoids become less effective with long-term use. Evidence that they may contribute to the development of laminitis makes long-term use undesirable. However, where stabling is not feasible, long-term corticosteroid administration becomes necessary for humane reasons. This should always be accompanied by vigorous insect control. In severe cases, oral prednisone at 0.5 mg per kg twice daily may be inadequate for initial control and more potent forms such as dexamethasone, 0.05 to 0.1 mg per kg given intramuscularly or orally once daily, may be necessary. Once the pruritus is controlled, the horse should be maintained on oral prednisone in order to diminish the side effects and allow for immediate withdrawal of medication should laminitis or other worrisome side effects become apparent. Ideally, the horse should be maintained at the lowest dose that controls the pruritus on an alternating or every third day basis. In some cases, 400 to 500 mg of prednisone on an alternate-day basis may be the best that can be achieved during the worst of the insect season. Corticosteroid treatment should be terminated gradually during cool weather over 2 to 3 weeks to allow adrenal function to return to normal.

Antihistamines are sometimes employed in the therapy of insect bite hypersensitivity but usually are not very effective. Hydroxyzine hydrochloride at 200 to 400 mg twice daily has been reported to be effective in some cases. Antihistamines may have a steroid-sparing effect and therefore may be helpful adjunctive therapy in cases that have responded incompletely to steroids.

Topical therapies other than daily to twice daily applications of insecticides and repellents include the use of antibacterial and antiseborrheic shampoos or sprays. Tar and sulfur shampoos or sprays formulated for animals are recommended for their antipruritic effects as well as mild antibacterial actions. Avon Skin so Soft, diluted 1:1 to 1:3 in water, is an effective repellent for some allergic horses. Lotions or oily preparations provide a mechanical barrier to gnats and may be beneficial, but are messy. A light-weight stable sheet altered to cover affected areas is most effective if use is begun before the onset of pruritus.

Specific immunotherapy (hyposensitization) provides no more benefit than placebo in Florida. There are several possible reasons for the lack of success, including inappropriate dosage or injection intervals, a dilution effect resulting from use of a whole body *Culicoides* spp. extract containing many unimportant antigenic moieties, and involvement of delayed (non-IgE-mediated) hypersensitivity reactions that do not respond to specific immunotherapy.

Supplemental Readings

Barbet, J. L., Bevier, D., and Greiner, E. C.: Specific immunotherapy in the treatment of *Culicoides* hypersensitive horses: A double blind study. Equine Vet. J., 22:232–235, 1990.
Broström, H., Larsson, Å., and Troedsson, M.: Allergic dermatitis (sweet itch) of Icelandic horses in Sweden: An epidemiologic study. Equine Vet J., 19:229–236, 1987.
Fadok, V. A., and Greiner, E. C.: Equine insect hypersensitivity: Skin test and biopsy results correlated with clinical data. Equine Vet. J., 22:236–240, 1990.
Foil, L. D., Foil, C. S., Corstvet, R. E., and Klimzcak C.: Studies on *Culicoides* hypersensitivity in Louisiana horses. In: Proceedings of the Annual Meeting of the American Academy of Veterinary Dermatology and the American College of Veterinary Dermatology, 1990, pp. 8–11.
Scott, D. W.: Immunologic Diseases. In: Large Animal Dermatology. Philadelphia, W. B. Saunders, 1988, pp. 284–333.

Ivermectin in Dermatologic Disorders

Thomas R. Klei, BATON ROUGE, LOUISIANA

Ivermectin, a mixture of two avermectin compounds, is an antiparasitic drug with a broad range of activity at relatively low dosages. Single treatments with this drug at the recommended dosage of 0.2 mg per kg are effective against most nematode and arthropod parasites of significance to equine dermatologic disorders.

Two formulations of the drug are currently available for use in horses. These are a 1.87 per cent wt./wt. paste for oral use, and a 1 per cent aqueous micellar formation that is easily dilutable and useful for nasogastric intubation or as an oral drench. Some differences have been described in the pharmacokinetics of the drug in these two formulations in the horse. Administration of the oral liquid by nasogastric tube results in peak drug levels in plasma at 4 to 5 hours, compared with 15 hours following administration of the paste formulations. The bioavailability of the drug following oral liquid administration is also 20 per cent higher than that following paste administration at the same dosage. Nonetheless, no difference in efficacy against any parasite has been noted where these two formulations have been compared. Many of the early studies of ivermectin efficacy against skin parasites used the injectable formulation of the drug, which is no longer available. The efficacy of ivermectin on specific parasite-associated dermatologic conditions is described below.

NEMATODES

ONCHOCERCIASIS

Onchocerca cervicalis, a filarial nematode, is common in horses throughout the world. The adult parasites live in the ligamentum nuchae and produce microfilariae that are found in the skin. Only a small portion of infected horses have skin lesions associated with the parasite. These lesions are considered to be the result of hypersensitivity responses to microfilariae. Although lesions are found on the face, withers, chest, and legs, they are most common on the ventral midline where microfilariae concentrations are greatest. Lesions may be characterized by depigmentation, alopecia, crusting, shallow ulceration, and scaling. Pruritus may occur, increasing the severity of the condition due to self-induced trauma. Horn flies, when present, are attracted to alopecic areas and in large numbers may exacerbate existing lesions. This phenomenon may obscure the effective treatment of onchoceriasis and lead to the conclusion that the drug is ineffective or that the original lesions were not *Onchocerca*-associated.

Ivermectin at the recommended dose of 0.2 mg per kg is 100 per cent effective in killing microfilariae in the skin within 24 hours. Lesions resolve with treatment within a month. The uniform success of ivermectin treatment against *Onchocerca* microfilariae has led to the practice of using this treatment to differentiate onchoceriasis from *Culicoides* hypersensitivity and thus aid in diagnosis of these conditions. Although ivermectin does not kill adult parasites, microfilariae do not quickly reappear in the skin and recurrence of lesions may be delayed for as long as 8 months. This result may be due to the effect of ivermectin on the reproductive organs of the female parasites.

Adverse reactions following ivermectin treatment in the form of ventral edema have been associated with the killing of large numbers of *Onchocerca* microfilariae. These reactions resolve without treatment within 2 to 3 days. At the time of introduction of ivermectin, this response was estimated to occur in 10 to 25 per cent of treated horses. Currently, this reaction is a rare occurrence, which is likely due to the widespread use of ivermectin and the resulting decrease in the number of horses with large quantities of skin microfilariae.

HABRONEMIASIS

The spirurid stomach worms of horses, *Habronema muscae*, *H. majus*, and *Draschia megastoma*, are common parasites of horses throughout the world. The adult parasites live in the stomach and produce larva-containing eggs that pass in the horse feces. These eggs are ingested by larvae of house flies and stable flies. The infective third stage larvae of the nematode are found in the adult flies. Normally, when these are ingested, the nematode life cycle is completed within the stomach. However, if third-stage larvae are deposited during fly feeding on mucus membranes or skin lesions, the larvae migrate into these aberrant sites and induce lesions that might be quite severe. These lesions can be characterized as ulcerative granulomas and most commonly occur in the lower limbs and prepuce. This seasonal occurrence had led to the term "summer sores." Single treatments with ivermectin at the recommended dose appear to be sufficient to kill larvae and induce lesion resolution. However, some reports indicate that second treatments may be necessary. The prevalence of summer sores, like cases of onchoceriasis, seems to be less since the introduction of ivermectin.

PINWORMS

The equine pinworm *Oxyuris equi* lives within the distal large intestine, but some stages of its life cycle produce a pruritus in the perianal region. The associated tail rubbing results in hair loss from the tail head region. It is assumed that a hypersensitivity reaction to the deposition of the eggs or ruptured female worms is responsible for this reaction. Removal of the parasites by any number of anthelmintics, including ivermectin, is suitable treatment. It should be noted that the killing and resulting expulsion of nematodes following ivermectin treatment is somewhat slower than that of other anthelmintics and thus pruritus may persist for a period of 2 weeks after treatment.

ACARINES

Mite infestations of horses are generally rare, but three mange mite genera may occur. These are *Sarcoptes scabiei* var. *equi*, *Psoroptes ovis*, *Psoroptes equi*, *Psoroptes cuniculi*, and *Choreoptes equi*. Sarcoptes organisms burrow into the skin and live in tunnels in the epidermis. *Psoroptes* spp. live on the surface of the skin but have piercing mouth parts that allow them to feed on tissue fluids. *Choreoptes* spp. also live on the surface but feed on skin debris. Lesions associated with these mites are described on page 692. Little information is available on the efficacy of ivermectin against infestations of these species of mites in horses. However, the few available published reports and efficacy of the drug against these species in other animal hosts both suggest that treatment with ivermectin at the normally recommended dosage is effective in the horse as well.

OTHER AGENTS

A number of other nematodes or arthropods are less frequently found as causitive agents of equine dermatitis. The efficacy of ivermectin against these agents is unreported in the horse. Free-living nematodes such as *Rhabditis* spp. may become facultative parasites as larvae in the skin. Although ivermectin is effective against most nematode species and stages, it is ineffective against some, notably adult filariae and *Micronema deletrix* in the horse. Thus, efficacy against these facultative nematodes is unknown and cannot be assumed. The biting louse *Haematopinus equi* is an uncommon parasite of horses. In swine, *H. suis* infestations are effectively treated with ivermectin. However, it should be noted that the registered ivermectin product for swine is an injectable formulation with a dose level above that of the equine products (300 μg per kg). Thus, efficacy of the drug against these lice in horses is unknown. Cattle grubs, *Hypoderma lineatum* and *H. bovis*, occasionally infect horses. It is likely that ivermectin is effective against these larvae. Recommendations for seasonal treatment of these infections as described for cattle should be followed.

Supplemental Readings

Campbell, W. C.: Ivermectin and Abamectin. New York, Springer-Verlag, 1989.
Foil, L., and Foil C.: Parasitic skin diseases. Vet. Clin. North Am. (Equine Pract. Parasitol.), 2:403–438, 1986.
Scott, D. W.: Parasitic Deseases. *In:* Large Animal Dermatology. Philadelphia, W. B. Saunders, 1988, pp. 207–283.

Dermatophytosis

Linda A. Frank, GAINESVILLE, FLORIDA

Equine dermatophytosis (ringworm, dermatomycosis, girth itch) is a fungal infection of the superficial keratinized layer of the epidermis, hair, and hooves. The fungi commonly involved in equine dermatophytosis are *Trichophyton equinum, T. mentagrophytes, T. verrucosum, Microsporum gypseum,* and *M. canis. T. equinum* and *T. mentagrophytes* account for the majority of infections seen in horses. Transmission of *T. mentagrophytes* involves rodents and cats. *T. verrucosum* infection in horses usually involves contact with infected cattle, and *M. canis* infection is usually associated with an infected or carrier cat in the barn. Of the zoophilic dermatophytes, *M. canis* is the most highly contagious. *M. gypseum* is a geophilic fungus that, under appropriate conditions, can cause cutaneous lesions.

Transmission of the zoophilic dermatophytes is by direct contact between animals or by contact with infected hair and crust on fomites or in the environment. Fungal spores can be infectious for greater than 12 months. In North America a large per centage of cases occur in fall and winter, when animals are in close contact in moist, dark environments. Wet, warm weather has also been associated with outbreaks of equine dermatophytosis. Abrasion of the skin surface is necessary for the establishment of a dermatophyte infection. This is why the more common locations for equine dermatophytosis are in the girth and saddle friction areas. The incubation period varies from 4 to 30 days depending on temperature, humidity, and geographic location. Young horses under 4 years of age are especially susceptible, apparently because of their lack of acquired immunity. Adult horses are less likely to become infected and, if infected, recover faster than young horses.

The diagnosis of dermatophytosis is often based on the history and clinical appearance of the lesions. A dermatophyte species cannot be identified from the clinical presentation. Growth on a commercial dermatophyte culture medium will confirm the diagnosis, and species identification by microscopic examination of the hyphae and conidia will help trace the source of infection. Vitamin enrichment medium is needed to culture *T. equinum* and *T. verrucosum. T. equinum* requires nicotinic acid and *T. verrucosum* requires thiamine and inositol for growth. Commercial dermatophyte culture media can support growth of these organisms when two drops of injectable B-complex are added to the medium.

THERAPY

Equine dermatophytosis is a self-limiting infection with lesions typically resolving in 1 to 3 months. The goal of treatment is to decrease the course and severity of the disease, prevent spread of the infection to other animals, and decrease environmental contamination. Based on the organism isolated, the source of the infection should be identified and eliminated, when possible, to prevent further outbreaks.

Treatment is directed at two areas: fungicidal therapy for the horse and decontamination of the environment. The first step is to isolate infected horses from noninfected ones until the lesions have resolved. Infected areas should be clipped with wide margins and the hair and crust disposed of to prevent environmental contamination with infectious material. The clippers must be disinfected prior to subsequent use. It is recommended that the horse not be worked under saddle as this will prolong the recovery period. All horses in contact with infected animals also need to be treated. An important part of the treatment program should include good nutrition, exposure to adequate sunlight, and endoparasite control. Vitamin and mineral supplementation, however, do not have any therapeutic effects.

Because of the self-limiting nature of the infection, the commonly recommended treatments for the horse involve use of topical fungicides. These medications include 3 per cent captan° (1 ounce of 50 per cent wettable powder in 1 gallon of water), 3 to 5 per cent lime sulfur, povidone–iodine preparations, 0.5 to 2 per cent chlorhexidine, and 0.5 per cent sodium hypochlorite (bleach). Captan is the most economical and least irritating of the topical solutions but should be applied with gloves since it can cause contact sensitization in people. The iodophors can discolor hair and may be irritating to the skin. Lime sulfur is a safe nonirritating product but can also stain the coat and has an objectionable odor.

°Orthocide, Ortho Products, Division of Chevron Chemical Co., San Francisco, CA

Topical fungicides should be applied daily with a sponge or brush to the *entire* body for 1 week, then twice weekly until clinical resolution of lesions occurs. Infected fungal elements may be recovered from resolving lesions if therapy is discontinued early. It is important to keep in mind that even with proper treatment, fungal infections may take 6 to 8 weeks to clear completely. Topical treatment may be preceded by an antifungal shampoo such as povidone–iodine or chlorhexidine to facilitate crust removal and allow better penetration of the topical agent.

Some fungicidal agents with apparent excellent efficacy against dermatophytes are not currently available in the United States. Enilconazole, a beta-substituted imidazole, is currently used in Europe as a topical and environmental fungicide for both large and small animals. It is applied as a topical spray or solution on the horse and as a spray or smoke generator in the environment. Natamycin, a nonirritating and odorless antifungal agent, is also useful for treating equine dermatophytosis as well as disinfecting the animal's environment. This broad-spectrum fungicidal agent is inactivated by sunlight; the animal must be treated in the barn or at night.

Spot treatment of local lesions can be attempted on an individual animal but is not recommended for dermatophyte outbreaks. Thiabendazole, when used as a 4 per cent solution in saline, is beneficial with improved efficacy when applied in 90 per cent dimethyl sulfoxide (DMSO). Most small animal antifungal preparations, such as miconazole,* and thiabendazole,† can be used for localized lesions in horses. However, due to the rapid spread of ringworm infections among horses, whole body treatment with a topical solution is more efficacious and economical.

Systemic therapy with griseofulvin has been used in the treatment of equine dermatophytosis; however, the therapeutic dose in the horse is not known. Griseofulvin orally dosed at 10 mg per kg once daily for 30 to 60 days has been used successfully to treat some horses. Massive weekly doses are not justified, because the drug has a short half-life of detection within the superficial epidermis. Contrary to what was once thought, griseofulvin does not become incorporated into the hair; therefore, infected hairs will still be present during treatment, necessitating concurrent topical therapy to decrease environmental contamination and spread. The actual efficacy of oral griseofulvin in the horse is unknown because of the high rate of self-cure seen over a 1-to 2-month course of treatment. This product is expensive and could be prohibitively costly if multiple horses are to be treated. Griseofulvin is teratogenic and should not be used in pregnant mares.

ENVIRONMENTAL DECONTAMINATION

Environmental decontamination is as important as equine therapeutics in the control of dermatophytosis because of the viability of fungal spores on fomites and in the environment. All brushes and tack must be cleaned and disinfected. Grooming equipment and tack from infected horses should not be used on noninfected ones. Better still, each horse should have its own equipment. It is best not to cover the lesions with blankets or tack. If blankets are used on infected animals, they should be washed and disinfected weekly. The stalls must be thoroughly cleaned and disinfected and the bedding destroyed. It is important to eliminate the predisposing factors such as overcrowding and damp, dirty environments.

Disinfection of the stalls, feeding utensils, tack, blankets, and grooming equipment can be accomplished with povidone–iodine, 6 per cent sodium hypochlorite, chlorhexidine solution, 3 per cent cresol, 5 per cent lime sulfur, benzalkonium chloride, 3 per cent captan, 1 per cent lime plus 1.5 per cent copper sulfate, and formaldehyde. Formaldehyde gas can be used to fumigate riding tack.

People can spread a dermatophyte infection by carrying infected hairs on their hands and clothing. For this reason, infected horses should be handled last and handlers should wash thoroughly between animals with a povidone–iodine or chlorhexidine scrub. Dermatophytosis is also highly contagious to people. Therefore, great care should be taken by all individuals who come in contact with infected animals.

PREVENTION

Prevention of outbreaks of dermatophytosis in the barn involves the routine application of many of the control methods discussed above. Overcrowding needs to be avoided and a good plane of nutrition and health maintained. Tack and grooming equipment should not be interchanged and require routine disinfection. Infected horses must be isolated and treated at the onset of clinical signs.

---

*Conofite, Pitman-Moore, Mundelein, IL
†Tresaderm, MSD Ag Vet, Division of Merck & Co., Rahway, NJ

Supplemental Readings

Desplenter, L.: Dermatophytosis in animals: Topical treatment and environmental control with enilconazole. First World Congress of Veterinary Dermatology, 1989.

McMullan, W. C.: The skin. In: Mansmann, R.A., and McAllister, E.S. (eds.): Equine Medicine and Surgery, 3rd ed. Santa Barbara, American Veterinary Publishing, 1982, pp. 789-843.

Mullowney, P. C., and Fadok, V. A.: Dermatologic diseases of horses: Part III. Fungal skin diseases. Compend. Cont. Educ. Pract. Vet., 6:S324, 1984.

Oldenkamp, E. P.: Treatment of ringworm in horses with natamycin. Equine Vet. J., 11:36, 1979.

Scott, D. W.: Fungal diseases. In: Large Animal Dermatology. Philadelphia, W. B. Saunders, 1988.

Stannard, A. A.: Equine dermatology. Proceedings of the 22nd Annual Convention of the American Association of Equine Practitioners, 1976, pp. 273-292.

Staphylococcal Skin Disease

Danny W. Scott, ITHACA, NEW YORK

Staphylococcus species are versatile pathogens of animals and humans. The organisms are gram-positive cocci, have a worldwide distribution, are prevalent in nature, and may gain entry into the animal host through any natural orifice and contaminated wounds. Localized disruption of normal host defenses facilitates development of infection. Maceration of skin by water, sweat, friction from skin folds, topical treatments, abrasions, cuts, punctures, insect bites, scratching, rubbing, tack, harness, or the introduction of a foreign body can all impair local defenses.

The coagulase-positive *Staphylococcus* most commonly isolated from equine infections is *Staphylococcus aureus*, with *S. intermedius* and *S. hyicus* less commonly recovered. There are apparently no significant differences in antimicrobial susceptibility patterns between these three staphylococcal species isolated from horses. In general, many strains are resistant to penicillin, ampicillin, and tetracycline.

FOLLICULITIS AND FURUNCULOSIS

Staphylococcal folliculitis and furunculosis are common in the horse. These conditions are also called acne, heat rash, summer rash, summer scab, sweating eczema of the saddle region, saddle scab, saddle boils, heat nodules, and heat pox. No age, breed, or sex predilections are evident. About 90 per cent of cases begin in spring and early summer. This period coincides with shedding of hair, heavy riding and work schedules, higher environmental temperature and humidity, and increased insect population densities. Poorly groomed horses may be at risk.

Skin lesions initially affect the saddle and tack areas. Frequently one first notices erect hairs over 2- to 3-mm papules that are more easily felt than seen. Some lesions enlarge to 6 to 10 mm in diameter and develop a central ulcer that discharges a purulent or serosanguinous material, then becomes encrusted. The chronic or healing phase is characterized by progressive flattening of the lesions and static or gradually expanding circular areas of alopecia and scaling. Some lesions progress to furunculosis, with varying combinations of nodules, draining tracts, ulcers, and crusts. Scarring, leukoderma, and leukotrichia may follow. The lesions are painful in up to 70 per cent of cases, rendering the horse unfit for riding or work, but rarely are pruritic. Whether or not immunity develops is unclear, but cases of chronically recurring lesions are well known. Less frequently, staphylococcal folliculitis and furunculosis are localized to the caudal aspect of the pasterns (pastern folliculitis) or tail (tail pyoderma). Affected horses are usually otherwise healthy.

The diagnosis of staphylococcal folliculitis and furunculosis is confirmed by microscopic examination of direct smears, skin biopsy specimens, and bacterial cultures. The differential diagnosis includes dermatophytosis, dermatophilosis, demodicosis, and pemphigus foliaceus.

Therapy varies with the severity and stage of the disease, the natural course of the infection, and economic factors. Mild cases may resolve spontaneously. More severe cases may require topical cleansing, drying, and antibacterial therapy. Iodophors* or chlorhexidine† is applied daily for 5 to 7 days, then twice weekly until the lesions are healed. Severe or progressive cases necessitate treatment with systemic antibiotics in addition to topical therapy. The systemic antibiotics should be chosen on the basis of culture

---

*Betadine shampoo or solution, Purdue Frederick Co., Norwalk, CT

†Nolvasan shampoo or solution, Fort Dodge Labs., Fort Dodge, IA

and sensitivity test results. In most instances, trimethoprim–sulfadiazine (15 mg per kg every 12 hours) or erythromycin (25 mg per kg every 6 hours) are effective oral antibiotics. Treatment is continued for 7 days beyond clinical cure. Severe cases of tail furunculosis may not respond to therapy. In horses with recurrent infections, antimicrobial shampoos such as iodophors or chlorhexidine, that are administered before and after work may be an effective preventive measure.

PSEUDOMYCETOMA

Staphylococcal pseudomycetoma (botryomycosis) is a rare granulomatous dermatitis of horses. No age, breed, or sex predilections are evident. About 75 per cent of cases follow a known local traumatic injury to the skin, such as a laceration, puncture, or surgery.

The majority of lesions occur on the leg, lip, or chin. Most horses have a solitary lesion or multiple lesions in a localized area. Rarely, multiple lesions appear to spread along lymphatics. The lesions are papular, nodular, or tumorous in size, firm, and usually ulcerated and replete with draining tracts. Small, whitish to yellowish sand-like granules or grains may be seen within the purulent discharge. Pain and pruritus are usually absent. Affected horses are usually otherwise healthy.

The diagnosis of staphylococcal pseudomycetoma is confimred by skin biopsy and bacterial culture. The differential diagnosis includes other bacterial and fungal granulomas, habronemiasis, sarcoid, squamous cell carcinoma, and exuberant granulation. The preferred therapy is complete surgical excision. Surgical debulking in conjunction with topical and systemic antibiotic therapy may also be curative. Antibiotics alone are rarely beneficial, presumably because the organism is protected within the granulomatous and fibrosing tissue reaction and within the tissue granules. Relapses or recurrences have not been reported.

CELLULITIS

Staphylococcal cellulitis is a rare equine dermatosis. No age or sex predilections are evident, but all reported cases have occurred in Thoroughbred racehorses in active training. Obvious trauma or infections have not been reported to precede the development of the dermatosis.

In most instances there is an acute onset of severe swelling and pain of one limb, usually a hind limb. The horse is extremely lame on the affected leg. All horses are febrile, and many develop tachycardia. Complications of staphylococcal cellulitis include cutaneous necrosis and slough, laminitis of the affected or contralateral limb, osteomyelitis and sequestrum formation, or bacteremia.

Therapy includes the immediate initiation of systemic antibiotics, phenylbutazone, hydrotherapy, and support bandages on the affected and contralateral limbs. Gentamicin sulfate (2 mg per kg every 8 hours given intravenously [IV] or intramuscularly [IM]) is administered in conjunction with potassium penicillin G (40,000 IU per kg IV every 6 hours) or procaine penicillin G (25,000 IU per kg IM every 12 hours) until healing has occurred. Relapses or recurrences have not been reported.

Supplemental Readings

Baggot, J. D., and Prescott, J. F.: Antimicrobial selection and dosage in the treatment of equine bacterial infections. Equine Vet. J., 19:92, 1987.
Biberstein, E. L., Jang, S. S., and Hirsh, D. C.: Species distribution of coagulase-positive staphylococci in animals. J. Clin. Microbiol., 19:610, 1984.
Devriese, L. A., Nzuambe, D., and Godard, C.: Identification and characteristics of staphylococci isolated from lesions and normal skin of horses. Vet. Microbiol., 10:269, 1984/85.
Devriese, L. A., Vlaminck, K., Nuytten, J., and De-Keersmaecker, P.: *Staphylococcus hyicus* in skin lesions of horses. Equine Vet. J., 15:263, 1983.
Markel, M. D., Wheat, J. D., and Jang, S. S.: Cellulitis associated with coagulase-positive staphylococci in race horses: Nine cases (1975–1984). J. Am. Vet. Med. Assoc., 189:1600, 1986.
Scott, D. W., and Manning, T. O.: Equine folliculitis and furunculosis. Equine Pract., 2:11, 1980.
Scott, D. W.: Bacterial pseudomyocisis (botryomycosis) in the horse. Equine Pract., 10:15, 1988.
Scott, D. W.: Large Animal Dermatology. Philadelphia, W. B. Saunders, 1988.

Cutaneous Mastocytosis

Karen A. Nyrop, PHOENIX, ARIZONA

Equine cutaneous mast cell lesions are relatively uncommon tumors. The lesion is characterized as hyperplastic, not neoplastic; mitotic figures are rarely seen, and the tumor has not been reported to metastasize.

CLINICAL SIGNS

Two forms of the disease have been described. In the first form, the typical lesion is a single cutaneous or subcutaneous nodule 2 to 20 cm in diameter located on the head, neck, or extremities. There is one report of a mastocytoma on the globe of a horse. Skin over the nodule may be normal, hairless, or in rare cases ulcerated. The larger masses can have central necrotic areas that are partially calcified. Male horses are more commonly affected; the mean age of affected horses is 7 years. Most nodules are freely movable under the skin, but occasionally the tumor can involve underlying musculature. Regardless, the mass is usually well encapsulated and noninvasive in nature. These lesions are neither painful nor hot to touch. They do not cause lameness if located on an extremity. The cause of cutaneous mastocytosis in the horse is unknown. *Onchocerca* infestation, chronic abscessation, and local antigen–antibody reactions have been suggested as possible etiologies but have not been proved.

The second form of the disease manifests with multiple cutaneous masses present at birth or shortly thereafter. Urticaria pigmentosa in humans closely resembles this generalized form in the horse. Nodules are found all over the body and range in size from several millimeters to 3 cm in diameter. The lesions are progressive and are first noticed as small firm nodules. As they become larger, the nodules develop a soft center that frequently ulcerates. The lesions then regress and heal, with new lesions forming in previously unaffected skin. This sequence repeats in approximately 30-day cycles.

DIAGNOSIS

Equine cutaneous mastocytoma is most easily diagnosed by histological examination of fine needle aspirates. Giemsa stain of the aspirate will reveal numerous mast cells filled with metachromatic granules and occasional eosinophils. These tumors are often diagnosed and treated at the same time by performing a total excision biopsy. Histological examination reveals a mass with loosely arranged collagen fiber bundles surrounded by clusters of mast cells and eosinophils, some of which have necrotic foci. The granular areas seen grossly and on cut section are necrotic debris surrounded by mineralization and an outer layer of macrophages. Generalized mastocytosis in foals has a similar histological pattern in the developing and ulcerated nodules. As the nodule regresses, it has fewer mast cells and more fibroblasts and collagen formation. Histological examination of bone marrow reveals focal areas of mast cells. Imprints of spleen and liver biopsies show increased numbers of mast cells. Peripheral blood studies of affected foals are normal.

Entities in the differential diagnosis include nodular necrobiosis, melanoma, calcinosis circumscripta, abscess, lymphadenopathy, or a cutaneous form of habronemiasis. Calcinosis circumscripta, like cutaneous mastocytosis, is often partially mineralized, which is readily noticed radiographically. Calcinosis circumscripta is a well-encapsulated lesion that usually occurs on the lateral aspect of the stifle, hock, or carpus, which is attached to a joint capsule or tendon sheath. These various entities present as firm, well-encapsulated subcutaneous nodules that can be ruled out by needle aspiration or total excision biopsy.

THERAPY AND PROGNOSIS

Total excision biopsy is the treatment of choice for equine cutaneous mastocytomas. This lesion is a hyperplastic disease and has never been reported to metastasize. Even when incomplete excision has been performed, the lesions do not recur. If total excision biopsy is not preferred, intralesional corticosteroids or radiotherapy may be effective. Spontaneous regression was observed in one foal with generalized cutaneous mastocytosis. The single cutaneous or subcutaneous nodules on adult horses are not known to regress spontaneously.

Supplemental Readings

Martin, C. L., and Leipold, H. W.: Mastocytoma of the globe in a horse. J. Am. Anim. Hosp. Assoc., 8:32–34, 1972.

McMullen, W. C.: Cutaneous mastocytoma. *In* Mansmann, R. A., and McAllister, E. S. (eds.): Equine Medicine and Surgery, 3rd ed., vol. 2. Santa Barbara, Calif., American Veterinary Publishing, 1982, p. 809.

Nyrop, K. A., DeBowes, R. M., Coffman, J. R., Johnson, J. W., and Leipold, H. W.: Equine cutaneous mastocytoma. Compend. Cont. Educ. Pract. Vet., 8:757–761, 1986.

Prasse, K. W., Lundvall, R. L., and Cheville, N. F.: Generalized mastocytosis in a foal, resembling urticaria pigmentosa of man. J. Am. Vet. Med. Assoc., 166:68–70, 1975.

Stannard, A. A.: Equine dermatology. *In:* Proceedings of the 22nd Annual Convention of the American Association of Equine Practitioners, 1976, pp. 273–292.

Stannard, A. A., and Pulley, L. T.: Mastocytoma of the horse. *In* Moulton J. E. (ed.): Tumors in Domestic Animals, 2nd ed. Los Angeles, University of California Press, 1978, page 32.

Anhidrosis

John Freestone, BATON ROUGE, LOUISIANA

Anhidrosis is defined as the inability to sweat in response to appropriate stimuli. A worldwide problem, anhidrosis occurs in areas where hot and humid conditions occur during the spring, summer, and fall. Anhidrosis initially was thought to affect horses moved from a cooler to a warmer environment, but it is now realized that indigenous horses also suffer from this condition. Apparently, exposure to high ambient temperatures and humidity throughout the day and night leads to anhidrosis. In North America, the disease is most common in the hot and humid Gulf Coast states, where anhidrosis is noted in horses of all ages, breeds, and sexes. Horses that are undergoing physical training are more frequently affected, and up to 25 per cent of Thoroughbred racehorses in training may be anhidrotic during the summer months. Pregnant and nonpregnant mares can suffer from anhidrosis, but nonpregnant mares appear to be more commonly affected. Stress may also predispose to the onset of the condition.

The etiology of anhidrosis remains undetermined. There are two main theories for its development: (1) ultrastructural alterations in the apocrine sweat glands, and (2) decreased numbers or downregulation of the sweat gland β_2-adrenoreceptors. Sweat gland ultrastructural alterations noted in anhidrotic horses include a reduced number of cytoplasmic vesicles, compacted intercellular spaces, and contracted ductal lumina. The sweat gland duct may be completely occluded by cellular debris. These findings suggest abnormal sweat production. Horses with anhidrosis have increased circulating plasma epinephrine concentrations, and it has been proposed that the β_2-adrenoreceptors may be downregulated as a result of constant stimulation.

Anhidrosis has been associated with hypothyroidism, but there are no differences in baseline T_3 and T_4 concentrations between normal and anhidrotic horses. Anhidrotic horses reportedly have significantly decreased urinary fractional excretion of chloride, while fractional excretion of sodium and calcium also tends to be lower.

PRESENTATION

Horses with anhidrosis may be referred because of failure to sweat, exercise intolerance, respiratory disease, or dermatologic abnormalities. Many owners fail to notice that a horse is not sweating but report inadequate performance, hard breathing after exercise (suggesting respiratory disease), and deterioration of the hair coat. Owners must be questioned carefully to ascertain if the horse's primary problem is anhidrosis or some other clinical disorder.

CLINICAL SIGNS

The clinical signs of anhidrosis result from inability to lose body heat by evaporation. Clinical findings include failure to sweat, tachypnea at rest, alopecia, elevated rectal temperature, and exercise intolerance. Horses may prefer to be near water or in the shade during the hot summer months. Anhidrotic horses may stand submerged in water troughs or attempt to splash water onto their bodies to cool themselves.

Horses can suffer from different degrees of anhidrosis ranging from partial sweat production to complete absence of sweating. Affected horses may sweat in patches under the mane, underneath the saddle, and between the axilla and hindlegs. These areas have large numbers of sweat glands and are the last areas to be affected prior to the onset of complete anhidrosis.

Performance horses presented for respiratory tract disease and exercise intolerance in the Gulf States should have anhidrosis ruled out as a potential cause of their clinical signs. Because anhidrotic horses rely on the respiratory tract for heat dissipation, they breathe very heavily, with marked flaring of the nostrils, for more than 60 minutes after exercise in an attempt to reduce body temperature.

Horses with long-standing anhidrosis develop dermatologic problems that may include a dry, sparse hair coat with excessive scaling, and alopecia of the face, neck, and shoulders.

DIAGNOSIS

The diagnosis of anhidrosis is based primarily on history and physical examination. Additional confirmation can be gained by intradermal skin testing using either epinephrine or terbutaline sulfate injected at increasing concentrations. The terbutaline sulfate challenge appears to be the test of choice as it directly stimulates the sweat gland β_2-adrenoreceptors. Terbutaline sulfate is injected intradermally at several sites at dilutions ranging from 1:1000 to 1:100,000,000. Epinephrine can be administered in doses of 0.5 ml intradermally at concentrations of 1:1000, 1:10,000, 1:100,000, and 1:1,000,000. Normal horses sweat at all epinephrine and terbutaline sulfate concentrations within 30 minutes. Horses with partial anhidrosis will sweat at only the highest epinephrine or terbutaline sulfate concentrations, while the completely anhidrotic horse will be refractory to stimulation. Horses receiving intravenous doses of epinephrine (1 ml of 1:1000) have been noted to sweat profusely, yet fail to sweat while exercising during high ambient temperatures and humidity. It therefore seems possible to stimulate the sweat glands to function with high concentrations of epinephrine.

THERAPY

Although many regimens have been suggested for the treatment of anhidrosis, none has been consistently effective. The most successful treatment is either to provide a cool environment for the horse or to move the horse to a cooler region of the country. When moving the horse is not an option, a combination of dietary and environmental control, coupled with electrolyte supplementation, may be successful. Concentrate rations should be limited. Fans in the horse's stall can aid in the movement of air and dissipation of heat. Four ounces of Lite salt sprinkled on the evening ration may be advantageous. Commercial electrolyte preparations containing sodium and potassium chloride have also been used with success. There have also been anecdotal reports that horses with a history of anhidrosis that are treated with electrolyte solutions before the onset of hot weather and throughout conditioning and racing do not develop anhidrosis. Other suggested medications include vitamin E and selenium preparations, adrenocorticotropin administration, iodinated casein, or T_4 supplementation.

Horses in training should be fit before the summer begins. Starting conditioning when environmental temperatures are already high may predispose to anhidrosis. Performance horses with anhidrosis that are rested through the hot summer months may compete without problems in the cooler months of the year. They seem to resume sweating once the nightime temperatures cool. Alternatively, a horse can be moved from the southern states during the summer to a cooler climate where sweating will begin.

Supplemental Readings

Beadle, R. W., Norwood, G. L., and Brencick, V. A.: Summertime plasma catecholamine concentration in healthy and anhidrotic horses in Louisiana. Am J. Vet. Res., 43:1446, 1982.

Jenkinson, D. M., Montgomery, I., Elder, H. Y., Mason, D. K., Collins, E. A., and Snow, D. H.: Ultrastructural variations in the sweat glands of anhidrotic horses. Equine. Vet. J., 17:287, 1985.

Mayhew, I. G., and Ferguson, H. O.: Clinical, clinicopathological, and epidemiological features of anhidrosis in central Florida thoroughbred horses. J. Vet. Intern. Med., 1:136, 1987.

Warner, A. E.: Equine anhidrosis. Compend. Cont. Educ. Pract. Vet., 4:S434, 1982.

Warner, A., and Mayhew, I. G.: Equine anhidrosis: A review of pathophysiological mechanisms. Vet. Res. Commun., 6:249, 1983.

Junctional Mechanobullous Disease in Belgian Foals

Catherine W. Kohn, COLUMBUS, OHIO

Junctional mechanobullous disease has been reported in three Belgian foals (two fillies and one colt) less than 2 weeks of age. Two of these foals were out of the same dam. Junctional mechanobullous disease is characterized by blister formation following minor trauma. Clinically, affected foals display separation of hoof walls from underlying corium at the coronet bands, areas of alopecia and superficial erosion over hocks, carpi, stifles, fetlocks, and bullae on mucous membranes. The disease may be heritable and in all reported cases has been fatal.

CLINICAL SIGNS

Although clinically normal at birth, within 2 days affected foals develop separation of dermal and epidermal laminae at the coronet band. A foal is reported to have sloughed one hoof at 30 hours of age. Initial signs of hoof wall separation may be misinterpreted by owners as trauma. By 10 days of age, foals are depressed, have bullae or ulcers on mucous membranes, and have areas of alopecia and erosion over pressure points on the limbs, such as the point of the hock and anterior surfaces of the carpi and fetlocks. Excessive salivation may be present due to oral ulceration. Septicemia, likely resulting from infection through ulcerated areas or contamination of the exposed corium, may complicate the clinical picture. Hoof wall separation progresses to sloughing associated with progressively more severe discomfort, depression, and poor appetite.

HISTOPATHOLOGY

Biopsy specimens should be taken from the junction of healthy skin or mucous membrane and erosion or bulla. Histological evaluation demonstrates cleft formation at the dermoepidermal junction, beneath the basal layer of the epidermis. Periodic acid-Schiff staining of tissue sections allows identification of the basement membrane attached to the dermis, thus forming the floor of the bulla or cleft. There is minimal inflammation in the adjacent dermis.

DIAGNOSIS

Clinical signs, age of affected foals, and breed allow a presumptive diagnosis of junctional mechanobullous disease. The diagnosis should be confirmed by finding typical histopathological signs in appropriate biopsy tissues. Junctional mechanobullous disease must be differentiated from other conditions resulting in bullae and ulcer formation in skin and on mucous membranes. The differential diagnosis includes bullous pemphigoid, pemphigus foliaceous, systemic lupus erythematosus (SLE), toxic epidermal neurolysis, dermatitis herpetiformis, and familial dermatomyositis. Of these conditions, bullous pemphigoid, pemphigus foliaceous, and systemic lupus erythematosus have been reported to occur in horses.

Subepidermal bullae or clefts that occur in skin or at mucocutanous junctions in bullous pemphigoid are characterized by deposition of immunoglobulin and the third component of complement at the basement membrane, demonstrated by fluorescent antibody testing. Bullous pemphigoid has rarely been reported in adult horses. In pemphigus foliaceous, subcorneal epidermal cleft formation and acantholysis are present. Fluorescent antibody testing shows intercellular deposition of immunoglobulin and, rarely, complement. Pemphigus foliaceous has never been reported in a neonatal foal. SLE has been infrequently documented in horses. Skin lesions in SLE may be characterized by cleft formation between the dermis and epidermis. Antigen–antibody complexes or sometimes complement deposited at the basement membrane are demonstrable by fluorescent antibody testing. Immunofluorescent testing of skin from foals with junctional mechanobullous disease does not show deposition of antibody, antigen–antibody complexes, or complement.

CLINICAL MANAGEMENT

Attempts at treating foals with junctional mechanobullous disease have been unsuccessful. The profound nature of the apparent underlying skin defect in these foals warrants a grave prognosis and euthanasia should be recommended. The disease may be heritable; it has been seen only in Belgian foals. Repetition of the breeding that produced the affected foal is unwise. Since two of the reported foals were out of the same dam, an autosomal recessive mode of inheritance is possible. However, proof of heritability is not currently available. The prevalence of the clinical condition appears to be low, as few cases have been reported, despite the popularity of the Belgian breed.

Supplemental Readings

Frame, S. R., Harrington, D. D., Fessler, J., and Frame, P. F.: Hereditary junctional mechanobullous disease in a foal. J. Am. Vet. Med. Assoc., *193*:1420–1424, 1988.

Johnson, G. C., Kohn, C. W., Johnson, C. W., Garry, F., Scott, D., and Martin, S.: Ultrastructure of junctional epidermolysis bullosa in Belgian foals. J. Comp. Pathol., *99*:329–336, 1988.

Kohn, C. W., Johnson, G. C., Garry, F., Johnson, C. W., Martin, S., and Scott, D.: Mechanobullous disease in two Belgian foals. Equine Vet. J., *21*:297–301, 1989.

Scott, D. W.: Large Animal Dermatology. Philadelphia, W. B. Saunders, 1988, pp. 306–317.

Chronic Eosinophilic Dermatitides

Malcolm C. Roberts, RALEIGH, NORTH CAROLINA

Chronic eosinophilic dermatitis, a generalized skin disease that has been described in five Canadian horses, appears to be similar to the skin manifestations of chronic eosinophilic gastroenteritis, an enteric disorder that has been reported in Western Australia, recognized for many years in Sweden, and encountered in Queensland and in parts of the United States. The etiology of the syndrome is unknown, although the sporadic condition most probably represents an allergic or immune-mediated reaction. The multisystemic nature of the condition is reflected in the spectrum of presenting clinical signs and the extent of involvement of the various affected epithelia.

Skin lesions have been associated with debilitating enteric conditions including granulomatous enteritis and eosinophilic gastroenteritis, and, to a much lesser extent, alimentary lymphosarcoma and severe parasitism. Many debilitated horses present with a dry, scurfy skin, dry staring hair coat, thin hair, or hair loss; dermatophilosis and secondary bacterial or fungal infections are not uncommon. However, chronic eosinophilic dermatitis is a generalized, largely symmetrical skin condition. Whether primary or subsequent to intestinal disease, it has distinctive clinical and pathological features. Affected animals are young (1 to 4 years old), with an upper age of 13 years. There is no sex predilection. Standardbreds predominated in the Swedish series; Thoroughbreds and Standardbreds have been represented in other reports.

CLINICAL SIGNS

Affected animals generally exhibit chronic weight loss, a variable, often ravenous, appetite, occasionally changes in fecal consistency to diarrhea, intermittent febrile episodes, ventral edema, and, rarely, abdominal discomfort. The dermatitis is frequently of several months' duration, and may have started as a dry, scaly, or fissuring and oozing inflammation around the coronets, face, head, or oral cavity. Subsequently it spreads over the entire body. Other findings include a dry exfoliative dermatitis, easily epilated hair, and focal alopecia. The lesions can progress rapidly to become cracked, excoriated, alopecic, ulcerated, exudative, and secondarily infected. There can be a pungent odor. Oral and lingual ulcers can further hinder feed intake. External nares can become ulcerated, cracked, and painful. Although some horses do not have pruritus, intense pruritus is likely to occur, accompanied by self-inflicted trauma, exudation, and secondary infection, particularly on the lower limbs and head. Movement may be restricted by edema, secondary infection, and dermal fibrosis. An exudative and ulcerative coronitis may be the first evidence of the problem or the most notable skin sign.

The Australian and Swedish cases were characterized by protein-losing enteropathy and malabsorption. Enteric protein loss was not reported in the Canadian series. None of the five horses had diarrhea, and only two had eosinophilic infiltration in the gastrointestinal tract. In the predominantly enteric cases, changes occurred through the alimentary tract, associated glands, ducts, and lymph nodes. The large intestine was affected more extensively than the small intestine, hence the diarrhea, although the lesions appeared segmented and multifocal.

PATHOLOGY

Skin lesions range from mild to severe, depending on complications of exudation, ulceration, excoriation, and secondary suppurative inflammation. All skin sections show acanthosis and hyperkeratosis, with foci of parakeratosis and crust and scale formation. Epidermal lesions progress to focal spongiosis with eosinophil exocytosis and subcorneal pustules. Areas of ulceration and exudation show a neutrophil-rich dermal response and focal eosinophilic or neutrophilic furunculosis. The dermal reaction is characterized by superficial and deep perivascular dermatitis replete with mononuclear cells and eosinophils. This progresses in severe cases to a lichenoid pattern; eventually, the whole dermis is infiltrated diffusely with eosinophils and lymphocytes, and diffuse dermal fibrosis is evident. Lesions similar to those in the skin are found throughout the alimentary tract of many horses. Intestinal sections are characterized by diffuse infiltration of the lamina propria, submucosa, and often the muscularis and serosa with eosinophils, mast cells, lymphocytes, macrophages, and plasma cells, and the formation of eosinophilic granulomas. Bowel wall thickening is predominantly mucosal and submucosal, although there are areas of transmural involvement with some marked serosal roughening. Villous atrophy is evident. The mucosal surface is often smooth; erosions and ulcers are not uncommon. Lesions elsewhere include nodular fibrosis of the pancreas, resulting in enlargement (in the Canadian series) or contracture, hepatic fibrosis, liver granulomas, and bile duct proliferation. Infiltrates occur in the draining lymph nodes, the liver and biliary system in most cases, the pancreas in some, and the salivary glands and respiratory tract in a few. Cholangitis and cholangiohepatitis are common features.

DIAGNOSIS

The diagnosis depends on a careful dermatologic investigation and recognition of a possible association with alimentary tract dysfunction. Skin biopsy should differentiate this from other generalized skin conditions such as pemphigus foliaceus and bullous pemphigoid. In the early stages of the disease, skin scrapings and cultures may yield positive results that could prove misleading. Bacteriology and virology have failed to identify any likely pathogen. The progressive nature of the disorder, together with signs referable to other organ systems, should aid diagnosis. A thorough investigation of chronic wasting should be undertaken in cases with predominant or suspected enteric signs. Laboratory features may include hypoalbuminemia, hypoproteinemia, and impaired small intestinal carbohydrate absorption (reduced or delayed oral glucose or d-xylose absorption). Elevated concentrations of γ-glutamyltransferase and alkaline phosphatase, especially the bile duct isoenzyme, indicate hepatic cholestasis. Hematological findings are variable; some animals have normocytic, normochromic anemia and slight neutrophilia. Peripheral eosinophilia is rare.

The differential diagnosis should include causes of coronitis at the outset and, subsequently, causes of generalized skin disease. Ulcerative coronitis has been associated with vasculitis, pemphigus foliaceus, grease heel, laminitis, exposure to irritants, and trauma. Horses with pemphigus foliaceus may appear depressed and have dependent edema, pyrexia, and pruritus, but alimentary tract signs are rare. Other generalized skin disorders to be excluded are dermatophilosis, dermatophytosis, seborrhea, sarcoidosis, cutaneous vasculitis, systemic lupus erythematosus, and toxicosis. The focal eosinophilic lesions are unlikely to be a response to migrating parasites because of the chronicity and absence of parasites in the lesions.

Extensive lesions on the lower limb, muzzle, head, and body are indicative of immune-mediated skin diseases, confirmatory diagnosis of which is usually made on the basis of both histological and immunofluorescent findings. However, the condition is different from known allergic or autoimmune conditions of horses. Direct immunofluorescence studies of skin or other tissue sections have proved nonspecific. The cause of the skin manifestations of inflammatory bowel disease, even in humans, is unsubstantiated but appears to be immune-mediated. Lesions in horses could be indicative of a chronic, ongoing immediate hypersensitivity reaction with a common antigen (or antigens) responsible for all manifestations. Such antigen(s) could be present systemically or may have penetrated the skin and gastrointestinal mucosa.

THERAPY

Therapy has not proved effective at arresting progress of the skin or enteric problems. Iodophor shampoos, insecticides, salves, antimicrobial, and/or corticosteroid-containing ointments have been applied topically, singly or in combination, to treat the skin lesions, often with systemic corticosteroid therapy. Immunosuppressive doses of corticosteroids have not influenced the progressive nature of the condition. The uncertain etiology precludes initiation of specific or selective therapy.

The prognosis is guarded to grave, depending on the stage of presentation. Recovery has not been reported. Thus, the investigation should be as thorough as possible to achieve a definitive diagnosis. The owner should be appraised of the natural course of the disease to avoid embarking on expensive and unrewarding supportive care and therapy. Management has included dietary support, especially high-energy protein feeds, to try to sustain the existing body condition. A necropsy should be conducted in the event of euthanasia. Attempts at therapeutically managing the diverse manifestations of this eosinophilic, epitheliotropic disease must await further work on the immunopathology of the skin and the alimentary tract.

Supplemental Readings

Lindberg, R., Persson, S. G. B., Jones, B., Thoren-Tolling, K., and Ederoth, M.: Clinical and pathophysiological features of granulomatous enteritis and eosinophilic granulomatosis in the horse. Zbl. Vet. Med. A., 32:526–539, 1985.
Nimmo Wilkie, J. S., Yager, J. A., Nation, P. N., Clark, E. G., Townsend, H. C. G., and Baird, J. D.: Chronic eosinophilic dermatitis: A manifestation of a multisystemic, eosinophilic, epitheliotropic disease in five horses. Vet. Pathol., 22:297–305, 1985.
Pass, D. A., and Bolton, J. R., Chronic eosinophilic gastroenteritis in the horse. Vet. Pathol., 19:486–496, 1982.
Roberts, M. C.: Protein-losing enteropathy in the horse. Compend. Cont. Educ. Pract. Vet., 5:S550–S556, 1983.
Roberts, M. C.: Malabsorption syndromes in the horse. Compend. Cont. Educ. Pract. Vet., 7:S637–S646, 1985.

Dermatologic Conditions of the Penis and Prepuce

Donna M. Gatewood, MANHATTAN, KANSAS

A variety of conditions, including neoplasia, parasitism, venereal disease, and physical injury, may manifest with dermatologic lesions on the penis and prepuce. Any of these conditions can result in acute obstruction of the penile urethra and cause subsequent dysuria, anuria, or secondary urinary tract problems. In breeding stallions, these can result in reluctance or inability to copulate even in the absence of obstruction. In any case, an accurate diagnosis of the problem is essential prior to initiation of therapy.

NEOPLASIA AND PARASITISM

Neoplasia and parasitism can be similar in appearance and must be differentiated before therapy is initiated. A punch biopsy sample or cytological impression for histological evaluation of the lesion is usually sufficient for establishing an etiological diagnosis. It is helpful to obtain a biopsy specimen composed of both abnormal and normal tissues.

SQUAMOUS CELL CARCINOMA

This is the most common tumor of the equine penis and prepuce; it has been reported that 45 per cent of equine squamous cell carcinomas occur at this site. Squamous cell carcinoma can develop from existing papillomas or may arise de novo.

The appearance of lesions varies with the location and stage of development. Early lesions may appear as reddened or pale plaques, while advanced lesions are typically granulomatous, cauliflowerlike growths and often multifocal. Histologically, the tumors consist of squamous epithelial cells that may or may not maintain the normal succession of layers. Epithelial columns, which extend into and out of the neoplastic mass in a disorganized manner, appear as epithelial pearls when examined histologically.

Cryosurgical removal is believed to be effective for small localized lesions; extensive involvement may require more radical surgical techniques. Although γ-radiation therapy has been used successfully to treat squamous cell carcinoma in other domestic animals, the current cost and risks make this modality impractical in horses. Strontium 90 beta therapy can be considered for lesions less than 2 mm thick; this therapy is probably most appropriate as an adjunct to surgical debulking.

Excision of the tumor should be followed by ancillary care as described for physical injuries later in this article. Squamous cell carcinomas rarely metastasize, and the prognosis for recovery following removal of the tumor is excellent.

Papillomas

Penile papillomas (warts) are caused by the equine papillomavirus and occasionally occur on the penis and prepuce, despite a predilection for other sites. In most cases, papillomas are self-limiting and regress spontaneously. Cryosurgery has been used effectively to hasten regression. Limited success in treating or preventing papillomas using autogenous vaccines (composed of ground papilloma tissue suspended in formalin) has been reported. A severe outbreak might warrant the prophylactic use of such a vaccine, but it should be used with caution, as there is a potential for anaphylactic reaction. Affected stallions should not be used for breeding if lesions are present, since the condition is considered transmissible.

Equine Sarcoidosis

Treatment of equine sarcoidosis lesions depends on their effect on copulation and urination. If these functions are not affected, the lesions can usually be left undisturbed. Because lesions may continue to increase in size, they should be reassessed periodically.

If immediate therapy is indicated, cryosurgical removal of lesions, including a 0.5 to 1.0 cm margin of unaffected tissue, might be effective. Topical application or injection of 5-fluorouracil or podophyllum can be used as adjunctive therapy to reduce recurrence.

If therapy is needed and time is not critical, Bacillus Calmette-Guerin (BCG) vaccine can be used. Protein cell wall derivatives of the bacillus have been used successfully to treat lesions as large as 6 cm in diameter. Therapy involves injecting the vaccine into and around the base of the tumor. The exact dose depends on the brand of BCG vaccine used; the reader is referred to the manufacturer's recommendations for details (see *Current Therapy in Equine Medicine 2*, p. 637).

Other Neoplastic Conditions

Melanoma, which is most common in aged gray horses, is occasionally observed on the penis or prepuce, but more frequently originates on other parts of the body. Excision is necessary only if the melanoma is extensive or interferes with reproductive or urinary activity. Cutaneous melanoma is often accompanied by extensive metastasis to adjacent areas; clinicians should advise clients of the potentially serious nature of the condition and the probability of recurrence.

Hemangiosarcoma of the penis and prepuce has been rarely reported. Surgical excision followed by careful monitoring for recurrence is regarded as the principal form of treatment.

Parasitism

Habronemiasis is the most common parasitic condition of the equine penis and prepuce, although *Onchocerca*, *Callitroga*, and *Setaria* spp. may produce similar lesions. Habronemiasis lesions ("summer sores") may closely resemble such neoplastic conditions as squamous cell carcinoma and sarcoidosis. A presumptive diagnosis can be made from the history and seasonal occurrence; definitive diagnosis requires the demonstration of larvae or characteristic eosinophilic response within tissue.

Early lesions are often responsive to systemic treatment with ivermectin. Oral ivermectin paste given at the manufacturer's recommended dosage has been shown to be useful, as has oral administration of the injectable product. Daily topical massage of lesions with a cream consisting of 10 ml (20 gm) of dexamethasone in 4 ounces of nitrofurazone may help reduce the inflammatory response to dying larvae after ivermectin therapy. Injection of corticosteroids into the lesion has been advocated, but corticosteroids should be used at minimal doses and with caution, since injectable corticosteroids have been associated with the development of laminitis.

Large lesions or those unresponsive to ivermectin therapy may require surgical debulking. Ancillary nursing care consisting of nonsteroidal anti-inflammatory drugs and daily hydrotherapy is indicated regardless of the specific therapy selected.

VENEREAL DISEASE

This discussion will be limited to dourine and coital exanthema, which have initial or major clinical signs that involve the skin of the external genitalia. Although equine viral arteritis, equine infectious anemia, and other diseases can cause lesions on the penis and prepuce, these are systemic diseases, and genital lesions are not usually a predominant feature in male horses.

DOURINE

Dourine has been eradicated in North America but is present in the Middle East, southern Africa, the Mediterranean coast of Africa, and South America. The causal agent of dourine is the protozoon *Trypanosoma equiperdum*, an organism that produces low morbidity but high mortality.

Initial clinical signs include mucoid urethral discharge and low-grade, recurrent pyrexia. This is followed by nonpainful, cold swelling of the prepuce, scrotum, and penis. Small (2 to 10 cm in diameter) raised plaques, which are considered pathognomonic, appear on the skin, particularly over lower body parts. Initial signs are transient and can spontaneously regress, sometimes within a few hours of appearance. Penile paralysis eventually occurs, and although libido may remain unaffected, penetration of the mare cannot be accomplished. As the disease progresses, emaciation and lameness occur and are usually followed by caudal incoordination, paralysis, and death.

In the United States, control of the disease is achieved by euthanasia and strict quarantine of contact animals; appropriate state and federal authorities should be contacted if dourine is suspected.

COITAL EXANTHEMA

Coital exanthema, or equine herpesvirus 3 infection, is characterized by the development of small vesicles on the shaft of the penis. Although the vesicles can result in temporary unwillingness to achieve penetration during breeding, affected stallions often have normal libido. Some stallions become depressed and pyretic and have nonspecific signs of systemic illness.

Shortly after their appearance the vesicles rupture and small (3 to 10 mm) ulcers develop. The lesions granulate and resolve in 10 to 21 days, frequently leaving small depigmented areas. Lesions can resemble the early stages of squamous cell carcinoma and can be differentiated by biopsy. Similar lesions occur on the vulvar mucosa of affected mares.

Treatment consists of 3 weeks of sexual rest and application of emollients or ointments such as nitrofurazone, lanolin, or petroleum jelly to prevent the formation of preputial adhesions. Recurrence can occur, often following periods of stress. The disease is self-limiting and usually follows an uncomplicated course, but affected horses should be isolated and not bred while lesions are present. Continued breeding activity will promote the spread of infection to susceptible mares and may prolong the course of the disease.

PHYSICAL INJURIES

GENERAL CONSIDERATIONS

Physical injuries such as lacerations, contusions, and thermal or chemical injuries most often result in inflammation, edema, and tissue necrosis. Therapy is symptomatic and is directed toward restoring the tissue to a normal state and proper anatomical configuration. Some injuries may be severe enough to warrant surgical procedures such as circumcision or penile amputation, but aggressive medical therapy should always be attempted before radical surgical intervention.

Several systemic diseases, such as equine viral arteritis, purpura hemorrhagica, and equine infectious anemia, can induce inflammation and edema of the preputial area and should be considered in the differential diagnosis when examining such lesions.

URETHRAL PATENCY

Urethral patency should be confirmed in all injuries accompanied by swelling of the penile or preputial tissue. If the urinary bladder appears distended on rectal palpation, obstruction should be suspected. If the patency of the urethra is in question, a urethral catheter should be passed to ensure adequate drainage of the bladder.

The use of sterile technique in passing a urinary catheter is essential because of the potential for introducing pathogenic bacteria into the upper urinary tract. The glans penis and fossa glandis should be thoroughly cleaned with a povidone–iodine solution. Sterile gloves and a sterile catheter should be used. The author prefers a 30 French, 150-cm canine feeding tube. A small amount of sterile, water-soluble lubricant may be applied to the tip of the catheter to ease passage through the urethra. If necessary, the catheter may be sutured in place and left for several days. In this case, the catheter should be monitored daily and replaced every 2 to 3 days until urination is normal.

TRAUMA

The most common physical injury to the penis is trauma caused by a kick from the mare while the stallion is dismounting after breeding. Resulting injuries usually include contusions, hemorrhage, and edema. The subsequent inflammatory response is usually severe and often results in acute paraphimosis accompanied by varying degrees of balanitis and posthitis.

Primary closure of lacerations of the penis and prepuce can be attempted if the wound is fresh. Antibiotic therapy and tetanus toxoid may be indicated, and ancillary medical therapy should be administered.

Immediate posttrauma therapy should include cold-water hydrotherapy and tissue massage (30 minutes per treatment, two to four times per day). Antibiotic ointments are indicated if there are lacerations. Once hemorrhage and fluid accumulation have ceased, warm-water hydrotherapy may be more effective for enhancing venous drainage and stimulating superficial granulation of lacerations. If the penis is adequately supported, mild exercise is beneficial for reducing peripreputial and ventral-midline swelling and edema. In severe cases, diuretics may be indicated for decreasing edema and fluid accumulation.

Nonsteroidal anti-inflammatory drugs should be considered to alleviate pain and reduce inflammation. Emollients may be of benefit if the mucosa of the penis or prepuce becomes dry and cracked.

Tranquilizers should be avoided if possible, since these agents tend to promote further penile prolapse and passive accumulation of additional edema. However, some stallions will not tolerate tissue massage, hydrotherapy, or application of medications without sedation. In these cases, mild tranquilization may be necessary, but phenothiazine-derived agents should not be used, as some have been implicated in cases of penile paralysis. Exposure to mares should also be avoided because sexual stimulation can exacerbate the problem by increasing penile engorgement.

If paraphimosis is present, the penis and prepuce should be elevated and supported to allow adequate venous and lymphatic drainage of injured tissue.

THERMAL AND CHEMICAL INJURIES

The principles of therapy described for trauma should be applied to thermal and chemical injuries, with several additional considerations.

Burn injuries warrant systemic therapy with broad-spectrum antibiotics in addition to the application of topical antibiotic creams. Silver sulfadiazine cream and aloe vera cream have been used extensively in human medicine for topical treatment of burns and have been successfully used to treat burned animals. Systemic and topical antibiotic therapy should continue until a healthy layer of granulation tissue is present.

Chemical injuries should be treated immediately with extensive rinsing to remove the irritant. Hydrotherapy and nonsteroidal anti-inflammatory drugs are indicated for patients with subsequent swelling and inflammation of the affected tissue.

Supplemental Readings

Bowen, J. M.: Venereal diseases of stallions. *In* Robinson, N. E. (ed.): Current Therapy in Equine Medicine 2. Philadelphia, W. B. Saunders, 1987, pp. 567–570.

Bridges, E. R.: The use of ivermectin to treat genital cutaneous habronemiasis in a stallion. Compend. Cont. Educ. Pract. Vet., 7:S94–S97, 1985.

Cotchin, E.: A general survey of tumours in the horse. Equine Vet J., 9:16–21, 1977.

Junge, R. E., Sundberg, J. P., and Lancaster, W. D.: Papillomas and squamous cell carcinomas of horses. J. Am. Vet. Med. Assoc., 185:656–659, 1984.

Larsen, R. E.: The stallion. *In* Mansmann, R. A., McAllister, E. S., Pratt, P. W. (eds.): Equine Medicine and Surgery, 3rd ed. Santa Barbara, American Veterinary Publishing, 1982, pp. 1384–1402.

Lasers in Dermatology
Lloyd P. Tate, Jr., RALEIGH, NORTH CAROLINA

The ruby laser invented by Theodore Maymen in 1962, was soon followed by the carbon dioxide (CO_2) laser. Lasers quickly became incorporated into various human medical specialties because of their biological effects on tissue (Table 1). In human medicine, ophthalmologists and dermatologists commonly use lasers in clinical practice, but in veterinary medicine these specialists have only recently begun to use lasers clinically.

The CO_2 laser achieves its thermal effect through absorption of infrared irradiation by water within cells that are superheated to the point of vaporization. Speedy transformation of laser energy into thermal energy is desired to decrease forward and lateral spread of heat, which causes thermal death of adjacent cells. It is advantageous for cutting to deliver this laser beam to a small focal spot. To decrease adjacent cell death and allow cooling of adjacent tissue between exposures, the continuous laser mode may be broken into pulses. The CO_2 laser may also be used to produce hyperthermia or a wide area of tissue coagulation by altering the focal distance.

TABLE 1. BIOLOGICAL EFFECTS OF LASER IRRADIATION BETWEEN WAVELENGTHS OF 400 NM AND 10,600 NM

1. Photopyrolysis: Direct conversion of irradiation to thermal energy (less than 100° C) to cause coagulation, hemostasis, or thermal necrosis.
2. Photovaporolysis: Rapid absorption and conversion to heat, resulting in vaporization of intra- and extracellular water, which mechanically disrupts cells.
3. Photochemolysis and photochemosynthesis: Produced by low-intensity irradiation to activate chemicals in tissues, causing lysis or synthesis.
4. Photoacoustic wave: Pressure wave resulting from laser beam impact damages cell structure.
5. Photoelectrolysis: Cell membrane destruction by electrical fields of high voltage, independent of mechanical and thermal effects of irradiation.
6. Photoexplosion: Mechanical damage caused by shock wave and blast effect resulting from expanding vapor in tissues heated in an ultra-short time.
7. Photoplasmolysis: Destruction of cellular architecture by altering electron orbits within atoms, caused by strong electrical fields from light that is pulsed extremely rapidly (nanoseconds).

Biological effects 1 through 3 are observed in laser dermatologic procedures using the CO_2, Nd:YAG, and Argon lasers. Procedures 4 through 7 require specific modulation of laser irradiation and increasing power densities.

Moving the focal point above or below the tissue surface will widen the laser beam, thus producing a generalized heating effect. This is advantageous in dermatology for sterilization of tissue or for general debulking of large areas of tissue.

Reflection of laser energy from instrumentation and smooth surfaces is a primary safety hazard that may inadvertently result in an unwanted laser burn. This hazard may be reduced by using anodized instruments. Protective goggles also prevent inadvertent burns to the cornea by reflected or direct exposure. Moist sponges should be used to shield adjacent tissues from accidental laser exposure.

Most laser procedures in large animal dermatology can be performed on the sedated standing animal following infiltration of the surgical site with local anesthetics. When a general anesthetic is required, the practitioner must remember that devastating airway fires can occur if the endotracheal tubes become ignited in the presence of a high oxygen flow. The smoke plume produced by the CO_2 laser may be irritating and have an offensive smell. Specialized filters and smoke evacuation equipment should be employed to capture as much of the plume as possible. In human dermatology masks are worn and particular care is taken to provide complete smoke removal when warts are the target tissue.

The CO_2 laser is used to remove sarcoids, especially those located in the ear. Other dermal tumors such as squamous cell carcinoma, particularly those located around the eye, can be resected with this laser. The laser provides a means of resection using a no-touch technique. The surgeon can visualize the depth of the incision simultaneous with its creation. Small blood vessels, lymphatics, and nerves are severed and sealed, which provides a clear field and may reduce pain and the recurrence of tumors. The laser may also be used in the defocused mode to thermally shave away layers of tissue until normal tissue is exposed. This is advantageous when the practitioner is working around the eye and ear, where underlying cartilage or other vital structures exist. Whether the procedure entails resecting with a focused beam or ablating with the defocused beam, the wound is generally left to heal by secondary intention. If suturing is indicated, laser incisions heal more slowly than steel scapel incisions but slightly faster than electrocautery incisions.

Large animals are frequently presented with injuries of the lower limbs in which large areas of dermis are lost. These often are allowed to heal by secondary intention or by applying a skin graft over a prepared bed of granulation tissue. The CO_2 laser may be used either to prepare a graft bed or to remove granulation tissue. In preparation of graft beds, the laser is used in defocused mode so that layers of granulation tissue may be shaved away to produce a smooth recipient surface. The tissue is simultaneously sterilized by the laser to minimize the possiblity of infection. The black residue of carbon particles is not detrimental to healing. Dermis is replaced by pinch grafting. The focused CO_2 laser beam creates pockets within granulation tissue, usually at approximately a 30- to 45- degree angle, in which the harvested segments of dermis are inserted. Best results occur when 12 to 24 hours elapse between creating pockets and placing harvested dermis. Revascularization of the pocket edges has begun and improves graft survival.

In human dermatology, the argon laser that produces a beam of irradiation between 488 and 514 nm is frequently employed for a multitude of dermatologic procedures because it is well absorbed by body pigments such as melanin and hemoglobin. This laser is generally used at low power settings but still produces good penetration. In large animal dermatology the potential use of this laser lies in the photochemical effect. The argon laser is employed as a pump source for a dye laser that can be tuned to produce a specific wavelength of irradiation. Chromophores injected into tissues are activated by the laser to produce a toxin, which results in cell death. Superoxide anion is the cell toxin most commonly produced by the laser chromophore reaction. The ideal chromatophore is retained at high concentrations in or around tumor cells and eliminated from the normal cell population. This allows selective destruction of tumor cells exposed to a laser irradiation. It is possible that photodynamic therapy will become a primary means of treating malignancies of the dermis such as squamous cell carcinoma, virus infections like sarcoids, and other infectious diseases.

Supplemental Readings

Goldman, L.: The Biomedical Laser: Technology and Clinical Applications. New York, Springer-Verlag, 1981, pp. 1–52.

Jennings, P. B.: The Practice of Large Animal Surgery. Vol. 1. Philadelphia, W. B. Saunders, 1984, pp. 318–319.

Ohshiro, T.: Laser treatment for nevi. Tokyo, Medical Laser Research Co., 1980, pp. 1–52.

Palmer, S. E.: Carbon dioxide laser removal of a verrucous sarcoid from the ear of a horse. J. Am. Vet. Med. Assoc., *195*:1123, 1989.

Regan, J. D, and Parish, J. A.: The Science of Photomedicine. New York, Plenum Press, 1982, pp. 1323–1340.

White, N. A., and Moore, J. N.: Current Practice of Equine Surgery. Philadelphia, J. B. Lippincott, 1990, pp. 26–33.

Section 17

NUTRITION

Edited by Sarah L. Ralston

Nutrient Requirements*

Harold F. Hintz, ITHACA, NEW YORK

A revision of the National Research Council's *Nutrient Requirements of the Horse* was published in 1989. The previous edition had been published in 1978. In the 11 years between publications considerable research was conducted into equine nutrition in many parts of the world, predominantly the United States, France, and Germany.

A major addition in the 1989 publication was the provision of equations for calculating energy, protein, calcium, phosphorus, magnesium, potassium, and vitamin A requirements for all classes of horses. An IBM diskette with the equations is provided with the publication. Thus, values can be quickly calculated for any size horse without the need to extrapolate from a table. Other changes are the inclusion of estimates for stallions and for heavy horses.

ENERGY

Several changes were made in the approach to defining energy requirements. In 1978 the maintenance requirement was defined as DE (kcal/day) = $155 \times W^{0.75}$, where DE is digestible energy and W is body weight (kg). This formula overestimated the energy requirements of ponies. Furthermore, Pagan and Hintz found no benefit from using metabolic body size when studying horses weighing 125 to 860 kg. They reported that the energy requirement for such horses confined to metabolism stalls could be defined by the formula DE (Mcal/day) = $0.975 + 0.021W$. The formula for zero body weight change plus normal activity of nonworking horses was calculated by Pagan and Hintz to be DE (Mcal/day) = $1.4 + 0.03W$. This equation is easy to use and seems to be reasonable for horses up to 600 kg and was adopted by the NRC. It overestimates the requirement of larger horses, probably because of the reduced voluntary activity of those animals. Therefore, the formula DE (Mcal/day) = $1.82 + 0.0383W - 0.000015W^2$ was used by NRC for the horses over 600 kg.

In the 1989 edition, the energy requirements for gestation are given for mares at 9, 10, and 11 months, respectively, rather than simply as during late gestation, as reported in the 1978 edition. This refinement was made possible because of the studies of chemical composition of the fetus at various stages of gestation conducted by Meyer and Ahlswede. The requirements were calculated by multiplying the DE maintenance requirements at 9, 10, and 11 months by 1.11, 1.13, and 1.20, respectively, based on increases in energy deposition.

The estimates for lactating mares were derived using the assumptions used in the 1978 edition,

---

*See also *Current Therapy in Equine Medicine 2* pages 387–421

i.e., that mares of light breeds produce milk equivalent to 3 per cent of body weight per day during early lactation (1 to 12 weeks) and 2 per cent of body weight during late lactation (13 to 24 weeks). Ponies were assumed to produce milk equivalent to 4 and 3 per cent of body weight per day during early and late lactation, respectively. The value for the conversion of DE into milk (792 kcal of DE per kg of milk) was the same as was used in 1978.

Changes were made in the requirements for growth. Several recent studies indicated that the 1978 edition significantly underestimated the requirements for yearlings. The daily DE for growing horses was calculated using the equation: DE (Mcal/day) = Maintenance DE + $[(4.81 + 1.17x - 0.023x^2)(ADG)]$, where ADG is the average daily gain in kg and x is the age in months. No conclusions were made as to optimal growth rate.

The energy requirements for the working horse are difficult to calculate. The 1978 values were reasonable for horses at light work but greatly underestimated the requirements at hard work. Several different equations have been developed, such as those of Anderson et al. and Pagan and Hintz, but they have limitations for practical applications. It was decided that requirements for light, medium, and intense work could be estimated by increasing the requirements by 25, 50, and 100 per cent above maintenance, respectively. Light work was considered to be represented by pleasure classes, hacking, and the like, medium work by roping, barrel racing, and jumping, and intense work by race training and polo.

PROTEIN

The protein requirements for maintenance and for working horses were calculated to be crude protein (CP) (gm/day) = 40 × Mcal DE/day. The requirement for pregnant mares is CP (gm/day) = 44 × Mcal DE/day. In the equation for lactating mares it was assumed that milk contained 0.21 per cent protein and the efficiency of conversion of CP to milk protein was 35.8 per cent. The CP (gm/day) for weanlings and yearlings was 50 and 45 per Mcal DE per day. The calculations resulted in slightly higher values for pregnant mares and lactating mares than in 1978, but values for growing animals and for maintenance were similar to those reported in 1978.

Lysine requirements (gm per day) were estimated as 2.1 and 1.9 per Mcal DE for weanlings and yearlings, respectively.

MINERALS

There were no large changes in the mineral requirements. It was noted that exercise would increase calcium losses in sweat and would perhaps increase bone density and therefore increase calcium requirements. However, it was assumed that if the calcium-to-calorie ratio fed was adequate for maintenance, the increased energy intake needed for exercise would satisfy the calcium requirements if the calcium-to-calorie ratio was maintained.

The 1989 values for the trace minerals are compared to the 1978 values in Table 1. The 1989 NRC decided that the statistical evidence did not warrant increasing the copper requirement to as high as that recommended by scientists at the Ohio State University.

VITAMINS

Vitamin A requirements were estimated to be 60 IU per day per kg body weight for pregnant and lactating mares and 30 IU per day per kg body weight for all other classes of horses. Thus, a 500-kg mare at maintenance or pregnant would require 15,000 or 30,000 IU per day, respectively. These values are slightly increased

TABLE 1. DIETARY CONCENTRATIONS° OF TRACE MINERALS ADEQUATE FOR HORSES: COMPARISON OF THE NATIONAL RESEARCH COUNCIL'S 1978 AND 1989 VALUES

Minerals	Growth or Maintenance (ppm)	
	1978	1989
Copper	9	10
Manganese	40	40
Zinc	40	40
Selenium	0.1	0.1
Iodine	0.1	0.1
Cobalt	0.1	0.1

°Dry matter basis.

TABLE 2. DIETARY CONCENTRATIONS° OF VITAMINS ADEQUATE FOR HORSES: COMPARISON OF THE NATIONAL RESEARCH COUNCIL'S 1978 AND 1989 VALUES

Vitamins	Maintenance		Growth	
	1978	1989	1978	1989
Vitamin D, IU/kg	275	300†	275	300†
Vitamin E, IU/kg	15	50	15	80
Thiamine, mg/kg	3	3	3	3
Riboflavin, mg/kg	2.2	2	2.2	2

°Dry matter basis.
†Recommendations for horses not exposed to sunlight or to artificial light with an emission spectrum of 280 to 315 nm.

over the 12,500 and 25,000 IU given in the 1978 edition.

Estimates of requirements for some other vitamins are compared in Table 2. The biggest change is for vitamin E. The vitamin E requirement was increased because of studies suggesting that higher levels would provide greater cell protection and increased resistance to disease. It was decided that data are insufficient to determine a requirement for pantothenic acid, B_6, B_{12}, folic acid, biotin, or ascorbic acid.

Supplemental Readings

Anderson, C. E., Potter, G. D., Kreider, J. L., and Courtney, C. C.: Digestible energy requirements for exercising horses. J. Anim. Sci., 56:91, 1983.
Gabel, A. A., Knight, D. A., Reed, S. M., et al.: Proceedings of the 29th Annual Convention of the American Association of Equine Practitioners, 1985, p. 163.
Knight, D.A., Weisbrode, S. E., Schmall, L. M., and Gabel, A. A.: Copper supplementation and cartilage lesions in foals. In: Proceedings of the 33rd Annual Convention of the American Association of Equine Practitioners, 1987, pp. 191-194.
Meyer, H., and Ahlswede, L.: The intrauterine growth and body composition of foals and nutrient requirements of pregnant mares. Animal Res. Devel. 8:86–102, 1976.
National Research Council: Nutrient Requirements of Horses, 4th ed. Washington, D. C., National Academy of Sciences–National Research Council, 1978.
National Research Council: Nutrient Requirements of Horses, 5th ed. Washington, D. C., National Academy of Sciences–National Research Council, 1989.
Pagan, J. D., and Hintz, H. F.: Equine energetics: II. Energy expenditure in horses during submaximal exercise. J. Anim. Sci., 63:815, 1986.

Diagnosis of Common Mineral Imbalances

Sarah L. Ralston, NEW BRUNSWICK, NEW JERSEY

The diagnosis of protein-energy malnutrition is often easily made from a complete dietary history and physical examination without additional diagnostic tests. The selection and interpretation of diagnostic tests are more important in cases of suspected mineral imbalances. Feed, blood, hair, and urine samples may provide information on the mineral status of a horse. The tests selected must be interpreted with recognition of both dietary and nondietary influences. This chapter discusses tests for the diagnosis of dietary imbalances of the most commonly imbalanced minerals in horse rations: calcium (Ca), phosphorus (P), copper (Cu), zinc (Zn), selenium (Se), and iron (Fe).

Clinical signs and regional forage characteristics should direct the selection of samples and tests. For example, a high incidence of poor reproductive performance in a herd would dictate investigation of potential imbalances in Ca, P, Cu, Zn, Se, protein, energy, and perhaps vitamin A. Regional trends in mineral content of forages, available from local extension agents or forage analysis laboratories, will aid in deciding which minerals are most likely to be a problem. However, mineral interactions are complex and imbalances may be present that are contrary to standard trends in a given area. For example, even in high Se regions, the list of differential diagnoses for chronic rhabdomyolysis in a horse should include Se deficiency. Excessive Cu supplementation, arsenic toxicity, and use of hay from a heavily irrigated field may all induce Se deficiency, even if dietary levels are adequate. Reasonable ranges of dietary minerals in feed are presented in Table 1.

CALCIUM

Clinical signs suggestive of Ca deficiency include abnormal bone and cartilage development and shifting leg lameness. In cases of acute deficiency (e.g., lactation and blister beetle toxicity), synchronous diaphragmatic flutter and tetany may be seen. Acute hypocalcemia, however, does not reflect a chronic deficit in dietary Ca. Instead, as in periparturient cows, acute hypocalcemia may be preceded by high dietary Ca intake. Clinical signs of Se deficiencies (see below) also may be seen if Ca intake is excessive.

Feed analysis is usually a reliable test for dietary Ca adequacy. Calcium in most forages is 50 to 60 per cent digestible. A reasonable dietary

TABLE 1. REASONABLE RANGES OF DIETARY MINERALS IN FEED OF ADULT HORSES

Mineral	In Dry Matter	Interference from Excessive Levels of:
Ca, %	0.25–1.5°	Zinc, aluminum, oxalate
P, %	0.15–6°	Aluminum, phytate
Cu, ppm	10–25	Iron, sulfur, molybdenum
Zn, ppm	40–100	Calcium, copper
Fe, ppm	40–250	Copper
Se, ppm	0.1–1.2	Copper, arsenic

Values in table are based on 1989 National Research Council's minima and author's experience.
°Calcium:phosphorus ratio in total ration must be greater than 1:1. Higher minimum amounts of both are necessary for late pregnant or lactating mares and horses more than one year old.

range is 0.15 to 1.5 per cent Ca in feed dry matter (DM) for adult horses (0.41 per cent minimum for late pregnant and 0.47 per cent minimum for lactating mares). *Setaria* spp. of grasses, green panic grass, and kikuyu, however, contain oxalates that inhibit Ca absorption and can cause signs of nutritional secondary hyperparathyroidism despite adequate Ca in the feed. A diet with Ca:oxalate below 0.5 may cause signs of nutritional secondary hyperparathyroidism. Other inhibiting factors include Zn (above 1000 mg per kg feed DM) and Ca:P ratio less than 1.0. High levels of dietary aluminum (Al) (4500 mg per kg feed DM) will enhance urinary excretion of Ca.

Because serum Ca is under homeostatic control it is not a reliable indicator of dietary Ca intake. Both ionized and total Ca concentrations are influenced by extraneous factors, such as the way the sample is handled after collection (e.g., use of cork stoppers, heparinized samples, or delay in separation of serum). Extreme caution should be used when interpreting serum Ca concentrations. Urinary Ca concentration is extremely responsive to dietary intake but also is difficult to interpret accurately.

In general, minerals in urine should be expressed either in relation to per cent creatinine clearance or total solids ratio (moles per mOsm). Urine Ca greater than 15 μmoles per mOsm or a Ca:creatinine per centage over 2.5 may indicate that Ca intake is adequate. However, the last meal consumed is reflected in urinary Ca for 3 to 6 hours. If a sample is obtained within 3 to 6 hours of alfalfa ingestion but before grain is fed, urine Ca may indicate adequate Ca availability, even though the total diet (hay plus grain) provides inadequate amounts of Ca in relation to P. This situation can occur if samples are taken before morning rations are fed. Urinary Ca concentrations are difficult to interpret unless all diet ingredients are fed at the same time and urine is obtained 3 to 6 hours later. Hair Ca does not reflect Ca intake and varies with coat color, age, sex, breed, and divalent mineral intake. (See also pages 119 and 566 and *Current Therapy in Equine Medicine 2*, p. 395, for clinical signs and therapy of Ca imbalances.)

PHOSPHORUS

Clinical signs suggestive of dietary P imbalances include shifting leg lameness, abnormal bone and cartilage development, spontaneous fractures (P excesses), and pica and angular limb deformities (P deficiencies).

Feed analysis is usually a reliable estimate of dietary P intake. A reasonable range would be 0.15 to 0.60 per cent P in feed DM for adult horses, 0.30 per cent minimum for lactating mares. However, excessive phytate-bound P or Al content (4500 mg Al per kg feed DM) will reduce P absorption. Serum inorganic P may be low if chronic severe deficiencies are present but is not a sensitive measure of dietary intake. If urine P is greater than 15 moles per mOsm and the creatinine clearance ratio is over 4.0 per cent, P intake may be excessive in relation to Ca. Urinary P is not as sensitive as Ca to recent meal intakes. Hair P does not reflect dietary intake of the mineral. (See *Current Therapy in Equine Medicine 2*, p. 395, for clinical signs and therapy of P imbalances.)

COPPER

Clinical signs suggestive of Cu deficiency in adult horses include ruptured aorta or uterine arteries, and perhaps anemia, recurrent bacterial infections, or depigmentation of skin and hair. Excesses may cause signs of Fe or Se deficiency.

Feed analysis is a good estimate of Cu intake. However, Fe or Zn over 1000 times the recommended amounts may inhibit availability. Ten mg Cu per kg feed DM is considered to be adequate for horses if energy, protein, and other minerals are within recommended ranges. Horses are tolerant of high Cu intakes (up to 200 mg per kg feed DM). Because of reported benefits of high copper intake, some feeds and supplements for horses contain in excess of 100 mg Cu per kg feed, a level toxic for sheep. Excessive Cu intake, 20 to 40 mg per kg body weight as a single dose, also enhances excretion of Se. In diets with marginal selenium, excessive Cu intake may cause signs of Se deficiency. Molybdenum and sulfur, which bind Cu in thiomolybdate complexes in ruminants, are well tolerated by horses. However, molybdenum levels in excess of 27 mg per kg feed DM will adversely affect Cu balance.

Serum Cu does not reflect subtle changes in dietary Cu intake in adult horses. Lactating mares fed a diet containing 4 mg Cu per kg feed DM for 4 weeks do not have low serum Cu levels. Ninety per cent of serum Cu is in the ferroxidase portion of ceruloplasmin; the rest is loosely bound to albumin. The former responds slowly; more than 4 weeks is required to change ceruloplasmin in response to dietary change. Superoxide dismutase also has been used to assess Cu status but has no apparent benefit over ceruloplasmin in the horse. Liver Cu stores are usually more than 50 per cent depleted before a change in serum concentrations is detectable. The risk of liver biopsy in horses outweighs the potential use of liver samples except in postmortem examinations. Urinary and hair Cu concentrations do not reflect dietary intake of the mineral. (See also *Current Therapy in Equine Medicine 2*, p. 400, for clinical signs of Cu deficiency.)

ZINC

The Zn requirements of horses are not well established. Although the NRC in 1989 recommended 40 ppm in the ration, the author has commonly seen adult horses fed diets as low as 20 ppm without apparent ill effects. Clinical signs of Zn excesses are usually those of deficiencies of Ca or Cu. Zn deficiency in other species causes parakeratosis, impaired wound healing, reduced immune competence, reduced glucose tolerance, and poor growth, but these have not been well documented in horses.

Feed analysis is a good estimate of Zn intake. Forty mg Zn per kg feed DM is considered adequate for growth and maintenance of the average horse, but up to 100 mg per kg feed DM is well tolerated. Ca intakes above the recommended range (see Table 1) may reduce Zn availability.

Serum Zn reflects gross excesses or deficiencies, but not short-term or subtle imbalances. Liver stores of Zn vary with diet but are not reflected in serum concentrations. Urinary and hair Zn do not reflect dietary intake of the mineral.

SELENIUM

Clinical signs suggestive of excessive Se intake in adult horses include loss of mane and tail hair, horizontal cracks in the hoof wall, and lameness. Exertional myopathies may indicate Se deficiency (see *Current Therapy in Equine Medicine 2*, p. 402).

Feed analysis is a reasonable estimate of Se intake. However, Se is not included in most forage analysis panels and must be asked for specifically. Elevated dietary concentrations of Cu, arsenic, sulfur and perhaps Ca, P, and Fe will inhibit absorption or retention of selenium. A reasonable range of Se is 0.1 to 1.0 mg Se per kg feed DM.

Serum Se and whole blood gluthathione peroxidase levels reflect dietary intake. Serum Se levels respond rapidly to dietary intake and are considered to be more accurate than whole blood levels. Glutathione peroxidase, an Se-containing enzyme, is measured in whole blood and responds slowly (10 to 11 weeks) to dietary changes. Glutathione peroxidase is very labile and blood samples must be rapidly chilled and frozen pending analysis. Glutathione peroxidase and whole blood Se levels are good indicators of chronic deficiencies. Serum Se will reflect both chronic and acute deficiencies and toxicities.

Urinary Se is not diagnostic, since Se is not excreted via the kidney. Hair Se levels reflect toxicity (greater than 5 mg Se per kg hair) and deficiency (less than 0.1 mg Se per kg hair). Hair Se is also affected by dietary Cu, Fe, arsenic, and perhaps other minerals.

IRON

Clinical signs of excess Fe intake may include those of induced Cu deficiency, such as recurrent bacterial infections or hepatic necrosis. Clinical deficiency is unlikely but theoretically may cause anemia. Feed analysis is a fair measure of Fe intake, though not all forms of Fe are available for absorption and only a small proportion is absorbed. Absorption is enhanced by low pH and ascorbic acid. Reasonable ranges are 40 to 250 mg Fe per kg feed DM. It is rare to find a forage deficient in Fe. Serum Fe is not a reliable measure of dietary adequacy, especially in clinically ill horses. Sepsis causes sequestration of Fe, reducing its availability to microbial populations but not to the horse. Anemia also is not a good indicator of Fe status in horses, as there are many other causes of low hemoglobin and low hematocrit unrelated to Fe status. Serum ferritin concentrations are more reliable and may reflect either deficiency or toxicity. Urinary and hair Fe levels do not reflect dietary intake of the mineral.

SUMMARY

Feed analysis is the most reliable test for dietary adequacy of all of the minerals discussed.

Blood samples may be taken to aid in the diagnosis of Cu, Se, Fe (serum ferritin), and Zn imbalances but are not reliable for Ca or P. Urinary ratios of Ca and P in relation either to total solutes or per cent creatinine clearance will reflect dietary imbalances, though Ca data should be interpreted with caution. Hair analysis currently is of use only in determining dietary excesses of deficiencies of Se.

Supplemental Reading

Caple I. W., Doake, P. A., Ellis, P. G.: Assessment of the calcium and phosphorus nutrition in horses by analysis of urine. Aust. Vet. J., 58:125–131, 1982.

Coombs, D. K.: Hair analysis as an indicator of mineral status of livestock. J. Anim. Sci., 65:1753–1758, 1987.

Mills, C. F.: Biochemical and physiological indicators of mineral status in animals: Copper, cobalt, and zinc. J. Anim. Sci., 65:1702–1711, 1987.

National Research Council: Nutrient Requirements of Horses. Washington, D. C., National Academy Press, 1989.

Schryver, H. F.: Mineral and vitamin intoxication in horses. Vet. Clin. North Am. (Equine Pract.) 6(2):295–318, 1990.

Ullrey, D. E.: Biochemical and physiological indicators of selenium status in animals. J. Anim. Sci. 65:1712–1726, 1987.

Nutritional Factors in Developmental Orthopedic Disease

Edgar A. Ott, GAINESVILLE, FLORIDA

Developmental orthopedic disease is a relatively new term. Previously referred to as metabolic bone disease, developmental orthopedic disease encompasses a number of definable orthopedic abnormalities that occur between birth and 18 months of age. Conditions considered to be part of the developmental orthopedic disease syndrome include: osteochondrosis, osteochondritis dissecans, subchondral cystic lesions, physitis (epiphysitis), acquired flexure deformities (contracted tendons), cervical vertebral malformation ("wobblers"), malformation of the cuboidal bones of the carpus and tarsus (angular limb deformity), and juvenile arthritis. The clinical manifestations of most of these conditions reflect inability of the growing skeletal system to tolerate stresses imposed on it. The cause of this failure, however, is controversial. Some authors suggest that all of the signs represent a single abnormality. However, there is also evidence that many different conditions may cause one or more developmental orthopedic disease problems.

There are basically three factors involved in these abnormalities: (1) Genetics. Genetically mediated conformational abnormalities result in excessive stress on one or more parts of the skeletal system and uneven growth patterns. Genetically mediated metabolic abnormalities in the utilization of nutrients, enzyme activity, or hormonal control of the growth process may also be involved. (2) Environment. Abnormalities may be caused by external stress or trauma imposed by voluntary or forced exercise, surface conditions of the ground, hoof trimming or shoeing, and excess body weight. (3) Nutrition. Nutritional deficiency, excess, or imbalance of key nutrients will adversely affect bone and cartilage because of alterations in the availability of components of skeletal structures or the enzymes and hormones that control the synthesis of these tissues.

This chapter describes the influence of nutrition on developmental orthopedic disease. However, in most cases at least two of the above factors are present, if not all three.

NORMAL CARTILAGE AND BONE STRUCTURE

Most developmental orthopedic diseases of the horse involve the growth, maturation, and ossification of cartilage. The lesions are located in the metaphyseal physis of the long bones, the epiphyseal physis, and the articular cartilages. Most lesions appear to originate near or at the osteochondral junction, suggesting errors in cartilage formation, vascularization, or mineralization.

Cartilage is a fibrillar matrix of collagen and

protoglycans produced by the chondrocytes. Collagen is a helical protein composed of three polypeptide chains, each consisting of about 1000 amino acid residues. The integrity of the helix is strengthened by intramolecular cross-links. Adjacent collagen molecules are joined by intermolecular cross-links. The organic portion of mature bone is 90 per cent collagen, most of which is type I. This collagen is composed of two $\alpha 1[I]$ chains and one $\alpha 2$ chain. Bone collagen accounts for the elastic and tensile strength of the structure. Cartilage, both epiphyseal and articular, is composed of primarily type II collagen, although up to 30 per cent type I may be present (Table 1). Type II collagen is composed of three $\alpha 1$ (II) chains.

FACTORS INFLUENCING DEVELOPMENTAL ORTHOPEDIC DISEASE

Energy

Energy intake, along with protein, is a primary factor influencing growth rate of the animal. There appear to be at least three concerns regarding the influence of energy intake on developmental orthopedic disease: (1) The rapidly growing animal puts more weight on the skeletal system at an early age, thus increasing the stress on immature bones. (2) Faster growth rates require higher concentrations of other nutrients critical to tissue synthesis. Nutrient concentrations appropriate for moderate growth may be inadequate at higher rates. (3) High energy intakes generally mean highly glucogenic diets that appear to alter normal hormone secretions, including insulin, triiodothyronine (T_3), and thyroxine (T_4). These hormones have been shown to influence cartilage cell growth and maturation.

Restricting the energy intake of a growing horse to less than the National Research Council's 1989 recommendations will reduce the growth rate of the animal and lower the animal's need for other critical nutrients. Reducing growth rates may be appropriate for animals with known genetic propensity for developmental orthopedic disease or to control an emerging problem. However, slowing the growth rate also slows down skeletal development. The commercial demand to maximize growth so that the individual will be competitive in the sale ring, show ring, or in the early 2-year-old competitions may make this approach impractical except in selected cases where individuals with special needs are identified. Maintenance of at least moderate growth rates is the most prudent approach.

Maximizing growth rates places a special demand on the dietary needs of the animal and nutrient interrelationships. The faster the animal grows, the more sensitive it is to variations in nutrient availability, as exemplified by the influence of rate of gain on the nutrient requirements of a weanling according to the NRC's 1989 equations. Increasing the average daily gain from 0.50 kg per day to 1.25 kg per day will require 63 per cent more energy, protein, zinc, and copper but 95 per cent more calcium and phosphorus (Table 2).

Highly glucogenic diets, that is, those that contain high concentrations of starch and other soluble carbohydrates such as sugar, may produce alterations in the insulin, T_3 and T_4 secretions after feeding that cause hormonal dissynchrony. Meals high in soluble carbohydrate result in a rapid glucose and insulin peak followed by an abrupt decrease. T_3 also increases rapidly and T_4 decreases. Alterations in the

TABLE 1. COLLAGEN IN THE SKELETAL SYSTEM

Type	Formula	Predominant Tissue	Characteristics
I	$[\alpha 1(I)]_2 \alpha 2$	Bone and tendons	Low hydroxylysine, few sites of hydroxylysine glycosylation
II	$[\alpha 1(II)]_3$	Cartilage	High hydroxylysine, heavily glycosylated

TABLE 2. INFLUENCE OF RATE OF GAIN ON THE DAILY NUTRIENT REQUIREMENTS OF A 230-KG, 7-MONTH-OLD WEANLING WITH EXPECTED MATURE WEIGHT OF 500 KG°

	Average Daily Gain (kg)			
	0.5	0.75	1.00	1.25
Digestible energy, Mcal	14.2	17.2	20.2	23.1
Crude protein, gm	712	860	1009	1157
Calcium, gm	25.2	33.2	41.2	49.2
Phosphorus, gm	14.0	18.4	22.9	27.3
Zinc, mg	196	237	278	319
Copper, mg	49.1	59.3	69.6	79.8

°According to the National Research Council's 1989 recommendations.

timing and relative concentrations of these hormones after each meal may alter the metabolic effects of these hormones on growing skeletal tissues. The final stages of chondrocyte differentiation and maturation depend on thyroid hormone levels, and alterations in cartilage tissue development caused by diets high in soluble carbohydrate have been demonstrated.

Protein

Although cartilage is composed primarily of protein, dietary protein appears to have little or no direct effect on developmental orthopedic disease. Protein intake will, however, influence the animal's growth rate and thus indirectly affect the amount of other nutrients required for optimum development. Conversely, restricting protein intake will slow the growth rate and reduce the weight stress on the skeletal system. If protein restriction is used to slow the growth of young horses, its restriction may also reduce skeletal development and mineralization.

Calcium and Phosphorus

Equine bone mineral is 34 to 35 per cent calcium and 17 to 18 per cent phosphorus. These two minerals are required for deposition of the hydroxyapatite crystal at the ossification sites. Inadequate cellular availability of either mineral will retard bone mineralization.

Inadequate calcium and phosphorus intakes or inappropriate ratios of these minerals (Table 3) may result in bone that is less mature than its chronological age, making it more vulnerable to traumatic stress. Excess phosphorus intake will stimulate parathormone production, which mobilizes bone calcium and stimulates urinary phosphorus excretion. This condition, called nutritional secondary hyperparathyroidism, is characterized in young horses by joint inflammation and lameness. The most severely affected bones, however, are those subjected to low levels of stress, especially facial bones, which become soft and bulge; hence the appellation "bighead." (see page 119)

Excess calcium intake, two or three times the requirement, may reduce phosphorus absorption. Therefore, young horses fed very high calcium diets require a dietary phosphorus intake above the requirement to ensure adequate phosphorus availability. High calcium intake may also reduce the availability of zinc and copper if phytic acid concentrations in the diet are elevated.

Copper

The major physiological effects of inadequate copper intake are expressed through the reduction of metalloenzymes dependent on copper. They include (1) lysyl oxidase, which is essential for the synthesis and perhaps maintenance of collagen and elastin, the major components of connective tissue, bones, and blood vessels; (2) the ferroxidase activity of ceruloplasmin, which is essential for hematopoiesis; (3) polyphenyloxidases, needed for the conversion of tyrosine to melanin; and (4) cytochrome oxidase, which apparently is required for phospholipid and superoxide dismutase (SOD) synthesis. Both may be involved in neurological function. SOD also affords protection from superoxide radical damage. There also appears to be a high correlation between serum copper and ceruloplasmin concentrations. The initial signs of copper inadequacy vary among species and with the age of the animal.

In the young growing horse, skeletal problems appear to be the most sensitive indicator of copper inadequacy. Lysyl oxidase, a copper-dependent enzyme, is essential for the oxidation of lysyl groups involved in cross-linking within the collagen molecule and between adjacent molecules. Inadequate copper, therefore, causes a reduction in cross-linkage within the collagen and increases the soluble collagen present in cartilage tissue.

It is possible that copper deficiency in utero may have a direct effect on subsequent skeletal development in growing horses. However, fetal liver copper concentrations are considerably higher than those in adult horses, suggesting that the mare preferentially provides for the needs of the fetus. Mean liver copper for ten foals at 5 to 11 months' gestation was 317 mg per kg DM ($\pm$ 153, SD) with a low of 145 and a high of 578 mg per kg DM. Serum copper concentrations at birth are quite low (13 to 36 μg per 100 ml) and increase to a plateau at about 28 days of age at 124 to 233 μg per 100 ml (Table 4).

Copper deficiency has been produced experimentally by feeding foals from 1 day of age a

TABLE 3. CALCIUM:PHOSPHORUS RATIOS FOR HORSES

Age	Minimum*	Optimum	Maximum†
Weanling	1:1	1.25:1	1.5:1
Yearling	1:1	1.50:1	2.0:1
2-year-old	1:1	2.00:1	2.5:1
Mature	1:1	2.00:1	5.0:1

*Phosphorus intakes above calcium intakes can result in nutritional secondary hyperparathyroidism and bone demineralization.

†High calcium intakes can cause hypercalcitonism, which may interfere with bone mineralization and reduce phosphorus absorption. High-calcium diets should be formulated with above-minimum phosphorus concentrations.

TABLE 4. NORMAL SERUM COPPER AND ZINC CONCENTRATIONS IN HORSES

Mineral	µg/100 ml	µmol/L
Copper		
Foals, birth	13–36	2.0–3.1
Foals, 1 mo.	124–233	19.5–36.7
Foals, 6 mo.	138–200	21.7–31.5
Mature	104–177	16.4–27.9
Zinc		
Foals, birth	75–130	11.5–19.9
Foals, 1 mo.	70–100	10.7–15.3
Foals, 6 mo.	70–100	10.7–15.3
Mature	80–122	12.2–18.7

Sources of data: Cymbaluk and Christison, 1989; Spais et al., 1977; Bell et al., 1987; Bridges et al., 1984; Bridges and Harris, 1988; Breedveld et al., 1988; Cymbaluk et al., 1986.

low-copper (1.7 mg per kg) diet. Serum copper decreased to 10 µg per 100 ml by 13 to 16 weeks. These foals developed osteochondritis dissecans, became lame, had a stilted gait, and had a 3- to 6-fold increase in soluble collagen in articular cartilage and aortic tissue. Foals with access to feed containing 14 mg Cu per kg did not develop osteochondritis dissecans.

ZINC

Zinc is an essential component of numerous enzymes, including alkaline phosphatase, carbonic anhydrase, and carboxyl peptidase A. These enzymes are involved in cartilage synthesis and mineralization and are essential for proper skeletal development. The zinc requirement for the growing horse is a 40 to 50 mg per kg diet. Although some authors suggest higher zinc concentrations to minimize developmental orthopedic diseases, no data have been published to support those recommendations.

Zinc toxicity due to zinc contamination of forages in areas adjacent to zinc smelters and similar industrial facilities results in lameness, osteochondrosis, and osteochondritis dissecans. Although intakes of zinc are difficult to establish under these conditions, feeding trials imposing zinc concentrations of 3600 mg per kg diet or higher result in elevated serum and liver zinc levels and reduced serum copper levels. The toxicity appears to manifest as induced copper inadequacy, probably due to competitive binding of the enzyme metallothionein. Some competitive effects of zinc on copper metabolism have been documented at dietary zinc concentrations as low as 150 mg per kg diet; however, other studies have been unable to demonstrate adverse effects at 500 and 1000 mg zinc per kg diet. Zinc–copper relationships in the growing horse need further elucidation.

CADMIUM

Normal dietary concentrations of cadmium do not appear to have any influence on developmental orthopedic disease. High cadmium intakes due to environmental contamination result in cadmium accumulation in the liver and kidney. Cadmium is often found in the emissions of zinc smelters and, like zinc, competes with copper for binding by metallothionein.

MOLYBDENUM

In ruminant animals, molybdenum reacts with sulfur in the rumen to produce thiomolybdates. These compounds chelate copper, reducing its absorption and metabolism and causing induced copper deficiency. Dietary molybdenum concentrations as low as 3 mg per kg diet will produce signs of copper deficiency in ruminants. Horses appear to be much less vulnerable to this interaction. Molybdenum intake of 27 ppm, which is considerably above normal dietary concentrations, reduced copper absorption from 38.5 per cent to 32.0 per cent and retention from 25.6 per cent to 17.7 per cent. Molybdenum at concentrations found in natural ingredients is unlikely to adversely affect copper absorption and metabolism in horses.

OTHER NUTRITIONAL AND PHYSIOLOGICAL FACTORS

Although ascorbic acid is not considered an essential dietary constituent for horses, this vitamin is an essential cofactor for the enzyme prolyl hydroxylase. Without this enzyme hydroxylated collagen will not form the triple helix essential for collagen stability. It has been shown in some species that young animals have an ascorbic acid requirement 25 times as high as adult animals, but no information is available on the ascorbic acid requirement of foals.

Estrogens and progesterone have been demonstrated to affect the rate of collagen synthesis. This may relate to the observation that colts are more likely to have developmental orthopedic disease than fillies.

In summary, developmental orthopedic diseases may be caused by genetics, conformational defects, trauma, or nutritionally induced abnormalities of cartilage or bone mineralization, and clinical cases usually involve two or more of these factors. Energy and protein intake influence the animal's growth rate and thus have a direct effect on its requirements for other nutrients. Highly glucogenic diets may alter hormone patterns and interfere with cartilage synthesis and maturation. Copper deficiency, simple or induced, will reduce the availability of copper-dependent enzymes and reduce the cross-linkages in collagen.

Supplemental Readings

Bridges, C. H. and Harris, E. D.: Experimentally induced cartilaginous fractures (osteochondritis dissecans) in foals fed low copper diets. J. Am. Vet. Med. Assoc., 193:215, 1988.

Eyre, D. R.: Collagen: Molecular diversity in the body's protein scaffold. Science, 207:1315, 1980.

Gunson, D. E.: Collagen in normal and abnormal tissues. Equine Vet. J., 11:97, 1979.

Knight, D. A., Weisbrode, S. E., Schmall, L. M., and Gabel, A. A.: Copper supplementation and cartilage lesions in foals. In: Proceedings of the 33rd Annual Convention of the American Association of Equine Practitioners, 1987, p. 191.

Kronfeld, D. S., and Donoghue, S.: Metabolic convergence in developmental orthopedic disease. In: Proceedings of the 33rd Annual Convention of the American Association of Equine Practitioners, 1987, p. 195.

Glade, M. J.: The control of cartilage growth in osteochondrosis: A review. Equine Vet. Sci., 6:175, 1986.

Pool, R. R.: Developmental orthopedic disease in the horse: Normal and abnormal bone formation. In: Proceedings of the 33rd Annual Convention of the American Association of Equine Practitioners, 1987, p. 143.

Rejno, S., and Stromberg, B.: Osteochondrosis in the horse: II. Pathology. Acta Radiol. Suppl., 358:153, 1978.

Stromberg, B.: A review of the salient features of osteochondrosis in the horse. Equine Vet. J., 11:211, 1979.

Thompson, K. N., Jackson, S. G., and Rooney, J. R.: The effect of above average weight gains on the incidence of radiographic bone aberrations and epiphysitis in growing horses. Equine Vet. Sci., 8:383, 1988.

Trotter, G. W., and McIlwraith, C. W.: Osteochondritis dissecans and subchondral cystic lesions and their relationship to osteochondrosis in the horse. J. Equine Vet. Sci., 1:157, 1981.

Enteral Nutritional Support of Sick Horses

William J. Burkholder, BLACKSBURG, VIRGINIA
Craig D. Thatcher, BLACKSBURG, VIRGINIA

The provision of adequate nutrition is an important component of comprehensive care in all fields of medicine. Nutrition affects all metabolic processes, but organs and cells with high rates of metabolism are more rapidly impaired by nutrient imbalances. The immune system is composed of cells that synthesize many different immune mediators and engage in dynamic cellular interactions. Nutrient deficiencies have been documented that compromise cellular and nonspecific immune function in as short a time as 3 to 5 days in several species, including the horse. Without a competent, functioning immune system, it is difficult to resolve disease, regardless of etiology.

The enterocytes of the intestinal mucosa are also metabolically dynamic cells with an average turnover rate of 3 days. Enterocytes are responsible for brush border digestion and absorption of nutrients and also provide a barrier against microbial translocation across the bowel wall into the systemic circulation. Anorexia causes intestinal mucosal atrophy, impaired digestion and absorption, and increased risk of infection from microbial translocation. Compromised enterocyte function persists for several days after refeeding begins if atrophy has occurred, with microbial overgrowth and diarrhea as likely consequences. Although other major organs require adequate energy, protein, vitamins, and minerals to function efficiently, the consequences of inadequate nutrition on the immune system and intestinal mucosa are reason enough to ensure adequate nutritional support of the sick horse.

PATIENT SELECTION

Hypophagic or dysphagic horses with infectious, inflammatory, metabolic, toxic, parasitic, or neoplastic conditions may be candidates for enteral nutritional support. The decision to initiate nutritional support can be made by integrating clinical and laboratory data that are routinely available to the veterinary practitioner. These include the dietary history, body condition score, physical examination findings, complete blood cell (CBC) count, and serum chemistries.

An accurate dietary history is necessary to determine whether the ration and the horse's consumption have been adequate in the recent past. Adequate nutrition is determined by the quality of feedstuffs and the quantity of feed consumed. A complete dietary history includes all of the ration components, the amount of feed offered and eaten, the feeding schedule, and the method of feed delivery. Water consumption and quality should also be evaluated.

The body condition of the horse is useful for determining the extent of malnutrition, the available tissue reserves, and the chances for metabolic derangements to occur if inadequate nutrition persists. Henneke et al. have proposed guidelines for assigning body condition scores of 1 to 9, where 1 represents emaciation and 9 represents extreme obesity. This scoring system is reproduced in the National Research Council's *Nutrient Requirements of Horses*, 5th rev. ed., 1989. Horses with scores of 1 to 3 have few reserves to sustain periods of high nutrient demands. Horses that are anoretic with body conditions of 8 or 9 are in danger of developing hyperlipidemia and subsequent liver dysfunction from hepatic lipidosis. Body condition scoring can easily be incorporated into the routine physical examination. Poor condition of the hooves, skin, hair coat, mucous membranes, and teeth and muscle atrophy can also indicate the presence of malnutrition.

Changes in the CBC and serum chemistries can occur if malnutrition is prolonged and severe. Anemia, lymphopenia, decreased plasma or serum total protein, decreased albumin, decreased serum electrolytes, and increased serum triglycerides coupled with other signs described above indicate the need for nutritional support. However, the appearance of these changes may be delayed for days to weeks after nutrient intake becomes inadequate. The hypophagic or anorectic horse will benefit from nutritional support before changes are observed in the CBC or serum profile; therefore, the practitioner should not delay instituting nutritional support in the absence of these changes. Persistent, insufficient consumption or anorexia for 3 to 5 days or longer is a good indication that nutritional support is required. The disease itself may be predictive of the need for nutritional support. Nutritional support should be instituted early if the clinician documents that the horse cannot or will not eat on its own.

The horse consuming an insufficient quantity of feed should be encouraged to meet daily nutrient requirements by increasing voluntary intake. Meeting nutrient requirements by increasing consumption is easier than force feeding nutrients to the horse. Hospitalized horses should be offered feeds similar to those fed at home. The dietary history is beneficial for ensuring that hospital and home rations are similar. However, if feeds similar to the home ration are offered and intake remains low, offering a variety of feedstuffs may help. Fresh pasture, leafy hays, rolled grains, and sweet feeds are examples of highly palatable feeds, although the horse may show preference for other feedstuffs. Consideration of whether the primary disease is aided or exacerbated by the type of ration eaten is important in the evaluation of alternate feeds (see p. 736).

Ration changes should be made gradually over several days. Sudden ration changes can result in laminitis, diarrhea, and colic. Increases in concentrates or grains should be limited to no more than 0.5 kg per day for a 500-kg horse. If alfalfa hay is substituted for grass hay, the alfalfa should gradually replace the grass hay over a 5-day period. Feed intake should be monitored to determine if voluntary consumption adequately meets the nutrient requirements of the horse. Requirements may be determined from the National Research Council's *Nutrient Requirements of Horses*, 5th rev. ed., 1989. Daily intake of energy, crude protein, calcium, and phosphorus should routinely be determined for all hospitalized equine patients and compared to nutrient requirements. Requirements are tabulated in increments of 100 kg of body weight for horses weighing between 400 and 900 kg. Maintenance digestible energy (DE) requirements for horses weighing 200 to 600 kg may be estimated from the equation $DE = 1.4 + 0.03 \times$ body weight (kg). Maintenance energy requirements for horses weighing 601 to 900 kg are estimated by the equation $DE = 1.82 + (0.0383 \times \text{body weight (kg)}) - (0.000015 \times \text{body weight}^2)$. Requirements for crude protein (CP) may be estimated by $CP = 40 \times DE$. Calcium requirements can be estimated using $Ca = 0.04 \times$ body weight (kg), and phosphorus from $P = 0.028 \times$ body weight (kg).

Nutrition should be provided by another route if voluntary intake of an acceptable ration is not adequate within 3 to 5 days after the onset of anorexia. Either enteral or parenteral routes can be used to provide sufficient quantities of nutrients to a horse not consuming enough feed to meet daily requirements. Enteral feeding via nasogastric, nasoesophageal, or esophagostomy tubes to provide nutritional support to the anoretic horse will be discussed in this chapter.

Enteral feeding has the advantages of being more physiologic with less potential for causing metabolic derangements than parenteral nutrition. Enteral nutrition is also less expensive and simpler to perform than parenteral nutrition. In addition, enteral nutrition maintains the function and structure of the gastrointestinal (GI) tract.

Hypophagic or anoretic horses that have a normally functioning GI tract from the stomach aborally are candidates for enteral alimentation. The horse undergoing tube feeding should be able to maintain sternal recumbency and hold its head above the level of its stomach to minimize the chance of gastric reflux and subsequent aspiration pneumonia. Clinical indications of a normally functioning GI tract include normal frequency and intensity of gut sounds on abdominal auscultation, lack of gastric reflux, and normal feces. Enteral feeding in the horse is contraindicated in several conditions. For example, lateral recumbency, head carriage below the level of the stomach, and dementia all increase the possibility of aspiration of refluxed food. Ileus and gastric reflux are also indications to avoid the enteral route for nutritional support. Horses with serum albumin levels less than 2.0 mg per dl may not be capable of absorbing nutrients from the GI tract and may develop diarrhea from hyperosmotic intestinal contents. Parenteral nutrition should be considered for nutritional support in patients that cannot tolerate enteral feeding (see p. 732).

PLACEMENT AND MAINTENANCE OF FEEDING TUBES

Slurries based on alfalfa meal, complete pelleted feeds, or commercial liquid products may be fed through nasogastric or esophagostomy tubes (Table 1). Placement of a large-bore stomach tube (internal diameter 12.7 mm or larger) facilitates administration of alfalfa meal or pellet slurries. An inexpensive marine bilge pump may be required to deliver the slurry through the tube. Commercial liquid diets can be gravity fed using a funnel and a smaller foal-size tube (internal diameter 6.35 mm). Enteral feeding tubes should be open-ended because closed-ended, fenestrated tubes are easily occluded and require higher pressure to force slurries and liquids through the openings. Open-ended feeding tubes are also easier to clear if they become obstructed.

Nasogastric intubation is the choice for enteral feeding tubes unless the nasal passages, pharynx, or proximal cervical esophagus need to be bypassed. A water-soluble lubricant should be applied to the tube before it is passed. The tube can be left in place or passed at each feeding. However, repeated tube passage is traumatic and may not be tolerated by the patient. The tube should be left in place if more than two feedings per day are required or if the horse objects to the tube being passed. A halter is used to secure the tube

TABLE 1. EXAMPLES OF RATIONS USED FOR TUBE FEEDING

Recipes for Slurries	
*Alfalfa/casein dextrose slurry**	*Pellet-vegetable oil slurry‡*
454 gm alfalfa meal	454 gm Complete Pelleted Horse Feed§
204 gm casein†	
204 gm dextrose	46 gm (50 ml) corn oil
52 gm electrolyte mixture (see below)	2–3 L water
5 L water	
Electrolyte Mixture for Alfalfa/casein dextrose slurry	*Commercial Enteral Products*
10 gm sodium chloride (NaCl)	Osmolite HN¶
15 gm sodium bicarbonate (NaHCO$_3$)	EquiCal¶
75 gm potassium chloride (KCl)	
60 gm potassium phosphate (dibasic anhydrous) (K$_2$HPO$_4$)	
45 gm calcium chloride (CaCl$_2 \cdot$ 2H$_2$O)	
25 gm magnesium oxide (MgO)	

*Adapted from Naylor, J. M., Freeman, D. E., and Kronfeld, D. S.: Alimentation of hypophagic horses. Compend. Cont. Educ. Pract. Vet., 6(2):S93–S100, 1984. (Reproduced by permission.)
†Casein (Sigma Chemical Co.) or dehydrated cottage cheese—82% crude protein with less than 2% lactose (American Nutritional).
‡Adapted from Hand, M. S.: Equine Critical Care Nutrition. Mark Morris Associates, Topeka, Kansas.
§Horse Chow 200, (Purina Mills, Inc.)
¶Ross Laboratories, Columbus, OH.

in place by passing the tube through the halter fittings and taping the tube to the cheek and gullet straps (Fig. 1). Indwelling tubes can cause rhinitis, pharyngitis, and erosion or ulceration of esophageal or gastric mucosa. Rhinitis may be reduced by relocating the tube to the alternate nostril every 2 or 3 days.

The proper location for the distal end of a nasal feeding tube in horses is presently debated. There are rationales for placing the tube either in the caudal thoracic esophagus or in the stomach. Advocates for stomach placement of the tube believe the equine thoracic esophagus is not efficient in propelling feed into the stomach without initiation of a contractile wave associated with normal swallowing. However, more reflux is observed in horses with esophagostomy tubes placed in the stomach rather than in the caudal thoracic esophagus.

Horses with trauma or inflammation of the nasal, pharyngeal, or proximal cervical esophageal areas and horses that have undergone surgical procedures in these areas may require an esophagostomy tube for enteral alimentation. Candidates for enteral feeding by cervical esophagostomy should be carefully selected because of the potential complications and the length of time the esophagostomy tube must be

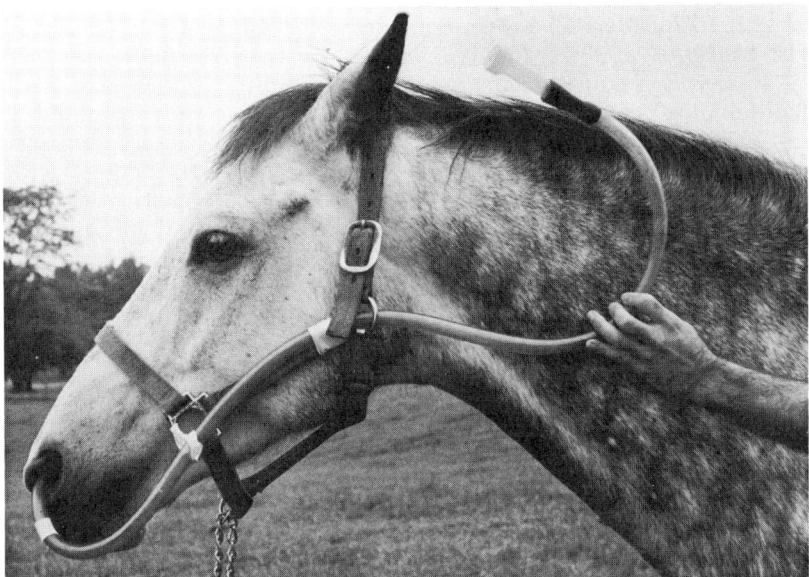

Figure 1. Placement of nasogastric tube for enteral nutrition. The tube is attached to the halter and is plugged with a syringe case.

maintained. Nasogastric feedings or parenteral nutrition offer more practical alternatives for short-term nutritional support of the equine patient.

Practitioners contemplating using an esophagostomy tube should refer to the articles by Freeman and Naylor and by Stick, Derksen and Scott in the supplemental readings list for complete details on the surgical procedure for placing the tube. Briefly, the esophagostomy is created at the junction of the middle and caudal thirds of the cervical esophagus. Depending on facilities, patient temperament, and clinician preference, the procedure can be performed with the patient under local or general anesthesia. A second stomach tube should be placed in the esophagus prior to the procedure to aid in identification and manipulation of the esophagus during surgery. An esophagostomy feeding tube should remain in place for at least 10 days to allow formation of a fibrous seal between the esophageal stoma and surrounding tissue. The esophagostomy tube should be passed into the stomach and securely sutured adjacent to the skin incision and on both sides of the neck to ensure that the tube is not prematurely dislodged. Attempts to replace an esophagostomy tube that is inadvertently removed can result in misdirection of the tube into the mediastinum and subsequent death of the horse from feed introduced into the thoracic cavity. Other potential complications include local swelling and infection, formation of draining fistulous tracts, mediastinitis and abscesses, damage to the recurrent laryngeal nerve, and delayed closure of the primary fistula after the tube is removed.

Tubes should be flushed with water following each feeding. The tube should be closed with a rubber stopper or plastic syringe case between feedings to prevent gastric distention from air (see Fig. 1). An obstructed tube should first be lavaged with water to attempt removal of the obstruction. Lavage at the obstruction can be accomplished by passing a small polyethylene tube down the feeding tube and flushing through the smaller tube. The feeding tube can be filled with a carbonated cola beverage, capped, and left for about 20 minutes if water lavage fails to clear the obstruction. The dilute carbonic acid in colas often digests food plugs sufficiently for the obstruction to be removed with lavage. Lastly, if these attempts fail, a probang can be used to push the plug from the tube. Care should be taken if using a probang because of possible trauma or puncture of the esophagus or stomach.

ESTABLISHING NUTRITIONAL GOALS

An estimate of the nutrient requirements for the horse is necessary to establish a reasonable enteral feeding protocol. A hypophagic horse may voluntarily consume a significant portion of its daily nutrient requirements, with the difference provided by tube feeding. However, the stress of tube feeding and the presence of increased food in the GI tract may cause the horse to become anoretic. The total daily requirements will then need to be delivered via the feeding tube.

The requirements of the sick horse should initially be based on the horse's present body weight. In most patients it is a challenge, even with multiple feedings, to administer more than the total volume of liquid or slurry to meet daily maintenance requirements for the patient's current body weight. Requirements for growth or to regain body tissue may be met after the primary disease has been corrected and adequate voluntary intake has returned. Furthermore, overfeeding can have as detrimental an effect on the course of disease as underfeeding or neglecting nutritional support entirely. Specific nutrient requirements have not been determined for sick horses; however, reasonable estimates may be derived using data from sick humans and the National Research Council's *Nutrient Requirements of Horses*. Humans with various illnesses have energy requirements between 60 and 100 per cent of normal maintenance requirements. For example, surgical patients without complications have energy requirements around 60 per cent of maintenance energy requirements, while cranial trauma or septic patients require maintenance energy levels. Horses confined to metabolism stalls have energy requirements that are 70 per cent of maintenance energy requirements for nonworking horses. No measurements have been made for sick horses using a metabolism stall to our knowledge. The sick horse is likely to benefit if sufficient feed can be provided to supply nutrient levels between 60 and 100 per cent of maintenance requirements based on the limited data cited above.

DIETS

Table 1 lists four diets that may be delivered through a nasogastric or esophagostomy tube. Two are commercially available products and two must be prepared from the constituent ingredients. Other complete pelleted horse feeds can be pulverized dry in a kitchen blender and mixed with water to make a slurry. Water should not be added to alfalfa or pellet meals until just before the slurry is administered. The cellulose in the meal will swell and produce a thick viscous mixture if water is added and the cellulose allowed to fully hydrate. Vegetable oil can be added to increase the energy density of slurried rations. Diets should be selected to ensure that nutrient levels are appropriate for the age and disease of the horse being fed. Products containing lactose should be avoided in adult horses because adult horses do not produce enough lactase to digest this sugar.

Alteration of the diet's nutrient profile may be beneficial in certain diseases. Energy sources from predominantly carbohydrates may be desirable in horses with hyperlipidemia, while high-fat diets may aid horses with respiratory disease. Horses with hepatic or renal dysfunction may benefit from protein sources containing higher contents of branched-chain amino acids and less aromatic amino acids. The level and type of fiber may be a concern in horses suffering from chronic diarrhea or recovering from intestinal resections. The reader is referred to page 737 for more in-depth considerations of altered nutrient profiles and diets for specific diseases. Table 2 shows the calculated nutrient profiles of the diets in Table 1 compared to maintenance nutrient requirements for a 500-kg adult horse.

DAILY FEED AMOUNTS AND FEEDING FREQUENCY

After a diet has been selected, the amount required per day is determined by dividing the nutrient requirement of the horse by the nutrient

TABLE 2. NUTRIENT PROFILE OF ENTERAL DIETS SUPPLYING DAILY MAINTENANCE ENERGY REQUIREMENTS FOR A 500-KG ADULT HORSE

Nutrient	Requirements*	Alfalfa/Casein/Dextrose Slurry	Pellet–Vegetable Oil Slurry	Osmolite HN†	Equical†
Energy (DE), Mcal	16.4	16.4	16.4	16.4	16.4
Protein, gm	656	1,710	682	688	742
Calcium, gm	20	81	32	11.7	32.8
Phosphorus, gm	14	41	20	11.7	22.4
Sodium, gm	8.2	16.2	10	14.4	25.9
Potassium, gm	25	159	—	24.2	29.3
Magnesium, gm	7.5	97	10	4.7	10.4
Copper, mg	82	35	122	23.6	120.8
Zinc, mg	328	100	438	264	414
Iron, mg	328	984	389	211	414
Selenium, mg	0.82	0.9	1.5	—	1.2

*Source: National Academy of Sciences: *Nutrient Requirements of Horses*, 5th rev. ed. Washington, D. C., National Academy of Sciences, National Research Council, 1989.
†Ross Laboratories, Columbus, OH.

content in the diet. Examples of calculations to determine the total feed required for the diets listed are provided in Table 3. Determining the amount of feed to meet the energy requirement automatically provides the required levels of all other nutrients *if* the diet has been balanced on an energy density basis. The daily amount of each ingredient in a multi-component slurry can be determined by multiplying the ingredient amount per recipe by the total recipes required per day. This calculation is shown in Table 4.

The number of feedings per day is determined after the total amount of ration required daily is calculated. Several factors limit the amount of diet that can be fed at any one feeding. The first is the small capacity of the equine stomach. A 500-kg adult horse has an average stomach capacity of 7 to 7.5 liters. The stomach capacity is smaller if the horse has not eaten for several days, and therefore the horse initially may not tolerate the expected volume. Second, the ration is likely to be a significant dietary change for the horse. As stated, ration changes should be made gradually. Third, large quantities of food introduced suddenly into the stomach of an anorectic horse may cause delayed gastric emptying. Delayed gastric emptying could result in movement of water into the GI tract, colic, and diarrhea, especially if the diet has an osmolarity of greater than 300 mOsm per liter. Incremental increases over 3 to 5 days are necessary to bring horses to the full amount of feed because of these three factors. One third of the calculated amount of feed should be administered the first day, two thirds the second day, and the full amount of feed may be fed on the third day if no adverse reactions have occurred. Hyperosmolar diets can initially be diluted with additional water to reduce the osmolarity. The additional water can gradually be withdrawn over the first 3 to 5 days. Mixing the feed for days 1 and 2 in the total volume of water required in the full amount of feed for day 3 achieves this dilution and gradual withdrawal. Table 5 lists the amounts of feed and water for the pellet–vegetable oil slurry that would be attempted with a 500-kg adult horse over the first 3 days of feeding. Liquid diets that are isosmolar such as Osmolite HN and EquiCal need not be diluted, but the horse should be gradually adapted to the full amount.

The final determination is how much volume to give at each feeding. Small volumes, from one quarter to one half of the expected stomach volume, should be fed at frequent intervals the first day. For example a 500-kg adult horse should initially receive 2 to 4 liters of slurry every 2 to 4 hours (Table 6). The volume can be gradually increased and the feeding frequency decreased if the horse tolerates the initial feedings. Commercial liquid diets can be fed as a constant infusion using a fluid administration pump. Continuous infusion, if possible, may be advantageous in horses that prove intolerant of bolus feedings. The volume of solution opened or reconstituted should be infused within a 12-hour period to avoid bacterial growth and spoilage. The horse

TABLE 3. QUANTITY OF DIETS REQUIRED PER DAY TO MEET DAILY ENERGY REQUIREMENT[*]

Diet	Energy Required	Energy per Recipe or Liter of Diet	Recipes or Liters Needed per Day
Alfalfa/casein/dextrose slurry	16.4 Mcal	2.77 Mcal/recipe	16.4/2.77 = 5.9 recipes
Pellet–vegetable oil slurry	16.4 Mcal	1.53 Mcal/recipe	16.4/1.53 = 10.7 recipes
Osmolite HN	16.4 Mcal	1.06 Mcal/L	16.4/1.06 = 15.5 L
EquiCal	16.4 Mcal	1.00 Mcal/L	16.4/1.00 = 16.4 L

[*]Daily energy requirement for a 500-kg adult horse = 16.4 Mcal of digestible energy.

TABLE 4. TOTAL FEED REQUIRED PER DAY TO MEET A 500 KG ADULT HORSE'S MAINTENANCE REQUIREMENTS[*]

Ingredient	Amount/Recipe	×	No. Recipes Needed/Day	=	Total Ingredients Needed/Day
Alfalfa/casein/dextrose slurry					
Alfalfa meal	454 gm	×	5.9	=	2679 gm alfalfa meal
Casein	204 gm	×	5.9	=	1204 gm casein
Dextrose	204 gm	×	5.9	=	1204 gm dextrose
Electrolyte mixture	52 gm	×	5.9	=	307 gm electrolyte mixture
Water	5 L	×	5.9	=	30 L water
Pellet–Vegetable Oil Slurry					
Complete Pelleted Horse Feed	454 gm	×	10.7	=	4860 gm complete pellet
Corn oil	46 gm	×	10.7	=	492 gm (535 ml) corn oil
Water	3 L	×	10.7	=	32 L water

[*]Total ingredients needed for 1 day are determined by multiplying the amount per recipe by the total recipes per day.

TABLE 5. AMOUNTS OF FEED AND WATER USED TO INITIATE ENTERAL FEEDING FOR A 500-KG ADULT HORSE USING THE PELLET–VEGETABLE OIL SLURRY

Ingredient	Day 1: ⅓ Food	Day 2: ⅔ Food	Day 3: Full Food
Complete Pelleted Horse Feed	1620 gm	3240 gm	4860 gm
Corn oil	164 gm (178 ml)	328 gm (357 ml)	492 gm (535 ml)
Water	32 L	32 L	32 L

TABLE 6. VOLUMES AND FREQUENCIES TO INITIATE ENTERAL TUBE FEEDING FOR A 500-KG ADULT HORSE

Day	Total Volume(L)	Volume per Feeding(L)	Feeding Frequency (hr)	Feedings per Day
Pellet–Vegetable Oil Slurry				
1	21	2–4	2–4	6–8
2	25	3–5	3–6	4–6
3	32	5–6	4–6	4–6
4	32	6–8	5–6	4–5
5	32	8	6	4
EquiCal				
1	5.5	1–2	5–6	4
2	11.0	2–3	5–6	5
3	16.4	3–5	5–6	4–5
4	16.4	4–6	6–8	3–4

must be monitored closely to avoid distention of the stomach, gastric reflux, and colic if the infusion is not tolerated.

Daily fluid requirements of the horse should be calculated. Horses on forced enteral nutritional support that are able to drink should have free access to good-quality water. Dietary water intake plus voluntary water consumption should be monitored to ensure adequate fluid intake. Additional water can be administered through the feeding tube if the horse does not consume enough water to meet its fluid requirements.

MONITORING

The equine patient should be monitored for complications from feeding after enteral nutritional support is initiated. Indications for discontinuing tube feeding include gastric reflux, GI ileus, abdominal distention, colic, and increased digital pulse. Tube feeding should be discontinued or the time between feedings increased if residual feed can be easily evacuated from the stomach into the feeding tube just before the next scheduled feeding. The next feeding should be postponed if 75 per cent or more of the previous meal is evacuated from the stomach. Half the volume of the next feeding may be given if 50 per cent of the previous meal remains. The total volume can be given if 25 per cent or less of the previous feeding is present.

Residual food should be replaced in the stomach to avoid depletion of hydrogen and chloride and to stimulate gastric emptying. Evacuation of large quantities of feed indicates poor gastric emptying and the lack of space in the stomach to accommodate additional food. The abdomen should be auscultated between feedings to assess GI activity and the abdominal contour observed for signs of distention. Results from feeding tube aspirations and GI activity can be integrated to assess potential ingesta flow through the digestive tract. The amount and character of the feces should also be recorded. Horses fed slurries or commercial enteral diets frequently develop loose or unformed stools. Diarrhea caused by enteral diets is generally accompanied by normal hemograms and normal body temperatures. The diarrhea readily resolves once tube feeding is stopped. Laminitis is also a potential complication, because slurries and other liquid diets usually contain relatively high levels of soluble carbohydrates. The character and strength of the digital pulse should be assessed between feedings and the feedings decreased or discontinued if strong bounding pulses are present.

Routine clinical and laboratory parameters useful in deciding that nutritional support is indicated are equally useful for assessing the effects of nutritional support, as well as the effects of other therapeutics on the patient. Serum and urine glucose levels can indicate whether carbohydrates are being utilized or wasted. Similarly, serum triglyceride levels may be useful in determining the energy balance of the patient. The combination of serum albumin, total protein, urea nitrogen, and ammonia levels can provide an assessment of nitrogen utilization. Packed cell volume can indicate the adequacy, deficit, or surplus of fluid provided by the diet. Serum electrolytes should be monitored and corrected as required, with either dietary manipulation of specific salts or appropriate provision of intravenous fluid therapy. A return of hematological and biochemical parameters to normal is always encouraging, but an improvement in general attitude, maintenance of body weight, and a return of appetite and voluntary feed consumption are important clinical indications of the effectiveness of enteral nutrition. Body weight should be measured twice weekly if scales are available. The willingness of the horse to eat should be determined 6 to 8 hours after the last forced feeding. At the time voluntary intake reaches an acceptable level, preferably 60 to 80 per cent of maintenance requirements, forced enteral feedings may be discontinued.

SPECIAL CONSIDERATIONS

Horses less than 2 years old present additional logistical and nutritional challenges. The smaller size of young growing horses further limits the volume per feeding and the size of tube that can be used. Neonatal foals will require mare's milk or milk replacer until weaning. The reader is referred to page 741 for in-depth information on feeding foals. Diets fed to young horses must be higher in nutrient concentrations than adult horse rations to maintain body weight. Protein usually is the limiting nutrient if commercially available feeds are used for enteral nutritional support of young horses. The addition of 10 gm of casein to 200 gm of EquiCal powder, or 30 gm per recipe of the pellet–vegetable oil slurry, provides enough protein to meet requirements for growing horses between 6 and 24 months old. Young growing horses are less tolerant of nutrient deprivation and, if anoretic, may deteriorate rapidly.

There are two exceptions to the general recommendation of providing maintenance requirements for the horse's present body weight. Mares in the last 3 months of gestation should be fed nutrient levels for their weight and stage of gestation to support normal development of the fetus. Mares that are lactating have the highest nutrient requirements of any category of horse. It is difficult to maintain lactation in a mare with a serious illness. Therefore, a more practical alternative may be to feed the foal as an orphan or graft the foal onto another mare. The higher requirements for lactation will need to be met if maintenance of lactation is an objective in the nutritional management of the sick mare nursing a foal.

Delays in implementing nutritional support may reduce the likelihood of a successful therapeutic outcome. Nutritional support should be considered and instituted early in the course of disease or disorder to optimize the chance for success of other therapeutic interventions. Normal animals are not expected to grow or perform to their potential without adequate nutrition. The expectation for the immune system to perform competently and for tissue repair to occur in the face of inadequate nutrition is contrary to the requirements of the underlying metabolism and physiology.

Supplemental Readings

Freeman, D. E., and Naylor, J. M.: Cervical esophagostomy to permit extraoral feeding of the horse. J. Am. Vet. Med. Assoc., 172:314–320, 1978.

Henneke, D. R., Potter, G. D., Kreider, J. L., and Yeates, B. F.: Relationship between condition score, physical measurements and body fat percentage in mares. Equine Vet. J., 15:371–372, 1983.

National Academy of Sciences: Nutrient Requirements of Horses, 5th rev. ed. Washington, D. C., National Academy of Sciences, National Research Council, 1989.

Naylor, J. M., Freeman, D. E., and Kronfeld, D. S.: Alimentation of hypophagic horses. Compend. Cont. Educ. Pract. Vet., 6(2):S93–S100, 1984.

Naylor, J. M., and Kenyon, S. J.: Effect of total calorie deprivation on host defence in the horse. Res. Vet. Sci., 31:369–372, 1981.

Rombeau, J. L., and Caldwell, M. D.: Enteral Tube Feeding. Philadelphia, W. B. Saunders, 1984.

Stick, J. A., Derksen, F. J., and Scott, E. A.: Equine cervical esophagostomy: Complications associated with duration and location of feeding tubes. Am. J. Vet. Res., 42:727–732, 1981.

Parenteral Nutrition

Shauna L. Spurlock, LOVETTSVILLE, VIRGINIA
Michael V. Ward, IRVINE, CALIFORNIA

The nutritional well-being of septic, traumatized, and postoperative patients has been the focus of increasing attention in both veterinary and human medicine. Enteral nutrition is inexpensive and serves as a direct source of nutrients for gastrointestinal (GI) mucosa (see page 724). However, there are disease conditions that preclude the use of the GI tract. Parenteral nutrition has been used successfully in such cases in humans for over 20 years and more recently in horses.

PATIENT SELECTION

The indications for parenteral nutrition include (1) inability to obtain access to the GI tract because of pharyngeal masses or other obstructions that prevent passage of food or a nasogastric tube, (2) intolerance of food in the GI tract as a result of dynamic or paralytic ileus caused by anterior enteritis, GI tract surgery, neonatal sepsis, or neonatal necrotizing enterocolitis, and (3) GI diseases, such as inflammatory bowel disease or severe diarrhea, that impair digestion and assimilation of nutrients.

Although a number of laboratory tests are available to evaluate nutritional status in horses, most cannot distinguish the effects of disease from those of nutrient deprivation and do not provide early indications of nutritional deprivation. Nutritional support is best directed at anticipating and thus reducing the severity of nutritional deficiencies. Therefore, the horse's clinical condition and the predicted course of the disease should be used as the major guidelines for nutritional support.

Parenteral nutrition should be considered if enteral nutrition is to be withheld from an adult horse for over 3 days or if a neonatal patient is to be deprived of food for more than 24 to 36 hours. The initiation of parenteral nutrition is not an emergency procedure. Any fluid or electrolyte deficits should be corrected first and the patient should be in stable condition before nutrient delivery is initiated.

ENERGY REQUIREMENTS

The energy requirements should be calculated for each patient. Controversy exists as to the level of caloric support needed by sick, confined animals. Some clinicians advocate the use of basal energy requirements, generally assumed to be one-half maintenance requirements. Others use maintenance requirements [DE (Mcal/day) = $0.075 + (0.021 \times$ body weight (kg))]. Another energy estimate is 33 kcal per kg per day, which has been shown to maintain body weight in normal adult horses fed intravenously (IV).

The patient's problems may increase metabolic rate and therefore energy expenditure. Elective abdominal surgery and extensive small intestinal resection increase maintenance energy requirements by 10 per cent or more. Major trauma increases requirements up to 20 per cent. Severe infections result in a 30 per cent increase, and burns may increase energy demands by as much as 100 per cent. Equine surgical patients fed IV according to these guidelines have an initial postsurgical weight loss with weight gain starting 10 to 14 days after the surgical procedure.

ENERGY SOURCES

Protein, lipid, and dextrose can all be used as energy sources. The caloric density of each varies. Protein provides roughly 4 cal per gm. Dextrose contributes 3.4 cal per gm when given IV. Lipids are the most calorie dense source, with roughly 9 cal per gm. In choosing the amount of each component to be included in the formulation, it is essential to consider not only the energy requirements of the patient and changes in nutrient utilization that accompany a specific disease but also the proper blend of nutrients to facilitate appropriate utilization. For example, the hypermetabolic state that follows trauma or infection is characterized by increased lipid utilization, breakdown of body proteins, and decreased peripheral utilization of glucose. Additional factors that influence nutrient utilization include hepatic or renal dysfunction and are discussed in the following article (see page 736).

SELECTION OF NUTRIENTS IN PARENTERAL MIXTURES

CARBOHYDRATE

Carbohydrate is a primary source of energy in the healthy animal. Despite reduced utilization of carbohydrates in severely injured or septic animals, dextrose is still necessary for the body to oxidize free fatty acids via the citric acid cycle.

Due to the relatively low caloric density of glucose, it is difficult to provide total caloric support with this energy source. Hypertonic dextrose solutions (greater than 10 per cent dextrose) are irritating to vascular endothelium and therefore in humans, hypertonic formulations are infused via a central venous catheter. In horses, dextrose concentrations up to 25 per cent of total formulation have been delivered safely via a peripheral jugular catheter without the development of phlebitis. To minimize this risk, however, catheters made of nonthrombogenic materials such as Silastic or polyurethane are essential (see p. 407).

Carbohydrate administration also preserves body protein, a primary goal of nutritional support. To take advantage of the nitrogen-sparing effects and to deliver adequate calories, a mixed-fuel system may be used, with 40 to 60 per cent of the nonnitrogen calories as dextrose and 50 to 60 per cent as lipid. In the majority of equine patients, this energy mixture is well tolerated.

Although some glucose is essential, excessive carbohydrate administration may be deleterious. Infusion of hypertonic glucose without protein or lipid is contraindicated because it induces hepatic lipidosis. Parenteral glucose administration elicits an insulin response that suppresses muscle catabolism, decreases the release of free fatty acids from adipose tissue, and enhances triglyceride clearance and tissue uptake through lipogenesis. Patients with sepsis or trauma have increased cortisol, adrenalin, and glucagon levels that cause a degree of insulin resistance, which reduces the inhibition of catabolism while continuing to suppress lipolysis. To minimize this potential complication, a stepwise increase in the level of glucose administered is advised, with periodic evaluation of serum and urine glucose concentrations.

If the renal threshold for glucose (approximately 200 to 220 mg per dl) is exceeded, glucosuria and an osmotic diuresis occur. If blood glucose levels exceed 150 mg per dl, the rate of glucose administration is decreased. If that fails to correct the hyperglycemia or leads to inadequate caloric intake, exogenous insulin may be given. However, in the likely presence of already elevated blood insulin levels, exogenous insulin may be of minimal use. In patients that have been tolerating a certain level of glucose administration, sudden intolerance may indicate the development of an infection or deterioration of the patient's clinical condition.

Once insulin levels are elevated, abrupt cessation of infusion may lead to profound hypoglycemia, coma, and seizures. This response is more likely to occur in debilitated patients. In human and canine patients that are well nourished, rapid decreases in glucose infusion rates do not produce hypoglycemia; however, in premature infants and malnourished or stressed patients, an 8- to 12-hour weaning period is recommended. This same protocol should be followed for equine patients.

LIPID

Lipid emulsions provide the most calorically dense nutrient and are a source of essential fatty acids. Commercial lipid emulsions contain long-chain triglycerides that are derived from either soybean or safflower oils. Glycerol, a carbohydrate energy source, is added to make these emulsions isotonic; egg phospholipid is added as an emulsifier. The resulting emulsion provides 9 cal per gm of lipid and 3.4 cal per gm of glycerol, or 1.1 and 2.0 kcal per ml in 10 per cent and 20 per cent lipid emulsions, respectively. These emulsions are isotonic and nonirritating to veins.

Metabolic clearance of lipid involves hydrolysis of triglyceride by lipoprotein lipase. Decreased lipid clearance related to prematurity and gram-negative sepsis has been observed in equine patients. Lipid emulsions should therefore be used with caution in dysmature foals or septic horses. Lipid clearance may be enhanced by the concurrent administration of heparin, dextrose, or insulin.

Lipid emulsions given in excess may overload the reticuloendothelial system, reducing the clearance of all particulate and cellular matter, and have an adverse effect on the function of the lung.

Factors to be considered when choosing the ratios of glucose to lipid in parenteral nutrition solutions include (1) concurrent disease processes and the anticipated ability of the patient to utilize glucose and fat, (2) the nitrogen-sparing effect of 40 to 50 per cent glucose calories, (3) the potential complications, (4) the ease of administration, (5) safety, (6) costs, and (7) anticipated duration of therapy. Parenteral nutrition mixtures containing lipid and minimal glucose might be considered for short-term administration in cases where pulmonary function is compromised or in patients experiencing glucose intolerance. Glucose-based parenteral nutrition is generally less expensive but requires the delivery of an extremely hypertonic formulation. It should be reserved for patients that have disorders of lipid metabolism.

PROTEIN

To maximize nitrogen retention in clinically ill patients, a combined, balanced amount of both energy and protein must be provided. However, the precise amount of protein required by the equine patient and the ideal amino acid ratios are unclear. In veterinary medicine, crystalline amino acid solutions have replaced the previously used protein hydrolysates as sources of nitrogen. Adverse anaphylactic reactions, commonly seen with the latter, have not been encountered with the crystalline solutions. In addition, pure crystalline amino acids are more effectively utilized than protein hydrolysates. Commercially available amino acid solutions range in concentration from 3.5 to 15 per cent, with an 8.5 per cent solution used most routinely for veterinary patients. These provide essential and nonessential amino acids in the easily utilizable L form.

As with other nutrients, excess protein may have detrimental effects. Excess protein leads to increasing urinary protein excretion, elevated plasma urea and amino acid concentrations, acidosis, osmotic diuresis, and an increase in metabolic rate. Impaired liver function or a relative deficiency of arginine, the rate-limiting substrate in urea synthesis, may result in the accumulation of ammonia in the blood. An increase in plasma urea is commonly observed prior to the appearance of increased blood ammonia levels. Protein administration requires periodic determination of blood urea nitrogen.

Protein requirements for adult horses have been estimated to be 0.49 to 0.68 gm per kg per day, with 0.60 appropriate for most healthy horses. Because of the increased demands for protein in the diseased horse, 1.0 to 1.5 gm per kg per day is typically delivered to adult equine patients.

The nonprotein calorie to gram of nitrogen ratio is used as an index to ensure that a favorable balance between protein and nonprotein calories is achieved. Applying this ratio theoretically allows optimal energy and protein utilization. A ratio between 150 and 300 has been adopted for equine patients. As the protein source is 16 per cent nitrogen, the number of grams of nitrogen available from an amino acid solution can be approximated by dividing the total number of grams of protein by 6.25.

FLUIDS AND ELECTROLYTES

Maintenance of fluid volumes and electrolyte concentration must also be considered in any patient with no oral intake of fluids. Correction of fluid deficits should be addressed before parenteral nutrition is initiated. Electrolytes may be delivered by using commercial crystalline amino acid solutions that contain electrolytes, by administering supplemental crystalloid solutions, or by specifically compounding fluids to meet the animal's requirements. Sodium, potassium, and chloride are compatible with most parenteral nutrition admixtures. Therefore, the necessary volume of crystalline solution usually may be added to the parenteral nutrition formulation. However, calcium and hypertonic solutions may "break" lipid emulsions and precipitate amino acids. If large amounts of electrolyte supplementation are necessary, particularly of calcium, caution should be used in mixing. To avoid this potential complication, a second peripheral venous line is recommended in patients requiring high levels of electrolyte supplementation.

Periodic laboratory evaluation of serum electrolyte levels is essential. Electrolyte imbalances most commonly encountered in the sick patient include increased or decreased calcium and phosphorus levels, increased or decreased potassium levels, and decreased magnesium levels.

Potassium deficits may be encountered because high levels of dextrose tend to drive potassium into the cells, or because intracellular potassium is liberated and then excreted during cell breakdown. Potassium and nitrogen deficits may therefore coexist during catabolic states. Increased serum potassium concentrations may be encountered with overly aggressive supplementation, decreased renal function, tissue necrosis, and sepsis. For these reasons, supplementation with potassium should be accompanied by laboratory monitoring of potassium levels as well as acid–base status. Acidosis causes potassium shifts that mask existing potassium deficits. For each 0.1 drop in pH, serum potassium levels may increase by 0.5 per cent.

Magnesium, which is not routinely measured in most clinical laboratories, may also be deficient in patients receiving parenteral nutrition because large quantities are required during anabolism. Hypomagnesemia may result in ileus and muscle weakness. It would be advisable to monitor magnesium levels in patients receiving parenteral nutrition.

TRACE ELEMENTS AND VITAMINS

Trace element deficits may be seen in patients with chronic diarrhea or in those with inadequate supplementation over a period of several months. Because of the relatively short duration of parenteral nutrition support in equine patients, clinical signs of deficiencies would be unlikely. A commercially available human IV supplement may be added directly to a parenteral nutrition mixture once a day if supplementation lasts more than 4 to 5 days. Although these supplements have been given to equine patients, the extent to which they satisfy specific requirements is not clear.

Patient ID _____ Weight _____(kg)__ Date _____

A. Anticipated level of nutritional support __(a)__ calories/kg/day.

  __(a)__ cal/kg/day × _____ kg body weight = __(b)__ total daily calories.

B. Nonnitrogen calorie distribution: __(b)__ × % dextrose = __(c)__ dextrose calories.

  __(b)__ × % lipid = __(d)__ lipid calories.

C. Protein provided: ratio of nonnitrogen cal/gm nitrogen __(e)__.

  (b)/(e) = __(f)__ gm of N.

  or

  __(g)__ gm protein/kg body weight × kg body weight = __(h)__ gm protein.

D. Compounding directions

  1. Amindo acids __(f)__ gm N/6.8 gm N = __(i)__ bottles 8.5% amino acid solution.

   or

   __(h)__ gm protein/42.5 gm = __(j)__ bottles 8.5% amino acid solution.

  2. Dextrose __(c)__ cal/850 = __(k)__ bottles 50% dextrose solution.

  3. Lipid __(d)__ cal/1000 = __(l)__ bottles 20% lipid emulsion.

NOTE: Mix amino acid solution and dextrose prior to adding lipids.

Figure 1. Parenteral nutrition work sheet.

COMPOUNDING

A worksheet for calculating amino acid, dextrose, and lipid requirements is provided in Figure 1. Table 1 provides some information on commercially available solutions. Few bacterial pathogens can survive in hypertonic amino acid or glucose solutions. Lipid emulsions and dextrose–amino acid solutions that are close to normal tonicity readily support the growth of bacteria and fungi. Therefore, to minimize the potential of contamination, compounding of nutrient solutions must be done with aseptic technique. Use of a laminar flow hood and well-trained personnel is ideal. However, less than ideal conditions are often used successfully if certain precautions are taken. A clean, dust- and draft-free environment is the first objective. Second, the transfer of nutrient solutions should not allow contaminated room air to enter the transfer system. A filtered compounding bag* has been used safely in the veterinary hospital setting. These bags have attachments for direct transfer of appropriate volumes of dextrose, amino acid, and lipid into one container for subsequent administration.

The order in which the products are combined is important. Undiluted amino acid or dextrose solutions can "crack" the emulsion of lipid. Thus, amino acid solutions should be well mixed with dextrose prior to adding lipid emulsion. Electrolytes, vitamins, and trace elements may

---

*1, 2, 3, or 4 liter Kabi All In One Bag, Clintec Nutrition Co., Deerfield, IL

TABLE 1. FACTS ON BOTTLES OF NUTRITIONAL PRODUCTS

20% Lipid emulsion: a 500-cc bottle contains 1000 calories
50% Dextrose: a 500-cc bottle contains 850 calories
8.5% Amino acid solution: a 500-cc bottle contains 42.5 gm protein, 6.8 gm nitrogen, 170 calories

then be added if desired. The compatibility of specific products should always be verified with the manufacturer. A freshly compounded bag may be stored in a refrigerator for up to 24 hours prior to hanging for administration. Any bag that is hung for administration should be discarded after 24 hours.

Delivery of the nutrient formulation is best done through an IV line used only for that purpose. However, it is not always practical to maintain multiple catheters to allow for the delivery of parenteral nutrition, supplemental fluids, and additional medication. One multilumen catheter may be used with different channels dedicated for delivery of the aforementioned solutions. As a third option, one IV line can be safely used for all these needs if aseptic technique is rigorously observed and the catheter is thoroughly flushed with saline between solutions. Recommended procedures include washing hands and swabbing the injection port with alcohol or an iodine solution and allowing it to air dry before invading the line (see p. 407). The delivery of nutrient should be discontinued during the administration of other medication and the line flushed with sterile solution before nutrient flow is started again.

Supplemental Readings

Dionigi, R., Cremaschi, R. E., Jemos, V., Dominioni, L., and Monico, R.: Nutritional assessment and severity of illness classification systems: A critical review on their clinical relevance. World J. Surg., 10:2–11, 1986.

Gideon, L.: Total nutritional support of the foal. Vet. Med. Small Anim. Clin., 72:1197–1207, 1977.

Gilbert, M., Gallagher, S. C., Eads, M., and Elmore, M.: Microbial growth patterns in a total parenteral nutrition formula containing lipid emulsion. J.P.E.N., 10:494–497, 1986.

Hansen, T. O.: Total parenteral nutrition in foals. In: Proceedings of the American College of Veterinary Internal Medicine Forum, Washington, D. C., May 1986, pp. 7/53–7/56.

National Research Council: Nutrient Requirements of Horses, 5th rev. ed. Washington, D. C., National Academy Press, 1989.

Spurlock, S. L., and Spurlock, G. H.: Experimental creation and treatment of short bowel syndrome in horses. In: Proceedings of the American College of Veterinary Internal Medicine Forum, San Diego, May 1987, pp. 469–471.

Spurlock, S. L., Spurlock, G. H., Parker, G., and Ward, M. V.: Long term jugular vein catheterization in horses. J. Am. Vet. Med. Assoc., 196:425–430, 1990.

Nutritional Management in Disease

Jonathan M. Naylor, SASKATOON, SASKATCHEWAN, CANADA

In recent years knowledge of the application of nutrition to the management of sick horses has improved. The effects of gut resection on nutrient digestion and absorption have been studied and different types of liquid diets for feeding horses have been investigated. Better nutrients have become available for intravenous (IV) nutrition. The effects of feeds and bedding on air quality have also been studied in more detail, making it easier to prevent and alleviate allergic lung conditions.

ASSESSMENT OF NUTRITIONAL STATUS

Evaluation of food intake and body condition should be part of the routine physical examination, improvement in voluntary food intake being one of the best indicators of recovery from illness. It is particularly important to establish whether cachexia is due to poor feed intake before one proceeds with more specialized tests of digestive or metabolic function. Prolonged starvation can lead to intestinal epithelial hypoplasia and malabsorption.

The quality of the feed must be evaluated before the adequacy of a given level of feed intake can be judged. Nutritional requirements may be elevated in sick horses because of fever, wound healing, and other factors. In some horses digestive derangements interfere with the efficiency of nutrient absorption.

Body condition allows an assessment of long-term nutritional adequacy. In mature horses negative energy balance results in loss of fat and muscle but not skeletal structures. Thus, flesh falls away from the bones. Body condition scoring is better than weighing in assessing fat stores because it is less affected by differences in body frame. The most reliable site for body condition scoring is the rump. Flesh cover over the shoulder also correlates reasonably well with total body fat. Contrary to popular opinion, the amount of flesh over the ribs correlates poorly with body condition.

In general, fat horses have a well-rounded rump, an invaginated crease along the backbone, and plenty of flesh over the shoulders. The inner thighs are thick with fat, and there is bulging fat around the tailhead. Pads of fat may be apparent over the ribs, neck, and shoulders. Horses in good (normal) condition have sufficient flesh over the loins to give a flat or convex surface between the dorsal spine and transverse vertebral processes without a crease. There is sufficient gluteal muscle that the surface joining the tuber coxae and tuber ischia is flat. The junction of the semitendinosus and biceps femoris should be clearly visible. Very thin horses have little flesh over the rump, the tuber coxae and tuber ischia are prominent, and the surface joining these points is concave. There is loss of thigh musculature and the semitendinosus is prominent on the plantar aspect of the limb. Flesh cover is poor over the spine, and the tips of the spinous and transverse processes of the lumbar vertebrae are visible. The scapula and ribs are also prominent. Growing animals show similar patterns of weight loss. Stunting as a result of severe nutritional restriction results in horses that are thin, with a large head and shallow thorax, because bone growth is not matched by soft tissue growth. Moderate nutritional restriction, however, results in slow growth, but body proportions are similar to those seen in normal animals of the same weight. Nutritional status in growing horses is best assessed using expected weight for age growth curves (see *Current Therapy in Equine Medicine 2*, Table 6, p. 418).

Blood chemistry offers some guidance to a horse's nutritional status. The best indices of food deprivation are plasma free fatty acid and glycerol concentrations, but techniques for measuring these indices are not routinely available. Some laboratories measure serum triglycerides and give a normal range of 60 to 780 mg per L; mild elevations in the range of 1000 to 5000 mg per L are usually consistent with a period of poor food intake. Normal serum triglyceride levels do not rule out poor food intake, since there is much variation in the triglyceride response to food deprivation. Also, a lag of more than 40 hours between the removal of food and an elevation in serum triglyceride levels is common. Fasted horses, and to a lesser extent ponies, also have elevated unconjugated bilirubin concentrations and may be icteric. Low serum albumin values usually reflect protein-losing enteropathy or renal or liver disease rather than long-term protein deprivation.

Studies in cattle indicate that changes in blood chemistry are most likely to be seen when very little food is eaten rather than when a prolonged low-grade undernutrition is present. Clinical experience suggests that horses with moderate undernutrition also show few changes in blood chemistry.

EFFECTS OF UNDERNUTRITION

Anorexia, a common response to infections, may initially enhance the ability to overcome acute bacterial infections. However, prolonged undernutrition adversely affects immune function. Host defenses are compromised by 3 to 5 days of complete food deprivation. Wound healing is poor, and there is greater susceptibility to postoperative problems.

In some chronic illnesses, cachexia is the cause of death. Losses of 20 to 35 per cent of normal body weight are incompatible with life. Cachexia can also limit the return of the horse to normal work. The equine gastrointestinal (GI) tract seems peculiarly sensitive to periods of starvation. Complete food deprivation for 3 to 5 days predisposes horses to diarrhea, which can be fatal. Cachectic adult horses can regain normal body condition, but growth restriction in young foals may have permanent consequences, particularly if the restriction is severe and occurs early in development. Pony foals that were not allowed to gain weight between 6 and 12 months of age had delayed epiphyseal closure and exhibited compensatory growth when subsequently fed an adequate diet. They grew best if they were allowed to eat as much as they wanted of a balanced diet high in energy and protein during the rehabilitation period. However, at 18 months of age they were still 20 to 40 kg lighter than normally fed control foals, which weighed around 300 kg.

DIETS FOR SICK HORSES

The following sections discuss dietary regimens that can be used in treating horses. When making dietary changes it is important not to disturb GI function with rapid changes of feed. Because the sudden introduction of alfalfa hay can cause diarrhea, alfalfa should be gradually introduced over a 5-day period. Rapid increments in grain feeding can result in founder; grain levels should not be increased faster than 0.5 kg a day for a 500-kg horse. Lush grass can also cause problems. Access should be gradually increased over a period of a week or more.

Hospitalized Horses

Many horses treated by veterinarians are in good body condition, have good appetites, and are suffering from minor wounds or are recuperating from infections. These horses do not require the high levels of feed often fed to working horses. They can be satisfactorily maintained on a diet composed primarily of hay fed at about 1.5 to 2.0 per cent of body weight daily. Both grass and legume hays are suitable for adult horses, provided they are of good quality. Alfalfa hay contains more protein and is particularly suitable for growing and lactating horses. It is also rich in minerals and usually only a salt block has to be provided to maintain mineral balance. In phosphorus-deficient areas a phosphate supplement may also be required. Heavily pregnant or lactating mares and weanling foals have high phosphate requirements and will also need dietary supplementation. Grass hays require salt and phosphate supplementation. If they are fed to pregnant, lactating, or growing horses, protein and calcium supplements are likely to be required.

Small amounts of grain, 0.5 to 1.0 kg twice a day, may be fed to maintain adaptation to grain and speed return to a high-grain diet when the horse returns to work.

Salt can be provided as a block on a free-choice basis. Phosphate supplements should either be incorporated into the salt or mixed with grain to ensure a consistent intake.

LAMINITIS

Overingestion of feeds containing rapidly fermentable carbohydrate, for example grains and lush grass, is one cause of laminitis. Animals with active laminitis should be fed average-quality hay and no grain. Obesity predisposes to laminitis and overweight horses should be *gradually* slimmed by restricting intake to small amounts (0.75 to 1.0 per cent of body weight per day) of good-quality hay.

CHRONIC OBSTRUCTIVE PULMONARY DISEASE

Horses with chronic pulmonary disease usually do best at pasture. Whenever possible, owners should be encouraged to keep affected horses out of doors. Open-sided sheds and blankets can be used to provide warmth and shelter when the weather is inclement. Waterproof blankets should be used if rain or wet snow is expected.

Horses kept indoors are exposed to allergens present in hays and bedding. Restricted ventilation prevents the venting of these allergens into the atmosphere and their replacement with fresh air. If hay or straw is baled moist or if it lies too long in a moist location in the field, thermophilic molds multiply. The spores of these fungi are small in size and are inhaled into the lung when dust is stirred up during feeding or by movement through the bedding. Because the fungi and spores are microscopic, a clean appearance does not guarantee freedom from molds.

If horses with chronic obstructive pulmonary disease must be kept indoors, they often improve if they are taken off hay, fed pelleted feeds, and placed in a well-ventilated stall. When hay has to be fed, it should be thoroughly soaked with water either with a hose or preferably placed in a net and completely immersed in a tub of water for at least 5 minutes. Soaked feed should be replaced frequently because it can easily mold. There will be less dust if hay cubes are fed in place of loose hay, but these should also be soaked. Feed should be fed on or close to the ground so that particles will tend to fall away from the horse's nose. Straw bedding is another source of molds. To avoid this, shredded paper or wood shavings should be used as bedding. Daily mucking out will reduce the build-up of molds. Since air quality depends on the management of the barn as a whole, adjacent horses should be treated in a similar manner.

CHOKE

Because esophageal obstruction may result in esophageal inflammation and spasm at the site of the obstruction, obstruction may recur if the horse is placed on a normal diet straight after treatment. Horses that have been treated for esophageal obstruction should be fed a soft mash for several days to allow the esophagus to heal.

Horses prone to obstruction should not be fed pellets. If the horse is a greedy eater, large round stones or a large salt block placed in the grain will slow down the rate of eating and decrease the probabilty of further episodes of choke.

GASTROINTESTINAL DISEASE

The nutritional principle involved in feeding horses with GI disease is to feed more grain when the large intestine is compromised, so that small intestinal digestion is maximized. When the small intestine is damaged, more hay should be fed to maximize fermentative digestion in the large intestine. Frequent feeding and use of highly digestible feeds should help maximize digestive capacity. Heavily lignified, overmature hays and grasses should be avoided. Higher protein, energy, and mineral densities may be needed in the diets to balance reduced digestive function. In some cases, the horse may compensate by increasing voluntary feed intake if free choice feed is available.

DIARRHEA

Large or small intestinal malfunction can produce diarrhea. Horses with acute diarrhea may lose more fluid and electrolytes in their diarrhea than are ingested. Oral electrolyte preparations designed for use in calves can help maintain these patients. Products that contain alkalizing agents—either as bicarbonate or metabolizable bases (e.g., acetate, citrate)—will help counteract the systemic acidosis that often develops in severely diarrheic horses. Glucose and glycine aid absorption of sodium and water, inclusion of acetate, citrate, or bicarbonate in the mix also improves fluid absorption. In addition to the role of glucose and glycine in aiding fluid and electrolyte absorption, these nutrients will also nourish the gut wall. Because the gut mucosa derives a major portion of its nutrients from the lumen, it is important that some enteral nutrition is available to help nourish the gut wall. The amount of energy present in many oral electrolyte solutions is too low to make a significant contribution to the animal's overall energy needs. High-energy oral electrolyte solutions contain more glucose (350 to 450 mmol per L) and can provide around 70 per cent of the maintenance energy requirements of a 50-kg foal if fed at the rate of 2 liters per feed, three times daily.

An old remedy for diarrheic horses is to reduce the amount of grain and increase the amount of hay fed. Fiber present in hay binds water and stimulates large intestinal contractions, which slow the flow of digesta through the large intestine. These changes should lead to a firmer appearing stool. Fiber may also favor the reestablishment of a normal cellulolytic microbial flora following grain overload or disturbances of the gut flora.

Some horses with diarrhea lose body condition. These cases require careful management. If diarrhea is primarily due to small intestinal malfunction, high-fiber diets should be fed. If small intestinal digestion is intact, grain should be fed. This will help support body condition even though grain will not improve fecal consistency.

Horses with small and large intestinal malabsorption are candidates for IV support if there is some hope that the underlying lesion is curable. Because of cost and potential complications this is only likely to be used at referral centers when severe diarrhea and malabsorption has persisted for more than 3 days. Horses fed IV may still benefit from small amounts of oral nutrients to help maintain the gut mucosa.

Small Intestinal Malabsorption/Resection

These horses should benefit from fiber-based diets. Alfalfa hay is probably the best choice of feed. Supplemental phosphate may be needed to help counteract reduced small intestinal phosphate absorption.

Ponies that have undergone extensive resection of the small intestine show a preference for roughage in the diet.

Large Colon Resection

These horses should benefit from grain diets with high-quality alfalfa hay or pellets. In general, forage digestion is depressed, but studies show that long-stem alfalfa hay is efficiently digested. This is the best forage source for these horses. The diet should contain at least 14 per cent protein and a phosphorus supplement should be fed to maintain phosphorus balance.

Colonic Impaction

Dietary management is useful in preventing recurrence of impaction colic. Fresh water should be freely available and the horse should receive regular exercise. Straw or excessively fibrous hays should be replaced with good-quality grass or legume hays. Some horses seem particularly prone to impaction and require a mildly laxative diet. Restricting hay intake and feeding a complete pelleted feed containing ground alfalfa softens the stool and decreases filling of the large intestine. The small particle size also reduces the resistance to flow through the gut. Young grass is another diet that often produces a soft stool. If it proves difficult to obtain soft feces by dietary manipulation, magnesium sulfate can be added to the diet at the rate of 100 gm a day for a 500-kg horse.

Hepatic Disease

In liver disease, conversion of ammonia to urea is impaired and in consequence ammonia, which is highly toxic, may accumulate in the blood. The liver also synthesizes glucose and helps regulate blood glucose concentration.

The diet should supply glucose as starches (or D-glucose) to minimize the need for hepatic glucose synthesis. Ammonia production can be reduced by ensuring the horse receives maintenance intakes of glucose precursors and proteins. Underfeeding, with a shortage of gluconeogenic nutrients in the diet, will result in catabolism of muscle proteins and release of amino acids. These will be presented to the liver for conversion to glucose with ammonia release. Overfeeding protein should also be avoided because excess amino acids are also deaminated. The ideal protein source has a high ratio of branched-chain to aromatic amino acids. Branched-chain amino acids are preferentially metabolized by muscle and other nonhepatic tissues.

One type of diet that would meet these requirements is small amounts of a corn–milo (sorghum) diet fed at frequent intervals. A 50:50 mix of ground corn cobs and milo meets maintenance protein requirements. Alternatively, corn cob meal contains adequate protein to satisfy maintenance requirements without milo supplementation. Grass hay can be fed for roughage. Legume hays, wheat, oats, and soybeans should be avoided. These products contain more aromatic amino acids than corn, milo, or grasses; alfalfa and soybean also contain excessive protein.

Vitamin supplementation of horses with liver disease is often practiced. Both water and fat-soluble vitamins can be given, preferably at the recommended daily intake on a daily basis.

Renal Disease

The common problems in horses with renal disease are calcium accumulation in serum due to inadequate renal excretion, excessive losses of sodium, (which is poorly available in the diet), and accumulation of urea.

The diet should contain required (usually maintenance) amounts of high biological value protein to minimize urea formation. A good-quality grass hay diet is probably the best feed. Legume hays rich in protein and calcium, calcium-containing mineral supplements, and protein supplements (soybean meal) should be avoided. If renal failure is chronic and there is a large degree of proteinuria it may be necessary to increase protein intake to help maintain serum albumin concentrations. A salt supplement should be available free-choice.

Cardiac Disease

Horses with chronic heart failure are rarely treated. The only dietary change that is likely to be required is salt restriction. Grain and forage-based diets are low in sodium and the only modification needed is to remove the salt block.

Cracked Hooves

Biotin is one of the nutrients required for normal horn formation. Some studies suggest that horses with weak, crumbly hoof walls with misshapen and cracked hooves may respond to biotin supplementation. Doses of 10 to 30 mg of biotin per horse per day are used. Treatment must be given for several months (up to 9 months) before growth of new horn completely replenishes the damaged horn. Many other causes of poor horn growth exist including laminitis and excessive drying in arid areas. Vertical cracks in otherwise strong hooves are unlikely to respond to supplementation.

Geriatric Patients

The major problems in geriatric patients are poor dentition and pituitary tumors. Poor teeth can interfere with the ingestion of any feed, particularly hay. Horses with pituitary tumors are likely to have impaired removal of glucose from their circulation. GI absorption of phosphorus is also reduced in older horses.

If dentition is good, a diet of grass hay and a 14 per cent protein, complete pelleted feed and grass hay is suitable for older horses. This provides plenty of protein and is less glucogenic than grain. Mashes will be beneficial in horses with poor, painful teeth.

ANOREXIA

Although sick horses often become anorectic, the time at which the clinician should begin supplemental feeding has not been established. Improving voluntary feed intake is usually tried early in the disease, while tube feeding is reserved for horses that are physically unable to ingest feed. IV nutrition is usually reserved for horses with nonfunctioning GI tracts. Methods of forced enteral nutrition (see p. 724) and IV nutrition (see p. 732) are covered elsewhere in this book.

IMPROVING VOLUNTARY FEED INTAKE

Palatable feeds are usually the first line of attack in improving voluntary feed intake. Young leafy grass is palatable and digestible and may be preferred by horses that refuse other foods. Alfalfa hay is more palatable than grass hay. Whole oats are more palatable than rolled oats. Sweet feeds—usually mixtures of molasses and rolled grains—can often increase palatability when added to grain feeds. However, some sick horses will reject a good alfalfa hay and grain and will eat poor hay or their bedding. For this reason, it is important to offer the sick horse its choice of a variety of feeds. There may be an initial preference for a novel feed such as apples or carrots, but this can soon diminish, and the person who feeds the horse should be constantly searching for feeds the horse will accept. The site at which feed is offered can be important, as some horses prefer to eat from the ground rather than from a manger or hay rack.

Bran mashes are a popular feed for sick horses, but bran has a low palatability. Palatability can be improved by mixing a quart of oats with a quart of bran. The mixture is steeped with boiling water and served warm but not hot. Molasses (up to 250 ml) and up to 20 gm of salt can be added for flavoring. Steamed oats, barley, and well-boiled linseed meal may be particularly palatable to some horses and can be substituted for part of the oats in the mash.

Fever and pain depress feed intake, and interleukin-1 (endogenous pyrogen) also stimulates catabolism of muscle protein. Nonsteroidal anti-inflammatory drugs can improve feed intake by blocking fever and reducing pain; they may also reduce degradation of muscle tissue. Anti-inflammatory drugs are not effective in improving feed intake in severely toxemic horses.

Feed stimulants such as diazepam directly stimulate feeding centers in the hypothalamus. My experience in sick horses suggests that the tranquilizing and ataxia-producing effects of diazepam often predominate, and I do not usually recommend its use. Anabolic steroids increase feed intake but because the effect may take up to 10 days they are unlikely to be of use in the immediate treatment of the sick horse. However, they can be useful in the convalescent period.

Vitamin supplementation may be beneficial to some horses. Normally the diet and synthesis of vitamins by the gut flora provides plenty of B vitamins, and the average horse has adequate stores of vitamins for short-term food deprivation. Horses that have been off feed for a number of days and horses that have disturbed gut function because of diarrhea or oral antibiotic therapy may benefit from vitamin B-complex administration.

FORCED FEEDING

There are two approaches to nutritional supplementation in sick horses unable or unwilling to eat. The first approach is to supplement part of the horse's requirements; the other is to provide all nutrients.

Partial supplementation, dosing with a high-protein food, is used in patients that are in fairly good body condition and still have some voluntary food intake. High-protein supplements improve the balance between protein requirements and protein intake and minimize catabolism of muscle protein. The horse is still in negative energy balance, and depot lipids are broken down to meet the energy deficit. One type of therapy involves the use of casein as a protein supplement. A dose syringe can be used to feed 50 gm of casein as a slurry three times a day. This provides less than a third of maintenance protein requirements but may convert a patient with marginal protein intake into positive protein balance. Casein is used as a supplement because it is 90 per cent digestible, its amino acid spectrum is particularly good, and the protein is likely to have a high biological value to the horse. Casein can either be used directly or, alternatively, some forms of dehydrated cottage cheese contain minimal lactose and fat and are rich in casein. We do not recommend the use of lactose-rich milk products because adult horses cannot digest lactose.

When horses cannot be fed orally because of derangements in GI fuction, adding 5 per cent dextrose to the IV fluids will provide a small amount of calories and may reduce catabolism of protein.

Supplemental Readings

Barcos, V., Rodemann, P., Dinarello, C. A., and Goldberg, A. L.: Stimulation of muscle protein degeneration and prostaglandin E_2 release by leukocytic pyrogen (interleukin-1). N. Engl. J. Med., 308:553, 1983.
Bertone, A. L., Ralston, S. L., and Stashak, T. S.: Fiber digestion and voluntary intake in horses after adaptation to extensive large-colon resection. Am. J. Vet. Res., 50:1628, 1989.
Della Fera, M. A., Naylor, J. M., and Baille, C. A.: Benzodiazepines stimulate feeding in clinically debilitated animals. Fed. Proc., 37:401, 1978.
Ellis, R. N. W., and Lawrence, T. L. J.: Energy and undernutrition in the weanling filly foal: 1. Effects on subsequent live-weight gains and onset of oestrus. Br. Vet. J., 134:205, 1978.
Hoffsis, G. F., Gingerich, D. A., Sherman, D. M., and Bruner, R. R.: Total intravenous feeding of calves. J. Am Vet. Med. Assoc., 171:67, 1977.
Kluger, M. J., and Rothenburg, B. A.: Fever and reduced iron: Their interaction as a host defense response. Science, 203:374, 1979.
Naylor, J. M., and Kenyon, S. J.: Effect of total caloric deprivation on host defense in the horse. Res. Vet. Sci., 31:369, 1981.
Ralston, S. L.: Equine clinical nutrition: Specific problems and solutions. Compend. Cont. Educ. Pract. Vet., 10:356, 1988.

Nutritional Management of the Critically Ill Neonate

Wendy E. Vaala, KENNETT SQUARE, PENNSYLVANIA

Proper nutritional support of the critically ill newborn foal is as crucial to its survival as the appropriate antibiotic selection or mode of ventilatory support. The neonate's diet must support the establishment of extrauterine homeostasis, a high basal metabolic rate, and rapid growth. Healthy, full-term foals nurse on average seven times an hour, consume between 20 and 30 per cent of their body weight in mare's milk daily, and gain approximately 1 to 3 pounds per day. If short gestational age, inability to nurse naturally, abnormal gastrointestinal (GI) function, and concurrent neonatal illness are superimposed, a sick foal's nutritional requirements become extremely difficult to calculate.

The rational use of nutritional supplementation requires criteria for assessing nutritional status, guidelines for estimating an individual's nutrient requirements, and a thorough understanding of the nutritional formulas and routes of administration available. Prolonged hyperalimentation demands further appreciation of the neonate's peculiar mineral and vitamin requirements in addition to energy and protein needs.

EFFECTS OF MALNUTRITION

Adequate neonatal nutrition is essential for maintaining normal function and growth. Malnutrition due to inadequate intake, abnormal absorption, or increased utilization results in weight loss, depressed growth rates, generalized muscle weakness, delayed wound healing, poor callus formation at fracture sites, GI atrophy and dysmotility, and impaired hepatic function. Ventilatory capacity and pulmonary function are reduced owing to loss of strength and function of diaphragmatic, intercostal, and abdominal muscles. The most devastating consequences of undernutrition for the neonate are impaired immune function and decreased resistance to infection. Protein–calorie malnutrition has been associated with depressed bone marrow activity, atrophy of the spleen, thymus, and other lymphoid tissues, decreased neutrophil chemotaxis and bactericidal activity, impaired antibody production, hypogammaglobulinemia, lymphopenia, depressed secretory and mucosal immunity, and depressed cell-mediated immune responses.

NUTRITIONAL ASSESSMENT

Recognition of protein–calorie malnutrition begins with the history and physical examination. A foal with a history of restricted oral intake, protracted nutritional losses, or increased metabolic demands (Table 1) is a candidate for nutritional support even before weight loss and other biochemical changes become evident. An acute weight loss of 5 per cent of body weight or a chronic weight loss of 10 to 15 per cent of body weight is an indication for supplemental nutritional therapy.

Physical examination findings suggestive of undernutrition include weight loss, reduced growth rate, lethargy, muscle wasting, dry scaly skin, glossitis, and reduced skin elasticity. Studies in neonates of other species have shown that catch-up growth following malnutrition is complete only if the period of undernutrition is relatively brief and has occurred after the hypothalamus and appetite center are fully functional. Standard growth curves using body weight, girth circumference, and withers height measurements for foals are available and can be used to identify individuals failing to maintain normal growth patterns.

TABLE 1. INDICATIONS FOR NUTRITIONAL SUPPLEMENTATION IN THE FOAL

Restricted oral intake
  Weak or absent suckle reflex
    Septicemia
    Neonatal maladjustment syndrome
    Prematurity/immaturity
  Gut immaturity/dysfunction
  Dysphagia
    Botulism
    Prematurity/immaturity
  Orphan foal
    Loss of dam
    Rejection by dam
  Gut dysmotility
    Peritonitis
    Enteritis
    Gastroduodenal reflux
    Necrotizing enterocolitis
    Gastroduodenal ulceration
Protracted nutritional losses
  Secretory diarrhea
    Salmonellosis
  Malabsorption
    Rotavirus diarrhea
    Lactose intolerance
Increased metabolic needs
  Septicemia
  Prematurity/immaturity
  Fever
  Localized infection

Measurements of skin fold thickness and body composition are not routinely available or practical for use in the foal. Biochemical indices of malnutrition include hypoalbuminemia and hypoproteinemia. In other species, serum albumin concentrations less than 4.0 gm per dl indicate inadequate protein intake. Unfortunately, the long, 20-day half-life of albumin renders this parameter less reliable during early stages of malnutrition. Total plasma protein concentrations may be misleading in newborn foals due to the wide range of presuckle protein values and the impact of colostrum ingestion on the globulin concentration. The sensitivity of other protein nutritional markers such as retinol-binding protein, transferrin, thyroxin-binding globulin, transthyretin (prealbumin), and fibronectin has not been evaluated in the foal. Clinically ill, hypophagic adult horses mobilize fat reserves and have elevated levels of total lipids, triglycerides, and cholesterol. Hypertriglyceridemia (greater than 500 mg per dl) in adult horses, without signs of pituitary adenomas, reflects inadequate caloric intake. These parameters have not been critically evaluated in foals. Hyperlipemia in neonatal foals also occurs during septicemia due to depressed lipoprotein lipase activity and impaired lipid clearance rather than simple malnutrition.

DIGESTION AND ABSORPTION

Within hours of birth, the foal must utilize milk lactose to extract the energy necessary for its survival. In the horse the development of brush-border disaccharidase activity follows a pattern similar to that of other mammals. Lactase, a β-galactosidase, reaches maximal levels at birth and declines steadily after 4 months of age. In contrast, the α-glucosidases maltase, sucrase, and trehalase are barely discernible in the equine fetus and increase after birth to reach adult levels by 7 months of age. Glucoamylase is detectable during the first week of life and attains adult levels by 10 months. This pattern of disaccharidase development suggests that newborn foals are incapable of maintaining acceptable growth on a diet containing sucrose, maltose, or polysaccharides as the primary carbohydrate source.

NUTRITIONAL REQUIREMENTS

Unfortunately, there are no specific nutritional recommendations for neonatal foals. Guidelines for caloric intake and most nutrients can be estimated based on a healthy foal's average milk consumption and the composition of mare's milk (Table 2). Consuming 20 to 25 per cent of its body weight as milk daily, a healthy 50-kg foal consumes 10 to 12.5 liters of milk per day to provide 120 to 150 kcal per kg per day, 5 to 6 gm protein per kg per day, and 4 to 5 gm fat per kg per day. Problems such as sepsis, surgery, and fever increase the neonate's resting energy expenditure (REE). Severe infection is associated with a 10 to 30 per cent increase in REE, and fever increases metabolic rate by 13 per cent for each degree Celsius rise in body temperature.

A healthy nursing foal ingests approximately 250 to 290 mg per kg of calcium daily. However, the calcium retention rate in foals and the intestinal absorption coefficient of calcium in mare's milk are not known, so that daily oral calcium requirements can only be estimated.

Neonatal foals have slightly higher mineral requirements than those listed for growing horses. Newborn foals are born with low serum levels of zinc (0.3 to 0.4 μg per ml) and copper (0.2 to 0.3 μg per ml). By 3 weeks of age, zinc and copper concentrations should be greater than 0.5 μg per ml and 1.0 μg per ml, respectively. Trace mineral deficiencies have been associated with anemia and metabolic bone diseases. Conservative supplementation is advised since excessive administration of trace minerals and fat-soluble vitamins can be detrimental.

Premature and growth-retarded foals have different and poorly defined nutrient requirements. Premature foals have blunted insulin responses and lower plasma glucose levels at birth than full-term neonates. In the absence of species-specific information, the nutritional needs of the premature infant can be considered when designing a feeding regimen for premature foals. Premature infants have higher energy (114 to 181 kcal per kg per day) and protein (4 to 6 gm per kg per day of enteral protein intake) require-

TABLE 2. COMPOSITION OF MARE'S, COW'S, AND GOAT'S MILK

	Mare*	Mare†	Cow†	Goat†
Milk constituent				
Gross energy	0.46 ± 0.004	0.6	0.67	0.67
Protein, gm/dl	2.16 ± 0.03	2.7	3.8	3.7
Fat, gm/dl	0.74 ± 0.04	1.6	4.4	4.1
Lactose, gm/dl	6.6 ± 0.03	6.1	4.9	4.2
Ca:P ratio	1.8	1.6	1.4	1.2
Ca, mg/dl	122 ± 2		130	129
P, mg/dl	66 ± 1		90	109
Total solids	10.4 ± 0.05	11	12–13	13.2
Ash, gm/dl	0.44 ± 0.01	0.5	0.7	0.8
Mineral composition	Mare‡	Mare§		
Iron (μg/gm)	0.86 ± 0.09			
Zinc (μg/gm)	3.7 ± 0.1	3.1 + 0.67		
Copper (μ/gm)	0.66 ± 0.07	0.85 + 0.40		

*Pagan, J. D., and Hintz, H. F.: Composition of milk from pony mares fed various levels of digestible energy. Cornell Vet., 76:139, 1986.
†Roberts, S. J.: Veterinary Obstetrics and Genital Diseases, 2nd ed. Ithaca, New York, Edwards Brothers, 1971.
‡Ullrey, D. E., Ely, W. T., and Covert, R. L.: Iron, zinc, and copper in mare's milk. J. Anim. Sci., 38:1276, 1974.
§Schryver, H. F., Offedal, O. T., Williams, J., et al.: Lactation in the horse: The mineral composition of mares milk. J. Nutr., 116:2142, 1986.

ments. Fat absorption is reduced owing to decreased bile salt synthesis and hepatic immaturity, resulting in inefficient lipid solubilization by micelle formation.

Premature and low birth weight infants have calcium and phosphorus requirements that cannot be met by human milk alone. Dysmature foals with incomplete skeletal ossification probably have higher calcium and phosphorus requirements as well. Parathyroid hormone stimulates calcium mobilization from bone to maintain normal levels of serum calcium even though dietary intake is inadequate. Therefore, serum calcium concentration is a poor indicator of the body's calcium needs. Adequacy of calcium intake can be better evaluated by periodic radiographic assessment of bone density. Abnormally elevated serum levels of alkaline phosphatase (higher than 1000 IU per L) are indicative of excessive calcium mobilization from bone in response to inadequate dietary intake.

SEPTICEMIA AND INTERMEDIARY METABOLISM

Gram-negative sepsis is the leading cause of death in critically ill neonatal foals. Sepsis disrupts intermediary metabolism, increases metabolic rate, and sequentially hinders utilization of carbohydrates, lipids, and finally protein for energy. Stress and endotoxin release precipitate a neurohormonal cascade of events mediated by leukocyte endogenous mediator and increased concentrations of catecholamines, glucocorticoids, and glucagon. Low perfusion states associated with septic shock are also accompanied by elevated levels of growth hormone, antidiuretic hormone, aldosterone, and thyroxin and inappropriately low levels of insulin.

The sepsis-induced increase in sympathetic activity results in glycolysis, hepatic gluconeogenesis, lipolysis, proteolysis, water, and sodium retention and increased urinary excretion of potassium and nitrogen. Elevated levels of catecholamines, glucagon, and glucocorticoids inhibit insulin secretion and increase peripheral insulin resistance, contributing to hyperglycemia and glucose intolerance. Lipid oxidation becomes the next preferential fuel source after carbohydrates. Triglyceride hydrolysis results in release of free fatty acids (FFA) and glycerol. During sepsis, a deficiency of the carrier peptide carnitine and decreased lipoprotein lipase activity impair FFA transport into mitochondria, block fatty acid oxidation, impair lipid clearance, and result in futile recycling of lipogenic substrates and lipemia. Protein degradation becomes the final fuel source. Branched-chain amino acids are catabolized to their respective ketoacids for oxidative metabolism in the tricarboxylic acid cycle. Excessive amino acid degradation eventually overwhelms hepatic metabolic capacity, resulting in uremia, the production of false neurotransmitters, and clinical signs of hepatoencephalopathy.

ENTERAL FEEDING

Foals can be fed orally or intravenously (IV). Enteral alimentation is more physiologic and less expensive, and facilitates normal gut maturation. Oral feedings stimulate the growth of intestinal villi and production of crypt cells, promote hepatic and biliary secretions, improve nitrogen retention, and induce brush-border disaccharidase activity. Enterocytes rely on absorption of glutamine, β-hydroxybutyrate, and other volatile fatty acids from the gut as their primary energy source. Parenteral alimentation alone cannot provide equivalent nutrition for these cells. Without enteral feeding, gut atrophy develops and the integrity of mucosal cell tight junctions is destroyed, predisposing to sepsis. Oral feeds also stimulate the release of enteroinsular hormones such as glucagon, gastrin, secretin, and cholecystokinin, which in turn have a tropic effect on gut maturation and differentiation.

Dysmature and growth-retarded foals often have poor tolerance for enteral feeds. In utero malnutrition results in a growth-retarded neonate with delayed GI development, abnormal disaccharidase activity, and depressed gut immunity characterized by decreased numbers of intestinal and intraepithelial lymphocytes. These changes help explain why many growth-retarded foals exhibit a variety of GI disturbances, including colic, diarrhea, and excessive intestinal gas production.

Routes of feeding include nursing from the foal's own dam or a nurse mare, nursing from a bottle or bucket, and nasogastric tube feeding. If a productive suckle and swallow reflex are present, bottle feeding is attempted with either infant or lamb nipples. The risk of aspiration when bottle feeding a foal can be reduced by avoiding overextension of the foal's head and neck. The foal should be encouraged to keep its nose below or level with its eyes to facilitate normal swallowing. Normal udder bumping and teat-seeking behavior can be stimulated by allowing the foal to approach the bottle from behind and under the handler's armpit. The nipple hole diameter should be small enough to prevent milk from streaming freely when the bottle is inverted. On-

TABLE 3. COMPOSITION OF MILK AND MILK SUBSTITUTES FOR FOALS

Product	Crude Protein (%)	Sugar (%)	Crude Fat (%)	Crude Fiber (%)
Foal-lac°	19.5	52.6	14.0	0.1
Nutri-Foal†	29.0	35.0	21.0	0.2
Nutrequin‡	22.0	NA	16.0	0.3
Mare's Milk Plus§	20.0	NA	14.0	0.15
Mare's Match‖	24.0	NA	16.0	0.15
Mare's milk	22.8	58.8	15.0	0.0
Goat's milk	25.0	31.0	34.0	0.0
Cow's milk	27.0	38.0	29.0	0.0
Acidified Cold Ad Libitum Formula¶	20.0	NA	14.0	NA

NA = not available.
°Foal-lac; Pet Ag, Inc., Elgin, IL
†Nutri-Foal; Ross Laboratories, Columbus, OH 43216
‡Nutrequin; Vetrepharm Inc., Athens, GA 30601
§Mare's Milk Plus; Buckeye Feed Mills Inc., Dalton, OH 44618
‖Mare's Match; Land O Lakes Inc., Fort Dodge, IA 50501
¶Acidified Cold Ad Libitum Formula; Milk Specialties Co., Deerfield, IL 60118

demand bottle feeding is ideal but often impractical and too labor intensive. An alternate schedule for newborn foals, less than 7 days of age, is regular feedings every 2 hours.

Bucket feeding allows the foal to drink with its head and neck flexed and should be considered for foals with a weak swallow reflex due to immaturity or foals destined to be hand-raised as orphans. Milk should be introduced initially in a hand-held, shallow bowl.

If ineffectual swallowing and suckling prevent bottle or bucket feeding, then nasogastric intubation is required. A small-bore, flexible silicone tube° (5 mm internal diameter) is preferred. Individual choice dictates whether to leave the tube indwelling or to pass the tube with each feeding. If the tube is left in place, the end can be positioned in the esophagus or stomach. Indwelling tubes should be sealed between feedings to prevent aerophagia and GI tympany. Depressed foals requiring nasogastric intubation should be maintained in sternal recumbency immedately after tube feeding to reduce the risk of gastroesophageal reflux and aspiration.

Enteral formulas used for foals include milk from the mare, goat, or cow, artificial replacers formulated for foals or calves, and human enteral products containing semielemental or elemental ingredients. The composition of some available formulas is listed in Tables 2 and 3. Mare's milk is preferred since it is the most physiologic. Goat's milk is a palatable and acceptable alternative that is higher in fat, total solids, and gross energy than mare's milk. Compared to cow's milk, goat's milk is composed of simpler fatty acids and smaller fat globules that are easier to digest. It is less acid and has better buffering capacity than cow's milk. Most foals readily accept a goat milk diet and exhibit satisfactory growth. Mild constipation is occasionally observed. Cow's milk can be substituted for mare's milk if addtional glucose is added and some of the fat is removed. This can be accomplished by purchasing 2 per cent fat skimmed milk and adding dextrose to the milk at the rate of 20 gm per L (40 ml of 50 per cent dextrose per L of milk).

A variety of powdered mare's milk replacers are commercially available. Ideally, a replacer should contain 22 per cent crude protein, 15 per cent fat, and less than 0.5 per cent fiber on a dry matter basis. Many of the manufacturers' directions for reconstituting milk replacers result in a concentrated milk formula with nearly double the dry matter content of mare's milk. This practice contributes to the development of constipation and dehydration occasionally observed in foals on milk replacer diets. A 12 to 15 per cent dilution is preferred and free access to water is essential. Many of these artificial replacers are designed to be fed with concentrates and roughage. The absence of these ingredients in the sick foal's diet may predispose to other GI disturbances such as diarrhea, flatulence, and mild colic.

Acidified Cold Ad Lib Formula (see Table 3) is a new type of calf milk replacer marketed under a variety of trade names. This product is designed to be fed free choice. Unlike other calf milk replacers, it contains no antibiotics or preservatives and stays fresh 3 days afer mixing because of the acidification. This formula is palatable, well tolerated by young foals, inexpensive, and meets the National Research Council's (NRC) requirements for growing horses.

Human enteral formulas have been used in

___
°Foal stomach tube, Bivona, Inc., Gary IN

foals. These formulas contain protein, carbohydrate, and fat in complex or simple forms such as peptides, amino acids, glucose oligomers, glucose, and long- and medium-chain triglycerides. One example of a liquid, semielemental formula is Carnation Peptamen (Table 4), an isotonic diet composed of readily absorbable ingredients present as peptides, medium- and long-chain triglycerides, starch, and maltodextrin. Peptamen provides a nonprotein calorie-to-nitrogen ratio of 131:1, with 33 per cent of the total calories contributed by lipids. Although not particularly palatable, Peptamen's high caloric density (1 kcal per ml) allows required calories to be supplied in small-volume feedings, which is often desirable in critically ill foals. Since the newborn foal has only low levels of maltase present immediately post partum, Peptamen, with the oligosaccharide maltodextrin as its primary carbohydrate source, should be introduced slowly to allow gut adaptation.

Complications associated with enteral feeding are listed in Table 5. The sicker the neonate, the more temperamental its GI function. Common GI disturbances include abdominal distention, flatulence, constipation, diarrhea, gastric reflux, and mild colic. In foals unaccustomed to oral feeds, enteral alimentation must be introduced slowly, beginning with small volumes of milk (50 to 100 ml) delivered via bottle or gravity flow through a nasogastric tube. If signs of feed intolerance develop, such as colic, abdominal distention, or reflux, enteral feeds should be reduced in volume or temporarily discontinued and parenteral nutritional therapy initiated.

Although healthy foals voluntarily consume in excess of 20 to 25 per cent of their body weight

TABLE 5. COMPLICATIONS ASSOCIATED WITH ENTERAL ALIMENTATION

Gastrointestinal intolerance
  Diarrhea
  Abdominal distention
  Gastric reflux
  Ileus, colic
  Constipation
Metabolic disturbances
  Electrolyte imbalances
  Hypoglycemia
Nasogastric tube–related problems
  Rhinitis
  Tube occlusion or dislodgment
  Nasopharyngeal trauma
  Gastric irritation
  Aerophagia, bloat, colic
  Aspiration pneumonia
Poor palatability

in milk daily, the provision of 10 per cent body weight (5 liters of milk per day for a 50-kg foal) will usually maintain a foal's weight and is a reasonable goal when tube feeding sick foals. At this rate, a 50-kg foal requires a minimum of 417 ml (14 ounces) of milk every 2 hours. All oral formulas should be fed as close to body temperature as possible. Overheating and uneven heating must be avoided. Microwave ovens denature protein and should not be used to heat colostrum. Powdered replacers should be diluted appropriately and thoroughly mixed with water to avoid sudden changes in concentration.

Gastric reflux due to bowel dysmotility and delayed gastric emptying has been associated with hypoxic gut damage following peripartum asphyxia, peritonitis associated with sepsis, bacterial or viral enteritis, gastroduodenal ulceration

TABLE 4. COMPOSITION OF CARNATION PEPTAMEN°

	% Total Calories	Gm/2000 Ml	% Lipid Energy	% Carbohydrate Energy
Fat	33	78		
MCT†			23	
LCT‡			10	
Sunflower oil			18	
Lecithin			6	
Milk fat			9	
Carbohydrate	51	254		
Maltodextrin				88
Starch				12
Protein	16	80		
Hydrolyzed whey peptides (average peptide length = 8 aaR§)				
Caloric density = 1 kcal/ml				
Osmolarity = 260 mOsm				
Nonprotein calories-to-nitrogen ratio = 131:1				

°Carnation Peptamen, Baxter Healthcare Corp., Deerfield, IL.
†Medium-chain triglycerides.
‡Long-chain triglycerides.
§Amino acid residues.

with or without stricture formation, and diet intolerance. Gastric emptying and gastroduodenal motility patterns can be improved in some patients with metoclopramide administered IV as a slow continuous infusion at a rate of 0.25 mg per kg per hour or orally at a dose of 0.6 mg per kg every 4 hours. Excitement can occur with overdosage. Metoclopramide is contraindicated if GI obstruction is suspected as the cause of the reflux.

Diarrhea can be treated symptomatically with oral bismuth subsalicylate (1.0 ml per kg PO every 4 to 6 hours) and/or loperamide (0.1 to 0.2 mg per kg PO every 6 hours). Diarrhea associated with broad-spectrum antibiotic therapy may respond to the administration of one of the commercially available probiotics or yogurt containing an active culture (1 to 2 ounces given three to four times per day) to help replenish normal intestinal flora.

Nasopharyngeal irritation from repetitive tubing or chronic nasogastric intubation can delay the return of normal suckling. Administration of a nasopharyngeal spray containing prednisolone (2000 mg; 50 mg per ml), furacin (750 ml), glycerin (1000 ml), and dimethyl sulfoxide (DMSO, 250 ml), helps reduce inflammation. Small (5 to 6 ml) volumes of this formulation are insufflated up the nares twice daily using a small-diameter nasopharyngeal tube inserted to the level of the medial canthus. During insufflation of the medication, the foal should be sternal or standing, with its head flexed, to prevent aspiration.

PARENTERAL ALIMENTATION

Parenteral nutrition (PN) describes the IV administration of sterile compound solutions containing dextrose, amino acids, lipids, vitamins, trace mineral, and electrolytes. Parenteral alimentation is indicated whenever feeding via the GI tract is inadequate because of anorexia, increased metabolic demands due to sepsis, or surgical stress; contraindicated because of gastric reflux, ileus or severe gastrointestinal disease; or impractical because of mechanical ventilation or esophageal disease. PN solutions are hypertonic and must be administered slowly and continuously through a large-diameter vein to maximize substrate utilization, avoid detrimental increases in plasma osmolarity, prevent osmotic diuresis, and minimize vessel irritation. Complications associated with PN are listed in Table 6.

Jugular vein catheters are the most common route of administration and should be as nonthrombogenic as possible. Polyurethane catheters are of low reactivity and can remain in situ for 3 weeks or longer. The 30-cm-gauge L-Cath* has been used extensively for IV nutrition in neonatal foals. All catheters should be inserted using aseptic technique. The venipuncture site is clipped with a No. 40 blade, cleansed with Nolvasan scrub for 5 minutes, sprayed with alcohol, and followed by dilute 2 per cent Nolvasan solution. Nolvasan preparations are preferred in foals to avoid the skin irritation encountered more frequently with Betadine preparations. Sterile gloves are worn for catheter insertion and the catheter hub is stabilized with sutures, tape butterflies, and occasionally Superglue. The venipuncture site and catheterized vessel are monitored daily for signs of thrombosis or phlebitis.

Volumetric infusion pumps such as the FloGard 6100† and Omni Flow‡ are recommended to ensure accurate infusion rates. A carefully regulated microdrip burrette§ can also be used to administer PN formulas. Monitoring techniques to help prevent some of the metabolic and catheter-related problems associated with PN therapy are listed in Table 7.

Products used for parenteral alimentation are presented in Table 8. The most commonly used stock solutions, 50 per cent dextrose, 10 per cent amino acids, and 10 per cent lipid emulsion, are used as the basis for sample calculations presented in Table 9. Other commonly used additives include potassium chloride solution, vitamins, and trace mineral mixtures. Parenteral

TABLE 6. COMPLICATIONS OF PARENTERAL ALIMENTATION

Metabolic disturbances
  Hyperglycemia/hypoglycemia
  Glucosuria/osmotic diuresis
  Hyperlipemia
  Hyperosmolar states
  Hyperchloremic acidosis
  Azotemia/uremia
  Electrolyte imbalances
  Cholestasis
Catheter-related problems
  Venous thrombosis
  Phlebitis
  Sepsis

---

*L-Cath, Lutner Medical Products, Tustin, CA
†FloGard 6100 Volumetric Infusion Pump, Baxter Healthcare Corp., Deerfield, IL
‡Omni Flow 4000, Omni Flow, Inc., Wilmington, MA
§Buretrol, Baxter Healthcare Corp., Deerfield, IL

TABLE 7. MONITORING PROCEDURES FOR PARENTERAL ALIMENTATION

Observation	Initial Monitoring Frequency	Monitoring After Stabilization
Vital signs	q. 4 h.	q. 8 h.
Catheter/vein inspection	q. 8 h.	q. 8 h.
Intake/output	q. 8 h.	q. 8 h.
Weight	Daily	Daily
Urine glucose	q. 6–8 h.	q. 8–12 h.
Serum glucose	q. 6–12 h.	q. 24 h.
Serum electrolytes	q. 24 h.	1–2/wk
Creatinine/blood urea nitrogen	q. 24 h.	2/wk
Triglycerides/cholesterol	Baseline	Weekly
Liver enzymes (GGT, LLDH, SAP)	Baseline	Weekly
Liver function tests (bilirubin)	Baseline	Weekly
Packed cell volume/total protein	q. 12–24 h.	q. 2–3 d.
White blood cell differential	Baseline	Weekly
Fibrinogen	Baseline	Weekly

TABLE 8. PRODUCTS FOR PARENTERAL ALIMENTATION

A. Dextrose Solution

Concentration (gm/dl)	Osmolarity (mOsm/L)	Calories (kcal/L)	L Required for Maintenance*
2.5	126	85	71
5.0	253	170	35
10.0	505	340	18
20.0	1010	680	9
50.0	2520	1700	4

B. Lipid Emulsions

Product	Concentration (gm/dl)	Osmolarity (mOsm/L)	Calories (kcal/L)
Intralipid†	10 (20)	280 (330)	1100 (2000)
Liposyn‡	10 (20)	276 (340)	1100 (2000)

C. Crystalline Amino Acids

Product (without electrolytes)	Concentration (gm/dl)	Total Nitrogen (gm/L)	Osmolarity (mOsm/L)
Aminosyn§	8.5 (10.0)	13.4 (15.7)	850 (1000)
Travasol‖	8.5 (10.0)	14.3 (16.8)	860 (1060)

D. Supplements

Multivitamin concentrate: M.V.C. 9 + 3 ¶				Trace elements: M.T.E. 5 # (1 ml vial)	
Ascorbic Acid	100 mg	Niacin	40 mg	Zinc	5 mg
Vitamin A	3300 IU	Pantothenic acid	15 mg	Copper	1 mg
Vitamin D	200 IU	Vitamin E	101 U	Manganese	0.5 mg
Thiamine (B_1)	3.0 mg	Biotin	60 µg	Chromium	10 µg
Riboflavin (B_2)	3.6 mg	Folic acid	400 µg	Selenium	20 µg
Pyidoxin (B_6)	4.0 mg	Vitamin B_{12}	5 µg		

*Maintenance for 50-kg foal = 120 kcal/kg/day = 6000 kcal.
†Intralipid, KabiVitrum Inc., Alameda, CA.
‡Liposyn, Abbott Labs., North Chicago, IL.
§Aminosyn, Abbot Labs., North Chicago, IL.
‖Travasol, Baxter Healthcare Corp., Deerfield, IL.
¶M.V.C. 9 + 3, Multivitamin Concentrate, Lypho Med Inc., Melrose Park, IL.
#M.T.E. 5, Trace Element Additive, Lypho Med Inc. Melrose Park, IL.

formulas should be compounded aseptically in a laminar flow hood. The use of sterile, empty 3- or 4-liter bags,§ with two or three lead transfer sets, facilitates sterile mixing of ingredients. Solutions should be added in order: glucose, amino acids, and lipid emulsion. This mixing sequence is required to maintain a suitable solution pH to allow lipid solubility. To ensure component compatibility it is advisable to use amino acids and lipids from the same manufacturer. Once compounded, PN solutions should be refrigerated

§Baxter All-in-One 4 liter bag, Baxter Healthcare Corp., Deerfield, IL; 3000 ml EVA Empty 3-in-1 Mixing Container with attached 3-Lead Transfer Set, Abbott Lab., North Chicago, IL.

TABLE 9. SAMPLE CALCULATIONS FOR A 45 KG FOAL RECEIVING PARENTERAL ALIMENTATION

Initial formulation:
  Glucose   10 gm/kg = 450 gm; 900 ml of 50% dextrose
  Amino acid   2 gm/kg = 90 gm; 900 ml of 10% amino acid
  Lipid   1 gm/kg = 45 gm; 450 ml of 10% lipid
Calories provided:
  Glucose   3.4 kcal/gm; 450 gm = 1530 kcal
  Amino acid   4.0 kcal/gm; 90 gm = 360 kcal
  Lipids   9.0 kcal/gm (emulsion contains glycerol and provides 11.0 kcal/gm); 45 gm = 495 kcal
  Total calories = 2385; 53 kcal/kg/day
Source of calories:
  Glucose = 64%   Amino acid = 15%   Lipids = 21%
Nonprotein calories per gram of nitrogen:
  Nonprotein calories = 2025
  6.2 gm protein = 1 gm nitrogen
  Nonprotein calories per gram of nitrogen = 139.6
Supplements:
  Multivitamin concentrate (M.V.C.—9 + 3), 10 ml
  Trace minerals (M.T.E.—5) 1 ml
  KCl: 20–40 mEq/L; marked hypokalemia requires additional supplementation

prior to use. Vitamins and trace elements are added shortly before administration.

Glucose solutions provide 3.4 kcal per gm and are hypertonic at concentrations greater than 5.0 per cent. Initial infusion rates begin at 10 gm per kg per day (7 mg per kg per min) and, if tolerated by the foal, can be increased slowly at the rate of 1 gm per kg per day to 15 gm per kg per day. Hypertonic glucose infusions should be started and stopped gradually to avoid sudden changes in glucose concentrations. Sepsis-induced glucose intolerance frequently limits glucose infusion rates in critically ill neonates, requiring additional calories to be supplied by lipids. Five and 10 per cent glucose solutions alone cannot provide adequate calories (see Table 8) and should not be used long term as the only nutrient source.

Lipid emulsions contain primarily long-chain triglycerides and provide a concentrated source of calories at 9 to 11 kcal per gm. Lipid emulsions are isotonic and help reduce total osmolarity when added to glucose and amino acid mixtures. A decreased incidence of vessel thrombosis has been observed following the addition of lipids to PN formulas. This observation may be due to a simple decrease in total osmolarity of PN infusions or to a protective effect of lipids on vascular endothelium. When insulin-resistant hyperglycemia restricts glucose administration, lipids can be used to provide 30 to 60 per cent of the nonprotein calories. Lipid infusion rates usually begin at 1 gm per kg per day and can be increased to 4 gm per kg per day in increments of 1 gm per kg per day. Lipid emulsions can be mixed with amino acids and glucose or administered separately. During lipid infusions, serum samples should be examined frequently for lipemia, and plasma triglyceride and cholesterol levels monitored routinely. During severe sepsis, impaired lipid clearance due to carnitine deficiency or reduced lipoprotein lipase activity results in lipemia. Heparin, which augments lipoprotein lipase activity, can be given at doses of 10 U per kg or added to the PN solution at a rate of 1 U per ml to reduce and improve lipid utilization. Marked prematurity has also been associated with lipid intolerance due to limited carnitine stores. The use of lipids in infants with hyperbilirubinemia is controversial. Kernicterus, the deposition of unconjugated bilirubin in brain cells, can occur when bilirubin levels exceed 18 to 20 mg per dl. FFA and bilirubin competitively bind to albumin. Elevated serum FFA concentrations have been associated with lipid administration in infants. Therefore, lipid emulsions are not routinely administered to infants with bilirubin levels above 8.0 mg per dl. Similar considerations are probably justified in foals. The use of lipids in patients with pulmonary compromise is also controversial because of concern that lipid emulsions interfere with pulmonary microcirculation and arterial oxygenation. Recent studies showed that oxygen diffusion in premature neonates was not affected by lipid infusions up to 4 gm per kg per day administered over 24 hours. Lipid infusions have been used successfully in foals receiving mechanical ventilatory support.

The hypermetabolic patient may benefit from the addition of lipids to PN formulas, for several reasons. The hormonal milieu responsible for sepsis-induced catabolism favors lipolysis and fat utilization while antagonizing insulin activity and glucose uptake. In the nutrient-depleted or hypermetabolic patient receiving hypertonic glucose or amino acid mixtures there is increased carbon dioxide (CO_2) production contributing to respiratory acidosis and increased oxygen consumption. In patients with pulmonary compromise, myocardial depression, and hypoperfusion, excessive glucose administration may precipitate respiratory distress and enhance cardiovascular deterioration. Excessive CO_2 production may interfere with weaning a patient from mechanical ventilatory support. Fat emulsions are oxidized with a lower respiratory quotient (RQ) than glucose (RQ of fat = 0.7, RQ of glucose = 1.0) and could prove beneficial under these circumstances by reducing metabolic CO_2 production and minute ventilation.

The most commonly used protein solutions contain free amino acids and provide approximately 4.0 kcal per gm of protein. The solutions are hypertonic and are available with or without electrolytes. The precise protein and amino acid requirements of term and preterm foals are not known. Protein requirements of term and preterm infants are approximately 2.2 gm per kg per day and greater than 3.0 gm per kg per day, respectively. The purpose of administering protein solutions is to provide amino acids and nitrogen for growth, healing, and cellular repair. The ratio of nonprotein calories to nitrogen should be approximately 100 to 200 to prevent catabolism of protein for energy. In foals, protein infusion rates usually begin at 2 gm per kg per day and are increased to 3 gm per kg per day.

The daily requirements of vitamins and trace elements are not available for neonatal term and preterm foals. Commercially available human preparations are used. Foals not receiving any enteral feeds require additional potassium chloride supplementation. Potassium is an intracellular ion. Depletion of total body potassium stores accompanies malnutrition and loss of cell mass. Osmotic diuresis secondary to hyperglycemia or diuretic-induced diuresis enhances renal potassium excretion. Between 40 and 60 mEq of potassium is routinely added to each liter of PN solution. Additional supplementation is required to treat severe hypokalemia.

Foals relying on chronic parenteral alimentation as their sole nutrient source require additional calcium and phosphorus supplementation. As discussed previously, precise requirements for neonatal foals are not known and there is no easily measured serum parameter to assess adequacy of calcium and phosphorus intake. Provision of sufficient quantities of these ingredients is hampered by the calcium and phosphorus solubility limitations of PN solutions. A conservative approach is to add calcium gluconate and potassium phosphate routinely to PN formulas when chronic IV alimentation without enteral support is anticipated. Calcium gluconate can be safely added to standard PN solutions at a rate of 25 to 50 mEq per L and potassium phospate at a rate of 5 to 15 mEq per L. This rate of supplementation is still inadequate for the growing foal and requires additional enteral supplementation if long-term PN support is necessary.

Sample calculations for PN formulation for a 50-kg foal are presented in Table 9. The dextrose, amino acid, and lipid requirements are calculated. Then vitamin, mineral, and electrolyte needs are determined. The total daily solution volume is divided by 24 to determine the hourly infusion rate. A foal is introduced slowly to the PN infusion to allow acclimation of neuroendocrine systems. It may take 12 to 18 hours to reach the target infusion rate. Parameters listed in Table 7 are used to determine the patient's tolerance of the formula. Increases in dextrose, protein, and lipid are made slowly according to the specialized needs of each foal. Often a combination of enteral and parenteral nutritional support is employed. Weaning from PN support must be gradual, with a slow reduction in dextrose, amino acid, and lipid concentrations over 2 to 3 days. To avoid rebound hypoglycemia, cessation of PN infusion is usually followed by 1 to 2 liters of 5 per cent dextrose to be certain glucose homeostasis is satisfactory. Ideally, a foal should be consuming a minimum of 10 per cent of its body weight in milk daily before all PN support is discontinued.

A foal's daily fluid requirements (100 ml per kg) are in excess of the fluid volume provided by most PN formulas. Other isotonic fluids used to meet fluid requirements can be piggy-backed into the main IV line together with the PN formula. To reduce the risk of catheter-related sepsis, injections into the main IV line should be minimized and blood sampling from the PN catheter forbidden. PN formulations should not be left hanging for longer than 36 hours. Systemic fungal infections have been associated with PN administration in humans and have been observed in foals receiving chronic PN support. Therefore, requests for fungal isolation should be included whenever blood or other body fluids are submitted for culture.

Supplemental Readings

Askanazi, J., Carpentier, Y. A., Elwyn, D. H., et al.: Influences of total parenteral nutrition on fuel utilization in injury and sepsis. Ann. Surg., 191·40, 1980.

Bozzetti, F.: Nutritional assessment from the perspective of a clinician. J.P.E.N., 11(suppl):115S, 1987.

Carpentier, Y. A., and Thonnart, N.: Parameters for evaluation of lipid metabolism. J.P.E.N., 11(suppl.):104S, 1987.

Cochran, E. B., Phelps, S. J., and Helms, R. A.: Parenteral nutrition in pediatric patients. Clin. Pharm., 7:351, 1988.

Dominioni, L., and Dionigi, R.: Immunological function and nutritional assessment. J.P.E.N.., 11(suppl.):70S, 1987.

Dudrick, S. J., MacFadyen, Jr., B. V., Van Buren, C. T.: Parenteral hyperalimentation: Metabolic problems and solutions. Ann. Surg., 176:259, 1972.

Gideon, L.: Total nutritional support of the foal. Vet. Med. Small Anim. Clin., 72:1197, 1977.

Gilder, H.: Parenteral nourishment of patients undergoing surgical or traumatic stress. J.P.E.N., 10:88, 1986.

Hansen, T. O.: Nutritional support: Parenteral feeding. In Koterba, A. M., Drummond, W. H., and Kosch, P. C. (eds.): Equine Clinical Neonatology. Philadelphia, Lea & Febiger, 1990, pp. 747–762.

Koterba, A. M.: Nutritional support: Enteral feeding. In Koterba, A. M., Drummond, W. H., and Kosch, P. C. (eds.):

Equine Clinical Neonatology. Philadelphia, Lea & Febiger, 1990, pp. 728–746.
Naylor, J. M. and Bell, R.: Raising the orphan foal. Vet. Clin. North Am. (Equine Pract.), 1:169, 1985.
Pereira, G. R., and Barbosa, M. M.: Controversies in neonatal nutrition. Pediat. Clin. North Am. (Newborn I), 33:65, 1986.
Roberts, M. C.: The development and distribution of mucosal enzymes in the small intestine of the fetus and young foal. J. Reprod. Fertil. Suppl., 23:717, 1975.

Section 18

EXOTIC DISEASES

Edited by William W. Laegreid

African Horse Sickness
William W. Laegreid, GREENPORT, NEW YORK

African horse sickness has been recognized for centuries. The disease, transmitted by biting midges, is highly fatal in susceptible populations. African horse sickness was originally confined to sub-Saharan Africa, where it was thought to exist as a relatively mild infection of wild animals. As domestic horses were introduced, the disease began to be recognized in its current form. Reports of a horse sickness-like disease in the Middle East are included in a document entitled "Le Kitab el-Akoua el-Kaflah Wa El Chafiah," dating back nearly 700 years. A similar disease was described by Western observers during early explorations of Africa in 1569. As European colonization of Africa progressed, reports of African horse sickness increased. Dr. Livingstone was reduced to walking rather than riding horseback during his years in Africa partly because of African horse sickness. Numerous reports of severe epizootics were recorded in colonial southern Africa as early as 1719. In recent times, numerous outbreaks have occurred in various regions of Africa and in the Mediterranean region. A severe outbreak occurred in Spain in 1966 and again in 1987, this time following importation of zebras from Namibia. This outbreak continued in 1988 and 1989, with extension into Portugal in 1989. At present, the outbreak on the Iberian peninsula is not yet under control. It is clear that African horse sickness presents a serious threat to the health of horses in Africa, the Near East, Middle East, and Southern Europe. With increasing international movement of horses, there is a greater likelihood that the disease might be introduced into areas far removed from those mentioned above.

AFRICAN HORSE SICKNESS VIRUS

African horse sickness virus, along with bluetongue, epizootic hemorrhagic disease, and Ibaraki viruses, is an orbivirus, family Reoviridae. The viral capsids are 70 μm in diameter, have icosahedral symmetry, and have a genome consisting of ten segments of double-stranded RNA. The coding assignments of the genome segments have not been determined. Hybridization and electrophoretic analyses of the genome have established a distinct relationship between African horse sickness virus and bluetongue virus. African horse sickness viral capsids are composed of seven structural proteins (VP 1 to 7). Two proteins, VP2 and VP5, form the outer layer of the capsid, which surrounds a core particle composed of proteins 1, 3, 4, 6, and 7, an arrangement that appears to be similar to that of bluetongue virus. Stripping the outer proteins from the virus particles reveals, under electron microscopy, the ring-shaped capsomeres that characterize the orbiviruses. It remains to be demonstrated, although it is likely by analogy to bluetongue virus, that VP2 is the protein that is recognized by neutralizing antibody and thus may define the serotype of African horse sickness virus. At least two nonstructural polypeptides, NS1 and NS2, are also identified in virus-infected cells. The role of the nonstructural polypeptides in viral replication is not known. NS1 is the major component of tubular structures that appear intracellularly during replication of African horse sickness virus. In bluetongue virus-infected cells, NS2 has mRNA binding activity and may have some role in virus assembly. NS2 in both blue tongue virus and African horse sickness virus is phosphorylated, but no functional role has been defined.

One property of the Reoviridae is the ability of the various segments of the genome to reassort. This phenomenon occurs when viruses of, for example, two separate serotypes infect the same cell at the same time. Some of the progeny virus from such an infection may have some segments of their genome from one of the parent viruses and some segments from the other, significantly altering their serological properties. Such reassortments have been shown to occur in nature, specifically within *Culicoides*. It may be speculated that reassortment might contribute to reversion to virulence of attenuated vaccine virus or to the development of viruses that could escape neutralization.

EPIZOOTOLOGY

African horse sickness virus is an arbovirus, a virus that replicates in and is transmitted by an arthropod vector(s). Direct animal-to-animal transmission of the virus does not occur between horses. The major vectors are biting midges of the genus *Culicoides*. These insects are widely distributed throughout the world, including the United States. *C. Imicola*, in Africa, and *C. variipennis*, a vector for bluetongue virus in the United States, are among the species known to be capable of transmitting African horse sickness virus. Other insects such as mosquitoes and ticks may act as mechanical vectors, but the significance of this mode of transmission is unknown.

The requirement of an insect vector for transmission of African horse sickness virus has several implications for the epizootology of the disease. First, the distribution of the disease will follow roughly the habitat of the vector. In the case of most *Culicoides* this means moist, low-lying areas such as river valleys, swamps, and coastal regions, areas where the standing water, rotting vegetation, and fecal matter required for *Culicoides* breeding tend to be found. Second, movement of the vector, either through the inadvertent activities of man or through meteorological events, may introduce African horse sickness into new areas. Some evidence indicates that outbreaks of African horse sickness occurred following unusual winds that blew clouds of midges from endemic areas in Africa and the Middle East into Spain, Cyprus, and the Cape Verde Islands, distances of up to 700 km. Third, the requirement for a vector explains the seasonal occurrence of African horse sickness outside sub-Saharan Africa. The disease is most common in mid- to late summer, corresponding to peak populations of *Culicoides*. The onset of cold weather in the fall is accompanied by a decline in the appearance of clinical cases of African horse sickness. However, the disease may reappear when climatic conditions are favorable for *Culicoides* multiplication or reintroduction.

Where the virus may reside over the winter is not known. Possibilities include vertical transmission in *Culicoides*, prolonged inapparent viremia in some equids, or infection of another mammalian reservoir. There is little evidence for vertical transmission in *Culicoides*, although this mechanism for viral overwintering cannot be ruled out. Species implicated as potential reservoirs for African horse sickness virus include elephants, camels, zebras, and dogs. Zebras can be infected with the virus, producing a prolonged viremic period and mild to sub-clinical disease. Infected dogs develop clinical signs similar to the disease in horses, and even die from African horse sickness. Identification of the viral reservoir is necessary to eradicate the disease from endemic areas.

DIAGNOSIS

CLINICAL SIGNS AND LESIONS

Four forms of African horse sickness were initially described by Theiler: a pulmonary form, a cardiac form, a mixed form, and a mild form known as African horse sickness fever. While these classifications are somewhat useful conceptually, lesions typical of any of the forms of African horse sickness may be found in various combinations in individual animals with the disease. There is no evidence to suggest that the different forms of African horse sickness are related to the viral serotype with which an animal is infected. However, owing to its common usage in the literature, Theiler's scheme will be adhered to in the following description of the clinicopathological signs and lesions of African horse sickness.

The pulmonary form is most common in naive

horses and in dogs. This is an acute disease occurring 3 to 5 days post infection. Affected animals have signs typical of severe pulmonary edema, including dyspnea, frothing at the nares, coughing, and a transient fever of up to 104° or 105° F (40° to 41° C). Mortality is reportedly high (greater than 95 per cent). Death may occur within hours of the onset of clinical signs. At necropsy, severe pulmonary edema and hydrothorax are the most pronounced lesions. The lungs fail to collapse completely when the thoracic cavity is opened. The interlobular septa are widened and, along with subpleural tissues, are filled with clear gelatinous fluid. Mediastinal edema is reportedly a common feature. The mucosal surfaces of the glandular portion of the stomach are often deeply reddened. There may be petechiation of many abdominal serosal surfaces. Histologically, pulmonary alveolar spaces and interlobular septa are filled with a variably cellular fibrin-rich exudate. Pulmonary vascular changes include congestion, increased numbers of intraluminal mononuclear cells, and nonsuppurative perivasculitis. Moderate congestion of the gastric mucosa is present. Lymph nodes are edematous with pronounced depletion of lymphocytes and karyorhexis within germinal centers.

The cardiac form has a more prolonged incubation period (7 to 14 days). This form is characterized clinically by pronounced edema of the head and neck, notably in the supraorbital fossae. In severe cases edema may extend well into the shoulders and chest. The febrile response is less severe than in the pulmonary form (104° F; 39° to 40° C). Mortality is about 50 per cent. Death occurs 4 to 8 days after the onset of clinical signs. Lesions typical of the cardiac form of African horse sickness include marked accumulations of gelatinous fluid in the subcutaneous tissues and intermuscular fascial planes in the head and neck. Hydropericardium and petechial to ecchymotic hemorrhages of the epi-and endocardium are present. Focal myocardial necrosis has been reported. As in the pulmonary form of disease, congestion of the gastric mucosa and lymphoid depletion are present.

The mixed form has an incubation period of 5 to 7 days. Clinical signs and lesions are a variable mix of those described in the pulmonary and cardiac forms. Death occurs within 3 to 6 days after clinical presentation in 80 per cent of affected horses.

Horse sickness fever is a mild form of the disease thought to result from the infection of partially immune horses from endemic areas with a heterologous serotype. An incubation period of 5 to 14 days is followed by a febrile episode of about 105° F (39° to 40° C), which lasts for several days. Few other clinical signs and no significant lesions are thought to be present. This form of African horse sickness is not fatal.

LABORATORY DIAGNOSIS

The presumptive diagnosis of African horse sickness, based on clinical signs, lesions, and history, is confirmed by virus isolation or serology. Samples for isolation include defibrinated blood, lung and spleen or other lymphoid organs. These are inoculated into cell culture or intracerebrally into suckling mice. Virus neutralization with specific reference antisera is used to identify the virus serotype. Immunofluorescence techniques have been applied to the demonstration of viral antigens in tissue sections.

Antibodies to African horse sickness virus may be detected by a variety of methods. These include group-specific tests: agar gel immunodiffusion, complement fixation (CF), indirect fluorescent antibody, enzyme-linked immunosorbent assay, and type-specific virus neutralization assay. The activity of CF antibodies is short-lived in circulation and thus is only thought to be indicative of recent infections. Virus neutralization antibodies are present for a longer period following infection. Type-specific serological tests that do not require as much time as virus neutralization are being developed.

IMMUNE RESPONSE, VACCINATION, AND CONTROL

There are nine recognized serotypes of African horse sickness virus. Horses that have recovered from infection are generally protected against challenge with homologous virus. Although few studies have been performed directly, this protection is probably antibody mediated, based on correlation of protection with in vitro neutralization by immune sera and transfer of protection from immune mares to foals via colostrum.

Recognition of solid protection against disease following recovery from infection led to the development of vaccines for African horse sickness. Early attempts at producing a killed vaccine were unsuccessful. In the 1930s, however, neurotropic, adult mouse–adapted, attenuated strains of African horse sickness virus were developed. Mixtures of serotypes of neurotropic murine-adapted virus were devised to create polyvalent vaccines that provided reasonably good immunity to infection under experimental and field conditions. These neurotropic murine strains were also adapted to grow in cell culture, but care had to be taken to ensure that immunogenicity was retained.

Both murine and cell culture vaccines have been used with success in endemic areas and in outbreaks in nonendemic regions. Unfortunately, the neurotropic murine vaccines were associated with numerous postvaccinal reactions such as encephalitis and blindness, resulting from vaccine virus replication in the brains of vaccinated horses. These reactions were reportedly less prevalent when the neurotropic murine strains were adapted to cell culture. Recent studies have indicated that horses vaccinated with the polyvalent attenuated vaccine may still become clinically infected with African horse sickness virus. Repeated vaccination was reported to result in a state of immunological nonresponsiveness or possibly hypersensitivity in a small percentage of animals. Failure of the polyvalent vaccine to protect against some serotypes, fears of reversion to virulence of the neuroadapted strains, and reluctance of countries without endemic disease to accept horses vaccinated with attenuated virus vaccines have continued to spur vaccine research and development. Current research is directed toward subunit and virus-vectored vaccines that may alleviate these problems.

In endemic areas, control measures such as annual vaccination prior to the *Culicoides* season, stabling animals in insect-proof stalls, and moving animals to higher elevations where the vectors are not prevalent have all been practiced to reduce the incidence of African horse sickness. In the event of an outbreak in a nonendemic area, slaughter of all infected animals, spraying of *Culicoides* breeding areas with insecticides, quarantine, and vaccination of all horses in a large area surrounding the outbreak are the only effective measures available.

The control and prevention of African horse sickness depend heavily on the quality and reliability of vaccination. Effective vaccines, polyvalent or cross-protective, that are acceptable to the international community are being developed to help control and eradicate this disease.

Supplemental Readings

Dardiri, A. H., and Salama, S. A.: African horsesickness: An overview. J. Equine Vet. Sci., 8:46–49, 1988.

Henning, M. W.: African Horsesickness, Perdesiekte, Pestis Equorum. In: Animal diseases in South Africa, 3rd ed. Johannesburg, Central News Agency, 1956, pp. 785–808.

Hess, W. R.: African Horsesickness. In Monath, T. P. (ed.): The Arboviruses: Epidemiology and Ecology. Vol. II. Boca Raton, Fla., CRC Press, 1988.

House, C., Mikiciuk, P. E., and Berninger, M. L.: Laboratory diagnosis of African horsesickness: Comparison of serological techniques and evaluation of storage methods of samples for virus isolation. J. Vet. Diagn. Invest., 2:44–50, 1990.

Newsholme, S. J.: A morphological study of the lesions of African horsesickness. Onderstepoort J. Vet. Res., 50:7–24, 1983.

Babesiosis
Donald P. Knowles, Jr., PULLMAN, WASHINGTON

Equine babesiosis, caused by *Babesia equi* or *Babesia caballi*, is a tick-borne hemoprotozoan blood disease affecting horses worldwide. Both species of *Babesia* are currently present in southern Florida. Ticks are the principal vectors of equine babesiosis. Potential tick vectors include species of the *Dermacentor*, *Hyalomma*, and *Rhipicephalus* genera.

Horses, donkeys, and their crossbreeds, as well as zebras, are susceptible to babesiosis. *B. caballi* apparently persists in its vectors for many generations, does not appear to persist for longer than 1 to 4 years in its vertebrate hosts, and is rarely transmitted from dam to fetus. For these reasons, tick vectors appear to be a major reservoir host of this parasite. By contrast, *B. equi* persists in its vertebrate host for many years (perhaps for life), and intrauterine transmission is common. The vertebrate host thus appears to be a major reservoir of *B. equi*.

CLINICAL SIGNS

Clinical disease is characterized by fever, anemia, and icterus arising from hemolysis caused by infection of erythrocytes by merozoites. In addition, *B. caballi* apparently sequesters in brain capillaries, occluding blood flow. Carrier horses with clinically inapparent disease are important in the dissemination of the disease. Clinical episodes occur under two conditions: when susceptible horses are moved into endemic areas, and when inapparent carrier horses are moved into nonendemic areas and appropriate tick vectors are present to spread equine *Babesia* spp. to susceptible horses.

DIAGNOSIS

In addition to the clinical signs listed above, a history of travel to areas endemic for *Babesia*, a history of tick infestation, or a history of blood transfusion support a diagnosis of babesiosis. The differential diagnoses of babesiosis include equine infectious anemia virus, purpura hemorrhagica, equine viral arteritis virus, equine ehrlichiosis, trypanosomiasis, leptospirosis, and poisoning. Definitive diagnosis currently depends on the identification of *Babesia* organisms in blood smears or by transfusion of blood into a susceptible animal. Direct parasitological verification of chronic *B. caballi* infection is almost impossible, but is occasionally successful with *B. equi* infection. The complement fixation (CF) test was adopted as the official serological test for equine babesiosis by the United States Department of Agriculture (USDA) in 1969. This test measures antibodies directed against *B. equi* or *B. caballi*. Horses that test positive on CF assay are restricted from entry into the United States. Serum submitted to state diagnostic laboratories is forwarded to the National Veterinary Services Laboratory, Ames, Iowa, for equine babesiosis testing.

THERAPY AND CONTROL

Since vaccines are currently not available, control of equine babesiosis in enzootic areas is most effectively aimed at tick elimination. It is hypothesized that in enzootic areas, horses acquire protective immunity to equine babesiosis through reinfections. Therefore, in enzootic areas, where reexposure is probable, drug therapy should be aimed at depressing parasitemia and effecting clinical remission without clearing the infection and the associated premunition. In general, *B. caballi* can be handled better with chemotherapeutic drugs than *B. equi*. Complete elimination of *B. equi* using drugs currently available is not possible. Drugs that have been shown to be useful in the treatment of equine babesiosis include diminazen (Berenil),* 4 to 5 mg per kg given once daily; imidocarb (Imazil),† 2 to 3 mg per kg given twice daily; amicarbalide (Diaprom)‡ single injection of 9 to 10 mg per kg; and quironium (Acaprin),§ 1.2 ml of 5 per cent solution per 100 kg administered in two subcutaneous injections 6 hours apart. Quironium frequently produces side effects of muscle tremor, salivation, defecation, restlessness, and dyspnea.

Supplemental Readings

Knowles, R. C.: Equine babesiosis: Epidemiology, control and chemotherapy. J. Equine Vet. Sci., 8:61–64, 1988.
Kuttler, K. L.: Chemotherapy of babesiosis: A review. *In* Ristic, M. and Kreier, J. P. (eds.): Babesiosis. New York, Academic Press, 1981, pp. 65–86.
Schein, E.: Equine babesiosis. *In* Ristic, M. (eds.): Babesiosis of Domestic Animals and Man. Boca Raton, Fla., CRC Press, 1988, pp. 197–208.

---

*Hoechst AG, Frankfurt, West Germany
†Wellcome Foundation, London, England
‡May and Baker, Dagenham, England
§Bayer AG, Leverkusen, West Germany

Contagious Equine Metritis

Peter J. Timoney, LEXINGTON, KENTUCKY

Contagious equine metritis (CEM) is a highly contagious venereal disease of the horse caused by *Taylorella equigenitalis*, a previously undescribed gram-negative coccobacillus with fastidious growth requirements. In the period since CEM was first reported and etiologically defined in 1977, the disease has been recorded in Europe, Japan, Australia, and North and South America. Currently available evidence indicates that CEM may be restricted solely to Equidae, since the causal agent, *T. equigenitalis*, has not been isolated from cases of natural infection in any species other than the horse. The disease has been reproduced in donkeys but not in cattle, sheep, pigs, or cats. Some species of laboratory animals are susceptible to experimental infection by the intrauterine route.

PATHOGENESIS

Although dissemination of CEM occurs principally by the venereal route, infection can also be spread by indirect means through the use of contaminated veterinary instruments and by stud farm personnel if strict hygienic measures are not observed when animals are being handled or examined.

Contagious equine metritis is a disease confined to the genital tract, with no attendant mortality. Clinical signs of infection have been observed in the mare but not in the stallion, in which *T. equigenitalis* exists as a surface commensal on the external genitalia without causing any local tissue reaction or stimulating any detectable serological response. Following an incubation period of 2 to 12 days, cases of natural or experimental infection in the mare may manifest with acute endometritis, cervicitis, vaginitis, a vulvar discharge, and a return to estrus after a shortened diestrous period. Many mares, however, experience an inapparent infection with *T. equigenitalis,* and although most barren mares fail to conceive after primary infection with this organism, the infertility is short term, lasting only a few weeks. Infection need not preclude a normal pregnancy. *Taylorella equigenitalis* has only very rarely been implicated in equine abortion.

There is evidence of variation in pathogenicity between strains of *T. equigenitalis,* most notably between those recovered from Thoroughbred and non-Thoroughbred breeds, the latter isolates often being nonpathogenic. Experimental studies have confirmed an association between certain colonial characteristics of the organism and strain virulence. Whereas large colonial variants caused typical CEM in mares and could be cultured from the cervix and clitoris, small colonial variants produced no clinical response and could only be recovered from clitoral and not cervical swabs during the experimental period.

Based on the findings in cases of natural and experimental CEM infection in the mare, it is evident that *T. equigenitalis* spreads rapidly and widely in the uterus and cervix for up to 14 days after exposure to the organism. This is associated with development of a moderately severe, diffuse, acute endometritis, cervicitis, and vaginitis that is characterized initially by edema and extensive neutrophilic infiltration of the endometrium. Extensive destruction of the luminal epithelium may follow in some cases. The edema decreases and there is increased cellular infiltration predominantly with lymphocytes, macrophages, and plasma cells. The acute inflammatory changes appear to peak at about 14 days, after which they subside and are succeeded by a mild diffuse or multifocal lymphocytic salpingitis, endometritis, cervicitis, and vaginitis that can persist for up to 4 months or longer. These changes are accompanied by a rapid decline in the number of *T. equigenitalis* organisms in the uterus and cervix. While the organism may subsequently be cultured infrequently from the ovarian surface, oviducts, uterus, cervix, and vagina, it is likely to be recovered much more frequently from the clitoral sinuses and fossa. Persistence of *T. equigenitalis* in the latter sites in the carrier mare is associated with the presence of scattered lymphoid nodules deep in the local connective tissue and some infiltration of the overlying tissue and epithelium with lymphocytes.

EPIDEMIOLOGY

Undoubtedly the most significant factor in the epidemiology of CEM is occurrence of the carrier state in the mare and the stallion. A clinically inapparent carrier state can develop in a variable per centage of mares after recovery from the acute phase of the infection. Two types of carriers have been described, uterine and clitoral. Uterine carriers are thought to be rare. The vast majority of mares persistently infected with *T. equigenitalis* are clitoral carriers. The organism is harbored in the clitoral sinuses and fossa for extended periods, even years. Such carriers can be variable shedders of the organism.

Carrier mares can become pregnant and may transmit *T. equigenitalis* to their offspring either during gestation or, more likely, at or shortly after parturition. The foals are exposed presumably through contact of their external genitalia with infective vaginal discharge or placental membranes. Such foals may harbor *T. equigenitalis* as part of the normal flora on their external genitalia until sexually mature and, in turn, constitute a potential reservoir of infection.

The inapparent carrier state can be established in a high per centage of stallions, in which the predilection sites for localization of *T. equigenitalis* are the urethral fossa and associated diverticulum, the urethral sinus. The organism can also be recovered from the terminal urethra and the internal surface of the prepuce. The carrier state may persist in the stallion for years, and such animals constitute a major risk in terms of national and international spread of CEM.

Dissemination of infection with *T. equigenitalis* within any horse population is greatly enhanced during the stud season by the practice of "walking in" or "vanning in" of nonresident mares for breeding purposes.

DIAGNOSIS

Contagious equine metritis is an exotic venereal disease that cannot be differentiated on clinical grounds alone from two other bacterial infections of the reproductive tract, *Klebsiella pneumoniae* and *Pseudomonas aeruginosa*, both commonly encountered infections in the domestic horse population. Isolation of *T. equigenitalis* in culture is currently the only absolute means of establishing a diagnosis of CEM in the mare or the stallion. The presence of gram-negative coccobacilli and numerous neutrophils in stained smears of cervical or vaginal discharge may suggest but not confirm infection in the acutely affected mare. Appropriate sites to culture in the barren, maiden, or postparturient mare include the uterus or cervix, clitoral fossa, and sinuses. Endometrial or cervical swabs should be taken during early estrus. The clitoral fossa and sinuses are the sites to be swabbed in pregnant mares. Suitably small swabs must be used for effective culturing of the clitoral sinuses. Vaginal discharge if present should also be cultured.

The sites to swab in the stallion or colt are the urethral fossa and sinus, the terminal urethra, prepuce, external surface of the penis, and, if possible, pre-ejaculatory fluid. Stallions or colts should be sampled when the penis is fully extruded. On occasion, it may be necessary to breed a suspect carrier stallion to a test mare and screen the mare bacteriologically and serologically to determine if transmission of CEM infection has occurred. In the case of both stallions and mares, swabs should not be taken for culture of *T. equigenitalis* within 7 days of treatment for a genital tract infection.

All swabs for culture of *T. equigenitalis* must be placed either in antibiotic-free Amie's or Stuart's transport medium, kept refrigerated, and dispatched to an approved testing laboratory within 24 hours of collection. Various selective media have to be used to isolate *T. equigenitalis*, strains of which may be sensitive or resistant to streptomycin, from heavily contaminated sites in the mare and the stallion. Isolates of *T. equigenitalis* are confirmed based on their morphological characteristics (nonmotile, gram-negative coccobacillus), positive reactions for catalase, oxidase, and phosphatase, nonfermentation of sugars, and reaction with specific rabbit antisera in the slide or tube agglutination test or by direct or indirect immunofluorescence tests. Determination of the cellular fatty acid profile of the organism by gas liquid chromatography can also be used as an adjunct to currently recommended identification procedures, where problems with autoagglutination of strains are encountered.

Serological confirmation of a diagnosis of CEM is only possible in the mare, as there is no evidence of a detectable antibody response in the stallion. Furthermore, serology can only be used in the identification of mares during the acute phase of the infection. Antibodies are detectable around 7 days, reach maximal titers at approximately 3 weeks, and decline between 6 to 10 weeks. A range of serological tests including serum rapid plate (RPA) and tube agglutination, complement fixation (CF), passive hemagglutination (PHA), enzyme-linked immunosorbent assay (ELISA), indirect immunofluorescence, and agar gel immunodiffusion tests have been used, of which the CF, ELISA, RPA, and PHA tests have been found of greatest value in detecting acutely infected mares. However, none of the currently available serological tests are reliable for detection of the carrier mare.

THERAPY

Although the causal organism of CEM, *T. equigenitalis*, is sensitive to a wide variety of antimicrobial agents in vitro, there is presently no completely effective treatment that will ensure both rapid clinical recovery and complete elimination of this organism from the reproductive tract of the chronically infected mare. Unlike the mare, clearance of the carrier state in the stallion can be readily achieved through local treatment of the external genitalia.

Opinions vary as to whether cases of acute CEM infection in the mare should be treated, and if so, whether treatment should be local and systemic or just local by intrauterine infusion. Affected mares will make spontaneous clinical recoveries from the disease, but a significant percentage may continue to harbor *T. equigenitalis* in the clitoral fossa and sinuses. The drugs used with greatest success and fewest toxic side effects in these cases have been penicillin, ampicillin, amoxycillin, nitrofurazone, cefotaxime, and the disinfectant chlorhexidine. Field experience has shown that acute endometritis is best treated by the intrauterine infusion of solutions or suspensions of penicillin, ampicillin, amoxycillin, or cefotaxime administered daily for 5 to 7 days. Daily infusion of 5 to 10 megaunits of penicillin in aqueous solution has been used successfully.

Systemic and local treatment with these drugs is recommended in instances of chronic endometritis, possibly complicated by salpingitis. Affected mares should be treated for 7 to 10 days with the recommended parenteral dosage of the selected antibiotic administered intramuscularly. Systemic treatment with procaine penicillin has been combined successfully with intrauterine infusion of 1 liter of 0.2 per cent chlorhexidine for 3 to 5 days.

Local treatment of clitoral carriers of *T. equigenitalis* requires thorough cleansing of the clitoral fossa and sinuses with a 4 per cent solution of chlorhexidine, care being taken to ensure that the sinuses are adequately irrigated and all smegmalike material removed. The fossa and sinuses should be dried and packed with a 0.2 per cent nitrofurazone soluble ointment daily for 5 days. Experience has shown that a single course of treatment may not necessarily be successful in eliminating the organism in every instance. Clitoral sinusectomy may have to be considered in exceptional cases where elimination of the carrier state has not been possible even after numerous courses of treatment.

Treatment of the CEM carrier stallion or colt initially involves the thorough cleansing of the external genitalia with a solution of not less than 2 per cent chlorhexidine. With the penis fully extruded, special care must be taken to ensure that all smegma is removed from the urethra fossa and sinus, sheath, and penis. After drying, a 0.2 per cent nitrofurazone soluble ointment is applied to the external genitalia. Treatment is repeated daily for 5 days. One course of treatment is usually successful in elimination of the carrier state. Repeated washing of the external genitalia of particular stallions may increase the frequency of *Klebsiella* and *Pseudomonas* infections.

PREVENTION

Programs developed by individual countries for the prevention and control of CEM have largely focused on the disease in Thoroughbreds. Fundamental to the success of such programs has been the decision to make CEM either a notifiable disease or a nonnotifiable but reportable condition. As a sequel to the 1977 epizootic in the United Kingdom and Ireland, codes of practice have been developed in many countries setting forth guidelines for veterinarians and horse breeders alike for the prevention and control of CEM.

Crucial to the efficacy of these programs is the availability of laboratories with proven competency to provide a rapid and accurate diagnostic service for this disease, with special reference to detection of the carrier state in the mare and the stallion. Aside from comprehensive bacteriological screening of stallion and mare populations to identify clinical and asymptomatic carrier animals, the codes stress the need for improved standards of hygiene on stud farms. Such hygienic practices, directed at the prevention of indirect spread of the disease between horses, include the greater use of disposable and sterile equipment by veterinarians and stud personnel.

Mares or stallions culture positive for *T. equigenitalis* must be isolated and precluded from breeding until successfully treated and confirmed free of this organism. Mares with a known history of CEM should be categorized as "high risk" and subjected to more rigorous bacteriological screening before breeding to identify possible carrier animals. It is recommended that such animals be swabbed from the clitoral fossa and sinuses on at least three occasions; one of these screenings should also include an endometrial swab taken during the estrous period prior to breeding. Surgical ablation of the clitoral sinuses and fossa is an additional prophylactic measure that may have to be resorted to in mares refractive to elimination of the carrier state by chemotherapeutic means.

Studies on the possible development of a vaccine against CEM have not been sufficiently successful to hold out hope that immunization is likely to provide an effective means of preventing this disease in the near future.

In the light of current difficulties in detecting certain carrier mares, artificial insemination would provide a means of reducing the spread of CEM and of preventing exposure of stallions to *T. equigenitalis*. It would eliminate the hazard associated with the natural breeding of high-risk mares. This is only feasible, however, in breeds in which artificial insemination is permissible under current rules of registration.

Considerable success has been achieved in preventing or reducing the incidence of CEM in countries in which a code of practice has been rigorously implemented over a period of years.

Supplemental Readings

A Common Code of Practice for the Control of Contagious Equine Metritis and Other Equine Reproductive Diseases for the 1990 Covering Season in France, Ireland and the United Kingdom. Horserace Levy Betting Board, 1989.

Mackintosh, M. E.: Contagious equine metritis. In O.I.E. Manual of Recommended Diagnostic Techniques and Requirements for Biological Products for Lists A and B Diseases. Vol. II. Paris, Office International Des Epizooties, 1990.

Platt, H., and Taylor, C. E. D.: Contagious equine metritis. In Easmon, C. S. F., and Jeljaszewicz, J. (eds.): Medical Microbiology. Vol. I. London, Academic Press, 1982, pp. 49–96.

Powell, D. G.: Contagious equine metritis. Adv. Vet. Sci. Comp. Med., 25:161, 1981.

Timoney, P. J., and Powell, D. G.: Contagious equine metritis—epidemiology and control. J. Equine Vet. Sci., 8:42, 1988.

Glanders

Linda K. Schlater, AMES, IOWA

Glanders is a contagious bacterial disease of horses, donkeys, and mules caused by *Pseudomonas mallei*. The disease is characterized by the formation of nodules and ulcers in the skin and respiratory tract.

Systematic control measures have eradicated glanders from the Americas and western Europe and have decreased the incidence in many other parts of the world. Endemic foci continue to persist in Asia, particularly India and Mongolia, Africa, and the Middle East.

Glanders is spread to healthy horses via the highly infectious nasal and skin discharges of infected horses. The usual mode of transmission is by ingestion of contaminated feed or water. The disease may also be acquired by inhalation of infectious aerosols or through cuts or abrasions in the skin.

After invasion, the organisms localize in the regional lymph nodes and lungs, where nodular, tuberclelike lesions develop. Metastasis to the upper air passages, skin, or other organs may occur as the disease progresses.

CLINICAL SIGNS

Acute glanders is characterized by high fever (39.5° to 41° C), shivering, depression, and rapid emaciation. There is ulceration of the nasal septum and turbinate bones with mucopurulent to hemorrhagic nasal discharge. The submaxillary lymph nodes are swollen, lobulated, and painless. Unlike what is seen in strangles, the nodes seldom rupture. There is inspiratory dyspnea due to edema of the glottis and obstruction of the air passages by nasal discharge. Death due to bronchopneumonia and septicemia occurs within a few days. Acute glanders rarely affects horses but is the most common form observed in donkeys and mules.

The usual form of the disease in horses is a chronic pulmonary infection that may be subclinical for months, detectable only by intradermal or serological testing. When clinical signs develop, they include intermittent cough, nasal discharge, malaise, and general loss of condition.

In some horses the upper respiratory tract and skin are affected. Nodules appear in the submucosa of the nasal cavity, particularly on the nasal septum and the turbinates. The nodules rupture to form shallow, craterlike ulcers that exude a thick, mucopurulent material. The ulcers heal slowly, leaving characteristic star-shaped scars in the mucous membrane.

In cutaneous glanders ("farcy") the typical nodules form along the lymphatics between affected lymph nodes. The lymph vessels radiating from the nodules become thickened and tortuous. Nodules often ulcerate, discharging a thick, viscid, brownish exudate. These ulcers are slow to heal and often reopen. Farcy lesions may appear on any part of the body, but they are more common on the inside of the thigh and hocks.

DIAGNOSIS

State and federal veterinary officials must be notified if glanders is suspected. Prompt diagnosis and investigation are critical to prevent further spread of the disease.

The most definitive method of diagnosis is isolation of the causative agent. In acute glanders, the organisms are relatively numerous in affected tissues, and isolation is not difficult. *Pseudomonas mallei* grows well but slowly on common laboratory media. Growth may be enhanced by the addition of glycerol or defibrinated horse blood to the medium. After 2 days of incubation on blood agar, colonies are small, round, and a glistening brownish gray in color. *Pseudomonas mallei* is gram-negative, nonmotile, and fairly inactive biochemically. The last two characteristics distinguish *P. mallei* from the related bacterium *P. pseudomallei*, the cause of melioidosis.

Attempts to isolate *P. mallei* from animals with chronic and latent glanders are usually unsuccessful. The intrapalpebral mallein test and the complement fixation (CF) test on serum are used to diagnose these forms of the disease.

Mallein, a glycoprotein produced by *P. mallei* cells grown in glycerol broth, produces a delayed hypersensitivity reaction in animals that have been sensitized by natural infection. The test is performed by injecting 0.1 ml of mallein into the skin close to the edge of the lower eyelid. A positive reaction is characterized by pain and swelling at the site of inoculation, purulent conjunctivitis, and photophobia.

The mallein test is very reliable for detection of inapparent carriers. It is routinely used in endemic areas for "test and slaughter" control programs.

The CF test is the most accurate of the serological methods used. Antibodies are first detectable 4 to 12 weeks following infection. Because of its sensitivity, the CF test is used for routine surveillance in countries where glanders has been eradicated.

DIFFERENTIAL DIAGNOSIS

Melioidosis must be considered in any differential diagnosis for glanders. Horses with melioidosis may have positive reactions on the mallein or glanders CF test, owing to the cross-reactivity of *P. mallei* and *P. pseudomallei*. Isolation of the respective etiological agents is the only definitive method of differentiating these two diseases (see below).

The differential diagnosis of glanders should also include epizootic lymphangitis, ulcerative lymphangitis, sporotrichosis, and strangles. These diseases may be ruled out on the basis of positive mallein or CF test results or confirmed by demonstration of the etiological agents in tissue or exudate.

THERAPY, CONTROL, AND PREVENTION

Sodium sulfadiazine has been used to treat glanders. However, since carrier states may develop following apparent recovery, treatment is contraindicated.

The most effective method of control is prompt quarantine of exposed animals and destruction of all animals with clinical disease. Contacts should be mallein tested at 3-week intervals until all reactors have been removed and destroyed. Removal of potentially contaminated feed and bedding and concurrent disinfection of stalls, mangers, buckets, and equipment are necessary to prevent transmission of infection during quarantine.

There is no effective vaccine. Prevention is aimed at the enforced restriction of importation of horses from endemic areas and surveillance of horses in international traffic. The United States Department of Agriculture requires that all equids entering the country be CF negative for glanders.

Humans are susceptible to glanders. Human infections are usually acquired through skin cuts and abrasions during contact with glanders exudates. Investigators should exercise extreme care to avoid exposure to exudates when examining horses with nasal discharge and when performing necropsies. Specimens submitted for laboratory diagnosis should be clearly identified as "glanders suspect."

Suppplemental Readings

Gaiger, S. H.: Glanders in man. J. Comp. Pathol. Ther., 21:223–236, 1913.
Hickman, J.: Glanders: A contribution to epidemiology. Equine Vet. J., 2:153–158, 1970.
Redfearn, M.S., and Palleroni, N. J.: Glanders and melioidosis. *In* Hubbert, W. T., McCulloch, W. F., and Schnurrenberger, P. R. (eds.): Diseases Transmitted from Animals to Man. Springfield, Ill., Charles C. Thomas, 1975, pp. 110–128.
Steele, J. H.: Glanders. *In* Steele, J. H. (ed.): CRC Handbook Series in Zoonoses. Vol. 1. Boca Raton, Fla., CRC Press, 1979, pp. 339–362.

Melioidosis

Linda K. Schlater, AMES, IOWA

Melioidosis, a glanders-like disease of humans and animals that occasionally occurs in horses, is caused by *Pseudomonas pseudomallei*. Melioidosis is a disease of the tropics and subtropics, particularly Malaysia and northern Australia. Endemic foci have been established in France and Iran, presumably through the introduction of carrier animals. Melioidosis has not been reported in horses or other domestic animals in the United States.

Pseudomonas pseudomallei is widespread in the soil and waters of endemic areas. The organisms usually enter the host through skin abrasions or by ingestion, but may also be inhaled. Direct transmission from animal to animal or animals to man is rare. After entry, the organisms invade the lymphatics with subsequent regional lymphangitis, lymphadenitis, and septicemia. Multiple nodular lesions develop in the lungs, lymph nodes, spleen, kidney, and skin. The typical lesion begins as a small granulomatous nodule with a caseous center. Some nodules become abscesses and contain greenish yellow pus. Lung lesions are similar to those found in glanders, tuberculosis, or fungal infections. Glanderslike nodules and ulcers may occur in the skin and nasal mucosa.

CLINICAL SIGNS

In man, melioidosis has been called the great imitator, because clinical signs may mimic many other diseases. The situation is no different in horses. Melioidosis has been associated with clinical disease that resembles bastard strangles, glanders, acute encephalitis, and enteritis.

Most cases in horses are diagnosed either clinically in the acute stage or at postmortem examination. Acute disease may be primary, but more often it is an exacerbation of underlying chronic infection. The most common clinical picture is sudden onset of acute bronchopneumonia. Clinical signs include high fever (39.5° to 41° C), depression, anorexia, and respiratory distress. Moist rales or harsh, wheezing lung sounds may be detected on auscultation. Mucous membranes are hyperemic; the conjunctivae, brick red. There may be purulent discharge from the mouth or nasal passages. Affected animals seldom respond to antibiotics and usually die within 7 days.

A subacute form with pulmonary and cutaneous involvement, clinically indistinguishable from glanders, has been reported. Clinical signs included purulent nasal discharge, anorexia, and rapid loss of weight. Nodules (1 to 2 cm diameter) and ulcers were present along the lymphatics of the legs and in the nasal cavity. Death occurred after a course of 1 month.

Melioidosis may also manifest as an enteritis, presumably as a result of ingestion of the organism. Colic, gut hypermotility, softened feces, and diarrhea are prominent clinical signs. Affected horses may also exhibit edema of the rear legs and abdomen, or lymphangitis.

Two cases of acute central nervous system disease due to melioidosis have been reported in horses. Affected animals were unable to stand and exhibited tetanic muscular spasms and convulsions.

DIAGNOSIS

Diagnosis may be difficult in areas where the disease is not endemic. A history of recent travel to the subtropics or tropics is an important consideration. A definite diagnosis can only be made by isolation of the causative agent. *Pseudomonas pseudomallei* may be cultured from abscesses, discharges, blood, and feces.

Pseudomonas pseudomallei is a small, gram-negative, bipolar staining, pleomorphic bacillus. The organism grows well on ordinary laboratory media. Colonies vary from smooth to rough and wrinkled in texture and from cream to orange in color. Motility is easily demonstrated in wet mount preparations. *Pseudomonas pseudomallei* is active biochemically. Strains produce acid from oxidation of glucose, reduce nitrate, liquefy gelatin, and peptonize litmus milk. Motility and biochemical activity differentiate *P. pseudomallei* from the glanders bacillus.

Serological testing, including complement fixation, enzyme-linked immunosorbent assay, or agglutination tests, may provide additional laboratory confirmation of melioidosis. However, it must be emphasized that to date, no serological test can differentiate between melioidosis and glanders.

THERAPY, PREVENTION, AND CONTROL

There is little information on the treatment of equine melioidosis. The choice of antimicrobial agent should be based on sensitivity tests. The organism is resistant to many drugs, including penicillin, ampicillin, gentamicin, tobramycin, polymyxin B, and first- and second-generation cephalosporins. Mild, subacute pulmonary infections in humans have responded to therapy with chloramphenicol, tetracycline, kanamycin, or trimethoprim-sulfamethoxazole.

Clients should be advised that antimicrobial therapy may be ineffective, particularly in disseminated infections. Massive dosages for prolonged periods are required to eliminate the organism from all tissues and prevent relapse. Treatment may be complicated by toxic drug reactions or the emergence of resistant strains during therapy. Surgical drainage of abscesses may be required in conjunction with antimicrobial therapy.

Vaccines for melioidosis are not available. Prevention is aimed primarily at reducing host contact with contaminated soil and water. Ordinary sanitary precautions such as prompt treatment of wounds, separating affected animals from healthy animals, and cleaning and disinfection of stalls may reduce the incidence of infections.

Humans are susceptible to melioidosis. Adequate measures must be taken to protect personnel handling affected horses, laboratory specimens, and cultures.

Supplemental Readings

Davie, J., and Wells, C. W.: Equine melioidosis in Malaya. Br. Vet. J., *108*:161–167, 1952.

Groves, M. G.: Melioidosis. *In* Steele, J. H. (ed.): CRC Handbook Series in Zoonoses. Vol. 1. Boca Raton, Fla., CRC Press, 1979, pp. 465–472.

Hower, C., Sampath, A., and Spotnitz, M.: The *pseudomallei* group: A review. J. Infect. Dis., *124*:598–606, 1971.

Ladds, P. W., Thomas, A. D., and Pott, B.: Melioidosis with acute meningoencephalomyelitis in a horse. Aust. Vet. J., *57*:36–38, 1981.

Japanese Encephalitis

Robert E. Shope, NEW HAVEN, CONNECTICUT

Japanese encephalitis is an acute, necrotizing mosquito-borne viral encephalomyelitis of horses and donkeys. The disease is most commonly encountered in epizootics in China, the maritime provinces of the eastern Soviet Union, Korea, and Japan, although the virus is distributed also in Nepal, India, Southeast Asia, the Philippines, and Taiwan. Sporadic cases occur in nonepizootic years. The causative virus is a member of the family Flaviviridae and is a 40-nm enveloped spherical particle containing RNA.

CLINICAL SIGNS AND DIAGNOSIS

The disease in horses is characterized by fever, often in excess of 40° C, reduced appetite, and listlessness, followed by encephalitic signs. These may include weakness, staggering gait, excitation, disorientation, blindness, recumbency, convulsions, violent struggling, and coma.

At necropsy, the brain is edematous. There may be widespread foci of glial proliferation, hyperemia, and perivascular mononuclear cuffing. Neurons exhibit chromatolysis and neuronophagia. Neither the clinical nor postmortem findings are specifc for Japanese encephalitis, but this disease should be suspected in acute encephalitis cases originating in Asia and the Pacific islands.

Specific diagnosis depends on isolation and identification of the causative virus, or demonstration of specific antigen or antibody in sera and tissues. Virus is isolated from brain samples taken as early as possible in the course of infection. Necropsy specimens also should be sampled and are often positive. Susceptible laboratory hosts include infant mice, embryonated eggs, and cell cultures such as Vero monkey kidney cells and the C6/36 clone of *Aedes albopictus* mosquito cells. The virus causes death or cytopathic effect and the isolate can be identified by serological tests such as complement fixation, enzyme-linked immunosorbent assay (ELISA), immunofluorescence, or hemagglutination inhibition. A standard diagnostic serum is available from the WHO/FAO Collaborating Centre for Arbovirus Research and Reference at Yale University.

Animals infected with Japanese encephalitis virus have a viremic phase that is usually clinically unrecognized. The encephalitic phase occurs later. Because encephalitis is a late phase of the disease, antibody is detectable by the time of onset of encephalitic signs in 80 per cent or more of horses. The complement fixation test was used formerly for diagnosis; ELISA is now recommended. The detection of IgM using the IgM capture technique permits reliable diagnosis with a single serum or cerebrospinal fluid specimen.

TREATMENT AND PREVENTION

There is no specific treatment for Japanese encephalitis. An inactivated vaccine is commercially available in Japan, and a live attenuated vaccine has been used in China in more than 500,000 horses, with 80 to 90 per cent seroconversion after a single inoculation.

Prevention of Japanese encephalitis depends on an understanding of its epizootiology. The virus is transmitted by *Culex tritaeniorhynchus* and other related mosquitoes. These mosquitoes breed primarily in rice paddies and feed on birds, pigs, horses, and people. In temperate Asia Japanese encephalitis is seasonal, occurring from late July through mid-September. The major vertebrate reservoir hosts are water birds such as the black crowned night heron, the little egret, and the plumed egret. Pigs serve as very efficient amplifying hosts and often abort as a result of infection. Horses develop viremia, but probably not in high enough titers or frequently enough to contribute significantly to the circulation of virus in nature. People also are dead-end hosts, although human encephalitis is a major problem in Asia.

Primary prevention depends on control of mosquitoes. The transmission of Japanese encephalitis virus has diminished remarkably in Japan since the second World War, attributed in part to the use of agricultural pesticides. In some areas pigs have been immunized or moved away from mosquito-breeding areas, and thus their role as amplifying hosts of the virus has been minimized. In most of Asia, however, Japanese encephalitis continues to be a formidable problem.

Supplemental Readings

Burns, K. F., Tigertt, W. D., and Matumoto, M.: Japanese equine encephalomyelitis: 1947 epizootic. II. Serological and etiological studies. Am. J. Hygiene, 50:27–45, 1949.

Rosen, L.: The natural history of Japanese encephalitis virus. Ann. Rev. Microbiol., 40:395–414, 1986.

Chen, B. Q., and Beaty, B. J.: Japanese encephalitis vaccine (2–8 strain) and parent (SA 14 strain) viruses in *Culex tritaeniorhynchus* mosquitoes. Am. J. Trop. Med. Hygiene, 31:403–407, 1982.

Venezuelan Equine Encephalomyelitis

Thomas E. Walton, LARAMIE, WYOMING

Venezuelan equine encephalomyelitis (VEE) is an infectious, zoonotic, mosquito-borne virus disease of Equidae and humans. The VEE complex of insect-transmitted viruses (arthropod-borne viruses, or arboviruses) is taxonomically classified in the alphavirus group of the family Togaviridae. These viruses have been isolated only in the Western hemisphere. The VEE complex viruses are antigenically related to the other equine encephalomyelitides, eastern (EEE) and western (WEE) equine encephalomyelitis viruses. The VEE virus complex is comprised of six antigenically related subtypes (I through VI); within subtype I are five variants. Epizootic VEE in equids is caused by variants A/B and C of subtype I; all other subtypes and variants of VEE virus appear to be nonpathogenic for equids and are found in sylvatic or enzootic, nonequine cycles. The epizootic variants are exotic to the United States. Many species of hematophagous insects have been incriminated in the transmission of epizootic VEE virus and no single genus or species is considered the primary vector. Epizootic activity has generally occurred in areas in which a definitive dry season occurs. Such areas are ecologically classified as tropical dry or tropical thorn forest.

Epizootic, equine pathogenic VEE virus variants caused recurring outbreaks in northern South America from the early years of the 20th century. Historically, outbreaks were reported almost annually in many of the countries of northern South America, including Colombia, Ecuador, Peru, Trinidad, and Venezuela. An outbreak reported in Argentina was ascribed to the use of an incompletely inactivated vaccine. In 1969, the virus was transferred from an ongoing epizootic in Ecuador by an unknown mechanism to Central America. During the next 3 years, clinical VEE was reported in equids and humans in Belize, Costa Rica, El Salvador, Guatemala, Honduras, Mexico, Nicaragua, and Texas. Epizootic VEE was last documented by isolation of virus from equids and mosquitoes during an outbreak in 1973 in Venezuela. During the succeeding 17 years, clinical encephalomyelitis and antibodies to epizootic VEE subtype I-ABC viruses have been reported periodically in equids in the United States and Central America. However, epizootic VEE virus has not been isolated anywhere in the hemisphere. While it is possible that epizootic VEE virus variants have persisted in these areas, the absence of overt epizootic activity and lack of viral isolates would suggest that the epizootic virus variants either have not persisted or that the epidemiology or pathogenicity of these viruses has changed. Equids experience very high viremias with epizootic VEE virus and are the most important amplifiers and indicators of epizootic VEE virus activity, unlike the low viremias reported with EEE and WEE virus. Epidemiological studies have confirmed that VEE epizootics terminate when susceptible horses are no longer available to support the outbreak. The interepizootic reservoir of epizootic VEE virus variants is unknown.

Enzootic VEE viruses are found annually in many areas of the tropical and subtropical countries of the Western hemisphere. These viruses are restricted to rodent– or bird–mosquito cycles in typical jungle or swampy environments with a high water table or constantly available fresh or brackish water. These areas are tropical wet forest ecological zones with no obvious dry season. The primary vector mosquitoes are members of the subgenus *Culex (Melanoconion)*. Horses infected with sylvatic VEE viruses may experience a low-titer viremia that is insufficient to infect vectors, but experience no clinical disease, and are therefore considered "dead-end" hosts, similar to the situation with WEE viruses. In the United States, sylvatic subtype II virus, Everglades, probably occurs annually in the Florida Everglades. A subtype III B virus, Bijou Bridge, has been reported occasionally in a bird (swallow)–insect cycle in the Rocky Mountain states. While these viruses are serologically related to and will cross-protect equids against infection with the epizootic variants, there is no known relationship between the sylvatic virus focus and VEE outbreaks from epizootic virus.

CLINICAL SIGNS

The clinical signs of VEE in an infected horse are difficult, if not impossible, to differentiate from those of infection with EEE or WEE viruses. Some experience subclinical or inapparent infections, while others have a mild to severe, and frequently fatal, clinical course of disease. For the first 5 days, the clinical syndrome is a nonspecific, febrile disease with no obvious neurological signs. Infected horses experience a fever of 41° C or more with leukopenia beginning ½ to 1½ days after infection and continuing for 3 to 6 days. They may stand quietly with their ears and head drooping and with a somnolent appearance. Inappetence and failure to drink water may be seen; weight loss can be dramatic. Clinical signs referable to the central nervous system are observed at approximately 5 days after infection, coincident with the first detection of neutralizing antibodies and the termination of detectable viremia. Some horses experience profound psychic depression and stupor, are unwilling to move, have difficulty in maintaining balance and stand with legs wide apart, support their head on fixed objects, and often fall and are unable to regain their feet. Others exhibit signs of excitation or stimulation, are hypersensitive to touch and sounds, may be aggressive or hyperactive, walk in circles or into obstacles, stand with heads pressed against obstacles or into dark corners, and chew aimlessly or froth from the mouth and nose. Horses may appear to be blind and exhibit nystagmus. When the horse falls down in terminal convulsions and coma, a characteristic paddling motion of the limbs is commonly seen. The fatality rate among infected animals that develop signs of encephalomyelitis may reach 80 per cent. During an epizootic, large numbers of susceptible horses develop clinical signs in a very short period of time.

DIAGNOSIS

Although a presumptive clinical diagnosis of encephalomyelitis can be made in the field, VEE cannot be diagnosed without laboratory confirmation. Seasonality of the disease during the months of vector activity with large populations of mosquitoes would suggest a diagnosis of arboviral encephalomyelitis. Initial signs of VEE may go undetected, and reports of sudden death in an apparently healthy horse are not uncommon. When clinical signs of encephalomyelitis predominate, the disease is indistinguishable from EEE or WEE. The differential diagnoses of VEE must include EEE, WEE, and other arboviral encephalitides; African horse sickness; rabies; intoxications; botulism; hepatoencephalopathy; and trauma and other causes of encephalitic signs.

A specific diagnosis can be made only by diagnostic laboratory procedures that include virus isolation and identification, or demonstration of a specific rise in antibody titer in paired acute and convalescent sera. Virus can be isolated from serum or plasma in intracranially inoculated suckling mice, weanling mice, guinea pigs, various cell cultures, or embryonating chicken eggs. Although VEE virus isolation from equine brains had been reported in experimentally and naturally infected horses, during the 1969 to 1972 outbreak VEE virus was rarely isolated from brain. The serum titer of epizootic VEE virus can exceed $10^{8.8}$ suckling mouse intracranial median lethal doses per ml. Persisting viremia after 5 to 6 days has not been shown and latent infections do not occur. By the time clinical encephalomyelitis is recognized, the viremia has generally ended. Therefore, most investigators recommend that serum for virus isolation be collected from febrile equids that appear normal and are located in the same or adjacent pastures as encephalomyelitic equids. Virus can be identified as VEE by using complement fixation (CF), hemagglutination inhibition (HI), neutralization, or antigen capture enzyme-linked immunosorbent assay (ELISA) tests. VEE virus isolates can be identified as to subtype and variant by using the short incubation HI test, HI with antiserum produced in rabbits to E_2 envelope glycoproteins, and RNA oligonucleotide fingerprinting.

The serological tests include HI, CF, neutralization, ELISA, and antibody capture enzyme immunoassay for immunoglobulin M. The interpretation of antibody or of an antibody titer rise must be made cautiously in horses located in or near an area in which sylvatic VEE subtypes and variants are located. Anti-VEE antibody in horses in these areas may not be a sound basis for a diagnosis of VEE, owing to serological cross-reactions between epizootic and sylvatic VEE viruses. Immunity after infection or attenuated virus vaccination is long-lasting, if not lifelong, and the presence of antibodies in such horses is evidence of solid immunity.

THERAPY

Only supportive therapy can be provided to an encephalitic horse with VEE. Specific antiviral agents are not currently available. The prognosis for an animal with clinical neurological disease from VEE virus is very poor. Death generally occurs 5 to 10 days after infection, or within 5 days after the onset of clinical signs of neurological disease. Supportive measures such as those recommended for treatment of EEE and WEE can be attempted and include administration of fluids, glucose, electrolytes, antipyretics, and corticosteroids. The use of anesthesia or tranquilizers to treat VEE has not been reported. Protection from injury due to recumbency and self-inflicted trauma can be provided by heavily padded bedding, padded stall, protective leg wraps, and a padded helmet.

PREVENTION AND CONTROL

Prophylaxis rather than therapy is the key to VEE prevention. A safe and effective trivalent, formalin-inactivated VEE vaccine is available with EEE and WEE viruses. The VEE fraction of this vaccine was produced using the attenuated strain TC-83 vaccine virus. Initial vaccination requires multiple injections and should be done according to the manufacturer's recommendations. A booster injection is recommended annually before onset of the vector season.

The attenuated VEE strain TC-83 vaccine has provided outstanding protection to equids. The immunity produced is probably lifelong in duration. Vaccine should be administered before the vector season. The vaccine is not recommended for use in pregnant mares, although adverse effects have not been documented. Foals may be vaccinated at 3 months of age, but should be revaccinated. Some vaccinated animals may have a viremia with vaccine virus and a febrile response of 1 to 2 days' duration. During an outbreak, protection to virulent virus infection develops in approximately 4 days; equine deaths generally cease 10 days after vaccine is used. This vaccine is no longer routinely used in the United States because of concerns about reversion to virulence and about vector transmission of vaccine virus, but it should be made available and used during a VEE emergency.

Formalin-inactivated VEE vaccines derived from equine virulent epizootic EEE virus should not be manufactured or used for immunizing equids. It has been demonstrated that residual virulent virus can remain after formalin treatment and can cause severe illness, high viremia, and death. Epizootics of VEE have occurred from the use of such formalin-treated viruses. While a new generation of vaccines is not currently available, studies are ongoing by a number of research groups using modern molecular biologic techniques. The nucleotide sequences of the genomes of an equine virulent, epizootic variant and of strain TC-83 vaccine virus have been determined. Nucleotide deletion and substitution is being used to produce infectious clones to immunize humans and equids. Preliminary studies in laboratory animals and equids hold great promise for new, safe, and effective vaccines in the near future.

Experiences during epizootics and epidemics with VEE and other arbovirus diseases have shown that the best control is an integrated disease management approach that includes vector suppression, physical protection of the susceptible host from the vectors, and vaccination. The 1969 to 1972 epizootic was not ultimately controlled until a massive aerial spraying with ultra-low-volume malathion was integrated into the campaign. The use of adulticides, larvicides, and physical disruption of the aquatic larval developmental habitats may help prevent or control epizootic VEE virus activity. Individual animals can be protected by the use of insect repellents or by screening them from the vectors.

Restricted movement or quarantine of equids should be required during an epizootic. Protection of febrile animals from the feeding of mosquitoes during an epizootic will almost certainly help to decrease the numbers of infected mosquitoes biting susceptible horses and humans.

PUBLIC HEALTH SIGNIFICANCE

Humans can be infected by both sylvatic and epizootic VEE virus subtypes and variants. The clinical syndrome can be mild to severe, and deaths have been reported primarily in children and the aged. Human disease has frequently been reported during equine epizootics, but the clinical course generally follows equine disease by approximately 2 weeks.

Numerous infections have been reported among laboratory workers as a result of aerosol infections from the handling of laboratory animals infected with sylvatic and epizootic variants and subtypes. The strain TC-83 virus vaccine was initially developed for use in at-risk laboratory workers. Vaccinated personnel should have demonstrable antibodies to the VEE virus variant or subtype with which they are working. Immunity to the more distantly related subtypes decreases more rapidly than immunity to the closely related variants. Many laboratory infections have occurred in previously vaccinated workers whose immunity had waned. Field veterinarians should be cognizant of the health risk from the bites of hematophagous vectors during epizootics or when working in typical sylvatic virus habitats.

Supplemental Readings

Acha, P. N., and Szyfres, B.: Venezuelan equine encephalitis. *In:* Zoonoses and Communicable Diseases Common to Man and Animals, 2nd ed. Science Publication No. 503. Washington, D.C., Pan American Health Organization, 1987, pp. 496–506.

Fenner, F., Bachmann, P. A., Gibbs, E. P. J., Murphy, F. A., Studdert, M. J., and White, D. O.: Togaviridae and flaviviridae. *In:* Veterinary Virology. New York, Academic Press, 1987, pp. 451–472.

Walton, T. E.: Venezuelan, eastern, and western equine encephalomyelitis. *In* Gibbs, E. P. J. (ed.): Virus Diseases of Food Animals: A World Geography of Epidemiology and Control. Disease Monographs, vol. 2. New York, Academic Press, 1981, pp. 587–625.

Walton, T. E., and Grayson, M. A.: Venezuelan equine encephalomyelitis. *In* Monath, T. P. (ed.): The Arboviruses: Epidemiology and Ecology. Vol. 4. Boca Raton, Fla., CRC Press, 1988, pp. 203–231.

Other Exotic Diseases

William W. Laegreid, GREENPORT, NEW YORK

GETAH

Getah virus infection was first shown to cause disease in horses during an outbreak at a racehorse training center in Japan in 1978. Prior to that the virus was known to infect mosquitoes, man, pigs, horses, and herons in Asia and Australia but was not associated with any clinical syndrome. Further epizootics occurred in Japan in 1979 and 1983. While serological evidence suggests that getah virus is distributed throughout much of Southeast Asia and Australia, association of the virus with disease is limited to Japan at this time.

Getah virus is an alphavirus of the family Togaviridae. It is an enveloped virus, 70 nm in diameter, with a positive-stranded RNA genome. Getah virus belongs to the Semliki Forest virus complex and serologically is closely related to the Sagiyama, Bebaru, and Ross River viruses. The virus infects many vertebrate hosts, including man and other primates, domestic livestock, especially pigs and horses, and birds. Many species of mosquitoes support replication of getah virus, with *Culex tritaeniorhynchus* the most significant vector in Southeast Asia and Japan. Several species of *Culex, Aedes,* and *Anopheles* mosquitoes, among others, are also thought to be capable of transmitting getah virus to vertebrates. Vectors are the primary means of transmission of getah virus, although infected horses shed virus in nasal secretions and may be experimentally infected by the intranasal route, suggesting that direct transmission is at least theoretically possible. However, in outbreaks the disease has appeared randomly in individuals with little discernible pattern of spread, indicating that vectors were probably the major means of transmission. In addition, the appearance of getah virus infection is seasonal in temperate regions, coinciding with the appearance of mosquitoes in the spring and summer months.

Getah virus infection in horses causes an acute febrile disease (39° to 40° C), which may be subclinical, 2 to 4 days following infection. The febrile episode is followed in one to several days by either rash of the extremities (25 per cent of cases), edema of the legs (17 per cent), or a combination of these two signs (26 per cent). Some horses show only the rash or edema without an episode of fever (18 per cent), while 32 per cent of cases have only fever. A serous nasal discharge and enlargement of submandibular lymph nodes may also be features of this disease. The signs resolve within a week of onset. The disease is not fatal, with full recovery approximately 1 week after onset of clinical signs.

Gross pathological changes include lymph node and splenic enlargement, subcutaneous edema and reddened, circumscribed thickened maculae in the dermis. Histologically, lymphoid hyperplasia with increased numbers of lymphocytes is present in the follicles of the spleen and lymph nodes. The dermal connective tissues contain perivascular and diffuse infiltrations of lymphocytes and histiocytes. Occasional hemorrhagic foci are also present. Perivascular cuffing by mononuclear cells and petechiation are present in the brain and spinal cord of some cases.

Diagnosis is made based on seasonal occurrence and clinical signs and is confirmed by virus isolation or serological confirmation of getah virus infection. The differential diagnoses include equine viral arteritis, mild forms of African horse sickness, and pupura hemorrhagica. Getah virus is isolated by inoculation of whole blood into suckling mouse brains or mammalian cell lines such as Vero. Virus neutralization, complement fixation (CF), and hemagglutination inhibition (HI) assays using specific reference antiserum define the isolate as getah virus. Virus neutralization, CF and HI, along with ELISA tests and dot immunobinding assays are also used in the serodiagnosis of getah virus infection. Cross-reactivity with other alphaviruses limits the use of CF and HI tests for getah virus identification. The virus neutralization test is more specific and is preferred for serodiagnosis.

The incidence of disease appears inversely related to the number of seropositive animals in an area. Vaccination with inactivated virus is practiced in Japan and is reported to be effective. Other control measures include reduction of insect vectors by the use of insect repellents, housing animals in enclosed stables, and eliminating mosquito breeding areas.

LOUPING ILL

Louping ill is primarily a disease of sheep in the border regions of Scotland and England, although it has been found elsewhere in Europe. Experimental and naturally occurring infections of horses with louping ill virus have been reported since the 1930s. The low seroprevalence and relative paucity of case reports suggest that the disease is relatively uncommon in horses.

Louping ill is caused by a virus of the family Flaviviridae. It is transmitted by the sheep tick *Ixodes ricinus*, which places it in the tick-borne encephalitides group of flaviviruses, a group that includes Omsk hemorrhagic fever, Kyasanur Forest disease, and Negishi, Powassan, and Central European encephalitis viruses. The virus appears to consist of only one strain that is differentiated only with difficulty from other members of the group. The virus infects and causes disease in many other vertebrate species in addition to sheep and horses, including man. However, in most species, including horses, the levels of viremia following infection are too low to efficiently transmit the virus to tick larvae or nymphs. Thus, the natural reservoir of louping ill virus and the enzootic cycle of infection are unknown.

There is considerable variability in the response of horses to infection with louping ill virus. Typically, there is a febrile episode 1 to 4 days after infection that coincides with the period of viremia. Progression to encephalitis is an occasional feature of the disease in horses. In other species, age, nutritional status, environmental factors, and presence of other infectious diseases have all been described as influencing the clinical presentation and development of central nervous system (CNS) disease with louping ill virus. Mortality is low but may increase with CNS involvement. There are no gross lesions associated with louping ill in the horse. Microscopically, the disease is characterized by a nonsuppurative meningoencephalitis.

The diagnosis of louping ill is made primarily by virus isolation and serology. Brain homogenates are inoculated onto cell cultures or intracerebrally in suckling mice, with confirmation by complement fixation, serum plaque reduction, or immunofluorescence assays. Hemagglutination inhibition is the serological test of choice. The differential diagnoses include other viral encephalitides and toxic or other causes of diffuse CNS damage.

Since the disease is usually not fatal in horses, supportive therapy may be effective. A cell culture–derived, formalin-inactivated vaccine is available in Europe. There are no reports of its use in horses. Vector control has been attempted. Logically, avoiding comingling of horses with sheep, either in barns or pasture, should reduce the chance of exposure to the tick. Vaccination of sheep may reduce the incidence of disease in other susceptible species.

EPIZOOTIC LYMPHANGITIS

Epizootic lymphangitis is a disease of horses, rarely cattle, caused by a fungus, *Histoplasma farciminosum*. The disease is most common in the countries of Europe, the Middle East, and North Africa that border the Mediterranean. In addition, epizootic lymphangitis is found in south, central, and east Africa, central Asia, the Soviet Union, and Colombia and Uruguay in South America. The disease was introduced elsewhere in Europe but was successfully eradicated.

Histoplasma farciminosum is present in tissue as an ovoid yeast structure approximately 3–4 μm in diameter. In culture, the organism forms sterile, thick-walled mycelia. Spores of *H. farciminosum* are fairly resistant and may remain viable for days in the soil or on bedding, grooming utensils, and the like. Transmission occurs by infection of cutaneous abrasions, coitally, or by inhalation of spores. Insects may be involved in the transmission of *H. farciminosum*, resulting in ocular manifestations of the disease.

The typical clinical presentation of epizootic lymphangitis is the appearance of subcutaneous granulomas in the head and cervical regions, extending later to the limbs. The granulomas often ulcerate and coalesce. Lymphatic vessels draining affected regions are commonly involved, leading to thickening or "cording" of these vessels. Early lesions may be unilateral but eventually there is progression to the opposite side. Keratoconjunctivitis has been reported in association with the cutaneous lesions. Inhalation of spores may result in upper and lower respiratory tract infections, possibly without cutaneous involvement. The liver, spleen, and joints have also been reported to be involved in some cases. In general, epizootic lymphangitis is a chronic disease with a 6- to 8-week incubation period followed by a prolonged period of clinical disease. Horses may have active lesions indefinitely although some cases resolve spontaneously. The disease is generally associated with a low mortality, except where there is visceral involvement.

Microscopically, the cutaneous lesions are characterized by organized granuloma formation with suppuration of some of the nodules. Large numbers of *H. farciminosum* yeast forms are present, both free and within macrophages. Lymphangitis, either suppurative or nonsuppurative, is usually present. Progressive interstitial pneumonia is reported with pulmonary forms of the disease.

Diagnosis is based initially on the clinical signs, lesions, and demonstration of the organism in smears of the exudate. The differential diagnoses include glanders, sporothricosis, other ulcerative lymphadenitides, and tuberculosis. Definitive diagnosis is based on culture of *H. farciminosum* from tissues or exudate. Samples should be collected into solution containing 500 units per ml penicillin and kept at 4° C until delivery to the laboratory. A direct fluorescent antibody technique for identification of *H. farciminosum* in exudate smears has been described. Complement fixation, passive hemagglutination, and skin hypersensitivity tests have been used to demonstrate the presence of specific antibody to the organism.

In many areas, diagnosis of epizootic lymphangitis results in the condemnation of affected animals. This is followed by destruction or disinfection of all bedding, tack and other material with which the animal may have been in contact. In some areas, treatment of less severely affected animals is practiced. Intravenous administration of sodium iodide, oral potassium iodide, or griseofulvin is effective. Topical application of tincture of iodine to ulcerated nodules may be of some use. Prevention of the disease by the use of a formalin-inactivated vaccine has been described.

Supplemental Readings

Getah

Kono, Y.: Getah virus disease. *In* Monath, T. P. (ed.): The Arboviruses: Epidemiology and Ecology. Vol. III. Boca Raton, Fla., CRC Press, 1988.

Kono, Y., Sentsui, H., and Ito, Y.: An epidemic of Getah virus infection among racehorses: Properties of the virus. Res. Vet. Sci., 29:162–167, 1980.

Wada, R., Kamada, M., Fukunaga, Y., Ando, Y., Kumanomido, T., Imagawa, H., Akiyama, Y., and Oikawa, Y.: Equine Getah virus infection: Pathological study of horses experimentally infected with the MI-110 strain. Jpn. J. Vet. Sci., 44:411–418, 1982.

Louping Ill

Reid, H. W.: Louping-Ill. *In* Monath, T.P. (ed.): The Arboviruses: Epidemiology and Ecology. Vol. III. Boca Raton, Fla., CRC Press, 1988.

Timoney, P. J.: Louping ill: A serological survey of horses in Ireland. Vet. Rec., 98:303, 1976.

Timoney, P. J.: Susceptibility of the horse to experimental inoculation with louping ill virus. J. Comp. Pathol., 90:73–86, 1980.

Epizootic Lymphangitis

Gabal, M.A., Hassan, F. K., Siad, A. A., and Karim, K. A.: Study of equine histoplasmosis farciminosi and characterization of *Histoplasma farciminosum*. Sabouraudia, 21:121–127, 1983.

Gabal, M. A., and Khalifa, K.: Study on the immune response and serological diagnosis of equine histoplasmosis (epizootic lymphangitis). Zbl. Vet. Med. B., 30:317–321, 1983.

Section 19

ASSESSMENT OF PERFORMANCE PROBLEMS

Edited by Elisabeth Morris

Introduction to Performance Evaluation

Elisabeth Morris, NORTH GRAFTON, MASSACHUSETTS

Peak performance of the athlete requires optimal functioning of all of the major body systems. Often, a single system breaks down, resulting in decreased performance. The causes of decreased performance may be indicated by the acute onset of joint swelling and lameness, indicative of a musculoskeletal problem; by a bilateral nasal discharge and exercise intolerance, indicative of a lower respiratory problem; or by an inappropriate respiratory noise during performance, indicative of upper respiratory tract obstruction. In other cases, the diagnosis of decreased or inadequate athletic performance may be a significant challenge, because many problems are subtle, apparent only at high speed, and involve more than one body system. For this reason, the evaluation of inadequate performance requires a detailed examination of all systems that affect optimum racing performance. Recent advances in equine sports medicine have resulted in the ability to combine traditional diagnostic methods with dynamic exercise testing and state-of-the-art imaging techniques to provide just such a comprehensive clinical evaluation. The aim of comprehensive testing is to determine the cause of exercise intolerance at a stage when treatment may still be effective.

What follows is a description of the newer diagnostic tests that can be used in evaluating inadequate performance in the equine athlete. Because the causes of poor performance are often multiple, a complete evaluation includes analysis of the respiratory, musculoskeletal, cardiovascular, and thermoregulatory system, a fitness evaluation, and routine hematology and clinical chemistry. Many of these tests are not available to the practitioner as they involve equipment available only at large universities or research centers. A knowledge of these tests will help the practitioner understand reports received from referral centers.

DIAGNOSTIC METHODS

A complete history and physical examination are the foundation of every diagnostic workup.

The history should include such information as the length of time the inadequate performance has been observed and the time during the race at which performance falls off. Suspicions of lameness (as indicated by gait asymmetry, the tendency to pull to one side, or reluctance to change leads) or of a respiratory problem (as indicated by abnormal noise) should be investigated. Exercise intolerance, including excessive time to cool out after the race or to resume normal respiratory or heart rate, is a nonspecific sign that could indicate pain as well as infectious or inflammatory processes. Routine blood work should include a complete blood cell count and a chemistry profile to evaluate electrolyte balance, enzyme measurements to detect organ dysfunction, and resting creatine kinase levels.

Before high-speed treadmills became available, performance evaluations were limited by the examiner's inability to evaluate the horse at racing speeds. Available field tests include a flexion test, observation of the horse during training under saddle or from behind in a jog cart, telemetered heart rate monitoring, and hematology and serum chemistry analysis immediately following exercise to evaluate dehydration, splenic contraction, and electrolyte balance, as well as several hours after exercise to diagnose abnormal creatine kinase elevations.

A high-speed motorized treadmill allows more specific diagnostic techniques to be used because the horse can be monitored by a stationary diagnostician during strenuous exercise. Many horses with uneven slow gaits will exhibit smooth stride at high speed, minimizing the significance of the gait asymmetry. Similarly, many horses that do not have gait asymmetries following flexion tests or at slow speeds will become progressively more lame at higher speeds. Hoof balance and gait analysis may be analyzed by direct visual observation as well as with high-speed video recordings and even cinematography. Upper airway function can be evaluated by endoscopy during strenuous exercise. Postexercise endoscopy with the aid of a long endoscope that reaches to the level of the carina may disclose pulmonary inflammation or exercise-induced pulmonary hemorrhage (EIPH). Telemetered electrocardiographs obtained during strenuous exercise may show exercise-induced arrhythmias. Finally, measurement of oxygen consumption and blood lactate levels during exercise allows the evaluation of metabolic efficiency and fitness.

Coupled with the high-speed analysis, diagnostic medical imaging techniques permit more specific identification of problems in equine athletes. High-resolution radiography is used to evaluate orthopedic disease in the limbs and axial skeleton and to identify respiratory disease. Soft tissue and bone scintigraphy is a sensitive means of localizing and quantifying injuries such as arthritis and stress-induced bone remodeling, which may be difficult to categorize from conventional radiographs. Since the radioisotope used in bone scintigraphy is also taken up in increased amounts by damaged muscle, the localization and quantification of exercise-induced myopathy is possible. Ventilation/perfusion scintigraphy is used to further evaluate the functional significance of structural abnormalities in the lung identified by radiography. Although presently only performed in the resting horse, future application of this technique may assist in determining the increase or decrease in ventilation/perfusion mismatch that may occur during strenuous exercise as a result of diseases such as chronic bronchitis or bronchiolitis and EIPH. Computed tomography can be used to image orthopedic lesions in three dimensions, enabling optimal understanding of the anatomical abnormality prior to surgical correction as well as adding tremendous information regarding the pathological process itself. Echocardiography allows the analysis of cardiac function and size. Ultrasonographic imaging of soft tissue can assist in the diagnosis of tendinous and ligamentous injury and the response of these structures to therapy. Thermography utilizes the imaging of infared radiation to detect increased heat production by soft tissue, indicating inflammation.

RESULTS OF THE COMPREHENSIVE CLINICAL EVALUATION

The various diagnostic modalities should be used to identify subtle, often multiple causes of inadequate performance in the elite equine athlete (Fig 1). Inadequate athletic performance is often caused by a constellation of abnormalities, thereby mandating a comprehensive approach in order to diagnose decreased athletic capability. Musculoskeletal impairments are the most common cause of suboptimal performance in the horse. Comprehensive evaluation indicates that the majority of horses suffer musculoskeletal pain from multiple sources; these sources are additive and result in inability to perform at maximal speeds.

The second most frequent cause of inadequate performance is upper respiratory dysfunction, which again may be the result of a second problem. Some cases of upper respiratory dysfunction are precipitated by musculoskeletal pain or inadequate fitness, resulting in early exhaustion of the muscles of the larynx and pharynx. In other cases the horse may have been performing

The Science of Racing

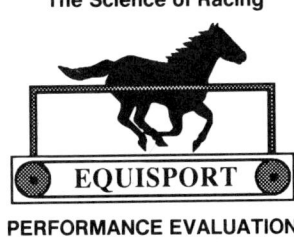

PERFORMANCE EVALUATION
SUMMARY REPORT

Signalment: 3 year old Standardbred Stallion

A. **Evaluation**
1. **Anamnesis**
   a. History of "breaking" after short distance of training speed work.
   b. Reports of loud gurgling noise and difficulty cooling down.
   c. History of myectomy as 2 year old.
2. **Weight:** 1110 lbs
3. **Temperature:** 99.8°
   Pulse: 32
   Respiration: 20
4. **Physical Examination**
   a. shaved areas over both carpi
   b. no other abnormalities
5. **Ophthalmological Examination**
   a. no abnormal findings.
6. **Neurologic Examination**
   a. no abnormal findings; no evidence of any neurologic deficits.
7. **Clinical Pathology Tests**
   a. CBC: within normal limits.
   b. chemistry screen: within normal limits
8. **Muscle Enzyme Evaluation**
   a. Pre-exercise CK: 222 U/L
   b. 6 hour Post-exercise CK: 442 (normal)
9. **Respiratory Examination**
   a. Upper Airway Examination:
      (1) *Resting Endoscopy*
         —mild left laryngeal paralysis at rest (grade 1 out of 4)
         —guttural pouches: NORMAL
      (2) *Treadmill Endoscopy*
         —Airway was examined during strenuous exercise to determine if an airway obstruction might be a contributor to the poor performance in the last race. During the first 2 attempts, the upper airway appeared normal. During the third evaluation, the horse was asked to trot at increasing speeds until he "broke" stride. **At this point, he was observed to dorsally displace his soft palate.**
      (3) *Post-Exercise Endoscopy*
         —no abnormal discharge; no evidence of exercise induced pulmonary hemorrhage following stress test: NORMAL
   b. **Lower Airway Examination:**
      (1) *Thoracic Radiographs*
         —within normal limits.
      (2) *Ventilation-Perfusion Scintigraphy*
         —within normal limits.
10. **Lameness Examination:**
    a. palpation: no abnormalities of peripheral skeleton.
    b. flexion tests:
       (1) **positive response to left front ankle flexion.**
       (2) **mild response to bilateral hind limb flexion.**
    c. hoof sensitivity: normal
    d. high speed: at a jog and at a gallop on the high speed treadmill, horse was observed to exhibit a significant **LH asymmetry** which worsened with increasing length of exercise. At a jog, he was seen to show a **left front** head bob. PLEASE SEE ACCOMPANYING VIDEO TAPE. The left front lameness was alleviated with intraarticular anesthesia of the fetlock joint.
11. **Bone Scan:**
    A short acting radiotracer which preferentially binds to active bone was injected and the horse was imaged with a gamma camera.
    Results:
       (1) Positive uptake bilateral medial aspect of middle carpal joints.
       (2) Increased uptake left front and hind distal cannon bone.
       (3) Increased uptake bilateral tarso-metatarsal joints.
12. **Radiography:**
    a. Bilateral sclerosis of the radial fossa of the third carpal bone.
    b. No abnormalities of the fetlocks.
    c. Mild periosteal proliferation evident in tarso-metatarsal joints.
13. **Stress Test**
    Not done due to identification of problems which would result in suboptimal performance.

B. **Comments**
These Are the Problems Found During the Evaluation of the Horse in Order of Significance:
1. Dorsal displacement of the soft palate during strenuous exercise.
2. Bilateral third carpal bone sclerosis.
3. Stress-induced remodeling of the distal epiphyses of the left third metacarpal and left third metatarsal bones.
4. Bilateral osteoarthritis of the tarso-metatarsal joints.

Figure 1. Results of a comprehensive sports medicine evaluation of a racehorse with a history of inadequate athletic performance.

adequately with dysfunctions such as dynamic collapse of the left arytenoid or vocal fold during the final seconds of strenuous exercise, but a new abnormality may have caused earlier onset of exhaustion and therefore earlier occurrence of the dysfunction.

Pulmonary radiography, coupled with ventilation/perfusion scintigraphy and cytological and microbiological analysis of transtracheal aspirates and bronchoalveolar lavage samples, has identified chronic bronchitis or bronchiolitis to be a relatively common problem in the equine athlete. This abnormality is the third most common cause of inadequate athletic performance. At present, antibiotic therapy followed by long-term management that combines increased exposure to fresh air (difficult at best at most training and racing facilities), bronchodilators, and mucolytics is the only option for treatment. When this condition becomes more easily identified and therefore more widely accepted as an important cause of poor performance and perhaps EIPH, management practices may be significantly altered in the early years of the horse's life, the time during which this chronic disease is most likely initiated.

In horses with no obvious medical cause of inadequate performance and in those that have never performed to expectation, exercise testing may disclose decreased metabolic efficiency as a result of individual deficiency or perhaps inadequate training. Finally, a small per centage of horses may have neurological disease, including cervical vertebral malformation, chronic abdominal pain due to gastric ulceration, or endocrine imbalances.

For optimal evaluation of the equine athlete with a history of inadequate performance, the analysis should be performed during active training or racing, when the abnormalities are most apparent. Management recommendations can then be applied during a potential layoff rather than after an attempt at return to work.

In summary, the clinical evaluation of the performance horse should include a comprehensive analysis, because inadequate performance of the elite athlete often results from the additive effects of multiple, subtle abnormalities that would not individually result in clinical signs. The addition of new technological advances to traditional diagnostic techniques in the field of equine sports medicine will undoubtedly increase the examiner's ability to diagnose problems and institute therapy at a time when appropriate management may result in a return to optimal performance.

Supplemental Readings

Morris, E. A., and Seeherman, H. J.: Clinical evaluation of poor performance in the racehorse: Results of 275 evaluations. Equine Vet. J., 23:169–174, 1991.

Morris, E. A., and Seeherman, H. J.: Evaluation of upper respiratory tract function during strenuous exercise in the horse. J. Am. Vet. Med. Assoc., 196:431–438, 1990.

Seeherman, H. J., Morris, E., and O'Callaghan, M. W.: The use of sports medicine techniques in evaluating the problem equine athlete. Vet. Clin. North Am., (Equine Pract.), 6:239–274, 1990.

Dynamic Endoscopy of the Upper Airway

Elisabeth Morris, NORTH GRAFTON, MASSACHUSETTS

Because many abnormalities of the upper airway are not apparent at rest, the definitive identification of upper airway dysfunction as a cause of decreased athletic performance has been a diagnostic challenge. Attempts to reproduce air flows occurring during exercise in order to observe upper airway function have included endoscopy during nasal occlusion and immediately following exercise. With the advent of the high-speed treadmill, the diagnostician can stand motionless by the side of the exercising horse and endoscopically observe the function of the upper airway.

EVALUATION OF THE UPPER AIRWAY AT REST AND DURING EXERCISE

For an accurate assessment of upper airway anatomy during situations most closely resembling those of performance, the exercise endoscopic evaluation should be done with the horse outfitted with the head gear worn during performance. Many horses with upper respiratory dysfunction exhibit abnormal noise or breathing difficulty only at the end of strenuous exercise. This is explained by the observation that many dysfunctions only occur during maximal ventilation coupled with exhaustion of the laryngeal and pharyngeal musculature. For this reason, the evaluation must be performed while the horse is exercising maximally at performance gait and until exhaustion is apparent, as determined by the horse's inability to maintain position at the front of the treadmill without the aid of the handlers. Although treadmills will approximate speeds maintained during racing, the horses do not have the added load of the rider or the harness-racing bike and driver. Therefore, to achieve comparable energy expenditure, the evaluation is performed while the horse works on an incline.

During exercise, the normal larynx will fully abduct as ventilation increases above resting levels and no movement of the arytenoid cartilages will occur until ventilation again returns to resting levels (Fig. 1). The horse is able to swallow during strenuous exercise and the reflex remains intact with full adduction of the arytenoids, which will then return to the fully abducted position. Normal horses may swallow several times during submaximal exercise, but repeated swallowing during strenuous exercise usually indicates an irritating stimulus often caused by abnormal anatomical location of laryngeal structures.

UPPER AIRWAY DYSFUNCTION AFFECTING PERFORMANCE

The most common upper respiratory dysfunction associated with exercise intolerance is continual or intermittent dorsal displacement of the soft palate (DDSP) during strenuous exercise. During endoscopic examination at rest, the irritation of the endoscope may induce DDSP, but during strenuous exercise this abnormality should not occur. Elevation of the soft palate above the epiglottis and into the airway as a result of DDSP redirects expiratory gases above and below the soft palate causing air flow through the mouth and nose of the exercising horse. The caudal border of the soft palate vibrates violently in the laryngeal orifice when expiratory air flow velocity increases during strenuous exercise, and the loud expiratory noise associated with DDSP occurs at this point in the respiratory cycle. In some cases the flapping of the caudal border is so violent as to damage the soft palate itself, with subsequent hemorrhage from this structure. In these cases, damage caused by the displaced palate may result in a ring of inflamed mucosa along the dorsal border of the pharynx immediately proximal to the rima glottidis. In all cases, the horse replaces the displaced palate immediately following the end of the exercise test, which emphasizes the difficulty of making this diagnosis without the ability to observe the structures during the exercise bout.

Video tape recordings show that different horses displace the soft palate at different points in the respiratory cycle. The most common factor initiating displacement is the tremendous increase in negative pressures during the inspiratory phase of respiration. This would result in ventral and medial collapse of the pharynx and dorsal displacement of the soft palate if this tendency were not counteracted by the action of the muscles of the pharyngeal area, including the palatopharyngeus, the pterygopharyngeus, and the tensor veli palatini muscles. In horses with DDSP during inspiration, the large negative pressures present in the upper airway during strenuous exercise result in displacement of the soft palate above the epiglottis when exhaustion of these pharyngeal muscles occurs (Fig. 2).

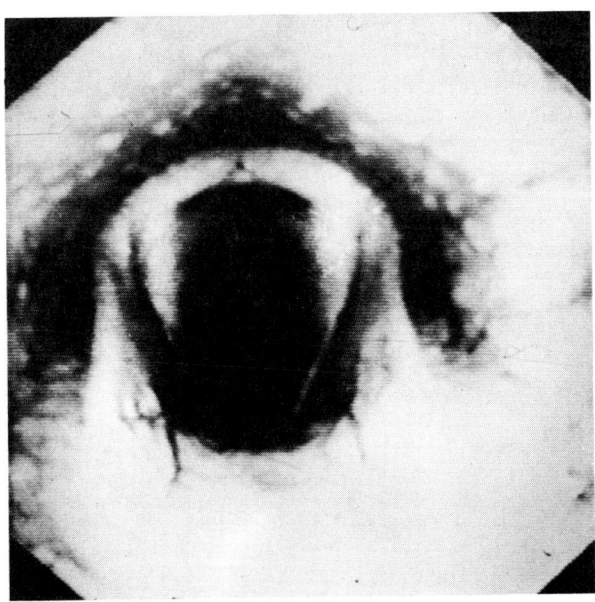

Figure 1. Normal upper airway during strenuous exercise. The arytenoids are symmetrically abducted and the vocal folds are out of the air stream. The epiglottis, which is ventral, is out of focus in this picture.

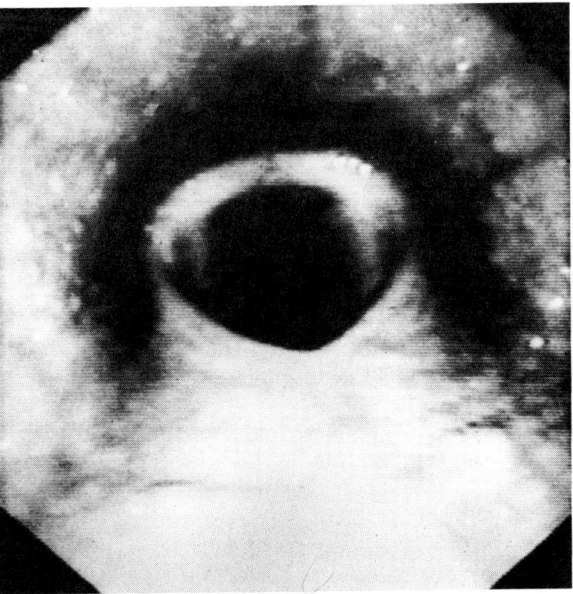

Figure 2. Dorsal displacement of the soft palate during strenuous exercise. The displaced palate hides the epiglottis and vocal folds.

In a second group of horses, displacement of the soft palate occurs during expiration. In contrast to the first scenario, the stationary position of the caudal border of the soft palate against the laryngeal structures becomes more and more lax, and as ventilation becomes maximal a portion of the expiratory air flow is redirected below the palate, resulting in elevation of the palate above the epiglottis.

A third group of horses that continually displace the soft palate during strenuous exercise do so as a result of inappropriate swallow. The swallow reflex includes the ventral and medial movement of the walls of the nasopharynx and the dorsal movement of the soft palate. If a swallow is initiated during strenuous exercise, when ventilation is maximal and muscular strength is decreased, the tendency toward DDSP is greatly increased. A hypoplastic epiglottis has been reported to predispose to this dysfunction.

Attempts to correct DDSP occurring during strenuous exercise include staphylectomy and/or resection of the sternothyroid or sternohyoid muscles. Less invasive management includes attempts to alter head carriage as well as "tongue tying." The success of these procedures may be evaluated by follow-up endoscopy of the upper airway during strenuous exercise.

Epiglottic entrapment results from envelopment of the tip of the epiglottis by the aryteno-epiglottic folds. Although occasionally an intermittent condition, epiglottic entrapment is most often diagnosed at rest by routine endoscopy. An attempt should be made to confirm the significance of the entrapment in each case, for the contribution of epiglottic entrapment to exercise intolerance appears to be variable. It is likely that this variability depends on the tightness of the arytenoepiglottic fold as it covers the epiglottis and the resulting variable degree of inspiratory and expiratory obstruction. Similarly, the presence or absence of an abnormal respiratory noise is variable and depends on the position and tightness of the arytenoepiglottic fold.

Complete paralysis of the left dorsal cricoarytenoid muscle (idiopathic laryngeal neuropathy) results in severe alterations of the airway during strenuous exercise. During peak inspiration, the paralyzed left arytenoid cartilage and the left vocal fold are drawn into the airway to appose the abducted right arytenoid cartilage, resulting in a momentary total obliteration of the rima glottidis. The characteristic inspiratory "roar" occurs at this point in the respiratory cycle. As soon as maximal exercise ceases and ventilation subsides, the roar dissipates and the left arytenoid cartilage returns to neutral position. The identification of complete laryngeal hemiplegia is usually possible in the resting horse, but the functional significance of partial laryngeal paresis is apparent only during observation of the larynx during exercise. The vast majority of horses with asymmetrical laryngeal function at rest can fully abduct the left arytenoid during exercise. But a very small percentage of horses will demonstrate progressive tiring of the abductors of the larynx during maximal exercise, and the left arytenoid will gradually be drawn into the rima glottidis during maximal inspiration. Although the dysfunction does not result in total occlusion of the rima, as is seen in cases of left laryngeal paralysis, the inability of the left arytenoid to fully abduct results in a slackening of the vocal fold, which is also drawn into the airway during inspiration. These horses will make an inspiratory roar during exercise.

CONCLUSION

The endoscopic identification of an upper respiratory tract abnormality in the resting horse does not necessarily indicate a clinical problem, nor does absence of an upper respiratory abnormality at rest rule out the possibility of intermittent obstruction during strenuous exercise. The clinical evaluation of dynamic upper respiratory tract function of the horse during treadmill exercise allows evaluation of upper respiratory tract function during conditions simulating those of competitive racing. Although many upper respiratory tract abnormalities may be diagnosed at rest (specifically, most cases of continual epiglottic entrapment and total laryngeal paralysis), the diagnosis of intermittent DDSP, intermittent epiglottic entrapment, and some cases of idiopathic laryngeal neuropathy necessitates observation of the upper respiratory tract during strenuous exercise. This diagnostic technique allows absolute verification that upper airway dysfunction is contributing to inadequate athletic performance in an individual horse. It also enables a precise description of the anatomical abnormalities resulting in the airway obstruction, thereby allowing an attempt at the most efficacious management technique.

Supplemental Readings

Derksen, F. J., Stick, J. A., Scott, E. A., Robinson, N.E., and Slocombe, R. F.: Effect of laryngeal hemiplegia and laryngoplasty on airway flow mechanics in exercising horses. Am. J. Vet. Res., 47:16, 1986.

Morris, E. A., and Seeherman, H. J.: Evaluation of upper respiratory tract function during strenuous exercise in the race horse. J. Am. Vet. Med. Assoc., 196:431, 1990.

Raphel, C. F.: Endoscopic findings in the upper respiratory tract of 479 horses. J. Am. Vet. Med. Assoc., 181:470, 1982.

Pulmonary Function Tests

Frederik J. Derksen, EAST LANSING, MICHIGAN

Tests of pulmonary function in athletic horses should be easily performed, sensitive to even subclinical levels of disease, and specific for the various lung conditions from which the athletic horse suffers. At present such tests are not available even in human medicine, where the patient is usually cooperative. However, two common, nonspecific tests of pulmonary function are available to the veterinarian: measurement of blood gas tensions and measurement of pleural pressure.

BLOOD GAS EVALUATION IN ATHLETIC HORSES

In disease, the lung fails to fully oxygenate the arterial blood, and hypoxemia results. Therefore, measurement of arterial blood gas tensions is a practical means of evaluating ventilation and quantitatively assessing the gas exchange efficiency of the lung. In the standing horse, arterial blood is readily obtained from the carotid or the facial artery. The sample must be heparinized and the syringe capped and stored on ice for transport to the laboratory.

Interpretation of arterial blood gas values in the resting horse has been discussed in detail elsewhere. Briefly, arterial carbon dioxide tension (Pa_{CO_2}) yields information regarding alveolar ventilation, because Pa_{CO_2} is inversely related to aveolar ventilation ($\dot{V}_A$) in the following manner:

$$\dot{V}_A = \frac{k \cdot \dot{V}_{CO_2}}{Pa_{CO_2}},$$

where $\dot{V}_{CO_2}$ is CO_2 production and k is a constant. Because CO_2 diffuses very rapidly across the alveolar–blood barrier, Pa_{CO_2} is rarely affected by diffusion limitations.

Pa_{O_2} is also influenced by alveolar ventilation as well as by inspired oxygen concentration. A third important determinant of Pa_{O_2} is the gas exchange efficiency of the lung. In normal resting horses breathing ambient air at sea level, the Pa_{O_2} is 90 to 100 torr. When Pa_{O_2} decreases and alveolar ventilation is normal, it may be concluded that there is lung disease and that the gas exchange efficiency of the lung has been impaired. The advantage of evaluation of gas exchange in the resting horse is that the technique allows a quantitative evaluation of lung function. The disadvantage of the technique is that it lacks sensitivity. That is, substantial lung disease must be present before Pa_{O_2} decreases.

It is likely that evaluation of gas exchange in exercising horses will allow detection of more subtle lung injury. Arterial blood is more difficult to obtain in exercising horses, but with the increased availability of high-speed treadmills, several reports have recently appeared in the literature describing gas exchange in the exercising horse. Evaluation of gas exchange in exercising horses may soon become a clinical tool to evaluate lung function in the athletic horse. At low to moderate levels of exercise, Pa_{O_2} remains at levels observed in resting horses. However, during near maximum exercise in apparently normal horses, Pa_{O_2} decreases significantly (Fig. 1). A similar decrease in Pa_{O_2} is observed in strenuously exercising humans but not in dogs. In normal horses exercise-induced hypoxemia has little effect on oxygen transport because of the flat slope of the oxyhemoglobin dissociation curve. In horses with lung disease, gas exchange abnormalities in the lung caused by disease and exercise-induced hypoxemia may combine to significantly affect oxygen transport to the tissues and performance. Diffusion limitation has been suggested as the most important cause of exercise-induced hypoxemia. During strenuous exercise, horses attain an enormous cardiac output (300 liters per minute), thereby increasing the velocity at which blood flows through the lung and decreasing the time available for each red blood cell to load oxygen. When this transit time becomes too short, insufficient oxygen is transferred (diffusion is limited) and hypoxemia results. Another cause of exercise-induced hypoxemia is relative hypoventilation. In ponies and other species, Pa_{CO_2} decreases during strenuous exercise.

In the horse at light and moderate exercise, Pa_{CO_2} decreases. However, during strenuous exercise Pa_{CO_2} rises significantly (but not above values encountered in the resting horse; see Fig. 1), indicating relative hypoventilation. The reason for this hypoventilation is unclear but may be related to mechanical factors limiting the enormous ventilation required by the exercising horse.

The fact that normal, strenuously exercising horses have a decrease in Pa_{O_2} and relative hypoventilation must be considered when evaluating horses with possible lung disease. It may

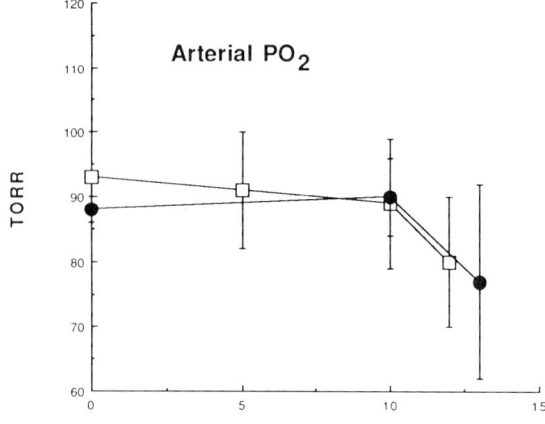

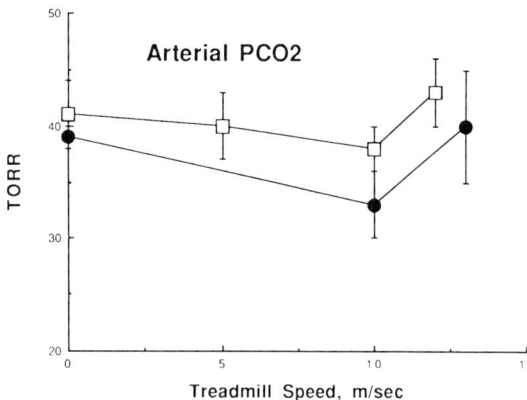

Figure 1. Arterial Po_2 and Pco_2 as a function of treadmill speed in two separate studies. Note the decrease in Pa_{O_2} and increase in Pa_{CO_2} at speeds greater than 10 meters per second. The decrease in Pa_{O_2} is only partially accounted for by the increase in Pa_{CO_2}. (From Wagner, P. D., Gillespie, J. R., Landgren, G. L., Fedde, M. R., Jones, B. W., Debowes, R. M., Pieschl, R. L., and Erickson, H. H.: Mechanism of exercise-induced hypoxemia in horses. J. Appl. Physiol., 66:1227–1233, 1989. Reproduced by permission.)

prove more useful to measure blood gas tensions at submaximal speeds

MEASUREMENT OF PLEURAL PRESSURE

The purpose of measuring pulmonary mechanics in athletic horses is to evaluate the horse's inspiratory and expiratory effort. If a horse has to expend too much effort to breathe, less energy is available for athletic performance. The work of breathing generated by the muscles of respiration is used to overcome the resistance to air flow in the airways, to neutralize the elastic recoil of the lung tissue, and to accelerate and decelerate the air mass. Using a model of the respiratory system analogous to electrical circuits, each one of these factors can be calculated if the air flow at the nose and the pleural pressure are known. Because of the requirements for specialized equipment, measurement of air flow is currently impractical in clinical practice. However, measurement of pleural pressure is easily achieved. Indeed, commercial equipment is available to facilitate this measurement.* A small tube is passed through the nares and into the thoracic portion of the esophagus and attached to a pressure transducer and physiograph. During breathing, the pressure swings in the thoracic portion of the esophagus represent pleural pressure. Pleural pressure swings are increased when the horse breathes deeper (increased tidal volume) and faster (increased respiratory frequency), and when the airways are narrowed (increased pulmonary resistance) or the lung is stiffer (decreased dynamic compliance). The latter two factors are relevant in horses with lung disease. Measurement of pleural pressure is valuable when performed in resting horses breathing with a predictable tidal volume and frequency. Under these circumstances, an increase in pleural pressure indicates airway obstruction or decreased lung compliance suggestive of lung disease. In normal horses at rest, the changes in pleural pressure during each breath range from 3 to 8 cm H_2O. In horses with severe lung disease, pleural pressure swings may be as high as 60 cm H_2O. Pleural pressure measurement in athletic horses allows quantitative lung function evaluation and more accurate diagnosis of pulmonary disease. In addition, measurement of pleural pressure is useful to monitor progress of therapy. The disadvantages of the technique are (1) it is relatively insensitive, so that subclinical pulmonary disease may be missed; (2) increases in pleural pressure swings during breathing can be caused not only by lung disease but also by changes in the pattern of breathing (tidal volume and respiratory frequency); and (3) the measurement is nonspecific, so that bigger changes in pleural pressure during tidal breathing occur with airway obstruction and decreased lung compliance resulting from a variety of lung diseases, including bronchopneumonia, chronic obstructive pulmonary disease, and pulmonary fibrosis.

The field of pulmonary function testing as it applies to the equine athlete is still in its infancy. Although techniques available to the practicing veterinarian can provide quantitative informa-

---

*Ventigraph Model PG/100 RC, Boehringer Ingelheim Vetmedica, Ingelheim, Germany

tion regarding lung function of the athletic horse, the techniques are nonspecific and insensitive. It is likely that in the future new tests will become available that will improve our ability to assess pulmonary abnormalities affecting performance horses.

Supplemental Readings

Bayly, W. M., Hodgson, D. R., Schulz, D. A., Dempsey, J. A., and Gollnick, P. D.: Exercise-induced hypercapnia in the horse. J. Appl. Physiol., 67:1958–1966, 1989.

Derksen, F. J., and Robinson, N. E.: Esophageal and intrapleural pressures in the healthy conscious pony. Am. J. Vet. Res., 41:1756–1761, 1980.

Jones, J. H., Longworth, K. E., Lindholm, A., Conley, K. E., Karas, R. H., Kayar, S. R., and Taylor, C. R.: Oxygen transport during exercise in large mammals: I. Adaptive variations in oxygen demand. J. Appl. Physiol., 67:862–870, 1989.

Wagner, P. D., Gillespie, J. R., Landgren, G. L., Fedde, M. R., Jones, B. W., Debowes, R. M., Pieschl, R. L., and Erickson, H. H.: Mechanism of exercise-induced hypoxemia in horses. J. Appl. Physiol., 66:1227–1233, 1989.

Imaging of the Lower Airways

Michael W. O'Callaghan, NORTH GRAFTON, MASSACHUSETTS

Radiography, scintigraphy, and ultrasonography are currently the only methods readily available for imaging the thorax of horses. Unfortunately, cross-sectional imaging modalities such as computed tomography, magnetic resonance imaging, single-photon emission computed tomography, and positron emission tomography are currently unsuitable, even if available, either because the gantry apertures containing the detectors are too small to accept a horse's thorax or because physical rotation of the detectors around a horse is impossible with existing equipment.

RADIOGRAPHY

Thoracic radiography remains the principal method for routinely evaluating the lungs of horses presented for evaluation of poor performance. In adult horses, radiographs of the entire lung field require x-ray equipment with at least 250 mA output. An output of 1000 mA is preferable to reduce movement artifact. Most portable x-ray units used in equine practice have maximum outputs in the 20 to 50 mA range. Such equipment is often available only in larger referral centers.

Radiographic technique is also important. Ideally, four radiographs, each taken with specific exposures for the different areas of the lung and repeated for both left and right sides of the thorax, are recommended. It is particularly important to avoid underexposure of the radiograph since the resulting apparent increase in interstitial opacity of the image mimics the appearance of infiltrative disease.

INDICATIONS

For evaluating poor performance the choice of diagnostic test is often more difficult than in cases of obvious respiratory disease. Thoracic radiography is one of many tests that may be used in evaluating respiratory disease; however, there are several specific indications for obtaining radiographs of the lung fields:

1. when the history, clinical findings, or other imaging techniques suggest lung lesions (e.g., exercise-induced epistaxis, bilateral nasal discharge, auscultatory evidence of lung disease, abnormal breathing patterns, coughing, history of recent anesthesia or long transport, ultrasonographic evidence of pleural fluid, and the like),

2. when upper respiratory tract signs are present but no abnormality is detected on examination of the upper airways,

3. when upper respiratory tract signs are severe and may have led to lung damage (e.g., soft palate dysfunction),

4. when upper respiratory tract lesions are accompanied by unaccountably severe signs possibly pulmonary in origin (e.g., lymphoid hyperplasia), and

5. when musculoskeletal causes of poor performance have been ruled out in cases with equivocal respiratory signs.

INTERPRETATION

Radiographs transmit primarily structural information, although some functional information can be gained if the pathogenesis of a particular process is well understood. Focal or localized alveolar infiltrates or filling provide the greatest contrast between normal and abnormal lung and are therefore the easiest to recognize. Thus, alveolar opacities or dense interstitial infiltrates associated with lung abscesses, localized bronchopneumonia, or recent exercise-induced pulmonary hemorrhage (EIPH) are readily diagnosed. The characteristic sites of some lesions (e.g., caudodorsal lung tip in EIPH, caudoventral lung in aspiration pneumonia, overlapping the diaphragmatic silhouette for some lung abcesses or as a ventrally distributed horizontal opacity in pleuritis) may be highly specific.

More commonly, varying degrees of diffuse interstitial, peribronchial, or combined bronchointerstitial infiltrates are present but are more difficult to recognize because the adjacent airways and alveoli remain partially air-filled. Contrast between normal and affected tissue is therefore less evident. Diffuse bronchointerstitial patterns can range from coarse, irregular, predominantly linear or reticulated opacities to the faintest of finely nodular patterns barely distinguishable from the vascular background. The former pattern is often seen in resolving bronchopneumonia when cellular material and fluid, previously in alveoli and the smallest airways, move into perilobular and interstitial spaces. The finely nodular pattern probably represents thickened small airways and infiltrate around secondary lung lobules in association with small airway disease.

Air trapping caused by small airway disease, particularly in horses with COPD, is recognized from thin, paired bronchial lines representing bronchial walls extending almost fully to the lung periphery contrasted by extra surrounding air (Fig. 1). These lines may persist even when interstitial infiltrate intervenes (e.g., in cases of COPD recently challenged by moldy hay). The pulmonary vessels in these cases may also appear small and spindly but are more clearly defined than expected because of the combined effect of compression and enhanced contrast. In cases of poor performance, the combination of a faint, finely nodular pattern and bronchial markings extending to the periphery suggests small airway disease, and is often confirmed by detection of mucopurulent or inflammatory debris in tracheal aspirates (Fig. 2).

Changes in vascular markings are highly variable but can be an important clue to lung pathology. Vessels in the caudodorsal lung may appear smaller than normal in some cases of EIPH and in others with local signs of small airway disease, suggesting either compression by air trapping or reflex reduction in blood flow to maintain ventilation/perfusion ($\dot{V}/\dot{Q}$) matching. In some cases of ventral lung disease such as pleuritis or ventral pneumonia, increased blood flow dorsally increases the prominence of vessels crossing the aorta. The opposite may occur in reactive airway disease such as allergic bronchitis, when air trapping compresses the lung vessels.

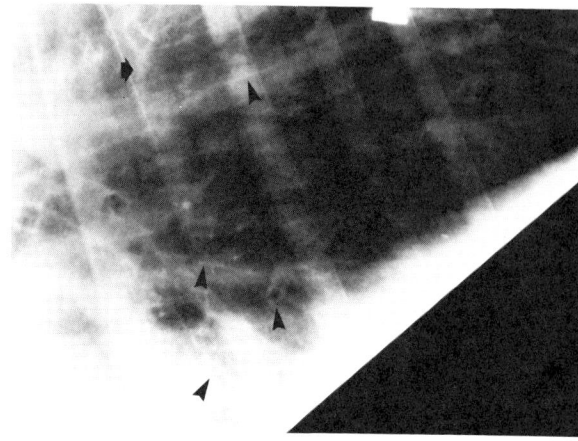

Figure 1. Thoracic radiograph showing the caudoventral lung of a horse with mild symptoms of COPD. The most notable feature is overaeration of the lung field, creating increased contrast. As a result, the larger and medium-sized airway walls *(arrowheads)* are clearly delineated well toward the lung periphery. Numerous clearly defined, thin-walled ringlike shadows are also noted *(lower right arrowhead)*. Vascular structures are also smaller than normal and difficult to identify *(small arrow)* as a result of compression.

While many of these more subtle changes can be appreciated by carefully evaluating the lung

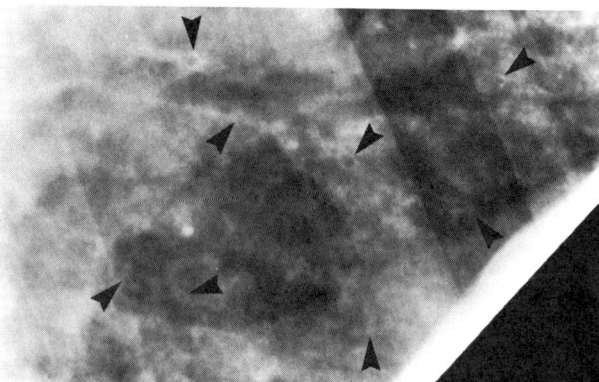

Figure 2. Caudal lung field of a 3-year-old Standardbred with a slight loss of form (2 to 3 seconds slower than most recent times) and intermittent cough. On thoracic radiographs there was a diffuse, fine "nodular bronchointerstitial" pattern, most prominent in the caudal lung field immediately dorsal to the diaphragm. Close examination of the so-called nodular opacities revealed they were composed of small (1 to 3 mm), ring opacities with fluffy outer margins (peribronchial cuffing) and relatively smooth inner margins around lucent centers *(arrowheads)*. True interstitial opacity is difficult to identify in this case. These findings are consistent with diffuse, low-grade small airways disease, without evidence of air trapping or extensive interstitial infiltrate except for the peribronchial cuffs. A transtracheal aspirate in this case revealed low-grade infection suggestive of bronchiolitis.

for signs of alveolar, interstitial, bronchial, and vascular components, their interpretation is often equivocal unless they are accompanied by some other correlative finding that supports the same diagnosis. Transtracheal aspiration and bronchoalveolar lavage are particularly helpful in identifying the pathological process, provided that cellular material is released to the airway surfaces. Functional impairment is more difficult to evaluate. Various lung function tests, some requiring a high-speed treadmill, allow global assessment of several useful parameters. However, to determine the regional distribution of lung fuction or impairment, a function-specific imaging modality such as scintigraphy is required.

SCINTIGRAPHY

Gamma cameras and the supporting equipment needed for scintigraphy are expensive to buy and maintain and require highly qualified operators. Currently, therefore, scintigraphy is readily available only in some university teaching hospitals, research institutions, and a few private referral centers.

Scintigraphy, based on the use of bone-seeking radiopharmaceuticals, has been most widely used to evaluate the musculoskeletal system. By contrast, lung scanning is still limited to a few imaging centers. For clinical purposes lung scintigraphy in horses is confined to pulmonary arterial perfusion imaging using ^{99m}Tc-MAA (macroaggregated albumin), administered by intravenous injection, and ventilation imaging using the radioactive aerosol ^{99m}Tc-DTPA (diaminetriaminepentaacetate) delivered by a closed face mask and filtered breathing circuit. Other ventilation agents, such as the noble gases ^{133}Xe, ^{81m}Kr, and aerosols of ^{111}In, have been employed in research but are unsuitable for clinical studies, for a variety of physical and logistic reasons. Ventilation/perfusion images can be read directly from images acquired with a multiformat camera. Alternatively, images can be stored on a computer system for later processing, including images of $\dot{V}/\dot{Q}$ ratio distribution over the entire lateral projection of each lung. Other functions of the lung such as mucociliary clearance rates of insoluble monodispersed aerosols, absorption clearance of ^{99m}Tc-DTPA, labeling of red blood cells to detect lung bleeding, and labeling of white cells to detect septic processes are possible but for the present are limited to research studies.

Indications

Experience with lung scintigraphy in horses is limited. Specific indications are therefore less well defined than for radiography, particularly as scintigraphy plays a complementary rather than a primary role in lung evaluation. In our experience, $\dot{V}/\dot{Q}$ scintigraphy has proved most useful in the following situations.

1. In horses with chronic, repetitive, or severe EIPH but few or negligible radiographic signs, scintigraphy has often demonstrated perfusion deficits in the caudodorsal lung.
2. When there is radiographic evidence of air trapping, vascular redistribution or unexplained bronchointerstitial infiltrate, matched ventilation and perfusion deficits have been demonstrated in the undercirculated or infiltrated lung.
3. In horses suspected of having reactive airway disease and overinflation of the lung on radiography, lung scans have demonstrated reduced peripheral ventilation and perfusion and a turbulent pattern of aerosol distribution in the major airways, similar to cases of confirmed COPD.
4. When lung function or treadmill step tests indicate $\dot{V}/\dot{Q}$ impairment but lung radiographs show either no evidence of lung pathology, or patterns indicative of EIPH or small airway disease.

Interpretation

Count densities recorded on the lung images reflect primarily the volume of lung subtended at the camera face and the degree of attenuation determined by tissue depth from the skin surface. Thus, on lateral views of the lungs in adult horses, count rates are heavily weighted in favor of lung tissue closest to the camera face, with negligible contribution from the opposite lung. Counts are therefore highest where the lung is thickest, i.e., cranial and dorsal to the diaphragm on the lateral image, and least where it is thinnest, i.e., in the costophrenic angle beneath the diaphragm, and cranially where the shoulder muscles overlie the thinnest sections of the lung, causing the greatest attenuation.

Aerosol-generated ventilation images display the sum of counts arising from aerosol deposited with each breath during aerosol administration. The resulting image is flow weighted, representing ventilation distribution. Areas of diminished aerosol deposition reflect local or generalized air flow reduction, the result of small airway disease or poorly compliant lung. The pattern of deposition of aerosols in the lung is also highly sensitive to airway turbulence. Thus, in the presence of small airway narrowing or inflammatory debris, turbulence causes deposition on the larger airways, a pattern seen characteristically in COPD. Peripheral underventilation is also characteristic in these cases (Fig. 3). Perfusion deficits reflect either reduced blood flow as a result

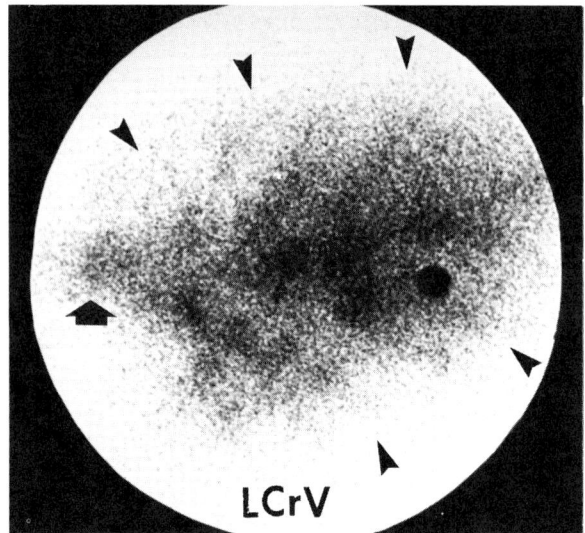

Figure 3. Left cranial ^{99m}Tc-DTPA aerosol ventilation scan of a horse with COPD. The head is to the left. The scan shows typical distribution of aerosol in horses with increased airway resistance and turbulence. Most of the aerosol has been deposited in the central airways and trachea *(arrow)*, whereas deposition in the periphery of the lung fields is considerably reduced *(arrowheads)*. The single circular photodense structure at the lower right, adjacent to the diaphragmatic margin, is a radioactive marker used for merging cranial and caudal images on the computer.

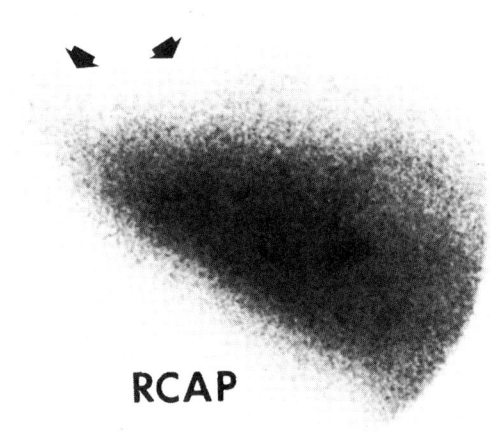

Figure 4. ^{99m}Tc-MAA perfusion scan of the right caudal lung of a horse with repeated incidents of exercise-induced hemorrhage. The head is to the right. Perfusion distribution over most of the lung is normal except for a large deficit *(arrows)* in the caudodorsal extremity of the lung. This finding closely correlates with pathological findings in horses with EIPH. In most horses demonstrating such a perfusion deficit, there is often only a mild change in ventilation to the same area, creating a ventilation/perfusion mismatch. $\dot{V}/\dot{Q}$ ratio images, created on the computer from these data, demonstrate high $\dot{V}/\dot{Q}$ ratios (2:1 to 4:1) in the affected area of the lung, whereas the remaining lung maintains a normal 1:1 ratio.

of hypoxic vasoconstriction to match $\dot{V}/\dot{Q}$, embolism, or competitive exclusion by the high-pressure bronchial circulation (e.g., in EIPH).

In cases of poor performance the most common pattern encountered has been an unmatched perfusion deficit in the caudodorsal lung fields. This pattern is seen to some degree in many horses with clinical EIPH and in a smaller proportion of horses with no history of bleeding (Fig. 4). We currently interpret this pattern as evidence of bronchial arterial dominance of the caudodorsal lung and a poor prognostic sign for long-term athletic performance in bleeders.

We have also seen mild but matched $\dot{V}/\dot{Q}$ deficits in the same area in both bleeders and poor performance horses, interpreted as probable evidence of reversible small airways disease. Similar irregular matched deficits have been seen along the thin section of the lung overlying the costophrenic margin, also interpreted as small airway disease since this pattern becomes accentuated and accompanied by turbulent deposition in the large airways in horses with COPD ("heaves"). Mildly increased turbulent deposition is seen in some of these cases. The most prominent lesions of this type have been seen in horses with clinically obvious heaves. These have included extensive, matched, reversible reductions in ventilation and perfusion to the periphery of the lung and severe turbulent deposition in the major airways. In horses with known reactive airways disease (reversible heaves) in remission, scintigraphy has proved to be a more sensitive indicator of disease than measurements of pleural pressure, since a mildly turbulent pattern of aerosol deposition remains even when pleural pressure has returned to normal levels.

ULTRASONOGRAPHY

A wide variety of ultrasound equipment is employed in equine practice and in referral institutions. For thoracic imaging real-time sector scanners are most valuable, particularly for echocardiography. For examination of the lung and pleural space, linear array scanners may also be used but can only be orientated vertically between rib spaces. The most useful scan head frequency is 3.0 MHz.

INDICATIONS

The main indications for ultrasound examination of the respiratory system are evaluation of the pleural space in cases of suspected pleural effusion, pleuritis, or pleuropneumonia and for evaluation of lung consolidation or lung masses suspected from prior radiographic, scintigraphic, or clinical examination. A discussion of these conditions is beyond the scope of this chapter since most cases are presented with overt signs of respiratory disease rather than for poor performance.

Supplemental Readings

Farrow, C. S.: Neck and thorax: Equidae. The lung. *In* Thrall, D. E. (ed.): Textbook of Veterinary Diagnostic Radiology. Philadelphia, W. B. Saunders, 1986, pp. 339–355.

Farrow, C. S.: Radiography of the equine thorax: Anatomy and technique. Vet. Radiol., 22:62–68, 1981.

Genereux, G. P.: Pattern recognition in diffuse lung disease: A review of theory and practice. Med. Radiog. Photog., 61:2–31, 1985.

Milne, E.N.C.: Some new concepts of pulmonary blood flow and volume. Radiol. Clin. North Am., 11:17–26, 1987.

O'Callaghan, M. W., and Seeherman, H. S.: New ways of looking at lung disease in the horses using radiography and scintigraphy. *In*: Proceedings of the 35th Annual Convention of the American Association of Equine Practitioners, 1989, 221–232.

O'Callaghan, M. W., Hornof, W. J., Fisher, P. E., and Raabe, O. G.: Ventilation imaging in the horse with 99m-technetium-DTPA radioaerosol. Equine Vet. J., 19:19–24, 1987.

O'Callaghan, M. W., Hornof, W. J., Fisher, P. E., and Pascoe, J. R.: Exercise-induced pulmonary hemorrhage in the horse: Results of a detailed clinical, post mortem and imaging study. VII. Ventilation/perfusion scintigraphy in horses with EIPH. Equine Vet. J., 19:423–427, 1987.

Rantanen, N. W., Gage, L., and Paradis, M. R.: Ultrasonography as a diagnostic aid in pleural effusion of horses. Vet. Radiol., 22:211–219, 1981.

Electrophysiologic Responses to Exercise

Frank S. Pipers, NORTH GRAFTON, MASSACHUSETTS

Although examination of the cardiovascular system of the resting horse is useful, many cardiovascular disturbances require exercise to induce a recognizable problem. Advances in technology such as cardiac telemetry, heart rate monitoring, and high-speed treadmills permit the acquisition of data before, during, and after maximal exertion.

Heart rate monitors record electrical signals from electrodes pasted to the chest wall and attached to a small electronic box, the size of a calculator, that is strapped with Velcro to the rider's thigh. The rider observes the average heart rate during various phases of exercise.

In telemetry, electrocardiography (ECG) information is transmitted from the horse to a system that displays and records the ECG. This has the advantage of not only indicating a problem but also of identifying the specific electrical disturbance.

Once a dysrhythmia has been identified, evaluation of structure and function is the next step in the cardiac evaluation. Echocardiography is an excellent means of acquiring this information in the resting horse but cannot be done during exercise, owing to excessive motion artifact. To acquire functional data during exercise one can record pressures as a catheter is passed from the jugular vein through the right atrium and ventricle into the pulmonary artery. Pressure is measured by a pressure transducer at the tip of the catheter. Blood samples may be removed from the right heart and pulmonary artery at various times during exercise for analysis of temperature and oxygenation. Placement of the catheter tip can be verified by ultrasonography before or after exercise.

Finally, scintigraphy is indispensable for studying myocardial perfusion during exercise. If a short-lived radioisotope is injected immediately after exercise and the heart is scanned with a gamma camera, the extent and intensity of blood flow can be determined and any defects in perfusion can be readily visualized. The cardiovascular changes that occur in the thickened athletic heart often are seen only during strenuous exercise, when blood flow to the heart may become compromised during diastole because of the high heart rate.

High-speed treadmills facilitate collection of these data because the clinician can stand beside an exercising horse while evaluating the heart rate, rhythm, and functional data. Treadmills also allow immediate postexercise scintigraphy, ultrasonography, and auscultation to be performed.

Cardiac dysrhythmias are often suggested as a cause of exercise intolerance, especially in horses with few problems detectable at rest. Studies at rest or under conditions that fail to replicate strenuous exertion may not rule in or rule out these potential disorders. In addition, in horses being exercise tested on a treadmill, dysrhythmias may be seen in animals free of clinical signs of cardiovascular disease. For these reasons it is necessary to have a controlled system whereby dysrhythmias can be evaluated while the horse is exercising, and to have some idea of the frequency of dysrhythmias in apparently healthy athletic horses. Much of the literature on cardiovascular responses to strenuous exercise in the normal horse is less than applicable, for it often reports data from horses not in the peak of condition or no longer pursuing an athletic career.

APPROPRIATE RESPONSES TO EXERCISE

Human athletes that perform isotonic exercise experience morphological changes such as an increase in the thickness and mass of the ventricular wall. Resting sinus bradycardia, sinus arrhythmia, a wandering atrial pacemaker, first- and second-degree heart blocks, and junctional rhythms are seen frequently and are attributed to elevations in vagal tone induced by conditioning. In addition to rate and rhythm modifications, ECG evidence of morphological alterations is frequently documented. T-wave alterations, ST segment changes, and ECG amplitude increases are typical examples and are related to the increases in cardiac muscle mass. Most electrophysiological and morphological changes noted in the human athlete have also been reported in the athletic horse. The numbers of horses studied, however, are small, and often the horses are less than optimally fit. These ECG changes are not pathological in man, and they may indicate an appropriate response to conditioning in the horse as well.

INAPPROPRIATE RESPONSES TO EXERCISE

Approximately 50 years ago reports in human medical literature began to appear suggesting that exercise might uncover cardiac rate and rhythm abnormalities inapparent at rest. Treadmill testing has been used extensively as a safe and effective method of monitoring human patients and provoking suspected cardiac disease.

In veterinary medicine we have long suspected exercise-induced cardiovascular problems. Frequently a horse experiences a bout of exercise intolerance that necessitates a clinical evaluation. The subsequent examination, usually performed at rest, often does not uncover any problem. The ECG may be recorded immediately after strenuous exercise but too late to capture the abnormal event. Telemetered ECG signals from a free-ranging animal can be very useful, but there are many technical problems with obtaining the data, and it may not be possible to work the animal strenuously enough to provoke the instability. It is for these reasons that treadmill telemetry testing is useful to reveal occult and transient episodes of electrical instability and correlate the instability with exercise intolerance.

Speculation on the mechanisms underlying exercise-induced dysrhythmias in the horse typically involves vascular occlusion or spasm resulting in ischemia, a potent trigger for malignant ventricular dysrhythmias. Spastic arterial disease is difficult to prove or disprove, and there is little evidence in the veterinary literature of atherosclerotic or occlusive heart disease in the horse. In a recent study of sudden death on midwestern racetracks, on postmortem examination 33 per cent of cases had only minor detectable lesions characteristic of ischemic changes.

It is more likely that dysrhythmias occur independent of ischemia and are the result of electrophysiological instability induced by neurohumoral mechanisms. These neurohumoral responses to exercise enhance diastolic depolarization (phase four), improve membrane conductivity, and shorten the refractory period in all cardiac tissues. In addition, catecholamine-stimulated β-adrenergic receptors activate the adenylate cyclase cyclic adenosine monophosphate pathway, which then increases transmembrane calcium influx. The net result of this cascade is that exercise can induce tachyarrhythmias by three prevalent mechanisms: reentry, automaticity, and triggered rhythmic activity. From human studies, tachyarrhythmic mechanisms are further delineated into those that are responsive to calcium blockers and those that are not, and those that can be stimulated by electrical pacing versus those that can be elicited by infusions of β-adrenergic agonists. Although there are no equivalent data available for the athletic horse, it is possible that electrophysiological instability rather than ischemic disease is the major cause of dysrhythmias.

EXERCISE-INDUCED ELECTROPHYSIOLOGICAL RESPONSES IN THE HORSE

Fifty-one racehorses were examined during a standardized maximal exercise test and the ECG was recorded by telemetry. All the horses were racing at the time of the evaluation and were referred for evaluation of poor performance. The cause of poor performance was subtle enough to have eluded diagnosis by traditional methods. The poor performance was attributed to mild upper or lower respiratory abnormalities or mild to moderate musculoskeletal pain at high speed in 26 of the horses. Twenty-five others had no identified problems.

NORMAL

All of the horses presented for performance evaluation had a resting heart rate within the previously published range (25 to 40 bpm). Once the horses were outfitted in racing gear, instrumented, and trained to use the treadmill, the preexercise heart rate varied between 25 and 100 bpm, presumably due to psychogenic factors. There was no correlation between preexercise data and subsequent maximal or recovery heart rates.

Maximal heart rate varied between 200 and 243 bpm in this group (mean, 218 ± 9 bpm). One minute after the end of exercise, heart rate averaged 195 ± 11 bpm; at 5 minutes the mean was 105 ± 14 bpm.

CLINICALLY UNIMPORTANT DYSRHYTHMIAS

One third of the horses tested had dysrhythmias judged to be of little clinical significance.

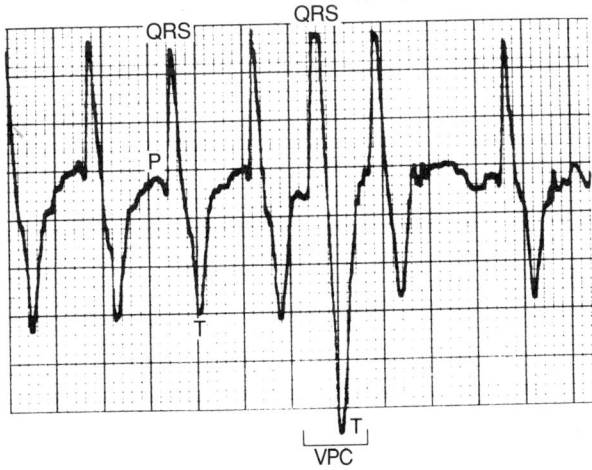

Figure 1. Electrocardiographic example of a seemingly benign exercise-induced ventricular dysrhythmia. VPC, ventricular premature contractions.

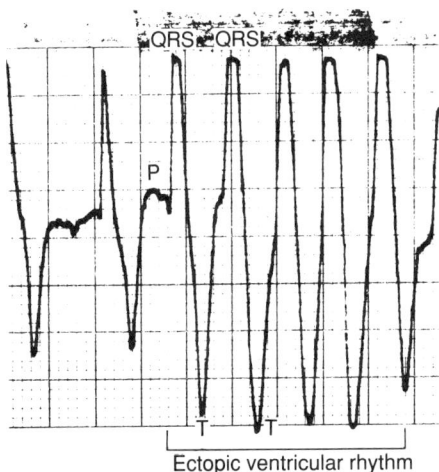

Figure 2. Example of paroxysmal ventricular tachycardia seen during exercise. The tachycardia was followed immediately by an abrupt change in exercise capacity.

These were single abnormal ECG events preceded and followed by normal beats (Fig. 1). None of these horses showed evidence of heart disease at rest. There was no difference in the frequency of occurrence of these clinically unimportant dysrhythmias between horses with identifiable causes of poor performance such as respiratory or musculoskeletal disease and those with no identifiable cause.

CLINICALLY IMPORTANT DYSRHYTHMIAS

Two horses (4 per cent) had sustained, potentially dangerous bouts of paroxysmal ventricular tachycardia during strenuous exercise (Fig. 2). These horses faltered and abruptly stopped exercising during these bouts. On 9-month follow-up, one of the two horses was destined to become a brood mare. The other, a gelding, had been rested for 4 months and was training successfully without signs of the previous problem.

Although this number is quite small, there is every evidence that electrophysiological instability rather than ischemic disease is a major contributor to the production of dysrhythmias during exercise. For this reason treadmill exercise coupled with ECG analysis is perhaps the most useful, effective, and efficient method to identify cardiac dysrhythmias contributing to poor performance.

Supplemental Readings

Hall, M. C., Steel, J. D., and Stewart, G. A.: Cardiac monitoring during exercise tests in the horse: 2. Aust. Vet. J., 52:1–5, 1976.

Maier-Bock, H., and Ehrlein, H. J.: Heart rate during a defined exercise test in horses with heart and lung diseases. Equine Vet. J., *10*:235, 1978.

Evans, D.: Cardiovascular adaptations to exercise and training. Vet. Clin. North Am., *1*:513–531, 1985.

Houston, T. P., Puffer, J. C., and Rodney, W. M.: The athletic heart syndrome. N. Engl. J. Med., *313*:24–32, 1985.

Ferst, J. A., and Chaitman, B. R.: The electrogram and the athlete. Sports Med., *1*:390–403, 1984.

Gait Analysis

Howard J. Seeherman, NORTH GRAFTON, MASSACHUSETTS

A number of advanced techniques have been developed to aid in the description of normal equine gait and the diagnosis of gait abnormalities. Use of these techniques includes research, clinical diagnosis of lameness, and quantitative analysis of the alternations in gait as a result of therapeutics. These techniques can be divided into two broad categories, kinematics and kinetics. Kinematic analysis utilizes high-speed cinematography, videography, electrogoniometry, and accelerometry to quantify the movements of the limbs and torso during exercise. Kinetic analysis utilizes instrumented shoes, force plates, and pressure-sensitive mats to evaluate weight-bearing profiles required to generate movement. A discussion of the available technology with an emphasis on the more accessible video-based systems follows.

QUANTITATIVE KINEMATICS

High-speed cinematography and videography have been used extensively to evaluate the kinematics of locomotion in normal and lame horses moving at a variety of gaits under different conditions, including racing and jumping. The effects of racetrack design on gait patterns has also been investigated with kinematic techniques. The main advantage of these techniques is slow motion capability allowing the detection of lameness and quantification of normal limb movement, which is difficult to visualize at racing speeds or during competitions. Computer-assisted digitization of the movement of the horse's limbs allows quantification of the gait patterns (Fig. 1). Kinematic analysis using cinematography has traditionally been the imaging mode of choice because of the high frame rate possible (100 to 250 frames per second is typical), short exposure times resulting in minimal blur, and the excellent resolution of the image. The disadvantages are the expense of the equipment and the need to process the film prior to analysis.

Recent advances in the field of video technology have made video competitive with film in kinematic gait analysis. Suitable low-cost video cameras designed for stop-action evaluation of racquet sports and golf techniques can be used to obtain high-quality kinematic evaluations of equine locomotion. These types of cameras use solid-state electronics to achieve shutter speeds up to $\frac{1}{1000}$th of a second. This short exposure time results in blur-free images of high speed motion. The limiting factor is the video data acquisition rate of 60 frames per second required for use with standard video recorders. The slow frame rate limits the number of images that can be acquired in a given time for detailed evaluation of rapid motion. No matter how sharp an image is obtained, there is still $\frac{1}{30}$th or $\frac{1}{60}$th of a second between frames. High-speed video is available at speeds of up to 2000 frames per second, but most of these systems are quite expensive and are not VHS compatible.

New computer systems enable relatively easy

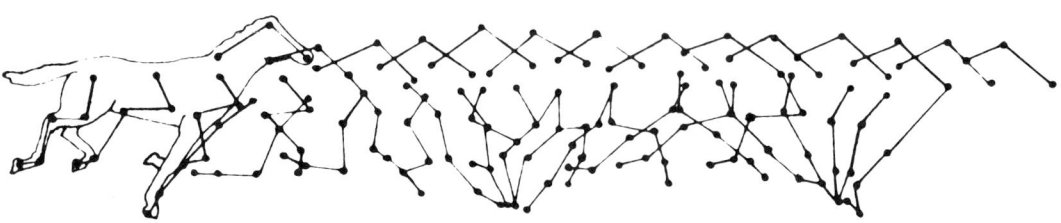

Figure 1. Stick figures generated from digitized kinematic analysis of the equine gallop.

frame by frame digitization of limb movements. Knowledge of frame rate and measurement of limb displacement allow calculation of velocity, angular velocity and acceleration. Applications of this technology include comparison of gait between subjects, comparison of the alterations in gait elicited by different ground surfaces, and evaluation of a single subject over time to see changes related to therapeutics or training.

Electrogoniometry and accelerometry have been used primarily as research tools to quantify changes in joint angles and mechanical energy changes in limb segments during locomotion in sound and lame horses. Routine clinical application of quantitative kinematics is limited by the expense of the equipment, the need to instrument the horse, and the time required for data acquisition.

QUALITATIVE KINEMATICS

In contrast to quantitative kinematic analysis, qualitative videography appears to be a valuable tool for routine clinical gait analysis. Video equipment is readily available and easy to use. Video tapes can be mailed so that details of lameness evaluations performed at referral clinics can be sent to veterinarians, owners, and trainers not present during the examination. Standard handheld video equipment can be used for routine evaluation of the movements of horse and rider.

Stop-action video cameras require the use of a tripod for improved image quality and supplemental video lighting for indoor recording. Equipping the camera with an auto-focusing, auto-zoom telephoto lens allows high-quality, whole-body imaging as well as close-up capability with a minimum of camera manipulation. Although the image quality is superior with ¾-inch video taping equipment, a ½-inch VHS format, portable video recorder (VCR) is recommended. The ½-inch VHS format is the most common type of video equipment found in the United States. Unfortunately, incompatibility with video tapes made for standard NTCS video monitoring devices in the United States makes it difficult to send video recordings to other countries, despite the widespread use of the ½-inch VHS video format throughout the world. Video "frame grabbing" hardware is also available for transmitting video images to computers for storage and for slide or print-making capability.

Treadmill Video Gait Analysis

The major advantage of treadmill lameness evaluations is the stationary position of the horse relative to the observer. The horse's gait can also be visualized from all angles and at a variety of speeds (Fig. 2). Abnormal or asymmetrical movements due to lameness are much more easily visualized because of the consistent, repetitive nature of treadmill exercise at a constant speed over the flat treadmill surface. Specific indications for treadmill video gait analysis include lameness not accentuated by flexion tests, vague or multiple lamenesses, and lameness that is evident only at high speed. The major disadvantage of treadmill gait analysis is that the motion of the horse during turns cannot be evaluated. In addition, treadmill evaluations should not be undertaken to judge the suitability of a normal horse's gait for racing or competitive showing. Although recent studies have indicated that steady-state exercise on a treadmill in trained horses is mechanically equivalent to exercise on the ground, horses will often increase the stride frequency and shorten their stride length until they become accustomed to the treadmill.

Following a suitable warm-up period, routine gait analysis for racehorses and sport horses includes video recording of the horse's motion from the front, the rear, and the side while the horse is moving at the walk, trot, and gallop. Standardbred racehorses are observed at the walk, slow and fast pace, or slow and fast trot in full racing gear. Most treadmills used for clinical evaluations are capable of velocities in excess of $14 \text{ m} \cdot \text{s}^{-1}$ (less than 2 minutes per mile), allowing visualization of the horse's gait up to racing speed. The recording of each gait from each angle begins with a whole-horse perspective; then the field of view is narrowed to evaluate distal limbs and finally hoof orientation as it contacts the tread surface (Fig. 3). A microphone mounted on the video camera records the sounds of the horse working on the treadmill.

Treadmill lameness evaluations are performed primarily at the trot or pace because of the symmetrical nature of these gaits. Although horses may have an inherent asymmetrical gait, most horses moving at the trot or pace will exhibit symmetrical side-to-side oscillations when observed from the front or rear. When observed from the side, most sound horses will have a relatively flat motion of the torso with minimal forward or backward oscillation of the spine. The pattern of sound generated by the sequence of the horse's feet contacting the tread surface is equally important in lameness diagnosis. The symmetrical limb movement of the trot and pace results in a distinctive two-beat sound generated by the ipsilateral or contralateral front and hind hooves contacting the tread surface at nearly the same time. Lameness is suspected if asymmetrical motion is observed from the front, rear, or

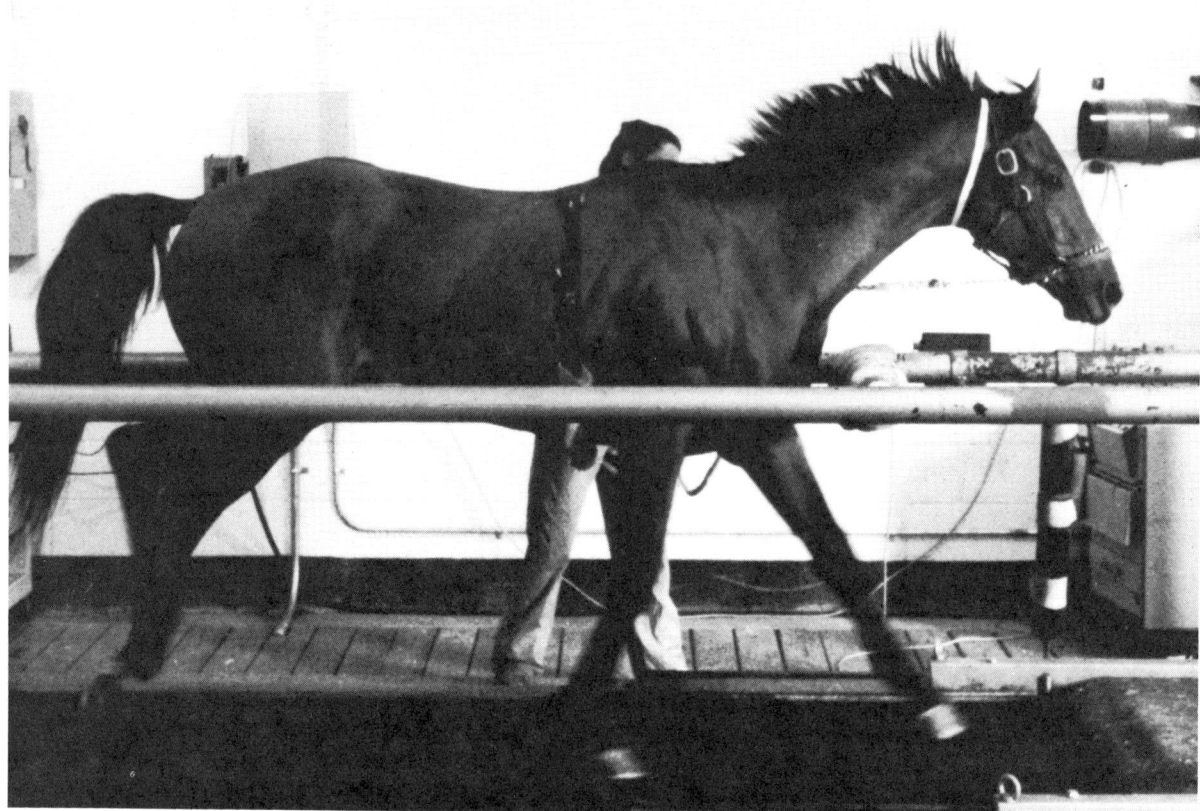

Figure 2. Side view of a horse cantering on the high-speed treadmill.

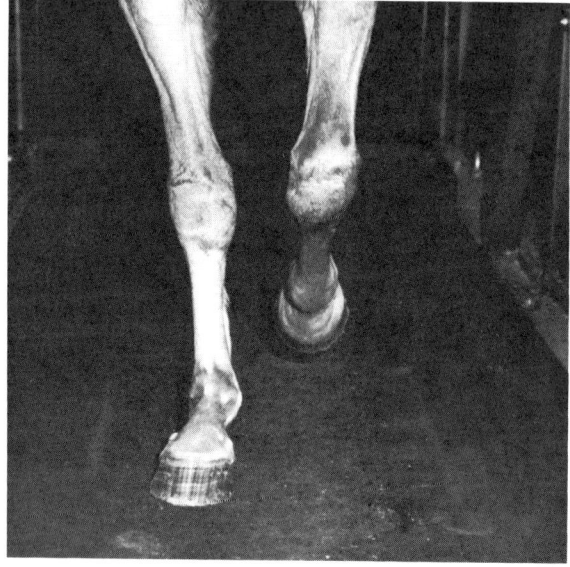

Figure 3. Orientation of the hoof as it strikes the tread surface. Note the obvious imbalance resulting in the outside surface of the hoof contacting the tread before the inside surface. This imbalance results in abnormal forces transmitted up the leg and predisposes to musculoskeletal injury.

side or if asymmetrical sounds of the hooves contacting the tread surface are detected.

Localization of the lameness to the forelimbs or hind limbs is the next step in the treadmill gait analysis. Primary forelimb lameness generally results in asymmetrical side-to-side motion of the front end of the horse, identifiable when the horse is observed from the front or rear at the trot or the pace. Forelimb lameness in an animal viewed from the side may appear as an apparent downward motion of the head and neck when the normal forelimb contacts the tread surface, accompanied by a shortened anterior stride of the lame forelimb. Primary hind limb lameness observed from the rear also results in an asymmetrical side-to-side motion at the trot or the pace. However, in contrast to forelimb lameness, hind limb lameness observed from the side of the horse allows identification of a rocking motion from back to front. Asymmetrical movements of the pelvis associated with hind limb lameness are also easier to detect when the horse is observed from the side. A reference marker placed above the level of the pelvis on the side of the treadmill opposite the observer can be used to compare differences in the movement of the pelvis of the lame versus the normal limb. In the normal horse, the pelvis reaches the highest point in the midstance portion of each half of the stride cycle, when the limb is directly under the horse's pelvis, resulting in symmetrical oscillation of the pelvis at the trot or pace. Slow-motion video gait analysis reveals that the apparent "hip hike" associated with hind limb lameness is the result of the pelvis on the lame side of the horse reaching its highest point when the foot on the lame hind limb contacts the tread surface. The upward motion of the pelvis appears to be initiated by a more powerful stride off the normal hind limb.

Once the lameness has been localized to the front or the rear, the evaluation is continued to determine which side of the horse is lame. The lame forelimb can appear stiff relative to the normal limb as a result of reduced joint motion associated with pain during the contact phase of the stride. The differences in joint movement and the redistribution of ground reaction forces alter the horse's motion to produce an asymmetrical downward rotation of the torso, head, and neck away from the lame forelimb and toward the normal limb when the sound forelimb contacts the tread surface. At low velocities the contact time for both limbs remains the same. However, as velocity increases there is a progressive shortening of the anterior phase of the stride and a decrease in the contact time of the lame forelimb relative to the normal limb. These differences disrupt the normal two-beat symmetry of the trotting or pacing gait, causing the horse to load the opposite forelimb sooner in the stride cycle. The asymmetrical movement generally results in a characteristic three-beat gait, depending on the severity of the lameness.

As was the case with forelimb lameness, the lame hind limb also can appear to be stiff relative to the opposite normal limb, resulting in uneven oscillations of the pelvis from side to side such that the pelvis appears to rotate away from the lame hind limb toward the normal limb when the sound foot contacts the tread surface. Contact time as well as the anterior phase of the stride are also reduced relative to the normal limb. In a horse with hind limb lameness, atrophy of the gluteal musculature on the lame side may contribute to the appearance of the pelvis being higher on the normal side. However, careful observation of the horse in motion will generally confirm that the pelvis is still rotating away from the lame hind limb and down onto the normal hind limb. Disruption of the symmetrical two-beat or four-beat gait can also be heard in cases of hind limb lameness.

Observing the position of the horse on the treadmill can be useful in characterizing lameness. Horses with forelimb lameness will usually lean away from the lame forelimb, causing increased tension on the lead rope on the lame side of the horse. This type of action is similar to a Standardbred racehorse being "on a line" at the racetrack. Horses with hind limb lameness will often trot or pace with the normal limb placed more directly beneath the body and the lame hind limb placed to the outside. In exaggerated cases the horse may actually lean on the rail of the treadmill opposite its lame side. Standardbred racehorses with hind limb lameness exhibit similar action on the racetrack, leaning on the shaft of the racebike.

The final step in the treadmill lameness evaluation entails diagnostic regional anesthesia to identify the anatomical site of the lameness. Based on the initial evaluation, a series of selective nerve blocking and intra-articular anesthetic agents is administered. Following each regional anesthetic procedure the horse is returned to the treadmill for evaluation of changes in the severity and location of the lameness. Successful elimination of lameness in one anatomical location may unmask additional lameness elsewhere. Video recordings made before and after regional anesthetic procedures are particularly useful in evaluating changes in the horse's gait in response to the regional anesthesia. Since both forelimb and hind limb lameness can be visualized from the side, only this view is used, to minimize the time necessary to obtain repetitive video recordings. If the severity of the lameness is successfully reduced, radiographs of the anatomical regions isolated by the use of regional anesthesia are taken. Additional diagnostic medical imaging modalities including ultrasonography and scintigraphy are used as needed.

KINETICS

Weight-bearing profiles obtained with instrumented shoes, force plates, and pressure-sensitive mats have been used to measure the forces of interaction between the limb and the ground (Fig. 4). This type of analysis has yielded valuable information relative to the magnitude and distribution of forces during normal locomotion and jumping. Alterations in the weight-bearing profiles and the pattern of redistribution of these forces to the remaining legs have allowed identification of the potential anatomical sites of sec-

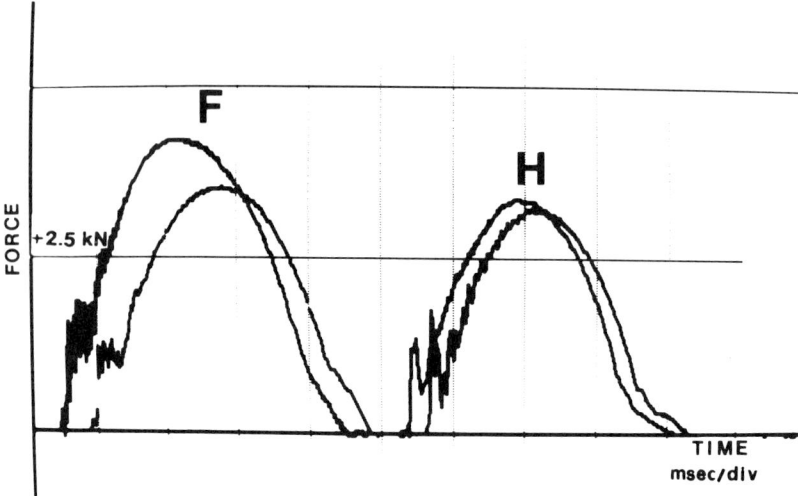

Figure 4. Peak vertical forces for the left and right forelimbs (F) and hind limbs (H) of a horse with a left front carpal lameness. The left forelimb and hind limb are offset to the right. Note the decrease in peak vertical forces in the force trace of the lame left front limb.

ondary lameness as a result of the redistribution of weight-bearing. Measuring weight-bearing profiles and recording the changes in these profiles in response to diagnostic anesthesia can aid in the clinical diagnosis of lameness. These measurements are particularly helpful in difficult cases of proximal front and rear limb lameness. Small improvements in weight-bearing profiles detected with kinetic measurements but not easily detected visually can be significant, due to the limited ability to completely desensitize orthopedic abnormalities in these anatomical locations. Routine clinical application of kinetic measuring systems is limited by equipment expense, complexity of the equipment, the prolonged time necessary to obtain sufficient data for analysis, and the extensive data reduction required to evaluate the results.

Strain gauges can be built into the shoes of the horse to measure vertical (weight-bearing) and horizontal (deceleration and acceleration) forces. Advantages include the ability to acquire data from every foot strike, but the equipment adds weight to the shoes and may therefore alter the characteristics of the stride. Force plates use either strain gauges or the deformation of piezoelectric quartz crystals to make continuous fast-time response measurements of vertical, horizontal, and lateral (side-to-side) forces exerted on the ground as the horse moves over the plate. With this type of equipment the peak vertical forces on each hoof have been determined to be 0.6 body weight at the walk, 1.0 body weight at the trot, and 1.75 body weight at the gallop. The primary disadvantage of the force plate is its small size, which allows only acquisition of data from one forelimb and the ipsilateral hind limb on each pass over the force plate. Force platforms have been used that can record information from foot falls over a length of 4 meters.

Computer-aided acquisition and analysis of data has vastly improved the usefulness of these techniques as research tools. Recent developments in computer modeling of limb function will undoubtedly improve the understanding of both normal and abnormal gaits. However, limited client understanding of this type of quantitative analysis remains an obstacle preventing the widespread use of these techniques for clinical lameness evaluations.

Supplemental Readings

Fredericson, I., Drevemo, S., Dalin, G., Hjerten, G., and Bjorne, K.: The application of high speed cinematography for the quantitative analysis of equine locomotion. Equine Vet. J., *12*:54–59, 1980.

Leach, D. H., and Dagg, A. I.,: A review of research on equine locomotion and biomechanics. Equine Vet. J., *15*:93–102, 1983.

Morris, E. A., and Seeherman, H. J.: Redistribution of ground reaction forces in experimentally induced equine carpal lameness. *In* Robinson, N. E., and Gillespie, J. R. (eds): Equine Exercise Physiology 2. Davis, Calif., ICEEP Publications, 1987, pp. 553–563.

Evaluation of Bone

Howard J. Seeherman, NORTH GRAFTON, MASSACHUSETTS

Lameness due to musculoskeletal injury is by far the most common cause of poor performance in horses. In a recent study, 74 per cent of racehorses evaluated for poor racing performance had significant musculoskeletal problems. Similar results were reported in a number of epidemiological studies evaluating wastage among Thoroughbred racehorses and racetrack breakdown injuries. For this reason, the musculoskeletal examination is a vital component of the comprehensive clinical evaluation of the equine athlete. Because the injury may be subtle or may involve multiple sites, it is often rewarding to supplement conventional lameness and radiographic evaluations with high-speed gait analysis.

Diagnostic medical imaging plays an extremely important role in the evaluation of orthopedic disorders. For the specific evaluation of bones and joints, the combination of radiography, computed tomography (CT), and radionuclide scintigraphy, along with the recent developments in the field of magnetic resonance imaging (MRI), allows visualization of both anatomical structures and physiological characteristics of the equine musculoskeletal system. Bone density and bone mineral content can be evaluated with a number of imaging techniques, including radiography, ultrasonography (US), CT, and single- or dual-photon absorptiometry. Changes in bone parameters in response to training and competition can be evaluated using these imaging parameters. The following is a discussion of the available means of obtaining an accurate diagnosis of subtle bone injury that will often result in poor performance.

All diagnostic evaluations should begin with a physical examination and a traditional lameness examination, including flexion tests. A positive response to flexion indicates the site of a lesion producing localized pain. Localization of the source of pain can be pursued by local anesthesia followed by radiography of the affected area.

RADIOGRAPHY

Radiography has been the traditional method for evaluating equine orthopedic disorders following localization of the site of lameness by physical examination and diagnostic studies under anesthesia. Standard radiographic equipment with various screen–film combinations can be used to evaluate the two-dimensional anatomy of bone. Xeroradiography allows better edge detection but increases the radiation exposure. However, determining the three-dimensional distribution of an abnormality is sometimes difficult, requiring multiple radiographic views. In addition, physiological activity such as the rate of bone remodeling can only be inferred from a series of radiographic evaluations repeated over an extended period of time. Lack of identifiable radiographic abnormalities or inability to localize a vague or multiple-site lameness is an indication for scintigraphic imaging.

RADIONUCLIDE SCINTIGRAPHY

Scintigraphy has proved to be an extremely important diagnostic method for imaging orthopedic lesions. Scintigraphy provides both anatomical and physiological information based on the distribution and intensity of uptake of a radiopharmaceutical. Indications for scintigraphic analysis of the musculoskeletal system include the following:

1. evaluation of specific anatomical locations in horses in which the site of the lameness has been determined but conventional radiography has not revealed a lesion;
2. survey of multiple locations when the location of the lameness cannot be determined with conventional methods;
3. imaging the axial skeleton and proximal limbs when fractures or osteoarthritis are suspected (scintigraphy has the advantage of not requiring general anesthesia);
4. locating developing orthopedic disease so that preventive measures can be instituted;
5. following the time course of healing after an orthopedic injury or surgical intervention, in order to establish a prognosis.

Orthopedic imaging is based on detection of a radiolabeled phosphate compound in soft tissue and bone. Intravenous injection of technetium phosphate compounds (MDP = technetium 99m methylene bisphosphonate, HDP = technetium 99m hydroxymethylene bisphosphonate) results in uptake by the mineral matrix of bone after the radiopharmaceutical passes through the vascular and extravascular fluid compartments. Blood flow and extraction efficiency (binding) are the two major factors that determine the degree of uptake of radiopharmaceutical in bone. The extraction efficiency is related to the amount of bone mineral turnover in the course of bone resorption or new bone formation. Radiation emitted by the radiopharmaceutical is detected with a gamma camera that is interfaced to a microdot imager for making hard copy images and to a dedicated computer system for storage and image analysis. Common orthopedic conditions associated with inflammation and increased bone remodeling such as infection, arthritis, and fractures appear as areas of increased activity on the scan. A notable exception is osteochondrosis dissecans (OCD). Lesions of OCD do not accumulate the radiolabeled phosphate compound unless there is reactive new bone formation. The same skeletal imaging radiopharmaceuticals are also taken up by damaged muscle tissue. The binding site for the radiopharmaceutical in muscle is unclear but may be related to the calcium release that occurs in damaged muscle or to binding to exposed protein macromolecules with calcium binding sites.

SCINTIGRAPHIC IDENTIFICATION OF NONADAPTIVE EXERCISE-INDUCED BONE REMODELING

Scintigraphic evaluation of a large number of horses has identified specific anatomical locations that may exhibit dramatic focal uptake of radiopharmaceutical at sites associated with lameness. Radiographs are often normal. The increased scintigraphic activity has been attributed to nonadaptive bone remodeling in response to exercise. Most horses with this condition have acute or chronic single-limb lameness. If bilateral or multiple regions are affected, the gradual onset of poor performance may occur without obvious lameness. This condition occurs most commonly in young Thoroughbred and Standardbred racehorses and may have an incidence as high as 50 per cent.

Lameness examination coupled with diagnostic anesthesia will often locate the anatomical regions involved. Affected horses usually exhibit pain on distal limb flexion or palpation of the diaphyseal region of affected long bones. Intra-articular anesthesia often eliminates the positive response to distal limb flexion and the associated lameness. When multiple sites are involved, the origin of the lameness may shift as each affected anatomical region is desensitized, making the lameness workup more complex.

The most common sites of increased focal radiopharmaceutical uptake are the distal third metacarpal and metatarsal epiphysis and the radial fossa of the third carpal bone (Fig. 1). Other common sites include the proximal and distal sesamoids and the third phalanx. Less commonly, the distal femur and proximal humerus may show increased focal uptake.

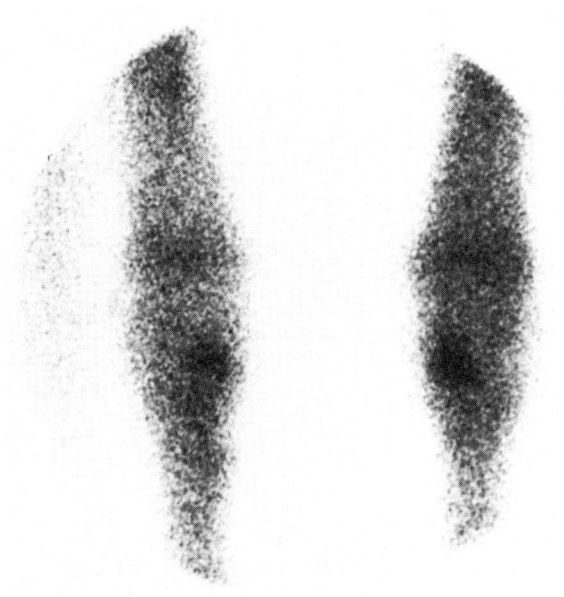

Figure 1. Anterioposterior scintigraph of the carpi of a 3-year-old Thoroughbred racehorse. Note bilateral focal uptake of radiopharmaceutical in the area of the radial fossa of the third carpal bones. Radiography of this area showed changes consistent with sclerosis.

Bone damage and bone remodeling are generally in equilibrium during training and racing, resulting in normal adaptation of bone density and bone architecture to exercise. An imbalance between these two processes can alter this adaptive response, resulting in bone damage, pain, and lameness. The increased uptake of radiopharmaceutical in these horses appears to result from excessive loading during exercise. The excessive loading may be attributable to intrinsic factors, such as poor foot and limb conformation, or to extrinsic factors, such as inappropriate training, a rigorous competition schedule, or abnormal footing. Abnormal excessive remodeling may result in decreased bone density or, alternatively, increased bone density (sclerosis) and increased bone stiffness.

The anatomical locations of nonadaptive exercise-induced bone remodeling correspond to common locations for fractures in racehorses. Stress fractures in Thoroughbred racehorses occur in areas of increased bone remodeling in the diaphysis of the third metacarpal bone (Fig. 2). Condylar fractures of the distal aspect of the third metacarpal and metatarsal bones, sesamoid fractures, and transverse and sagittal slab fractures of the radial fossa of the third carpal bone

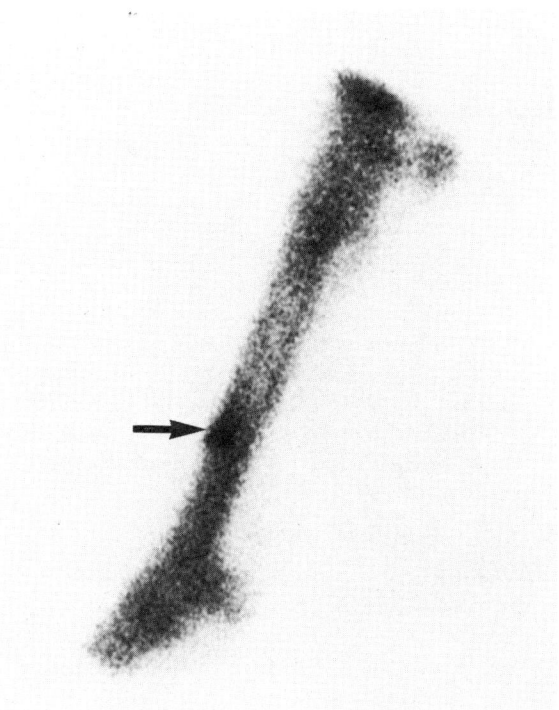 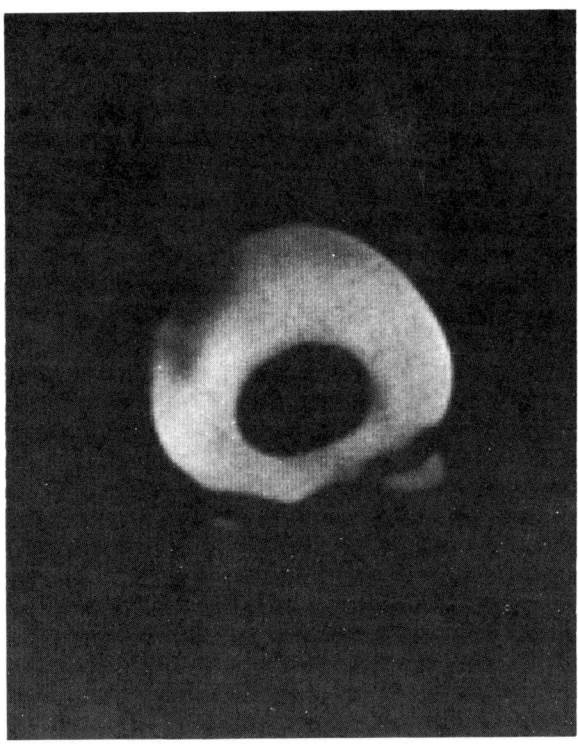

Figure 2. (a) Lateral scintigraph of the third metacarpal bone of a Thoroughbred racehorse showing focal increased uptake of radioisotope in the dorsal cortex due to active bone remodeling consistent with nonadaptive exercise-induced remodeling. (b) CT scan of the same third metacarpal bone of a Thoroughbred racehorse showing a focal area of decreased density due to active bone remodeling.

occur in corresponding areas of nonadaptive exercise-induced bone remodeling. Lateral and medial wing fractures of the third phalanx also occur in areas of increased activity. These common racetrack fractures may be occurring in areas that are structurally weakened by nonadaptive bone remodeling.

A 2- to 3-month period of reduced exercise will usually resolve the lameness associated with this condition and repeat scintigrams are usually within normal limits. Chronic diaphyseal stress fractures of the third metacarpal bone may require cortical osteostixis (cortical drilling) to resolve the problem. Adjunctive therapy such as intra-articular polysulfated glycosaminoglycans and intra-articular hyaluronan (see p. 128) can be used when articulations are involved. Oral isoxuprine can be administered on the theoretical basis that increased peripheral blood flow will aid remodeling. Rest is contraindicated unless lameness is severe, because the rest-induced reduction in bone remodeling will result in a recurrence of the condition as soon as exercise is resumed. Proper foot balance is maintained to limit abnormal forces on bones and joints. Since these areas of nonadaptive exercise-induced bone remodeling resolve with a period of controlled exercise, it is possible that early detection of the condition may prevent subsequent injuries that might occur with continued racing.

Scintigraphic Identification of Axial Skeletal and Proximal Limb Lameness

Because of the difficulty of diagnostic regional anesthesia, the diagnosis of lameness originating in the proximal limb or axial skeleton is often greatly facilitated by the use of nuclear imaging. Scintigraphy yields detailed images with which to evaluate the pelvis and proximal limbs for suspected fractures and subluxation, eliminating the need for general anesthesia to obtain diagnostic radiographs. Areas of increased uptake of radiopharmaceutical have been identified in the distal femur, proximal tibia, proximal humerus, and distal scapula that appear normal on radiographic evaluation. Based on the scintigraphic appearance, the etiology of the increased activity is likely to be similar to that of nonadaptive exercise-induced bone remodeling in the distal limbs or, alternatively, the increased activity may result from compression fractures or incomplete fractures of the subchondral or metaphyseal cancellous bone. These types of fractures may not be apparent on radiographs because of insufficient demineralization of the affected bone or because of the limited number of views that can be taken of proximal limbs.

Horses with vague signs of lameness may have nonspecific back pain. Scintigraphic evaluation of these animals reveals active remodeling of bone in the midlumbar region. Radiographs may reveal lytic and proliferative bone causing the dorsal spinous processes to impinge on one another. This type of disorder is observed primarily in jumping horses. Thoroughbred racehorses with back pain have also been observed with the same problem.

SCINTIGRAPHIC IDENTIFICATION OF AVULSION OF SOFT TISSUE ATTACHMENTS TO BONE

Lameness associated with damage in the region of soft tissue attachments to bone can also be localized with scintigraphy. Elimination of the lameness by regional anesthesia or local infiltration with anesthetic agents may be difficult because of inaccessibility of the site or variations in the nerve supply to the region. Areas of increased uptake of radiopharmaceutical are commonly observed at the origin of the suspensory ligament (the proximal palmar metacarpal bone), the origin of the long plantar ligament (plantar aspect of the calcaneus), the insertion of the cruciate ligaments (proximal tibia), the insertion of the peroneus tertius muscle (dorsal surface of the third metatarsal bone), and the insertions of the distal sesamoidean ligaments (palmar or plantar aspect of the first phalanx). Increased uptake of radiopharmaceutical in the proximal sesamoid bones may also be due to disruption of the insertion of the suspensory ligament or the origin of the distal sesamoidean ligaments. Radiographically, these regions often appear normal. However, in some cases multiple views demonstrate new periosteal bone associated with tearing of Sharpey's fiber attachment to the bone or avulsion fractures.

SCINTIGRAPHIC DIAGNOSIS OF MUSCLE DISORDERS CAUSING OBSCURE LAMENESS

Exercise-induced muscle damage may be difficult to diagnose because some horses will not exhibit signs of muscle stiffness, muscle hardness may not be palpable, and there may be no myoglobinuria. The serum creatine kinase (CK) concentration generally peaks 6 hours after exercise, then rapidly decreases to preexercise levels. It is therefore the best indicator of acute muscle damage. Concentrations in the range of 1,000 to 30,000 IU per L obtained 6 to 8 hours after training or racing are consistent with localized exercise-induced muscle damage. Concentrations of serum CK in excess of 50,000 to 200,000 IU per L are more indicative of generalized muscle disorders. The AST/SGOT concentrations peak 24 to 48 hours after exercise and may remain elevated for a week following the initial muscle damage. The radiopharmaceutical used to image bone disorders is also taken up by acutely injured muscle, enabling localization of damaged muscles within 24 to 48 hours of injury (Fig. 3). Uptake abates after this time, indicating that cells are no longer dying. The muscle groups most commonly damaged during intense exercise appear to be the gluteals, semimembranosus, semitendinosus, and the quadriceps femoris. Bilaterally symmetrical uptake of the radiopharmaceutical is the most common finding; however, unilateral distribution has also been described.

SCINTIGRAPHY OF FRACTURES

When careful palpation and flexion cannot identify the source of the lameness in quite lame horses, scintigraphy is extremely valuable for locating fractures. Diagnostic evaluation under regional anesthesia is usually contraindicated because the fracture may destabilize while the horse is exercising on a partially desensitized limb. Survey radiographs can be used to locate the fracture if there is displacement or sufficient demineralization of the fracture site to produce a visible defect in the bone. However, nondis-

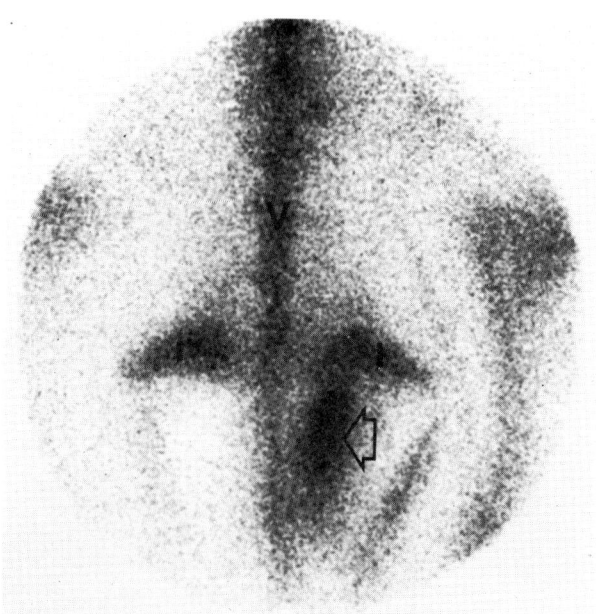

Figure 3. Scintigraphic image of the pelvis of a horse showing focal uptake of radioisotope by the left gluteal muscle *(arrow)*. The camera was positioned over the back of the horse and aimed in an anteroventral direction. Other areas of uptake are the vertebral column and the tuber ischii.

placed fractures, fractures associated with growth plates, or fractures that have not demineralized adequately may be difficult to visualize on survey radiographs. Sufficient bone remodeling occurs within 48 hours of the injury to cause an increased uptake of radiopharmaceutical. Nondisplaced fractures that initially may be difficult to visualize with radiography but can be identified with scintigraphy include maleolar fractures of the distal tibia, fractures of the tibial tuberosity, and sagittal fractures of proximal first phalanx, distal third metacarpal, and metatarsal bones. Scintigraphy is particularly useful for early diagnosis of wing fractures of the third phalanx, which may require up to 2 weeks to demineralize sufficiently to be visible on radiographs. Nondisplaced middiaphyseal fractures have also been diagnosed with scintigraphy before they produced radiographic abnormalities.

COMPUTED TOMOGRAPHY

Cross-sectional imaging CT provides a very accurate, three-dimensional image of bone. Since most CT scanners are designed for horizontal data acquisition, images must be obtained with the horse in lateral recumbency and under general anesthesia. This requires a specially designed gantry and table to hold the horse and control its position in the scanner (Fig. 4). Alternatively, the horse can be imaged while being supported on a padded movable forklift palette. CT in horses is limited by the requirement for lateral recumbency under general anesthesia and by the diameter of the scanner, which allows only images of the limbs and head to be made. However, CT can be used to reconstruct the three-dimensional orientation of bone fractures or bone cysts prior to surgery. This type of imaging has been used in conjunction with scintigraphy to characterize the physiological activity and three-dimensional configuration of stress fractures in the third metacarpal bone in Thoroughbred racehorses (see Fig. 2b). Cross-sectional imaging has also been used to locate the optimal orientation of the cortical drill holes used in the surgical correction of chronic stress fractures. Adequate distal limb images can be obtained in a reasonable amount of time (approximately 45 minutes) to allow surgical correction of the abnormality under the same anesthesia.

MAGNETIC RESONANCE IMAGING

Three-dimensional MRI of structure and function has proved valuable in human medicine. MRI is based on the absorption of radio-frequency energy by the magnetic moments of atomic nuclei in tissue placed in a strong magnetic field. In mammalian tissue, the most abundant nuclei are the protons of hydrogen in water and fat. Tissue of different atomic structure as well as normal versus pathological tissue differ in their response to applied magnetic fields. Since MRI images are based on events occurring at the molecular level, these images provide both the anatomical information of CT and the physiological information of scintigraphy without the det-

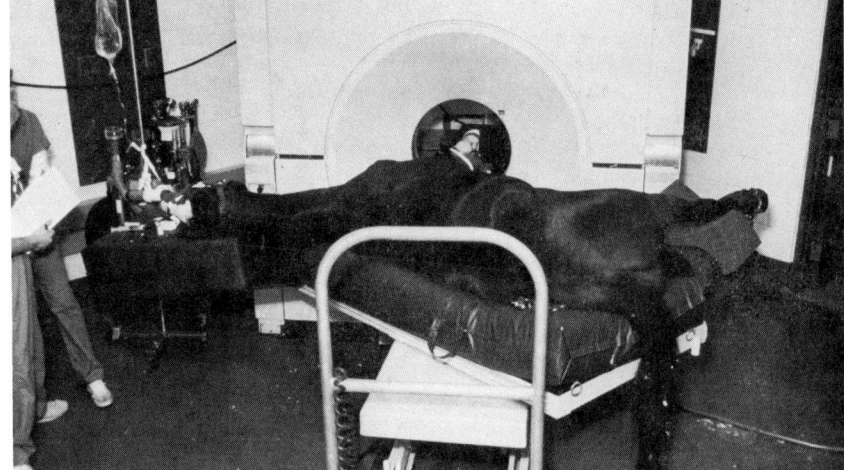

Figure 4. A CT scanner being used to image a horse's leg.

rimental effects of ionizing radiation. Although imaging of the central nervous system is the primary use of MRI, imaging of the musculoskeletal system may also yield valuable information. While it is true that MRI does not show cortical bone, other components of the musculoskeletal system (including cancellous bone) image very well. MRI is especially useful for orthopedic soft tissue imaging because fat, fibrous tissue, muscles, articular cartilage, nerves, and vessels have very different imaging characteristics, resulting in excellent soft tissue image contrast. For this reason MRI has become a noninvasive alternative to diagnostic arthroscopy for detecting intra-articular pathology. The potential applications of this imaging modality in horses are undefined; limitations include cost, physical design of the imaging system, and the prolonged imaging times necessary with currently available scanners. Small, flexible surface coils that conform to the area imaged may be available in the future for investigation of musculoskeletal injury.

NONINVASIVE BONE DENSITOMETRY

There are a number of noninvasive methods for determining bone density. The most common techniques are single-photon absorptiometry, dual-photon absorptiometry, monoenergetic x-ray densitometry, and dual-energy projection radiography. Single- and dual-photon absorptiometry is based on detecting the differential attenuation of a narrow beam of photons from either a monoenergetic or bienergetic radionuclide source using a scintillation detector system. Single-photon absorptiometry is suited for evaluating bone in regions without significant overlying soft tissue structures. Dual-photon absorptiometry takes into account the differential attenuation of the photon beam by soft tissue versus bone at the two photon energy levels and is therefore less affected by surrounding soft tissue. The major disadvantages of these two techniques are long scan times, short half-life of the radionuclide source, and Nuclear Regulatory Commission licensing for access to the radionuclide. Monoenergetic x-ray densitometry and dual-energy projection radiography eliminate most of these disadvantages. However, the cost and availability of the equipment may be prohibitive for routine use.

Noninvasive bone densitometry in horses is currently limited to research on the effects of training on bone density and bone strength. Ultimately, noninvasive bone densitometry will be used to detect alterations in bone properties in response to exercise, with the goal of avoiding traumatic failure. Widespread use of noninvasive bone densitometry awaits the development of newer techniques that can be used reliably in the field on large numbers of horses.

Supplemental Readings

Barbee, D. D., and Allen, J. R.: Computed tomography in the horse: General principles and clinical applications. *In:* Proceedings of the 32nd Annual Convention of the American Association of Equine Practitioners, 1986, p. 483.

Koblick, P. D., Hornof, W. J., and Seeherman, H. J.: Scintigraphic appearance of stress-induced trauma of dorsal cortex of the third metacarpal bone in racing Thoroughbred horses: 121 cases (1978–1986). J. Am. Vet. Med. Assoc., 192:390, 1988.

Lamb, C. R., and Koblick, P. D.: Scintigraphic evaluation of skeletal disease and its application to the horse. Vet. Radiol., 29:16, 1988.

Evaluation of Tendons and Ligaments

Virginia B. Reef, KENNETT SQUARE, PENNSYLVANIA

Tendon and ligament injuries are common causes of lost training time, lost racing time, and career changes in horses. They are most common in horses performing at high intensity, such as horses that race on the flat (Thoroughbred, Standardbred, Arabian, Quarter Horse), horses that race over fences, upper level combined training horses, cutting horses, barrel racers, and polo ponies. These injuries occur less frequently in dressage horses, jumpers, hunters, endurance horses, driving horses, pleasure horses, and other types of show or competition horses. The injury most frequently occurs during a fast work or race; however, clinical signs often are not apparent for 24 to 48 hours or more.

The most common clinical sign in horses with

flexor tendon or ligament injuries is swelling of the affected tendon or ligament and the surrounding soft tissue structures. Local heat and sensitivity of the area on deep palpation are also frequently noted. Lameness occurs in approximately 50 per cent of the horses examined at our hospital with flexor tendon or ligament injuries. Aggressive therapy for the flexor tendon or ligament injury often results in dramatic improvement in the clinical signs in a few days. Horses with severe injuries to the flexor tendons or ligaments may have abnormal angulations of the limb such as a dropped fetlock or subluxation of the pastern. Diagnostic ultrasonography (US) accurately demonstrates damage to the tendinous or ligamentous structures and is indicated in all horses with swelling or thickening of a tendinous or ligamentous structure. If lameness is detected in the absence of tendon or ligament swelling, a complete lameness examination including diagnostic nerve blocks, if appropriate, and radiographic evaluation may be indicated before US is performed. Lameness in the absence of tendinous or ligamentous swelling is infrequently associated with tendon or ligament damage.

ULTRASONOGRAPHY

A thorough knowledge of the anatomy of the structures under investigation and their interrelationships is crucial for the accurate interpretation of the sonogram. Patient preparation is also important in obtaining a quality US image. The hair over the structures to be scanned should be clipped closely with a No. 40 clipper bade and the skin cleaned. Shaving the hair over the affected structures may be necessary for optimal image quality. After the skin has been cleaned, US transmission gel is applied liberally to achieve an air-free interface between the transducer and the skin surface. A high-frequency transducer with a fluid offset, either hand-held or built into the transducer, is necessary for optimal imaging of the structures immediately beneath the skin surface. Without this hand-held or built-in offset, a transducer artifact will appear superimposed on the structure immediately beneath the skin surface. A 7.5-MHz transducer is ideal for obtaining quality images of the flexor tendons or ligaments in the horse and allows visualization of structures up to 4 or 5 cm from the skin surface. Optimal images are obtained with the transducer held perpendicular to the structures being evaluated. This maximizes the amount of reflected ultrasound from these structures. The tendons and ligaments should be scanned in two mutually perpendicular planes from their origin to insertion. The limb is scanned transversely initially (the scan plane perpendicular to the structure's long axis). The tendon or ligament is displayed in its short-axis cross-section and the location of the lesion can easily be visualized. The cross-sectional area of the lesion and tendon can be measured, or mutually perpendicular diameter measurements of the lesion and tendon can be made. The sagittal imaging plane (the scan plane parallel to the long axis of the structure) can then be used to evaluate the pattern of fiber alignment. The extent of injury can be measured from the point of the accessory carpal bone, point of the hock, or any other permanent reference point. The exact length of the lesion as well as the lesion's cross-sectional area and the per centage of the tendon or ligament affected can provide important prognostic information. Reevaluation of the tendon or ligament as it heals and reassessing the tendon and lesion cross-sectional area at the precise site of the previous measurement are also useful in evaluation of tendon and ligament healing. The limb can also be divided into zones, each zone measuring approximately 8 cm in length. The forelimb is divided into three major zones, beginning from just below the accessory carpal bone and ending at the fetlock joint. Each zone is divided into two parts, A and B. The zones are labeled 1A and 1B, 2A and 2B, and 3A and 3B. An additional zone, 3C, has been used to describe the portion of the flexor tendons as they pass over the fetlock joint region. The hind limb can be similarly divided into zones 1A and 1B, 2A and 2B, 3A and 3B, and 4A and 4B from the distal portion of the hock to the fetlock joint.

ULTRASONICALLY DETECTED ABNORMALITIES OF THE FLEXOR TENDONS OR LIGAMENTS

An anechoic core lesion or hole is the most common lesion visualized on sonograms of the flexor tendons or ligaments (Fig. 1). This lesion is most frequently located in the central portion of the affected structure, but any portion of the tendon or ligament may be involved. In most horses only one area of tendon or ligament injury is seen, but multiple lesions are occasionally detected. The anechoic core lesions represent an acute area of fiber tearing with hemorrhage and fluid accumulation. The core lesion usually remains anechoic for the first few weeks and then becomes hypoechoic as graulation tissue and immature fibrous tissue repair the injury. As the healing progresses and the fibrous tissue matures, the echogenicity of the core approaches

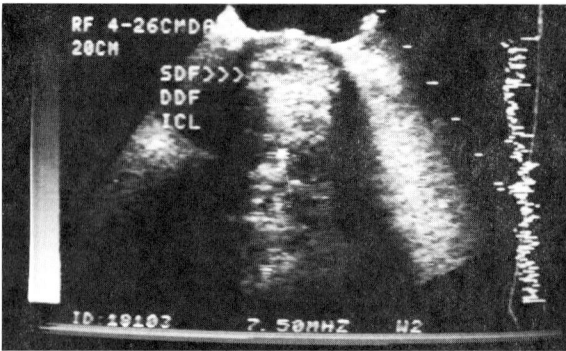 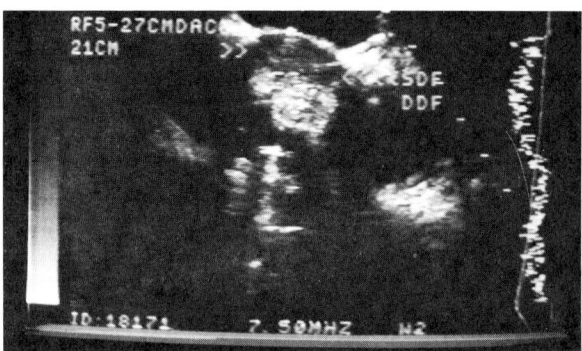

Figure 1. Transverse (short-axis) sonogram obtained from a 10-year-old Trakehner stallion (advanced combined training horse) with an acute core lesion sustained 4 days earlier during a competition. *Arrows* point to the core lesion in the medial and central portion of the tendon. The core lesion was visible from 4 to 26 cm distal to the accessory carpal bone in the right foreleg. This image was obtained at 20 cm distal to the accessory carpal bone. The lesion measured 0.4 sq cm and the tendon measured 1.8 sq cm at this location. SDF, superficial digital flexor tendon; DDF, deep digital flexor tendon; ICL, inferior check ligament.

Figure 2. Transverse (short-axis) sonogram of a 4-year-old Standardbred colt with an acute diffuse tendon injury. *Arrows* point to the diffuse injury in the palmar and lateral portion of the superficial digital flexor tendon (SDF) in the right foreleg. This lesion was visible from 5 to 27 cm distal to the accessory carpal bone; this image was obtained at 21 cm. The affected portion of the tendon measured 1.3 sq cm and the entire tendon measured 1.7 cm at this location. DDF, deep digital flexor tendon.

the echogenicity of the normal tendinous or ligamentous tissue. The core lesion often remains quite distinct from the uninjured area during the healing process. As the lesion heals the linearity of the lesion will gradually improve, returning to a more normal parallel fiber alignment. Occasionally calcification may occur in a chronic tendon or ligament injury. Calcification appears as a bright, hyperechoic area casting an acoustic shadow. The acoustic shadow is caused by the relatively high acoustic impedance of bone compared to soft tissue, reflecting the majority of the ultrasound beam.

In some horses a discrete core lesion cannot be visualized even in the acute stage of the injury. In these horses the tendon or ligament appears swollen and has a heterogeneous echogenicity consistent with multifocal injury and scattered areas of fiber disruption (Fig. 2). Other types of tendon or ligament injury such as splits or cleft-type injuries separating one portion of the tendon or ligament from another occur infrequently and are most commonly seen in the suspensory ligament. Complete disruption of a tendinous or ligamentous structure occurs infrequently. The severity of the injury is characterized by the type of lesion seen, the size or cross-sectional area of the lesion, the extent or length of the lesion, and the per centage of the structure affected. The echogenicity of the lesion is related to the age and severity of the injury. More severe injuries involve a large per centage of the structure in its cross-sectional area and extend for most of the length of the structure from origin to insertion. In some horses no tendinous or ligamentous damage will be detected, only an anechoic or hypoechoic space in the soft tissues (peritendinitis) or flexor tendon sheath (tenosynovitis).

FREQUENCY OF TENDON OR LIGAMENT INJURIES

Bowed tendons are the most common flexor tendon or ligamentous injuries seen in our hospital, both in Thoroughbred and Standardbred racehorses and in all other horses performing at speed. Injuries to the superficial digital flexor tendon are most common in the Thoroughbred racehorse, whereas suspensory ligament injuries are more common in the Standardbred racehorse. Injuries are most common in the left forelimb in the Thoroughbred and Standardbred racehorses, whereas they occur with equal frequency in both forelimbs in horses that race over fences, combined training horses, jumpers, and other types of performance horses. Most flexor tendon and ligament injuries occur in the forelimb; however, suspensory ligament injuries occur frequently in the hind limb of Standardbred racehorses.

THERAPY

Conservative treatment includes stall rest with hand walking, cold water hydrotheraphy, application of ice and poultices, and anti-inflammatory drugs (see p. 146). A controlled exercise program of walking and jogging for progressively longer times can often be initiated 2 to 3 months after injury. US reevaluation of tendon healing guides the progression of the controlled exercise program. Tendon splitting surgery is indicated in acute core lesions to drain the central hematoma and may improve tendon healing. Superior check ligament desmotomies are indicated for the treatment of bowed tendons, effectively lengthening the tendon and possibly reducing tendon strain. The initial US examination results can be used to determine the best treatment for the tendon or ligament injury.

PROGNOSIS

The prognosis for a horse with a tendon or ligament injury to return successfully to work varies with the severity of the original injury, the type of work performed by the horse, and the breed of the horse. The majority of Standardbred or Thoroughbred racehorses with tendon or ligament injuries are able to return successfully to racing if given adequate time for tendon healing. Horses with larger tears and extensive injuries that involve the majority of the length of the affected tendon or ligament are more likely to return to performance at a lower level and are more likely to have a recurrence of the injury. Thoroughbred racehorses with bilateral bowed tendons are less likely to return to racing successfully than those with unilateral tendon injuries, whereas there is no difference in the prognosis for Standardbred racehorses, horses that race over fences, or horses that perform at lower levels of competition with bilateral bowed tendons.

Supplemental Readings

Genovese, R. L., Rantanen, N. W., Hauser, M.L., and Simpson, B. S.: Diagnostic ultrasonography of equine limbs. Vet. Clin. North Am. (Equine Pract.), 2:145, 1986.

Genovese, R. L., Rantanen, N. W., and Simpson, B. S.: The use of ultrasonography in the diagnosis and management of injuries of the equine limb. Compend. Cont. Educ. Pract. Vet., 9:945, 1987.

Hauser, M. L., and Rantanen, N. W.: Ultrasound appearance of the palmar metacarpal soft tissues of the horse. J. Equine Vet. Sci., 3:19, 1983.

Hauser, M. L., Rantanen, N. W., and Genovese, R. L.: Suspensory desmitis: Diagnosis using real-time ultrasound imaging. J. Equine Vet. Sci., 4:258, 1984.

Pharr, J. W., and Nyland, T. G.: Ultrasonography of the equine palmar metacarpal soft tissues. Vet. Radiol., 22:265, 1984.

Evaluation of Muscle

Stephanie J. Valberg, DAVIS, CALIFORNIA

CLINICAL EVALUATION OF SKELETAL MUSCLE

Approximately 50 per cent of horses suffer from musculoskeletal disorders at some point in the racing season. About 10 per cent of these disorders are due to muscular problems. Muscle disorders that may affect performance include trauma, exertional myopathies, inflammation following intramuscular injections, atrophy, myotonia, and hyperkalemic periodic paralysis. In addition, many young horses never race due to lack of ability, and a proportion of these losses may be due to insufficient training adaptations in skeletal muscle. A number of horses also develop, at some point in their career, premature signs of fatigue during exercise that may be of muscular origin.

Evaluation of muscle disorders includes a lameness examination as well as careful visual inspection of the entire musculature with the horse standing perfectly square. The contralateral muscles of each limb should be palpated and compared for signs of pain, inflammation, and atrophy. Ancillary diagnostic aids for evaluating areas of inflammation include serum aspartate transaminase and creatine kinase (CK) determinations, thermography, and ultrasonography. Electromyography of neck, trunk, and limb muscles provides supplemental information about the extent of muscle atrophy, the sarcolemmal conductance (which may be abnormal in myotonia and hyperkalemic periodic paralysis), and the extent of focal necrosis in exertional myopathies. Percutaneous needle biopsies of skeletal muscle can also aid in establishing a definitive diagnosis. A more detailed description of muscle diseases in the horse is provided elsewhere in the text (see pp. 113 and 571). Evaluation of potential skeletal muscle limitations to performance requires muscle biopsies as well as exercise tolerance testing.

MUSCLE BIOPSY

The percutaneous muscle biopsy technique greatly facilitates the routine evaluation of skeletal muscle in performance horses. Biopsy specimens from standardized sites in the gluteus medius and semitendinosus muscle are commonly examined. Standardization is necessary because muscle fiber compositions vary along the length and depth of a muscle. After a ¼-inch incision is made through a local skin block, muscle tissue is obtained using a 5-mm outer diameter biopsy needle. Samples for biochemical analyses are frozen immediately in liquid nitrogen, whereas samples for histochemical analysis are frozen in freon or isopentane suspended in liquid nitrogen. Muscle biopsies can be analyzed for their contractile, metabolic, and morphometric properties.

CONTRACTILE PROPERTIES

The per centage of fast and slow twitch muscle fibers in a biopsy specimen (muscle fiber composition) can be determined using histochemical stains for myosin adenosine triphosphatase (ATPase) activity. Muscle fibers are classified as either slow twitch (type I fibers) or fast twitch (type IIA and IIB fibers). In some species type IIA fibers have been found to contract faster than type IIB fibers, but this has not been investigated in the horse. The major propulsive muscles in the horse have a high per centage of fast twitch fibers. In general, breeds that perform over short distances at speed (Quarter Horses and Thoroughbreds) have over 90 per cent fast twitch fibers (largely type IIB), whereas endurance breeds such as Arabians have about 75 per cent fast twitch fibers. There are wide variations in the muscle fiber composition of individuals within breeds, and considerable overlap exists between breeds. When the breed differences in muscle fiber composition were first discovered, it was hoped that fiber composition would be an indicator of potential racing speed. However, because a number of factors are important to performance, a single factor such as fiber composition does not stand alone as a predictor of performance.

The effect of training on contractile properties of muscle remains controversial. Only small changes in the ratio of slow to fast twitch fibers seem to occur with training in the horse. In racehorses that undergo several months of high-intensity training, the proportion of fast twitch type IIA fibers in muscle appears to increase and that of type IIB fibers decreases. It is not clear whether these changes actually affect the speed of muscle contraction.

METABOLIC PROPERTIES

The oxidative capacity of muscle can be quantitatively determined by measuring the activity of enzymes such as citrate synthase and succinate dehydrogenase. The oxidative capacity of fast and slow twitch fibers can be estimated using histochemical stains such as nicotinamide dinucleotide dehydrogenase (NADH-DH) and succinate dehydrogenase. When both myosin ATPase stains and oxidative stains are used, muscle fibers can be classified as slow twitch (high oxidative), fast twitch oxidative, and fast twitch glycolytic fibers. The metabolic properties of muscle fibers have important bearing on the amount of glycogen utilized and lactate produced during exercise. A high per centage of type IIB fibers with a low oxidative capacity in a biopsy specimen has been corrrelated with high glycogen utilization and lactate accumulation during near-maximal exercise. Training increases the oxidative capacity of skeletal muscle. This change is selective for those fiber types which are recruited during exercise. Thus, in fit racehorses all muscle fiber types have a high oxidative capacity, whereas in dressage horses type IIB fibers often have a much lower oxidative capacity than type I and IIA fibers. The oxidative capacity of muscle in horses is so high that histochemical staining for oxidative capacity in types I and IIA fibers is often maximal in untrained horses. It is important, therefore, to obtain both a quantitative measurement of muscle oxidative capacity as well as a histochemical estimate of the oxidative capacity of the different fiber types when assessing training status.

MUSCLE MORPHOMETRY

Assessment of muscle biopsy specimens should also include evaluation of muscle morphology. Fiber types are normally randomly distributed in muscle fascicles, with a tendency for some type IIB fibers to localize at the periphery of fascicles. Fiber sizes vary with the age of the horse and the state of training. In young and untrained animals, type IIB fibers are much larger than type IIA and type I fibers. During race training, type IIB muscle fibers become smaller in size and fiber sizes appear to be uniform across all types. The density of capillaries in muscle fibers can be evaluated by alkaline phosphatase or α-amylase–periodic acid–Schiff stain. The greatest capillary density is found around type I fibers, followed by type IIA and IIB fibers. With at least 4 months of race training, an increase in the density of capillaries in skeletal muscle can be observed. A decrease in fiber size and an increase in capillary density with training are believed to enhance the delivery of oxygen and the removal of deleterious waste products from muscle.

The ideal muscle morphology, fiber composition, and metabolic properties have yet to be determined for each type of performance event. Muscle biopsy specimens from successful racehorses have been examined; all showed the training adaptations discussed above. In racehorses, a balance of oxidative characteristics (smaller fiber sizes, increased capillary density, high oxidative enzyme capacities) and characteristics of high power output (large cross-sectional area of muscle, high proportion of fast-twitch fibers, high glycolytic enzyme activities) is important. While further training of an individual may increase its endurance, at some point it may be at the risk of losing power output. Defining the particular balance between oxidative characteristics and power output that meets the peak capacity of an individual is a major challenge when assessing fitness.

Horse owners are frequently interested in evaluating muscle biopsy specimens from yearlings prior to purchase. This has not proved profitable because muscle fiber compositions are not proportional to an individual's speed and because marked metabolic changes occur in muscle with training.

EXERCISE TOLERANCE TESTING

Blood parameters, determined during and after exercise, can be used as indices of muscle metabolism. These parameters also reflect the ability of the cardiopulmonary system to deliver oxygen to the tissues and to remove deleterious byproducts formed during exercise. Plasma lactate concentrations reflect the production of lactate by some muscle fibers, oxidation of this lactate by other fibers, and release of the lactate into the bloodstream. During an incremental exercise test, blood lactate concentrations are proportional to muscle lactate concentrations. As training progresses, glycogen utilization and lactate accumulation during a standardized near-maximal exercise test should decrease. Excessive lactate production during standardized exercise would indicate poor training adaptation or possibly a metabolic defect. Excessive elevations in blood lactate levels during submaximal exercise have been observed in a horse with a respiratory enzyme deficiency (complex I) in muscle mitochondria.

Plasma ammonia concentrations can also be measured as an indicator of the limitations of oxidative metabolism in skeletal muscle. During maximal exercise, muscle pH decreases, the availability of ATP for contraction falls, and the purine nucleotide cycle is activated. In this process adenosine phosphates are deaminated and ammonia as well as inosine monophosphate is formed. Elevations in plasma ammonia concentrations may complement plasma lactate as a marker for limitations in muscle oxidative capacity. Blood parameters that can be used to monitor muscle damage during exercise include plasma CK activities determined before and 4 to 6 hours after exercise. Most horses have less than a fivefold increase in CK activity following short, near-maximal exercise or even after 1 hour of endurance-type exercise.

Submaximal exercise testing has particular application for endurance horses. In endurance performance, one of the limiting factors in skeletal muscle is the availability of energy substrates such as glycogen and blood-borne substrates. Oxidative utilization of fuels by skeletal muscle is much more energy efficient than anaerobic glycolysis and also permits the utilization of blood-borne substrates. One of the benefits of training in endurance performance is that the muscle is able to utilize fuels, including blood glucose, free fatty acids, and glycogen, more efficiently, and this has a sparing effect on muscle glycogen. If muscle metabolism is of specific interest, histochemical and biochemical analyses of pre- and postexercise muscle biopsy specimens for glycogen, lactate, creatine phosphate, and ATP concentrations may be done. Horses show substantially less glycogen utilization during a standardization exercise test following endurance-type training and minimal increases in bood lactate. The utilization of fatty acids by skeletal muscle during exercise has not been extensively studied in the horse, although plasma free fatty acid concentrations are known to increase after about 15 minutes of trotting.

In conclusion, evaluation of skeletal muscle in performance horses requires a thorough history, physical examination, and prudent use of diagnostic tests such as serum chemistries, muscle biopsies, and exercise testing. Test results should always be interpreted in conjunction with other findings on a comprehensive examination of all body systems important for performance.

Supplemental Readings

Lindholm, A., and Piehl, K.: Fiber composition, enzyme activities and concentrations of metabolites and electrolytes in muscles of Standardbred horses. Acta Vet. Scand., 15:287, 1974.

Snow, D. H.: Skeletal muscle adaptations: A review. In Snow, D. H., Persson, S. G. B., and Rose, R. J. (eds.): Equine Exercise Physiology. Cambridge, England, Granta Editions, 1983, pp. 160–183.

Valberg, S. J., Essen Gustavsson, B., Lindholm, A., and Persson, S.: Blood chemistry and skeletal muscle metabolic responses during and after different speeds and durations of trotting. Equine Vet. J., 21:91, 1989.

Valberg, S. J., Essen Gustavsson, B., Lindholm, A., and Persson, S.: Energy metabolism in relation to skeletal muscle fiber properties during treadmill exercise. Equine Vet. J., 17:439, 1985.

Fitness Testing
Elisabeth Morris, NORTH GRAFTON, MASSACHUSETTS

Exercise performance testing is a diagnostic procedure used to determine the level of metabolic fitness of the athlete. Maximal exercise testing is a primary diagnostic tool for the evaluation of exercise intolerance and level of fitness in the human athlete. The recent availability of high-speed treadmills has allowed the inclusion of exercise testing as a routine part of the evaluation of inadequate performance in the horse. The standardized incremental step test is an integral part of the clinical evaluation of poor performance, the determination of performance potential, and the analysis of the effects of training on the metabolic capability of the athletic horse. Because the instrumentation necessary for the evaluation is relatively simple and noninvasive, the standardized exercise test is easily tolerated by the horse and therefore may be used in the clinical setting. Many abnormalities, such as musculoskeletal pain and upper or lower respiratory dysfunction, will result in suboptimal results during an exercise test, and therefore exercise testing is only one component of the evaluation of racing performance. A complete evaluation should also include a thorough physical examination, a lameness evaluation, an upper airway examination at rest, during exercise, and during the postexercise period, hematological and serum chemistry analysis, routine thoracic radiographs, and an analysis of nutrition. More advanced diagnostic tests include radiography, echocardiography, tendon and bone ultrasonography, thermography, and radionuclide scintigraphy of soft tissue, bone, and lung.

INDICATIONS FOR PERFORMING AN EXERCISE TEST IN THE EQUINE ATHLETE

Optimal athletic performance depends on the peak function of all physiological systems. Any musculoskeletal pain will result in abnormal compensatory alterations in gait and therefore increased metabolic cost of locomotion. Upper respiratory obstruction will result in increased metabolic cost of breathing as well as decreased delivery of oxygen to the lungs. Pulmonary pathology may result in decreased ventilation, impaired diffusion of gases, alterations in perfusion, shunting, or ventilation/perfusion ($\dot{V}/\dot{Q}$) mismatch. An exercise test can be of diagnostic benefit in the following situations:

1. In horses with inadequate or decreased performance with no detectable abnormalities localized to any physiological system. The results of the exercise test may be compared to the normal exercise values for age- and breed-matched individuals. Deficiencies in aerobic or anaerobic efficiency (fitness), musculoskeletal strength, or the presence of functional cardiovascular pathology during maximal exercise may be identified.

2. Young horses with inferior performance potential may be identified by less than expected peak metabolic parameters during an exercise test. In this situation the exercise test is being used as a screening procedure.

3. To assess the effects of training, a standardized exercise test may be repeated over time to monitor changes in fitness.

4. To assist in identifying whether a specific abnormality results in impaired athletic performance, the results of a standardized exercise test on individuals with known abnormalities may be compared with results of exercise testing in normal age- and breed-matched individuals.

PROTOCOLS FOR PERFORMANCE TESTING ON A TREADMILL

Treadmill performance testing allows precise control over the velocity used in the test, exercise of the horse in close proximity to physiological testing equipment, and evaluation of a wide range of exercise-related parameters. Two types of exercise tests commonly used for equine performance testing are constant work rate tests and incremental step tests. The constant work rate test is used to evaluate the response to exercise as a function of time at a constant velocity. These tests are best suited for obtaining steady-state measurements and for determining the time required to reach steady state at a given exercise level. The major disadvantage of the constant work rate tests for clinical evaluations is that the test must be repeated several times, usually over several days, at increasing exercise levels in order to determine peak levels of measured variables.

The standardized incremental exercise test evaluates the metabolic response to exercise during intervals of increasing exercise intensity. Incremental work rate step tests are best suited for determining peak values, since a wide range of exercise intensities can be evaluated in a single exercise bout. The typical standardized exercise test consists of ten intervals of increasing velocity run with the high-speed motorized treadmill inclined to a slope of 6 degrees. The velocity of the treadmill is increased sequentially in 1-minute intervals to velocities of 1.8, 2.7, 3.4, 4.5, 5.4, 6.8, 9.0, 10.8, 12, and 13 meters per second, corresponding to times of 15, 10, 8, 6, 5, 4, 3, 2.5, 2.25, and 2 minutes per mile. The exercise test is terminated when the horse shows signs of exhaustion, manifested by inability to maintain position at the front of the treadmill without the aid of the holders. The treadmill is then returned to the horizontal position and the horse is allowed to walk for a period of 15 minutes at 1.8 meters per second. In racehorses, peak values for exercise variables are generally attained during one of the final three exercise intensities. Once the horse is trained to run on the treadmill, the entire standardized incremental step test can be completed as a single exercise bout. In addition, the same incremental protocol can be used to compare horses with varying physical ability.

The standardized exercise test involves the measurement of oxygen consumption ($\dot{V}O_2$), carbon dioxide production ($\dot{V}CO_2$), respiratory exchange ratio, venous blood lactate concentration, heart rate, hematocrit, and total plasma protein during the exercise protocol and at 1, 5, and 15 minutes after exercise (Table 1). To be effective as a clinical diagnostic tool, the instrumentation used for the exercise test must be minimally invasive, easily tolerated by relatively "untrained" horses, and generate the results as rapidly as possible. $\dot{V}O_2$ and $\dot{V}CO_2$ are measured continuously during the exercise test using either a closed mask system or an open flow respirometry system. The open flow system is accurate, relatively simple, and therefore easy to use in a clinical setting on horses inexperienced on the treadmill. The horse wears a loose-fitting mask, which captures all of the expired gases due to the constant maintenance of negative pressures within the mask. A small sample of the expired gases is diverted through oxygen and carbon dioxide analyzers, enabling the calculation of $\dot{V}O_2$ and $\dot{V}CO_2$ (Fig. 1).

Blood samples for determining hematocrit, total plasma protein, and venous blood lactate concentrations are taken at 1-minute intervals during the exercise test via an intravenous catheter placed in the left jugular vein prior to the initiation of the test. Heart rate is measured by a telemetered electrocardiograph (ECG) monitor or a telemetered heart rate monitor. Serum samples obtained from clotted, centrifuged blood samples are taken prior to the exercise test and 6 hours following completion of the test and assayed for creatine kinase (CK) to evaluate exercise-induced muscle damage.

TABLE 1. MAXIMAL EXERCISE TEST MEASUREMENTS FOR ADULT STANDARDBRED AND THOROUGHBRED RACEHORSES DURING A STANDARDIZED INCREMENTAL EXERCISE TEST

Parameter	Standardbred (Mean ± SD)	Thoroughbred (Mean ± SD)
$\dot{V}O_2$ (ml/kg/min)	165.0 ± 2.0	164.6 ± 3.0
$\dot{V}CO_2$ (ml/kg/min)	198.9 ± 2.5	196.6 ± 4.0
R ($\dot{V}CO_2/\dot{V}O_2$)	1.33 ± 0.02	1.30 ± 0.03
LAC (mmol/L)	16.1 ± 0.8	15.8 ± 1.6
HR (bpm)	227.0 ± 2.0	228.0 ± 3.0
Hematocrit (%)	59.0 ± 1.0	64.0 ± 1.0
STEPmax (steps)	9.1 ± 0.1	8.6 ± 0.1
Δ CK (IU/L)	42.0 ± 69.4	73.0 ± 14.8

$\dot{V}O_2$ = oxygen consumption, $\dot{V}CO_2$ = carbon dioxide production, R = respiratory quotient, LAC = lactate production, HR = heart rate, ΔCK = change in creatine kinase values, STEPmax = number of incremental steps completed.

INTERPRETATION OF RESULTS OF THE INCREMENTAL EXERCISE TEST

Metabolic power required by the contractile proteins of muscle to generate movement is derived from energy released by the hydrolysis of adenosine triphosphate (ATP) to adenosine diphosphate (ADP) within the muscle cells. In mammalian skeletal muscle, ADP is rephosphorylated to maintain the supply of ATP during exercise by three metabolic pathways: phosphocreatine (PC) reaction, anaerobic glycolysis, and aerobic metabolism. These three metabolic path-

OPEN FLOW RESPIRATORY GAS ANALYSIS

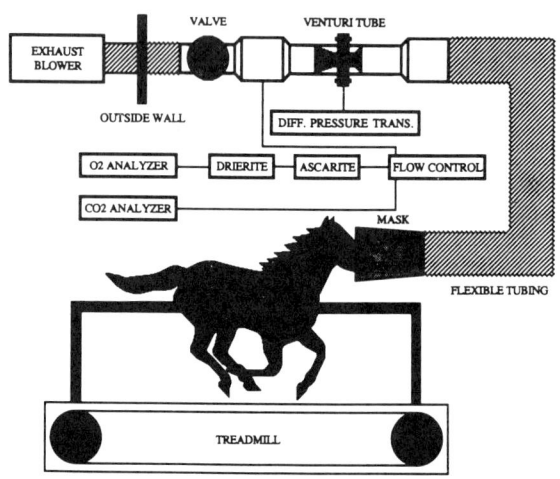

Figure 1. The open flow respirometry gas analysis system for measurement of oxygen consumption ($\dot{V}O_2$) and carbon dioxide production ($\dot{V}CO_2$) during exercise. (From Seeherman, H. J. and Morris E. A.: Methodology and repeatability of standardized treadmill exercise test for clinical evaluation of fitness in horses. Equine Vet. J., Suppl. 9:20–25, 1991. Reproduced by permission.)

ways interact to ensure a constant supply of ATP for sustained exercise of different intensities and duration. The primary source of ATP during the initial period is the conversion of PC and ADP to ATP and creatine in the muscle. Although the PC reaction can increase the rate of ATP production instantaneously to very high rates, the concentration of this high-energy phosphate compound stored in the muscle is sufficient for only a few seconds of maximal activity. The assessment of energy production from creatine phosphate necessitates muscle biopsies, which are not practical in a clinical setting. Continued muscle activity requires additional regeneration of ATP from anaerobic glycolysis and aerobic metabolism.

Anaerobic glycolysis regenerates ATP during the metabolism of muscle glycogen to lactic acid. Maximal rates of ATP regeneration from anaerobic glycolysis in the muscle cytosol can be achieved in 10 to 20 seconds and are limited by the availability of glycogen stored in the muscle and the associated metabolic acidosis and muscle fatigue resulting from the accumulation of lactate. As a result of these limitations, maximum rates of exercise can only be sustained for approximately 60 seconds if anaerobic glycolysis is the only source of metabolic power. The contribution of anaerobic power to total energy output is evaluated by analysis of venous blood lactate values at the end of each incremental step during the exercise test and the highest levels of blood lactate tolerated at the end of exhaustive exercise. The lactate generated during each incremental step is an indicator of the speed with which aerobic metabolism can respond to the additional energy requirements, for during the time when the aerobic pathways are working to increase energy production required at the new treadmill velocity, the anaerobic pathways will supply the required energy. At the end of exhaustive exercise, when energy requirements exceed those supplied by maximal oxygen consumption, the increase in blood lactate concentration is a measure of sustained anaerobic power output. The ability to tolerate high concentrations of lactate during exhaustive exercise is a means of evaluating anaerobic endurance and is dependent on the buffering capacity of the blood and the efficient export of lactate out of the muscle into the circulation.

The third major metabolic pathway for regenerating ATP is aerobic metabolism. This complex metabolic pathway regenerates ATP by the chemical oxidation of glycogen and triglycerides stored in the muscle. Additional substrate for this reaction is delivered to the muscle via the circulation as glucose derived from glycogen stores in the liver and free fatty acids derived from adipose tissue. Oxygen required for this process is supplied by the cardiopulmonary transport system. The aerobic metabolic pathway requires 45 to 60 seconds to reach maximal rates of ATP regeneration in the horse and becomes the sole source of metabolic power for sustained submaximal exercise. At higher exercise intensities, aerobic metabolism continues at the maximal rate and anaerobic glycolysis supplies the additional metabolic power input until maximum concentrations of lactate and associated metabolic acidosis are achieved. Parameters involved in aerobic energy production are evaluated by measurement of $\dot{V}O_2$ and $\dot{V}CO_2$ (Fig. 2). $\dot{V}O_2$ is simply oxygen uptake from the lungs and therefore reflects oxygen consumed by the cells. Peak aerobic power, or the maximal energy production possible to be generated from aerobic metabolism, can be measured directly by analysis of maximal oxygen consumption ($\dot{V}O_2$max). During the incremental exercise test, $\dot{V}O_2$max is usually reached during the last two steps. This value is determined when, despite increased energy demands (an increase in the treadmill velocity), there is no increase in $\dot{V}O_2$, signifying that the added energy production is being generated from anaerobic metabolism. In addition to increased energy production with maintenance of the same oxygen consumption, criteria for determination of $\dot{V}O_2$max also include a continued increase in $\dot{V}CO_2$, resulting in a respiratory quotient

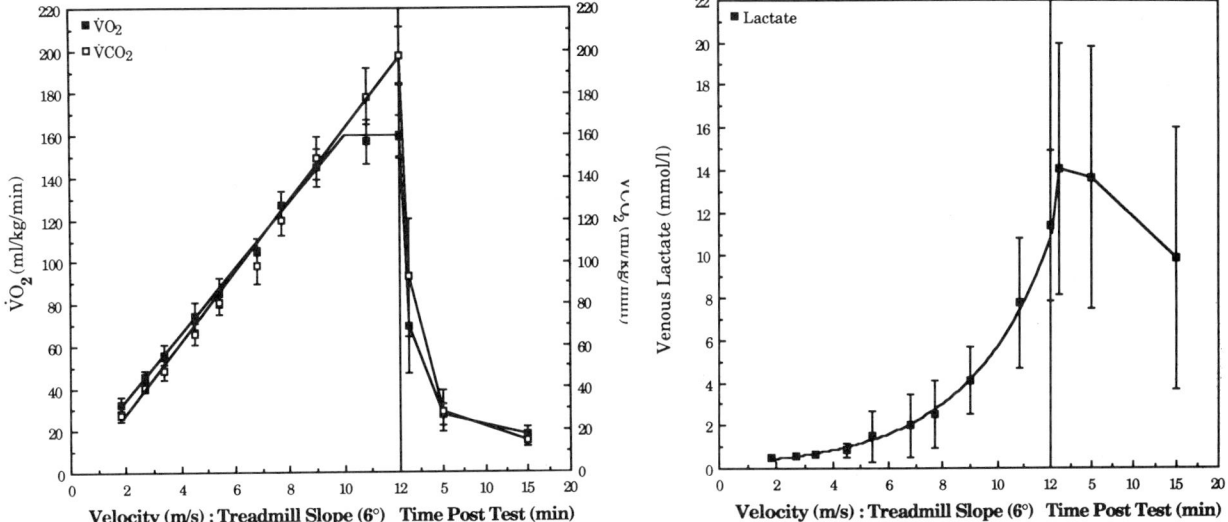

Figure 2. Results of the standardized incremental exercise test performed by adult Thoroughbred racehorses. (*a*) Oxygen consumption ($\dot{V}o_2$) and carbon dioxide production ($\dot{V}co_2$) as a function of treadmill velocity. $\dot{V}o_2$max is achieved when an increase in running velocity does not result in an increase in $\dot{V}o_2$. $\dot{V}co_2$ continues to increase as a response to metabolic acidosis. (*b*) Venous blood lactate levels as a function of treadmill velocity. Venous lactate levels rise abruptly near the end of the exercise test, indicating a substantial contribution to energy production by anaerobic glycolysis.

($R = \dot{V}co_2/\dot{V}o_2$) above 1.2. This increase in the respiratory exchange ratio serves as an indicator of acute metabolic acidosis during exercise. The slope of the line describing velocity versus oxygen consumption is an indicator of metabolic efficiency, as a lower slope indicates more efficient use of oxygen to achieve a similar velocity or power output (Fig. 3).

During the exercise test, peak heart rates are achieved during the last two incremental steps. The relationship between heart rate and exercise intensity closely approximates the relationship between $\dot{V}o_2$ and treadmill velocity. Unlike man, the horse does not significantly increase stroke volume during exercise, so the increase in heart rate is the most important means of increasing cardiac output. The increase in heart rate, coupled with the capacity of the horse to increase the number of circulating red blood cells during exercise by up to 40 per cent via splenic contraction, results in a tremendous increase in oxygen delivery to the tissues. These additive physiological adaptations to strenuous exercise prevent a decrease in arterial oxygen content despite a measurable degree of exercise-induced hypoxemia. During the incremental step test,

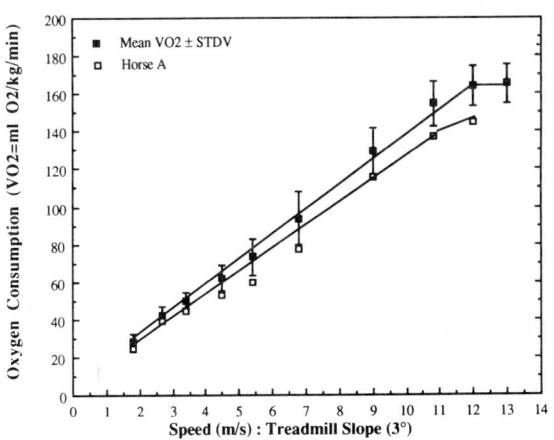
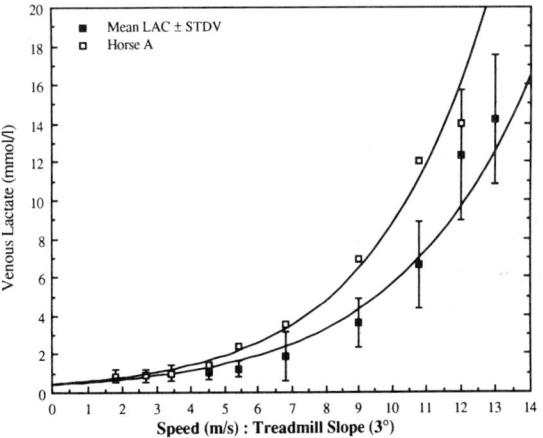

Figure 3. Results of the standardized exercise test on a 3-year-old Standardbred racehorse with inadequate athletic performance. Results in this individual are compared with mean values in age- and breed-matched individuals. (*a*) $\dot{V}o_2$max for this individual is less than the mean. (*b*) The blood lactate levels of this individual indicate a greater reliance on anaerobic energy production early in the exercise test.

the heart rate is recorded at the end of each step, and blood samples are taken each minute to be analyzed for hematocrit.

Following muscle damage, muscle cell contents are released into the general circulation. A relatively specific and sensitive indicator of skeletal or cardiac muscle damage is an increase in serum CK values. In the normal racehorse, serum CK does not increase significantly following exhaustive exercise during the incremental step test. But in horses with obvious as well as subclinical muscle damage, or in horses that have sustained trauma to a muscle group (including a muscle tear), serum CK values rise following strenuous exercise. Because serum CK values peak approximately 6 hours following muscle damage, a 6-hour postexercise serum sample is routinely taken from each horse following the exercise test and CK levels are compared to those found in the pre-exercise sample.

FIELD PROTOCOLS FOR PERFORMANCE TESTING

Most field tests use a constant work rate protocol. In these types of tests, the horse is instrumented with the desired physiological measuring devices and either data are telemetered to a remote recording device or instruments are connected directly to a recorder carried by the rider or driver. Data are collected during the time interval when the horse passes through a measured distance at different velocities controlled by the rider or driver. The most common measurements made in field tests include heart rate, venous lactate levels, rectal temperature, and respiratory rate. The main indication for measuring heart rate in field tests is to assess changes in cardiopulmonary fitness in response to training. The first step in this process is to determine maximum heart rate and heart rate as a function of exercise intensity at the beginning of the training period using a heart rate monitor or telemetered ECG. The initial measurements can then be compared to similar measurements taken periodically during the training program. With increased cardiopulmonary and musculoskeletal fitness, the heart rate at any given exercise intensity decreases. Similarly, the velocity eliciting a particular percentage of maximum heart rate (%HRmax) will increase with increased fitness.

In contrast, maximum heart rate does not change in response to training. When no change occurs in the measurements between successive exercise tests, either the training program has reached its maximum effectiveness or the horse has reached a maximum level of cardiopulmonary fitness. To distinguish between these two possibilities, the intensity or duration of the training program should be increased. If heart rate at a given velocity does not continue to decrease or the velocity at a given %HRmax does not continue to increase, then maximal cardiopulmonary fitness has been attained and further increases in the training intensity are probably not useful. If these measurements continue to change, then the training program was not capable of eliciting maximum cardiopulmonary fitness.

Changes in lactate concentrations before and after exercise can be used in a similar manner to evaluate the efficiency of aerobic metabolism. As the rate of increase in aerobic metabolism accelerates in response to training, the lactate concentration at the end of a given exercise intensity will decrease. Changes in peak lactate concentrations after exhaustive exercise can also be used as an indicator of changes in peak anaerobic power input and anaerobic endurance in response to training. Measurement of blood lactate is technically more difficult than measurement of heart rate. It is difficult to standardize the sampling times, and blood samples must be obtained.

Supplemental Readings

Bayly, W. M., Schulz, D. A., Hodgson, D. R., and Gollnick, P. D.: Ventilatory responses of the horse to exercise: effect of gas collection systems. J. Appl. Physiol., 63:1210–1217, 1987.

Evans, D. L., and Rose, R. J.: Method of investigation of the accuracy of four digitally-displayed heart rate meters suitable for use in the exercising horse. Equine Vet. J., 18:129–132, 1986.

Rose, R. J., and Evans, D. L.: Cardiovascular and respiratory function in the athletic horse. In Gillespie, J. R., and Robinson, N. E. (eds.): Equine Exercise Physiology 2. Davis, Calif., ICEEP Publications, 1987, pp. 1–24.

Seeherman, H. J., and Morris, E. A.: Comparison of yearling, two year old and adult Thoroughbreds using a standardized exercise test. Equine Vet. J., 23:175–184. 1991.

Seeherman, H. J., and Morris, E. A.: Methodology and repeatability of standardized treadmill exercise test for clinical evaluation of fitness in horses. Equine Vet. J. Suppl. 9:20–25, 1991.

Hematological and Endocrine Changes During Exercise

Jonathan H. Foreman, URBANA, ILLINOIS

Considerable hematological and serum electrolyte changes occur in the normal athletic horse during and after a single bout of exercise. It is important to recognize such normal alterations in order to interpret possible abnormalities in horses that are no longer racing or performing up to their potential. Such horses have been termed exercise intolerant.

COMPLETE BLOOD CELL COUNT

The complete blood cell count (CBC) helps to assess the horse's oxygen-carrying capacity (hematocrit, hemoglobin, red blood cell [RBC] count, and indices) and recent exposure to an inflammatory process or stress (white blood cell [WBC] count, differential). Immediate submission of blood samples for a CBC is ideal. However, if overnight storage is necessary before analysis, blood should be kept refrigerated. Storage at room temperature allows RBCs to imbibe fluid from the plasma, resulting in increased hematocrit and mean corpuscular volume and sometimes in decreased RBC counts due to hemolysis. Differential WBC counts are altered in stored blood, because WBCs continue to mature and degenerate despite refrigeration.

Resting hematocrits in racehorses usually range between 35 and 45 per cent, but values as low as 30 per cent may not be abnormal because the horse can mobilize the stored RBCs from the spleen during exercise. Thoroughbreds and previously trained horses tend to have higher hematocrit, hemoglobin, and RBC counts than untrained or non-Thoroughbred horses. Resting hematocrit is most helpful in detecting anemia when values are less than 30 per cent.

The horse's unique ability to sequester RBCs in the spleen and then to release them is under sympathetic control. Increasing levels of fear, excitement, and exercise cause the release of increasing numbers of RBCs. The most accurate measurements of blood, plasma, and RBC volume are made during sympathetic stimulation, that is, immediately after exercise or after administration of exogenous epinephrine (0.4–1.0 mg/100 kg IV as 0.1 per cent solution). These measurements require intravenous (IV) administration of dyes such as Evans blue or indocyanine green.

The CBC can reflect a recent bout of exercise and indicate whether exercise was mild or severe. Exercise raises the hematocrit dramatically and proportionate to the speed of exercise. Immediate postexercise hematocrits in racehorses may be as high as 65 to 70 per cent and should decrease to 50 to 55 per cent by 15 minutes and to resting values by 30 minutes. This increase in apparent circulating RBC mass is due to splenic "dumping" of stored RBCs as well as to fluid shifts from the intravascular to the extracellular space. Failure of an exercise-intolerant horse to manifest this exercise-induced increase in hematocrit is not common.

The stress of a single bout of exercise may lead to mild neutrophilia and moderate lymphocytosis. This relative decrease in neutrophil/lymphocyte ratio can be normal if intermittent and transient, but if present in the same horse chronically may be indicative of overtraining. Overtraining is a syndrome in which the subject is training or racing so hard and so frequently that it is not being allowed sufficient time to recover. Approximately 30 days of small paddock or pasture rest is often sufficient to allow such a horse to recover from overtraining without losing a measurable amount of previously achieved fitness. In the absence of infection, a pronounced neutrophilia, especially with a left shift for several hours after endurance exercise, is usually indicative of severe stress in an exhausted horse.

SERUM ELECTROLYTES

Remarkable shifts in serum electrolyte values can be seen after normal exercise and may not be the result of organic disease. In sprinting work such as is performed by Standardbred and most Thoroughbred racehorses, 2 minutes of 5-degree inclined treadmill cantering at 720 meters per minute raises serum potassium to as much as 10 mEq per L, a level often thought to be incompatible with life. In normal horses, these potassium values return to normal or near normal within 2 to 5 minutes after cessation of exercise. Sodium and chloride levels often remain relatively unchanged after sprinting work in racehorses. Mild increases have been reported and are thought to be due primarily to fluid shifts into the extracellular compartment.

A number of Quarter Horses have been reported with periodic hyperkalemic paralysis, a familial disease in which high serum potassium levels occur at rest or after light levels of exercise such as lunging. In these horses potassium values may take hours to return to normal following cessation of exercise (see p. 117).

Endurance horses exercising over longer distances (25 to 100 miles) at slower paces exhibit different electrolyte shifts than do sprinters. The sweating of considerable amounts of sodium and chloride results in anion shifts manifested by measurable elevations in serum bicarbonate concentration. This hypochloremic metabolic alkalosis becomes most important when selecting a fluid for IV support of the exhausted endurance horse. Isotonic saline and not an alkalinizing solution such as bicarbonate or lactated Ringer's solution should be the fluid of choice in such a horse. Low sodium and chloride levels after endurance exercise will also be corrected by the administration of saline.

Hypocalcemia is occasionally seen in endurance but not sprinting horses and has been associated with exertional myopathy, generalized muscle weakness, and synchronous diaphragmatic flutter. IV calcium supplementation in addition to volume fluid replacement is usually corrective (see p. 566).

SERUM ENZYMES

Creatine kinase (CK), aspartate aminotransferase (AST, previously SGOT), or lactate dehydrogenase (LDH) levels are not significantly elevated after exercise in fit horses performing exercise to which they are accustomed. Chronically elevated muscle enzyme levels, especially following a period of enforced rest, are evidence of myopathy. Exercise-induced myopathy may be diagnosed by the measurement of serum CK levels before and 6 hours after exercise. A significant increase in postexercise levels indicates exercise-induced muscle damage. Because CK is cleared from the serum by 24 hours, whereas AST will remain elevated for up to 7 days following muscle damage, analysis of CK enables the identification of muscle damage due to a specific exercise bout.

Liver enzymes such as AST, succinate dehydrogenase, γ- glutamyltranspeptidase, and alkaline phosphatase should not be elevated in normal horses even after severe exercise. Such hepatobiliary enzyme elevations may, however, be seen in athletic horses if they are also receiving anabolic steroids while in training. These liver enzyme changes should be reversible after the anabolic steroid effects diminish within 6 to 8 weeks of administration.

ENDOCRINE DISORDERS

Hypothyroidism

Endocrine disorders are uncommon in sedentary or exercising horses. However, a relationship has been shown to exist between deficiencies in thyroid hormone and myopathies ("tying-up") in some horses. Because the origin of myopathies may be multifactorial, the veterinarian must examine each subject for other problems such as a lameness, which may cause an altered gait resulting in muscle soreness. The diagnosis of hypothyroidism is complicated by the fact that phenylbutazone administration for 5 days will markedly decrease serum concentrations of thyroid hormones. Thus, a single resting determination of serum thyroid levels without an adequate history of drug administration is not the best way to document hypothyroidism in horses. Further, normal thyroid hormone values may vary considerably between laboratories owing to differences in measurement methods.

In addition to measurements of muscle enzymes at rest and after exercise, we routinely perform thyroid-stimulating hormone (TSH) tests to assess thyroid function in horses with possible myopathy. We administer 5 IU TSH° IV at 9 A.M. Administration at 9 A.M. takes into account the normal circadian variations in the serum levels of triiodothyronine (T_3) and thyroxine (T_4). T_3 peaks at 8 A.M. and T_4 peaks at 4 P.M. Venous serum samples are drawn before TSH administration and hourly for 6 hours after challenge. In a nonhospital setting, sampling 4 hours after administration of TSH is sufficient to detect the peak level of T_3, the active form of thyroid hormone. We routinely assess the serum values at 6 hours, because T_4 peaks at that point. Peak T_3 and T_4 values should be two to four times greater than resting values.

Horses with low resting thyroid hormone levels or poor TSH responses often respond to exogenous thyroid supplementation. We routinely add 30 grains (1.95 gm) thyroid hormone† twice a day to the feed of such horses. While not all respond, some horses perform more effectively, have less muscle-origin unsoundness, and maintain or gain weight more easily. If there is no response within 6 weeks to 30 grains administered per os twice a day, the dosage can be increased to as much as 60 grains per os twice a day.

Addison-like Disease

A different manifestion of hormonal abnormalities may be seen in the racing athlete when

---

°Dermathycin, Coopers Animal Health, Kansas City, KS
†Thyroid U.S.P., Rugby Labs., Long Island, NY

turned out for a rest on pasture. Sudden withdrawal of exogenously administered corticosteroids may result in "steroid letdown" or an addisonian crisis. Such horses are excessively lethargic, lifeless, and chronically thin. They continue to lose weight rather than gaining weight when out on pasture and not exercising as heavily.

Documentation of such a syndrome is difficult, because the trainer may be reluctant to discuss corticosteroid administration. Resting cortisol levels are decreased and do not increase following exogenous adrenocorticotropin stimulation (1 unit per kg IV), because the adrenal glands are iatrogenically suppressed by chronic corticosteroid administration.

Supplemental Readings

Bayly, W. M.: The interpretation of clinicopathologic data from the equine athlete. Vet. Cin. North Am. (Equine Pract.), 3:631–647, 1987.

Carlson, G. P.: Hematology and body fluids in the equine athlete: A review. In Gillespie, J. R., Robinson, N. E. (eds.): Equine Exercise Physiology 2. Davis, Calif., ICEEP Publications, 1987, pp. 393–425.

Foreman, J. H., Bayly, W. M., Grant, B. D., and Gollnick, P. D.: Standardized exercise test and daily heart rate responses of Thoroughbreds undergoing conventional race training and detraining. Am. J. Vet. Res., 51:914–920, 1990.

Harris, P., and Snow, D. H.: The effects of high intensity exercise on the plasma concentration of lactate, potassium and other electrolytes. Equine Vet. J., 20:109–113, 1988.

Koterba, A. M., and Carlson, G. P.: Acid-base and electrolyte alterations in horses with exertional rhabdomyolysis. J. Am. Vet. Med. Assoc., 180:303–306, 1982.

Spier, S. J., Carlson, G. P., Pickar, J., Snyder, J. R., Holliday, T. A., and Cardinet, G. H.: Hyperkalemic periodic paralysis in horses: Genetic and electrophysiologic studies. In: Proceedings of the 35th Annual Convention of the American Association of Equine Practitioners, 1990, pp. 399–402.

Waldron-Mease, E.: Hypothyroidism and myopathy in racing Thoroughbreds and Standardbreds. J. Equine Med. Surg., 3:124–128, 1979.

Ergogenic Diets and Nutrients

Pamela L. Ferrante, BLACKSBURG, VIRGINIA
David S. Kronfeld, BLACKSBURG, VIRGINIA

Ergogenic aids enhance work output and theoretically can improve performance in the athlete. The term may refer to specific diets that are optimal for athletic tasks. More commonly, ergogenic nutrients are supplements to diets formulated to meet minimal requirements. This article discusses four types of diets for athletes, routine ration evaluation, and claims made for certain allegedly ergogenic supplements, especially in horses.

The optimal diet for an athletic horse should provide the required energy and the minimum nutrient requirements, supply optimal amounts and proportions of fuels, facilitate the utilization of fuels, minimize the weight and bulk of bowel contents, maintain hydration, and buffer acids produced in the lower bowel and in muscle. In practice, diets for athletes are variations on four themes: (1) more of the maintenance ration, (2) less bulky, nutrient-dense diets, (3) diets enriched for work with more carbohydrate or fat, and (4) diets enriched for both work and stress.

NUTRIENT-DENSE DIETS

In choosing or evaluating a diet, the practitioner should consider energy density first, since energy requirement is determined by the amount of exercise performed and lack of energy may be limiting. The increase in need for energy can be met by several methods. One is to increase the daily ration in line with the caloric requirements while keeping the proportion of the ingredients the same as for maintenance. In this approach, the increased need for essential nutrients is met by the increased food intake. It assumes no increased need for specific nutrients relative to calories.

Hard-working horses cannot obtain the necessary energy from bulky feeds such as hay without developing a "hay belly" or rotund abdomen and carrying extra weight of intestinal contents. Nutrient-dense diets with more energy are made by reducing the forage or fiber content and increasing the soluble carbohydrate or fat content.

Food fiber resists hydrolytic digestion in the

small intestine and is then fermented in the large intestine. As a result, the bulk of the large bowel contents consists of dry matter residues and water. Fiber also depresses the digestibility of dietary energy and dry matter. Diminishing the bulk of intestinal contents and improving digestibility of feeds is often the only means of improving the performance of athletes engaged in maximal or supramaximal efforts.

Low-fiber diets have two potential limitations. They may reduce the capacity of the large bowel and its contents to act as a reservoir for water and electrolytes. This is particularly important in endurance horses, especially under hot ambient conditions during which horses are more vulnerable to dehydration. The other limitation is carbohydrate overload (not to be confused with carbohydrate loading). Low fiber implies high levels of soluble carbohydrate, which may overload the hydrolytic capacity of the small intestine. If so, excess soluble carbohydrates reach the large bowel and favor rapid fermentation. This leads to production of excess gas and lactic acid, which is less readily absorbed than acetic acid. Possible results are digestive upsets, flatus, and osmotic diarrhea. Worse are the prospects of colic and laminitis.

Diets enriched for work are rich in carbohydrates or, alternatively, fats. These represent two alternative nutritional strategies: carbohydrate loading, which raises muscle glycogen content before exercise, or fat adaptation, which spares glycogen utilization during exercise.

Carbohydrate-Rich Diets

Carbohydrate loading originally involved supercompensation or overswing in glycogen concentration. Human athletes trained on a medium-carbohydrate diet engaged in a maximal effort a few days before the target event to deplete muscle glycogen, then rested and consumed a high-carbohydrate diet to boost muscle glycogen. Good results were demonstrated in events lasting 30 minutes to 3 hours but, since the participants were aware of the diet received, these studies were open to bias. Some of these athletes died of focal myocardial necrosis following carbohydrate loading. Others suffered from rhabdomyolysis, and a few developed fatal kidney failure following carbohydrate loading. A more moderate form of carbohydrate loading is now recommended: simply training and racing on a high-carbohydrate diet.

Carbohydrate ingestion during submaximal exercise also attempts to spare muscle glycogen. It appears to help performance in humans if the muscle glycogen levels are either low at the start, or if exercise is prolonged so that hepatic glycogenolysis and gluconeogenesis are needed to replenish blood glucose. One problem with this approach is that blood glucose levels are elevated for only about 60 minutes following glucose ingestion and fall to normal levels and then below after 2 or 3 hours. This is due to overcompensation by insulin. Fructose, an isomer of glucose, does not initiate an insulin response in humans and has been proposed as an alternative carbohydrate source to glucose prior to endurance events.

Training on a high-carbohydrate diet has induced rhabdomyolysis (tying-up) in racing sled dogs. An analogy was made to "Monday-morning" disease in draught horses. Traditional diets for hard-working horses are rich in soluble carbohydrates. How much they contribute to tying-up in light horses is unclear. The condition in dogs was prevented by replacing grain with meat and fat. These observations led to the strategy of fat adaptation as an alternative to carbohydrate loading.

Fat-Rich Diets

Most diets for horses contain 2 to 4 per cent fat, but horses will consume and digest rations containing up to 15 to 20 per cent fat. One problem encountered with high-fat diets is palatability. Corn oil and vegetable oil blends seem to be accepted by most horses. Attempts at altering the performance of horses by feeding high-fat diets have not yielded conclusive results.

Studies of muscle glycogen in horses fed high-fat diets have yielded both anticipated and bizarre results. One study indicated that horses fed a high-fat diet for 3 to 4 weeks had lower than normal glycogen muscle stores. This difference was not seen, however, when the adaptation period was longer. In another study, horses were fed a mixed diet containing 0 or 10 per cent added fat for 12 weeks of aerobic training consisting of trotting on an inclined treadmill at speeds up to 9 miles per hour but not exceeding a heart rate of 160 bpm. This regimen reduced muscle glycogen before exercise but spared muscle glycogen during exercise. Also, horses fed the high-fat diet improved more during training than those fed the control diet.

More difficult to reconcile with known regulation of muscle metabolism are studies from Texas. Horses were sprint trained when fed diets containing 0 or 10 per cent added fat. Surprisingly, muscle glycogen content was increased in horses fed the high-fat diet. During a 600-meter sprint, muscle glycogen declined more and blood lactate increased more in horses fed the high-fat diet. Moreover, mean sprint times were 59.0 and 56.7 seconds in horses fed the control and high-fat diets, respectively. The situation invites further study.

Part of the adaptive response to a high-fat diet may involve increased storage of triglycerides in the muscles, ensuring a constant fuel supply for active muscle, especially in low-intensity work. Lower muscle glycogen stores may not be of concern if the fat adaptation has a glycogen-sparing effect during submaximal effort.

RATION EVALUATION

Veterinarians are frequently asked opinions on a particular food or product. The prudent answer is that the whole ration needs to be evaluated, because how good or bad, suitable or unsuitable, a food or product may be depends on its interactions with the rest of the diet. Our usual procedures range from simple and imprecise to quantitative and more expensive.

Labels are read to review ingredients and to identify sources of starch, fiber, protein, and fat. Usually only the first few ingredients are quantitatively important. If salt is on the list, it is usually less than 1 per cent. Cereal grains and soybeans are deficient in calcium, so a calcium supplement is needed.

Calculations of caloric and nutrient contents can be made from tables of composition if a whole diet or the formula of a product is known. A weighted average for calories and each nutrient of interest is calculated. Tables contain representative values of analysis but do not reflect ranges, especially for roughages.

More precision is achieved by analyzing samples of each feedstuff. Samples are sent to a commercial laboratory with a request for proximate analysis plus minerals, including trace minerals. Many laboratories no longer routinely measure ash and crude fiber, but these should be requested for horses, to allow calculation of nitrogen-free extract, an approximation of soluble carbohydrate.

Amounts of each feedstuff that are fed to individuals or groups of horses are determined by questioning. Farm staff usually use volumes, and representative volumes must be weighed. If the weight consumed and the analysis for each feedstuff are known, the daily ration can be calculated as weighted averages.

Amounts of concentrates and hays are usually well determined. Intakes of available pasture, however, usually call for assumptions. One approach is to assume the National Research Council's estimates of total dry matter intake, subtract the known amounts of feeds, and assign the remainder to pasture.

SUPPLEMENTS

SODIUM BICARBONATE

Oral sodium bicarbonate administration prior to exercise has improved human performance in the 800-meter run and in spring repetitions. Muscle fatigue during anaerobic exercise is in part caused by accumulation of hydrogen ions within the muscle cell. Increased extracellular buffering increases the efflux of lactic acid from the muscle cell and presumably delays the onset of fatigue.

The effective dose of sodium bicarbonate must raise blood bicarbonate by about 6 mEq per L. Such a large dose of sodium bicarbonate has side effects of urgency and diarrhea in humans.

Sodium bicarbonate administration to horses has led to inconsistent results. In one study, an oral dose of 300 mg per kg of body weight improved times in 8 of 14 horses racing for at least 2 or more minutes. As in studies on humans and other species, the effectiveness of "soda loading" appears to be limited and to require further delineation.

Daily supplementation with sodium bicarbonate at 1 per cent dietary dry matter has been found to produce metabolic alkalosis and reduce clinical and cardiovascular effects of carbohydrate overloading in horses. Daily supplementation at this level could mitigate the adverse effects of low-fiber, high-carbohydrate diets through both systemic and local buffering in the gastrointestinal tract.

The use of sodium bicarbonate is contraindicated in situations conducive to hypochloremic alkalosis due to heavy sweating in endurance events or hot climates. It also should be avoided in conjunction with potassium depletion, for example, with chronic furosemide administration.

CARNITINE

This conditional nutrient is a cofactor or carrier for transporting long-chain fatty acids into the mitochondria. It may spare muscle glycogen by enhancing β-oxidation of fatty acids. Under certain circumstances, carnitine may become limiting, for example at exercise intensities about half-maximal where glucose may be preferred to free fatty acids for oxidation as a power source, but free fatty acids are available.

An oral dose of 10 gm of carnitine is effective in doubling the plasma concentration of free carnitine. Its influence on exercising horses has not been evaluated, but this prospect retains much interest, because carnitine may delay fatigue under restricted exercise conditions.

Ascorbic Acid

Vitamin C is a cofactor for several hydrolases, including those involved in the synthesis of carnitine and steroid hormones. Thus, it may affect carnitine availability, especially in animals trained on high-fat diets for long-distance events.

Stress depletes ascorbic acid in many species, including the horse, and strenuous exercise, like all other extra demands on the body, causes stress. Low plasma ascorbic acid levels have been found in horses in training for racing. Although the bioavailability of ascorbic acid after oral administration is poor, plasma concentrations can be increased by oral administration of 20 gm of ascorbic acid daily to horses.

B Vitamins

There is consensus in human nutrition that deficiencies in several vitamins will impair work performance. Whether "supercharging" with these vitamins will improve performance remains in question. Moreover, it is not known whether exercise increases the requirements for any of the vitamins.

Vitamins play a role in exercise by acting as coenzymes for many reactions in intermediary metabolism. A crucial point in carbohydrate metabolism is the pyruvate dehydrogenase reaction. This is dependent on thiamine pyrophosphate, flavin adenine nucleotide (FAD) derived from riboflavin, nicotinamide adenine nucleotides, a pyridoxyl derivative, and acetyl-CoA derived from pantothenic acid. Pyridoxyl phosphate (B_6) also has a role in transamination of amino acids, yielding ketoacids for oxidation.

Vitamins are also involved in the production and protection of red blood cells. Both folic acid (folacin) and cyanocobalamin (B_{12}) are involved in the synthesis of erythrocytes. Pyridoxyl phosphate is also involved in hemoglobin synthesis.

Requirements for most B vitamins should be met by dietary intake and bacterial synthesis in the cecum and large intestine. Maintenance levels of thiamine, however, may not be aequate for exercising horses. To ensure adequate levels, the National Research Council recommends that diets should contain 5 mg thiamine per kg of dietary dry matter.

Intensive exercise significantly decreases serum folate concentration. Bioavailability from oral administration of folic acid is very poor in the horse.

Dimethylglycine

N,N-dimethylglycine (DMG) is used as a nutritional supplement for athletes in the hope of reducing lactate accumulation and delaying fatigue. Proponents have claimed that oral DMG administration (about 1 mg per kg twice daily) enhances phosphagen stores in muscle, decreases lactate production, decreases blood lactate after exercise, and improves speeds of Greyhounds and horses.

An Australian study on racing Greyhounds compared time trials over long and short distances without and with DMG (0.8 mg per kg twice daily) or dichloroacetic acid (DIPA, 1.5 mg per kg once daily). Times for the longer distance (510 meters) were improved by both DMG and DIPA. No differences were observed at 200 meters. These results are consistent with DMG and DIPA having no effect on the phosphagens, but favoring oxidation of pyruvate derived from muscle glycogen rather than blood glucose. In contrast, a crossover study of DMG administration to exercising horses showed no improvement in oxygen transport or in plasma, blood, or muscle lactate concentrations after exercise. It was concluded that DMG had no beneficial effects on cardiorespiratory function or lactate production in the exercising horse.

Vitamin E

α-Tocopherol protects membranes by preventing the formation of peroxides, hydroperoxides, and other radicals from polyunsaturated fatty acids. Intense exercise produces lipid peroxidation products and free radicals that affect the integrity of mitochondria, endoplasmic reticulum, and sarcoplasmic reticulum within the cell. The National Research Council recommends that diets for exercising horses should contain 80 to 100 IU of vitamin E per kg of dietary dry matter, corresponding to about 400 to 1000 mg per day for a light horse, depending on its activity. Vitamin E appears to be relatively harmless, one common first sign of toxicity being hypertriglyceridemia. The general tolerance range has been suggested to be up to 20 times the minimum level, but it may be less in the horse, which is prone to hyperlipidemia.

Other

Various nutritional or pseudonutritional agents have been proposed as ergogenic aids, usually with appealing rationales and many testimonials but no supporting data from properly designed trials.

Octacosanol is a 28-carbon alcohol found in

small amounts in some vegetable oils and waxes, notably wheat germ oil. It may be an enhancer of vitamin E. It has been proposed as an ergogenic aid, to be used daily for many weeks in physical training programs.

Superoxide dismutase (SOD) is an enzyme that generates hydrogen peroxide, which is used by glutathione peroxidase to oxidize reduced glutathione. Thus, SOD is important in a number of oxidative functions in many cells, including red blood cells, white blood cells, and muscle cells. Various preparations are available for oral or parenteral use. Their value for athletes is uncertain. It is unlikely that this protein can remain intact throughout the processes of digestion, absorption from gut into blood, transport in the circulation, and absorption into muscle cells.

γ-Hydroxybutyrate is a free radical scavenger. By analogy with vitamin E and SOD, it has been proposed as an ergogenic aid.

γ-Oryzanol is a ferulic acid ester of triterpenyl alcohols. It also has been proposed to be a natural antioxidant that prevents membrane damage during anaerobic exercise.

Bioflavanoids are naturally occurring antioxidants. They are not essential nutrients but may be enhancers of vitamin C availability, i.e., less vitamin C may be needed to reach the optimal range in a diet rich in bioflavanoids.

Iron salts have been proposed to combat sports anemia but have been shown to be ineffective for this purpose in racehorses. Most are irritative to the gastrointestinal tract, so care must be taken to determine the total iron salts in feed ingredients and supplements.

Methyl-sulfonyl-methane (MSM), a derivative of dimethyl sulfoxide, has been claimed to promote healing and recovery from disease, athletic injuries, and stress. Some zealous proponents claim much greater efficacy of MSM in curing lameness in hindquarters than in forequarters. The FDA has questioned its safety and efficacy as a feed additive.

Probiotics are fermentation products of bacteria or yeast that contain potentially beneficial amino acids, B vitamins and active enzymes. They are claimed to improve digestibility, but data in horses have been conflicting. A number of expert owners of show dogs and horses have attested to improvements in coat, which is difficult to quantify, hence document, but remains, nevertheless, one of the better indications of improved nutrition.

Several of the above substances can be isolated from common foods and consequently have been claimed by manufacturers and distibutors to be classified as feed ingredients. In our view, isolated pure substances should not be covered by such a claim without demonstrated safety, because many substances found in the body in small concentrations are potentially harmful when purified and administered by mouth. Examples include potassium, adenosine triphosphate, arginine, tryptophan, and testosterone.

PRERACE TREATMENTS

The value of prerace treatment of horses with intravenous solutions of ergogenic nutrients remains undocumented by comparative trials. Thiamine has been claimed to have a calming effect and to strengthen the heart, but these claims remain unsupported in the literature. Anaphylactic reactions have been induced by intravenous administration of thiamine in humans and cyanocobalamin in humans and horses. Vasodilation is caused by intravenous nicotinic acid but not nicotinamide.

Amino acids may be simply an expensive source of fuel, for synthesis of protein is reduced during exercise and amino acids are metabolized as fuel. Amino acids may release hormones; for example, valine causes insulin release and arginine causes growth hormone release. Inosine also has been claimed to have an ergogenic effect.

Glucose is an efficient fuel, but its rate of uptake by muscle cells is dependent on insulin. The insulin response is less to intravenous glucose than to oral glucose. A reduction in insulin diminishes glucose uptake by muscle and use of glucose as a source of power. Because glucose is important in exercise more intense than half-maximal, oral glucose may be better for more intense events, and intravenous glucose may be better, paradoxically, for lower intensity events. These comments are based on accepted metabolic regulation, but the time course of events has not been determined in horses.

Supplemental Readings

Gannon, J. R., and Kendall, R. V.: A clinical evaluation of DMG and DIPA on the performance of racing Greyhounds. Canine Pract., 9:7–13, 1982.

Kronfeld, D. S., Atkins, T. O., and Downey, R. L.: Nutrition, anaerobic and aerobic exercise, and stress. In Burger, I. H., and Rivers, J. P. W. (eds.): Nutrition of the Dog and Cat. Cambridge, England, Cambridge University Press, 1989, pp. 133–146.

Kronfeld, D. M., and Ferrante, P. L.: Diets for athletic horses. In: Proceedings of the 6th Annual Forum of the American College of Veterinary Internal Medicine, 1988, pp. 533–536.

Lawrence, L. M.: Nutrition and fuel utilization in the athletic horse. Vet. Clin. North Am., 6:393–418, 1990.

McGilvrey, R. W.: The use of fuels for muscular work. *In* Howald, H., and Poortmans, J. R. (eds.): Proceedings of the 2nd International Symposium on the Biochemistry of Exercise, Magglingen. Basel, Birkhauser, 1975, pp. 12–30.

Meyer, H.: Nutrition of the equine athlete. *In* Gillespie, J. R., and Robinson, N. E. (eds.): Equine Exercise Physiology 2. Davis, Calif., ICEEP Publications, 1987, pp. 644–673.

National Research Council: Nutrient Requirements of Horses, ed. 5. Washington, D.C., National Academy of Sciences, 1989.

Rose, R. J., Schlierf, H. A., Knight, P. K., et al.: Effects of N,N-dimethylglycine on cardiorespiratory function and lactate production in Thoroughbred horses performing incremental treadmill exercise. Vet. Rec., 125:268–271, 1989.

Section 20

APPENDICES

Table of Drugs: Approximate Doses
N. Edward Robinson, EAST LANSING, MICHIGAN

Drug	Dose	Route
Acepromazine	0.03–0.066 mg/kg for sedation	IM
	0.033–0.055 mg/kg followed by 0.055–0.066 mg/kg butorphanol	IV
	0.04 mg/kg followed by 0.6 mg/kg meperidine	IV
	0.02–0.055 mg/kg t.i.d. for α-receptor blockade	IM
Acetazolamide	2.2 mg/kg b.i.d. or t.i.d.	PO
Acetylcysteine (10%)	2–5 ml/50 kg q.i.d.	Aerosol
Albendazole	25 mg/kg b.i.d. for 5 days for *D. arnfieldi*	PO
	50 mg/kg b.i.d. for 2 days for *S. vulgaris* larvae	PO
	4–8 mg/kg b.i.d. for 1 month for *Echinococcus*	PO
Alfaprostol	3 mg/450 kg for luteolysis; 2 doses 14–18 days apart	IM
Allopurinol	5 mg/kg	IV
Altrenogest	0.044 mg/kg s.i.d. for 8–12 days; for estrous synchronization, follow with luteolytic dose of prostaglandin $F_{2\alpha}$	PO
	11–44 mg/450 kg s.i.d. for pregnancy maintenance	PO
Aluminum hydroxide (antacid)	200–250 ml t.i.d.	PO
Aluminum hydroxide	60 mg/kg	PO
Amicarbalide	9–10 mg/kg single injection	IM or SC
Amikacin	3.5–7.5 mg/kg b.i.d. to q.i.d.	IM or SC
	1–10 mg/kg b.i.d. for foals	Slow IV or IM
	75–100 mg	Subconj.
	125 mg	IA
Aminophylline	5–10 mg/kg b.i.d.	PO
Aminopropazine fumarate	0.5 mg/kg b.i.d.	IM or IV
Aminopyrine	2.5–10 mg/450 kg	IV or IM
Ammonium chloride	20–520 mg/kg s.i.d. (acidifier)	PO
	0.3 gm/50 kg q.i.d. (expectorant)	PO
Amoxicillin trihydrate	10–22 mg/kg t.i.d.	IM
Ampicillin sodium trihydrate	25–100 mg/kg t.i.d. to q.i.d.	IV or IM
	11–22 mg/kg b.i.d. or t.i.d.	IM
	50 mg	Subconj.
Aspirin	15–100 mg/kg b.i.d.	PO
Atracurium	0.04–0.07 mg/kg	IV
Atropine	0.01–0.1 mg/kg	IV, IM, or SC
	1%, q. 3–24 h.	Ophthalmic

Table continued on following page

TABLE OF DRUGS: APPROXIMATE DOSES—*continued*

Drug	Dose	Route
Azlocillin	25–75 mg/kg q.i.d.	IV
Betamethasone	0.02–0.1 mg/kg	IM or PO
Bethanechol	0.025–0.075 mg/kg t.i.d. or q.i.d.	SC
	0.3–0.4 mg/kg t.i.d. or q.i.d.	PO
Bismuth subsalicylate	0.5–1 ml/kg q. 4–6 h. in foals	PO
	1–2 L/450 kg b.i.d.	PO
Boldenone undecylenate	1 mg/kg, repeated at 3-week intervals	IM
Botulinum antitoxin (100–150 IU/ml)	200 ml (foal)	IV or IM
	500 ml (adult)	IV or IM
Buparvaquone	4–6 mg/kg, single dose	IV
Butorphanol tartrate	0.05–2 mg/kg (see xylazine, detomidine, and acepromazine)	IV or IM
Calcium borogluconate (23%)	0.2–0.4 ml/kg in 1–2 L of 5% dextrose	Slow IV
Calcium chloride	1–2 gm/450 kg	IV slowly to effect
Cambendazole	20 mg/kg for *S. westeri*	PO
Captan	3% solution	Topical
Carbenicillin sodium (indanyl ester)	50–80 mg/kg b.i.d. or t.i.d.	IV or IM
	200 mg	Subconj.
Carbon disulfide	24 mg/450 kg	PO
Casein (iodinated)	5 gm s.i.d.	PO
Cefaclor	20–40 mg/kg t.i.d.	PO
Cefadroxil	22 mg/kg b.i.d.	PO
Cefamandole	10–30 mg/kg q. 4–8 h.	IV or IM
Cefataxime sodium	20–30 mg/kg q.i.d.	IV
Cefazolin sodium	15 mg/kg b.i.d. or t.i.d.	IV or IM
	50 mg	Subconj.
Cefixime	400 mg/kg t.i.d.	PO
Cefonicid	10–15 mg/kg s.i.d.	IV or IM
Cefoperazone	30–50 mg/kg b.i.d. or t.i.d.	IV or IM
Ceforanide	5–10 mg/kg b.i.d.	IV or IM
Cefotaxime	25–50 mg/kg b.i.d. to t.i.d.	IV or IM
Cefotetan	15–30 mg/kg b.i.d.	IV or IM
Cefoxitin	30–40 mg/kg t.i.d. or q.i.d.	IM
Ceftazidime	25–50 mg/kg b.i.d.	IV or IM
Ceftiofur	1–2 mg/kg s.i.d. to b.i.d.	IM
Ceftizoxime	25–50 mg/kg b.i.d. or t.i.d.	IV or IM
Ceftriaxone	25–50 mg/kg b.i.d.	IV or IM
Cefuroxime axetil	25–50 mg/kg t.i.d.	IV or IM
	250–500 mg/kg b.i.d.	PO
Cephadroxil	25 mg/kg q. 4–6 h. (foals)	IV
Cephalexin	10–30 mg/kg t.i.d. to q.i.d.	PO
Cephalothin sodium	20–40 mg/kg t.i.d. to q.i.d.	IV or IM
	100 mg	Subconj.
Cephapirin	30 mg/kg q. 4–6 h.	IV or IM
Cephoxitin	20 mg/kg q.i.d.	IV
Charcoal (activated)	1–3 gm/kg as slurry (1 g in 5 ml water), repeat if necessary in 8–12 hours	PO
Chloral hydrate	60–200 mg/kg for foal restraint	IV
	40–100 mg/kg	PO
Chloramphenicol palmitate	4–10 mg/kg t.i.d. or q.i.d. (foal)	PO
	25–50 mg/kg t.i.d. or q.i.d. (adult)	PO
Chloramphenicol succinate	25 mg/kg t.i.d. to q.i.d.	IV or IM
	50–100 mg	Subconj.
Chlorhexidine	0.5%–2%	Topical
Chlorpromazine	1 mg/kg	IM
Cimetidine	6.6 mg/kg q. 4–6 h.	IV or PO
Clenbuterol	0.8–3.2 μg/kg b.i.d.	PO
	0.8 μg/kg b.i.d.	IV
	200 μg for uterine relaxation	IM or Slow IV
Cloxacillin	10–30 mg/kg q.i.d.	IM
Colistin	2,500 U/kg q.i.d.	Slow IV
Corticotropin	1 U/kg	IM
Coumaphos	0.06% wash, 0.1% dust	Topical
Cromolyn sodium	200–300 mg	Insufflated into pharynx
Danthron	15–30 ml/kg	PO
Dantrolene sodium	10 mg/kg loading dose	PO
	2.5 mg/kg q. 2 h. maintenance	PO
	1.9 mg/kg in saline for acute myopathy	Slow IV
	2 mg/kg s.i.d. to prevent myositis	PO

TABLE OF DRUGS: APPROXIMATE DOSES—continued

Drug	Dose	Route
Dembrexine	0.3 mg/kg	PO
Demecarium bromide	0.25% b.i.d.	Ophthalmic
Detomidine	0.005–0.02 mg/kg	IV
	0.01–0.02 mg/kg followed by 0.044–0.066 mg/kg butorphanol	IV
	0.02–0.04 mg/kg followed by 2.2 mg/kg ketamine	IV
Dexamethasone	0.02–0.2 mg/kg s.i.d.	IV, IM, PO
	0.5–2 mg/kg for septic shock	IV
Dexamethasone phosphate suspension	0.1% q. 3–8 h.	Ophthalmic
Dextran (6% solution)	8 gm/kg s.i.d. for up to 3 days	IV
Diazepam	0.05–0.5 mg/kg; repeat in 30 minutes if necessary	Slow IV
Dichlorvos	35 mg/kg	PO
	0.93% solution	Topical
Dicloxacillin	10 mg/kg q.i.d.	IM
Diethylcarbamazine	1 mg/kg s.i.d. for 21 days for onchocerciasis	PO
	50 mg/kg s.i.d. for 10 days for verminous myelitis	PO
Digoxin	0.002 mg/kg b.i.d.	IV
	0.01 mg/kg b.i.d.	PO
Dihydrostreptomycin	11 mg/kg b.i.d.	IM or SC
Dimercaprol	2.5–5 mg/kg as 10% solution in oil q. 4 h. for 2 days, then b.i.d. until recovery	IM
Dimethyl glycine	1–1.6 mg/kg s.i.d.	PO
Dimethyl sulfoxide	0.5 mg/kg to 1.0 gm/kg (10% solution in 5% dextrose); repeat lower doses q. 6–12 h.	IV
	50% solution	Topical
Diminazene	4–5 mg/kg s.i.d.	SC
Dinoprost tromethamine	10 mg/450 kg	IM
Dioctyl sodium sulfosuccinate (DSS) 5% solution	10–20 mg/kg q. 48 h.	PO
	10 ml in warm water as enema for retained meconium	
Dipyrone	5–22 mg/kg	IV or IM
Dioxathion	0.15% wash	Topical
Diphenylhydantoin (phenytoin)	1–10 mg/kg q. 2–4 h.	IV, IM, PO
Dobutamine	1–5 μg/kg/min (250 mg in 500 ml saline infused at 0.45 ml/kg/hr)	IV
Dolophine hydrochloride	0.2–0.4 mg/kg	IM
Domperidone	0.2 mg/kg	IV
Dopamine	1–5 μg/kg/min (200 mg in 500 ml saline infused at 0.45 ml/kg/hr)	IV
Doxapram	0.5–1.0 mg/kg q. 5 min. (do not exceed 2 mg/kg in foals)	IV
	0.02–0.05 mg/kg/min for neonatal foal resuscitation	IV
Doxycycline	3 mg/kg b.i.d.	PO
Ecothiophate iodide	0.03% b.i.d.	Ophthalmic
EDTA calcium disodium	75 mg/kg/day in divided doses for lead poisoning	Slow IV
	6.6% solution (1.1 ml/kg) q. 8–12 h.	IV (see p. 363)
Ephedrine sulfate	0.7 mg/kg b.i.d.	PO
Epinephrine 1:1000	4–8 ml/450 kg	IM or SC
Erythromycin estolate	25 mg/kg b.i.d.	PO
Erythromycin lactobionate	2.5–5 mg/kg t.i.d. or q.i.d.	IV
	20–40 mg	Subconj.
Estradiol	0.004–0.008 mg/kg q. 2 d. for urinary incontinence	IM
Ethyl alcohol (50%)	5–10 ml/50 kg	Aerosol
Ethylenediamine dihydriodide	0.5–1.5 gm/450 kg s.i.d.	PO
Famotidine	4.0 mg/kg t.i.d.	PO
Febantel	6 mg/kg	PO
Fenbendazole	5 mg/kg	PO
	10 mg/kg for *P. equorum*	PO
	50 mg/kg s.i.d. for 3 days for verminous arteritis	PO
	50 mg/kg for *S. westeri*	PO
Fenprostalene	0.5 mg/450 kg	SC
Floxacillin	10 mg/kg q.i.d.	IM
Flumazenil	0.5–2.0 mg	Slow IV
Flumethasone	0.002–0.008 mg/kg	PO
Flunixin meglumine	0.25–1.1 mg/kg s.i.d. to t.i.d.	PO, IM, IV
Fluoroprednisolone acetate	5–20 mg/450 kg	IM
Fluprostenol	250 μg/450 kg	IM
Flurbiprofen sodium	t.i.d. or q.i.d.	Ophthalmic
Folic acid	75 mg (foal)	IM
Follicle-stimulating hormone	10–50 mg/450 kg	IV, IM, SC
Furazolidone	4 mg/kg t.i.d.	PO

Table continued on following page

TABLE OF DRUGS: APPROXIMATE DOSES—*continued*

Drug	Dose	Route
Furosemide	1–3 mg/kg b.i.d.	IV or IM
Gentamicin	2–4 mg/kg b.i.d. to q.i.d.	IV, IM, SC
	10–40 mg	Subconj.
	q. 2–6 h.	Ophthalmic
	150 mg (unbuffered)	IA
Glucagon	25–50 mg/kg	IV
Glycerin	1 gm/kg	PO
Glycerol (5%)	2–5 ml/50 kg	Aerosol
Glycerol guaiacolate	110 mg/kg for convulsions	IV
	0.1–0.2 gm/50 kg q.i.d. (expectorant)	PO
Glycerol	0.5–2 gm/kg for brain edema	IV
Glycopyrolate	0.01 mg/kg	IV
Glycosaminoglycan, polysulfated	250 mg once weekly	IA
	500 mg q. 4 d.	IM
Gonadotropin-releasing hormone	0.05 mg, 2 and 0.5 hours before breeding for low libido	SC
	0.04 mg, 6 hours before breeding to induce ovulation	IM
Griseofulvin	10 gm/450 kg s.i.d. for 2 weeks, then 5 gm/450 kg s.i.d. for 7 weeks	PO
Guaifenesin (5%–10%)	To effect (approx. 110 mg/kg needed for induction)	Slow IV
	5% with 4.4 mg/kg thiamylal	Rapid IV
Heparin	10 U/kg loading dose	IV
	15 U/kg/hr maintenance	Slow IV
	40–100 U/kg b.i.d. or q.i.d. for acute laminitis	IV
	20–90 U/kg for peritonitis prevention	SC
Human chorionic gonadotropin	2,000 IU to synchronize ovulation	IV
Hyaluronate sodium	10–50 mg/joint (see manufacturer's recommendations)	IA
Hyaluronic acid	20–120 mg	Locally around inflamed tendon
Hydralazine	0.5 mg/kg	IV
Hydrochlorothiazide	250 mg/450 kg s.i.d.	PO
Hydrocortisone sodium succinate	1–4 mg/kg	IV Drip
Hydroxyzine hydrochloride	0.5–1 mg/kg b.i.d.	IM or PO
Idoxuridine	q. 4–6 h.	Ophthalmic
Imidocarb diproprionate	2 mg/kg s.i.d. for 2 days for *B. caballi*	IM
	4 mg/kg q. 3 d. for 4 treatments for *B. equi*	IM
Imipramine	100–600 mg b.i.d. for 2 weeks to improve ejaculation	PO
	0.55 mg/kg t.i.d.	IM or IV
	1.5 mg/kg t.i.d.	PO
Indanyl carbenicillin	20–30 mg/kg t.i.d.	PO
Insulin-protamine zinc	0.15 IU/kg b.i.d.	IM or SC
Insulin	0.4 U/kg	IM or SC
Iodide sodium	20–40 mg/kg s.i.d. for several weeks	PO
Iodochlorhydroxyquin	10 gm/450 kg (repeat for 3–4 days, then gradually reduce dose if response obtained)	PO
Iron cacodylate	1 gm	IV
Isoniazid	5–20 mg/kg s.i.d.	PO
Isoproterenol hydrochloride	0.4 µg/kg by slow infusion (discontinue when heart rate doubles)	IV
	0.05–1 µg/kg/min for foal resuscitation	IV
Isoproterenol (0.05%)	5–10 ml/50 kg q.i.d.	Aerosol
Isoxsuprine hydrochloride	0.6–1.8 mg/kg b.i.d.	PO
Itraconazole	3 mg/kg b.i.d. for up to 2 mo.	PO
Ivermectin	0.2 mg/kg	PO
	0.2 mg/kg twice at 4-day intervals for lice and mange	PO
Kanamycin	7.5 mg/kg t.i.d.	IV or IM
Kaopectate	2–4 qt/450 kg b.i.d.	PO
Ketamine	(See xylazine and detomidine)	
Ketoconazole	30 mg/kg s.i.d. or b.i.d. (dissolve in 0.2N HCl)	PO
Levallorphan tartrate	0.02–0.04 mg/kg	IV
Levamisole	8 mg/kg	PO
Levothyroxine	10 mg in 70 ml Karo syrup s.i.d.	PO
Lidocaine	0.5 mg/kg bolus q. 5 min. until 2–4 mg/kg total	IV
Lime sulfur	3%–5%	Topical
Lindane	3% spray	Topical
Loperamide	0.1–0.2 mg/kg q.i.d.	PO
Magnesium sulfate	0.2–1 gm/kg dissolved in 4 L warm water s.i.d.	PO
Magnesium hydroxide (antacid)	200–250 ml t.i.d.	PO

TABLE OF DRUGS: APPROXIMATE DOSES—continued

Drug	Dose	Route
Malathion	0.5% wash, 5% dust	Topical
Mannitol (20%)	0.25–2.0 gm/kg	Slow IV
Mebendazole	8.8 mg/kg	PO
	20 mg/kg s.i.d. for 5 days for *D. arnfieldi*	PO
Meclofenamic acid	2.2 mg/kg b.i.d.	PO
Megestrol acetate	65–85 mg/kg s.i.d.	PO
Meperidine	(See acepromazine)	
Methadone	0.05–0.1 mg/kg	IV
Methetharimide	10–20 mg/kg	IV
Methicillin	25 mg/kg q. 4–6 h.	IM
	100 mg	Subconj.
DL-Methionine	20–50 mg/kg	PO
Methocarbamol	15–25 mg/kg q.i.d.	IV
	40–300 mg/kg for convulsions	
Methoxychlor	0.5% wash	Topical
Methylcellulose flakes	0.25–0.5 kg/450 kg in 10 L water	PO
Methylprednisolone acetate	0.2–0.7 mg/kg	IM
Methylprednisolone sodium succinate	2–4 mg/kg	IV
Methylsulfonylmethane	0.5–1.0 gm/450 kg s.i.d.	PO
Methylsulfmethoxine	30 gm/450 kg s.i.d.	PO
Metoclopramide	0.25 mg/kg t.i.d. or q.i.d.	IV Drip or SC
	0.6 mg/kg q. 4 h.	PO
Metronidazole	15 mg/kg q.i.d.	IV or PO
Mezlocillin	25–75 mg/kg q.i.d.	IV
Miconazole IV (1%)	q. 2–4 h.	Ophthalmic
Mineral oil	10 ml/kg s.i.d.	PO
Minocycline	3 mg/kg b.i.d.	PO
Morphine sulfate	0.2–0.4 mg/kg	IM
	0.02–0.04 mg/kg	IV
Moxalactam	50 mg/kg t.i.d.	IV or IM
Nafcillin	10 mg/kg q.i.d.	IM
Naloxone	0.01–0.02 mg/kg	IV
Naproxen	10 mg/kg s.i.d. or b.i.d.	PO or IV
Natamycin	q. 2–4 h.	Ophthalmic
Neomycin	1 gm q.i.d.	PO
	2 gm b.i.d.	PO
	0.5 gm q.i.d. (foal)	PO
	1.5 gm b.i.d. (foal)	PO
Neostigmine	0.02 mg/kg	SC
Netilmicin	2 mg/kg b.i.d. to t.i.d.	IV or IM
Niclosamide	100 mg/kg	PO
Nitrofurantoin	3 mg/kg b.i.d.	IM
Nizatidine	6.6 mg/kg t.i.d.	PO
Norepinephrine	0.01 mg/kg	IM
Omeprazole	0.5–2 mg/kg s.i.d. or b.i.d.	IV
Ouabain	2.5–3 mg/450 kg q. 2 h. until heart rate slows or intoxication develops; not to exceed 10 gm total	IV
Oxacillin	25–50 mg/kg b.i.d. or t.i.d.	IV or IM
Oxfendazole	10 mg/kg	PO
Oxibendazole	10–15 mg/kg	PO
	15 mg/kg for *S. westeri*	PO
Oxymorphone	0.02–0.03 mg/kg	IM or IV
Oxytetracycline	10–20 mg/kg s.i.d.	IV
Oxytocin	2.5–5 U/450 kg as bolus q. 20 min.	IV
	80–100 U in 500 ml saline	Slow IV
	20–150 U/450 kg	IM
	1–3 U/450 kg for milk letdown	IV
Pancuronium	0.04–0.066 mg/kg	IV
Penicillamine D	3–4 mg/kg q.i.d. for 10 days	PO
Penicillin G procaine	20,000–50,000 IU/kg b.i.d. or t.i.d.	IM
Penicillin G benzathine	10,000–40,000 IU/kg q. 48–72 h.	IM
Penicillin sodium	10,000–50,000 IU/kg q.i.d.	IV or IM
Penicillin K	10,000–50,000 IU/kg q.i.d.	IV or IM
	20,000 IU/kg q.i.d.	PO
Penicillin V	110,000 mg/kg b.i.d. to q.i.d.	PO
Pentazocine	0.8 mg/kg	IV
Pentobarbital	2–20 mg/kg for convulsions	IV

Table continued on following page

Drug	Dose	Route
Pentosan sulfate	250 mg q. 7–10 d.	IA
Pentoxylline	7 mg/kg s.i.d.	PO
Pentylenetetrazol	6–10 mg/kg	IV
Perphenazine	0.5 mg/kg s.i.d.	PO
Phenobarbital	5–25 mg/kg in 30 ml saline for convulsing foals	IV over 30 min
	9 mg/kg t.i.d. for maintenance	IV
Phenothiazine	55 mg/kg	PO
	27.5 mg/kg with piperazine	PO
Phenoxybenzamine hydrochloride	0.7–1 mg/kg in 500 ml saline t.i.d. or q.i.d.	IV
Phenylbutazone	2–4.4 mg/kg s.i.d. or b.i.d.	PO or IV
Phenylephrine	10%	Ophthalmic
Phenytoin	5–10 mg/kg for convulsing foals	IV
	1–5 mg/kg q. 4 h. for maintenance	IV, IM, PO
	10–22 mg/kg b.i.d. for digoxin-induced arrhythmias	PO
Physostigmine	0.1–0.6 mg/kg	IM or Slow IV
Pilocarpine hydrochloride	4% gel b.i.d. to q.i.d.	Ophthalmic
Piperazine	88–110 mg/kg	PO
Pipercillin	15–50 mg/kg b.i.d. to q.i.d.	IV or IM
Polymixin B or E	10,000 U/kg q.i.d.	PO
Potassium chloride	40 gm in 4–6 L water b.i.d.	PO
Potassium iodide	1 gm/50 kg q.i.d.	PO
Potassium permanganate	1% solution for mouthwash	
Pralidoxime chloride	20–50 mg/kg (20 mg/ml)	Slow IV or IM
Prednisolone acetate	1% q. 3–8 h.	Ophthalmic
Prednisolone sodium succinate	0.2–3 mg/kg s.i.d. or b.i.d.	PO or IM
	2–5 mg/kg for septic shock	IV
Prednisone	0.02–1.0 mg/kg b.i.d.	IM
Primidone	1–2 gm b.i.d. to q.i.d. (foal)	PO
Progesterone	150 mg s.i.d. to suppress estrus	IM
	300 mg s.i.d. to maintain pregnancy (see p. 637 for synchronization of ovulation)	
repositol	1000 mg/450 kg once weekly for abortion prevention	IM
Promazine	0.5–1 mg/kg	IV
	1–2 mg/kg granules	PO
Propantheline bromide	0.014 mg/kg	IV
Proparacaine	0.5%	Ophthalmic
Propranolol	0.38–0.78 mg/kg t.i.d.	PO
	0.05–0.16 mg/kg b.i.d.	IV
Propylene glycol (5%)	3 ml/50 kg	Aerosol
Prostaglandin F$_{2\alpha}$	10 mg to short-cycle mares	IM
Prostalene	2 mg/450 kg, 2 doses 2 weeks apart	SC
Psyllium mucilloid	1 gm/kg s.i.d. to q.i.d.	PO
Pyrantel pamoate	6.6 mg/kg	PO
	13.2 mg/kg for tapeworms	PO
Pyrantel tartrate	2.64 mg/kg s.i.d. for control of intestinal nematodes	PO
Pyrilamine maleate	1 mg/kg	IV, IM, SC
Pyrimethamine	0.25 mg/kg b.i.d. for 3 days, then s.i.d. for 27 days (for equine protozoal myeloencephalitis)	PO
Quinidine sulfate	0.02 mg/kg q. 2–6 h.	PO
gluconate	2.2 mg/kg q. 10 min. until 8–10 mg/kg total	IV
	0.064% solution, 0.5–2 L/hr	
Ranitidine	6.6 mg/kg t.i.d.	IV or PO
Rifampin	10–20 mg/kg s.i.d.	PO
	3–5 mg/kg b.i.d. with erythromycin for R. equi	PO
Ronnel	2.5% spray	Topical
Saline (hypertonic)	7.5%, 4 ml/kg for hypovolemia	IV over 20 min
Selenium (Sodium selenite)	5.5 mg/450 kg	IM
Sodium bicarbonate	30 gm b.i.d.	PO
Sodium hypochlorite	0.5%	Topical
Sodium iodide	20–40 mg/kg s.i.d.	PO
Sodium sulfate	1 gm/kg dissolved in warm water	PO
Sodium thiosulfate (20%)	0.22 ml/kg	Slow IV
Spectinomycin	20 mg/kg t.i.d.	IM
Stanozolol	0.5 mg/kg, up to 4 doses q. 1–2 wk.	IM
Stilbestrol	30 mg/450 kg	IM
Stirofos	1% wash	Topical
Streptomycin	11 mg/kg b.i.d.	IM or SC

TABLE OF DRUGS: APPROXIMATE DOSES—*continued*

Drug	Dose	Route
Sucralfate	2–4 gm/450 kg b.i.d. to q.i.d.	PO
Sulfonamides	100–200 mg/kg on day 1, 50–100 mg/kg subsequently (check labels on each product)	IV, IM, SC
Sulfonamides, potentiated	30 mg/kg b.i.d. or t.i.d.	PO
Terbutaline	0.02–0.06 mg/kg b.i.d.	IV
Tetanus antitoxin	100 IU/kg q. 3–5 d. for therapy	IM, SC, IV
Tetracycline	6.6–11 mg/kg b.i.d.	IV
Tetramethrin	0.4% solution, wipe-on	Topical
Theophylline	1 mg/kg q.i.d.	PO
Thiabendazole	44 mg/kg	PO
	88 mg/kg for *P. equorum*	PO
	440 mg/kg s.i.d. for 2 days for verminous arteritis	PO
	4% solution in saline or 90% DMSO	Topical
Thiamine hydrochloride	0.5–5 mg/kg	IM
Thiamylal sodium	2–4 mg/kg	IV
Thiopental	8–12 mg/kg	IV
Thyroxine (1)	0.01 mg/kg s.i.d.	PO
Ticarcillin	40–80 mg/kg t.i.d.	IV or IM
Timolol maleate	0.5% b.i.d.	Ophthalmic
Tobramycin	1–1.7 mg/kg t.i.d. (human dose)	IV or IM
	10–30 mg	Subconj.
Tocopherol acetate	6,000 IU/250–500 kg s.i.d.	PO
Toxaphene	0.5% wash	Topical
Triamcinolone	0.02–0.1 mg/kg	IM
	(40 mg/ml), 0.25 ml, q. 2–4 d.	Subconj.
Trichlorfon	40 mg/kg	PO
Trichlormethiazide	200 mg/450 kg	PO
Triflupromazine	0.2–2.0 mg/kg	IV
Trifluridine	q. 2–3 h.	Ophthalmic
Trimethoprim–sulfadiazine	15 mg/kg b.i.d.	IV
	15–30 mg/kg b.i.d.	PO
	2.5–5 gm s.i.d.	Intrauterine
Tromethamine	300 mg/kg	IV
Tripelennamine hydrochloride	1 mg/kg b.i.d. to t.i.d.	IV or IM
Tropicamide	0.5%–1%	Ophthalmic
Tylosin	10 mg/kg b.i.d.	IM
Vancomycin	20–40 mg/kg b.i.d. to q.i.d.	IV or PO
Vinegar	250 ml/450 kg s.i.d. for enterolith prevention	PO
Vitamin E	1500–2000 IU s.i.d. (foal)	PO
Vitamin K_1	0.5–1 mg/kg q. 4–6 h. for warfarin toxicosis	SC
	1–2 mg/kg (divided at several sites) for sweet clover poisoning	SC
	0.5–2 mg/kg (foals)	IM
Warfarin	Begin with 0.018 mg/kg s.i.d. (see p. 153)	PO
Xylazine	0.2–1.1 mg/kg	IV
	0.33–0.44 mg/kg followed by 0.033–0.066 mg/kg butorphanol	IV
	1.1 mg/kg followed by 1.76–2.2 mg/kg ketamine	IV
	0.6 mg/kg with 0.02 mg/kg acepromazine	IV
	0.66 mg/kg to ejaculate ex-copula	IV
Yohimbine	0.12 mg/kg for xylazine or detomidine antagonism	Slow IV
	0.075 mg/kg to restore intestinal motility	IV

NOTE—This table was composed from doses recommended by authors in this and previous editions of *Current Therapy in Equine Medicine*. It is recommended that the manufacturer's literature be checked before a drug is used. Many drugs have not been approved for use in horses. IA = intra-articular, IM = intramuscular, IV = intravenous, PO = per os, SC = subcutaneous.

Clinical Pathology Data

Desmond P. Leadon, NAAS, IRELAND

Differential diagnosis is fundamental to the successful practice of veterinary medicine. History taking and clinical examination are essential to diagnosis and can never be replaced by the submission of samples for laboratory examination. Those who attempt this substitution will inevitably be disappointed in the quality of the service available to their practice and to their clients from the diagnostic laboratory. Laboratory data of good quality, used in the appropriate context, can be enormously useful in narrowing the differential diagnosis, confirming the diagnosis, suggesting a prognosis, and assessing response to therapy. The usefulness of laboratory data is heavily dependent on various factors, including appropriate sampling, sample handling, laboratory methodology and quality control, test selection, and subsequent interpretation. Some important features of these factors are outlined below.

SAMPLING

Timing of sample collection and the method of restraint are important considerations in equine blood sampling. In cases of overt clinical disease, the most important consideration is pretreatment sampling. This is obviously of primary importance in fluid and electrolyte therapy and blood culture. Pre-exercise sampling may be essential in the investigation of subclinical disease entities, such as those that may contribute to poor or reduced performance in competition or racehorses. Minimal restraint is essential if the effects of splenic contraction on blood composition are to be avoided.

Venous blood is usually collected from the jugular vein in foals and adult horses. In animals in which occlusion of the jugular veins has occurred, the lateral thoracic vein is usually an appropriate alternative. It is prudent, in an era of ever-increasing litigation, to prepare the site of venous or arterial puncture using an alcohol or other bactericidal impregnated swab. This procedure is clearly vital if blood culture is to be carried out. An 18- or 20-gauge, 1.5-inch-long needle is usually used for the collection of venous blood samples, either into a syringe for subsequent transfer to other containers or, alternatively, using an evacuated tube system. Evacuated tube systems for venous blood collection are usually color coded and labeled to illustrate their usage, as outlined in Table 1.

Color-coding systems for nonevacuated containers may differ from those used in evacuated systems. If artifacts due to inappropriate blood-to-anticoagulant ratio are to be avoided, proper filling of the sample tube to the level indicated by the manufacturer must be achieved in both systems. Thorough mixing of the blood sample and anticoagulant is essential.

Arterial blood gas estimations are useful in the assessment of pulmonary function in the adult horse, essential to equine neonatal intensive care, and of considerable value in many other clinical situations. In adult horses, arterial blood samples may be obtained from the facial, carotid, or great metatarsal arteries. In foals, samples are taken from the great metatarsal, brachial, radial, carotid, or facial arteries. Arterial blood should be collected into a preheparinized syringe or arterial blood sampler.

Blood culture is of particular value in the diagnosis and treatment of septicemia, especially in the neonate and, perhaps somewhat surprisingly, in the confirmation of a diagnosis of *Rhodococcus equi* infection in a limited number of foals. Several blood culture systems are commercially available. Some require separate blood culture bottles for aerobic and anaerobic culture. Others are suitable for both.

TABLE 1. COLOR CODES AND USE OF VENOUS BLOOD EVACUATION CONTAINER SYSTEMS

Stopper Color	Tube Contents	Use
Violet	EDTA	Hematology
Blue	Sodium citrate (3.8%)	Fibrinogen (Clauss method) and coagulation studies
Black	Sodium citrate (3.1%)	Erythrocyte sedimentation rate
Gray	Sodium fluoride, potassium oxalate	Glucose
Red	Plain (no anticoagulant)	Serum biochemistry
Green	Lithium heparin	Plasma endocrinology; fibrinogen (heat precipitation method)

SAMPLE HANDLING

All samples should be analyzed as soon as possible. In serum and plasma samples left at room temperature, changes in soft tissue enzymes, electrolytes, and glucose levels occur within an hour or so of collection. Neutrophil counts become unreliable within a few hours of collection of EDTA samples. Insulated containers are inexpensive and should be included, with a supply of crushed ice, in the equipment routinely carried by those in veterinary clinical practice. This equipment is essential if extremes of heat are likely or if the pattern of calls prevents regular return to the veterinary practice.

Blood films or cytological smears can readily be prepared and fixed on glass slides using any one of the many commercially available fixative aerosols. A small, light, portable centrifuge (hand or electrically operated) is another valuable item of practice equipment if long-distance travel is an essential feature of the working day. Although separation of plasma is achieved easily in equine blood samples under the influence of gravity, the time gained by centrifugation is valuable and the few minutes necessary for this procedure can be a valuable investment for both the client and the practice. To ensure optimal clot formation and retraction, serum samples should be collected into glass containers rather than plastic ones. Serum should always be permitted to clot before refrigeration or cold storage, and again, separation and storage are advantageous.

LABORATORY METHODS

Clinical pathology studies can be conducted at a basic but nevertheless useful level on the premises where the horse or horses are kept, at a practice laboratory, or at some form of referral laboratory. The results obtained from each of these three distinct sources of information are seldom directly comparable, due to differences in methods and equipment. There is, for example, little point in comparing serum aspartate transaminase and creatine kinase values obtained from a horse with rhabdomyolysis on day 1 using a dry chemistry system with those obtained on day 2 in a practice laboratory that uses a spectrophotometer and those obtained on day 3 in a referral laboratory in which an automated multichannel analyzer is used. These different items of equipment result in different normal value ranges. Furthermore, different analytic methods may be used by different laboratories, even where identical equipment is installed. It is therefore essential to be familiar with the normal ranges used by the specific laboratory to which the clinical pathology samples are submitted.

Sources of potential error within the laboratory must also be taken into account. Commercial referral and the more substantial practice laboratories will all incorporate quality control procedures into their daily work outline. Quality control systems are used to control the day-to-day variation in results that occurs from instrument-related error. Quality control is important not only in the relatively sophisticated laboratory but also in the simple procedures that can be carried out elsewhere. The need for quality control is not confined to biochemistry analyzers. Many veterinarians now own or have access to cell counters. These instruments are also subject to drift and error and should be included in a quality assurance program from a referral source of acknowledged status, on a regular, planned basis.

TEST SELECTION

Seldom is there a comprehensive set of tests to assist with the diagnosis of specific disease entities; economic considerations usually must be taken into account as well. Hematology is often included in clinical pathology examinations in cases of infection, parasitism, anemia, and clotting disorders. Serum biochemistry studies can assist in the investigation of infection, parasitism, inflammation, and specific organ and multiorgan dysfunction. Blood gas analysis is valuable in the management of pulmonary disorders and metabolic disorders. A combination of hematology and serum biochemistry in the investigation of systemic disease may often provide a deeper insight into the disease process than the use of either alone. Investigation of particular organ systems may require the use of more specific techniques; for example, respiratory disease may be better evaluated with transtracheal aspiration or bronchoalveolar lavage specimens than with hematology and serum biochemistry studies. Urinalysis and creatinine clearance studies may be more valuable in cases of urinary tract disease than measurement of serum urea and creatinine levels.

INTERPRETATION

The interpretation of laboratory data in a diagnostic context is based on the concept of a normal range for hematological and biochemical measurements. Normal ranges for these and other clinical pathology data are usually recorded as a mean ± 2 SD. It is essential to bear in mind that this will result in the exclusion of 5 per cent of individuals or samples from the normal range, i.e., 2.5 per cent of normal individuals will be beyond the upper limit and 2.5 per cent of normal individuals will be below the lower limit. It can be extremely difficult to be certain that a single value in a single sample from a horse that is presented to a clinician for the first time is a reliable indicator of disease. It is also important to realize that even values within the normal range may be abnormal for some individuals. Clinical signs and other laboratory results with, where necessary, further diagnostic techniques such as radiography or other forms of imaging are thus indispensable. Other laboratory results also must be interpreted with caution, as the statistical probability of obtaining an abnormal value increases with the number of laboratory tests performed, and serum enzyme values have a skewed, not a normal, distribution.

Interpretation of laboratory data is therefore an art as well as a science. Although a series of normal values that have been derived from a variety of sources appears below, these data should be taken to provide approximate guidelines, not absolute diagnostic criteria.

Supplemental Readings

Bauer, J. E.: Normal blood chemistry. *In* Koterba A. M., Drummond W. H., and Kosch, P. C. (eds.): Equine Clinical Neonatology. Philadelphia, Lea & Febiger, 1990, pp. 602–614.

Blackmore, D. J., and Brobst, D.: Biochemical Values in Equine Medicine. Newmarket, England, Animal Health Trust, 1981.

Brewer, B. D.: Renal disease. *In* Koterba A. M., Drummond W. H., and Kosch P. C. (eds.): Equine Clinical Neonatology. Philadelphia, Lea & Febiger, 1990, pp. 446–461.

Brobst, D. F., and Parry, B. W.: Normal Clinical Pathology Data. *In* Robinson, N. E. (ed.): Current Therapy in Equine Medicine 2. Philadelphia, W. B. Saunders, 1987, pp. 725–729.

Coffman, J. R.: Equine Clinical Chemistry and Pathophysiology. Bonner Springs, Kansas, Veterinary Publishing Co., 1981.

Cohn, C. W., and Chew, D. J.: Laboratory Diagnosis and Characterization of Renal Disease in Horses. Vet. Clin. North Am. (Equine Pract.), 3:585, 1987.

Fogarty, U., and Leadon, D.: "Poor Performance" syndrome: A review of the literature and some data on the haematological and blood biochemical changes in two groups of thoroughbred horses performing below expectation. Ir. Vet. J., 41:203, 1987.

Harvey, J. W.: Normal Hematologic Values. *In* Koterba, A. M., Drummond, W. H., and Kosch, P. C. (eds.): Equine Clinical Neonatology. Philadelphia, Lea & Febiger, 1990, pp. 561–570.

Jain, N. C.: The horse: Normal hematology with comments on response to disease. *In* Schalm's Veterinary Hematology, 4th ed. Philadelphia, Lea & Febiger, 1986, pp. 140–177.

Mayhew, I. G.: Large Animal Neurology. Philadelphia, Lea & Febiger, 1989, pp. 49–55.

Ricketts, S. W.: The laboratory as an aid to clinical diagnosis. *In* Vet. Clin. North Am. (Equine Pract.) 3:445, 1987.

Rose, R. J., Rossdale, P. D., and Leadon, D. P.: Blood gas and acid-base status in spontaneously delivered, term induced and induced premature foals. J. Reprod. Fertl. Suppl., 32:521, 1982.

Rossdale, P. D., Falk, M., Jeffcott, L. B., Palmer, A. C., and Ricketts, S. W.: A preliminary investigation of cerebrospinal fluid in the newborn foal as an aid to the study of cerebral damage. J. Reprod. Fertil. Suppl., 27:593, 1979.

TABLE 2. HEMATOLOGY VALUES—RED BLOOD CELLS OF NEONATAL FOALS

Parameter	Age	Range	Units	Source
Red cell count	<12 hours	9.0–12.0	$\times 10^6/\mu l$	Harvey, 1990
	1 day	9.2–11.0	$\times 10^6/\mu l$	Harvey, 1990
	<36 hours	7.8–11.9	$\times 10^6/\mu l$	Ricketts, 1987
	3 days	7.8–11.4	$\times 10^6/\mu l$	Harvey, 1990
Packed cell volume	<12 hours	37–49	%	Harvey, 1990
	1 day	34–46	%	Harvey, 1990
	<36 hours	0.31–0.45	L/L	Ricketts, 1987
	3 days	30–46	%	Harvey, 1990
Hemoglobin	<12 hours	12.6–17.4	gm/dl	Harvey, 1990
	1 day	12.0–16.6	gm/dl	Harvey, 1990
	<36 hours	11.6–14.6	gm/dl	Ricketts, 1987
	3 days	11.5–16.7	gm/dl	Harvey, 1990
Mean corpuscular (cell) volume	<12 hours	36–45	fl	Harvey, 1990
	1 day	36–46	fl	Harvey, 1990
	<36 hours	31.7–41.5	fl	Ricketts, 1987
	3 days	35–44	fl	Harvey, 1990
Mean corpuscular (cell) hemoglobin concentration	<12 hours	32–40	gm/dl	Harvey, 1990
	1 day	32–40	gm/dl	Harvey, 1990
	<36 hours	31.0–36.6	gm/dl	Ricketts, 1987
	3 days	34–40	gm/dl	Harvey, 1990

TABLE 3. HEMATOLOGY VALUES—WHITE BLOOD CELLS OF NEONATAL FOALS

Parameter	Age	Range	Units	Source
White cell count	<12 hours	6.9–14.4	$\times 10^3/\mu l$	Harvey, 1990
	1 day	4.9–11.7	$\times 10^3/\mu l$	Harvey, 1990
	<36 hours	3.7–12.1	$\times 10^3/\mu l$	Ricketts, 1987
	3 days	5.1–10.1	$\times 10^3/\mu l$	Harvey, 1990
Neutrophils (segmented)	<12 hours	5.55–12.38	$\times 10^3/\mu l$	Harvey, 1990
	1 day	3.36–9.57	$\times 10^3/\mu l$	Harvey, 1990
	<36 hours	51–91	%	Ricketts, 1987
	3 days	3.21–8.58	$\times 10^3/\mu l$	Harvey, 1990
Lymphocytes	<12 hours	0.46–2.54	$\times 10^3/\mu l$	Harvey, 1990
	1 day	0.67–2.12	$\times 10^3/\mu l$	Harvey, 1990
	<36 hours	10–30	%	Ricketts, 1987
	3 days	0.73–2.17	$\times 10^3/\mu l$	Harvey, 1990
Monocytes	<12 hours	0.04–0.43	$\times 10^3/\mu l$	Harvey, 1990
	1 day	0.07–0.39	$\times 10^3/\mu l$	Harvey, 1990
	<36 hours	0–3	%	Ricketts, 1987
	3 days	0.08–0.58	$\times 10^3/\mu l$	Harvey, 1990

TABLE 4. BLOOD BIOCHEMISTRY VALUES—NEONATAL FOALS

Parameter	Age	Range	Units		Source
Total protein	<12 hours	4.0–7.9	gm/dl	Serum	Bauer, 1990
	<12 hours	5.1–7.6	gm/dl	Plasma	Harvey, 1990
	1 day	5.2–8.0	gm/dl	Plasma	Harvey, 1990
	<36 hours	31–59	gm/dl	Serum	Ricketts, 1987
	3 days	5.3–7.9	gm/dl	Plasma	Harvey, 1990
Albumin	<12 hours	2.7–3.9	gm/dl	Serum	Bauer, 1990
	1 day	2.5–3.6	gm/dl	Serum	Bauer, 1990
	<36 hours	17–33	gm/dl	Serum	Ricketts, 1987
	3 days	2.8–3.7	gm/dl	Serum	Bauer, 1990
Globulin	<12 hours	1.1–4.8	gm/dl	Serum	Bauer, 1990
	1 day	1.5–4.6	gm/dl	Serum	Bauer, 1990
	<36 hours	8–32	gm/dl	Serum	Ricketts, 1987
	3 days	1.6–4.5	gm/dl	Serum	Bauer, 1990
Fibrinogen	<12 hours	100–350	mg/dl	Plasma	Harvey, 1990
	1 day	100–400	mg/dl	Plasma	Harvey, 1990
	1 day	104–389	mg/dl	Plasma	Bauer, 1990
	<36 hours	0.5–6.0	gm/L	Plasma	Ricketts, 1990
	<36 hours	0.9–1.4	gm/L	Coagulometry (citrated plasma)	Leadon (unpublished)
	3 days	150–500	mg/dl	Plasma	Harvey, 1990
Creatine kinase	<12 hours	65–380	IU/L	Serum	Bauer, 1990
	1 day	40–909	IU/L	Serum	Bauer, 1990
	<36 hours	20–107	IU/L	Serum	Ricketts, 1987
	3 days	21–97	IU/L	Serum	Bauer, 1990
Aspartate aminotransferase	<12 hours	97–315	IU/L	Serum	Bauer, 1990
	1 day	146–340	IU/L	Serum	Bauer, 1990
	<36 hours	30–130	IU/L	Serum	Ricketts, 1987
	3 days	80–580	IU/L	Serum	Bauer, 1990
Glucose	<12 hours	108–190	mg/dl	Serum	Bauer, 1990
	1 day	121–233	mg/dl	Serum	Bauer, 1990
	<36 hours	1.1–5.1	mmol/L	Serum	Ricketts, 1987
	3 days	101–226	mg/dl	Serum	Bauer, 1990
Bilirubin (Total)	<12 hours	0.9–2.8	mg/dl	Serum	Bauer, 1990
	1 day	1.3–4.5	mg/dl	Serum	Bauer, 1990
	<36 hours	16–94	μmol/l	Serum	Ricketts, 1987
	3 days	0.5–3.9	mg/dl	Serum	Bauer, 1990
Urea	<12 hours	12–27	mg/dl	Serum	Bauer, 1990
	1 day	9–40	mg/dl	Serum	Bauer, 1990
	<36 hours	4.3–9.3	mmol/l	Serum	Ricketts, 1987

Table continued on following page

TABLE 4. BLOOD BIOCHEMISTRY VALUES—NEONATAL FOALS—Continued

Parameter	Age	Range	Units		Source
Creatinine	3 days	2–29	mg/dl	Serum	Bauer, 1990
	<12 hours	1.7–4.2	mg/dl	Serum	Bauer, 1990
	1 day	1.2–4.3	mg/dl	Serum	Bauer, 1990
	<36 hours	98–252	μmol/L	Serum	Ricketts, 1987
	3 days	0.4–2.1	mg/dl	Serum	Bauer, 1990
Sodium	<12 hours	133–163	mEq/L	Serum	Bauer, 1990
	1 day	123–159	mEq/L	Serum	Bauer, 1990
	<36 hours	126–146	mmol/L	Serum	Ricketts, 1987
	3 days	123–161	mEq/L	Serum	Bauer, 1990
Potassium	<12 hours	3.4–5.4	mEq/l	Serum	Bauer, 1990
	1 day	3.6–5.6	mEq/l	Serum	Bauer, 1990
	<36 hours	3.7–5.4	mmol/L	Serum	Ricketts, 1987
	3 days	3.4–5.2	mEq/L	Serum	Bauer, 1990
Chloride	<12 hours	93–117	mEq/L	Serum	Bauer, 1990
	1 day	90–114	mEq/L	Serum	Bauer, 1990
	<36 hours	100–108	mmol/L	Serum	Ricketts, 1987
	3 days	90–112	mEq/L	Serum	Bauer, 1990

TABLE 5. HEMATOLOGY VALUES—RED BLOOD CELLS OF ADULT HORSES

Parameter	Range	Units	Source
Red blood cells	6.8–12.9	$\times 10^6/\mu l$	Jain, 1986
	6.5–12.3	$\times 10^6/\mu l$	Ricketts, 1987
Packed cell volume	32–53	%	Jain, 1986
	0.33–0.49	L/L	Ricketts, 1987
Hemoglobin	11.0–19.0	gm/dl	Jain, 1986
	11.2–16.2	gm/dl	Ricketts, 1987
Mean corpuscular (cell) volume	37.0–58.5	fl	Jain, 1986
	36.2–49.3	fl	Ricketts, 1987
Mean corpuscular (cell) hemoglobin content	31.0–38.6	%	Jain, 1986
	29.9–36.7	gm/dl	Ricketts, 1987

TABLE 6. HEMATOLOGY VALUES—WHITE BLOOD CELLS OF ADULT HORSES

Parameter	Range	Units	Source
White blood cells	5,400–14,300	$\times 10^3/\mu L$	Jain, 1986
	3.7–11.3	$\times 10^3/\mu L$	Ricketts, 1987
	6.6–10.8	$\times 10^3/\mu L$	Fogarty and Leadon, 1987
Neutrophils (segmented)	22–72	%	Jain, 1986
	39–71	%	Ricketts, 1987
	44–74	%	Fogarty and Leadon, 1987
Lymphocytes	17–68	%	Jain, 1986
	27–59	%	Ricketts, 1987
	26–51	%	Fogarty and Leadon, 1987
Monocytes	0–14	%	Jain, 1986
	0–4	%	Ricketts, 1987
	0–2	%	Fogarty and Leadon, 1987
Eosinophils	0–10	%	Jain, 1986
	0–3	%	Ricketts, 1987
	0–3	%	Fogarty and Leadon, 1987

TABLE 7. BLOOD BIOCHEMISTRY VALUES—ADULT HORSES

Parameter	Range	Units	Source	
Total protein	47–67	gm/L	Serum	Ricketts, 1987
	50–68	gm/L	Serum	Fogarty and Leadon, 1987
	5.5–7.9	gm/dl	Serum	Bauer, 1990
Albumin	27–40	gm/L	Serum	Ricketts, 1987
	25–38.5	gm/L	Serum	Fogarty and Leadon, 1987
	2.8–4.8	gm/dl	Serum	Bauer, 1990
Globulin	17–34	gm/L	Serum	Ricketts, 1987
	20.7–36.1	gm/L	Serum	Fogarty and Leadon, 1987
	1.9–3.8	gm/dl	Serum	Bauer, 1990
Fibrinogen	0.5–4.0	gm/L	Plasma	Ricketts, 1987
	1.2–1.5	gm/L	Coagulometry (citrated plasma)	Fogarty and Leadon, 1987
	100–600	mg/dl	Plasma	Harvey, 1990
Creatine kinase	50–150	IU/L	Serum	Ricketts, 1987
	23–220	IU/L	Serum	Fogarty and Leadon, 1987
	69–272	IU/L	Serum	Bauer, 1990
Aspartate aminotransferase	70–250	IU/L	Serum	Ricketts, 1987
	101–290	IU/L	Serum	Fogarty and Leadon, 1987
	149–267	IU/L	Serum	Bauer, 1990
Bilirubin (Total)	12–39	μmol/L	Serum	Ricketts, 1987
	0.5–1.8	mg/ml	Serum	Bauer, 1990
Urea	3.5–7.3	mmol/L	Serum	Ricketts, 1987
	12–24	mg/dl	Serum	Bauer, 1990
Creatinine	90–200	μmol/L	Serum	Ricketts, 1987
	0.9–2.0	mg/dl	Serum	Bauer, 1990
Sodium	134–143	mmol/L	Serum	Ricketts, 1987
	131–147	mEq/L	Serum	Bauer, 1990
Potassium	3.3–5.3	mmol/L	Serum	Ricketts, 1987
	3.2–5.2	mEq/L	Serum	Bauer, 1990
Chloride	89–106	mmol/L	Serum	Ricketts, 1987
	95–107	mEq/L	Serum	Bauer, 1990

TABLE 8. ARTERIAL BLOOD GAS/ACID–BASE VALUES

Parameter	Age	Value	Units	Source
pH	Foals 1–12 hours	7.378 ± 0.011	pHa	Rose et al., 1982
	Foals 12–48 hours	7.374 ± 0.004	pHa	Rose et al., 1982
	Foals 2–7 days	7.384 ± 0.014	pHa	Rose et al., 1982
	Adults	7.411 ± 0.032	pHa	Blackmore and Brobst, 1981
Pa_{CO2}	Foals 1–12 hours	42.2 ± 1.8	mm Hg	Rose et al., 1982
	Foals 12–48 hours	44.5 ± 1.2	mm Hg	Rose et al., 1982
	Foals 2–7 days	42.4 ± 1.0	mm Hg	Rose et al., 1982
	Adults	5.43 ± 0.35	KPa	Blackmore and Brobst, 1981
Pa_{O2}	Foals 1–12 hours	77.3 ± 3.1	mm Hg	Rose et al., 1982
	Foals 12–48 hours	83.2 ± 3.1	mm Hg	Rose et al., 1982
	Foals 2–7 days	88.2 ± 5.9	mm Hg	Rose et al., 1982
	Adults	12.8 ± 1.06	KPa	Blackmore and Brobst, 1981
Base excess	Foals 1–12 hours	−0.3 ± 1.2	mmol/L	Rose et al., 1982
	Foals 12–48 hours	0.4 ± 0.5	mmol/L	Rose et al., 1982
	Foals 2–7 days	−0.2 ± 1.1	mmol/L	Rose et al., 1982
	Adults	1.1 ± 1.4	mmol/L	Blackmore and Brobst, 1981

TABLE 9. URINALYSIS AND CREATININE CLEARANCE RATIOS

Parameter	Age	Value	Units	Source
pH (urine)	Foal (neonatal)	5.5–8.0		Brewer, 1990
	Adults	7.5–8.5		Cohn and Chew, 1987
Specific gravity (urine)	Foals (neonatal)	1.001–1.027		Brewer, 1990
	Adults	1.008–1.012		Coffman, 1981
Creatinine clearance ratios				
Na^+	Foal (neonatal)	0.31 ± 0.18	%	Brewer, 1990
	Adult	0.02–1.0	%	Ricketts, 1987
K^+	Foal (neonatal)	13.26 ± 4.49	%	Brewer, 1990
	Adult	15–65	%	Ricketts, 1987
Cl^-	Foal (neonatal)	0.42 ± 0.32	%	Brewer, 1990
	Adult	0.04–1.6	%	Ricketts, 1987
PO_4^-	Foal (neonatal)	3.11 ± 3.81	%	Brewer, 1990
	Adult	0–9	%	Ricketts, 1987

TABLE 10. CEREBROSPINAL FLUID VALUES

Parameter	Age	Value	Units	Source
Appearance	Foals	Clear	—	Rossdale et al., 1982
	Foals	Xanthochromia (slight)	—	Mayhew, 1989
	Adults	Clear	—	Brobst and Parry, 1987
Red blood cells	Foals	<500	per μl	Rossdale et al., 1982
	Foals	0	per μl	Mayhew, 1989
White blood cells	Foals	<5	per μl	Rossdale et al., 1982
	Adults	<8	per μl	
	Adults	<6	per μl	Mayhew, 1989
Total protein	Foals	100	mg/dl	Rossdale et al., 1982
	Adults	32–48	mg/dl	Brobst and Parry, 1987
Creatine kinase	Foals	5.2–9.2	IU/L	Rossdale et al., 1982
	Adults	0–8	IU/L	Blackmore and Brobst, 1981
Na^+	Foals	142.6 ± 2.8	mmol/L	Rossdale et al., 1982
	Adults	140–150	mmol/L	Blackmore and Brobst, 1981
K^+	Foals	3.6 ± 2.1	mmol/L	Rossdale et al., 1982
	Adults	2.5–3.5	mmol/L	Blackmore and Brobst, 1981
Cl^-	Foals	109 ± 3.4	mmol/L	Rossdale et al., 1982
	Adults	95–123	mmol/L	Blackmore and Brobst, 1981

TABLE 11. OTHER BODY FLUID VALUES

Fluid	Parameter	Value	Units	Source
Synovial fluid	Appearance	Viscous		
		Clear		
		Yellow		
	Cell count	0.2–0.9	$\times 10^9$/L	Blackmore and Brobst, 1981
		<500 (nucleated)	cells/μl	Brobst and Parry, 1987
	Total protein	8.3 ± 2.7	gm/L	Blackmore and Brobst, 1981
		0.6–2.0	gm/dl	Brobst and Parry, 1987
Peritoneal fluid	Appearance	Clear/yellow		
	Cell count	0.2–9.0	$\times 10^9$/L	Blackmore and Brobst, 1981
		2.0–4.0	$\times 10^3$/μl	Brobst and Parry, 1987
	Total protein	1–34	gm/L	Blackmore and Brobst, 1981
		0.7–2.0	gm/dl	Brobst and Parry, 1987
Pleural fluid	Appearance	Clear/yellow		
	Cell count	1–10	$\times 10^3$/μl	Brobst and Parry, 1987
	Total protein	0.2–4.0	gm/dl	Brobst and Parry, 1987

Interstate Shipment of Horses

N. Edward Robinson, EAST LANSING, MICHIGAN

In general, horses being shipped between states must be accompanied by a health certificate issued by a licensed, accredited veterinarian. In some states, horses consigned for slaughter are exempt from many of the requirements. The health certificate must include a description of the animal, including breed, color, age, sex, and any identifying marks, brands, or tatoos, and must state that the animal is free of infectious and contagious diseases of Equidae. Some states require the recording of body temperature at the time of examination. The majority of states require a negative agar gel immunodiffusion test (Coggins test) for equine infectious anemia. This test must be performed at a laboratory approved by the U.S. Department of Agriculture. The name and location of the laboratory, the accession number, and the date of the negative test are required on most health certificates.

The following table summarizes the interstate health requirements as of February 1, 1991. An update can be obtained from the USDA Voice Response Service (1-800-234-8732). When this service is used, a code number is used to access the information for a particular state. This code number is listed in parentheses after the name of each state.

INTERSTATE HEALTH REGULATIONS

State (Code No.)	Telephone Number	Health Certificate?	Permit Number?	Special Instructions
Alabama (25)	205-242-2647	Yes	No	EIA test within 12 months.
Alaska (25)	907-745-3236	Yes	Yes	EIA test within 180 days; all animals over 6 months.
Arizona (21)	602-542-4293	Yes	No	
Arkansas (27)	501-225-5138	Yes	No	EIA test within 12 months; foals less than 6 months accompanying negative dam exempt.
California (22)	916-445-4191	Yes	No	EIA test within 6 months; foals less than 6 months accompanying negative dam exempt; special regulations for CEM.
Colorado (26)	303-239-4161	Yes	No	EIA test within 12 months; foals less than 6 months accompanying negative dam exempt.
Connecticut (28)	203-566-4616	Yes	No	EIA test within 12 months.
Delaware (33)	302-739-4811	Yes	No	EIA test within 6 months; health certificate must include body temperature, measured within 10 days of entry; horses with body temperature >102° F cannot enter.
Florida (35)	904-488-7747	Yes	No	EIA test within 12 months; horses cannot enter within 21 days of live rhinopneumonitis vaccine; special regulations on piroplasmosis.
Georgia (42)	404-656-3671	Yes	No	EIA test within 12 months; foals less than 6 months accompanying negative dam exempt; health certificate must include body temperature; horses with body temperature >102° F cannot enter.
Guam (48)	671-734-3940	Yes	No	EIA test within 90 days; health certificate must state no equine encephalitis in area of origin within 6 months; vaccinate for equine encephalitis more than 15 days before shipping.
Hawaii (44)	808-487-5351	Yes	Yes	EIA test within 90 days; health certificate must state no equine encephalitis in area of origin within 6 months; vaccinate for equine encephalitis more than 15 days before shipping; sponge with 0.5% malathion or other approved insecticide within 7 days of shipping.
Idaho (43)	208-334-3256	Yes	No	

Table continued on following page

INTERSTATE HEALTH REGULATIONS—continued

State (Code No.)	Telephone Number	Health Certificate?	Permit Number?	Special Instructions
Illinois (45)	217-782-4944	Yes	No	EIA test within 12 months.
Indiana (46)	317-232-1346	Yes	No	EIA test within 12 months; foal accompanying negative dam exempt.
Iowa (42)	515-281-5305	Yes	No	EIA test within 12 months.
Kansas (57)	913-296-2326	Yes	No	
Kentucky (59)	502-564-3956	Yes	No	EIA test within 6 months; show horses within 12 months; foal accompanying negative dam exempt.
Louisiana (52)	504-925-3980	Yes	No	EIA test within 12 months.
Maine (63)	207-289-3701	Yes	No	EIA test within 6 months; foal accompanying negative dam exempt.
Maryland (63)	301-841-5810	Yes	No	EIA test within 12 months; all horses over 9 months.
Massachusetts (62)	617-727-3018	Yes	No	EIA test within 6 months.
Michigan (64)	517-373-1077	Yes	No	EIA test within 180 days.
Minnesota (66)	612-296-2942	Yes	No°	EIA test within 12 months; foal accompanying negative dam exempt; trail ride, exhibition, and slaughter animals exempt.
Mississippi (67)	601-354-6089	Yes	No	EIA test within 12 months.
Missouri (66)	314-751-3377	Yes	No†	EIA test within 12 months; foal accompanying negative dam exempt.
Montana (68)	406-444-2976	Yes	Yes	EIA test for horses from Texas, Oklahoma, Louisiana, Mississippi, Alabama, Florida, Georgia, North and South Carolina, Kentucky, Tennessee, and Arkansas within 6 months.
Nebraska (63)	402-471-2351	Yes	No	EIA test within 1 year unless entering from Montana, Minnesota, Wyoming, North Dakota, South Dakota, Colorado, Kansas, and Iowa; foals less than 6 months exempt.
Nevada (68)	702-789-0180	Yes	No	
New Hampshire (64)	603-271-2404	Yes	No	EIA test within 6 months; foal accompanying negative dam exempt.
New Jersey (65)	609-292-3965	Yes	No	EIA test within 12 months.
New Mexico (66)	505-841-4000	Yes	No	EIA test within 12 months; foals less than 6 months exempt.
New York (69)	518-457-3502	Yes	No	EIA test within 12 months; foals less than 6 months exempt.
North Carolina (62)	919-733-7601	Yes	No	EIA test within 12 months.
North Dakota (63)	701-224-2655	Yes	No	EIA test if horses or mules originating from Alabama, Arkansas, Florida, Georgia, Kansas, Kentucky, Louisiana, Mississippi, Missouri, North Carolina, Oklahoma, South Carolina, Tennessee, Virginia, West Virginia, and Texas.
Ohio (64)	614-866-6361	Yes	No	EIA test within 6 months; all animals over 12 months; special regulations on VEE.
Oklahoma (65)	405-521-3891	Yes	No	EIA test within 6 months; all horses over 6 months.
Oregon (67)	503-378-4710	Yes	Yes	EIA test within 6 months.
Pennsylvania (72)	717-783-5301	Yes	No‡	EIA test within 12 months; foals less than 6 months accompanying negative dam exempt.
Puerto Rico (77)	809-725-1685	Yes	No	EIA test within 6 months; piroplasmosis test within 6 months.
Rhode Island (74)	401-277-2781/2/3	Yes	No	
South Carolina (72)	803-788-2260	Yes	No	EIA test within 6 months.
South Dakota (73)	605-773-3321	Yes	No	EIA test within 12 months.
Tennessee (86)	615-360-0120	Yes	No	EIA test within 6 months for sale, within 12 months for any other purpose; foals less than 6 months exempt.
Texas (89)	512-479-6841	Yes	Yes§	EIA test within 6 months; fever tick and screwworm requirements as for cattle.

INTERSTATE HEALTH REGULATIONS—Continued

State (Code No.)	Telephone Number	Health Certificate?	Permit Number?	Special Instructions
Utah (88)	801-533-6060	Yes	No	EIA test within 12 months.
Vermont (88)	802-828-2421	Yes	Yes	EIA test within 12 months; all animals over 6 months.
Virginia (82)	804-786-2483	Yes	No	EIA test within 12 months; special regulations on CEM.
Virgin Islands (84)	809-778-0991	Yes	No‖	EIA test within 6 months; foal accompanying negative dam exempt; WEE and EEE vaccination required.
Washington (92)	206-753-5040	Yes	No	EIA test within 6 months; all animals over 6 months; EIA test not required on horses from Oregon.
West Virginia (98)	304-348-2214	Yes	No	EIA test within 12 months.
Wisconsin (94)	608-266-3481	Yes	No	EIA test within 12 months; foal accompanying negative dam exempt.
Wyoming (99)	307-777-7515	Yes	No	EIA test within 12 months; foal accompanying negative dam exempt.

Excerpted from information provided by the United States Department of Agriculture Veterinary Services

CEM = contagious equine metritis; EIA = equine infectious anemia; EEE = eastern equine encephalomyelitis; WEE = western equine encephalomyelitis; VEE = Venezuelan equine encephalomyelitis.

°Unless EIA test results are pending.

†Unless equids are entering from states in which VEE has been diagnosed within the preceding 12 months. For permits, telephone 314-751-4359

‡Unless state of origin is quarantined for VEE or other infectious or contagious diseases of horses.

§If for slaughter or treatment at a veterinary clinic.

‖Unless from state banning EEE vaccination.

INDEX

Note: Page numbers in *italics* refer to illustrations; page numbers followed by the letter "t" refer to tables. Page numbers following II refer to pages in *Current Therapy in Equine Medicine 2*.

Abdomen, drainage of, 243
  pain in. See *Colic*.
  paracentesis of, 169, 193, 238–241
Abdominocentesis, 193, 238–241
Abducens nerve, function of, 523t
Abortion, II:520–525
  from herpesvirus infection, 319
  of one twin fetus, 659, 659t
Abscess, 421
  cranial, 553
  inguinal, 161
  of foot, II:266–272
  of liver, 253
  of lung, 300, 304, 780
  of retropharyngeal lymph nodes, 175
  of submandibular node, 325
  pectoral, 161
  treatment of, 4t
Absorption, tests of, 170–171
Acarines, control of, 691–692, 697
Accessory nerve, function of, 523t
Accessory sex glands, 678–681
Accreditation, USDA, 73
Acer spp., toxicity of, 373, 375, 498
Acetylpromazine, 95–96
Acid-base imbalance, 18
  in colic, 194
Acidosis, 19
  renal tubular, 627–628, II:722–724
  treatment of, 349
Acinetobacter calcoaceticus, 114
Actinobacillus spp., antibiotics for, 471t
  in septicemia, 435, 438
Actinobacillus equilli, 400
Actinomyces bovis, 111
Actinomycetes, culture of, 313, 313t
Activated charcoal, 340, 346
Addison-like disease, 807–808
Adductor myopathy, 100
ADH (antidiuretic hormone), 620
ADH (antidiuretic hormone) response, 622
α-Adrenergic receptor blockade, 24
  for laminitis, 86
β_2-Adrenoceptor agonists, 306–307
Aflatoxicosis, 253
Aflatoxin, 369–370
African horse sickness, 753–756
Agalactia, 369
Aganglionosis, ileocolonic, 448
α_2-Agonists, 22–23
Air, sampling of, 312–313

Airway, function of, measurement of, 293
  hyperresponsiveness of, 329
  lower, endoscopy of, 299–301
    radiography of, 780–781, *780*
  patency of, 481
    testing for, 32
  radiography of, 779–781
  scintigraphy of, 781–782
  ultrasonic imaging of, 782–783
  upper, dynamics of flow in, 291–292, *292*
    endoscopy of, 287–288, 774–776, *775*
    measurement of pressure in, *293*
    obstruction of, 292–293
Alar fold obstruction, 266
Albumin, in adult blood, 827t
  in foal blood, 825t
Alimentary tract, II:1–122. See also
  Gastrointestinal system.
  biopsy of, 169–170
  endoscopy of, 167–168
  neoplasia of, II:107–109
  radiography of, 168
  ultrasonic imaging of, 168–169
Alkali disease, 125
Alkaloids, antidotes to, 347t
Alkalosis, 19
  treatment of, 349
Allergic bronchitis, 780
Alloantibodies, 429–430
Alphavirus, 547
Alveoli, periostitis of, 271
Alyssum, toxicity of, 373, 374
Amikacin, 9
Aminoacetyl penicillins, 12
Aminoglycosides, 8–9
  dosages of, 6t
  nephrotoxicosis caused by, 356, 624
Ammonia, in stables, 315
Amphetamines, antidotes to, 350t
Amphotericin B, nephrotoxicosis caused by, 355
Ampulla, impaction of, 199
  ultrasonic imaging of, 678–679, *679*
Amsinckia spp., toxicity of, 254, 375
Anaerobic bacteria, 32
Anal atresia, 448
Analeptics, 308, 310
Analgesics, 201–203, 202t
Anaphylaxis, vaccination and, 49
Anemia, aplastic, 494–495
  blood loss, 490, 492–493, II:300–303

Anemia *(Continued)*
  Coggins test for, 38
  from lead poisoning, 363
  hemolytic, 490–491, 495–501, II:295–300
  hypoproliferative, 491, 494–495, II:303–305
  iron and, 719
  myelophthisic, 495
  nutritional, 494
  of chronic disease, 494
  physiological, of newborn, 474
  symptoms and diagnosis of, 487–492
  tests for, 489t
Anemic hypoxia, 493
Anesthesia, complications of, 100
  dosages of, for draft animals, 96, 98t
  epidural, 25–26, 27–28
    in donkeys, 102
  evaluation before, 97
  general, 28–31
    for draft animals, 97–101
  inhalation, for draft animals, 98, 99–100
    for mules and donkeys, 104
  injectable, 25–26, *27, 28*
    for mules and donkeys, 102–103
  local, 25–26
  of draft horses, 95–101
  of foals, 476–478, *477*, 482–483, II:203–205
  of mules and donkeys, 101–104
  regional, 26–28, *27, 28*, 102
  topical, 26
Angular limb deformities, 88, 105–106
  acquired, 463
Anhidrosis, 703–704, II:187–188
Ankylosis, 129
Anorexia, 725, 737, 740
Antacids, for gastric ulcer, 189
Anterior uveitis, 585, 589
  in septicemia, 441
  postsurgery, 602
  prognosis for, 592
  recurrent, 592
  symptoms of, 592
  treatment of, 592–594, 595t
Anthracene, toxicity of, 361
Anthrax, vaccination against, 39, 49
Anti-inflammatory agents. See *Corticosteroids; Nonsteroidal anti-inflammatory agents*.
Antiarrhythmic therapy, 386–389, 391, 392t
Antibiotic-associated colitis, 355–368

833

Antibiotics, choice of, 3–8, 4t, 471t
  dosages of, 6t–8t, 305t
    for foals, 460t
  duration of treatment with, 305–306
  for abscesses, 4t
  for corneal ulcer, 596–599, 597t
  for gastrointestinal disorders, 4t
  for lymphatic disorders, 4t
  for peritonitis, 242
  for pleuropneumonia, 327–328
  for pneumonia, 471–473
  for reproductive disorders, 4t
  for respiratory disorders, 4t, 304–306
  for septicemia, 440–441, 440t
  for skin disorders, 4t
  for uveitis, 594, 595t
  for vascular disorders, 4t
  in colitis, 249–250
  susceptibility tests and, 5
  toxicity of, 355–356, 367–368
Antibodies. See also *Immunity.*
  colostral, 37, 38, 422
  indirect fluorescent test for, 251
Anticoagulants, antidotes to, 350t
  in blood therapy, 519–520
  toxicity of, 354–355, 371
Anticonvulsants, dosages of, 564t
Antidiuretic hormone (ADH), 620
Antidiuretic hormone (ADH) response, 622
Antidotes, 347t, 350t–352t
Anthelmintics, 51
  daily administration of, 53–54
  dosage of, 52t
  drug resistance and, II:332–334
  for lung parasites, 333–334, 334t
  for prophylaxis, II:328
  rotation of, 51
Antipyretic agents, 16
Antisecretory therapy, for colitis, 250
Antitussives, 310
Aortic insufficiency, 397–398, *398*
Aortic regurgitation, 397–398
Aortoiliac thrombosis, 383
Aplastic anemia, 494–495
Apnea, 479, 481
Arachidonate metabolism, *231*
Arrhythmias, 383–393, II:154–164
  exercise-induced, 784–785
  myocardial disease and, 393
  pathological, 385–393
  physiological, 384–385
  supraventricular, 385–390
  ventricular, 390–393
Arsenic, antidotes to, 347, 350t
  toxicity of, II:668–670
Arterial blood gas, 822, 827t
Arteritis, equine viral, 322–324, 511
  vaccination against, 39, 48
  verminous, 190
Arthritis, degenerative, 107
  plasmacytic, 134
  septic, in foal, 441, 455–462, *456, 459, 461,* II:225–230
Arthrodesis, 90
Arthropathy, steroid-induced, 128
Arthroscopic debridement, 133
Arthrotomy, 133
Artificial insemination, 676–677
Arytenoid cartilage, asymmetry of, 286
  movement of, during exercise, 288
Arytenoid chondritis, 92, 289–291, *290*
Arytenoid depression, 92
Arytenoidectomy, 291
Ascarid impaction, 190
  ultrasonic findings of, 420
Asclepias spp., toxicity of, 374
Ascorbic acid, dietary supplementation with, 812
  in normal diet, 723

Aspartate aminotransferase, 255
  in adult blood, 827t
  in foal blood, 825t
  in myopathy, 90, 114
Aspergillus spp., 268, 369
  causing corneal ulcer, 596, 597
Aspergillus nidulans, 279
Aspiration, transtracheal, 301
Aspiration pneumonia, 181t, 182, 363
AST. See *Aspartate aminotransferase.*
Aster xylorrhiza, 125
Astragalus spp., toxicity of, 376
Asystole, emergency drugs for, 29t
Ataxia. See *Vestibular disease.*
Atheroma, 265
Atlanto-occipital site, collection of CSF from, 528
Atresia, anal, 448
  choanal, 269
  tricuspid, 448, 449
Atrial fibrillation, 383, 387–389, *388,* 401
Atrial premature depolarization (APD), 385–386, *385, 386*
Atrial tachycardia, 386–387, *386, 387*
Atrioventricular (AV) block, 384
  advanced, 389–390
Atrioventricular valvular insufficiency, 398
Atropine, 593
  antidotes to, 350t
Auditive tube diverticulum, diseases of, II:612–618, 93–94, 275–280
Auditory tubes, 275
Auriculopalpebral nerve, blocking of, 26
Azlocillin, 12
Azoturia, 90, 114

Babesia spp., anemia caused by, 499
Babesiosis, 499–500, 692, 756–757
Bacillus piliformis, 254, 442
Bacteria, airborne, 314
  anaerobic, 3
  colonization of, 1
  conjunctivitis caused by, 585
  cystitis caused by, 616
  diarrhea from, 451–452
  endocarditis caused by, 399–402, 421
  growth of, 2
  meningitis caused by, 552–553
  relation with host, 1–2
Bacteroides spp., 237
Bacteroides fragilis, antibiotics for, 471t
  diarrhea from, 452, 454
Balance, loss of. See *Vestibular disease.*
Barbiturates, 98
  antidotes to, 350t
Barium salts, antidotes to, 347t
Barn, construction of, 37, 310–311, 311t
Basal ganglion, lesions of, 173
Basophilic stippling, 363–364
Bastard strangles, 325, 553
Bedding material, COPD from, 331
  particle release from, 331t, 332t
Behavior, abnormal maternal, 636
  problems of, 636, 642, II:123–138
    in trailers, II:135–138
    progesterones for, II:129–131
    stereotypic, II:131–134
Benzimidazole, 51
Berteroa incana, toxicity of, 374
Bicarbonate ion, 19
  supplementation of, 20, 811
Biceps reflex, 526
Bighead, 119, 270
Bile, acids in, 256
Bile duct, distended, 257
  obstruction of, 253
  stones in, 259
Bilirubin, in adult blood, 827t
  in foal blood, 825t

Bilirubinemia, 256
Bioassay, types of, 340
Bioflavinoids, 813
Biopsy, indications for, 683–684
  interpretation of, 685–686
  of alimentary tract, 169–170
  of liver, 257, 262
  of lung, 302–303
  of muscle, 800
  of rectal mucosa, 170
  of skin, 684–685, 684t
  synovial, 132, 136
  techniques for, 684–685
Biotin, 740
Bismuth salts, antidotes to, 347t
Black walnut wood, and laminitis, 155, 337–338, 373, 374
Blackflies, control of, 688
Bladder, displaced, II:715–717
  effects of cystitis on, 616
  infections of, I:708–712
  paralytic, II:712–713
  ruptured, 419, *419,* II:717–718
  ultrasonic imaging of, 418–419
Blastomycosis, 162t
Blindness, causes of, 574–575
  CSF tap to determine cause of, 575
  from trauma, 33, *591*
  in foal, 609–610
  night, 574
  signs and diagnosis of, 573–574
Blister beetle, toxicity of, 358, 368–369, II:120–122
Blood, carbon dioxide in, 20
  characteristics of, in anemia, 488–490
  collection of, 822, 822t
  complete cell count (CBC), 807
  culturing, 400, 437–438, 822
  effects of exercise on, 807–808
  evacuated container color codes for, 822t
  hematocrit of, 807
  in cerebrospinal fluid, 529, 828t
  in feces, 170
  nitrogen in, 19, 254
  of foal, 417
  red cell count (RBC), 824t, 826t
  transfusion of, 33, 517, 520
  typing of, laboratories that perform, 667
  white cell count (WBC), 132, 807, 825t, 826t
Blood biochemistry values, for adult horse, 827t–828t
  for newborn foal, 475, 825t–826t
Blood gas analysis, 19–20, 479–480
  arterial, 822, 827t
  in athletic horses, 777–778
  variables in, 480t
  venous, 822
Blood loss anemia, 490, II:300–303
  acute, 492–493
  chronic, 493
Blood pressure, monitoring of, 31
  of foal, 474
Blood tests, for colic, 193
  in exercise testing, 803–804, 803t
Blood therapy, II:317–372
  anticoagulants in, 519–520
  collection techniques in, 519
  donor selection for, 518–519
  transfusion in, 33, 517, 520
Blood urea nitrogen (BUN), 19, 256, 825t, 827t
Blowflies, 691
Bobtail disease, 125
Bone, collagen in, 721
  computed tomography of, 110, 795
  densitometry of, 796
  fracture of. See *Fracture.*
  radiography of, 791
  scintigraphy of, 144, 791–795
Bone density, 122

Bone marrow, differential count of, 491
Borborygmi, 191
Bordetella bronchiseptica, 471t
Borrelia burgdorferi, 131, 692
Bot infestation, 52, 691
Botryomycosis, 162
Botulism, 338, 370–371, 542–544, II:367–370
 antitoxin for, 352t
 vaccination against, 39, 48
Bougienage, 183
Bowed tendon, 798
Bradyarrhythmias, 383
Bradycardia, emergency drugs for, 29t
Brain, examination of, 524
 hemispheres of, 522–524
 lesions of, 521–522
 necrosis of, caused by *Fusarium*-infested feed, 377, 558–559
 trauma to, 173, 536–538, *537*
Brain stem, dysfunction of, 521
Bran disease, 119
Breeding season, exogenous control of, 643, II:493–494
Bromides, antidotes to, 350t
Bronchiolitis, 304
Bronchitis, allergic, 780
Bronchoalveolar lavage, 301
Bronchodilators, 308
 for respiratory disorders, 306–307
Bronchomucotropic agents, 308
Bronchointerstitial pneumonia, 473
Bronchopneumonia, radiographic diagnosis of, 780, 301, *302*
Brood mares, nutrition of, 108, 108t
Brucella abortus, 111
Bruxism, 185
BSP clearance test, 256
Bucked shins, 143–144
 prevention of, 144
Buffel grass, 121
Bulbourethral glands, ultrasonic imaging of, 679–680, *680*
BUN (blood urea nitrogen), 19, 256, 825t, 827t
Burns, II:639–641
Butorphanol, 30

Cachexia, 737
Cadmium, toxicity of, 365–366, 723
CaEDTA (edetate calcium disodium), 364
Calcification, dystrophic, 139
Calcium, deficiency of, 566–568, 717–718
 dietary supplement of, 108, 568t
 excretion of, 121–122
 in cerebrospinal fluid, 530
 metabolic disorders of, II:189–192
 nutritional requirements for, 121t, 718t, 722
 orthopedic disorders and, 464, 722
 phosphorus and, 722t
 plasma concentration of, 119–120
Calculi, biliary, 259
 urinary, 613–615
Campylobacter jejuni, diarrhea from, 452
Candida parapsilosis, 400
Canker, 87–88
 of foot, II:266–272
Cantharidin, 368
 toxicity of, II:120–122
Capillary refill time, 19
Carbamate poisoning, 338
Carbohydrate. See also *Energy*.
 loading of, 810
 overload of, 113, 155
 in parenteral nutrition, 732–733
Carbon dioxide, in blood, 20
Carbon dioxide laser, 295, 711–712
Carbon fiber tow implantation, 148
Carbon monoxide, antidotes to, 350t
Carbon tetrachloride, antidotes to, 347t
 toxicity of, II:665

Carboxypenicillins, 12
Cardiac. See also *Heart*.
Cardiac chamber enlargement, 382
Cardiac glycosides, 373, 374
Cardiac tamponade, 403
Cardiovascular diseases, 381–410, II:139–180
Carnitine, dietary supplementation with, 811–812
Carpal bones, distal radial, 137
 scintigraphy of, *792*
Cartilage, 720–721
 erosion of, 129
Cartilage flaps, 107
Castor bean, toxicity of, 358
Cataplexy, 562, 565
Cataracts, 601–602, 609, II:456–458
Catarrhal strangles, 325
Cathartics, 346
Catheterization, of jugular vein, 407
Cattle grubs, 697
Cauda equina neuritis, 577, 579, 619
Caudal epidural injection, 25–28
Caudal thigh myopathy, 115
CBC (complete blood cell count), 807
Cecum, dilation of, 198
 impaction of, 198
Ceftiofur, 10
Cefoxitin, 10
Cellulitis, 701
CEM (contagious equine metritis), 757–760
Cenchrus ciliaris, 121
Central nervous system, edema in, 34
 trauma to, 33–34
Cephalosporins, 9–10
 dosages of, 6t
Cephoxitin, 10
Cerebellum, abiotrophy of, 534–535
 dysfunction of, 522
 examination of, 524
Cerebrospinal fluid, 527
 analysis of, 528–530
 bacteria in, 3
 clinical norms for, 828t
 collection of, 527–530, II:341–345
 hydrocephalus and, 530–531
 in trauma, 539
 of foal, 416–417, 417t
 pressure of, 33
Cerebrum, edema of, 524
 hemispheres of, 522–524
 lesions of, 521–522
 trauma to, 173, *537*
Cervical lesions, of foal, 415–416
Cervical myelopathy, 532, 533
Cervical spinal cord, compression of, 111, *534*
 fracture of, *536*
 lesions of, 526
Cervical vertebrae, instability of, 527
 malformation of, 463, 532–534
Cervix, abnormalities of, II:516–518
 ultrasonic imaging of, 650
Cesarean section, II:542–544
Cestrum diurnum, 126
Chain of custody, 343
Charcoal, activated, 340, 346
Chemical restraint, α_2-agonists for, 22–23, 23t
 clinical use of, 24–25
 during mechanical ventilation, 483t
 of draft horse, 95–97, 96t
 opioid antagonists for, 23t
 phenothiazines for, 23t
Chemotherapy, 1–3. See also specific drugs and drug groups.
 antibiotic choice in, 3–8
 clinical field trials in, 74–75
 drug dosages in, 815t–821t
Chest tubes, indwelling, 328, 405
Chiggers, control of, 691
Chip fractures, 129
Chloramphenicol, 10

Chloride, in adult blood, 827t
 in cerebrospinal fluid, 530
 in foal blood, 826t
Chlorophenol, 362
Choanal atresia, 269
Choke, 179–180
 diet for, 738
Choking, 363
Choking down, 283
Cholangiohepatitis, 254
Cholangitis, 263
Choledocholithiasis, 259–263
Choledochotomy, 262
Cholelithiasis, 259–263, *257, 261*
 liver failure from, 254
Cholelithotripsy, 262
Cholestasis, 263
Cholinergic agents, antidotes to, 350t
Cholinesterase inhibitors, antidotes to, 350t
Chondritis, of arytenoid cartilage, 92, 289–291, *290*
Chondroids, 277
Chondroprotective agents, 127–131
Chordae tendineae, rupture of, 397
Chorioptic mange mites, 692, 697
Chorioretinal scars, 610
Chorioretinitis, 610
Chronic obstructive pulmonary disease (COPD), 300, 304, II:596–603
 diet for, 738
 etiology and pathology of, 329
 radiographic image of, *780*
 scintigraphic diagnosis of, 781–782, *782*
 symptoms and diagnosis of, 329–330
 treatment and prevention of, 330–331
Cicatrix, of nasopharynx, 282–283
Cilia augmenters, 318
Cimetidine, for gastric ulcer, 188
Circling, in cerebral lesions, 522
Cirrhosis, 255
Claviceps, 369
Cleft palate, 174, II:1–3
Clostridial infections, 162
 diarrhea from, 451
 intestinal, II:97–99
Clostridium botulinum, 48, 370–371, 542
Clostridium cadaveris, 245
Clostridium difficile, 356
Clostridium perfringens, 212, 245
Clostridium tetani, 540
Clover, toxins in, 371
Coagulation cascade system, 431
Coagulative necrosis, 123
Coal tar, toxicity of, 361
Cobalt, requirement of, 716t
Coccidiodes immitis, 268
Coggins test, 38
Colic, analgesics for, 201–203, II:27–29
 anesthesia and, II:38–41
 cardiovascular function and, 205
 death risk from, 208t
 diet for, 738–739
 difficult treatment of, II:30–32
 distention and, II:41–44
 epizootiology of, II:15
 examination for, 191–200
 from sand, II:55–58
 gastrointestinal motility and, 203–205
 laxatives for, 205–206, 205t
 perioperative management of, II:33–38
 physical exam for, II:19–22
 prognosis of, 207–210, 209t
 prognostic factors in, II:15–19
 risk factors for, 206–207, II:15–19
 surgery for, 195
 symptoms and diagnosis of, 190–191
 treatment for, 201–206
 ultrasonic findings in, 420, *420*
Colistin, 13

Colitis, 2, 190
  pathogenesis of, 244–245
  preacute toxemic, II:94–97
  pseudomembranous, 356
  symptoms and diagnosis of, 245–247
  treatment of, 247–250
Collagen, 720, 721, 721t
Collateral sesamoidean ligament, calcification of, 151
Colon, atresia of, 448
  displaced, *199*, 200, 220–221, II:60–65
  endoscopy of, 167
  flexion of, 199
  fluid in, 192
  gaseous distention of, 192, 197
  impacted, 190, 191, 198, *198*, 218–219, II:53–55
    diet for, 739
  intussusception of, 222, II:66–68
  nephrosplenic entrapment of, 190, 192
  obstruction of, *200*, 219–220, II:68–70
  pseudoimpaction of, 199
  resection of, diet for, 739
  strangulation of, 198, 199
  torsion of, 199, *199*
  volvulus of, 190, 191, 221–222, II:66–68
Colostral antibodies, 37, 38
Colostrum, 422–424, 435
Competitive rides, 80
Compressive neuropraxia, 524
Computed tomography (CT), 795, *795*
Confidentiality, 59
Congestive heart failure, 399
Conidiobolus coronatus, 268
Conjunctivitis, 585–586
Conoglossum officinale, toxicity of, 375
Consent for treatment, 58
Constrictive pericarditis, 403
Convulsions, treatment of, 349
COPD. See *Chronic obstructive pulmonary disease (COPD)*.
Copper, antidotes to, 347t
  deficiency of, 125, 687, 718–719, 722
  in serum, 723t
  orthopedic disorders and, 464, 722
  requirement of, 716t, 718t, 722
Copulatory dysfunctions, 669–670
Cornea, damage to, 589–590
  edema in, 589
  stromal abscess of, 594–596
  ulceration of, 596–599
    antibiotics for, 597t
Corpus luteum, ultrasonic imaging of, 652, *652*
Corticosteroids, 14–16
  for anterior uveitis, 593
  for endotoxemia, 231
  for respiratory disorders, 306
  for tendinitis, 147
  intra-articular use of, 127–128, 128t
  preparations of, 128t
  side effects of, 128
Corynebacterium equi, in foal, II:230–232
Corynebacterium pseudotuberculosis, 161
Coughing, 310
  in COPD, 329
Coumarin, antidotes to, 350t
  toxicity of, 354, 502–503, II:305–306
Cranial nerves, 523t
  dysfunction of, 521, 577–578
  evaluation of, 415
  examination of, 522
  proximity patterns of, 524t
Cranium, abscess of, 553
  fracture of, 538
  trauma to, 33, II:377–380
Creatine kinase, in adult blood, 827t
  in foal blood, 825t
  myopathy signaled by, 90, 114, 806, 808

Creatinine, 19
  clearance of, clinical norms for, 828t
  in adult blood, 827t
  in foal blood, 826t
Cresols, antidotes to, 347t
  toxicity of, 361
Cricoarytenoidus dorsalis, 286
Crotalaria spp., toxicity of, 254, 375
Croup myopathy, 115
Cryptococcus neoformans, 268
Cryptorchidism, I:571–573
Cryptosporidium, diarrhea from, 453
Crystalloid solutions, 20–21
  composition of, 21t
CSF. See *Cerebrospinal fluid*.
CT (computed tomography), 795, *795*
Culicoides, dermatitis from, 689, 693–696, II:624–626
Curare, antidotes to, 350t
Curvularia geniculata, 162t
Cutaneous vasculitis, 164
Cyanide, antidotes to, 351t
Cyclooxygenase, inhibition of, 14, 16
Cycloplegic therapy, 593
Cystic calculi, 614–615
Cystic sinus disease, 273
Cystitis, 616–617, II:708–712
Cysts, 421

Dallas grass, 121
Dantrolene sodium, 91, 100–101
Darting, of wild burros, 103
DDSP (dorsal displacement of the soft palate), 283–284, 775–776
Deep digital flexor tendon, injury of, 146
Degenerative arthritis, 107
Degenerative joint disease, 89–90, 134, 524
  etiology of, 137–138, *138*
  symptoms and diagnosis of, 138–139
  treatment for, 15, 17, 139–140
Degenerative myeloencephalopathy, 559–561, II:353–355
Degenerative myelopathy, 525, 527
Dehydration, 19
Demineralization, 121
Demodex spp., 692
Demodicosis, II:626–627
Dental care, 49–50. See also *Teeth*.
Dental conditions, and sinus disorders, 271
Dental enamel, fluorosis and, 126
Dental repulsion, 272
Deposition, 63–65
Depression, CNS, 349
Dermatitis, *Culicoides*-caused, 689, 693–696
  eosinophilic, 706–708
  from vitamin deficiency, 687
Dermatology, lasers in, 711
Dermatomycosis, 698
Dermatophilosis, II:630–632
Dermatophilus congolensis, 162
Dermatophytosis, 698–699
Descemetocele, 596
Desmitis, distal accessory ligament, 141
  suspensory, 141–143, *142*, 151
Desmotomy, medial patellar, 88
  superior check ligament, 148
Detomidine, 23, 96–97
Deviated septum, 266
Deworming, 52, 52t
  seasonal, 53, 53t
Dextrose therapy, 21
Diabetes insipidus, 620–622
Diabetes mellitus, II:181–185
Dialysis, for kidney failure, 625–626
Diaphragm, synchronous flutter of, 82, 113, 114, II:485–486
Diarrhea. See also *Colitis*.
  bacterial, 451–452
  chronic, II:100–102

Diarrhea *(Continued)*
  foal heat, 449, II:87–88
  in septicemia, 441
  nutritional, 449
  parasitic, 452–453
  treatment of, 453–454
  viral, 449–450
Diazepam, 434
DIC. See *Disseminated intravascular coagulation (DIC)*.
Dicoumarol, toxicity of, 371
Dictyocaulus arnfeldi, 300, 301, 332–333
Diets, 726, 728–729. See also *Nutrition*.
  for pregnant mares, 665t
  for sick horses, 737–740
  low-fiber, 810
  maintenance, 728t
  nutrient-dense, 809–811
Digestion, tests of, 170–171
Digital flexor tendon, injury to, 146
Digitalis, antidotes to, 351t
  toxicity of, 374
Digoxin, for fibrillation, 388–389
  for tachycardia, 392t
  toxicity of, 356
Dihydrostreptomycin, 8
Dimethyl sulfoxide (DMSO)
  anemia caused by, 501
  for colic, 204–205
  for endotoxemia, 232
  for seizures, 564
  for tendinitis, 147
Dimethylglycine, dietary supplementation with, 812
Dioctyl sodium sulfosuccinate, for colic, 205, 206
Dioxin, toxicity of, 362
Disease, control programs against, 39
  development of, 1–2
Disk diffusion, 3
Diskospondylitis, 109–111
Disseminated intravascular coagulation (DIC), 504–507, II:306–309
Distal phalanx, displacement of, 155, *156*, 157
  sinking of, 155
Diuretics, to treat poisoning, 348
Diverticulum, 177
  urachal, 419
DMSO. See *Dimethyl sulfoxide (DMSO)*.
Documentation, 57–59
Donkeys, lungworm in, 332
  sedation and anesthesia of, 101–104
Doppler echocardiography, 382
  color flow, 396
Dorsal metacarpal disease, 143–146
Dorsal spinous processes, crowding and overriding of, 110, 112
Dourine, 710
DPJ (duodenitis-proximal jejunitis), 90, 211–214
Draft horse, anesthesia of, 95–101
  lameness problems of, 85–91
  postanesthesia complications of, 100
  respiratory problems of, 92–95
Draschia megastoma, 556, 697
Drug sampling, II:689–692
Drugs. See also specific drugs and drug groups.
  dosages of, 815t–821t
  for emergency use, 29t
DSS (dioctyl sodium sulfosuccinate), 205, 206
Duodenal ulcer, 184, 253
  in foal, 186
  in yearling, 186
Duodenitis-proximal jejunitis, 90, II:44–45
  complications of, 213–214
  laboratory findings in, 212t
  histological lesions in, 212
  symptoms and diagnosis of, 211–212
  treatment for, 212–213
Duodenoscopy, 167, 186

Dust, as pathogen, 312–313
  photomicrograph of, *314*
Dysphagia, 171–175
  from esophageal obstruction, 175
  in guttural pouch mycosis, 278
  in strangles, 325
  muscular causes of, 174–175
  neurologic causes of, 173–174
  of foal, 415
  types of, 176t
Dysplasia, physeal, 106–107
  retinal, 609
Dyspnea, 363
Dystocia, 412

Eastern equine encephalitis (EEE), 547–550, *548*, II:345–347
Echinococcus granulosus, 333
Echocardiography, 387, 393, *394, 397, 398*, 403, 408, *409, 410*, 421, II:139–147
  color flow Doppler, 396
  Doppler, 382
Ectoparasites, II:622–624
  control of, 688–692
Edema, central nervous system, 34
  cerebral, 524
  corneal, 589
  dependent, 397
  pulmonary, 382
  in vasculitis, 512
Edetate calcium disodium, 364
EEE (eastern equine encephalitis), 547–550, *548*, II:345–347
Effusion, pleural, *404*, 405, 421
Ehrlichiosis. See *Potomac horse fever*.
EHV-1. See also *Herpesvirus infection*.
  control of, 321
  isolation of, 320
  serology of, 320
EHV-3, 710
EHV-4, 319, 320, 322
EIA. See *Hemolytic anemia, infectious*.
Eicosanoids, inhibition of, 14
EIPH. See *Exercise-induced pulmonary hemorrhage*.
Ejaculatory dysfunctions, 669–670, 670t, II:562–563
Ejection fraction, 393
Electrocardiography, 384–394, *785*
  during exercise, 783
  fetal, II:152–154
Electrolyte therapy, 18
Electrolytes, in cerebrospinal fluid, 530
  exercise and, 807–808
  in parenteral nutrition, 734
Electromyography, 526
  of foal, 416
  of hyperkalemic periodic paralysis, 117
  tail alteration detected by, 580–581
Embolic disease, 402
Embryo, loss of, 644–647, *646*
  shape of, *655*
Embryo transfer, II:573–578
  donor of, 637–638
  recipient of, 638
  technique of, 638–640
Embryonic vesicle, 654, *654*
Emergency care, drugs for, 29t
Empyema, guttural pouch, 276–278
Encephalitis, causing dysphagia, 173
  CSF findings in, 529
  eastern, 547–550, II:345–347
  epizootiology of, 547–548
  Japanese, 764–765
  pathogenesis of, 548
  signs and diagnosis of, 548–549
  therapy and prognosis for, 549–550
  vaccination against, 39, 550
  Venezuelan, 547, 548, 765–768

Encephalitis *(Continued)*
  vestibular disease in, 575
  western, 547–550, II:348–349
Encephalomalacia, 558–559
Encephalomyelitis. See *Encephalitis; Myeloencephalitis*.
Endocardial cushion defects, 410
Endocarditis, bacterial, 399–402, 421
  echocardiogram of, *400*
  leading to myocardial disease, 393
  prognosis for, 402
Endochondral ossification, 105
Endocrine system, diseases of, II:181–192
  orthopedic diseases and, 464
Endometritis, fungal, II:511–513
Endophytes, toxicity of, 369
Endoscopy, 167–168
  laser surgery and, 296
  of esophagus, 178–179, 187
  of lower airway, 299–301
  of stomach, *185*, 187, *187, 188*
  of upper airway, 287–288, 774–776
  video, 288, 292
Endotoxemia, 17, 155, 216, 225–226, 504–508, II:81–87
  colic and, 203
  laminitis and, 85, 156
  mediators of, 226
  pathophysiology of, 226–228
  symptoms and diagnosis of, 228–229
  treatment for, 229–232
Endotoxic shock, 16
Endotoxin antiserum, 230, 249
Endurance horses, II:465–490
Endurance rides, 80
Energy requirements, in diet, 715–716, 721–722, 729, 732–733
Enteral feeding, 729–730, 730t
  complications associated with, 746t
  nasogastric intubation for, 726–727, *727*, 745
  of foal, 744–747
  rations for, 726t
  nutritional profile of, 728t, 748t
Enterobacter spp., 471t
Enterocolitis, drug-induced, 356, 367–368
  necrotizing, 454–455
Enterolithiasis, 191, 199, *200*, 223–224
  prevention of, 224
Enteroliths, II:68–70
Entropion, 584–585
Environment, as respiratory disease factor, 310–315, 330–331
  parasite control in, 54
  ventilation of, 311–312, 330–331
Enzyme immunoassay test, 425
Enzyme-linked immunosorbent assay (ELISA), for rotavirus, 170
Enzymes, in cerebrospinal fluid, 529–530
Eosinophilic dermatitis, 706–708
Eosinophilic synovitis, 134, 136
Epicauta beetle, toxicity of, 358, 369–369
Epidural anesthesia, 25–26, 27–28
  in donkeys, 102
Epiglottis, cysts under, 281–282, 293
  displacement of, *284*, 285
  entrapment of, 281, 293
  hypoplastic, 92
Epilepsy, II:349–353
Epiphora, 271, 583, 584t
  in foal, 584
Epiploic foramen, strangulated bowel within, 214
Epistaxis, 274, 278
  in dicoumarol poisoning, 371
  unilateral, 274
Epizootic lymphangitis, 769–770
EPM (equine protozoal myeloencephalitis), 527, 554–556, 575, 578
Equine viral arteritis, 322–324, 511

Equipment, for trail rides, 81t
Ergogenic diets, 809–813
ERU (equine recurrent uveitis), 592
Erysipelothrix rhusiopathiae, 400
Erythrocytosis, 516, II:316–317
Erythromycin, 11
Erythron, 488t, 489t, II:291–295
Erythropoiesis, inadequate, 491–492, 494–495, II:303–305
Escherichia coli, antibiotics for, 471t
  diarrhea from, 452
  in endocarditis, 400
  in peritonitis, 237
  in septicemia, 435
  testing for, 170
Esophagitis, 177
  reflux, 183
Esophagus, bougienage of, 183
  contrast radiography of, 177–178, *178*
  diseases of, 176t, II:12–15
  endoscopy of, 178–179
  lavage of, 180
  obstruction of, 180–182, 181t
  perforation of, 183, 236
  stricture of, 181t, 182
  surgery on, 182
  treatment of obstruction, 179–182
Estrogen, and collagen synthesis, 723
Estrous cycle, *654*
  performance problems in, 635
Estrus, excessive, 634–635
  exogenous control of, I:493–494
  failure of, 633–634, 643–644
  irregular, 634
  persistent, 641–642
  pregnancy and, 635
  prolonged, 634
  synchronization of, II:495–498
  ultrasonic imaging of, *653*
  winter, 635
Ethics, 57
Ethmoid turbinates, hematoma of, 274–275, 297
Ethylene glycol, antidotes to, 351t
Eumycotic mycetoma, 162t
Eupatorium rugosum, toxicity of, 374
Euthanasia, 35, 67
EVA (equine viral arteritis), 322–324, 511
Exanthema, coital, 710
Exercise, appropriate response to, 784, *785*
  blood effects of, 807–808
  blood gases and, 777–779, II:479–481
  bone remodeling caused by, 792–793
  cardiovascular problems and, II:176–180
  clinical problems with, II:465–490
  electrolyte balance in, 807–808
  electrophysiologic responses to, 783–785
  for tendinitis, 149
  glycolysis during, 804
  heart parameters during, 805
  inappropriate response to, 784, *785*
  incremental testing of, 803, 803t, *805*
  lameness caused by, 793–794
  laryngeal movements during, 283, 288
  nasopharyngeal movements during, *284*
  respiration during, 803–804, 803t, *805*
  spleen in, 807
Exercise-induced pulmonary hemorrhage (EIPH), 300t, 304, 335–336, II:603–605
  radiographic diagnosis of, 780
  scintigraphic diagnosis of, 781–782, *782*
Exercise intolerance, 265
  arrhythmias and, 784
  in COPD, 329
Exercise tolerance testing, 801
Exercise training, II:465–469
Exertional myopathy, 90, 113–115
Exertional rhabdomyolysis, 113, 114, II:487–490
Exhausted horse syndrome, 81–82, II:482–485
Exhaustion, 113

Export, certificates for, 73
Extracellular fluid (ECF), 18
Extrasystoles, atrial or ventricular, 383
Eye, blindness in, 573–575
    from trauma, 591
  of foal, 609–610
  cancer of, 605–606, 607
  cataracts in, 601–602, 609, II:456–458
  discharge from, 583–586
    causes of, 584t
  diseases of, 574, II:427–463
    adnexal, II:440–445
    conjunctival, II:440–445
    corneal, 596–600, II:450–456
    differential diagnosis for, II:433–436
    optic nerve, 574, 610–611, II:458–460
    retinal, 610, II:458–460
    therapeutic techniques for, II:436–439
  emergency treatment of, 588t, II:460–464
  examination of, 574, 583–584, 588t, II:427–433
  funduscopic examination of, 574
  impaired function of, 608–611
  inflammation of, II:445–450
  injury to, 587–591, 590, 591, 610
  medication of, 588t
  neoplasia of, 604–608
  pressure in, 603
  rupture of fibrous tunic, 590
Eyelid, injury to, 588–589, 589
  melanoma of, 606

Face, analgesia of, 26–27
Face flies, control of, 690–691
Facial asymmetry, 265
Facial deformity, 271, 273
Facial nerve, disorders of, 578
  function of, 523t
  paralysis of, 266
Facial paralysis, 172
Facial swelling, 265
Fainting disease, 565
False nostril, 266
Fat, added to diet, 810–811
  dietary, 686
  in parenteral nutrition, 733
Fatigue, 81–82, II:474–476
  postexercise, 113
Feces, bacteria in, 3
  blood in, 170
  culture of, 170
  parasite examination of, 54, 54t, 170
  rotavirus in, 450
  Salmonella in, 247, 451
  sand in, 192, 219
Feed, poisoning from, 338, 339, 366–371
  types of, 740
Feed impaction, 180t
Feed stimulants, 740
Feeding, problems of, 171–175, II:123–126
Feeding tubes, placement and maintenance of, 726–727
  rations for, 726t
Femoral nerve, paralysis of, 578
Fertility, evaluation of, in stallion, 668–681, II:555–558
Fescue, toxicity of, 369
Fetal death, II:525–528
Fetal hypoxia, 412
Fetal membrane, abnormalities of, II:528–531
Fetlock joint arthrodesis, 143
Fetlocks, locked, 139
  osteoarthritis of, 140
Fetus, gender of, 660–663, 660, 661, 662, 663
  certainty of determination of, 663t
  susceptibility of, to warfarin, 354
Fibrillation, atrial, 383, 387–389, 388, 401
Fibrin, 504
Fibrinogen, in adult blood, 827t
  in foal blood, 825t

Fibrinous pericarditis, II:171–172
Fibronectin, 428
Fibrosis, pericardial, 403
Fiddleneck, toxicity of, 375
Fistulous withers, 109, 110, 111–112
Flank, analgesia of, 27
Flatweed, toxicity of, 571, 579
Flavivirus, 547
Fleas, 691
Flexor tendon, anomalies of, 88, 797–798
  contracture of, 125
Flexor tendinitis, 140
Flexure deformity, acquired, 463
Flies, control of, 688–691
Floors, construction of, 37
Fluid, deficit of, 20
  requirements of, 19–20
  route and rate of administration of, 21–22
Fluid balance, maintenance of, in parenteral nutrition, 734
Fluid therapy, 18
  equipment for, 248
  intravenous, 247–248, 248t
  for colitis, 247–248
  for diarrhea, 450
  for pneumonia, 471
  for renal failure, 624–625
  for septicemia, 439–440
  for shock, 33, 492–493
  for vasculitis, 512
Flunixin meglumine, 17
  for colic, 201–202
Fluoracetate, antidotes to, 351t
Fluoride, antidotes to, 347, 351t
  toxicity of, 358–359
Fluoroquinolones, 10
Fluorosis, 126
Flutter, synchronous diaphragmatic, 82, 113, 114, II:485–486
Foal, anesthesia of, 203–205, 476–478, 477, 482–483
  antibiotic dosages for, 460t
  behavior of, 412t
  birth of, 412
  blindness in, 609–610
  blood chemistry values for, 825t–826t
  botulism in, 542, 543, 544
  cerebrospinal fluid of, 416–417, 417t
  CNS disorders in, 530–535
  congenital eye defects of, 610
  cystitis in, 616
  deficiency of immunity in, 423–425, 423t, II:215–219
  diseases of, 427–484, II:193–253
  endoscopy of, 167
  eye discharge in, 584–585
  gastric acid secretion of, 184
  gastrointestinal problems in, 445–455, II:232–241
  hematology values for, 824t–825t
  hemostasis in, 427–431
  hepatic disease in, II:232–241
  high-risk, 411–412, II:193–199
    diagnostic procedures for, 412–413
    management of, 413–414
  interval deworming of, 52, 52t
  iodine deficiency in, 687
  isoerythrolysis in, II:244–247
  jaundice of, 430t
  junctional mechanobullous disease in, 705–706
  lung abscesses in II:230–232
  malnutrition of, 742
  neonatal maladjustment syndrome of, 432–434, II:219–222
  neurological examination of, 414–417, II:199–202
  nutrition of, 88, 107t, 108–109, 720–724, II:205–209
    in critical illness, 741–750
    supplemental, 742t

Foal *(Continued)*
  orthopedic diseases in, 105–109, 462–465, 720–724
  osteomyelitis in, 455–462, II:225–230
  parenteral feeding of, 749, 749t
  physical examination of, 37, 415–417
  physiology of, 474–475
  pneumonia in, etiology and pathogenesis of, 466–468
    symptoms and diagnosis of, 468–470
    treatment and prevention of, 470–473
  premature, 743
  prenatal care of, 412
  rejection of, II:126–128
  renal failure in, 624
  respiratory failure in, 479t
  respiratory support of, 478–484, 483t, II:247–253
  restraint of, 483t, II:203–205
  sedation of, 475–476, 482–483
  sepsis evaluation of, 413t, 452
  septic arthritis in, 441, 455–462, II:225–230
  septicemia in, 435–442, II:222–225
  transfer of immunity to, 422–427, II:210–215
  ulcers in, 185–186
  ultrasonic evaluation of, 417–421
  white muscle disease of, 113, 123
  zinc deficiency in, 687
Foal heat diarrhea, 449, II:87–88
Follicle mites, 692
Folliculitis, 700
Foot, abscesses of, II: 266–272
  anatomy of, II: 255–260
  canker in, II:266–272
  diseases of, II:255–289
  orthopedic problems of, II:282–289
  radiology of, II:260–265
  thrush of, II:266–272
  wounds of, II: 266–272
Foot trimming, for laminitis, 158–159
Forage, and COPD, 331
  poisoning from, 542
Forced feeding, 741
Fore limb flexor tendon, injury of, 146
Foreign body, in airway, 300
  in nose, 274
  in throat, 180t
Forensic medicine, 341–342, 344–345
Formaldehyde, antidotes to, 347t
Fossae, synovial 151
Foxglove, toxicity of, 374
Fractional excretion of phosphorus (FEP), 121
Fracture, 794–795
  chip, 129
  cranial, 538
  emergency treatment of, 34
  manibular, 173
  maxillary, 173
  metacarpal, 141, 145
  of cervical cord, 536
  of lateral cartilages, 87
  of temporal bone, 537
  osseous, 524
Frontal lobe, lesions of, 522
Fumonisin B$_1$, 378
Fungi, aflatoxins from, 369–370
  airborne spores of, 314
  culture of, 313, 313t
  endophytic, 369
  leukoencephalomalacia caused by, 377–379, 558–559
  nose disorders caused by, 268–269
  skin diseases caused by, 698–699
  stachybotryotoxicosis caused by, 379
Furosemide, for EIPH, 336
Furunculosis, 700
Fusarium spp., 558
Fusarium moniliforme, 377

INDEX

Gait, examination of, 414, 415, 416, 786–790, *786, 788, 790*
Gallstones, 254, 259–262
Gaseous distention, 168, 192, 197
Gastric diseases, II:41–44
  diet for, 738
Gastric reflux, 191
Gastric ulcer, 184
  in adult, 186–187
  in foal, 185–186
  NSAIDs causing, 187, 355
  treatment for, 188–189
Gastrointestinal system. See also specific organs.
  congenital defects of, 448
  infections in, treatment of, 4t
  problems of, in foal, 445–455, II:232–241
Gender, determining fetal, 660–663
General anesthesia, agents of, 29–30
  by inhalant, 30–31
  for draft animals, 97–101
  monitoring of, 31
  of foal, 476–478
  preoperative assessment for, 28–29, 97
Gentamycin, 9
Getah, 768–769
Girth itch, 698
Glanders, 162t, 761–762
Glaucoma, 602–604
  medication for, 604t
Globe, trauma to, 589–590, *590*, 610
Globulin, in adult blood, 827t
  in foal blood, 825t
Glomerulonephritis, 136, II:702–703
Glossopharyngeal nerve, disorders of, 578
  function of, 523t
Glucocorticoids, 14–16
  dosages of, 15t
  duration of action of, 15t
  for vasculitis, 512
  indications for, 15
Glucose, absorption tests of, 171
  in adult blood, 827t
  in cerebrospinal fluid, 530
  in foal blood, 825t
γ-Glutamyl transferase, 255
Gluteal nerves, disorders of, 578
Glycosaminoglycan, polysulfated, 16, 17
  intra-articular use, 127, 129–130
Glycosaminoglycan-peptide complex (Rumalon), 131
Goiter, 687
Goldenrod, toxicity of, 373, 374
Gonitis, 88
Graft, laser preparation of bed for, 712
Grain overload, and laminitis, 85
Gram stain, 3
Granulation tissue, excessive, II:642–645
Granuloma, of nose, 268
Granulomatous disease, generalized, II:645–646
Grindelia squarrosa, 125
Griseofulvin, for sporotrichosis, 162–163
Groundsel, toxicity of, 375
"Grunt" test, 92
Guaifenesin, 30, 98–99
Guttural pouch, diseases of, 93–94, 172, 175, 275–280, II:612–618
  endoscopy of, 93, 279
  lavage of, 94, 277
  mycosis of, 278
  radiography of, 94
  surgical drainage of, 278

Habronema, 333, 606–607, 697, 709
Habronemiasis, 163
  conjunctivitis caused by, 586
Halicephalobus deletrix, 556, 557
Halitosis, 271
Hallucinogens, antidotes to, 351t
Halothane, hypotension induced by, 100
Health certificate, for international transport, 72
  for interstate transport, 829t–831t
Heart. See also *Cardiac* entries.
  arrhythmias of, 382–393, II:154–164
  arrhythmias of, monitoring, 784. See also specific arrhythmias.
  blood flow disorders in, acquired, II:164–166
    congenital, II:167–170
  congenital disease of, 381–382
  enlargement of, 382
  isoenzyme determinations in, 395
  murmurs of, 396, 397, 409
  myocardial disease, 382, 393–395
  pericardial disease, 382
  valves of, lesions, 396, 399
    stenosis of, 396–397
  valvular insufficiency of, 397–399
Heart block, types of, 383–385
Heart failure, congestive, 399
Heart rate recovery, 81
Heart sounds, 386
Heart volume overload, 409
Heavy metal poisoning, 339, 347, 363–366, 501
  antidotes to, 350, 364
Heliotropum spp., toxicity of, 375
Hemangiosarcoma, 709
Hemarthrosis, 135
Hematocrit, 807
Hematology values, for adult horse, 826t
  for newborn foal, 824t–825t
Hematomas, 421
Hematopoietic diseases, 487–520, II:291–322
Hemiparesis, 523t
Hemodialysis, for kidney failure, 625–626
Hemoglobin, of adult blood, 826t
  of foal blood, 824t
Hemolytic anemia, 490–491, II:295–300
  immune-mediated, 495–497
  infectious (EIA), 497–498, 511
  microangiopathic, 500
  miscellaneous causes of, 501
  oxidant-induced, 498–499
  parasitic, 499–500
  treatment of, 496–497, 498
Hemophilia, 429, 501–502, II:309–310
Hemorrhagic myopathy, postanesthetic, 100
Hemorrhagic shock, 32
Hemosiderophages, 335
Hemostasis, colic and, 194
  disorders of, 428–431
    laboratory findings in, 431t
  factors affecting, 429–430, 429t
  mechanism of, 427–428
  normal ranges for, 428t
Hemothorax, 492
Heparin, antidotes to, 351t
  for disseminated intravascular coagulation, 506
  for endotoxemia, 231
  for laminitis, 156
  for peritonitis, 217, 243–244
Hepatic disease, 253–259. See also *Liver*.
  diet for, 739
  differential diagnosis of, 444t
  etiology of, 253–254
  signs and diagnosis of, 254–258
  treatment of, 258–259
Hepatitis, from herpesvirus, 443
  tetanus antitoxin and, 39
Hepatoencephalopathy, 254
  vestibular disease in, 575
Hepatomegaly, 257
Hepatotoxins, 443t
Herbicide poisoning, 346
Hernia, congenital, 448
  inguinal, 190, 191, 197
  scrotal, 191, *419*
Hernia *(Continued)*
  ultrasonic imaging of, 418
  umbilical, 216
  strangulating, 190
Herpesvirus infection, abortion, 319
  CSF findings in, 529
  diagnosis of, 320–321
  epizootiology of, 319–320
  hepatitis from, 443
  myeloencephalopathy with, 550–552, II:365–367
  treatment and control of, 321–322
  vaccination to, 39, 47
  vasculitis from, 619
Hexachlorobenzine (HCB), toxicity of, 361
Hind limb flexor tendon, injury of, 146
Histamine type 2 receptor antagonists, 188–189
Histoplasma farciminosum, 268, 769–770
Histoplasmosis, 162t
Hoof, avulsions of, II:275–277
  cracks in, 87, II:272–275
    dietary correction of, 740
  lacerations of, II:275–277
  laminitis in, 154–160, *159, 160*, II:277–281
Hoof trimming, for tendinitis, 147
Hoof wall, detachment of, 155
  resection of, 86, 158
Horn flies, control of, 690
Horner's syndrome, 270, 280, 522, 525
Horse show, attending veterinarian duties, 77
  testing veterinarian duties, 77
  veterinarian duties, 77
Hound's tongue, toxicity of, 375
Houseflies, control of, 690–691
Hyaluronic acid, for tendinitis, 147
Hydration, assessment of, 247t
Hydrocephalus, 530–531, *531*
γ-Hydroxybutyrate, 813
Hypercalcemia, 113
Hypercapnia, 480
Hyperchloremia, 627
Hyperesthetic leukotrichia, II:647–648
Hyperkalemia, 19, 113
Hyperkalemic periodic paralysis, 117–118, 573
Hyperlipidemia, II:114–116
  in ponies, 254
Hypermagnesemia, 113
Hypermetria, 415, 525
Hypernatremia, 18, 113
Hyperostosis, fluoride and, 359
Hyperparathyroidism, calcium homeostasis and, 119–120, 270
  signs and diagnosis of, 121
  treatment of, 122
Hyperphosphatemia, 119
Hypertension, pulmonary, 382, 397
Hyperthermia, malignant, 100, 113
  treatment of, 348
Hypertonic saline, 33, 248, 492
Hyphema, 590–591
Hyphomyces destruens, 163, 268
Hypocalcemia, 113
  in rhabdomyolysis, 90
  preparturient, 530
  tetany in, 566–568
Hypocapnia, 480
Hypochaeris radicata, toxicity of, 571, 579
Hypochloremia, 19
Hypochromotricia, 687
Hypoderma spp., 556, 557, 697
Hypoglossal nerve, function of, 523t
Hypoglycemia, in foal, 433
Hypokalemia, 19, 113
Hypomagnesemia, 113
Hyponatremia, 18–19, 113
Hypoproliferative anemia, 491, 494–495, II:303–305
Hypotension, emergency drugs for, 29t
  halothane-induced, 100
  postoperative myositis and, 31

Hypothermia, treatment of, 348
Hypothyroidism, 808, II:185–188
Hypovolemia, in colic, 191
 treatment of, 348
Hypovolemic shock, 19, 32, 248, 492–493
Hypoxemia, 480
Hypoxia, anemic, 493
 fetal, 412

Icterus, 253
Ileocecal intussusception, 198
Ileocolonic aganglionosis, 448
Ileum, impacted, 198, II:53–55
Ileus, 447–448
 postoperative, 203
Imipenem, 10–11
Immune-mediated synovitis, 134–136
Immunity, evaluation of, 424–425, 424t
 passive transfer of, 422–423
 failure of, 423–424, 423t
 management of, 425–427
Immunization. See *Vaccination*.
Immunoglobulins, 422–424
Impaction, ascarid, 190
 from feed, 180t
 from sand, 192, 219
 of colon, 198, *198*, 218–219, II:53–55
 pelvic flexure, 192
Incontinence, urinary, 618–620
Incremental exercise test, 803, 803t
Indicator plants, 125
Infection, process of, 2
Infectious diseases, prevention of, 37–49
Infertility, 644
Inflammation, etiology of, 162t
 glucocorticoid treatment of, 15
Influenza, epizootiology of, 317–318
 isolation of virus, 317
 myopathy from, 114
 pathogenesis of, 317
 prevention and treatment of, 318–319
 serology of, 317
 subtypes of, 316–317
 vaccination to, 39, 47
Infraorbital nerve, blocking of, 26
Inguinal abscess, 161
Inguinal hernia, 190, 191, 197
Inhalation anesthesia, 30–31
 dosages for draft animals, 98
 for draft animals, 99–100
 for mules and donkeys, 104
Insecticides, 688–691, II:656–660
 antidotes to, 350t
 for control of ectoparasites, 689, 689t
 poisoning by, 338, 346
Insects, control of, 688–691, 689t
Insemination, artificial, 676–677
Inspiratory noise, 285
Insurance, equine mortality, *66*, 341
 examinations for, 65
Interphalangeal joint, proximal, 90
Interstate shipment, health regulations
 regarding, 829t–831t
Interstitial lung infiltrates, 300t
Intervertebral disks, degeneration of, 112
Intestine. See also *Colon; Small intestine*.
 infarcted nonstrangulated, II:70–73
 obstruction of, 192, 197–198
 volvulus of, 420
Intra-articular medication, 127–131
 antimicrobial, 133
 corticosteroids in, 128t
 sodium hyaluronate in, 129t
Intracellular fluid (ICF), 18
Intracranial pressure (ICP), 530
Intraluminal obstruction, 179–182, 216
Intraocular pressure, 603
Intravenous catheter, 22
Intravenous fluid replacement, 18, 247–248, 248t

Intraventricular septum, 394
Iodide therapy, for sporotrichosis, 162
Iodine, deficiency of, 687
 requirement of, 716t
Ionophores, toxicity of, 366–378
Iron, antidotes to, 347t
 deficiency of, 719
 dietary supplementation with, 813
 excess of, 719
 requirements of, 718t
Iron fumarate, toxicity of, 443
Ischemia, causing blindness, 574
Isocoma wrightii, toxicity of, 374
Isoerythrolysis, in foal, 429–430, II:244–247
Ivermectin, 51
 for nematode control, 696–697

Japanese encephalitis, 764–765
Jasmine, toxicity of, 126
Jaundice, 429–430
 agglutination test for, 430t
Jejunitis. See *Duodenitis-proximal jejunitis*.
Joint, degeneration of. See *Degenerative joint disease*.
 drainage of, 133
 effusion of, 88, 107, 125, 135
 fluid in, bacteria in, 3
 trauma to, 134
Juglans nigra, toxicity of, 155, 337–338, 373, 374
Jugular vein, catheter for, 407
 distention of, 397, 409
 thrombophlebitis of, 406–408
 thrombosis of, 22, 383
 ultrasonic imaging of, 406
Junctional mechanobullous disease, 705–706

Kanamycin, 9
Keratinization, improper, 125
 promotion of, 157
Keratitis, 585, 596–599
 punctate, 599–600, *600*
Kerosene, toxicity of, 362
Ketamine, 29, 99
Ketoconazole, for sporotrichosis, 163
Kidney, diseases of, 613–631, II:693–712, II:722–734
 disseminated intravascular congestion in, 505
 function in colic, 194
 necrosis of, 355
 pyelonephritis of, 617–618
 stones in, 613–614
 toxicosis caused by drugs, 355–356
 ultrasonic imaging of, 419
Kidney failure, acute, 623–626, II:693–698
 causes of, 623–624, 628
 chronic, 628–630, II:698–702
 diet for, 739–740
 polyuria in, 621, 629
 signs and diagnosis of, 624, 629–630
 treatment and prognosis of, 624–626, 630
Kinematics, qualitative, 787–789
 quantitative, 786–787
Kinetics, 789–790
Klebsiella spp., antibiotics for, 471t
 in septicemia, 435, 438
Kleingrass, toxicity of, 373, 376

Lactate dehydrogenase, 256
 in myopathy, 114
Lactate, in aerobic metabolism, 806
 in anaerobic metabolism, *805*
Lactation, 412
 premature, 412, 423
Lactose tolerance, 171
Lameness, causes of, 124t
 differential diagnosis of, 123–126
 evaluation of, 787–789

Lameness *(Continued)*
 of draft horse, 85–91
 prevention of, 50
Laminar necrosis, 86
Laminitis, 128, 524, II:277–281
 acute, 154–155
 chronic, 86, 155
 colic and, 191
 diet for, 738
 etiology of, 85
 glucocorticoid treatment of, 15
 grades of, 154
 predisposing factors for, 154, 155t
 prognosis of, 160
 radiograph of, *156*
 refractory, 86, 155
 selenium toxicity distinguished from, 125
 signs of, 85
 subacute, 155
 support, 155
 surgery for, 159–160, *159, 160*
 signs and diagnosis of, 154–156
 treatment of, 86, 156–158, 157t
Lantana, toxicity of, 373, 376–377
Laparoscopy, 169
Laryngeal hemiplegia, 280, 578
 arytenoid chondritis distinguished from, 289
 etiology of, 286
 in draft horse, 92
 incidence of, 285–286
 treatment for, 92–93
Laryngeal nerve, recurrent, paralysis of, 363
Laryngeal prosthesis, 92
Laryngeal sacculectomy, 92
Laryngoplasty, 92, 289
Larynx, asynchronous function of, 286–287
 diseases of, II:607–612
 grading of function of, 287, 288–289
 movements during exercise, 283, 288
Lasalocid, toxicity of, 366
Laser, effects of, *712*
 in dermatology, 711–713
 sacculectomy by, 93
 surgery with, 294–297
Late agglutination test, 425
Lateral cartilages, fracture of, 87
 ossification of, 86–87
Lateral geniculate body, lesions of, 575
Lathyrism, 571
Lathyrus hirsutus, toxicity of, 376
Laxatives, 205–206
 for colic, 205t
LDH (lactic dehydrogenase), 256
Lead, analysis for, 364
 antidotes to, 347, 351,363
 toxicity of, 173, 363–364, II:667–668
Legal considerations, chain of custody in, 343
 confidentiality in, 59
 expert witness testimony in, 62–63, 343
 fact witness testimony in, 61–62, 343
 guidelines for testifying and, 63
 malpractice actions and, 61
 postmortem investigations and, 340–341
 subpoenas of medical records and, 59–60
Leptospira interrogans, 592
Lethal white foal syndrome, 448
Leukemia, myelogenous, 514–515, II:316
Leukoencephalomalacia, 173, 253, 377–379, 558–559
Leukotrichia, hyperesthetic, II:647–648
Lice, 691, 697
Lidocaine, 25
 for arrhythmias, 392t
Ligament, evaluation of, 796–798
 injury to, 798–799
 splitting of, 143
Limb nerves, disorders of, 578–579
Lincosamides, 11
Lipid emulsions, for parenteral nutrition,

Liver, abscess of, 253
  acute failure of, II:110–112
  aflatoxin in, 369
  biopsy of, 257, 262
  chronic disease of, II:112–113
  cirrhosis of, 255
  congenital diseases of, 254
  diseases of. See *Hepatic disease.*
  disorders of, in foal, II:272–244
  distended, 257
  enzymes in, 255–256
  failure of, 253, 254, 254–255
    in foal, 442–445. See also *Tyzzer's disease.*
  fibrosis of, 254
  function of, in colic, 194
  function tests of, 256
  neoplasia of, 253
  of foal, 475
  test norms for, 444t
  ultrasonic imaging of, 257–258, *257, 258, 260,* 261, *261,* 420–421
Local anesthesia, 25–26
Locoweed, toxicity of, 338, 373, 376
Louping ill, 769
Lumbosacral space, collection of CSF from, 527–528
Lung. See also *Pulmonary* entries.
  abscess of, 300, 304, 780
  biopsy of, 302–303
  cancer of, 300
  edema in, 382
  function of, 777–778
  hemorrhage of, 300, 304, 780
  parasites of, 300, 332–333, 334t
  pleural pressure in, 778
  radiography of, 301, *302,* 780
Lungworm, 300, 332–333
Lupus erythematosus, 134, 162, 164
  synovitis and, 136
Lyme disease, 131
Lymph nodes, abscesses of, 175, 325
Lymphadenopathy, 182
Lymphangitis, epizootic, 769–770
  ulcerative, 161
Lymphocyte count, of adult blood, 826t
  of foal blood, 825t
Lymphosarcoma, 513–514, 607, II:314–316
Lysine, requirement of, 716

Macrolides, 11
  dosages of, 6t
Magnesium sulfate, for colic, 205, 206
Magnetic resonance imaging (MRI), 795–796
Maintenance diet, 728t, 729, 729t
Malabsorption syndromes, II:102–107
  diet for, 739
Malignant hyperthermia, 100, 113
Malnutrition, 742
Malpractice, 61
Mandible, fracture of, 173
Manganese, requirement of, 716t
Mange, 692
Maple, toxicity of, 373, 375, 498
Mare, aberrant maternal behavior in, 636
  age-related ovulatory dysfunction in, 643–644
  embryo transfer to, 637–640
  estrous cycle of, 635–636
  infertility of, 644
  maiden, 411
  nutrition of, 108, 108t, 412
  prefoaling management of, 664–667
  reproductive tract abnormalities of, 656–657
  sexual dysfunction in, 633–636
  stallionlike behavior in, 636, 642
  subfertility of, 644
Mast cell lesions, 702

Mast cell tumor, of eye, 606–607
Mastication, painful, 271
Mastocytosis, 702
Maxilla, fracture of, 173
McMaster's technique, 54
Mean corpuscular hemoglobin, of adult blood, 826t
  of foal blood, 824t
Mean corpuscular volume, of adult blood, 826t
  of foal blood, 824t
Mechanical ventilation, 482–484, 483t
Meconium, impacted, 168
  retained, 446–447, II:117–118
Medical records, 57–59
  confidentiality of, 59
  control over, 58
  release of, 59
  subpoenas of, 59–60
Melanoma, intraocular, 607
  of eyelid, 606
  of penis, 709
Melioidosis, 762–763
Menadione, 355
Meningitis, 111
  bacterial, 552–553
  CSF findings in, 529
  in foal, 433
  septicemia and, 441
Meningoencephalitis, 417
Mental nerve, blocking of, 26
Mercury, antidotes to, 347, 350t
  toxicity of, 359–360
Mercury chloride, toxicity of, 346
Metabolism, of calcium, II:189–192
Metacarpal bones, fractures of, 141, 145
  pain in, 141
  scintigraphy of, *793*
Metacarpal disease, dorsal, 143–146
Metatarsal pain, 141
Metaldehyde, antidotes to, 351t
Methanol, antidotes to, 351t
Methemoglobinemia, 498
  treatment of, 352t
Methylsulfonyl methane, 813
Methylxanthine derivatives, 307
  toxicity of, 356
Metritis, contagious equine (CEM), 757–760
Metronidazole, 11
Mezlocillin, 12
Microsporum spp., 698
Micturition, testing of, 619–620
Midges, 693–696
  control of, 688–689
Milk, composition of, 743t, 745t
  substitutes for, 745, 745t
Milkweed, toxicity of, 373t
Miller's disease, 119
Miller's itch, 692
Mineral oil, for colic, 205
Minerals, deficiency of, 88, 125
  dietary, 687
  in parenteral nutrition, 734
  requirements of, 716, 716t
  suggested intake of, 107t
  toxicity of, 125
Miniature horses, colic in, 190
Minimal inhibitory concentrations, 3
Mites, 691, 692, 697
Mitral regurgitation, 382, 387, *397*
Molybdenum, in diet, 718, 723
Monday morning sickness, 90, 114
Monensin, and myocardial disease, 393
  poisoning by, 337, 366
Moniliformin, 378
Monocyte count, of adult blood, 826t
  of foal blood, 825t
Morphine, antidotes to, 352t
Mosquitoes, control of, 690
Motility, disorder of, 179
  gastrointestinal, 203–204

Motility *(Continued)*
  of sperm, 672–673, 676
  of small intestine, 217
Motor cortex, lesions of, 522–523
Motor neurons, dysfunction of, 525, 526
Mouth-to-nose resuscitation, 481
MRI (magnetic resonance imaging), 795–796
Mucokinesis, 308
  agents of, 309t
Mucolytic agents, 308, 309
Mucosal brush border disaccharidase-related maldigestion, 171
Mule, sedation and anesthesia of, 101–104
Murmur, heart, 396, 397, 409
Muscarinic antagonists, 306
Muscle, biopsy of, 800
  contractile properties of, 800
  damage to, 806
  disorders of, 113–116
  evaluation of, 799–801
  metabolism in, 800
  morphology of, 800–801
Muscle strain, 115–116
Mycetoma, 162t
Mycotoxicosis, 377–379, 558–559
Mydriatic therapy, 593
Myelitis, verminous, 556–557
Myeloencephalitis, equine protozoal (EPM), 173, 527, 554–556, II:359–363
  CSF findings in, 529, 555
  nerve involvement in, 578
  vestibular disease in, 575
Myeloencephalopathy, degenerative, 559–561, II:353–355
  herpesvirus, 550–552, II:365–367
Myelogenous leukemia, 514–514, II:316
Myelography, indications for, 526
  procedures for, 526–527
Myeloma, 515–516, II:316
Myelopathy, cervical, 532, 533
  degenerative, 525, 527
Myelophthisic anemia, 495
Myiasis, 691
Myocardial disease, 382, 393–395
Myoglobinuria, 114
Myopathy, adductor, 100
  croup, 115
  dysphagia caused by, 174
  exertional, 90, 113–115
  from influenza, 114
  postanesthetic, 100, 572
  treatment of, 115, 174
Myositis, 86
  postoperative, 31, 90
Myotonia, 571

NADA (New Animal Drug Application), 74
Naphthalene, toxicity of, 361
Naracin, toxicity of, 366
Narcolepsy, 562, 565–566, II:349–353
Narcotics, for colic, 202–203
Nasal cavity, diseases of, 266–270
Nasal discharge, 271, 304
  bloody, 273
Nasal passages, diseases of, 265–270
Nasal polyps, 269
Nasal septum, 265
  amyloid deposition in, 267
  cysts of, 267
  deviated, 266
  necrosis of, 268
  neoplasms in, 267
  resection of, 267
Nasal sinuses. See *Sinuses.*
Nasal turbinates, 265
  necrosis of, 270
Nasogastric intubation, 726–727
  complications associated with, 746t
  of foal, 744–747
  rations for, 726t, 746t

Nasogastric reflux, 211
Nasolacrimal duct, catheterization of, 586t
  dysgenesis of, 585
  insufficiency of, 586
  obstruction of, 271
Nasopharynx, cicatrix of, 282–283
  displacement of, during exercise, 284–285, *284*
Nasotracheal intubation, 32
Navicular syndrome, 149–150
  radiographic changes in, *152*
  signs and diagnosis of, 150–151, *150, 152*
  treatment for, 130, 151, 153–154
Nd:YAG laser, 295–297
Nebulization, 472
Necroscopy, forensic, 341, 344–345
Necrosis, coagulative, 123
  laminar, 86
  of brain, 377, 557–558
  of kidney, 355
  of nasal turbinates, 270
  of septum, 268
Necrotic pododermatitis, 87–88
Necrotizing enterocolitis, 454–455
Nematodes, control of, 696–697
Neodymium:yttrium-aluminum garnet (Nd:YAG) laser, 295–297
Neomycin, 9
Neonatal maladjustment syndrome, 432–434, II:219–222
Neonatal respiratory distress, 479–484
Neoplasia. See names of individual tumor sites.
Nephrolithiasis, 613–614
Nephropathies, II:704–708
Nephrosplenic entrapment of colon, 190, 192
Nephrotoxicosis, drug-induced, 355–356
Nerium oleander, toxicity of, 338, 374
Nervous system, central, 33–34
  diseases of, 521–561, II:339–386
  examination of, 521–527, II:339–341
Netilmycin, 9
Neuroleptanalgesia, 97
Neurologic diseases, 521–561, II:339–386
  EHV-1 and, 319
Neurological examination, 521–527
  of foal, 414–417
Neuropathy, peripheral, II:380–386
  postoperative, 100
Neuropraxia, compressive, 524
Neutrophil count, of adult blood, 826t
  of foal blood, 825t
New Animal Drug Application (NADA), 74
Night blindness, 574
Nightshade, toxicity of, 373, 376
Nitrofurantoin, 11
Nodular skin disease, II:634–637
Nonpurpuric vasculitis, 162
Nonsteroidal anti-inflammatory agents, 14, 16–17
  dosages of, 16t
  for colic, 201–202, 204–205
  for colitis, 249
  for endotoxemia, 230–231
  for respiratory disorders, 306
  for tendinitis, 147
  for vasculitis, 512
  gastric ulcer caused by, 187, 355
  toxicity of, 355
Nonstrangulating obstruction, 190, 218–221
Nose, congenital deformities of, 266, 269
  diseases of, 265–266
  foreign body in, 274
  intranasal diseases of, 266–270
  neoplasms of, 268
Nostrils, diseases of, 265–266
  laceration of, 266
NSAIDs. See *Nonsteroidal anti-inflammatory agents*.

Nutrition, 715–750, II:387–426. See also *Diets*.
  anemia from inadequate, 494
  assessment of status of, 736–737
  calcium and phosphorus requirements in, 121t, 722
  convalescent, 724–731, II:421–426
  developmental orthopedic disease and, 720–724
  energy requirements and, 715–716, 721–722, 729t, 732–733
  enteral, 726–727, 726t, *727*, 729–730, 730t, 744–747
  ergogenic, 809–813
  feed types in, 740
  forced feeding and, 741
  hyperparathyroidism and, 120–121
  in management of disease, 737–740
  in septicemia, 439
  maintenance, 728t, 729, 729t
  mineral requirements in, 716, 716t, 718t
  of critically ill neonate, 741–750
  of geriatric patient, 740
  of neonate, 743–744
  orthopedic disorders and, 464
  parenteral, 249, 747–750. See also *Parenteral nutrition*.
  prerace, 813
  protein requirements in, 716, 722
  ration evaluation in, 811
  skin health and, 686–687
  suggested daily intake for weanlings, 109, 465t, 721t
  suggested daily intake for mares, 108t
  suggested daily intake for yearlings, 107t, 109, 465t
  suggested daily intake for foals, 107t, 108–109
  supplemental, 108, 740, 811–813
  tube feeding and, 726–727, 726t, *727*
  vitamin requirements in, 716–717, 716t
Nutritional secondary hyperparathyroidism, 119–122, 270
Nutritional therapy, after esophageal obstruction, 183
  for colitis, 249

Obstruction, removal of, 180–182
Obstructive gastrointestinal disease, 447–448
Occipital lobe, lesions of, 523t
Occipito-atlantoaxial malformation, 531–532, *532–533*
Octacosanol, 812–813
Oculomotor nerve, function of, 523t
Odontoid process, fracture of, *538*
Oil, toxicity of, 362, II:666–667
Oleander, antidotes to, 351t
  toxicity of, 338, 373, 374
Olfactory nerve, function of, 523t
Onchocerca cervicalis, 111, 592
Onchocerciasis, cutaneous, 696–697, II:627–629
Onions, toxicity of, 498
Open flow respirometry, *804*
Ophthalmic nerve, function of, 523t
Ophthalmology, anesthesia in, 26
Ophthalmoscopy, 609
Opioid antagonists, 23t
Opioids, 24
Optic nerve, atrophy of, 611
  disorders of, 574
  hypoplasia of, 609
  trauma to, 591
Optic neuritis, 610–611
Orbit, disorders of, 574
  injury to, 587–588, 588t, 610
  neoplasia of, 607–608
Organophosphate poisoning, 338
  antidotes to, 350t

Orthopedic disease, developmental, 105–109, 462–465
γ-Oryzanol, 813
Ossification, endochondral, 105
  of lateral cartilages, 86–87
Ossifying spondylosis, 110, 112
Osteitis, pedal, 151
Osteoarthritis, 135
  of fetlock joint, 140
Osteoarthrosis, 89–90
Osteochondral fragments, 107
Osteochondritis dissecans, 88, 107–108, 463
  genetic predisposition to, 463–464
Osteochondrosis, 88–89, 107–108, 125, 462–463
Osteochondrosis dissecans, in zinc poisoning, 365
Osteodystrophia fibrosa, 119, 270, 271
Osteomyelitis, 132, *456, 458, 459, 461*
  in foal, 455–462, II:225–230
  septicemia and, 441
  vertebral, 109, 110–111, *111*
Osteophytes, 129, 139, 151
  vertebral, 112
Osteostixis, 145
Otitis media, 175, 575
Ovary, abnormalities of, II:500–503
  tumors of, 642
  ultrasonic imaging of, 650–652, 656
Overcirculation, pulmonary, 409
Ovulation, delayed, 643
  double, 656
  failure of, 633–634, 643–644, 656
  management of, II:498–500
  ultrasonic imaging of, 651–652, *651*
Oxalates, antidotes to, 352, 347t
  poisoning by, 119, 121
Oxygen therapy, 481–482
  in pneumonia, 471
  intranasal administration of, 32
Oxytropis spp., toxicity of, 376
Oxyuris equi, 697

Pacemaker, wandering atrial, 384–385
Packed cell volume (PCV), 19
  of adult blood, 826t
  of foal blood, 824t
Paddocks, construction of, 37
Pain, abdominal. See *Colic*.
  metatarsal or metacarpal, 141
Pancreas, disease of, 253
Pancreatitis, acute, II:46–47
Panicum spp., toxicity of, 121, 376
Panniculus reflex, 526
  defect of, 525
Papilloma, penile, 709
Papular urticaria, 164
Paracentesis, abdominal, 169, 193, 238–241
  of guttural pouches, 276
Paralysis, in botulism, 370
  hyperkalemic, 117–118, 573
Paralytic bladder, II:712–713
Paranasal sinuses, 265
  diseases of, 271–274
Parascaris equorum, 333
Parasite control, 49, 51–54, II:336–337
  environmental, 54
  evaluation of, 54–55
  interval, 52–53
  of ectoparasites, 688–692, 689t
Parasites, 163–164
  causing CNS disorders, 556–557
  conjunctivitis caused by, 586
  control of, 49, 51–54, II:336–337
  diagnosis of, II:323–327
  diarrhea from, 452–453
  ectoparasites, 688–692
  external, II:622–632
  gastrointestinal, 697

Parasites *(Continued)*
  in pastures, II:334–336
  internal, II:323–337
  myocardial disease and, 393
  of lung, 332–334
  penile, 709
  vestibular disease caused by, 575
Parasitism, 191
Parasympatholytics, 306
Parathyroid hormone, function of, *120*. See also *Hyperparathyroidism*.
Paravertebral nerve, blocking of, 27
Parenteral nutrition, 249, 747–750
  complications of, 747t
  compounding of, 735, 735t
  monitoring of, 748t
  nutrients for, 732–735, 735t
  of foal, 749, 749t
  products for, 748t
Parietal lobe, lesions of, 523t
Parotid gland, swelling of, 93
Parturition, 666
  complications of, II:537–542, II:544–547
  induction of, 667, II:533–537
  injuries during, II:550–555
Pasteurella spp., 161
  antibiotics for, 471t
Patella, upward fixation of, 88
Patellar reflex, 526
Patent ductus arteriosus, 410
Pathology, procedures in, 823–824
  sampling for, 822
PBBs (polybrominated biphenyls), toxicity of, 360
PCBs (polychlorinated biphenyls), toxicity of, 360
PCP (phencyclidine), antidotes to, 351t
Pectoral abscesses, 161
Pedal bone, rotation of, *156*
  sinking of, 85
Pedal osteitis, 151
Pelvic flexure impaction, 192
Pelvic plexus, lesions in, 526
Pelvic urethra, ultrasonic imaging of, 680–681, *680*
Pelvis, scintigraphic imaging of, *794*
Penicillins, 11–12
  dosages of, 7t
Penis, lesions of, 709
  neoplasia of, 708–709
  parasitism of, 709
  physical injuries to, 710–711
Pentachlorophenol, toxicity of, 361, 362
Pentachlorothiophenol, toxicity of, 361
Pentosan sulfate, 17, 131
Performance, estrus and, 635–636
  evaluation for, 771–774, 773t
  heart and, 381–383
  testing of, 802–806
Performance horses, 771–814, II:465–490
  clinical assessment of, II:476–477
Pericardial disease, 382
Pericardial effusion, 403, 421
Pericardial fibrosis, 403
Pericardial friction rub, 403
Pericardiocentesis, 404–405
Pericarditis, 402–405, 421
  constrictive, 403
  fibrinous, II:171–172
  indwelling drains for, 405
  leading to myocardial disease, 393
  prognosis for, 405
Perineum, abnormalities of, II:518–520
  analgesia of, 27–28
Periosteal transection and stripping, 106
Periostitis, chronic ossifying alveolar, 271
Peripheral vascular disease, II:173–176
Peritoneal effusion, 241t

Peritoneal fluid, 193, 239
  analysis of, 240t
  clinical norms for, 828t
Peritoneum, adhesions of, 216
  dialysis of, 243
    for poisoning, 348
  lavage of, 243
Peritonitis, *186*, 190, 455, II:79–81
  anaerobic bacteria in, 237
  conditions associated with, 237t
  differential diagnosis of, 241t
  diffuse, 200
  diffuse septic, 236
  fibrinous, *186*
  localized, 236
  signs and diagnosis of, 237–238
  treatment for, 217, 241–242
  ultrasonic findings in, 420
Persistent fetal circulation, 410
Petroleum products, toxicity of, 362, II:666–667
pH alteration, to treat poisoning, 348
Phalanx, distal, displacement of, 155, *156,* 157
  sinking of, 155
Pharynx, cicatrix of, 282–283
  collapse of, 283–285
  compression of, 94
  diseases of, II:607–612
  lymphoid hyperplasia of, 282, 293
  neoplasia of, 174
  paresis of, 100
  trauma to, 174
PHBs (polyhalogenated biphenyls), toxicity of, 360
Phencyclidine, antidotes to, 351t
Phenobarbital, 434
Phenol, antidotes to, 347t
  toxicity of, 360–361
Phenothiazine tranquilizers, 23–24, 23t
  antidotes to, 352t
  toxicity of, 498, II:665–666
Phenylbutazone, 17
  toxicity of, II:118–119
Phenytoin, 434
Phosphorus, antidotes to, 347t
  calcium and, 722t
  deficiency of, 718
  dietary supplement of, 108
  fractional excretion of, 121
  nutritional requirements of, 121t, 718t, 722
  orthopedic disorders and, 464, 722
Photoactivated vasculitis, 162, 164–165, II:646–647
Photoperiod, and reproduction, 643, II:491–492
Photosensitization, 164–165, II:632–633
  in liver failure, 255
Phycomycosis, 162
Physeal dysplasia, 106–107
Physitis, 88, 106, 125, 463
Phytonadione, 355
Picornavirus, 324
Pigeon chest, 161
Pinworm, 697
Piperazine, 51
Piroplasmosis, 499–500, 692
Pituitary, tumors of, 574, II:182–185
Placenta, 412
  retained, 85, II:547–550
Placental insufficiency, 412
Placentitis, 412
Plants, toxic, 372–377, II:672–682
Plasma, calcium concentration in, 119–120
  protein in, 19
  replacement of, 20
  triglycerides in, 256
Plasma therapy, 248–249, 517–518, II:317–322
  for septicemia, 439
Plasma volume, 18

Plasmacytic arthritis, 134
Pleura, biopsy of, 302–303
Pleural cavity, anaerobic infection of, 327
  drainage of, 328
Pleural effusion, 405
  in foal, 421
  ultrasonic imaging of, *404*
Pleural fluid, clinical norms for, 828t
  in pleuropneumonia, 327
  ultrasonic imaging of, 421
Pleural friction rubs, 403
Pleural pressure, 778–779
Pleuritis, 300t, 421
Pleuropneumonia, 327–328, II:592–596
Pleuroscopy, 303
Plumber's pitch, toxicity of, 361
Pneumocystis carinii, 333
Pneumonia, 300
  aspiration, 181t, 182, 363, 780
  bronchinterstitial, 473
  in foals, 466–473
  meconium aspiration, 412
  septicemia and, 441
  ultrasonic findings in, 420
Pneumothorax, 32
Pododermatitis, necrotic, 87–88
Poisoning, 337
  agents of, II:649–653
  aminoglycoside, 356
  amphotericin B, 355
  antidotes to, 347, 350–353
  arsenic, II:668–670
  blister beetle, 358
  cadmium, 365–366
  carbamate, 338
  carbon tetrachloride, II:665
  castor bean, 358
  coal tar derivative, 361
  dicoumarol, 371
  digitalis, 356
  drug, 353–358
  elimination of toxicant in, 346, 348
  endophytic, 369
  feed-associated, 366–371
  fluoride, 358–359
  fungicide, 361
  heavy metal, 339, 347, 363–366, 501
  herbicide, 361
  industrial agents of, 358–362
  insecticide, 338, 346
  ionophore, 366–367
  lead, 173, 363–364, II:667–668
  liver involvement in, 443
  mercury, 359–360
  mercury chloride, 346
  methylxanthine, 356
  monensin, 337, 366
  oleander, 338, 373, 374
  onion, 498
  organophosphate, 338
  oxalate, 119, 121
  petroleum product, 362, II:666–667
  phenolic, 360–361
  phenothiazine, II:665–666
  plant, 372–377, II:672–682
  polyhalogenated biphenyl, 360
  quinidine, 356
  selenium, 125, II:670–671
  sesbania, 358
  strychnine, 346
  theophylline, 356
  treatment of, 340–353, 373, II:653–656
  vitamin D, 126
  warfarin, 502–503, II:305–306
  yew, 338, 373, 375
  zinc, 125, 364–365
Polyarthritis, 131
Polydipsia, 620–621, 629
  differential diagnosis of, 621t

Polyhalogenated biphenyls (PBBs, PCBs, PHBs), 360
Polymorphonuclear leukocytes, 3
Polymyxin B, 13
Polyneuritis equi, 172, 569–570
  vestibular disease in, 575
Polyuria, 620–622, 642
  differential diagnosis of, 621t
  in kidney failure, 629
Poor performance syndrome, II:469–474
  heart and, 381–383
Portal vein, thrombosis of, 253
Positive end-expiratory pressure (PEEP), 32
Postanesthetic myopathy, 100, 572
Postexercise fatigue, 113
Postmortem examination, 67
  forensic, 341–342, 344–345
  legal considerations of, 340–341
  specimen collection for, 68t, 339t, 342–343, 342t, 345
Potassium, exchangeable, in ICF, 18
  in adult blood, 827t
  in foal blood, 826t
  supplementation of, 20
Potassium chloride challenge test, 118
Potentiated sulfonamides, 13
  dosages of, 7t
Potomac horse fever, 191, 692, II:92–93
  diarrhea in, 245
  serology of, 251
  signs and diagnosis of, 251–252, 500
  treatment and prevention of, 252–253, 500
  vaccination against, 39, 48
  vasculitis after, 511
Precordial thrill, 409
Pre-excitation, 389, *389*
Pregnancy, diet in, 665t
  estrus in, 635
  rates of, *645*
  twin, 657–659, II:532–533
  ultrasonic imaging of, 653–656
Prehension, 172–173
Premolars, retained 173
Preoperative assessment, 28–29
  of donkeys and mules, 101
Prepurchase examination, 36, 68–71, *70*
Preventive medicine, 35–36
  client education, 36–37
  dental care, 49–50
  infectious disease prevention, 37–49
  parasite control, 49
Probiotics, 813
Progesterone, and collagen synthesis, 723
Progesterone therapy, 647
Progestins, behavioral uses of, II:129–131
Proliferative synovitis, 134, 135
Propranolol, for tachycardia, 392t
Proprioception, defects of, 525
Prostaglandins, inhibition of, 14
Prostate, ultrasonic imaging of, 679, *680*
Protein, dietary, 686
  for parenteral nutrition, 733–734
  in adult blood, 827t
  in cerebrospinal fluid, 529
  in foal blood, 825t
  in plasma, 19
  requirements of, 716, 722
Protein-vitamin-mineral supplements, 108
Proteus spp., 471t
Prothrombin time, 256
Proximal splint bone periostitis, 141
Pseudoallescheria boydii, 268
Pseudomembranous colitis, 356
Pseudomonas spp., causing keratitis, 596–598
Pseudomonas aeruginosa, 9, 400
  antibiotics for, 471t
Pseudomonas mallei, 162t, 761–762
Pseudomonas pseudomallei, 762
Pseudomycetoma, 701

Pseudotruncus arteriosus, 410
Psoroptes spp., 697
Psyllium mucilloid, for colic, 205–206
Pulmonary. See also *Lung.*
  artery, rupture of, 397
  edema, 382
  function testing, 777–779, *778*
  hemorrhage. See *Exercise-induced pulmonary hemorrhage (EIPH).*
  hypertension, 382, 397
  overcirculation, 409
  thromboembolism, 406
Pulmonic regurgitation, 398
Pulmonic valvular insufficiency, 398–399
Pulse, in laminitis, 155
Punch biopsy, 684–685
Punctate keratitis, 599–600, *600*
Pupil, response of, to light, 33, 609
Purpura hemorrhagica, 162t, 164, 326, 511
Pyelonephritis, 617–618, II:708–712
Pyemotid mites, control of, 691–692
Pyrogens, 16
Pyrrolizidine toxicity, 254, 338, 373, 375–376
Pythiosis, 162
Pythium spp., 162t, 163

Queensland itch, 689
Quidding, 271
Quinidine sulfate, as antiarrhythmic, 386, 387, 388, 389, 391, 392t
  toxicity of, 356
Quinolones, 10

Rabies, 525, 545–546, II:364–365
  diagnosis of, 526, 545–546
  dysphagia caused by, 172, 173
  vaccination against, 39, 546
Racetrack, racing association veterinarian at, 79–80
  racing commission veterinarian at, 79
Radiography, contrast, 168
  in prepurchase examination, 71
  of alimentary tract, 168
  of bone, 791
  of esophagus, 177–178, *178*
  of guttural pouch, 94
  of lower airway, 779–781
  of navicular syndrome, 151, 152
  of spine, 110, 527
  thoracic, 301–302, *302*, 470, 470t
Radionuclide scintigraphy. See *Scintigraphy.*
Ranitidine, for gastric ulcer, 188–189
Rectal tear, 197
  classification of, 233
  diagnosis of, 233
  packing for, 234, *234*
  prevention of, 235–236
  treatment and management of, 233–235, *234*
Rectum, biopsy of mucosa of, 170
  endoscopy of, 167
  examination of, 192, 218
    normal findings in, 196, *197*
    pathological findings in, 197–200, 218
  technique for, 196
  prolapsed, II:73–75
  tears in, 197, 233–236, II:75–79
Red blood cell count (RBC)
  of adult, 826t
  of neonate, 824t
Reflexes, of foal, 416
Reflux, 183, 191
  nasogastric, 211
Reflux esophagitis, 183
Regional anesthesia, 26–28
  of thoracic limb, 102

Regurgitation, 363. See also *Aortic regurgitation; Mitral regurgitation; Pulmonic regurgitation; Tricuspid regurgitation.*
Renal failure. See *Kidney failure.*
Renal tubular acidosis, 627–628, II:722–724
Reproduction, 633–681, II:491–577
  photoperiod and, 643, II:491–492
Reproductive disorders, of mares, 633–636
  of stallions, 668–670
Reproductive tract, infections of, treatment of, 4t
Respiration, noisy, 265
  normal, 480
  of foal, 474
Respiratory disorders, II:579–603
  caused by herpesvirus, 319
  cultures for, 304
  laser surgery for, 294–297
  of draft horse, 92–95
  of foal, 479–484, 479t
  of lower tract, 299–303, 300t
  treatment of, 4t, 303–310
  viral, 304, 316–324, II:581–590
Respiratory system, evaluation of, II:579–581
  open flow respirometry, *804*
  of foal, 479–480, 480t
  stimulants of, 308, *308*
Rest, for respiratory disorders, 303–304
Restraint, chemical, 22–23, 23t. See also *tranquilizers.*
  during mechanical ventilation, 483t
  of draft horse, 95–97, 96t
  pre-anesthesia, 101–102
Retained placenta, II:547–550
  and laminitis, 85
Retina, dysplasia of, 609
Retrograde ejaculation, 670
Rhabditis spp., 697
Rhabdomyolysis, 90–91, 524
  exertional, 113, 114, II:487–490
Rhinitis, 270
Rhinopneumonitis, vaccination against, 39, 47–48
Rhinosporidium spp., 268
Rhodococcus equi, 161, 304, 421
  antibiotics for, 471t
  diarrhea for, 452
  pneumonia from, 466–470
Rhododendron spp., toxicity of, 374
Riboflavin, requirement of, 716t
Ricinus communis, toxicity of, 358
Rifampin, 13
Ringbone, articular, 89
  nonarticular, 89
Ringworm, 698
Roaring, 363
Rodenticides, II:660–663
Rostral thalamus, lesions of, 522
Rotation, third phalanx, 85
Rotavirus, 449–450
  testing for, 170
Russian knapweed, 173

Sacculectomy, 92
  laser, 93
Sacrococcygeal spinal cord, lesions of, 526
Sacroiliac subluxation, 110, 112–113
Salinomycin, toxicity of, 366
Salivary glands, disease of, II:3–6
Salmonella spp., 191, 245, 247
  antibiotics for, 471t
  diarrhea from, 451–452, 454
  in septicemia, 435, 437
  testing for, 170
Salmonellosis, 191, 245, 247, II:88–92
Sample, collection of, 822, 822t
  handling of, 823
Sand, colic from, II:255–258
  impaction with, 192, 219

Sarcoid, 606
  immunotherapy for, 637–639
  laser removal of, 712
Sarcoidosis, 709
Sarcoptic mange mites, 692, 697
Scab mites, 692
Schiff-Sherrington syndrome, 538
Scintigraphy, during exercise, 783
  of airway, 781–782
  of bone, 144, 791–795, *792, 793, 794*
  of navicular syndrome, 151
  of spine, 110
Sclerosis, subchondral, 139
Scratch certificates, 76
Screwworm, 691
Scrotal hernia, 191, *419*
SDH (sorbitol dehydrogenase), 255
Sedatives, 22–25
  colic treated by, 202
  for foal, 475–476, 482–483
  for mules and donkeys, 102
Seedy toe, 155
Seizures, 33, 561
  causes of, 563t
  etiology and pathogenesis of, 562
  in foal, 433–434, 563t
  signs and diagnosis of, 562, 564
  treatment of, 564–565, 564t
Selenium, deficiency of, 113, 123, 718, 719
  excess of, 125, 719
  for myopathy, 115, 174
  requirement of, 716t, 718t
  toxicity of, II:670–671
Semen, abnormalities of, II:564–566
  collection of, 674–675, 675t
  evaluation of, 675–676
  physical characteristics of, 671–674, 672t
  preservation of, 677
Semen extenders, 676, 676t
Semitendinosus strain, 116
Semitendinosus tenectomy, 116
Senecio spp., toxicity of, 254, 375, 443
Sepsis, 417
  hemolysis and, 430–431
Sepsis scoring, 413t, 452
Septic arthritis, 441, *456, 459, 461,* II:225–230
  pathogenesis and findings of, 459–460
  treatment and prognosis of, 460–462
  types of, 455–458
Septic shock, 442
Septicemia, 406
  antibiotics for, 440t
  blood analysis for, 437–438, 822
  etiology and pathogenesis of, 435–436
  in foal, 435–442, 744, II:222–225
  meningitis and, 441
  signs and diagnosis of, 436–438
  treatment and prognosis for, 438–442
Septum, 265
  amyloid deposition in, 267
  cysts of, 267
  deviation of, 266
  intraventricular, 394
  necrosis of, 268
  neoplasms of, 267
  resection of, 267
Sesamoid fracture, 140
Sesamoiditis, 140–141, *141*
Sesbania spp., toxicity of, 358
Setaria spp., 556
Setaria sphacelata, 121
Sexual dysfunction, in mare, 633–636
  in stallion, 668–670, 669t
SGOT. See *Aspartate aminotransferase*.
Shaker foal syndrome, 542, 543, 544
Shave biopsy, 685
Shivers, 90, 572
Shock, 19
  emergency drugs for, 29t
  from trauma, 32, 492–493

Shock *(Continued)*
  hemorrhagic, 32
  hypertonic saline for, 21
  hypovolemic, 19, 32, 248, 492–493
Shoeing, for laminitis, 158–159
  for navicular syndrome, 151
Sick sinus syndrome, 383
Sidebone, ossification of, 86
Silver nitrate, antidotes to, 347t
Single radial immunodiffusion assay (SRID), 423, 424–425
Singletary pea, toxicity of, 373, 376
Sinoatrial arrest, 385, *385*
Sinoatrial block, 385
Sinocentesis, 272
Sinoscopy, 272
Sinus arrhythmia, 385
Sinus tachycardia, *391*
Sinuses, 265
  cancer of, 273–274
  diseases of, 271–274
  trauma to, 272
  trephination of, 272
Sinusitis, 272–273, II:605–607
Skeletal system, collagen in, 721t
  infections of, treatment of, 4t
Skin, biopsy of, 683–686, 684t
  deficient sensation in, 525
  diseases of, 683–713, II:619–648
    treatment of, 4t
  ectoparasites of, 688–697
  eosinophilic dermatitis of, 706–708
  fungal disorders of, 698–699
  nodular disease of, II:634–637
  staphylococcal infection of, 700–701
Skull, demineralization of, 121
Slap test, 92
SLE. See *Systemic lupus erythematosus*.
Small intestine, motility of, 217
  obstruction of, 197, *198*, 214
    laboratory findings in, 215t
    signs of, 215
    treatment of, 215–217
  resection of, 216
    diet after, 739
  strangulated obstruction of, 214, II:47–51
  volvulus of, 420, 447
Snake bite, 501, II:663–664
  antidotes to, 352t
Snakeroot, toxicity of, 373, 374
Sodium, exchangeable, in ECF, 18
  in adult blood, 827t
  in cerebrospinal fluid, 530
  in foal blood, 826t
Sodium bicarbonate, dietary supplementation with, 811
  precursors of, 20
Sodium chlorate, toxicity of, 361
Sodium cromoglycate, 307–308
Sodium fluoroacetate, toxicity of, 359
Sodium hyaluronate, 16, 17
  dosages of, 17t
  for traumatic synovitis, 135
  intra-articular use of, 127, 128–129, 129t
Sodium iodide, for sporotrichosis, 162
Soft palate, displacement of, 283–284, *284,* 775–776, *775*
  paresis of, 283
Solanum spp., toxicity of, 376
Sole, bruised, 155
  penetration by distal phalanx, 155
Solutions, crystalloid, 20–21
  composition of, 21t
Sorbitol dehydrogenase, 255
Sorghum, toxicity of, 373, 376, 610
Spasm, esophageal, 180t
Spavin, 89
Spavin test, 89
Spectrophotometry, of cerebrospinal fluid, 528

Sperm, characteristics of, 673–674
  morphology of, 673
  motility of, 672–673, 676
Spider bite, antidotes to, 352t
Spinal cord. See also *Cervical spinal cord; Sacrococcygeal spinal cord; Thoracolumbar spinal cord.*
  compression of, 538–539, *538, 539*
  dysfunction of, 522
  examination of, 524–526, 525t
  lesions of, 525–526, 619
  trauma to, 33, *536*, 538–539, II:374–376
Spine, disorders of, 109–113
Spiramycin, 11
Spleen, 807
Spondylosis, ossifying, 110, 112
Sporothrix schenkii, 162
Sporotrichosis, 161, 162–163
Squamous cell carcinoma, of eye, 605–606
  of penis, 708–709
Stable, air filtering of, 315
  dimensions of, 310–311, 311t
  disinfection of, 314–315
  noxious gases in, 315
  ventilation of, 311–312, 311t, *312*
Stable flies, control of, 690
Stachybotryotoxicosis, 379
Stallion, accessory sex glands of, 678–681
  copulatory dysfunction in, 669–670
  genital abnormalities of, II:558–562
  low libido in, 668–669, 669t
  seminal characteristics of, 671–674, 672t
  sexual dysfunction in, 668–670, 669t
  unruly or savage, 670
Staphylococcus spp., antibiotics for, 471t
  skin infection caused by, 700–701
Steatitis, 123
Stenosis, 527
Steroid flare, postinjection, 128
Steroids. See *Corticosteroids.*
Stillbirth, 369
Stimulants, for respiratory disorders, 308, 310
Stomach, dilation of, 198
  endoscopy of, *185,* 187, *187, 188*
Stomoxys calcitrans, 163
Stones, in biliary tract, 259
  in urinary tract, 613–615
Stool. See *Feces.*
Strangles, 93, 164, 175, II:590–592
  etiology of, 324–325
  signs and diagnosis of, 325
  therapy and control of, 325–326
  vaccination against, 39, 48, 326
  vasculitis and, 511
Strangulating lipoma, 190
Strangulating umbilical hernia, 190
Straw itch mites, 691
Streptococcus spp., antibiotics for, 471t
  in guttural pouch empyema, 277
  in vasculitis, 511
Streptococcus equi, 164, 175, 324. See also *Strangles.*
  vaccination against, 326
Streptomycin, 8
Stress, monitoring, 81
  signs of, 81–82
  treatment of, 82
Stress fractures, 144–146
Stress tetany, 113, 114
Stridor, 265, 283
Stringhalt, 571, 579
Strongyles, 51
  benzimidazole-resistant, 51
  chemotherapy for, 51–55, II:331–332
  egg counts of, 55
Strongyloides westeri, 52, 161, 170
  diarrhea from, 452
Strongylus edentatus, 51

Strongylus vulgaris, 51
   diarrhea from, 452
   myelitis from, 556
Strychnine, antidotes to, 352t
   toxicity of, 346
Subchondral sclerosis, 139
Subepiglottic cyst, 174
Submandibular nodes, abscesses of, 325
Subpoena ad testificandum, 59
Subpoena duces tecum, 59
Sudden death, 340–341
   causes of, 341t
   diagnosis of, II:685–689
Sulfobromophthalein clearance test, 256
Sulfonamides, 13
   dosages of, 7t
Sulfur, in diet, 718, 723
Summer pasture-associated obstructive pulmonary disease, 306, 330
Superficial digital flexor tendon, injury of, 146
Superior check ligament desmotomy, 148
Superoxide dismutase, 130–131, 813
Supraorbital nerve, blocking of, 26
Suprascapular nerve, paralysis of, 578
Supraventricular arrhythmias, 385–390
Supraventricular tachycardia, 386–387
Surfactants, 308
Surgery, abdominal, complications of, 216
   esophageal, 182
   for colic, 195
   for degenerative joint disease, 139
   for ethmoidal hematoma, 275
   for laminitis, 159–160
   laser, 294–297
   of nasal septum, 267
Suspensory desmitis, 141–143, *142*, 151
Suspensory ligament, 140
   ultrasonic imaging of, 142t
Swallowing, difficulty in. See *Dysphagia*.
Swamp cancer, 163
Sweeny, 578
Sweet itch, 689
Swellings, 421
Sympathomimetics, 306–307
Synovial biopsy, 132, 136
Synovial effusion, 107, 125
Synovial fluid, cell count in, 135, 136
   clinical norms for, 828t
Synovial fossae, enlarged, 151
Synovitis, 456, 457
   eosinophilic, 134, 136
   immune-mediated, 134, 135–136
   infectious, 131–133
   noninfectious, 134–136
   proliferative, 134, 135
   SLE-like, 136
   traumatic, 134–135
   villonodular, 135
Systemic lupus erythematosus, 134, 162, 164
   synovitis and, 136

Tabanids, control of, 688
Tachycardia, 383
   atrial, 386–387, *386, 387*
   emergency drugs for, 29t
   sinus, *391*
   supraventricular, 386–387
   ventricular, 391, *391*, 393, 785
Taeniae, 197
Tail, alteration of, 580
   electromyography of, 580–581
   examination of, 581
   function of, 579
Tapeworm, 52
   control of, 54
Tarpaper, toxicity of, 361
Tarsitis, 89
Tarsocrural joint, 89
Taxus spp., toxicity of, 338, 375

Taylorella equigenitalis, 757–758
Teeth, care of, 49–50, II:6–12
   disease of, related to sinus disorders, 271
   eroded and pitted, 126
   loose, 121
   pitted, 359
   retained deciduous, 173
Temporal bone, fracture of, *537*
Tendinitis, acute, 146–147
   exercise regimen for, 149
   flexor, 140
   subacute, 147–148
   treatment of, 146–149
Tendon, 146
   bowed, 798
   evaluation of, 796–798
   flexor, 88, 125, 797–798
   injury to, 798–799, *798*
   remodeling of, 148–149
   splitting of, 148
   transplantation of, 148
Tennessee Walking Horse, soring of, 77
Tenotomy, deep digital flexor, 86
   at midpastern, 159
Tetanus, 540–541, II:370–373
   39, 541
Tetany, hypocalcemic, 566–568
   stress, 113, 114
Tetrachlorodibenzodioxin (TCDD), 362
Tetracyclines, 13
   dosages of, 7t
Tetralogy of Fallot, 409, 410
Thalamus, rostral, lesions of, 522
Theiler's disease, 254, II:110–112
Theophylline, 307
   toxicity of, 356
Thermography, for diagnosis of myopathy, 116
   of navicular syndrome, 151
Thermoregulation, II:477–479
Thiamine, requirement of, 716t
Thiamylal, 30
Thigh, myopathy of, 115
Thoracic limb, regional anesthesia of, 102
Thoracic radiography, 301–302, *302*, 470, 470t
Thoracocentesis, 32, 302, 328
Thoracolumbar spinal cord, lesions of, 526
Thorax, examination of, 302, *302*
Thrombocytopenia, 507–510, II:310–312
Thromboembolism, pulmonary, 406
Thrombophlebitis, 400, 406–408
   prevention of, 407
Thromboxanes, inhibition of, 14
Thrush, of foot, II:266–272
Ticks, control of, 692
Tie back, 92
Tiletamine, 30
Tilmicosin, 11
Tobramycin, 9
Tocopherol. See *Vitamin E*.
Toe, excessive wear on, 89
Togavirus. See *Encephalitis*.
Tongue, dysfunction of, 173
   lacerations of, 173
   paralysis of, 173
Topical anesthesia, 26
Total body water (TBW), 18
Total plasma protein (TPP), 19
Toxicology, 337–377, II:649–691. See also *Poisoning*.
   analytical, 339–340
   diagnostic, 337–339
   feed sampling for, 338
   postmortem samples for, 68t, 339t, 342–343
   samples for, 339t
Trace minerals, 687, 716t
   deficiency of, 88, 125
   in parenteral nutrition, 734

Trace minerals *(Continued)*
   suggested intake of, 107t
   toxicity of, 125
Trachea, aspiration of, 301
   deformity of, 300t
Tracheobronchial aspirates, 301
Tracheobronchial foreign bodies, 300
Trail rides, 80–83
   equipment for, 81t
Tranquilizers, 22–25
   for mules and donkeys, 102
Transphyseal bridging, 106
Transport, international, 72–73
Transposition of the great vessels, 410
Transtracheal aspiration, 301
Transtracheal washes, 3
Trauma, CSF findings in, 529, 539
   examination for, 32–33
   fracture, 34
   intracranial, II:377–380
   orthopedic disease caused by, 464
   superficial, 34–35
   to brain, 536–538
   to central nervous system, 33–34
   to eye, 587–591
   to penis, 710–711
   to sinuses, 272
   to spine, 538–539, II:377–380
   vestibular disease caused by, 575
Traumatic synovitis, 134–135
Treadmill, for cardiac testing, 783–784
   for gait analysis, 787–789
   for performance testing, 802–806
Trephination, of sinuses, 272
Triceps reflex, 526
Trichophyton spp., 698
Tricuspid atresia, 409, 410
Tricuspid insufficiency, 398
Tricuspid regurgitation, 382, 398, *398*
Trigeminal nerve, disorders of, 577–578
   function of, 523t
Trochlear nerve, function of, 523t
Truncus arteriosus, 410
Tuber sacrale, prominence of, 112
Tuberculosis, 300t
Turbinate congestion, 100
Twins, abortion of, 659t
   carrying of, 657–659
   examination for, 658
   ultrasonic imaging of, 655–656
Tying up, 90, 114, 808
Tylosin, 11
Tympanic membrane, 275
Tympany, 276
   laser surgery for, 297
Tyzzer's disease, 254, 433, 442–445

Ulcer. See also *Duodenal ulcer; Gastric ulcer*.
   pathogenesis of, 184–185
   signs and diagnosis of, 185–188
   treatment of, 188–189
Ulcerative lymphangitis, 161
Ultrasound, for colic, 420, *420*
   gender determination by, 660–663
   of alimentary tract, 168–169
   of cervix, 652–653
   of embryo, 644
   of heart, 382, 387, 393, 403, 408, 421, II:139–147
   of hernia, 418
   of jugular vein, 406
   of kidney, 419
   of liver, 257–258, *257, 258, 260, 261, 261*, 420–421
   of lower airway, 782–783
   of ovaries, 650–652
   of pleural effusion, *404*
   of pleuritis, 327
   of pregnancy, 653–656

Ultrasound (Continued)
  of stallion accessory sex glands, 678–681, *679, 680*
  of suspensory ligament, 142t
  of swellings and masses, 421
  of tendons and ligaments, 146, 797–798, *798*
  of thorax, 302
  of umbilicus, 417–418
  of uterus, 652
  techniques and equipment for, 648–650, *649*
Umbilical hernia, 190, 216
Umbilical infection, 417–418
Urachal diverticulum, 419
Urachus, patent, 419
  ultrasonogram of, *418*
Urea, in adult blood, 827t
  in foal blood, 825t
Ureter, stones in, 613–614
Urethra, diseases of, 615, II:719–720
  patency of, 710
  pelvic, ultrasonic imaging of, 680–681, *680*
  stones in, 614–615
Urinalysis, clinical norms for, 828t
Urinary incontinence, 618–620
Urinary tract, diseases of, 418–419, 613–630, II:693–734
  malformations of, II:720–722
  neoplasia of, 623, II:720–722
  obstruction of, 613–615, II:713–715
  stones in, 613–615
Uroperitoneum, 419, *419*
Urticaria, papular, 164
  recurrent, II:619–621
Uterus, abnormalities of, II:503–508
  cysts of, 657
  disorders of, II:508–511
  torsion of, 190, 191
  ultrasonic imaging of, 650, *653*, 656–657
Uveitis. See *Anterior uveitis*.

Vaccination, anaphylaxis from, 49
  combination, 44t–45t
  efficacy of, 38
  for African horse sickness, 756
  for Herpesvirus, 39, 47
  for influenza, 318
  for Japanese encephalitis, 765
  for strangles, 326
  for Venezuelan encephalitis, 767
  schedules for, 46t
  types of, 40t–43t
Vagus nerve, disorders of, 578
  function of, 523t
Valvular abnormalities, 382
Valvular insufficiency, 382, 393, 396
Vancomycin, 13
Vasculitis, 510–513, 619, II:312–314
  cutaneous, 164
  nonpurpuric, 162
  photoactivated, 162, 164–165, II:646–647
  treatment of, 4t
Vasoactive drugs, for navicular syndrome, 153
Vasodilation, for laminitis, 158
Vectorcardiography, II:147–151

Venereal diseases, of mares, 757, II:513–516
  of stallion, 709–710, II:567–570
Venezuelan equine encephalomyelitis (VEE), 547, 548, *548*, 765–768
Ventilation, 311–312
  adequacy of environmental, 37
  mechanical, 482, 483t
  of foal, 481–484, II:247–253
Ventilatory support, 32
Ventricular arrhythmias, 390–393, *785*
Ventricular dilation, 382
Ventricular enlargement, right, 393
Ventricular pre-excitation, 389, *389*
Ventricular premature depolarization (VPD), 390–391, *390*
Ventricular septal defect, 381–382, 409–410, *410*
Ventricular tachycardia, 391, *391*, 393
  exercise-induced, 785, *785*
Verminous arteritis, 190
Verminous myelitis, 556–557
Vertebrae, instability of, 527
  malformations of, 463, 532–534, II:355–359
Vertebral osteomyelitis, 109, 110–111
Vertebral osteophytes, 112
Vesicular glands, ultrasonic imaging of, 678, *679*
Vestibular disease, 575
  nerve damage causing, 578
  signs and diagnosis of, 576
  treatment for, 576–577
Vestibulocochlear nerve, disorders of, 578
  function of, 523t
Veterinarian, accredited, 73
  attending, 77
  horse show, 76–78
  racetrack, 78–80
  testing, 77
  trail ride duties of, 80–83
Villonodular synovitis, 135
Virus, A/equine 1, 316, 317
  A/equine 2, 316–317
  airborne, 314
  conjunctivitis caused by, 585–586
  diarrhea caused by, 449
  equine herpesvirus. See *Herpesvirus*.
  isolated from cerebrospinal fluid, 529
  isolation of, 317, 320
  respiratory disease caused by, 316–324. See also names of diseases.
Visceral pain, 201–203. See also *Colic*.
Visceral distention, 168
Visceral larva migrans, CSF findings in, 529
Vision, assessment of, 608–609, 611
Vitamins, in parenteral nutrition, 734
  supplementation with, 740–741, 812
Vitamin A, 464
  deficiency of, 574, 687
  requirement of, 716
Vitamin B-complex, deficiency of, 687
  dietary supplementation with, 812
Vitamin C, dietary supplementation with, 812
  in diet, 723
Vitamin D, 464
  calcium metabolism and, 119
  deficiency of, 126
  excess of, 126
  requirement of, 716t

Vitamin E, 123, 464
  deficiency of, 560, 687
  dietary supplementation with, 812
  for myopathy, 115, 174
  requirement of, 716t
Vitamin K, 355, 371
Volvulus, 190
  of colon, 190, 191, 221–222, II:66–68
  of small intestine, 420, 447

Wandering atrial pacemaker, 384–385, *384*
Warfarin, antidotes to, 350t
  drug interactions of, 153t
  toxicity of, 354, 502–503, II:305–306
Warts, penile, 709
Water deprivation testing, 621–622
Water. See also *Fluid therapy*.
  distribution in body, 18
  quality of, II:682–685
WBC (white blood cell count), 132, 807
  of adult, 826t
  of neonate, 825t
Weanling, nutrition of, 109, 465t, 721t
  overfeeding of, 109
Wedge biopsy, 685
WEE (western equine encephalitis), 547–550, *548*, II:348–349
Wenckebach block, 384, *384*
Western equine encephalitis (WEE), 547–550, *548*, II:348–349
White blood cell count (WBC), 132, 807
  of adult, 826t
  of neonate, 825t
White foal syndrome, 448
White muscle disease, 113, 123
Withers, fistulous, 109, 110, 111–112
Wobblers, 559–560
Wounds, care of, II:642–645
Wry nose, 266

Xanthochromia, in cerebrospinal fluid, 528, 529
Xeroradiography, of bucked shins, 144
X-rays. See *Radiography*.
Xylazine, 23, 28, 29, 96, 99
  for colic, 202
Xylazine-ketamine-guaifenesin, 30
Xylose, absorption tests of, 171

Yearling, duodenal ulcer in, 186
  nutrition of, 109, 465t
  overfeeding of, 109
Yellow star thistle, 173
Yew, toxicity of, 338, 373, 375

Zinc, deficiency of, 125, 687
  excess of, 125, 723
  in serum, 723t
  orthopedic disorders and, 464, 723
  requirement of, 716t, 718t, 719
  toxicity of, 364–365
Zinc sulfate turbidity test, 425
Zolazepam, 30